Adult and Pediatric Urology

VOLUME 3

Adult and Pediatric Urology

THIRD EDITION

EDITORS

Jay Y. Gillenwater, M.D.
Hovey S. Dabney Professor
Department of Urology
University of Virginia Health Sciences Center
Charlottesville, Virginia

John T. Grayhack, M.D.
Professor
Department of Urology
Northwestern University Medical School
Chicago, Illinois

Stuart S. Howards, M.D.
Professor
Department of Urology
University of Virginia Health Sciences Center
Charlottesville, Virginia

John W. Duckett, M.D.
Professor of Urology
University of Pennsylvania School of Medicine;
Director, Pediatric Urology
Children's Hospital of Philadelphia
Philadelphia, Pennsylvania

With 1642 illustrations

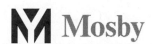 Mosby

St. Louis Baltimore Boston Carlsbad Chicago Naples New York Philadelphia Portland
London Madrid Mexico City Singapore Sydney Tokyo Toronto Wiesbaden

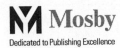

Mosby
Dedicated to Publishing Excellence

A Times Mirror
Company

Publisher: Anne S. Patterson
Editor: Susie Baxter
Developmental Editor: Anne Gunter
Project Manager: Peggy Fagen

THIRD EDITION

Printed in the United States of America
Composition by Graphic World, Inc.
Project management by Graphic World Publishing Services
Printing/binding by Maple-Vail Book Manufacturing Group

Mosby–Year Book, Inc.
11830 Westline Industrial Drive
St. Louis, Missouri 63146

ISBN: 0-8151-4008-8
96 97 98 99 / 9 8 7 6 5 4 3 2

Contributors

Vaseem Ali, M.D.
Division of Urology
The University of Texas Medical School
Houston, Texas

Frederick C. Ames, M.D.
Department of Surgical Oncology
The University of Texas MD Anderson Cancer
  Center
Houston, Texas

Richard J. Andrassy, M.D.
Professor of Surgery and Pediatrics
Chief, Division of Pediatric Surgery
Department of Surgery
University of Texas Medical School
Houston, Texas

David M. Barrett, M.D.
Professor and Chair
Department of Urology
Mayo Clinic
Rochester, Minnesota

Laurence S. Baskin, M.D.
Assistant Professor of Pediatrics and Urology
Department of Urology
University of California School of Medicine
San Francisco, California

Mark F. Bellinger, M.D.
Associate Professor
Division of Urology
University of Pittsburgh School of Medicine;
Director, Department of Pediatric Urology
Children's Hospital of Pittsburgh
Pittsburgh, Pennsylvania

George S. Benson, M.D.
Professor
Division of Urology
University of Texas Medical School
Houston, Texas

David A. Bloom, M.D.
Professor
Department of Surgery
Section of Urology
Chief of Pediatric Urology
University of Michigan School of Medicine
Ann Arbor, Michigan

Bruce Blyth, M.D.
Clinical Assistant Professor
Department of Surgery
University of Colorado Health Sciences Center
Denver, Colorado

Michel A Boileau, M.D.
Bend Urology Associates
St. Charles Medical Center
Bend, Oregon

Wade Bushman, M.D., Ph.D.
Assistant Professor
Department of Urology
Northwestern University Medical School
Chicago, Illinois

Anthony A. Caldamone, M.D.
Professor of Surgery
Department of Urology
Brown University School of Medicine;
Director of Pediatric Urology
Rhode Island Hospital
Providence, Rhode Island

Douglas A. Canning, M.D.
Assistant Professor of Urology
Department of Surgery
University of Pennsylvania School of Medicine
Philadelphia, Pennsylvania

William J. Catalona, M.D.
Professor and Chief
Division of Urologic Surgery
Washington University School of Medicine
St. Louis, Missouri

Marc Cendron, M.D.
Section of Urology
Dartmouth-Hitchcock Medical Center
Lebannon, New Hampshire

Peter L. Choyke, M.D.
Professor
Department of Radiology
Uniformed Services University of the Health
  Sciences;
Chief, MRI
Henry M. Jackson Foundation at the Clinical
  Center
Bethesda, Maryland

Ralph V. Clayman, M.D.
Professor of Urology and Radiology
Departments of Surgery (Urology) and Radiology
Washington University School of Medicine
St. Louis, Missouri

Bo L.R.A. Coolsaet, M.D.
Professor of Urology
State University of Utrecht
Utrecht, The Netherlands

Douglas E. Coplen, M.D.
Assistant Professor
Division of Urologic Surgery
Washington University School of Medicine
St. Louis, Missouri

Joseph N. Corriere, Jr., M.D.
Professor of Surgery
Division of Urology
University of Texas Medical School
Houston, Texas

Barbara Y. Croft, Ph.D.
Associate Professor
Department of Radiology
University of Virginia Health Sciences Center
Charlottesville, Virginia

Jean B. deKernion, M.D.
Professor of Surgery
Division of Urology
UCLA School of Medicine
Los Angeles, California

William C. DeWolf, M.D.
Urologist-in-Chief
Urologic Oncology and Director
Urology Research Laboratories
Beth Israel Hospital
Boston, Massachusetts

John P. Donohue, M.D.
Distinguished Professor and Chairman
Indiana University School of Medicine
Indianapolis, Indiana

John W. Duckett, M.D.
Professor
Department of Urology
University of Pennsylvania School of Medicine;
Director, Pediatric Urology
Children's Hospital of Philadelphia
Philadelphia, Pennsylvania

Richard F. Edlich, M.D., Ph.D.
Distinguished Professor of Plastic Surgery and
    Biomedical Engineering
Department of Plastic Surgery
University of Virginia Health Sciences Center
Charlottesville, Virginia

Jack S. Elder, M.D.
Division of Urology
Rainbow Babies Children's Hospital
Cleveland, Ohio

Gary J. Faerber, M.D.
Assistant Professor
Section of Urology
University of Michigan School of Medicine
Ann Arbor, Michigan

R. Sherburne Figenshau, M.D.
Division of Urology
Washington University School of Medicine
St. Louis, Missouri

Loulie M. Fisher, M.D.
Private Practice
Pensacola, Florida

Stuart M. Flechner, M.D.
Department of Urology
Cleveland Clinic Foundation
Cleveland, Ohio

Richard S. Foster, M.D.
Associate Professor
Department of Urology
Indiana University School of Medicine
Indianapolis, Indiana

Jackson E. Fowler, Jr., M.D.
Professor of Surgery and Chief
Division of Urology
University of Mississippi School of Medicine
Jackson, Mississippi

Inderbir S. Gill, M.D.
Department of Surgery
Division of Urology
University of Kentucky School of Medicine
Lexington, Kentucky

Jay Y. Gillenwater, M.D.
Hovey S. Dabney Professor
Department of Urology
University of Virginia Health Sciences Center
Charlottesville, Virginia

John T. Grayhack, M.D.
Professor
Department of Urology
Northwestern University Medical School
Chicago, Illinois

Marko Gudziak, M.D.
Division of Urology
The University of Texas Medical School
Houston, Texas

M. Craig Hall, M.D.
Department of Urology
The University of Texas MD Anderson Cancer
    Center
Houston, Texas

Faruk Hadziselimovic, M.D.
Director
Institute of Andrology
Listal, Switzerland

Terry W. Hensle, M.D.
Professor
Department of Urology
Columbia University College of Physicians and
    Surgeons;
Director of Pediatric Urology
Babies Hospital–Columbia Presbyterian Medical
    Center
New York, New York

Ernest E. Hodge, M.D.
Department of Urology
Cleveland Clinic Foundation
Cleveland, Ohio

Stuart S. Howards, M.D.
Professor
Department of Urology
University of Virginia Health Sciences Center
Charlottesville, Virginia

Robert Huben, M.D.
Chief, Urologic Oncology
Roswell Park Cancer Institute
Buffalo, New York

M'Liss A. Hudson, M.D.
Assistant Professor
Division of Urologic Surgery
Washington University School of Medicine
St. Louis, Missouri

Dale Huff, M.D.
Professor of Pathology
University of Pittsburgh School of Medicine
Director
Developmental Perinatal Pathology
Magee-Womens Hospital
Pittsburgh, Pennsylvania

Alan D. Jenkins, M.D.
Associate Professor
Department of Urology
University of Virginia Health Sciences Center
Charlottesville, Virginia

Scott B. Jennings, M.D.
Fellow in Urologic Oncology
Surgery Branch, National Cancer Institute
Bethesda, Maryland

Judith M. Joyce, M.D.
Associate Director
Nuclear Medicine
The Western Pennsylvania Hospital;
Director
Nuclear Medicine
Suburban General Hospital
Pittsburgh, Pennsylvania

Panayotis P. Kelalis, M.D.
Anson L. Clark Professor of Pediatric Urology
Chairman, Department of Urology
Mayo Clinic and Mayo Foundation
Rochester, Minnesota

Charles D. Kellum, M.D.
Department of Radiology
HCA Colliseum Park Hospital
Macon, Georgia

Stephen A. Koff, M.D.
Professor of Surgery
Division of Urology
Ohio State University College of Medicine;
Chief, Pediatric Urology
Children's Hospital
Columbus, Ohio

Stanley Kogan, M.D.
Professor of Urology
New York Medical College;
Codirector
Section of Pediatric Urology
Westchester County Medical Center
New York, New York

Harry P. Koo, M.D.
Assistant Professor
Section of Urology
University of Michigan School of Medicine
Ann Arbor, Michigan

James M. Kozlowski, M.D.
Associate Professor of Urology, Surgery, and Tumor
    Cell Biology
Director, Genitourinary Oncology Program
Northwestern University Medical School
Chicago, Illinois

John N. Krieger, M.D.
Professor
Department of Urology
University of Washington School of Medicine
Seattle, Washington

Robert M. Levin, M.D.
Research Professor
Division of Urology
Department of Pharmacology
University of Pennsylvania School of Medicine
Philadelphia, Pennsylvania

W. Marston Linehan, M.D.
Head, Urologic Oncology Section
Surgery Branch, National Cancer Institute
Bethesda, Maryland

Marguerite C. Lippert, M.D.
Associate Professor
Department of Urology
University of Virginia Health Sciences Center
Charlottesville, Virginia

Larry I. Lipshultz, M.D.
Professor
Scott Department of Urology
Baylor College of Medicine
Houston, Texas

Fray F. Marshall, M.D.
Professor of Urology
Director, Division of Adult Urology
Johns Hopkins University School of Medicine
Baltimore, Maryland

Jack W. McAninch, M.D.
Professor and Chief
Department of Urology
University of California School of Medicine
San Francisco, California

David L. McCullough, M.D.
Professor and Chairman
Department of Urology
Bowman Gray School of Medicine
Winston-Salem, North Carolina

W. Scott McDougal, M.D.
Professor of Surgery
Department of Urology
Harvard Medical School;
Chief of Urology
Massachusetts General Hospital
Boston, Massachusetts

Elspeth M. McDougall, M.D.
Assistant Professor
Division of Urologic Surgery
Washington University School of Medicine
St. Louis, Missouri

Edward J. McGuire, M.D.
Professor and Director
Department of Urology
University of Texas Medical School
Houston, Texas

Kevin T. McVary, M.D.
Assistant Professor
Department of Urology
Northwestern University Medical School
Chicago, Illinois

Randall B. Meacham, M.D.
Assistant Professor
Division of Urology
University of Colorado Health Sciences Center
Denver, Colorado

Douglas F. Milam, M.D.
Assistant Professor
Department of Urology
Vanderbilt University School of Medicine
Nashville, Tennessee

H. Norman Noe, M.D.
Professor
Department of Urology
University of Tennessee College of Medicine;
Chief of Pediatric Urology
LeBonheur Children's Medical Center
Memphis, Tennessee

Andrew C. Novick, M.D.
Chairman
Department of Urology
Cleveland Clinic Foundation
Cleveland, Ohio

Helen O'Connell, M.D.
Division of Urology
University of Texas Medical School
Houston, Texas

Robert A. Older, M.D.
Associate Professor of Radiology
Chief, Section of Uroradiology
Department of Radiology
University of Virginia Health Sciences Center
Charlottesville, Virginia

Jayashree Parekh, M.D.
Assistant Professor
Department of Radiology
University of Virginia Health Sciences Center
Charlottesville, Virginia

Raymond E. Poore, M.D.
Department of Urology
Bowman Gray School of Medicine
Winston-Salem, North Carolina

Ronald Rabinowitz, M.D.
Professor of Urology and Pediatrics
University of Rochester School of Medicine and
    Dentistry;
Chief of Pediatric Urology
Strong Memorial Hospital
Chief of Urology
Rochester General Hospital
Rochester, New York

John F. Redman, M.D.
Professor and Chairman
Department of Urology
University of Arkansas for Medical Sciences;
Chief, Urology Service
University Hospital and Arkansas Children's
    Hospital
Little Rock, Arkansas

Martin I. Resnick, M.D.
Lester Persky Professor and Chairman
Department of Urology
Case Western Reserve University School of
    Medicine;
Director, Department of Urology
University Hospitals of Cleveland
Cleveland, Ohio

Michael L. Ritchey, M.D.
Associate Professor of Surgery and Pediatrics
Department of Surgery (Urology)
University of Texas Medical School;
Chief, Pediatric Urology
Hermann Children's Hospital
Houston, Texas

George T. Rodeheaver, Ph.D.
Research Professor of Plastic Surgery
University of Virginia Health Sciences Center
Charlottesville, Virginia

Randall G. Rowland, M.D., Ph.D.
Professor
Department of Urology
Indiana University School of Medicine
Indianapolis, Indiana

Grannum R. Sant, M.D.
Professor and Vice-Chairman
Department of Urology
Tufts University School of Medicine
Boston, Massachusetts

Anthony J. Schaeffer, M.D.
Herman L. Kretschmer Professor and Chairman
Department of Urology
Northwestern University Medical School
Chicago, Illinois

Seth Schulman, M.D.
Assistant Professor
Department of Pediatrics
University of Pennsylvania School of Medicine
Philadelphia, Pennsylvania

Curtis A. Sheldon, M.D.
Associate Professor of Surgery
Division of Urology
University of Cincinnati College of Medicine;
Director, Pediatric Urology
Children's Hospital Medical Center
Cincinnati, Ohio

Grahame H. H. Smith, M.D.
Formerly, Fellow
Department of Pediatric Surgery
The Children's Hospital of Philadelphia
Philadelphia, Pennsylvania
Royal Alexandra Children's Hospital
Sydney Australia

Joseph A. Smith, Jr., M.D.
William L. Bray Professor and Chairman
Department of Urology
Vanderbilt University School of Medicine
Nashville, Tennessee

Brent W. Snow, M.D.
Associate Professor of Urology/Pediatrics
University of Utah Health Sciences Center
Salt Lake City, Utah

Howard McC. Snyder, III, M.D.
Division of Urology
Children's Hospital of Philadelphia
Philadelphia, Pennsylvania

R. Ernest Sosa, M.D.
Associate Professor
Department of Urology
Cornell University Medical College
New York, New York

J. Patrick Spirnack, M.D.
Associate Professor
Department of Urology
Case Western Reserve University School of
   Medicine;
Director of Urology
Metrohealth Medical Center
Cleveland, Ohio

William D. Steers, M.D.
Associate Professor
Department of Urology
University of Virginia Health Sciences Center
Charlottesville, Virginia

Gerald Sufrin, M.D.
Professor and Chairman
Department of Urology
State University of New York at Buffalo
School of Medicine and Biomedical Sciences
Buffalo, New York

Charles D. Teates, M.D.
Professor and Vice-Chairman
Department of Radiology
University of Virginia Health Sciences Center
Charlottesville, Virginia

Charles J. Tegtmeyer, M.D.
Professor of Radiology and Anatomy
Director, Division of Angiography, Interventional
   Radiology and Special Procedures
Department of Radiology
University of Virginia Health Sciences Center
Charlottesville, Virginia

John G. Thacker, Ph.D.
Professor of Mechanical Engineering
Department of Mechanical and Aerospace
   Engineering
University of Virginia Health Sciences Center
Charlottesville, Virginia

Joseph G. Trapasso, M.D.
Department of Urology
Graduate Hospital
Philadelphia, Pennsylvania

E. Darracott Vaughan, Jr., M.D.
James J. Colt Professor of Urology
Department of Urology
Cornell University Medical College
New York, New York

Robert L. Vogelzang, M.D.
Associate Professor
Department of Radiology
Northwestern University Medical School
Chicago, Illinois

Andrew C. von Eschenbach, M.D.
Professor and Chairman
Department of Urology
The University of Texas MD Anderson Cancer
   Center
Houston, Texas

R. Dixon Walker, III, M.D.
Professor of Surgery
Division of Urology
University of Florida College of Medicine;
Chief of Pediatric Urology
Shands Hospital
Gainesville, Florida

Steve W. Waxman, M.D.
Fellow, Reconstructive Urology and Urodynamics
Department of Surgery
Division of Urology
Duke University School of Medicine
Durham, North Carolina

George D. Webster, M.B., F.R.C.S.
Professor
Department of Surgery
Division of Urology
Duke University School of Medicine
Durham, North Carolina

Alan J. Wein, M.D.
Professor and Chairman
Division of Urology
University of Pennsylvania School of Medicine;
Chief of Urology
Hospital of the University of Pennsylvania
Philadelphia, Pennsylvania

Jeffrey P. Weiss, M.D.
Clinical Associate Professor of Urology
Temple University School of Medicine
Philadelphia, Pennsylvania

Robert M. Weiss, M.D.
Professor and Chief
Section of Urology
Yale University School of Medicine
New Haven, Connecticut

B. Dale Wilson, M.D.
Assistant Professor
Department of Dermatology
Roswell Park Cancer Institute
State University of New York at Buffalo
School of Medicine and Biomedical Sciences
Buffalo, New York

Henry A. Wise, II, M.D.
Clinical Professor
Department of Surgery
Ohio State University College of Medicine;
Chief, Section of Urology
Riverside Methodist Hospital
Columbus, Ohio

Arthur W. Wyker, Jr., M.D.
Professor
Department of Urology
University of Virginia Health Sciences Center
Charlottesville, Virginia

Stephen A. Zderic, M.D.
Assistant Professor
Division of Urology
University of Pennsylvania School of Medicine;
Attending Surgeon
The Children's Hospital of Philadelphia
Philadelphia, Pennsylvania

Preface

The text of the third edition of *Adult and Pediatric Urology* has again been revised after five years because of the rapid introduction of new information about urological disease. The text was written to serve as a reference for residents and practicing urologists. We have attempted to make the text readable and user-friendly and to provide a complete description of the subject (rather than an all inclusive dissertation). The authors have tried to assimilate all the important information about each subject and to evaluate it in order to reach to the best conclusion or consensus. Practicing urologists and residents alike have commented favorably on the content and presentation of the material in the previous editions. We believe the new edition continues to present excellent coverage of the topics in a clear and concise manner.

The edition consists of three volumes. The first two volumes cover adult urology, and all of the pediatric section is now contained in the third volume. In order to update the text by including new developments in urologic care, many chapters have been rewritten by new contributors, and new chapters have been added on laparoscopy and the kidney in pregnancy. Those contributors who have written for previous editions have extensively revised their material.

For residents preparing for the boards, as well as practicing urologists seeking recertification, this edition also has an accompanying question and answer book, *Review of Adult and Pediatric Urology*, edited by Stuart Howards. The text will also soon be available on Bibliomed® Urology CD-ROM.

All textbooks contain dated information. For this text we have addressed this problem in two ways. First, most of these chapters were written less than a year before publication. Second, we will be updating *Adult and Pediatric Urology* annually in the YEAR BOOK OF UROLOGY. The YEAR BOOK OF UROLOGY has been reorganized to function as a supplement to this textbook, in addition to being an annual survey of the year's best urological literature.

Any text is no better than its editors, authors, and publishers. Working with Jack Grayhack, Stuart Howards, and John Duckett has been both pleasant and intellectually stimulating. Each of the editors has worked closely with his authors to ensure the best coverage possible for a wide array of subjects. The authors enthusiastically responded and produced scholarly, critical, and informative chapters. Anne Gunter, Susie Baxter, and the Mosy–Year Book staff have also been invaluable partners in this enterprise. I know of no other group who could have transformed so much manuscript into a completed textbook in such a compressed time frame. The result is an up-to-date, thorough, and eminently-readable textbook of general urology.

For the editors

Jay Y. Gillenwater

Contents

PART II

PEDIATRIC UROLOGY

Adult and Pediatric Urology

PART II

Pediatric Urology

CHAPTER 43

General Considerations of Congenital Anomalies

Ronald Rabinowitz

To a great extent, pediatric urology deals with the care of infants and children with congenital anomalies. Many of these anomalies are external and obvious and are recognized at birth. Others are internal and may be discovered because of evaluation of urologic signs or symptoms or by association with a pattern or syndrome of anomalies. More recently, congenital anomalies are being diagnosed in a fetus by maternal ultrasonography. In the past two decades, developments and advances in neonatology, genetics, pediatric anesthesia, pediatric radiology, neonatal intensive care nursing, dysmorphology, obstetrics, and instrumentation have had great impact on the care of infants with congenital urologic anomalies. They have contributed to the evolution of pediatric urology as a "subspecialty or superspecialty depending upon one's bias . . ." (Williams, 1984). In his address to the Royal College of Surgeons in 1983, David Innes Williams described the development of the surgery of urologic congenital anomalies. He reviewed the progress of knowledge from an isolated report of an anomaly to its pathologic description, classification, and evaluation. In conjunction with the advancement in knowledge have come surgical advances allowing early intervention and reconstruction.

As in all aspects of medicine, the importance of the history and physical examination cannot be overemphasized. Because the fetus is unable to undergo a direct hands-on evaluation, diagnostic ultrasonography acts as the fetal physical examination in the diagnosis of congenital anomalies.

Congenital anomalies may be classified according to their pathogenesis. These anomalies may be characterized as malformations, deformations, or disruptions. Malformations occur during formation of a structure and thus usually are present by 8 weeks gestational age. Organs whose development continues beyond this time are obviously at risk for malformation later in gestation. These systems include the central nervous system (CNS) and genitalia. The underlying etiology may be genetic or environmental. Deformations result from mechanical molding of an often normally developed organ. Disruptions also occur in normally formed organs and are usually environmental in etiology, but they may be genetic (Stevenson and Hall, 1993). The majority of the congenital anomalies discussed in this chapter are malformations.

Approximately 2% to 3% of live newborns will have a major congenital anomaly. By 5 years of age an additional 2% to 3% will be found to have such an abnormality. Minor structural abnormalities are noted in approximately 15% of live newborns. The risk of a major malformation is only 1%, if the infant has no minor anomalies. The risk increases to 3% in the presence of one minor anomaly, 10% in association with 2 minor anomalies, and 20% when there are 3 or more minor defects (Stevenson and Hall, 1993).

HISTORY
Familial

Many congenital urologic anomalies are familial, including external anomalies, such as hypospadias (Bauer et al., 1981) and cryptorchidism (Jones and Young, 1982). These external anomalies may be isolated or part of a syndrome. Family history is important in children with renal disease, including both infantile and adult polycystic kidney disease (Blyth and Ockenden, 1971). A family history of a previous stillborn or early death from pulmonary hypoplasia of Potter syndrome may be important. Polycystic disease also has been described in association with microcephaly and polydactyly (Hsia et al., 1971; Seller, 1981). Hydronephrosis secondary to ureteropelvic junction obstruction also has been seen in families (Kelalis et al., 1971). More than one study has shown the increased risk for vesicoureteral reflux in siblings (Dwoskin, 1984; Jerkins and Noe, 1982). Last, a family history of genital ambiguity may be seen in familial enzymatic disorders, such as adrenogenital syndrome (New et al., 1983). In fact, a detailed family history of any congenital anomalies may yield important information because urologic anomalies often are seen in conjunction with nonurologic abnormalities in many familial syndromes.

In addition to the family history of siblings, lost pregnancies, and associated anomalies, history of ethnic background and consanguinity may be important. Increasing parental age also may be associated with a higher risk for congenital anomalies.

Gestational

A detailed gestational history may provide clues in the family of a child with a congenital anomaly. In addition to such obvious information as the correlation of gestational age by both dates and examination, the history of fetal movement and activity, maternal weight gain, and a history of any illnesses in the mother may be important. Maternal illness includes both chronic disease and an acute process, either viral or bacterial. Other important historical factors include use of medications, alcohol, tobacco, and psychotropic drugs. The use of drugs or radiation therapy may be teratogenic.

Congenital renal anomalies are associated with oligohydramnios (Potter, 1965) and also may be seen with polyhydramnios (Blank et al., 1978). Information regarding the delivery also may be important.

PHYSICAL EXAMINATION
Urologic

Although the emphasis is on urologic congenital anomalies, the urologic examination is relatively straightforward for the urologist. The abdomen is observed for muscle laxity and asymmetry. Gentle palpation will help identify the kidneys and any abnormal mass. The kidney is the most common organ of origin of an abdominal mass in the neonate. Palpation and transillumination will help to characterize the mass as being solid or cystic, smooth or irregular, and to assess its mobility. The number and position of abdominal masses also are important.

The genitalia also are examined visually and palpated. The penis is examined for size, completeness of foreskin, presence of chordee, and position of urethral orifice. The size and position of gonads are noted. Urethral and vaginal orifices in the female along with the labia and inguinal areas are examined. Clitoral size is determined. Rectal examination may be extremely helpful in palpating an abdominal or pelvic mass, uterus, and inguinal hernia or gonad.

Nonurologic

Although the urologic examination is of utmost importance to the urologist dealing with congenital anomalies, the nonurologic examination may provide invaluable clues to the presence or increased risk of a urologic congenital abnormality (see Specific Congenital Anomalies Associated with Renal Malformations or Renal Insufficiency). The presence of abnormalities of the ears, eyes, chest, gastrointestinal (GI) system, and skeletal system may lead to the diagnosis of a urologic abnormality. Ear abnormalities were found to be associated with genitourinary malformations more than 30 years ago (Hilson, 1957). Abnormal facies and pulmonary findings are associated with oligohydramnios and renal dysplasia or obstruction (Thomas and Smith, 1974). Vertebral anomalies in the cervicothoracic area often are seen with renal agenesis or renal ectopy (MURCS* association) (Duncan and Shapiro, 1979). Vertebral defects in the lumbosacral spine also are associated with urinary malformations (VATER association) (Duncan and Shapiro, 1979). In addition to obvious neural tube defects, such as myelomeningocele, there also can be clues to occult spinal dysraphism. A surface finding over the sacrum should be searched for, which may vary from a dimple to a tuft of hair to a skin tag. It can be a clue to the development of tethering of the spinal cord (Higginbottom et al., 1980). Children found to have aniridia, hemihypertrophy, or Beckwith-Wiedemann syndrome are all at significant risk for the subsequent development of Wilms' tumor (Cohen et al., 1971; Haicken and Miller, 1971; Miller et al., 1964). Gastrointestinal anomalies, such as tracheoesophageal fistula, are associated with renal abnormalities in the VATER association (Duncan and Shapiro, 1979). Urinary abnormalities also are associated with imperforate anus (Belman and King, 1972). A vaginal orifice in females must be identified because there is a significant incidence of urinary abnormalities associated with congenital absence of the vagina (Chawla et al., 1966). Neurofibromatosis (von Recklinghausen disease) has urologic manifestations with an increased risk for renovascular hypertension, pheochromocytomas, and vesical neurofibromas (Carlson and Wilkinson, 1972; Fienman and Yakovac, 1970; Tilford and Kelsch, 1973). Many infants with multiple congenital anomalies have a single umbilical artery, the presence of which may lead one to suspect a renal anomaly (Altschuler et al., 1975).

DIAGNOSTIC STUDIES

The urologist should be intimately involved in the decision to evaluate a child for a congenital urologic anomaly and to decide which diagnostic studies are indicated. In addition, in instances of familial congen-

---

Acronyms are defined in the lists of congenital anomalies that appear at the end of this chapter.

ital anomalies, the urologist may recommend prenatal diagnostic studies.

When the infant or child is suspected of having an underlying urologic structural anomaly, screening ultrasonography is commonly the initial diagnostic study (Shkolnik, 1985). With ultrasonography one can examine the kidneys, liver, great vessels, ureters, urinary bladder, and pelvic organs and gonads. This extensive screening can then act as a guide to further investigations. In those instances in which a nonurologic anomaly has a high risk for associated urinary tract obstruction, the presence of an entirely normal ultrasonographic study of the urinary tract including normal parenchyma with equal-size kidneys may reassure the urologist. In evaluating siblings for uropathology, ultrasonography may be an excellent diagnostic tool. Siblings of those with obstructed kidneys are easily evaluated in this way. Concerning siblings of refluxers, some would be content with a normal sonogram and would not evaluate the sibling further unless symptoms occur. Others would do a more extensive screening and include a nuclear cystogram as part of the evaluation. Siblings or children of patients with adult polycystic kidney disease can be followed up with interval ultrasound studies. Children who are at increased risk for the development of malignant renal tumors because of aniridia, hemihypertrophy, or Beckwith-Wiedemann syndrome are screened with frequent renal sonograms. If the ultrasound study is not entirely normal, further diagnostic evaluation must be carried out in the form of radiographic or nuclear medicine studies.

In addition to evaluating neonates and children, an increased family risk for urologic malformation or gestational suspicions may lead to studies of the fetus with the use of prenatal ultrasonography (Sabbagha, 1980). Various genetic syndromes associated with renal malformation may be diagnosed in this fashion. The fetal kidneys may be visualized as early as 9 weeks gestational age (Green and Hobbins, 1988). Syndromes associated with renal agenesis and renal cystic diseases may be diagnosed by fetal ultrasonography (Hirata et al., 1990).

Another common tool for the study of the fetus is amniocentesis (Gerbie and Elias, 1980). Amniocentesis has been extremely helpful in the prenatal diagnosis of chromosomal anomalies (Simpson, 1980), metabolic disorders (Burton and Nadler, 1980), and neural tube defects (Cowchock and Jackson, 1980). The use of amniocentesis to obtain fetal cells from the amniotic fluid for chromosomal analysis is indicated in increasing maternal age, as all trisomies have an increased incidence after the maternal age of 35 years. Prenatal chromosomal analysis is also indicated when there has been a previous child with a chromosomal anomaly, especially a trisomy. Additionally, those families at risk for X-linked recessive disorders might consider aborting males (Motulsky and Fraser, 1980). Many metabolic disorders inherited as autosomal recessive or X-linked recessive may now be diagnosed by biochemical assays of various components in the amniotic fluid. The finding that alpha-fetoprotein levels are elevated in the amniotic fluid when the fetus has an open neural tube defect has allowed this to be used as a screening study in high-risk patients and families with a previous diagnosis of a neural tube defect. Amniocentesis is, of course, used in conjunction with prenatal ultrasonography to confirm as accurately as possible any diagnosis.

In a few instances, early prenatal ultrasonography (at approximately 20-weeks' gestational age), progressive dilatation of the urinary tract, and a decrease in amniotic fluid volume may indicate a role for fetal intervention using indwelling catheter shunts (Glick et al., 1985).

GENETIC FACTORS

Approximately 3% of live newborns will be found to have a congenital anomaly associated with a chromosomal abnormality (0.5%), a single gene defect (0.7%), or an abnormality of polygenic inheritance (1.8%) (Gordon, 1976).

Chromosomal Anomalies

Since the description of Down syndrome as the first cytogenetic syndrome to be clinically identified in 1959 (Lejune et al., 1959), a number of chromosomal syndromes have been identified, many with urologic abnormalities (see Specific Congenital Anomalies Associated with Renal Malformation or Renal Insufficiency and Specific Congenital Anomalies Associated with Genital Malformations). These now include those with complete extra autosomes, those with duplication of a portion of an autosome (long arm, or "q," or short arm, or "p" monosomies), and sex chromosomal abnormalities.

Among the trisomies, Down syndrome (trisomy 21) is the most common. Males are hypogonad, often having a small penis, and approximately one fourth will have cryptorchidism (Bergsma, 1979; Jones, 1988). Whereas trisomy 18 syndrome (Edwards' syndrome) has a high incidence of urologic anomalies, including horseshoe kidney and hydronephrosis in approximately 50% and hypospadias and cryptorchidism in others, 90% die within the first year of life, usually of cardiopulmonary etiology (Bergsma, 1979; Edwards et al., 1960; Jones, 1988). Likewise, although trisomy 13 syndrome (Patau syndrome) will have a renal anomaly in three fourths of cases (cystic kidneys, hydronephrosis, horseshoe kidney, duplication anomalies) and all will have undescended testes, only 5% will survive 3 years. These newborns have severe neurologic defects with midline defects of the face, eye, and brain (Bergsma, 1979; Jones, 1988; Patau et al., 1960). In trisomy 8 syndrome, the diagnosis may be very important because these children can survive into adulthood. In addition to their mental deficiency, eye, ear, and CNS abnormalities are found. From a urologic standpoint, these children have been found to have hydronephrosis, vesicoureteral reflux, and cryptorchidism (Bergsma, 1979; Cassidy et al., 1975; Jones, 1988). These patients with trisomy 9 syndrome not only have renal malformations, cryptorchidism, and micropenis, but also major CNS abnormalities, and they commonly do not survive the postnatal period (Jones, 1988). The chromosome 22 syndrome (cat-eye syndrome) will commonly have inferior coloboma of the iris and/or anal atresia. From a urologic standpoint renal agenesis, horseshoe kidney, hydronephrosis, and vesicoureteral reflux all have been identified. There is a high risk for cardiac abnormalities, as well as varying degrees of mental retardation (Bergsma, 1979; Jones, 1988).

A complete extra set of chromosomes (triploidy syndrome) is reported to be responsible for approximately 20% of spontaneous abortions secondary of chromosomal abnormalities. Those infants that survive to birth are developmentally profoundly retarded and have CNS, eye, ear, skeletal, and cardiac defects. There is a high incidence of genital ambiguity and hypospadias, micropenis, and cryptorchidism seen in the external genitalia. Renal anomalies include hydronephrosis and dysplasia (Bergsma, 1979; Jones, 1988; Wertelecki et al., 1976).

Among the partial trisomies, there can be an extra long arm (q) of a chromosome or an extra short arm (p) of a chromosome. The trisomy 10q syndrome has a high incidence of renal anomalies and cryptorchidism in addition to severe mental retardation, microcephaly, and eye, ear, skeletal, and cardiac anomalies. Hypospadias also may be seen in this condition in which 50% do not survive the first year of life (Jones, 1988). Partial trisomy 11q syndrome includes micropenis as one of the major abnormalities, associated with growth retardation, microcephaly, and ear abnormalities. Urinary malformations also may be found. Only half survive the first year of life (Bergsma, 1979). Trisomy 4p has a high incidence of cryptorchidism, micropenis, and hypospadias in association with microcephaly and severe mental retardation. Renal anomalies and agenesis may be found. Approximately two thirds of these infants will survive the first year of life (Gonzalez et al., 1977; Jones, 1988). Trisomy 9p has multiple skeletal anomalies in conjunction with severe mental retardation. Most survive, and many have hypospadias, small penis, cryptorchidism, or renal anomalies (Centerwall et al., 1976; Jones, 1988). The trisomy 20p syndrome has micropenis and crypt-

orchidism in association with skeletal, eye, and ear abnormalities. Renal and cardiac anomalies also may be seen in this syndrome (Jones, 1988).

In addition to duplications or partial duplications of autosomes, there may be partial deficiencies or deletions (monosomies). These often also have associated renal and genital malformations. Prader-Willi syndrome has been found to have partial deletion of the long arm of chromosome 15 (monosomy 15q). These obese, hypotonic, retarded children come to the attention of the urologist because of hypogonadism and cryptorchidism (Jones, 1988). Monosomy 13q (13q–) syndrome is associated with mental and growth retardation, as well as eye, ear, cardiac, and skeletal anomalies. Males have hypospadias and cryptorchidism. Renal anomalies are occasionally found in this condition. Some patients with this chromosomal anomaly develop retinoblastoma (Jones, 1988). Patients with monosomy 18q (18q–) syndrome of facial, eye, and ear anomalies, mental and growth retardation, and skeletal anomalies also are found to have cryptorchidism. Horseshoe kidney also may be seen in these children (Jones, 1988). Hypospadias and cryptorchidism are commonly seen in monosomy 4p (4p–) syndrome, also characterized by marked mental and growth retardation and facial anomalies (Bergsma, 1979; Jones, 1988). The abnormal laryngeal development of infants with monosomy 5p (5p–) syndrome has caused this to be called the cat's-cry syndrome. The children are slow to develop and profoundly mentally retarded. They have multiple facial anomalies and occasional cryptorchidism and renal anomalies, such as agenesis (Bergsma, 1989; Jones, 1988). Monosomy 9p (9p–) syndrome is associated with cryptorchidism, micropenis, and hydronephrosis. These children have craniofacial anomalies, profound mental retardation, and cardiac anomalies (Jones, 1988).

In addition to chromosomal abnormalities of autosomes, sex chromosomal abnormalities commonly have associated urologic anomalies. Turner syndrome (XO syndrome) is characterized by short stature and dysgenic ovaries. There is often a broad chest with webbing of the posterior neck. Renal anomalies are present in more than half, horseshoe kidney being the most common (Bergsma, 1979; Jones, 1988; Persky and Owens, 1971). Klinefelter syndrome (XXY syndrome) is the most common cause of male hypogonadism. These males are usually tall and slim. Almost half have gynecomastia, and virilization is diminished. They are mentally slow. Penis and testes are small (Caldwell and Smith, 1972; Jones, 1988). More severe changes are seen with increased aneuploidy to XXXY and XXXXY. The greater degree of aneuploidy correlates with more severe degrees of growth retardation, mental retardation, and testicular and penile hypoplasia. Although cryptorchidism is seen occasionally with Klinefelter syndrome, almost one third of those with XXXY syndrome have cryptorchidism (Jones, 1988). The XYY syndrome also is associated with cryptorchidism, small penis, or hypospadias. These boys have abnormal facies and tall stature, but are mildly mentally deficient (Jones, 1988).

A large number of patients with chromosomal anomalies will come to the attention of the urologist. The association of cryptorchidism with hypospadias or micropenis should lead to chromosomal investigation. Many of these chromosomal abnormalities also have associated ear, eye, facial, neurologic, cardiovascular, skeletal, or GI anomalies, singly or severally. Many have familial tendencies, and these parents can undergo genetic evaluation and counseling. Virtually all of these conditions can be diagnosed prenatally by amniocentesis.

Single Gene Defects

Single gene defects occur with a frequency of approximately 0.7% (Gordon, 1976). These include autosomal dominant, autosomal recessive, and X-linked disorders, transmitted by mendelian patterns of inheritance (McKusick, 1992). There has been a rapid increase in the number of these conditions diagnosed. In 1958, there were 285 autosomal dominant single gene defects recorded (Verschuer, 1958). By 1983, this number had increased to 934 proven and an additional 893 suspected autosomal dominant single gene disorders, for a total of 1827. By 1988, there were 1442 proven and 1117 suspected autosomal dominant single gene disorders (total 2559). In 1992, 2470 proven and 1241 suspected autosomal dominant single gene disorders (total 3711) had been reported (McKusick, 1992). There were 89 documented autosomal recessive single gene disorders documented in 1958 (Verschuer, 1958) compared with 588 proven and an additional 710 suspected autosomal recessive conditions (total 1298) listed in 1983. By 1988, these numbers had increased to 626 proven and 851 suspected autosomal recessive conditions (total 1477). In 1992, 647 proven and 984 suspected autosomal recessive single gene defects (total 1631) had been reported (McKusick, 1992). Similarly, the number of X-linked single gene disorders has increased from 38 in 1958 (Verschuer, 1958) to 115 proven and an additional 128 suspected (total 243) in 1983. These numbers had increased to 139 proven and 171 suspected X-linked single gene disorders by 1988 (total 310). In 1992, 190 proven and 178 suspected X-linked single gene disorders (total 368) had been reported (McKusick, 1992). Many of these single gene defects have urologic manifestations (see Specific Congenital Anomalies with Renal Malformations or Renal Insufficiency and Specific Congenital Anomalies Associated with Genital Malformations).

Although autosomal dominant (adult) polycystic kidney disease usually presents in the adult, it can present in childhood or even in infancy (Ross and Travers, 1975). It may even present as a unilateral abdominal mass (Farrell et al., 1984). It is being diagnosed in childhood more frequently using ultrasonography (Wolf et al., 1978). Alport syndrome (hereditary nephritis with nerve deafness) is the most common hereditary form of nephritis and commonly presents in childhood with microhematuria and proteinuria. Many have associated sensorineural hearing loss, and progression to renal failure may occur in young adulthood (McCrory et al., 1966). Autosomal dominant renal tubular acidosis (type I; distal) may present in early childhood with growth retardation, nephrocalcinosis, and nephrolithiasis (Morris and Sebastian, 1983). The nail-patella syndrome of hypoplastic nails (especially thumbnail) and hypoplastic or absent patella is associated with nephropathy in approximately one third of cases. The syndrome may be recognizable at birth, and nephritis, which may occur in one third, may present in childhood (Similä et al., 1970). Hematuria also may be the presenting and only finding of benign familial hematuria, a condition that is not progressive and not associated with any other abnormalities (McConville et al., 1966).

Tuberous sclerosis is an autosomal dominant disorder characterized by mental retardation, epilepsy, and angiofibromatous skin lesions. One half to three fourths of children will develop renal hamartomas or cysts (Stapleton et al., 1980). Renal hamartomas also may occur in neurofibromatosis (von Recklinghausen disease), but this condition, characterized by multiple café-au-lait spots, is more commonly associated with pheochromocytoma and renal artery stenosis (Bergsma, 1979; Jones, 1988). Von Hippel-Lindau syndrome usually does not present until young adulthood, commonly with retinal and cerebellar hemangiomas. This condition also is associated with renal cysts, renal cell carcinoma in one third of cases (many of which are multiple or bilateral), and pheochromocytoma (Levine et al., 1983).

Some autosomal dominant disorders commonly have associated genital anomalies (See Specific Congenital Anomalies Associated with Genital Malformations). Cryptorchidism, hypospadias, and hypogonadism are commonly seen in multiple lentigines (LEOPARD) syndrome and Noonan syndrome. In LEOPARD syndrome, the diagnosis is commonly made in early childhood by the skin lesions (Sommer et al., 1971). Children with Noonan syndrome usually have short stature, mental retardation, and webbed neck similar to Turner syndrome (Collins and Turner, 1973). Hypospadias and hypertelorism are seen in Opitz syndrome in conjunction with cryptorchidism. This is probably related to the Opitz-Frias syndrome, which also includes dysphagia (Cordero and Holmes, 1978). Isolated deficiency of gonadotropin has been associated with hyposmia or anosmia in Kallmann syndrome. Cryptorchidism may be present, but these children are often first seen because of failure to undergo secondary sexual development at puberty (Santen and Paulsen, 1973).

Last, urologists must be acutely aware of the often fatal autosomal dominant condition, malignant hyperthermia, which occurs in approximately 1 in 15,000 pediatric anesthetic administrations (Nelson and Flewellen, 1983). This pharmacogenetic disorder of calcium binding and transport is most commonly triggered by halothane and succinylcholine. Important factors include a family history of anesthetic difficulties or myopathy. Many of the males have cryptorchidism. Most have elevated levels of creatinine phosphokinase. If this condition is suspected preoperatively, patients can be pretreated with dantrolene sodium (Britt et al., 1977; Ellis, 1981; King et al., 1972; McKusick, 1992).

There are many autosomal recessive disorders associated with renal or genital malformations. Autosomal recessive (infantile) polycystic kidney disease presents in the newborn with massive bilateral renal enlargement and is commonly associated with oligohydramnios, pulmonary hypoplasia, and Potter facies. Patients have associated and characteristic cystic disease of the liver with periportal fibrosis (Blyth and Ockenden, 1971). Juvenile nephronophthisis usually presents in childhood or adolescence (Chamberlain et al., 1977) and has been found to be associated with retinitis pigmentosa (Avasthi et al., 1976). These patients present with salt-losing nephropathy and progressive renal failure. Cystinosis, a metabolic disorder of impaired renal tubular reabsorption, commonly presents by 1 year of age with growth retardation, renal rickets, and progressive uremia (Schneider and Schulman, 1983). Another metabolic disorder, oxalosis, commonly presents in childhood with nephrocalcinosis and urolithiasis secondary to high urinary oxalate excretion. Progressive renal failure commonly develops in childhood or adolescence (Williams and Smith, 1983). The sickling syndromes may present with or have associated hematuria, renal infarction, or papillary necrosis. Hematuria may be the presenting sign of a sickling syndrome (Strauss and McIntosh, 1978). The Jeune thoracic dystrophy syndrome is characterized by a small thorax and respiratory distress in the first few months of life. Renal cystic dysplasia and renal insufficiency are common in surviving children (Herdman and Langer, 1968; Okerklaid et al., 1977). Renal cysts, dysplasia, and renal insufficiency are seen in Zellweger (cerebrohepatorenal) syndrome. This condition, which is fatal during the first year of life, includes developmental defects of the brain and hepatomegaly with hepatic fibrosis and insufficiency (Danks et al., 1975).

Some autosomal recessive syndromes have both renal and genital involvement. The Meckel-Gruber syndrome of posterior encephalocele and other craniofacial anomalies is associated with polycystic dysplastic kidneys, cryptorchidism, and hypoplastic external genitalia. This condition is fatal in infancy secondary to renal or pulmonary insufficiency (Hsia et al., 1971; Seller, 1981). The cryptophathalmos syndrome, which consists of developmental defects of the eyes and other facial anomalies, is associated with hypospadias, cryptorchidism, and developmental anomalies of the uterus and vagina. Renal anomalies also may be seen in this condition (Azevedo et al., 1973; Fraser, 1962). The Smith-Lemli-Opitz syndrome of microcephaly, cranial facial anomalies, and limb abnormalities also is associated with cryptorchidism, hypospadias, and occasionally renal anomalies (Smith et al., 1964). The Laurence-Moon-Biedl syndrome of obesity, mental retardation, retinitis pigmentosa, and digital anomalies also includes genital or gonadal hypoplasia. Some also have renal abnormalities (Bauman and Hogan, 1973; Hurley et al., 1975).

Some autosomal recessive disorders are commonly associated with genital abnormalities. The adrenogenital syndrome, which includes various enzymatic disorders of steroidogenesis, usually presents with genital ambiguity as female pseudohermaphroditism, but males also may be affected (New et al., 1983). A form of male pseudohermaphroditism, pseudovaginal perineoscrotal hypospadias, is secondary to deficiency of 5 α-reductase (Peterson et al., 1979). Cystic fibrosis has associated male infertility secondary to abnormalities or changes in the vas deferens (Kaplan et al., 1968; Oppenheimer and Esterly, 1969). The syndrome of XX gonadal dysgenesis consists of phenotypically normal females who have streak gonads and no secondary sexual characteristics (Simpson, 1979).

From an anesthesia standpoint, deficiency of pseudocholinesterase may be important, especially in the homozygote because this results in prolonged apnea following neuromuscular blockade with succinylcholine (Hodgkin et al., 1965; Viby-Mogensen, 1981).

X-linked disorders are often associated with genital anomalies, but some also have significant renal abnormalities as well (see Specific Congenital Anomalies Associated with Genital Malformations and Specific Congenital Anomalies Associated with Renal Malformations or Renal Insufficiency). Fabry syndrome consists of multiple cutaneous angiokeratomas, corneal opacification, and progressive renal insufficiency. Symptoms of severe burning pain in the extremities usually begin in childhood or adolescence (Desnick et al., 1983). Lowe (oculocerebrorenal) syndrome is another metabolic disorder, characterized by mental retardation, hypotonia, bilateral cataracts, cryptorchidism, and renal tubular dysfunction, resulting in progressive renal insufficiency during childhood or adolescence (Abbassi et al., 1968).

In many X-linked disorders, genital anomalies are very prominent. Aarskog syndrome consists of short stature, facial and digital anomalies, and cryptorchidism with partial penoscrotal transposition (Aarskog, 1970). Swyer syndrome of XY gonadal dysgenesis is characterized by female external genitalia and bilateral streak gonads that have a high risk of undergoing malignant degeneration (Espiner et al., 1970; Simpson, 1976). The syndromes of androgen insensitivity may be complete or incomplete. Also called testicular feminization, discovery is often made in childhood by the presence of a testis in a hernia sac in a phenotypic female. These children are genetic males (46, XY). In the complete syndrome, florid feminization occurs at puberty. In the incomplete form, varying degrees of masculinization occur, and the external genitalia may be phenotypically ambiguous (Migeon et al., 1979).

Polygenic

Some urologic disorders are not necessarily associated with a single chromosomal abnormality or single gene defect, yet their increased predisposition in some families makes them genetically predetermined (Carter, 1969). In a large review of the familial aspects of hypospadias, Bauer and associates (1981) reported on some 300 families with this condition. In 21% of the families there was a second individual with hypospadias, and in 5% of the families there was a third affected family member. Fourteen percent of boys with hypospadias had a sibling with hypospadias. This significantly increased incidence is much greater than normal (0.32%), demonstrating the increased risk in some families. In addition, the more severe the degree of hypospadias present, the greater the incidence of hypospadias in a sibling. Although the risk in these families is significantly greater than normal, the risk is significantly less than expected for mendelian patterns of inheritance in single gene defects.

Similarly, although cryptorchidism occurs in approximately 0.8% of children (Scorer and Farrington, 1971), the incidence of cryptorchidism in siblings of boys with cryptorchidism was 6% to 10% and the incidence of cryptorchidism of their fathers was 4% (Czeizel et al., 1981; Jones and Young, 1982). Thus, although cryptorchidism often accompanies multiple malformation syndromes and many chromosomal and single gene defects, isolated cryptorchidism is likely of polygenic inheritance.

The syndrome of müllerian aplasia (Rokitansky sequence; Rokitansky-Küster-Hauser syndrome) consists of absent or rudimentary müllerian structures in 46, XX females with normal female phenotype and normal ovaries. There is a very high incidence of associated renal ectopia or solitary kidney. The increased risk to siblings is consistent with polygenic inheritance (Simpson, 1976).

Primary vesicoureteral reflux also likely has a polygenic mode of inheritance. The incidence of vesicoureteral reflux is less than 1% (Ransley, 1978). However, the siblings of children with vesicoureteral reflux have been reported to have reflux in 33% (Jerkins and Noe, 1982) and 23% (Dwoskin, 1984).

Other urologic conditions that also may have a polygenic mode of inheritance include unilateral and bilateral renal agenesis, ureteral duplication anomalies, and ureteropelvic junction obstruction (Burger and Burger, 1974).

ENVIRONMENTAL FACTORS

Some congenital anomalies result from environmental exposure to substances known as teratogens. These teratogens may interfere with the growth, proliferation, migration, and/or differentiation of fetal cells (Hoyme, 1990). Some teratogens can damage a developing system throughout gestation, whereas for others the time duration of susceptibility may be very brief. Teratogens do cross the placenta, and fetal thresholds for toxicity are likely significantly lower than those for adults. These environmental teratogens, many of which can be avoided, include infection, drugs, and irradiation (Wilson, 1977).

Infection

It was first recognized in 1941 that a maternal infection (Rubella) can cause fetal malformation (Gregg, 1941). The fetal rubella syndrome may have renal anomalies, hypospadias, and cryptorchidism (Jones, 1988; Menser et al., 1967). Most maternal infections that cause fetal malformations result in intrauterine growth retardation and CNS abnormalities. These include the TORCH infections (toxoplasmosis, rubella, cytomegalovirus, herpes simplex I and II, and syphilis) (Bergsma, 1979; Hoyme, 1990; Jones, 1988). Congenital varicella also has been reported to be associated with urogenital anomalies (Klauber et al., 1976). Maternal immunization during pregnancy has not been shown to be teratogenic (Hoyme, 1990).

Although not an infectious agent, maternal diabetes has a two- to three-fold increased incidence of congenital anomalies (Mills, 1982). There is a significantly increased risk for neural tube defects in insulin-dependent diabetic mothers. There is also an increased risk for both renal and genital malformations in these infants (Hoyme, 1990).

Maternal fever also has been reported to be teratogenic. The malformations commonly include growth retardation and CNS abnormalities, including neural tube defects (Hoyme, 1990).

Drugs

Malformations also can be caused by various drugs. The teratogenic potential of a chemical attracted worldwide attention 35 years ago with the discovery of limb defects secondary to maternal ingestion of thalidomide. The epidemic from 1959 to 1962 resulted in approximately 10,000 neonates with thalidomide embryopathy, some of whom also had renal malformations (Bergsma, 1979; Lenz, 1966; McBride, 1961). The first association of anticonvulsants with congenital anomalies was reported in 1968 (Meadow, 1968), and multiple studies confirmed what is now known as the fetal hydantoin syndrome. Whereas growth deficiency, craniofacial anomalies, and hypoplasia of the distal phalanges are common, hypospadias, cryptorchidism, micropenis, genital ambiguity, and renal malformations also are seen (Hanson and Smith, 1975). All anticonvulsants have been reported to be teratogenic (Hoyme, 1990).

There appears to be an increased risk to the male genital system in the offspring of mothers who took diethylstilbestrol (DES) while pregnant. There is also an increased risk of hypospadias (Aarskog, 1979; Mau, 1981; Schardein, 1980), but this does not appear to be statistically significant. Gill and associates (1979) found that one third of men who were exposed to DES in utero had testicular hypoplasia or epididymal cysts. Two thirds of those with testicular hypoplasia also had cryptorchidism. In daughters of mothers who took DES while pregnant, there is an increased risk for cervical and vaginal dysplasia and premalignant abnormalities (Robboy et al., 1984). These females have an increased risk for vaginal, cervical, and fallopian tube defects (Hoyme, 1990).

Although the fetal alcohol syndrome was not reported in the medical literature until 1973 (Jones et al., 1973), alcohol is probably the most common teratogenic drug causing significant fetal risk. The effects may be seen in up to 0.9% and the syndrome in up to 0.3% of live births (Hoyme, 1990). The major defect of the fetal alcohol syndrome is on growth and CNS development. Additionally, however, renal anomalies also have been reported (Clarren and Smith, 1978).

In utero exposure to cocaine has been reported to cause intrauterine growth retardation (Chouteau et al., 1988), premature labor, abruptio placentae (Chasnoff et al., 1987), and genitourinary defects (Chasnoff et al., 1988). These genitourinary defects include hydronephrosis, hypospadias, and urethral obstruction sequence. The etiology is believed to be secondary to the constrictive effect of cocaine on the fetal, placental, and/or uterine vasculature. Thus, the fetus is always at risk for the teratogenic effects of cocaine, even after organ development because the pathogenesis is disruption (Jones, 1991).

In 1985, Lammer and co-workers reported a constellation of malformations (CNS, craniofacial, cardiac, and thymic) associated with the drug isotretinoin used to treat acne. Another vitamin A congener, etretinate (used to treat psoriasis) has an extremely long half-life and has been associated with malformations when gestation began months after cessation of this drug (Hoyme, 1990).

Aromatic hydrocarbons used as solvents have been evaluated in occupational settings where, if carefully controlled, they have been considered safe. The solvent toluene, a paint thinner, has been used as a psychotropic inhalation agent and found to cause CNS abnormalities in the user. Recently, toluene has been confirmed as teratogenic, causing growth retardation, microcephaly, and craniofacial anomalies. Cryptorchidism and renal anomalies also have been reported (Hersh et al., 1985).

Cigarette smoking also has been reported to cause intrauterine growth retardation, but no specific defects have been reported (Abel, 1980).

Irradiation

In utero exposure to radiation increases the risk for CNS abnormalities and the subsequent increased likelihood of development of neoplasia (Sweet and Kinzie, 1976). Although other abnormalities, including genital malformations and hypoplasia, may be seen, when the malformations are documented to be secondary to intrauterine radiation exposure, there is always concomitant CNS abnormality and growth retardation (Brent, 1980).

SPECIFIC CONGENITAL ANOMALIES ASSOCIATED WITH RENAL MALFORMATIONS OR RENAL INSUFFICIENCY

Renal malformations are associated with many varied syndromes and anomalies. The specific details of each individual condition listed in this section can be found in *Smith's Recognizable Patterns of Human Malformation* (Jones, 1988). The mode of inheritance, if known, is included. These lists are taken from *Smith's* and modified by Bergsma (1979), Zonana and DiLiberti (1990), McKusick (1992), and van Allen (1993).

Renal malformations frequently are seen in the following conditions:

Early urethral obstruction sequence (includes prune belly)

Jeune thoracic dystrophy syndrome (autosomal recessive)

Johanson-Blizzard syndrome (autosomal recessive)

Meckel-Gruber syndrome (autosomal recessive)

Melnick-Fraser syndrome (autosomal dominant)

MURCS association (*m*üllerian duct aplasia, *r*enal aplasia, *c*ervicothoracic *s*omite dysplasia)

Oligohydramnios sequence (Potter syndrome)

Orofacial-digital syndrome

Partial trisomy 10q syndrome

Rokitansky sequence (Rokitansky-Küster-Hauser syndrome)

Rubinstein-Taybi syndrome

Townes syndrome (autosomal dominant)

Triploidy syndrome

Trisomy 8 mosaic syndrome

Trisomy 9 mosaic syndrome

Trisomy 13 (Patau) syndrome

Trisomy 18 (Edwards) syndrome

Trisomy 22 (cat-eye) syndrome

VATER association (*v*ertebral defects, *a*nal atresia, *t*racheal-*e*sophageal fistula, *r*adial and *r*enal dysplasia)

XO (Turner) syndrome

Zellweger syndrome (cerebrohepatorenal syndrome) (autosomal recessive)

4 p– syndrome

18 q– syndrome

Renal malformations occasionally are seen in the following conditions:

CHARGE association (*c*oloboma, *h*eart disease, *a*tresia choanae, *r*etarded growth, *g*enital anomalies, *e*ar anomalies)

Cryptophthalmos syndrome (autosomal recessive)

EEC syndrome (*e*ctrodactyly, *e*ctodermal dysplasia, *c*left lip and palate) (autosomal dominant)

Ehlers-Danlos syndrome (autosomal dominant)

Facioauriculovertebral spectrum

Fetal alcohol effects

Fetal hydantoin effects

Fetal trimethadione effects

Opitz-Frias syndrome (autosomal dominant)

Poland sequence

Radial aplasia–thrombocytopenia syndrome (autosomal recessive)

Roberts syndrome (autosomal recessive)

Russell/Silver syndrome

Saethre-Chotzen syndrome (autosomal dominant)

Thanatophoric dysplasia syndrome

Trisomy 4p syndrome

Trisomy 9p syndrome

Trisomy 20p syndrome

Trisomy 21 syndrome

13q– syndrome

18 ring syndrome

Renal insufficiency is a frequent component in the following conditions:

Early urethral obstruction sequence (includes prune belly)

Fabry syndrome

Jeune thoracic dystrophy syndrome (autosomal recessive)

Lowe syndrome (oculocerebrorenal syndrome) (X-linked)

Nail-patella syndrome (autosomal dominant)

Occult spinal dysraphism sequence (tethered spinal cord)

Zellweger syndrome (cerebrohepatorenal syndrome) (autosomal recessive)

Renal insufficiency also may be seen in the following conditions:

Johanson-Blizzard syndrome (autosomal recessive)

Laurence-Moon-Biedl syndrome (autosomal recessive)

Russell/Silver syndrome

Williams syndrome

SPECIFIC CONGENITAL ANOMALIES ASSOCIATED WITH GENITAL MALFORMATIONS

Genital malformations often are associated with various syndromes and conditions. These are described in detail in *Smith's Recognizable Patterns of Human Malformation* (Jones, 1988), and are listed in the following paragraphs in association with various syndromes, along with the mode of inheritance, if known. These lists are taken from *Smith's* and modified by McKusick (1992) and Bergsma (1979).

Hypospadias or ambiguous genitalia frequently are seen in the following conditions:

Aniridia/Wilms' tumor association

Cryptophthalmos syndrome (autosomal recessive)

Fetal trimethadione effects

Laurence-Moon-Biedl syndrome (autosomal recessive)

Opitz-Frias syndrome (autosomal dominant)

Rapp-Hodgkin ectodermal dysplasia syndrome (autosomal dominant)

Rieger syndrome (autosomal dominant)

Robinow syndrome (fetal face syndrome) (autosomal dominant)

Smith-Lemli-Optiz syndrome (autosomal recessive)

Triploidy syndrome

4p– syndrome

13q– syndrome

Hypospadias or ambiguous genitalia also may be seen in the following syndromes:

Aarskog syndrome (X-linked)
Beckwith-Wiedemann syndrome
Dubowitz syndrome (autosomal recessive)
Ellis-van Creveld syndrome (epispadias) (autosomal recessive)
Fanconi pancytopenia syndrome (autosomal recessive)
Fetal hydantoin effects
Johanson-Blizzard syndrome (autosomal recessive)
Multiple lentigines syndrome (LEOPARD *l*entigines, *e*lectrocardiograph abnormalities, *o*cular hypertelorism, *p*ulmonic stenosis, *a*bnormalities of genitalia, *r*etardation of growth, *d*eafness syndrome) (autosomal dominant)
Partial trisomy 10q syndrome
Popliteal web syndrome (autosomal dominant)
Roberts syndrome (autosomal recessive)
Russell/Silver syndrome
Shprintzen syndrome (autosomal dominant)
Trisomy 4p syndrome
Trisomy 9p syndrome
Trisomy 13 (Patau) syndrome
Trisomy 18 (Edwards) syndrome
XXXXY syndrome
XXY (Klinefelter) syndrome
XYY syndrome

Micropenis and hypogenitalism often are found in the following conditions:

Carpenter syndrome (autosomal recessive)
CHARGE association (*c*oloboma, *h*eart disease, *a*tresia choanae, *r*etarded growth, *g*enital anomalies, *e*ar anomalies)
Kallmann syndrome (autosomal dominant)
Meckel-Gruber syndrome (autosomal recessive)
Noonan syndrome (autosomal dominant)
Popliteal web syndrome (autosomal dominant)
Prader-Willi syndrome
Robinow syndrome (fetal face syndrome) (autosomal dominant)
Triploidy syndrome
Trisomy 4p syndrome
Trisomy 9 mosaic syndrome
Trisomy 20p syndrome
XXY (Klinefelter) syndrome
9p– syndrome
18q– syndrome

Micropenis and hypogenitalism also may be seen in the following:

Acrodysostosis syndrome
de Lange syndrome
Fanconi pancytopenia syndrome (autosomal recessive)

Fetal hydantoin effects
Fibrodysplasia ossificans congenita syndrome (autosomal dominant)
Hallermann-Streiff syndrome
Trisomy 9p syndrome
Trisomy 21 (Down) syndrome
XYY syndrome

Cryptorchism is frequently found in the following syndromes:

Aarskog syndrome (X-linked)
Carpenter syndrome (autosomal recessive)
Cryptophthalmos syndrome (autosomal recessive)
de Lange syndrome
Early urethral obstruction sequence (include prune belly)
Escobar syndrome (autosomal recessive)
Freeman-Sheldon syndrome (autosomal dominant)
Frontometaphyseal dysplasia syndrome
Kallmann syndrome (autosomal dominant)
Laurence-Moon-Biedl syndrome (autosomal recessive)
Lowe syndrome (oculocerebrorenal syndrome) (X-linked)
Meckel-Gruber syndrome (autosomal recessive)
Miller-Dieker syndrome (autosomal recessive)
Multiple lentigines syndrome (autosomal dominant)
Noonan syndrome (autosomal dominant)
Optiz-Frias syndrome (autosomal dominant)
Partial trisomy 10q syndrome
Pena-Shokeir I syndrome (autosomal recessive)
Popliteal web syndrome (autosomal dominant)
Prader-Willi syndrome
Roberts syndrome (autosomal recessive)
Robinow syndrome
Rubinstein-Taybi syndrome
Ruvalcaba syndrome
Seckel syndrome (autosomal recessive)
Senter syndrome
Smith-Lemli-Opitz syndrome (autosomal recessive)
Triploidy syndrome
Trisomy 4p syndrome
Trisomy 13 (Patau) syndrome
Trisomy 18 (Edward) syndrome
Trisomy 20p syndrome
XXXXY syndrome
4p– syndrome
9p– syndrome
13q– syndrome
18q– syndrome

Cryptorchidism occasionally is seen in the following conditions:

Amyoplasia congenital disruptive sequence

Cockayne syndrome (autosomal recessive)
Coffin-Siris syndrome
Diastrophic dysplasia syndrome (autosomal recessive)
Distal arthrogryposis syndrome (autosomal dominant)
Dubowitz syndrome (autosomal recessive)
Ellis-van Creveld syndrome (autosomal recessive)
Fanconi pancytopenia syndrome (autosomal recessive)
Femoral hypoplasia–unusual facies syndrome
Hallermann-Streiff syndrome
Saethre-Chotzen syndrome (autosomal dominant)
Shprintzen syndrome (autosomal dominant)
Steinert myotonic dystrophy syndrome (autosomal dominant)
Treacher-Collins syndrome (autosomal dominant)
Trisomy 8 syndrome
Trisomy 9p syndrome
Trisomy 21 (Down) syndrome
XXY (Klinefelter) syndrome
XYY syndrome
5p– (cat's-cry) syndrome
Zellweger syndrome (cerebrohepatorenal syndrome) (autosomal recessive)

Hypoplasia of the labia majora is a frequent component of the following syndromes:

Escobar syndrome (autosomal recessive)
Popliteal web syndrome (autosomal dominant)
Robinow syndrome (fetal face syndrome) (autosomal dominant)
Trisomy 18 (Edwards) syndrome
9p– syndrome
18q– syndrome

It also is occasionally seen in:

Amyoplasia congenita disruptive sequence
de Lange syndrome
Fetal alcohol effects

Uterine and/or vaginal abnormalities often are found in the following conditions:

Cryptophthalmos syndrome (autosomal recessive)
Johanson-Blizzard syndrome (autosomal recessive)
Rokitansky sequence (Rokitansky-Küster-Hauser syndrome)
Trisomy 13 (Patau) syndrome

In addition, uterine and/or vaginal anomalies occasionally may be seen in the following syndromes:

Roberts syndrome (autosomal recessive)
Trisomy 18 (Edwards) syndrome

REFERENCES

Aarskog D: A familial syndrome of short stature associated with facial dysplasia and genital anomalies. *J Pediatr* 1970; 77:856.

Aarskog D: Maternal progestins as a possible cause of hypospadias. *N Engl J Med* 1979; 300:75.

Abbassi V, Lowe CU, Calcagno PL: Oculo cerebro-renal syndrome—a review. *Am J Dis Child* 1968; 115:145.

Abel EL: Smoking during pregnancy: a review of effects on growth and development of offspring. *Hum Biol* 1980; 52:593.

Altschuler G, Tsang RC, Ermocilla R: Single umbilical artery. *Am J Dis Child* 1975; 129:697.

Avasthi PS, Erickson DG, Gardner KD: Hereditary renal-retinal dysplasia and the medullary cystic disease–nephronophthisis complex. *Ann Intern Med* 1976; 84:147.

Azevedo ES, Biondi J, Ramalho LM: Cryptophthalmos in two families from Bahia, Brazil. *J Med Genet* 1973; 10:389.

Bauer SB, Retik AB, Colodny AH: Genetic aspects of hypospadias. *Urol Clin North Am* 1981; 8:559.

Bauman ML, Hogan GR: Laurence-Moon-Biedl syndrome. *Am J Dis Child* 1973; 126:119.

Belman AB, King LR: Urinary tract abnormalities associated with imperforate anus. *J Urol* 1972; 108:823.

Bergsma D: *Birth Defects Compendium*, ed 2. New York, Alan R. Liss, Inc, 1979.

Blank E, Neerhout RC, Burry KA: Congenital mesoblastic nephroma and polyhydramnios. *JAMA* 1978; 240:1504.

Blyth H, Ockenden BG: Polycystic disease of kidneys and liver presenting in childhood. *J Med Genet* 1971; 8:257.

Brent RL: Radiation teratogenesis. *Teratology* 1980; 21:281.

Britt BA, Kwong RHF, Endrenyi B: The clinical and laboratory features of malignant hyperthermia management—a review. In Henschel EO (ed): *Malignant Hyperthermia: Current Concepts*. New York, Appleton-Century-Crofts, 1977, pp 9-45.

Burger RH, Burger SE: Genetic determinants of urologic disease. *Urol Clin North Am* 1974; 1:419.

Burton BK, Nadler HL: Antenatal diagnosis of metabolic disorders. *Clin Obstet Gynecol* 1980; 7:27.

Caldwell PH, Smith DW: The XXY (Klinefelter's) syndrome in childhood: detection and treatment. *J Pediatr* 1972; 80:250.

Carlson DH, Wilkinson RH: Neurofibromatosis of the bladder in children. *Radiology* 1972; 105:401.

Carter CO: Genetics of common disorders. *Br Med Bull* 1969; 25:52.

Cassidy SB, McGee BJ, Van Eys J, et al: Trisomy 8 syndrome. *Pediatrics* 1975; 56:826.

Centerwall WR, Miller KS, Reeves LM: Familial 'partial 9p' trisomy: six cases and four carriers in three generations. *J Med Genet* 1976; 13:57.

Chamberlain BC, Hagge WW, Stickler GB: Juvenile nephronophthisis and medullary cystic disease. *Mayo Clin Proc* 1977; 52:485.

Chasnoff IJ, Burns KA, Burns WJ: Cocaine use in pregnancy: perinatal morbidity and mortality. *Neurotoxicol Teratol* 1987; 9:291.

Chasnoff IJ, Chisum GM, Kaplan WE: Maternal cocaine use and genitourinary tract malformations. *Teratology* 1988; 37:201.

Chawla S, Bery K, Indra KJ: Abnormalities of the urinary tract and skeleton associated with congenital absence of vagina. *Br Med J* 1966; 1:1398.

Chouteau M, Namerow PB, Leppert P: The effect of cocaine abuse on birth weight and gestational age. *Obstet Gynecol* 1988; 72:351.

Clarren SK, Smith DW: The fetal alcohol syndrome. *N Engl J Med* 1978; 298:1063.

Cohen MM Jr, Gorlin RJ, Feingold M, et al: The Beckwith-Wiedemann Syndrome. *Am J Dis Child* 1971; 122:515.

Collins E, Turner G: The Noonan syndrome—a review of the clinical and genetic features of 27 cases. *J Pediatr* 1973; 83:941.

Cordero JF, Holmes LB: Phenotypic overlap of the BBB and G syndromes. *Am J Med Genet* 1978; 2:145.

Cowchock FS, Jackson LG: Use of alpha-fetoprotein for diagnosis of neural tube and other anomalies. *Clin Obstet Gynecol* 1980; 7:83.

Czeizel A, Erodi E, Joth J: Genetics of undescended testis. *J Urol* 1981; 126:528.

Danks DM, Tippett P, Adams C, et al: Cerebro-hepato-renal syndrome of Zellweger. *J Pediatr* 1975; 86:382.

Desnick RJ, Sweeley CC: Fabry's disease: Alpha galactosidase. A deficiency. In Stanbury JP, Wyngaarden JB, Fredrickson DS, et al (eds): *The Metabolic Basis of Inherited Disease*, ed 5. New York, McGraw-Hill, 1983; pp 906-944.

Duncan PA, Shapiro LR: The VATER and MURCS associations: vertebral and genitourinary malformations with distinct embryologic mechanisms. *Teratology* 1979; 19:24A.

Dwoskin JY: The siblings of the child with reflux. In Johnston JH (ed): *Management of Vesicoureteric Reflux*. Baltimore, Williams & Wilkins, 1984; pp 236-240.

Edwards JH, Harnden DG, Cameron AH, et al: A new trisomic syndrome. *Lancet* 1960; 1:787.

Ellis FR: Malignant hyperpyrexia. In *Inherited Disease and Anaesthesia*. Amsterdam, Excerpta Medica, 1981, pp 163-199.

Espiner EA, Veale AMO, Sands VE, et al: Familial syndrome of streak gonads and normal male karyotype in 5 phenotypic females. *N Engl J Med* 1970; 283:6.

Farrell TP, Boal DK, Wood BP, et al: Unilateral abdominal mass: an unusual presentation of autosomal dominant polycystic kidney disease in children. *Pediatr Radiol* 1984; 14:349.

Fienman NL, Yakovac WC: Neurofibromatosis in childhood. *J Pediatr* 1970; 76:339.

Fraser GR: Our genetical 'load.' A review of some aspects of genetical variation. *Ann Hum Genet* 1962; 25:387.

Gerbie AB, Elias S: Amniocentesis for antenatal diagnosis of genetic defects. *Clin Obstet Gynecol* 1980; 7:5.

Gill WB, Schumacher GFB, Bibbo M, et al: Association of diethylstilbestrol exposure in utero with cryptorchidism, testicular hypoplasia and semen abnormalities. *J Urol* 1979; 122:36.

Glick PL, Harrison MR, Golbus MS, et al: Management of the fetus with congenital hydronephrosis: II. Prognostic criteria and selection for treatment. *J Pediatr Surg* 1985; 20:376.

Gonzalez CH, Sommer A, Meisner LF, et al: The trisomy 4p syndrome: case report and review. *Am J Med Genet* 1977; 1:137.

Gordon H: Genetics. In Kelalis PP, King LR, Belman AB (eds): *Clinical Pediatric Urology*. Philadelphia, WB Saunders, 1976, p 1068.

Green JJ, Hobbins JC: Abdominal ultrasound examination of the first-trimester fetus. *Am J Obstet Gynecol* 1988; 159:165.

Gregg NM: Congenital cataract following German measles in the mother. *Trans Ophthalmol Soc Aust* 1941; 3:35.

Haicken BN, Miller DR: Simultaneous occurrence of congenital aniridia, hamartoma, and Wilms' tumor. *J Pediatr* 1971; 78:497.

Hanson JW, Smith DW: The fetal hydantoin syndrome. *J Pediatr* 1975; 87:285.

Herdman RC, Langer LO: The thoracic asphyxiant dystrophy and renal disease. *Am J Dis Child* 1968; 116:192.

Hersh JH, Podruch PE, Rogers G, et al: Toluene embryopathy. *J Pediatr* 1985; 106:922.

Higginbottom MC, Jones KL, James HE, et al: Aplasia cutis congenita: a cutaneous marker of occult spinal dysraphism. *J Pediatr* 1980; 96:687.

Hilson D: Malformation of ears as sign of malformation of genitourinary tract. *Br Med J* 1957; 2:785.

Hirata GI, Medearis AL, Platt LD: Fetal abdominal abnormalities associated with genetic syndromes. *Clin Perinatol* 1990; 17:675.

Hodgkin WE, Giblett ER, Levine H, et al: Complete pseudocholinesterase deficiency: genetic and immunologic characterization. *J Clin Invest* 1965; 44:486.

Hoyme HE: Teratogenically induced fetal anomalies. *Clin Perinatol* 1990; 17:547.

Hsia YE, Bratu M, Herbordt A: Genetics of the Meckel syndrome (dysencephalia splanchnocystica). *Pediatrics* 1971; 48:237.

Hurley RM, Dery P, Nogrady MB, et al: The renal lesion of the Laurence-Moon-Biedl syndrome. *J Pediatr* 1975; 87:206.

Jerkins GR, Noe HN: Familial vesicoureteral reflux: a prospective study. *J Urol* 1982; 128:774.

Jones IRG, Young ID: Familial incidence of cryptorchidism. *J Urol* 1982; 127:508.

Jones KL, Smith DW, Ulleland CN, et al: Pattern of malformation in offspring of chronic alcoholic mothers. *Lancet* 1973; 1:1267.

Jones KL: *Smith's Recognizable Patterns of Human Malformation*, ed 4. Philadelphia, WB Saunders, 1988.

Jones KL: Developmental pathogenesis of defects associated with prenatal cocaine exposure: fetal vascular disruption. *Clin Perinatol* 1991; 18:139.

Kaplan E, Shwachman H, Perlmutter AD, et al: Reproductive failure in males with cystic fibrosis. *N Engl J Med* 1968; 279:65.

Kelalis PP, Culp OS, Stickler GB, et al: Ureteropelvic obstruction in children: experiences with 109 cases. *J Urol* 1971; 106:418.

King JO, Denborough MA, Zapf PW: Inheritance of malignant hyperpyrexia. *Lancet* 1972; 1:365.

Klauber GT, Flynn FJ Jr, Altman BD: Congenital varicella syndrome with genitourinary anomalies. *J Urology* 1976; 8:153.

Lammer EJ, Chen CT, Hoar RM, et al: Retinoic acid embryopathy. *N Engl J Med* 1985; 313:837.

Lejune J, Gautier M, Turpin R: Étude des chromosomes somatiques de neuf enfants mongoliens. *CR Seances Acad Sci III* 1959; 248:1721.

Lenz W: Malformations caused by drugs in pregnancy. *Am J Dis Child* 1966; 112:99.

Levine E, Weigel JW, Collins DL: Diagnosis and management of asymptomatic renal cell carcinomas in von Hippel-Lindau syndrome. *Urology* 1983; 21:146.

Mau G: Progestins during pregnancy and hypospadias. *Teratology* 1981; 24:285.

McBride WG: Thalidomide and congenital abnormalities. *Lancet* 1961; 2:1358.

McConville JM, West CD, McAdams AJ: Familial and nonfamilial benign hematuria. *J Pediatr* 1966; 69:207.

McCrory WW, Shibuya M, Worthen HG: Hereditary renal glomerular disease in infancy and childhood. *Adv Pediatr* 1966; 14:253.

McKusick VA: *Mendelian Inheritance in Man: Catalogs of Autosomal Dominant, Autosomal Recessive, and X-Linked Phenotypes*, ed 10. Baltimore, Johns Hopkins University Press, 1992.

Meadow SR: Anticonvulsant drugs and congenital abnormalities. *Lancet* 1968; 2:1296.

Menser MA, Robertson SEJ, Dorman DC, et al: Renal lesions in congenital rubella. *Pediatrics* 1967; 40:901.

Migeon CJ, Amrhein JA, Keenan BS, et al: The syndrome of androgen insensitivity in man: its relation to our understanding of male sex differentiation. In Vallet HL, Porter IH (eds): *Genetic Mechanisms of Sexual Development*. New York, Academic Press, 1979, pp 93-128.

Miller RW, Fraumeni JF, Manning MD: Association of Wilms' tumor with aniridia, hemihypertrophy and other congenital malformations. *N Engl J Med* 1964; 270:922.

Mills JL: Malformations in infants of diabetic mothers. *Teratology* 1982; 25:384.

Morris RC, Sebastian AA: Renal tubular acidosis and Fanconi syndrome. In Stanbury JB, Wyngaarden JB, Fredrickson DS, et al (eds): *The Metabolic Basis of Inherited Disease*, ed 5. New York, McGraw-Hill, 1983, pp 1080-1843.

Motulsky AG, Fraser GR: Effects of antenatal diagnosis and selective abortion on frequencies of genetic disorders. *Clin Obstet Gynecol* 1980; 7:121.

Nelson TE, Flewellen EH: The malignant hyperthermia syndrome. *N Engl J Med* 1983; 309:416.

New MI, Dupont B, Grumbach K, et al: Congenital adrenal hyperplasia and related conditions. In Stanbury JB, Wyngaarden JB, Fredrickson DS, et al (eds): *The Metabolic Basis of Inherited Disease*, ed 5. New York, McGraw-Hill, 1983, pp 973-1000.

Okerklaid F, Danks DM, Mayne V, et al: Asphyxiating thoracic dysplasia. *Arch Dis Child* 1977; 52:758.

Oppenheimer EH, Esterly JR: Observations on cystic fibrosis of the pancreas: V. Developmental changes in the male genital system. *J Pediatr* 1969; 75:806.

Patau K, Smith DW, Therman E, et al: Multiple congenital anomaly caused by an extra chromosome. *Lancet* 1960; 1:790.

Persky L, Owens R: Genitourinary tract abnormalities in Turner's syndrome (gonadal dysgenesis). *J Urol* 1971; 105:309.

Peterson RE, Imperator-McGinley J, Gautier T, et al: Hereditary steroid five alpha-reductase deficiency: a newly recognized cause of male pseudohermaphroditism. In Vallet HL, Porter IH (eds): *Genetic Mechanisms of Sexual Development*. New York, Academic Press, 1979, pp 149-167.

Potter EL: Bilateral absence of kidneys and ureters: a report of 50 cases. *Obstet Gynecol* 1965; 25:3.

Ransley PG: Vesicoureteric reflux: continuing surgical dilemma. *Urology* 1978; 12:246.

Robboy SJ, Noller KL, O'Brien P, et al: Increased incidence of cervical and vaginal dysplasia in 3980 diethylstilbestrol-exposed young women. *JAMA* 1984; 252:2979.

Ross DG, Travers H: Infantile presentation of adult-type polycystic kidney disease in a large kindred. *J Pediatr* 1975; 87:760.

Sabbagha RE: Ultrasonic evaluation of fetal congenital anomalies. *Clin Obstet Gynecol* 1980; 7:103.

Santen RJ, Paulsen CA: Hypogonadotropic eunuchoidism: I. Clinical study of the mode of inheritance. *J Clin Endocrinol Metab* 1973; 36:47.

Schardein JL: Congenital abnormalities and hormones during pregnancy: a clinical review. *Teratology* 1980; 22:251.

Schneider JA, Schulman JD: Cystinosis. In Stanbury JB, Wyngaarden JB, Fredrickson DS, et al (eds): *The Metabolic Basis of Inherited Disease*, ed 5. New York, McGraw-Hill 1983, pp 1844-1866.

Scorer CG, Farrington GH: *Congenital Deformities of the Testis and Epididymis*. London, Butterworths, 1971.

Seller MJ: Phenotypic variation in Meckel syndrome. *Clin Genet* 1981; 20:74.

Shkolnik A: Ultrasonography of the urogenital system. In Kelalis PP, King LR, Belman AB (eds): *Clinical Pediatric Urology*, ed 2. Philadelphia, WB Saunders Co, 1985, pp 181-219.

Similä S, Vesa L, Wasz-Höckert O: Hereditary onychoosteodysplasia (the nail-patella syndrome) with nephrosis-like renal disease in a newborn boy. *Pediatrics* 1970; 46:61.

Simpson JL: Müllerian aplasia. In *Disorders of Sexual Differentiation*. New York, Academic Press, 1976, pp 342-345.

Simpson JL: Gonadal dysgenesis and sex chromosome abnormalities: Phenotypic-karyotypic correlations. In Vallet HL, Porter IH (eds): *Genetic Mechanisms of Sexual*

Development. New York, Academic Press, 1979, pp 365-405.

Simpson JL: Antenatal diagnosis of chromosomal disorders. *Clin Obstet Gynecol* 1980; 7:13.

Smith DW, Lemli L, Opitz JM: A newly recognized syndrome of multiple congenital anomalies. *J Pediatr* 1964; 64:210.

Sommer A, Contras SB, Graenen JM, et al: A family study of the Leopard system. *Am J Dis Child* 1971; 121:520.

Stapleton FB, Johnson D, Kaplan GW, et al: The cystic renal lesion in tuberous sclerosis. *J Pediatr* 1980; 97:574.

Stevenson RE and Hall JG: Terminology. In Stevenson RE, Hall JG, Goodman RM (eds): *Human Malformations and Related Anomalies*, vol I. New York, Oxford University Press, 1993; pp 21-30.

Strauss J, McIntosh RM: Sickle cell nephropathy. In Edelmann CM Jr (ed): *Pediatric Kidney Disease*. Boston, Little, Brown and Co, 1978, pp 776-788.

Sweet DL, Kinzie J: Consequences of radiotherapy and antineoplastic therapy for the fetus. *J Reprod Med* 1976; 17:241

Thomas IT, Smith DW: Oligohydramnios, cause of the nonrenal features of Potter's syndrome, including pulmonary hypoplasia. *J Pediatr* 1974; 84:811.

Tilford DL, Kelsch RC: Renal artery stenosis in childhood neurofibromatosis. *Am J Dis Child* 1973; 126:665.

van Allen MI: Urinary tract. In Stevenson RE, Hall JG, Goodman RM (eds): *Human Malformations and Related Anomalies, vol II*. New York, Oxford University Press, 1993; pp 501-550.

Verschuer O: *Lehrbuch der Humangenetik*. Munich, Urban and Schwarzenberg, 1958.

Viby-Mogensen J: Succinylcholine neuromuscular blockade in subjects heterozygous for abnormal plasma cholinesterase. *Anesthesiology* 1981; 55:231.

Wertelecki W, Graham JM, Sergovich FR: The clinical syndrome of triploidy. *Obstet Gynecol* 1976; 47:69.

Williams DI: Pediatric urology in the evolution of surgery. *Ann R Coll Surg Engl* 1984; 66:159.

Williams HE, Smith LH Jr: Primary hyperoxaluria. In Stanbury JB, Wyngaarden JB, Fredrickson DS, et al (eds): *The Metabolic Basis of Inherited Disease*, ed 5. New York, McGraw-Hill, 1983, pp 204-228.

Wilson JG: Current status of teratology. In Wilson JG, Fraser FC (eds): *Handbook of Teratology, vol I*. New York, Plenum Press, 1977; pp 47-74.

Wolf B, Rosenfield AT, Taylor KJW, et al: Presymptomatic diagnosis of adult onset polycystic kidney disease by ultrasonography. *Clin Genet* 1978; 14:1.

Zonana J, DiLiberti JH: Congenital and hereditary urinary tract disorders. In Emery AEH, Rimoin DL (eds): *Principles and Practice of Medical Genetics, vol II*, ed 2. Edinburgh, Churchill Livingstone, 1990; pp 1273-1289.

CHAPTER 44

Perinatal Urology

Marc Cendron
Jack S. Elder
John W. Duckett

The last 20 years have brought about dramatic changes in the evaluation and management of urologic problems encountered in the neonatal period. Prenatal ultrasound has revolutionized the approach to congenital anomalies, in particular, those involving the genitourinary tract. Current technology allows the detection of urinary tract and renal lesions as early as 12 to 14 weeks' gestation and has provided insight regarding the natural history of these lesions before birth. The majority of pregnant women undergo sonography, allowing the fetus to be evaluated before it becomes sick. The development and use of experimental animal models have further expanded our understanding of the pathophysiology of certain disorders, such as obstructive uropathy. Combined with refinements in surgical and anesthetic techniques, early prenatal diagnosis has provided the pediatric urologist with the opportunity to counsel parents and subsequently to offer specialized high quality care for the newborn diagnosed prenatally with a congenital abnormality of the urinary tract.

This chapter presents an overview of the embryology and ontogeny of renal function, an understanding of which is paramount in the evaluation of the fetal urinary tract. Prenatal ultrasound screening is discussed as it pertains to the urologist. The urologic evaluation of the newborn with prenatally diagnosed genitourinary lesions is reviewed with special consideration to hydronephrosis, the most common entity diagnosed on prenatal ultrasound screening. Finally, common urologic problems encountered in the neonatal period are discussed, including conditions that are being seen with increasing frequency in children who have been in the pediatric intensive care for prolonged periods of time.

DEVELOPMENTAL ASPECTS OF RENAL PHYSIOLOGY IN THE FETUS AND NEWBORN

Embryology of the Kidney

Until recently, little information was available regarding developmental renal physiology. With the survival of extremely premature infants and the study of fetal animal models, a better understanding of the functional development of the fetal kidney has emerged (Brocklebank, 1992). Although the placenta functions as the main hemodialyzer for the fetus, the fetal kidneys play a significant role in blood pressure regulation, fluid and electrolytes homeostasis, acid-base balance, and the synthesis of certain hormones.

Before attaining its functional status at about 14 weeks' gestation, the kidney has undergone three stages of morphogenic and physiologic development (Cameron and Chambers, 1983). The first stage of formation of the kidney is the pronephros, a nonfunctional organ, which involutes by 5 weeks' gestation. The mesonephros is the second stage of kidney formation, consisting of about 20 pairs of glomeruli and thick-walled tubules, which secrete urine. The mesonephros degenerates but contributes to the formation of the ureteral bud, which arises from the dorsal aspect of the mesonephric duct. During the fifth week of gestation, the ureteral bud elongates and penetrates the mesonephric blastema, an area of undifferentiated mesenchyme located at the caudal end of the nephrogenic ridge, causing differentiation into the excretory system of the kidney during the seventh week.

The molecular mechanisms regulating renal organogenesis currently are being studied in animal models and in cell-culture line systems. Metanephric organ

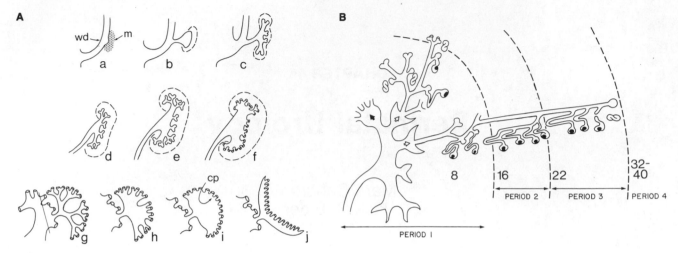

FIG. 44-1

A, Embryology of the upper urinary tract: the ureteral bud. *A,* bud arises from the wolffian duct *(wd)* and penetrates the metanephric mesenchyme *(m). b,* the mesenchyme caps the expanded end of the bud. *c,* the bud develops polar, hilar, and ampullary projections, which dichotomize. *d* and *e,* more dichotomous divisions, and *f,* confluence of the lumens of the divisions forming the pelvis and major calyces. *g,* second series of ampullary divisions to form the minor calyx (shown in one only). *h,* confluence of lumens except first division which forms the infundibulum. *i,* expansion of the lumen to form rounded minor calyx with orifices of the papillary ducts in the convex cribriform plate, *(cp). j,* inversion of the plate to form the papilla. **B,** Embryology of the upper urinary tract: the nephronic components. The minor calyces are shown in the early spherical shape with cribriform plate *(solid arrow)* and later indented forming papilla *(open arrow).* Nephrons develop in periods according to the nature of ampullary activity. *Period 1,* 8 to 15 weeks, temporary nephrons induced by dichotomizing ampullae of branching collecting ducts; *period 2,* 16 to 21 weeks, the ampulla induces nephrons that are linked by a common duct to a collecting duct—the so-called arcades in the inner cortex. *Period 3,* 22 to 32 weeks, the ampulla advances toward the capsule, inducing nephrons that connect independently to its newly formed collecting duct in the outer cortex. *Period 4,* 32 to 40 weeks, the ampullae rarely divide, and the already established nephrons mature. (Courtesy of F. Douglas Stephens, M.D.)

culture systems have aided in elucidating the regulation of growth and branching of the ureteral bud, the changes in extracellular matrix composition, and the cell adhesion events that occur during nephrogenesis. Some of the growth factors controlling cellular proliferation and differentiation following induction also have been characterized better (Fouser and Avner, 1993). Branching of the ureteral bud, for instance, is regulated by the mesenchyme and by growth factors provided by other surrounding tissues. The specific mechanisms have not been clearly identified, but recent experimental data suggest that chondroitin sulfate proteoglycans may be important factors in branching morphogenesis (Klein, 1989). To date, few peptide growth factors have been identified as responsible for metanephric development. However, recent studies suggest that postinductive nephrogenesis may be regulated by a finely tuned balance of local autocrine and/or paracrine growth factors. Alterations in the balance between positive growth factors and negative growth factors may result in abnormal nephrogenesis.

As the kidney develops under the influence of both the inductive process and under the influence of various growth factors and gene products, dividing branches of the ureteral bud penetrate the mesenchyme, compressing it and fragmenting it into sepa-

rate aggregate islands of cells. These oval masses elongate to form tubular structures that become sinuous and establish connections with the ampullae of the ureteral bud. Subsequently, the ureteral bud undergoes a series of approximately 15 generations of divisions, always in two branches. As described, this branching process is regulated by certain growth factors. Early in nephrogenesis, the polar aspect of the ureteral bud divides more rapidly than its midportion. The first four or five polar and two or three interpolar branches coalesce to form the renal pelvis (Fig. 44-1, *A*). The next three to five branches organize to form the major calyces (Osathonondh and Potter, 1963). Further divisions of the ureteral bud result in the formation of the minor calyces. First-generation collecting tubules develop at the papillary ducts and represent branching distal to the minor calyces. The collecting tubules represent five to seven additional generations of tubules. By 20 weeks, approximately 30 million tubules have developed, and differentiation of the renal collecting system is complete. (Potter, 1972).

The nephron arises from differentiated cells of the metanephric blastema, which becomes the glomerulus, Bowman's capsule, proximal and distal convoluted tubules, and loop of Henley (Fig. 44-1, *B*). Simultaneously, the nephron becomes vascularized by an in-

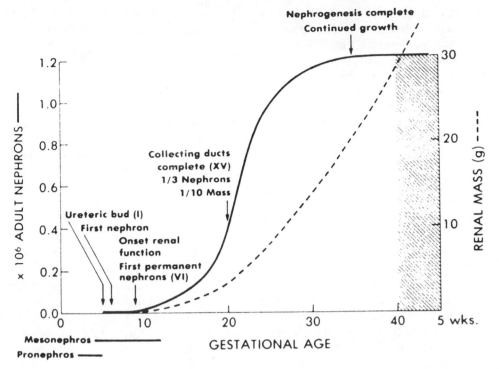

FIG. 44-2
Fetal renal development. The branching of the collecting system is complete by 20 weeks, but the majority of nephrons and most of the functional mass form in the cortex after 20 weeks. (From Harrison MR, Golbus MS, Filly RA, et al: *J Pediatr Surg* 1982c; 17:728.)

growth of capillaries that arise from the middle sacral and common iliac arteries. Experimental evidence suggests that differentiation imparts angiogenesis—stimulating activity to the metanephric blastema. Recently, a specific heparin-binding angiogenesis factor has been isolated and characterized from the embryonic mouse metanephros (Risaun and Ekblom, 1986). In addition, fibronectin has been found to have an important role in the guided migration of capillary endothelial cells into the primitive S-shaped tubules (Sariola et al., 1984). Formation of the renal unit (or nephron) is, therefore, the result of close interaction between three distinct cell types brought together by organized migration. These cell types are the epithelium of the wolffian-duct-derived ureter, the mesenchyme of the metanephric blastema, and the endothelial cells (Saxen and Sariola, 1987). Further nephron development occurs at nearly an exponential rate as the ureteral bud continues to divide.

In summary, the ureteral bud forms the collecting system, namely the ureter, renal pelvis, calyces, papillary ducts, and collecting system, whereas the metanephric blastema forms the entire excretory system (i.e., the nephrons). By 20 weeks' gestation, the ureteral bud has completed its series of divisions and the ductal system is complete. At this point, approximately one third of the ultimate number of nephrons are present; these nephrons form the juxtamedullary zone of the future renal cortex (Oliver, 1968). Elab-

TABLE 44-1

Nephrogenesis in the Human

Week of Gestation	Number of Nephrons	%
8	20-200	0.01
20	350,500	43
24	680,000	83
28	767,000	93
36*	822,000	100

From Potter EL: *Normal and Abnormal Development of the Kidney.* Chicago, Year Book Medical Publishers, 1972.
*Completion of nephrogenesis.

oration of the nephrons progresses along vertical extensions in the ends of the collecting ducts. Nephron formation is actually completed by 36 weeks' gestation (Fig. 44-2; Table 44-1). From then, until the child is two to three years of age, the nephrons undergo maturation, and hypertrophy occurs through 12 years of age.

Morphology of the Kidney

The human kidney has multiple lobes, whereas the kidney in the rat, rabbit, and cat is unipapillary with a single calyx (Potter, 1972). At 10 weeks, three to four lobes have developed. As branching of the ureteral bud continues, the number of lobes gradually increases, and by the end of the fourth month, approximately 15 are present. Each papilla forms a renal lobe, with one or two papillae opening into one calyx.

The lobes are hemispheric, with the calyx in the center and the tubules radiating outward with their attached nephrons, capped by the residual undifferentiated blastema. As vascular development proceeds, large blood vessels in the papillae become fixed in position, and in these areas, further peripheral growth is impaired. As a result, tubules lateral to the blood vessels may protrude from the surface of the kidney, forming secondary lobulation. At 36 weeks, when nephron formation is complete, approximately 30 lobes and lobulations may be seen (Potter, 1972) (Fig. 44-3). As renal maturation occurs and the nephrons increase in length and tortuosity, the demarcation of the surface of the kidney becomes less distinct. However, the lobar structure is permanent.

Initial renal morphogenesis occurs at the level of the upper sacral segments. The vertebral column of the embryo straightens as it grows, and the kidneys undergo growth in a cranial direction. During the eighth week, the kidney comes into contact with the large fetal adrenal gland, and by the end of the eighth week, renal ascent is nearly complete. The renal pelvis initially forms on the ventral surface of the kidney. As the kidney ascends, the kidneys rotate medially 90 degrees.

In summary, three events appear to be crucial to the development of two normal kidneys: (1) development of a single ureteral bud from each mesonephric duct during the fifth week of gestation; (2) induction of differentiation of the metanephric blastema by precise directional growth of the ureteral bud into the

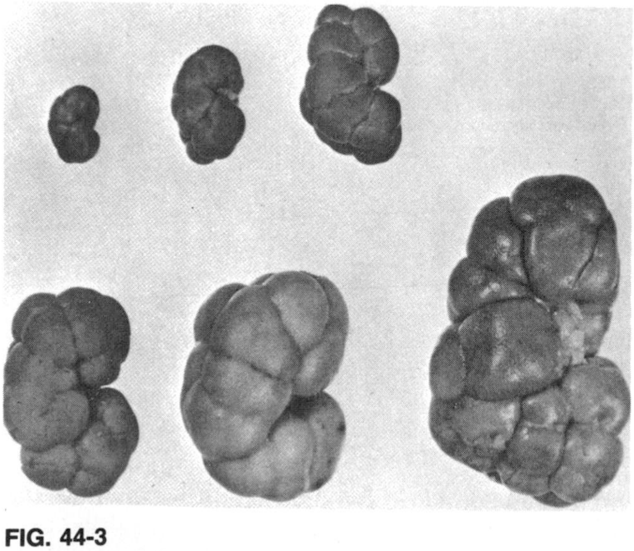

FIG. 44-3
The lobes of the kidney gradually increase in number and size during fetal development. Weight of kidneys and fetuses from which they were removed: 0.4 g and 93 g, 0.9 g and 254 g, 1.6 g and 508 g, 3.7 g and 1065 g, 7.5 g and 2080 g, 11.2 g and 3070 g. (From Potter EL: *Normal and Abnormal Development of the Kidney.* Chicago, Year Book Medical Publishers, 1972.)

blastema; and (3) ascent of the kidneys during the sixth, seventh, and eighth weeks.

Renal Function in the Fetus

The developing fetal kidney is very different functionally from the newborn kidney (Smith and Robillard, 1989). Throughout normal gestation, the placenta is the major regulatory organ of the fetal environment. Urine formation by the fetal kidney begins between nine and twelve weeks of gestation. Evidence for early urine production is documented by distention of the renal pelvis (Potter, 1972). Hydrostatic pressure generated by the accumulation of urine in the collecting system in the early stages appears to be influenced by the development of Chwalla's membrane at the caudal end of the ureteral bud (McCrory, 1980). This phenomenon may be responsible for the early canalization and dilatation of the collecting system. Subsequent rupture of Chwalla's membrane at nine weeks of gestation allows the urine to flow into the bladder. Others have demonstrated kinks and folds in the early ureteral development resulting from recanalization of the ureteral bud that may be precursors of obstructions at the ureteropelvic junction and ureterovesical junction (Alcaraz et al., 1991; Ostling, 1942, 1991).

Renal Blood Flow in the Fetus

Despite the fact that the kidneys constitute a larger percentage of body weight in the fetus than later in life, the fetal kidneys receive only 2% to 4% of the total cardiac output (Alexander and Nixon, 1961; Gilbert, 1980; Rudolph and Heyman, 1974). Approximately 40% to 60% of the fetal cardiac output travels through the placenta.

Autoregulation, a phenomenon by which the kidney is able to preserve its blood flow at a constant level during major changes in perfusion pressure may exist in the fetus (Smith and Robillard, 1989). At birth, following clamping of the umbilical cord, the cardiac output increases accompanied by a substantial rise in the renal vascular resistance, which maintains the intrarenal blood flow at rates similar to those late in gestation. As renal vascular resistance gradually decreases, an increasing proportion of the cardiac output is directed to the kidney for glomerular filtration, such that 15% to 18% of total output is received by the newborn kidneys. Renal blood flow, as estimated by *p*-aminohippuric (PAH) clearance, doubles by 2 weeks of age and reaches adult levels by 2 years of age (corrected for body surface area) (Rubin et al., 1949).

Several factors are known to influence fetal renal hemodynamics. These include the renin-angiotensin system (RAS), arginine vasopressin, atrial natriuretic factor, certain prostaglandins, kallikrein-kinin, and the sympathetic nervous system (Alexander and Nixon,

1962; Robillard et al., 1994). In the human fetus, renin has been localized in the mesonephros and in the metanephros by 8 weeks of gestation (Celio et al., 1985). A role for the RAS has been postulated in the process of angiogenesis, since renin also has been identified in the mesonephric and renal arteries (Jones et al., 1989). In addition, the high serum renin level found in the human newborn may account for the high renal vascular resistance (Arant, 1981; Gomez et al., 1988; Kotchen et al., 1972; Sulyok et al., 1979). The intrarenal distribution of blood flow in the fetus differs quantitatively from that of the newborn (Robillard et al., 1981). In the latter stages of gestation, glomerular blood flow appears to shift toward the superficial cortex, whereas no change in the medullary nephron perfusion occurs. This trend continues after birth and reflects diminishing vascular resistance in the outer cortex (Olbing et al., 1973). This centrifugal pattern of changing distribution of intrarenal blood flow appears to parallel the changes in glomerular maturation (Table 44-2). In the newborn, the volume of outer cortical glomeruli is proportionately less than that of the middle and inner cortical glomeruli, but in adulthood the size of the glomeruli from these three regions is similar (Fetterman et al., 1965; Spitzer and Brandis, 1974).

Throughout gestation, renal blood flow appears to be regulated by both humoral and neural factors. Changes in vascular resistance, after birth, allow greater perfusion of the kidney, which results in an increasing glomerular filtration rate. The decrease in renal vascular resistance might be due to decreases in circulating levels of vasoconstrictor catecholamines, vasopressin, and angiotensin, or to concomitant increases in levels of vasodilator prostaglandins (Corey and Spitzer, 1992; Gleason, 1987; Nakamura et al., 1986). Most of the increase in renal blood flow occurs in the outer zone of the cortex and is critical in urine production and glomerular filtration.

Glomerular Function in the Fetal Kidney

Urine is excreted by the fetal kidney as early as the fifth week of gestation when the mesonephros is capable of making urine. Renal tubular function begins in the metanephric kidney between 9 and 12 weeks'

gestation. By 14 weeks, the loop of Henle is functional and tubular reabsorption occurs. At term, urine flow rate average is more than 1 liter per day (Fig. 44-4). Urine production in the fetus has been estimated by ultrasound measurements of bladder dimensions and frequency of fetal micturition (Brace et al., 1994).

Glomerular filtration rate (GFR), which reflects the kidney's ability to filter blood, increases progressively with gestational age (Smith et al., 1993) (Fig. 44-4). Fetal GFR is dependent on several factors, including the permeability of the glomerular wall, the surface area available for filtration, and the ultrafiltration pressure, which depends on efferent arteriolar resistance, capillary blood flow, and the protein concentration in arterial plasma (Guignard and John, 1986). However, relatively little information is actually available on fetal GFR (Smith and Robillard, 1989).

Estimation of glomerular filtration in the perinatal period is based on determination of inulin clearance, which has been studied in neonate and premature, low birth weight infants (Coulthard, 1985; Wilkins, 1992). These methods are not entirely accurate and may vary, but they have been improved by the use of constant infusion techniques and by factoring in body weight as opposed to body surface area. (Coulthard, 1983; Wilkins, 1992). GFR is dependent on the following factors:

1. Ultrafiltration pressure
   —hydrostatic pressure within the glomerular capillary (P_{GC})
   —oncotic pressure within the capillary (Onc_{gc})
   —hydrostatic pressure within the proximal tubule (P_{pt})
   —ultrafiltration pressure $= P_{gc} - (Onc_{gc} + P_{pt})$
2. Permeability of the glomerular wall
3. Surface area of the filtration membrane

Wilkins (1992) confirmed that from gestational age 26 weeks to 40 weeks, GFR quadruples. After birth, GFR continues to mature slowly and progressively for about 4 months after birth. During the first 2 years of life, the rate of increase in GFR is much greater than that of somatic growth. It remains constant thereafter in the range of 90 to 100 ml/min/1.73 m². Studies in very low birth weight infants have to shown that, as early as 26 weeks' gestation, the fetal kidney has the capacity to assume excretory function, and this capacity can be achieved 2 days after birth (Wilkins, 1992). The mechanisms responsible for the rapid increases in GFR are not well understood. Since 80% to 90% of nephrons are formed by 26 weeks' gestation, their functional potential may be stimulated by the redistribution of blood flow through the kidneys, which occurs following removal of the fetus from the intrauterine environment.

TABLE 44-2

Nephron Glomerular Filtration Rate in the Guinea Pig

Age (Days)	Cortical* (nl/minute)	Juxtamedullary† (nl/minute)
1	0.9	17.2
15	4.1	43.2
30	19.3	42.1

From Spitzer A, Brandis M: *J Clin Invest* 1974; 53:279. Used by permission.
*Eighty percent of all glomeruli.
†Twenty percent of all glomeruli.

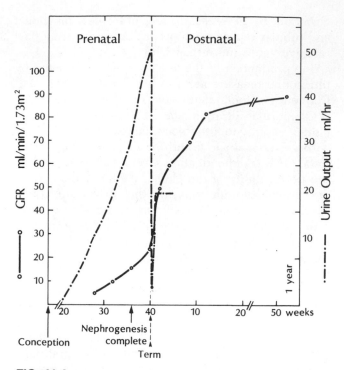

FIG. 44-4
Changes in glomerular filtration rate (GFR) and urine output during fetal development and infancy. A report (Robinowitz et al: *Am J Obstet Gynecol* 1989; 161:1264) suggests that urine output at term may be 50 ml/hr.

The ontogeny of the three primary parameters affecting GFR has been studied carefully in animal models. In the newborn guinea pig, it appears that a relatively small increase in the ultrafiltration pressure occurs, which can account for 10% of the increase in overall GFR (Spitzer and Edelman, 1971). The permeability of the glomerular capillaries also increases causing a slight increase in GFR. Finally, there is a progressive increase in the filtering surface area (Spitzer, 1992). In the newborn kidney, the glomeruli are larger relative to the tubules when compared with their relative sizes in infants and children (Fetterman et al., 1965). With renal growth and maturation, there is a modest increase in glomerular size, but the capillary network within the glomerulus continues to develop, with a resultant increase in the total surface area for filtration. A twenty- to twenty-fivefold increase in capillary surface area has been demonstrated in various species (John et al., 1980; Savin, 1983), and it accounts for 85% of the rise in total GFR.

Renal development and maturation occur in a centrifugal pattern. Thus, at any stage, the most mature nephrons are located in the deep (juxtamedullary) cortex, and the most immature nephrons are in the outer cortex. Although the majority of nephrons are located in the outer cortex, at birth the blood flow is directed primarily to the deeper cortical nephrons, whereas in the adult kidney, blood flow to the inner and outer cortex is equal. Thus there is a similar changing pattern of distribution of glomerular filtration with an increasing ratio of outer cortical GFR to inner cortical GFR with age (Olbing et al., 1973; Tavani et al., 1980). Table 44-2 reflects the early centrifugal changes in glomerular filtration in the deep cortical and outer cortical nephrons.

Tubular Function

The proximal convoluted tubule, loop of Henle, distal convoluted tubule, and collecting ducts are responsible for handling the filtrate from the glomerulus. Tubular functions include regulation of fluid volume, electrolyte balance, acid-base balance, and excretion of nitrogenous waste products. In the fetus, tubular function is reduced compared to that in postnatal life. Maturation of tubular function does occur in parallel to the increase in prenatal GFR (Table 44-3).

Transport of filtrate from the tubular lumen to interstitial fluid or peritubular capillaries is called *reabsorption*, and transport from the capillary to the tubular lumen is termed *secretion*. Transport may be active (against an electrochemical gradient and requiring metabolic energy) or passive (along an electrochemical gradient). Substances that are passively transported include water, certain organic acids, and urea. Substances that are actively reabsorbed include sodium, glucose, and amino acids. Other substances, such as organic bases and PAH, are secreted actively.

There are two types of active transport mechanisms in the kidney: systems that cannot be saturated and systems that are limited by a transport maximum (T_m). An example of a transport system that cannot be saturated is sodium transport. Characteristically, a relatively constant fraction of these substances is transported and excreted. In contrast, transport of glucose, bicarbonate, and PAH are limited. In systems limited by a T_m, all of the substance is reabsorbed or secreted until the maximum amount that can be transported, the T_m, is reached. The T_m for a substance must be distinguished from the plasma threshold for that substance. For example, the plasma threshold for glucose is the plasma concentration at which glucose first appears in the urine. In contrast, the T_m for glucose is the maximum amount that the tubules can reabsorb and is measured in milligrams per minute.

Although the plasma osmolality in humans is relatively constant at approximately 300 mOsm/L, the osmolality of the urine varies from 50 to 1500 mOsm/L depending on hydration, age of the patient, and state of maturation of the tubular system. Urine is concentrated as a result of a solute concentration gradient in the renal medulla. The solute concentration in the cortex and at the corticomedullary junction is isosmotic with arterial plasma, whereas at the tip of

TABLE 44-3

Functional Development of the Kidney

	Premature Infant	Full-Term Infant	Adult	Age of Maturation (months)
GFR (ml/min/1.73 m²)	8-10	20-30	120	12-24
Renal plasma flow (ml/min/1.73 m²)		120-150	630	3-6
Filtration fraction (%)		30-40	20	6-36
T$_m$ glucose (mg/min/1.73 m²)		35-100	300	12-24
Urinary dilution (mOsm/L)	50	50	50	—
Maximum urinary concentration (mOsm/L)	400-600	400-600	1,200-1,400	3
Maximum urine–plasma osmolar ratio	2.5		4	3
Ammoniogenesis	Lowered	Normal		
Urinary acidification	Normal*	Normal*		2
Hydrogen ion excretion	Normal or lowered	Lowered		

Modified from Royer P: The kidney in the newborn. In Royer P, Habib R, Mathieu H, et al (eds): *Pediatric Nephrology*. Philadelphia, WB Saunders Co, 1974, pp 116-127.
*Except in metabolic acidosis.

the papilla, solute concentration is extremely hypertonic compared with arterial plasma.

The concentration gradient is created by active transport of sodium out of the ascending limb of the loop of Henle. The extent of the gradient is directly proportional to the length of the loop of Henle. Blood flow through the medullary region of the kidney permits maintenance of the concentration gradient. The vasa recta loop up and down through the medulla, preventing dissipation of the concentration gradient created by active sodium transport out of the loop of Henle. As plasma travels down the descending limbs of the vasa recta, water leaves and solutes enter plasma since the plasma is going from a lesser to a more concentrated environment. As the plasma enters the ascending limb of the vasa recta, water enters and solutes leave the plasma passively, since the plasma is going from a concentrated to a more dilute environment. The ultimate effect is that plasma leaving the vasa recta is slightly hypertonic compared with plasma entering the vasa recta, resulting in some dissipation of the concentration gradient. If blood flow through the medulla is slowed, the dissipation is lessened; if blood flow increases, dissipation is increased.

Approximately half of the concentration gradient is provided by active reabsorption of sodium. The additional solute that allows the mature kidney to concentrate urine to 1500 mOsm/L is urea.

The concentration of solutes in the tip of the papilla of the mature kidney is approximately 1500 mOsm/L. As urine traverses the collecting tubules and collecting ducts that run through the medulla, it becomes more concentrated. If the walls of the collecting tubule are permeable to water, the fluid in the collecting tubules has the same solute concentration as that in

the deepest portion of the medulla, that is, it is quite concentrated. On the other hand, if the collecting duct and distal convoluted tubules are impermeable to water, the urine remains dilute. Antidiuretic hormone (ADH), produced by the posterior pituitary gland, regulates the permeability of the collecting duct and distal convoluted tubule.

In summary, urinary concentration is dependent on the ability of the ascending limb of the loop of Henle to transport sodium actively out of the tubular lumen into the interstitium, the length of the loop of Henle, permeability of the distal convoluted tubule and collecting duct to water, availability of ADH, ability of the kidney to respond to ADH, excretion of urea, solute load, and blood flow through the vasa recta.

All mammalian fetuses normally excrete urine hypotonic to plasma. Although the mechanisms for hypotonic urine in the fetus are not entirely understood, one reason is that fetal urea is cleared through the maternal circulation, preventing the development of a high concentration gradient. Thus, urinary sodium and chloride concentrations are substantially lower than plasma levels.

At birth, the neonate is able to concentrate urine to a maximum osmolality of 400 to 600 mOsm/L. The neonatal kidney gradually increases its concentrating ability and achieves an adult level at approximately 3 to 6 months. The inability of the newborn to concentrate urine is related to an inefficient countercurrent multiplier system with diminished accumulation of urea in the medulla, increased medullary blood flow, decreased tubular responsiveness to circulating ADH, and a relatively short loop of Henle (Yared et al., 1984).

The major limitation in concentrating ability is the low rate of urea excretion, which results because the infant is in a substantially anabolic state and uses most of its dietary nitrogen intake for growth. Infants fed a high protein diet demonstrated a rapid increase in urinary concentrating ability, with the increase being entirely attributable to increased urinary urea (Edelmann et al., 1960). In the normal infant, with increasing length of the loop of Henle and increasing blood flow to the outer cortex, higher concentrations of urea in the renal papilla result, allowing improvement in concentrating ability.

Another reason for the limited urine-concentrating ability of the newborn kidney is the low ADH activity. Bioassayable ADH is low or absent in infants less than 2.5 months of age (Janovsky et al., 1965), and there is also evidence of a relative insensitivity of the distal tubule to ADH (Schlondorff et al., 1978).

The newborn infant is able to dilute the urine as well as an adult, lowering urinary osmolality to 50 mOsm/L. Premature infants can decrease the osmolality to levels as low as 25 to 35 mOsm/L (Aperia et al., 1974). Furthermore, infants from 3 weeks to 13 months have a better urine-diluting capacity than adults, but it diminishes with age (Rodriguez-Soriano et al., 1981).

However, the newborn is unable to excrete a water load as well as an adult. For example, infants given a water load of 3% of their body weight excrete only 10% of the load in the first 3 hours, whereas an adult excretes all of it during this time (Ames, 1953; McCance et al., 1954). Furthermore, the infant has a maximum urinary flow of 6 to 8 ml/min/1.73 m² compared with 12 ml/min/1.73 m² in the adult (Barnett et al., 1952). Thus, although an infant's kidney is able to dilute urine as well as an adult's, its diuretic capacity is limited. Nevertheless, the immature kidney can double its urine output following administration of furosemide (Kurjak et al., 1981). In the rat, there is experimental evidence that there is an unelucidated factor in adult blood not present in infant rats that allows the kidney to generate a full diuretic response (Solomon et al., 1979).

The ability of the infant to reabsorb and excrete sodium is dependent in large part on its gestational age. The healthy term infant usually is in positive sodium balance regardless of the amount of salt in the diet (Spitzer, 1982). The fractional sodium excretion (Fe_{Na}) is determined by the formula:

$$Fe_{Na} = (U_{Na}/P_{Na})/(U_{Cr}/P_{Cr})$$

where $\quad U_{Na}$ = urinary sodium concentration

$\qquad P_{Na}$ = plasma sodium concentration

$\qquad U_{Cr}$ = urinary creatinine concentration

$\qquad P_{Cr}$ = plasma creatinine concentration

In the term infant, fractional sodium excretion is low, approximately 0.1% to 0.2% (Siegel and Oh,

1976). This low sodium excretion is probably secondary to the high plasma renin and aldosterone concentrations that are five to ten times higher in the neonate than in the adult (Arant, 1981). It has been speculated that constant sodium removal is used for the development of new bone in the neonate and that the removal of sodium serves as a constant stimulus for renin release (McCurdy, 1983).

Although term infants retain sodium easily, they have a limited ability to excrete a salt load compared with adults (Goldsmith et al., 1979). Since experimental aldosterone blockade does not alter the fractional sodium excretion in rats (Elinder and Aperia, 1983), it has been hypothesized that this limited ability to excrete a salt load may be secondary to an inability to elaborate natriuretic factors, such as oxytocin and kallikrein (Stewart and Jose, 1985).

In contrast, premature infants less than 35 weeks of gestation have a natriuresis resulting in a negative sodium balance (Sulyok, 1976), with fractional sodium excretion varying between 0.8% and 6.0% (Siegel and Oh, 1976). During this period, the premature infant reduces its high total body water content (approximately 80%) and extracellular fluid compartment (approximately 50%). The negative sodium balance is probably secondary to mutiple factors, including inefficient absorption in the gastrointestinal tract, short length of the proximal convoluted tubule in preterm infants, and a decreased sensitivity of the distal convoluted tubule to aldosterone (Siegel and Oh, 1976). Appropriate recognition of this physiologic loss of sodium is important, because aggressive replacement of the sodium loss can result in sodium and fluid retention, which could increase the risk of a symptomatic patent ductus arteriosus or necrotizing enterocolitis (Bell et al., 1979, 1980).

An important buffering mechanism in the maintenance of acid-base balance is the excretion of hydrogen ions by the kidney. The normal newborn has a relative metabolic acidosis. The urine in the neonate, and especially in preterm infants, is alkaline during the first week of life and becomes acidic during the second week (Edelmann, 1967). Furthermore, premature newborns are unable to acidify their urine as well as full-term infants. Urinary pH often is more than 6 in premature infants (Sulyok et al., 1972). The early production of alkaline urine is normal and evaluation for renal tubular acidosis need not be undertaken (Arant, 1984b).

Although term newborns ultimately excrete an acidic urine, they have a diminished capacity for excreting hydrogen ions compared with adults. One explanation for this limited capacity may be that the renal excretion of ammonia is less, particularly in the premature infant (Siegel and Oh, 1976).

In addition, the renal threshold for bicarbonate reabsorption in the fetus and neonate is lower than in the adult and is altered by changes in the extracellular fluid volume (ECFV) (Robillard et al., 1977). The expanded ECFV in the normal fetus and neonate depresses proximal tubular bicarbonate reabsorption. However, as the ECFV falls during the first few weeks of life, increasing bicarbonate reabsorption occurs, resulting in a rise in plasma bicarbonate and serum pH and a decrease in urine pH. Thus, although the infant is able to excrete usual acid loads, in the presence of a metabolic acidosis the newborn may require supplemental bicarbonate.

Another example of tubular immaturity is glucose excretion. Urinary glucose concentrations in premature infants less than 34 weeks' gestation are significantly higher than in older infants. Similarly, fractional excretion of glucose is high before 34 weeks' gestation (Arant, 1978). Thus, sick premature infants under 34 weeks' gestation receiving hyperalimentation for maintenance of sufficient caloric intake may be at risk for significant glycosuria. If unrecognized, this situation could result in an osmotic diuresis and dehydration. Consequently, infants receiving solutions of 10% dextrose should have their urine monitored frequently for the presence of glucose, particularly if they are less than 34 weeks' gestation.

Determination of Renal Function in the Fetus

Evaluation of GFR is important in infants with structural or functional abnormalities of the urinary tract or if nephrotoxic medications are being used. Traditionally, GFR has been based on a determination of creatinine clearance by the following formula:

$$C_{Cr} = [(U_{Cr} \times V)/P_{Cr}] \times (1.73/SA)$$

where
C_{Cr} = creatinine clearance ($ml/min/1.73\ m^2$)
U_{Cr} = urine creatinine concentration (mg/dl)
V = urine volume (ml/min)
P_{Cr} = plasma creatinine concentration (mg/dl)
SA = surface area (m^2)

The GFR in infants and children is compared with adult levels by using a correction factor, that is, the GFR is expressed as milliliters per minute per 1.73 m^2.

Creatinine is filtered, as well as reabsorbed and secreted. Using creatine may overestimate the GFR compared with measurements using inulin, which is neither reabsorbed nor secreted. However, although inulin clearance is a more precise method of determining GFR, it is impractical. In children between 1 and 12 years of age, a simple formula has been derived

that estimates GFR from the plasma creatinine and a child's length (Schwartz et al., 1976):

$$GFR = (0.55 \times L)/P_{Cr}$$

where L = length (cm). This formula is similar to the one derived earlier by Barratt (1974) and also applies to females between 13 and 21 years of age. However, in males between 13 and 21 years of age, the formula results in a significant underestimation of GFR, and in this group, a more accurate formula (Schwartz and Gauthier, 1985) is:

$$GFR = 1.5\ (\text{age in years}) + 0.5\ (L/P_{Cr})$$

A third formula is used for determination of GFR in full-term infants between 1 week and 1 year of age (Schwartz et al., 1984):

$$GFR = (0.45 \times L)/P_{Cr}$$

The third formula is not applicable to infants less than 1 week of age, since serum creatinine during this period is a reflection of the maternal renal status, and it takes approximately 1 week for the term newborn with normal renal function to reach a baseline creatinine level. In addition, the formula has not been verified in premature infants.

Another technique of measuring renal function in infants uses a radionuclide, such as technetium 99m diethylenetriamine pentaacetic acid (^{99m}Tc DTPA), which is cleared by glomerular filtration:

$$GFR = Vd \times (0.693/T_{1/2})$$

where
Vd = volume of distribution
$T_{1/2}$ = half-time of disappearance of the radionuclide

When this system is used, it is possible to determine the GFR by drawing a single specimen of blood at a specified time following injection of the radionuclide.

Although formulas using serum creatinine and body weight or height are relatively accurate in children with normal renal function, they are not very accurate in children with renal insufficiency.

In a preliminary report, Chandhoke and colleagues (1990) presented a newer and presumably more accurate method of assessing GFR using iothalamate that is infused subcutaneously with an insulin pump. After 24 to 48 hours of infusion, the distribution of the iothalamate reaches an equilibrium, and serum and urine samples are obtained, allowing one to derive the GFR. The technique has been compared to inulin clearance in adults with normal and abnormal renal function and has been extremely accurate. Extensive trials in children are underway.

Periodic determination of GFR in the sick neonate, particularly the premature infant, is important when the dosages of drugs that are excreted primarily by the kidney are calculated. When nephrotoxic drugs, such as aminoglycosides, are used, serial measurements of serum creatinine and trough drug levels should provide sufficient information to be certain that dosage is appropriate. Furthermore, in infants born earlier than 34 weeks' gestation, serum creatinine concentration often remains unchanged from maternal levels until 34 to 35 weeks of conceptional age is reached because the GFR is too low to clear creatinine from the plasma. The contribution to serum creatinine by maternal creatinine, ongoing creatinine production, rate of creatinine excretion, conceptional age, hemoconcentration or hemodilution associated with postnatal weight loss or fluid therapy, and the influence of nonrenal factors on GFR vary independently in any given infant (Arant, 1984a). However, regardless of renal or conceptional age, if the serum creatinine rises, the clinician should be alerted to renal dysfunction secondary to a structural or functional renal abnormality or to nonrenal factors, such as mechanical ventilation, that may alter the GFR in the neonate (Tulassay et al., 1983).

With the ability to image the fetal urinary tract came the opportunity of assessing renal function before birth. At the present time, direct measurement of renal function in utero is not technically feasible. However, fetal renal function can be inferred from (1) measurements of fetal urine outputs, (2) sonographic appearance of the kidneys, and (3) analysis of fetal urine composition after percutaneous aspiration.

Fetal urine output has been studied in a variety of animal models. In 1964, Chez and associates studied urinary flow in utero in rhesus monkeys using indwelling catheters placed in the urethra or bladder. They demonstrated that average urine flow was 5 ml/kg/hr.

In 1973, Campbell and co-workers studied human fetal urine output by measuring the size of the bladder in three dimensions by ultrasound (bladder size $= 4/3 \times \pi \times$ length $\times$ width $\times$ breadth $\div 2$) and determining the number of times the fetus voids per hour. In a series of patients between 32 weeks' gestation and term, the fetal bladder cycle varied from 50 to 155 minutes with a mean of 110 minutes. The bladder volumes were noted to increase from 11 ml at 32 weeks to 40 ml at term. Rabinowitz and colleagues (1989) have shown that fetal urine output increases from 5 ml/hr at 20 weeks to 51 ml/hr at term. Data from other studies have shown that (1) in the small fetus, urine output is lower, corresponding to fetal size rather than gestational age; (2) the fetus of a diabetic mother has an increased urine output; and (3) the fetus with anencephaly and polyhydramnios has a normal urine output (Kurjak et al., 1981; Wladimiroff and Campbell, 1974; Wladimiroff et al., 1976). In addition, administration of intravenous (IV) furosemide to the mother during the last trimester doubles fetal urine output (Kurjak et al., 1981; Wladimiroff, 1975). Therefore it appears that the volume of amniotic fluid is not a reliable indicator of fetal renal function except at the extremes of oligohydramnios.

The sonographic detection of cortical cysts and increased cortical echogenicity has been associated with irreversible renal damage in the fetus (Mahoney et al., 1984). Normal fetal kidneys beyond 30 weeks' gestation exhibit an echotexture similar to that of liver, with an internal architecture showing a differentiation between cortex and medulla. The medulla containing tubules and fluid appears darker. In contrast, a dysplastic kidney exhibits no internal architecture and may have increased echogenicity caused by a disruption in normal histology. The dysplastic fetal kidney is characterized by the presence of disorganized metanephric structures surrounded by fibrous tissue, which may be associated with cortical cysts (Hill, 1988). More than 90% of dysplastic kidneys with cortical cysts are associated with an obstructive process occurring during nephrogenesis. Mahoney and associates (1984) studied the kidneys of 49 fetuses with obstructive uropathy and found that the presence of cortical cysts had 100% specificity and a positive predictive value of 100% for the presence of renal dysplasia. However, the absence of cortical cysts cannot ensure the absence of renal dysplasia. Of the dysplastic kidneys, only 44% had cortical cysts. Increased echogenicity of the kidneys alone also was shown to be less specific and to have a lower positive predictive value than the presence of cortical cysts. The evaluation of renal function solely on the basis of renal echogenicity is further limited by the subjective nature of this feature. Ultrasonographic examination of the fetal kidneys may provide prognostic information if cortical cysts and increased echogenicity are detected, but is less specific in their absence (Crombleholme et al., 1990).

Fetal urine is an ultrafiltrate of fetal serum. Glick and co-workers (1985) observed that fetuses with congenital hydronephrosis and normal renal function produce hypotonic urine, whereas those with poor function made urine that was isotonic. In this study from the fetal treatment program in San Francisco, 20 fetuses with bilateral hydronephrosis were evaluated, 18 of which had percutaneous drainage of fetal urine prior to birth. In an attempt to determine prognostic criteria of renal function, urine electrolytes were studied. Prognostic features for "good" renal function included urinary sodium less than 100 mEq/L, chloride less than 90 mEq/L, osmolality less than 210 mOsm/L, and urine output greater than 2 ml/hr. Other reported prognostic criteria for good renal function were normal to moderately decreased amniotic fluid and a normal echogenic appearance of the kidneys. These criteria were established as a means to select those fetuses with sufficient renal function to have a favorable postnatal outcome if in utero decompression of an obstructive process was carried out early enough to prevent the sequelae of obstructive uropathy. These criteria have been questioned by several groups since normal controls in normal fetuses were not provided. In addition, they failed to take into account variation in urine electrolytes during gestation (Elder et al., 1990; Nicolini et al., 1992a; Wilkins et al., 1987).

In a follow-up study, Crombleholme and associates (1990) evaluated a series of 40 fetuses with bilateral hydronephrosis and found that the prognostic criteria accurately predicted a good outcome after intervention, showing a statistically significant difference in survival in the good versus poor prognosis group (81% vs. 12.5%). In addition to measuring the levels of fetal urine Na, Cl, and osmolarity, other groups have evaluated urine Ca^{++}, PO_4, and β_2-microglobulin to assess fetal renal function (Muller et al., 1993; Nicolini et al., 1992a and b) Nicolini and colleagues (1992b) found that fetal urinary calcium and sodium were significantly elevated in fetuses with renal dysplasia compared with those fetuses noted to have lower urinary tract obstruction but normal renal histology and normal clinical outcome (Nicolini, 1992b). Urinary calcium levels were reported to be the most sensitive indicators of renal dysplasia (100%), but they lacked specificity (60%). Urinary sodium was slightly less sensitive (87%) but was found to be the most specific (87%). Urinary PO_4, creatinine, and urea were not helpful in confirming renal dysplasia. Muller and coworkers (1993) found that β_2-microglobulin levels were significantly elevated in patients with an elevated creatinine (>0.56 mg/dl at 1 year of age) and recommended its use as a predictor of renal function at 1 year of age. It has been suggested that β_2-microglobulin may allow the identification of fetuses at risk for renal damage from unrelieved obstruction of the urinary tract.

FETAL MEMBRANES

The extraembryonic or fetal membranes include the chorion, amnion, yolk sac, and allantois (Gray and Skandalakis, 1972; Moore, 1982; Tuchmann-Duplessis, 1972). These membranes are intimately related to the placenta, which develops from (1) the chorion (fetal portion) and (2) the endometrium (maternal portion). The fetal membranes and placenta are essential to fetal growth and development by providing several important functions, such as protection by cushioning, nutrition, respiration, and excretion.

Implantation of the blastocyst on the uterine wall begins on the sixth or seventh day following fertilization. The trophoblast rapidly proliferates and differentiates into the cytotrophoblastic and syncytiotro-

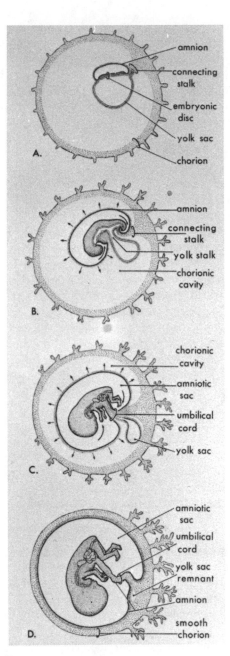

FIG. 44-5
Drawings illustrating how the amnion becomes the outer covering of the umbilical cord and how the yolk sac is partially incorporated into the embryo as the primitive gut. At 3 weeks **(A)**, 4 weeks **(B)**, 10 weeks **(C)**, and 20 weeks **(D)**. (From Moore KL: *The Developing Human. Clinically Oriented Embryology,* ed 3. Philadelphia, WB Saunders Co, 1982.)

phoblastic layers of the placenta. In addition, lacunar networks develop, creating a primitive uteroplacental circulation. Finally, primary villi form on the outer surface of the chorionic sac. By the end of the second week, the conceptus is completely embedded within the endometrium. Concurrently, the yolk sac and the amniotic cavity develop (Fig. 44-5). The allantois appears during the third week.

The yolk sac serves several important functions during embryogenesis. First, it appears to provide nutrients to the embryo during the second and third weeks while the uteroplacental circulation is being established. Second, angiogenesis begins in the yolk sac during the third week and persists until hematopoietic activity in the liver begins in the sixth week. Furthermore, germ cells form in the yolk sac and subsequently migrate to the gonadal ridge. Finally, the dorsal aspect of the yolk sac is incorporated into the embryo during the fourth week as an endodermal tube, the primitive gut. This structure gives rise to the epithelium of the gastrointestinal tract, trachea, bronchi, and lungs. By 12 weeks, the yolk sac is quite small but may still be identified. The stalk of the yolk sac usually is detached from the gut during the fifth week; persistence of the yolk stalk results in a diverticulum from the ileum, known as Meckel's diverticulum, with an incidence approximating 2% (Moore, 1982).

The allantois appears during the third week as a small fingerlike diverticulum from the caudal wall of the yolk sac. Although this structure functions as a reservoir for excretory products or as a respiratory chamber in some vertebrates, in the human it does not function. However, hematopoiesis occurs on its walls during the first 2 months, and its blood vessels become the umbilical vein and arteries. The allantois itself connects the urinary bladder to the umbilicus. As the bladder increases in size, the allantois becomes much smaller and forms the urachus. After birth, the urachus becomes the median umbilical ligament and extends from the dome of the bladder to the umbilicus.

The amnion, the innermost of the fetal membranes, is derived from the cytotrophoblast adjacent to the dorsal aspect of the germ disc. As the amnion grows, it gradually obliterates the chorionic cavity, concurrent with ventral longitudinal folding of the embryo. The primary junction of the amniotic cavity with the embryo is on its ventral surface. The amnion provides the epithelial covering for the umbilical cord. The amnion therefore lines the expanding amniotic cavity, which holds increasing volumes of fluid. Early in pregnancy the amniotic fluid appears to be a transudate of maternal plasma (Berman et al., 1967). During the first trimester, amniotic fluid production results from the active transport of electrolytes and other solutes across the amnion, which is composed of a single layer of cells. There is passive diffusion of water along the osmotic gradient thus generated (Wallenburg, 1977). As the fetal kidneys start to produce urine, and as flow through the urinary tract occurs, fetal urine is the major source of amniotic fluid. It is also likely that prior to keratinization of fetal skin at about 17 weeks, some of the amniotic fluid may be derived from water transport across the highly permeable fetal

TABLE 44-4

Amniotic Fluid Volume During Pregnancy

Gestation (weeks)	Volume (ml)	Fetal Urine Output (ml/24 hr)
14	100	—
16	185	—
18	360	—
20	380	—
24	450	—
28	800	230
32	850	293
36	850	439
40	800	655

Data from Haswell GL, Morris JA: *Obstet Gynecol* 1973; 42:725; Queenan JT, Thompson W, Whitfield CR, et al: *Am J Obstet Gynecol* 1972; 114:34. Used by permission.

skin (Abramovich et al., 1974; Parmley and Seeds, 1970).

The volume of amniotic fluid increases at a relatively constant rate during pregnancy until the end of the second trimester. Regulation of amniotic fluid volume depends not only on urine production by the fetus, but also on fetal swallowing, which starts between 8 and 11 weeks' gestation (Tomoda et al., 1985). By the end of the second trimester (24 weeks), the volume of amniotic fluid has increased steadily to approximately 800 ml, with this volume remaining relatively constant throughout the remainder of gestation. A mild decrease in volume is seen just prior to term (Table 44-4). Normally, amniotic fluid volume ranges from 500 to 2000 ml. During the first half of gestation, the amniotic fluid has an electrolyte composition and osmolality similar to that of fetal and maternal blood (Lotgering et al., 1986). Later, amniotic fluid osmolality progressively decreases with advancing age, reaching values of 250 to 260 mOsm/kg of water near term. The amniotic fluid composition of various electrolytes parallels the variations in osmolality. Later in gestation, sodium and chloride concentrations decrease, and urea and creatinine concentration increase (Wallenburg, 1977). Regulatory mechanisms of amniotic fluid volumes have not been completely studied, but there are three possible mechanisms involved: (1) water and solute transport across fetal membranes, (2) regulation of excretion and absorption by the fetus, and (3) maternal influences via the placenta over the fetus' fluid status.

The amniotic fluid provides several functions; it (1) allows symmetric growth and development of the fetus, (2) allows the fetus to move freely, (3) cushions the embryo and fetus against external forces, (4) aids in maintaining body temperature of the embryo and fetus, and finally (5) may have a role in lung development (Brace and Wolf, 1989).

An excessive amount of amniotic fluid (over 1.5 to 2 L) is termed *polyhydramnios* (or hydramnios) and a significantly diminished fluid volume is termed *oli-*

gohydramnios (less than 0.5 L). Throughout gestation, the circulation of amniotic fluid is a very dynamic event. The fetus swallows up to 500 ml per day as the urine output increases (Saunders and Rhodes, 1975). The placenta also may play an important role in the turnover of amniotic fluid, and the biological half-life of water in amniotic fluid has been reported to be as low as 90 minutes (Hutchinson et al., 1959; Seeds, 1985).

Obstetric evaluation of the fetus by ultrasound includes an assessment of amniotic fluid volume, particularly in the second and third trimesters. Several methods have been proposed. These include subjective assessment, measurement of the single, deepest pocket of fluid seen, amniotic fluid index, planning metric measurement of total intrauterine volume, and several mathematical formulae. In clinical practice, variability for all of these methods is low and is too similar to provide a basis for choosing one over the other (Doubilet and Benson, 1994; Moore and Coyle, 1990). Currently, the amniotic fluid index seems to be the most widely used criteria to evaluate amniotic fluid volume.

Polyhydramnios

As previously noted, polyhydramnios refers to the presence of an excessive amount of amniotic fluid. It occurs in 0.25% to 0.67% of pregnancies. Greater than 2000 ml of amniotic fluid during the third trimester constitutes polyhydramnios. The diagnosis may be suggested by maternal symptoms including excessive abdominal pressure, a protuberant or rapidly increasing size of the abdomen, excessive uterine contractions, or dyspnea. Physical signs include evidence of a disproportionate increase in uterine fundal height, abdominal girth, weight gain, and abdominal striae. Although the fetal head may be ballotted, the extremities often are difficult to identify with certainty. In addition, it may be difficult to hear the fetal heart tones.

In 2% of patients with polyhydramnios, the excessive amniotic fluid accumulates acutely, usually by 23 to 25 weeks' gestation, resulting in a very tense and tender uterus (Queenan, 1983). Chronic polyhydramnios is much more common and is diagnosed during the third trimester by abdominal examination or abdominal ultrasound.

Associated conditions and fetal malformations associated with polyhydramnios are shown in Table 44-5 (Behrman and Kliegman, 1983; Queenan and Gadow, 1970). Approximately one third are idiopathic. In women with diabetes mellitus, polyhydramnios is more common when the diabetes is severe. The most common associated congenital anomaly is anencephaly; approximately one half of pregnancies associated with anencephaly have polyhydramnios. In addition,

TABLE 44-5

Associated Conditions and Fetal Malformations Associated with Disorders of Amniotic Fluid Volume

Polyhydramnios (% of Total)	Oligohydramnios
Diabetes mellitus (25)	Bilateral renal agenesis
Anencephaly (20)	Posterior urethral valves
Erythroblastosis fetalis (11) (usually associated with hydrops fetalis)	Prune-belly syndrome
Multiple gestation (8)	Urethral atresia
Meningocele or encephalocele	Bilateral renal dysplasia
Tracheoesophageal fistula	Pulmonary hypoplasia
Esophageal or duodenal atresia	Growth retardation
Pyloric stenosis	Amnion nodosum
Klippel-Feil syndrome	Amniotic fluid leak
Cleft palate, cleft lip, or both	Limb defect
Achondroplasia	Fetal demise
Diaphragmatic hernia	Abdominal pregnancy
Multiple anomalies*	
Trisomy 18	
Idiopathic (34)	

*Not central nervous system.

abnormalities of formation of the upper gastrointestinal tract, such as tracheoesophageal fistula or esophageal or duodenal atresia, also have a high incidence of hydramnios.

The prognosis in a pregnancy complicated by polyhydramnios is poor. Perinatal mortality is 35% to 40%, and the incidence of stillborn infants is 10% to 20%. Perinatal mortality associated with twin gestations, erythroblastosis fetalis, and diaphragmatic hernia is quite high.

Recently, a small number of mothers with polyhydramnios have been treated with indomethacin, which reduces fetal urine output and consequently diminishes amniotic fluid volume considerably. This treatment has been reported to result in significant neonatal renal dysfunction in a few cases (Simeoni et al., 1989).

Oligohydramnios

Oligohydramnios occurs in approximately 0.4% to 5.0% of pregnancies, depending on the sonographic criteria and source of patients, and carries an increased risk of fetal abnormality and morbidity (Mercer et al., 1984; Philipson et al., 1983). Since the daily turnover of amniotic fluid depends in large part on adequate fetal urinary output, oligohydramnios often is associated with obstructive lesions of the urinary tract. Usually the diagnosis is made during prenatal ultrasound examination. In some cases, the diagnosis is subjective and may require serial ultrasound examinations to assess more accurately the true amniotic fluid volume.

If oligohydramnios is found or suspected and there is an associated urinary tract abnormality, one of two patterns generally is seen. In bilateral renal agenesis, neither the kidneys nor bladder are identified. The sonographic diagnosis of this condition is highly accurate (Romero et al., 1985). Bilateral renal agenesis usually results in oligohydramnios, but cases of normal amniotic fluid volume associated with this condition have been reported (Thomas and Smith, 1974). On the other hand, if oligohydramnios results from bladder outlet obstruction secondary to posterior urethral valves or prune-belly syndrome, characteristically a distended bladder is seen associated with bilateral hydronephrosis. Small cysts in the kidneys may be detected by ultrasound and indicate renal dysplasia. The fetal mortality rate for pregnancies complicated by oligohydramnios is high, particularly when it is detected prior to 27 to 30 weeks' gestation (Mercer et al., 1984; Sivit et al., 1986). Further discussion of the diagnosis and management of these conditions is presented elsewhere in this chapter.

When the urinary tract is normal in the presence of oligohydramnios, fetal growth often is retarded. Other associated conditions include amnion nodosum and a chronic amniotic fluid leak (Nimrod et al., 1984) (see Table 44-5).

Since amniotic fluid normally cushions the fetus, oligohydramnios often results in compression abnormalities. When oligohydramnios is secondary to bilateral renal agenesis, the phenotypic condition is referred to as *Potter's syndrome* (Fig. 44-6). Characteristically, such a fetus has external features suggestive of intrauterine compression, including a flattened nose, a recessed chin, low-set aberrantly folded ears, spadelike hands, talipes equinovarus, and hypoplastic lungs. Currently, it is thought that amniotic fluid is important in allowing normal lung development, largely by its cushioning effect. Support for this hypothesis is provided by reports of monozygotic twins,

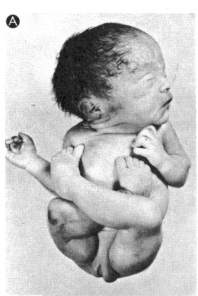
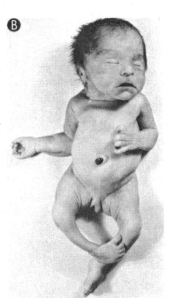
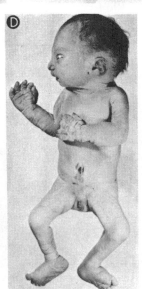

FIG. 44-6
Infants with Potter's syndrome. **A** and **B,** Infant with renal agenesis in intrauterine position and with legs extended showing how intrauterine fixation causes bowing of legs. Note low-set ears. **C,** Bowing of legs and deformity of chest from intrauterine fixation resulting from oligohydramnios. **D,** Excessive amount of skin causing enlargement of the hands often associated with renal agenesis. All infants appear remarkably senile. (From Potter EL: *Normal and Abnormal Development of the Kidney.* Chicago, Year Book Medical Publishers Inc, 1972.)

one of whom had renal agenesis (Marras et al., 1983; Thomas and Smith, 1974). Both fetuses were cushioned by the normal amniotic fluid and were born with normally developed lungs and without the secondary features of Potter's syndrome. The possible role of amniotic fluid in directly stimulating pulmonary development is unclear at this time.

Umbilical Cord

The site of attachment of the umbilical cord to the placenta is determined at implantation and is usually near the center of the placenta. If the blastocyst does not attach to the placenta at the embryonic pole, the connecting stalk (i.e., the umbilical cord) attaches to the placental margin or to the chorion. The cord is usually 55 cm in length and 1 to 2 cm in diameter. Excessively long or short cords are infrequent (Miller et al., 1981; Naeye, 1985). Usually there are two arteries and one vein encased in a mucoid substance called *Wharton's jelly*, which is rich in mucopolysaccharides. The umbilical vein is longer than the arteries, and the vessels are longer than the cord, resulting in significant tortuosity of the cord vessels and looping of the cord itself.

Approximately 1% of newborns have only one umbilical artery, which is associated with a variety of fetal anomalies, including the urinary tract (Bourke et al., 1993). In the past, it was believed that such neonates deserved routine radiographic imaging of the genitourinary tract. A recent study of screening renal ultrasound in 27 infants with a single umbilical artery showed that 5 (19%) had a renal anomaly (Leung and Robson, 1989). Consequently, imaging of the urinary tract by ultrasonography is advisable if there is a single umbilical artery.

Fetal circulation differs from postnatal circulation. In the fetus, well-oxygenated blood is provided by the placenta through the umbilical vein. Approximately half of this blood travels through the portal sinus and hepatic sinusoids, and the other half bypasses the liver, passing through the ductus venosus into the inferior vena cava. After passing through the heart, which has its own unique fetal circulatory pattern, blood of medium oxygen saturation travels down the aorta. Blood that is to return to the placenta travels through the umbilical arteries, which are large branches of the hypogastric arteries. The umbilical arteries have a branch, the superior vesical artery, at the level of the bladder, and then continue on to the umbilicus adjacent to the urachus. At birth, following the development of the neonatal circulatory pattern, the umbilical vein fibroses and becomes the ligamentum teres. The umbilical arteries distal to the branch of the superior vesical artery become the lateral umbilical ligaments. Near the base of the bladder, the obliterated umbilical artery is an important landmark in the identification and dissection of the distal ureter.

ENDOCRINE FUNCTION OF THE PLACENTA

The placenta represents the site of exchange between maternal and fetal circulation. In addition to its filtering role, the placenta appears to have an active metabolic role and an important endocrine function, which contributes to the maintenance of the pregnancy and growth of the fetus (Fig. 44-7). (Carter et al., 1991; Jones, 1988; Ohlsson, 1989). Furthermore, it serves as an immunologic barrier, allowing the fetus to grow and develop with the maternal autogenically different environment. The trophoblast that forms the epithelium through which the exchanges occur possesses the important property of allowing the passage of certain macromolecules. Active transports, as well as exchanges, over concentration gradients also are known to occur. Interestingly, it appears that the intimate relationship between trophoblast and fetal capillaries is due to the influence of the trophoblast itself on fetal capillary growth. The exact controls that the placenta exerts on fetal growth are unknown, however. Certain influences, such as that of human chorionic gonadotropins (hCG), are recognized with regard to sexual differentiation and adrenal gland development. Fetal hCG plasma levels influence fetal testosterone secretion from the testis. Peak secretion of fetal testosterone occurs at about 12 weeks' gestation

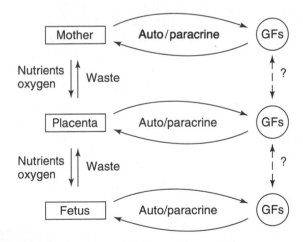

FIG. 44-7
The transfer of substrates and waste between mother and fetus is, for the most part, unidirectional. Adequate transfer of substrates (nutrients and oxygen) from the mother to the fetus via the placenta, and efficient removal of waste from the fetus to the mother are essential for normal fetal growth. Growth factors (GFs) are synthesized in the maternal reproductive tissues, placenta, and fetus and act locally in an autocrine/paracrine manner. Endocrine transfer of growth factors between the mother, placenta and fetus has not been shown to occur. (From : Growth factors in fetal growth. In Thorburn GD, Harding R (eds): Textbook of Fetal Physiology. Oxford, England, Oxford University Press, 1994.)

concomitantly with wolffian duct development and differentiation of the external genitalia (Conley and Masson, 1994). In addition, hCG may have a role in maintaining the fetal zone of the adrenal gland early in gestation.

The placenta has a very important endocrine role and throughout pregnancy secretes certain hormones, such as placental I-lactogens, progesterone, and estrogen, the regulation of which is poorly understood. Later in pregnancy, glucocorticoids produced by the fetus induce placental estrogen production, which in turn induces parturition. The placenta may influence fetal growth early, but later the fetus appears to become more autonomous and have a role in regulating placental function. Fetal growth factors originate from the fetus, but fetal growth itself depends on the normal development and function of the uterus and placenta. Placental growth factors also have been identified, but their role on the fetus is unclear (Ohlsson, 1989). The placenta is known to contain a high concentration of epidermal growth factor (EGF) receptors. EGF is a direct stimulator of DNA synthesis and may regulate fetal growth mainly by its influence on placental development. In order for fetal growth to occur, different cellular processes, specifically, proliferation and differentiation, are regulated by intercellular communications. There appears to be no central regulatory process but rather an integrated system where cell-to-cell and cell-to-matrix interactions are mediated by effector molecules within the extracellular matrix, by peptide growth factors, and by intercellular recognition molecules. The exact role of the placenta with regard to fetal growth remains to be determined precisely. The weight of the placenta has been demonstrated to increase with gestational age, and fetal weight is directly correlated to placental weight (Molteni et al., 1978).

PRENATAL ULTRASOUND OF THE URINARY TRACT

Since its introduction in the 1950s, ultrasonographic evaluation of the fetus has undergone significant improvement. Technological advances have allowed for earlier and more precise identification of congenital anomalies. The safety of ultrasound has been studied extensively, leading to the American Institute for Ultrasound in Medicine (AIUM) Bioeffects Committee to conclude that, with judicious use of ultrasound screening in pregnancy, the benefits outweigh any potential risks (American Institute for Ultrasound in Medicine, 1993).

The first report of the use of ultrasonography in pregnancy was published in 1958 and the first reported ultrasound diagnosis of a fetal urologic anomaly was published in 1970 (Donald et al., 1958; Garrett et al., 1970). The introduction of this diagnostic modality

heralded in a new era in medicine: an era in which a noninvasive diagnostic technique could reveal congenital anomalies in the fetus, thus allowing for prenatal counseling, early management, and possible intervention should the lesion be amenable to treatment. Availability of sonographic screening in the fetus has increased dramatically, such that several European countries have instituted programs for routine prenatal screening. Controversies do exist with regard to the indications and extent of use of ultrasound in pregnancy, as well as to when it should be administered (Garmel and D'Alton, 1994). Prenatal ultrasonography has become an important component of the fetal evaluation. Suspected anomalies can be precisely delineated and a team of specialists can offer expert advice and counseling. Options in the management and treatment can be discussed in order to plan for delivery and care of the newborn under optimal conditions (Lorenz and Kuhn, 1989).

With the increasing availability and use of ultrasonography, indications for screening of the fetus have been better defined: determination of gestational age by biparietal head diameter; suspicion of a gestational abnormality and strong family or maternal histories of prior congenital anomalies. Practice guidelines have been formulated and proposed by the American College of Obstetrics and Gynecologists (American College of Obstetrics and Gynecologists, 1993).

Although routine prenatal ultrasound has been advocated (Ellis and Bennett, 1984), a recent multicenter, randomized study of screening ultrasound in more than 15,000 low-risk pregnant women failed to demonstrate conclusively a significant difference in adverse outcome as defined by fetal death, preterm labor and delivery, significant neonatal morbidity, and neonatal death (Ewigman et al., 1993). Unfortunately, studies such as this one, designed to evaluate the efficacy of ultrasound as a diagnostic tool that is possibly helpful in improving clinical outcomes, fail to take into account the fact that the natural history of certain congenital anomalies has not been investigated fully and that, in turn, standardized management protocols do not exist for these prenatally diagnosed conditions. At the present time, current recommendations are to offer the options of a routine ultrasound to any pregnant patient following in a discussion of the potential risks and benefits (Garmel and D'Alton, 1994).

The overall incidence of detectable fetal anomalies is approximately 1%. The diagnostic accuracy depends on the expertise of the ultrasonographer, the quality of the equipment, the extent of the malformation, and timing of the study. The type of institution reporting rates of congenital anomaly diagnosed prenatally influences the reported incidence of fetal anomalies: tertiary centers may include anomalies that have been

TABLE 44-6

Genitourinary Anomalies Detectable by Prenatal Ultrasonography

Condition	Sex (Ratio)	Frequency	Kidney(s)	Ureter(s)	Bladder	Amniotic Fluid	Prognosis
Ureteropelvic junction obstruction (unilateral)	M/F (3-4:1)	1:2,000	Hydronephrosis	Not seen	Normal	Normal	Good after surgical correction
Multicystic kidney (unilateral)	M/F (1:1)	1:3,000	Large with cysts of variable size	Not seen	Normal	Normal	Normal
Primary obstructive megaureter	M/F (3:1)	1:10,000	Hydronephrosis	Dilated	Normal	Normal	Good after surgical correction
Ectopic ureterocele or ureter	M/F (1:6)	1:10,000	Large cyst; possible duplex kidney	Dilated	Normal or enlarged	Normal	Good after surgical correction
Posterior urethral valves	Male	1:8,000	Bilateral hydronephrosis; possible cortical cysts	Dilated	Enlarged	Variable; diminished or absent in severe obstruction	Usually good after surgical correction or drainage; poor if oligohydramnios is present
Prune-belly syndrome	Nearly always male	1:40,000	Bilateral hydronephrosis; possible cortical cysts	Dilated	Enlarged	Variable; diminished or absent if severely affected	Usually fair to good; may need surgical drainage; poor if oligohydramnios is present
Vesicoureteral reflux	M/F (1:5)	1:100	Hydronephrosis if reflux high grade	Variable	Normal; dilated if reflux high grade	Normal	Good; may need surgical correction
Infantile polycystic kidney disease	M/F	1:6,000-1:14,000	Large, echogenic	Not seen	Small or not seen	Usually absent or severely diminished	Poor
Renal agenesis	M/F (2.0-2.5:1)	1:4,000 (bilateral) 1:1,500 (unilateral)	Not seen	Not seen	Not seen	Severely diminished or absent	Stillbirth
			Not seen	Not seen	Normal	Normal	Normal
Hydrocolpos	Female		May have hydronephrosis	Not seen	Normal	Normal	Good after surgical correction
Ovarian cyst	Female		Normal (cyst may be confused with kidney or bladder)	Not seen	Normal	Normal	Good after surgical correction

referred from obstetricians and radiologists, significantly increasing the frequency of various anomalies.

The incidence of urologic anomalies detected in utero is approximately 1 in 500. In addition, a wide spectrum of dilatation of the urinary tract can be seen, making hydronephrosis the most commonly detected congenital condition that is observed by prenatal ultrasound. It may represent up to 50% of all abnormalities detected by prenatal ultrasound. By pooling a number of reports, it has been calculated that the incidence of detectable urinary tract dilatation in utero is 1 per 100 pregnancies, but of these only 1 in 500 is felt to represent a significant urologic problem (Thomas, 1990). Thus, the urologist must be familiar with prenatal ultrasound diagnoses and with the information one should expect to obtain at different times in gestation, as well as the accuracy of ultrasound in detecting urogenital abnormalities.

Table 44-6 lists the primary structural anomalies and conditions of urologic significance that may be revealed during a prenatal ultrasound examination. In all of these conditions, with the exception of primary vesicoureteral reflux and cloacal exstrophy, prenatal ultrasound usually demonstrates an abnormality, although a specific diagnosis can only be made on postnatal evaluation. Most of the obstructive anomalies occur primarily in males.

Normal Ultrasound Findings

In the normal fetus, current diagnostic capabilities allow for the detection of urinary tract anomalies as early as 12 to 14 weeks' gestation (Bronshtein et al., 1990; Patten et al., 1990). The role of ultrasound in the evaluation of the fetal urinary tract is twofold: (1) to identify the fetuses with any anomalies involving the urinary tract and (2) to monitor these lesions and characterize their impact on the overall health of the fetus. Variables that must be considered in the evaluation of the fetal urinary tract are gestational age at diagnosis, area of the urinary tract where lesions are identified, degree of dilatations of the urinary collecting system, evidence of obstruction, and associated anomalies elsewhere in the fetus.

Normal fetal anatomy can be identified very early in gestation. The bladder is visible at 14 weeks and appears as an echolucent area at the base of the fetal trunk. The size of the bladder may vary as it fills and empties in a cyclical manner. The maximum bladder capacity typically is 10 ml at 30 weeks and 50 ml at term. The presence of a filled bladder and normal kidneys gives presumptive evidence of adequate renal function. Conversely, nonvisualization of the urinary bladder, particularly in association with oligohydramnios, suggests poor renal function and poor prognosis (Bronshtein et al., 1993).

Although the kidneys may be visualized by 12 to 13 weeks, they should be identified in 90% of cases by 17 weeks (Lawson et al., 1981). The fetal kidneys are seen in transverse section just below the level of the umbilical vein early in gestation. They may be recognized by their typical shape and by the presence of a central echo from the intrarenal portion of the collecting system (Fig. 44-8). The renal collecting system (calyces and pelvis) should not be seen. The renal pelvis, when visible, is indicative of hydronephrosis. According to Hoddick, distention of the renal pelvis may range in anteroposterior (AP) diameter from 3 to 11 mm in up to 18% of normal fetuses studied after 24 weeks' gestation (Arger et al., 1985; Hoddick et al., 1985). It was suggested that a pelvic diameter larger than 10 mm or a ratio of the AP pelvic diameter to the AP renal diameter of greater than 0.5 indicated significant fetal hydronephrosis. These criteria were subsequently modified by Kleiner and associates (1987) with the addition of caliectasis as an additional indicator of significant hydronephrosis. The renal parenchyma appears to have a similar echo texture to that of the liver, and later in development the corticomedullary junction may be visible. Standards for normal renal size have been established in the fetus (Grannum et al., 1980; Jeanty et al., 1982; Lawson et al., 1981; Samparo and Aragio, 1989; Scott et al., 1991). The kidney circumference can be estimated to be equal to one third of the abdominal circumference throughout gestation. A formula to determine normal fetal kidney length has been proposed: kidney length (m m) = 16 + .06 × gestational age in weeks (Jeanty et al., 1982). Normally, the fetal ureter should not be seen.

The fetal adrenals may be recognized after the thirtieth week and appear as relatively hypoechoic ovoids or triangular structures superior to the upper poles of the kidneys. They are approximately half as large as the normal kidney. Later in gestation, the kidneys are surrounded by retroperitoneal fat, which assists greatly in their visualization.

Fetal sex also can be determined early in gestation. Determination of sex requires unequivocal visualization of the penis or scrotum or both, or of the labia majora. Birnholz (1983) demonstrated the sexual identity of 40% of fetuses under 24 weeks' gestation. Misdiagnosis occurred in 3%. 100% accuracy was reported in another study of second trimester examinations (Stephens and Sherman, 1983). Nonvisualization of the genitalia during the second trimester generally is due to a prone or complete breech fetal position or may be related to impaired imaging secondary to maternal obesity or oligohydramnios (Birnholz, 1983).

Determination of fetal sex is important primarily in patients whose fetuses are at risk for X-linked genetic disorders, such as hemophilia, chromic granulomatous disease, and Lesch-Nyhan syndrome. In addition, sonographic imaging of the fetal external genitalia might help in assessing the result of maternal steroid

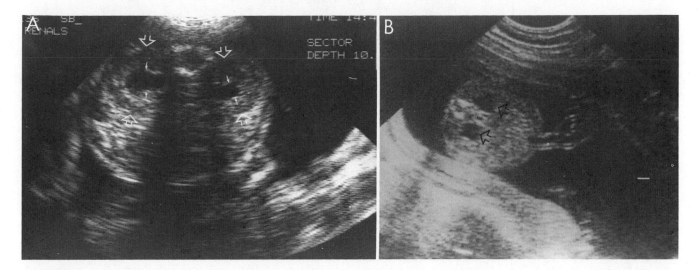

FIG. 44-8

A, Normal kidneys. Transverse section through both fetal kidneys shows bilateral prominence of renal pelvis (right, 8 mm; left, 6 mm) *(tiny arrows)*. Transverse anteroposterior renal width (right, 21 mm; left, 20 mm) *(open arrows)*. RP/RD ratio: right, 38%; left, 30%. Both kidneys were normal with extrarenal pelvis on postdelivery follow-up. **B,** Normal kidneys. Renal pelvis prominence bilaterally (right, 9 mm; left, 8 mm) *(open arrows)* in fetus at 22 weeks' gestation. Four subsequent examinations showed less prominence of the renal pelvis. At 32 weeks' gestation and 3 days after delivery, no renal pelvic dilatation was present. (From Arger PH, Coleman BG, Mintz MC, et al: *Radiology* 1985; 156:486.)

therapy in the female fetus with congenital adrenal hyperplasia.

Prenatal Detection of Genitourinary Anomalies

Genitourinary anomalies detectable by prenatal ultrasonography are summarized in Table 44-6.

Bilateral renal agenesis occurs in approximately 1 out of 4000 pregnancies (Potter, 1965). Unilateral renal agenesis is two to three times more common. Renal agenesis is thought to occur from an abnormality of the mesonephric duct or ureteral bud, resulting in failure of the metanephric blastema to differentiate. In such cases, the kidney and ureter are absent. Approximately 40% of infants with bilateral renal agenesis are stillborn, and those born alive die rapidly from pulmonary hypoplasia. Morphologic features in bilateral renal agenesis include low-set ears, prominent epicanthic folds, hypertelorism, and pulmonary hypoplasia (Potter, 1972). If the diagnosis of renal agenesis is made early in gestation, therapeutic abortion should be considered. If the diagnosis is made later in gestation, management of the associated complications, including breech presentation and intrapartum fetal distress, may be facilitated and neonatal resuscitation avoided.

Diagnosis of bilateral renal agenesis is made by the findings of oligohydramnios, absent kidneys, and nonvisualization of the urinary bladder. The most reliable indicator is the inability to visualize the urinary bladder because the adrenal glands in these fetuses tend to be ovoid and may resemble fetal kidneys (Bronshtein et al., 1993; Potter, 1965). The diagnosis of renal agenesis can be confirmed by imaging the

bladder intermittently over a period of at least 2 hours. If the bladder continues to remain nonvisualized, 10 ml of furosemide should be infused intravenously into the mother to confirm fetal anuria (Harrison et al., 1984; Kurjak et al., 1984).

The prenatal diagnosis of bilateral renal agenesis has been quite accurate at experienced centers. Romero and co-workers (1985) reported on 49 patients who were being evaluated for possible bilateral renal agenesis. The diagnosis was made and confirmed in 18 patients. There was only one false-negative ultrasound and no false-positive studies in their original report. However, in an addendum, the authors reported that three false-positive diagnoses were made. In these three newborns, kidneys reportedly were present and morphologically normal in two and abnormal in one. Apparently, these infants experienced severe intrauterine growth retardation, and the authors were less certain about their ability to establish the diagnosis of renal agenesis prenatally with 100% accuracy.

Bilateral renal agenesis has a polygenic inheritance pattern with a recurrence rate of 2% to 5%. In the series by Romero and associates (1985), 3 of 16 (19%) fetuses in whom there was a family history of bilateral renal agenesis were found to have this diagnosis. In a study of parents and siblings of index patients with bilateral renal agenesis, severe dysgenesis, or both, 9% had an asymptomatic renal malformation, most frequently unilateral renal agenesis (Roodhooft et al., 1984).

Very early in gestation, amniotic fluid may be present in association with bilateral renal agenesis, but it diminishes rapidly during the second trimester. Bilateral renal agenesis may be associated with normal amniotic fluid if there is another defect that impairs the normal flow of amniotic fluid, such as esophageal atresia, or if the fetus is part of a monoamniotic twin pregnancy with a normal twin (Thomas and Smith, 1974).

Hydronephrosis, or dilatation of the upper urinary tract, is the most common urologic abnormality found by prenatal ultrasound. Dilatation of the renal collecting system and/or ureter may be caused by either an obstructive process, such as ureteropelvic junction (UPJ) obstruction, ureterovesical junction (UVJ) obstruction, or bladder outlet obstruction, or it may be secondary to vesicoureteral reflux (Blane et al., 1983). Physiologic or nonobstructive dilation of the upper urinary tract refers to mild hydronephrosis for which no eitology can be determined (Blyth et al., 1993). Other anomalies, such as multicystic dysplastic kidney or a distended loop of bowel, may be misinterpreted as hydronephrosis.

The causes of fetal hydronephrosis are many but can be divided broadly into obstructive and nonobstructive dilatation. This distinction can usually not be made unequivocally on prenatal ultrasonography but is very important with regard to the ultimate effect on renal function. A distended renal pelvis alone does not imply that high intrapelvic pressures exist that might impair renal development and thus cause a reduction in function. The fetal and neonatal renal pelvis is extremely compliant and therefore may accommodate greater volumes at lower pressures. However, as renal pelvic distention increases so do the chances of having a functionally deleterious lesion. Furthermore, unilateral distention will not, in general, impact significantly on overall kidney function, whereas bilateral hydronephrosis may be associated with abnormal renal development.

The development of sonographic criteria that help in distinguishing physiological from pathological hydronephrosis has greatly contributed to the ability to assess the information provided by prenatal ultrasound (Arger et al., 1985; Fernbach et al., 1993; Grignon et al., 1986; Hoddick et al., 1985; Kleiner et al., 1987; Mandell et al., 1992b). Appropriate clinical management requires an accurate delineation of the abnormality(ies), as well as an appreciation of the natural history of untreated lesions and their impact on the developing fetus. Over the last 15 years, much progress has been made in defining the natural history of various forms of obstructive uropathy by careful follow-up of untreated cases and by the establishment of certain animal models that re-create fetal hydronephrosis (Blachar et al., 1994; Bronshtein et al., 1990; Burbige et al., 1992; Harrison and Filly, 1991; Nakayama et al., 1986; Reznick et al., 1988; Wilson et al., 1988).

A complete understanding of the natural history of fetal hydronephrosis is still evolving, especially in cases of upper urinary tract dilatation detected prior to 20 weeks' gestation. A recent report by Bronshtein and co-workers (1990) that describes the use of transvaginal ultrasound screening in the early stages of pregnancy found that fetal hydronephrosis may vary greatly over the course of gestation. In fact, out of 27 cases of fetal hydronephrosis (renal pelvis >3 mm) diagnosed between 13 and 17 weeks' gestation, only six displayed any evidence of urinary tract dilation postnatally; ten cases of unilateral hydronephrosis disappeared between 15 weeks' gestation and term. Parameters of abnormal renal pelvic dilatation in fetuses less than 20 weeks' gestation need to be further defined.

In order to better define fetal hydronephrosis and its impact on the developing urinary tract, ultrasonographic features must be evaluated systematically, including a measurement of overall growth and development of the fetus, amniotic fluid index, gender, renal parenchymal appearance, extent of dilatation of the collecting system, unilateral or bilateral involvement, bladder size and emptying, bladder wall thickness, and external genitalic anomalies. Because of the increased incidence of associated malformations, the fetus should be evaluated for extrarenal anomalies. The fetus with hydronephrosis should be scanned several times during gestation to monitor the evolution of the process.

Several series have reviewed the accuracy of diagnosing fetal hydronephrosis by ultrasound (Avni et al., 1985; Blane et al., 1983; Sholder et al., 1988; Watson et al., 1988). False-positive scans have been noted in 9% to 22% of prenatally suspected uropathies (Noe and Magill, 1987; Reznick et al., 1988). The incidence of physiologic or minimal hydronephrosis has not been well ascertained. However, progression of mild or physiologic hydronephrosis occasionally can be seen later in gestation or postnatally. In a recent study Morin and associates (in press) showed that 6.5% of patients initially thought to have mild fetal hydronephrosis required postnatal surgical treatment for a significant urologic lesion. Progression to pathological levels of hydronephrosis is most often associated with UPJ obstruction or vesicoureteral reflux (Mandell et al., 1991; Noe and Magill, 1987; Watson et al., 1988; Zerrin et al., 1993).

Fetal renal dimensions measured by ultrasound are important in diagnosing lesions that may impact on renal functional development. Later in gestation, a fetal renal pelvis AP diameter greater than 10 mm after 24 to 26 weeks' gestation usually is associated with an obstructive process (Arger et al., 1985; Johnson et al., 1992; Mandell et al., 1991). In many series, no abnormalities were found postnatally if the renal pelvis was less than 10 mm in diameter (Grignon et al., 1986). More recently, however, anecdotal reports of progression of fetal hydronephrosis and subsequent documented pathologic dilatation of the upper urinary tract have been described in fetuses with pelvic diameters less than 10 mm (Cendron et al., 1994b; Flashner et al., 1993).

With ultrasound screening being performed earlier in gestation and with improvements in sonographic resolution, dilatation of the upper urinary tract is being diagnosed more frequently. Certain sonographic criteria appear to have some prognostic significance, including caliectasis, worsening hydronephrosis, and increased cortical echogenicity (Cendron et al., 1994a). Other specific sonographic criteria, such as AP renal pelvis diameter, AP renal pelvis to kidney ratio, transverse diameter of renal pelvis to kidney ration, renal parenchymal thickness, and caliectasis, have been analyzed by Corteville and colleagues (1991). Of the criteria, caliectasis correlated best with functionally significant renal lesions. Current recommendations are that fetuses found to have an AP diameter of the renal pelvis >10 mm, an AP pelvic to renal cortex ratio >0.5, or fetuses with evidence of caliectasis after 24 weeks' gestation be evaluated postnatally.

Mild fetal hydronephrosis and transient dilatation of the urinary tract are issues that have clouded postnatal management. The etiology and significance of mild fetal hydronephrosis (AP diameter of the renal pelvis <10 mm after 24 weeks' gestation) have not been fully elucidated. Hoddick and co-workers (1985) demonstrated that the degree of maternal hydration had no significant influence on the fetal urinary tract. These findings were later confirmed by Allen and associates (1987). Potential causes for mild dilatation of the fetal urinary tract include transient obstruction, vesicoureteral reflux, and natural kinks and folds that may occur early in development (Blyth et al., 1993; Homsy et al., 1986; Najmaldin et al., 1990; Zerrin et al., 1993). The hormonal milieu of the fetus, as well as the degree of fetal bladder distention, also may influence renal pelvic diameter. Maternal hydronephrosis is seen commonly in pregnancy, and progesterone, a smooth muscle relaxant, also may play a role in mild fetal hydronephrosis.

Obstructive uropathy refers to urologic lesions that impact significantly on the development of renal function and are caused by a fixed obstruction within the urinary tract. Careful sonographic evaluation of the dilated fetal urinary tract may accurately localize the level of obstruction. The three most common causes of obstructive uropathy in the fetus are ureteropelvic junction obstruction, ectopic ureterocele, and posterior urethral valves (PUV).

UPJ obstruction is the most common cause of neonatal hydronephrosis (Lebowitz and Griscom, 1977). This lesion may vary in its severity, cause very large distention of the renal pelvis, and may be bilateral.

Although the pathogenesis is not well understood, partial ureteral obstruction early in pregnancy (first or second trimester) may result in pelvicaliectasis and renal dysplasia, whereas late partial obstruction may only cause pelvicaliectasis. Complete ureteral obstruction occurring prior to 10 weeks' gestation may be the cause of multicystic dysplastic kidney and contralateral hydronephrosis in the newborn (Gonzales et al., 1990; Schmitmeijer and Van der Harten, 1975). UPJ obstruction is felt to be an abnormality in the development of the UPJ or proximal ureters with disorganization in the smooth muscle and connective tissue elements resulting in a narrowed ureteral lumen (Hanna et al., 1976b).

In general, UPJ obstruction is secondary to an intrinsic obstruction caused by an aperistaltic segment at the UPJ, but a second renal artery supplying the lower pole is often an associated finding and has been implicated in the pathogenesis of hydronephrosis. UPJ obstruction usually occurs unilaterally, although in 21% of patients diagnosed in infancy, the condition is bilateral (Fig. 44-9; see also Table 44-12). In the presence of unilateral UPJ obstruction, the amniotic fluid and bladder are normal, and the ipsilateral ureter is

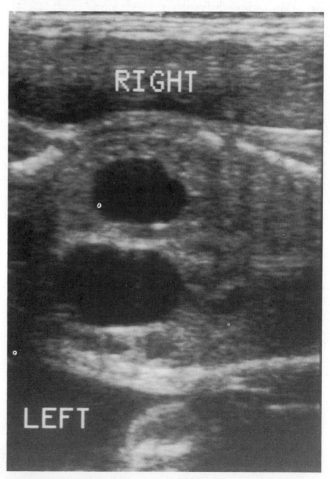

FIG. 44-9
Bilateral ureteropelvic junction obstruction in fetus at 26 weeks' gestation.

not visualized by ultrasound. The degree of renal pelvic and calyceal dilatation and thickness of renal cortex are variable. A distended renal pelvis alone does not imply that kidney function is reduced, because the fetal and neonatal renal pelvis are extremely compliant.

The diagnosis of UPJ obstruction prenatally is dependent on fulfilling the echographic criteria for significant pelviectasis, in the absence of a dilated ureter, distended bladder, ectopic ureterocele, and posterior urethra. The prenatal sonographic diagnosis of UPJ obstruction is thus a diagnosis of exclusion that can be achieved with a good degree of reliability (Kleiner et al., 1987). In general, the prognosis of unilateral UPJ obstruction is good because of the normal contralateral kidney. Cases of bilateral UPJ obstruction are at risk for poor outcome because of compromise in both kidneys (Flake et al., 1986).

In complete ureteral duplication the ureter draining the upper pole opens into the bladder caudal and medial to the lower pole ureter. The upper pole ureter commonly ends in an expansion between mucosa and muscle of the bladder known as a ureterocele. Hydronephrosis is common in the upper pole, as is obstruction-induced dysplasia (Caldamone et al., 1984). Every fetus exhibiting hydronephrosis should undergo careful inspection of the bladder to exclude a ureterocele as a cause. Ectopic ureterocele obstructing the bladder outlet may result in bilateral hydronephrosis (Reitelman and Perlmutter, 1990). Obstructing ectopic ureterocele is the third leading cause of neonatal hydronephrosis (Lebowitz and Griscom, 1977). More than 80% of affected neonates are female and the condition is bilateral in 10% to 15% of patients. In male patients, 40% have a single system drained by the ureterocele.

Megaureter may be detected by prenatal ultrasound and is characterized by a dilated kidney and ureter and usually a normal bladder. *The condition may be bilateral and may or may not be obstructive.* In nonobstructed cases, the megaureter may be secondary to vesicoureteral reflux, physiologic (secondary to high urinary flow in the fetus), or result from a mild functional obstruction at the ureterovesical junction. Complete evaluation of the condition is deferred until after birth, and early delivery is not warranted. When bilateral hydroureteronephrosis is detected, a distended bladder suggests bladder outlet obstruction secondary to posterior urethral valves, prune belly syndrome, urethral atresia, or high-grade reflux.

Posterior urethral valves is the second most common cause of neonatal hydronephrosis (Fig. 44-10). This condition is of particular concern because bladder outlet obstruction often has a very deleterious effect on both bladder and kidney development (Parkhouse et al., 1990). Infants born with this condition exhibit a spectrum of disease; in the most severe cases, pre-

natal sonographic findings include oligohydramnios, a dilated urinary bladder and posterior urethra, bilateral hydronephrosis, and subcortical renal cyst formation indicative of renal dysplasia. In addition, ascites and abdominal wall distention may be present. The sonographic features of PUV may vary considerably in the fetus depending on the gestational age and severity of obstruction. Thickening of the bladder wall with trabeculation and a dilated posterior urethra may be detected later in pregnancy (Cendron et al., 1994a).

The most important prognostic feature in the fetus with bladder outlet obstruction is the presence or absence of sufficient amniotic fluid. Oligohydramnios or anhydramnios detected during the second trimester, associated with bilateral hydronephrosis, is indicative of severe bladder outlet obstruction and nearly always is fatal (Mandell et al., 1992b). The primary cause of neonatal mortality is an inability to ventilate the lungs because of severe pulmonary hypoplasia. Many of these infants also have such severe renal dysplasia that even if the infant were to survive from a respiratory standpoint, renal function would be extremely poor or nonexistent (Coplen et al., in press). Infants with bladder outlet obstruction associated with oligohydramnios have external morphologic features characteristic of Potter's syndrome. In the fetus with bladder outlet obstruction, the degree of hydronephrosis may be less than with primary UPJ obstruction, but the bladder is dilated in the former condition.

The fetus with *prune belly syndrome* also has a sonographic appearance similar to that described for posterior urethral valves and the two conditions cannot be distinguished prenatally. However, prune belly syndrome is less common, and the chances of a viable newborn with either condition depend primarily on the presence or absence of amniotic fluid. An occasional female with this condition and impaired gastrointestinal motility has been reported (Glick et al., 1985); it may be a forme fruste of the megacystis-microcolon-hypoperistalsis syndrome.

Although *multicystic dysplastic kidney* is the most common cause of an abdominal mass in the neonate, it is less common than UPJ obstruction. Grossly, the reniform contour of the kidney is lost. A grapelike cluster of cysts of varying size replaces the renal cortex, and these kidneys do not function. The prenatal diagnosis is based on these macroscopic findings (Fig. 44-11). Characteristically, multiple cysts of varying size are seen unilaterally without identifiable parenchyma. However, the presence of one central dominant cyst with peripheral cysts of similar size can cause confusion in trying to distinguish this from UPJ obstruction. Indeed, a number of reports evaluating prenatal ultrasonography have not indicated an ability to distinguish UPJ obstruction from multicystic kidney. Multicystic kidney occurs bilaterally in 20% and is fatal. Hydronephrosis of the contralateral kidney oc-

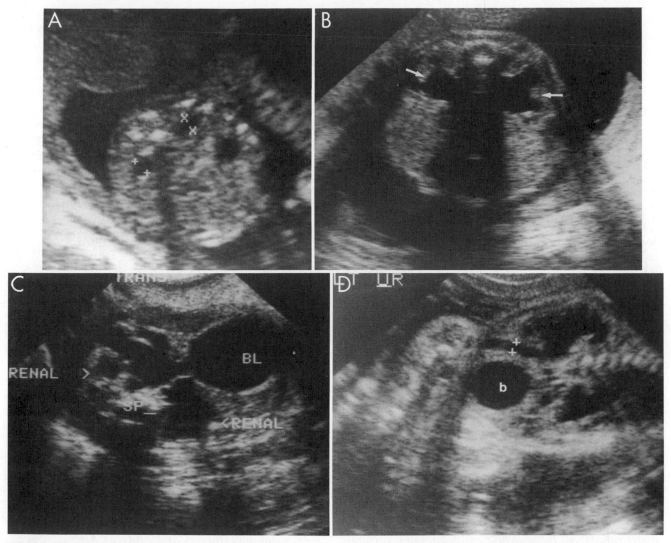

FIG. 44-10
Posterior urethral valves. **A,** Transverse section at 21 weeks' gestation shows minimal bilateral pelvic prominence (+, ×). Right and left pelves measure 5 mm. **B,** Transverse section shows bilateral hydronephrosis (right, 14 mm; left, 21 mm) at 33 weeks' gestation *(arrows)*. **C,** Oblique sagittal section shows prominent bladder *(BL); SP* = spine. **D,** Longitudinal section through left kidney shows hydronephrosis plus dilated ureter (+); *b* = bladder. (From Arger PH, Coleman BG, Mintz MC, et al: *Radiology* 1985; 156:487.)

curs in 10% and is usually due to UPJ obstruction (DeKlerk et al., 1977).

Infantile polycystic kidney disease is an autosomal recessive disorder that affects the kidneys and liver. In this condition, the kidneys undergo cystic dilatation of the collecting tubules. In contrast to the adult form of the disorder (autosomal dominant with large cysts), the cysts generally are 1 to 2 mm in diameter. The liver demonstrates periportal fibrosis and bile duct proliferation. One of the earliest reports of successful in utero diagnosis of polycystic kidney disease was by Garrett and colleagues (1970). Romero and associates (1984) reported a series of 10 fetuses with infantile polycystic kidney disease, and the diagnosis was made correctly prenatally in nine. Characteristically seen was oligohydramnios, nonvisualization of the urinary

bladder, bilateral renal enlargement (kidney circumference–abdominal circumference greater than 2 SD above the mean), and a typical highly echogenic appearance secondary to sound reflection off the wall of the numerous dilated tubules. Nephromegaly may not be demonstrated until 24 weeks' gestation. Thus, an ultrasound performed before 24 weeks in patients at risk should be repeated at 24 weeks to be more certain of the correct diagnosis. Although most infants with this disorder are stillborn or die within the first few weeks of renal failure, pulmonary hypoplasia, or both, an occasional patient survives only to succumb to the complications of periportal fibrosis later in childhood.

Adult polycystic kidney disease is an autosomal dominant disorder that occasionally presents in infants and has been detected prenatally (McHugo et al.,

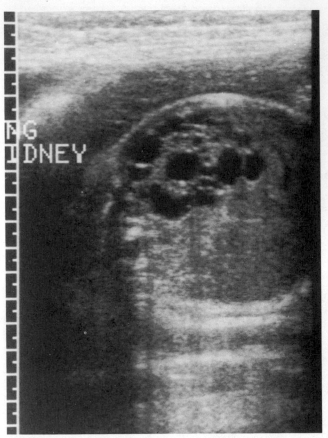

FIG. 44-11
Multicystic kidney at 31 weeks' gestation. Note multiple cysts of varying size without identifiable parenchyma.

1988). Typically the kidneys are enlarged and abnormally reflective, macroscopic cysts are often present. In addition, there is accentuation of the corticomedullary junction. In contrast, in autosomal recessive (infantile) polycystic kidney disease, the corticomedullary junction typically is not seen and the kidneys are highly echogenic without macroscopic cysts

At present, prenatal detection of hydronephrosis should impact positively on the postnatal outcome by allowing prenatal consultation by the pediatric urologist and the formulation of a management plan geared towards the prevention of further renal deterioration. The site of delivery may be changed to a tertiary care setting for early postnatal intervention. In general, however, postnatal management can be organized in a nonemergent basis. Only in rare cases is prenatal intervention indicated to prevent fatal consequences of obstructive uropathy.

FETAL INTERVENTION

The ability to identify congenital lesions in the fetus has increased our understanding of the natural history of the lesions prenatally and also has introduced new therapeutic options. In the fetus diagnosed with bilateral dilatation of the upper urinary tract and suspected of having obstructive uropathy, intervention has been proposed. However, fetal intervention is an area that has generated tremendous controversy not only because of medical concerns but also because of the ethical and legal issues at hand (Diamond et al., 1984; Elder et al., 1987; Gruppe, 1987; Marwick, 1993; Stestes et al., 1992). The goal of management of a fetus with congenital hydronephrosis is to prevent the sequelae of the obstructive process. These sequelae include renal maldevelopment as seen in renal dysplasia causing renal failure and oligohydramnios caused by urinary retention and pulmonary hypoplasia. However, at the root of medical concerns regarding treatment of fetal hydronephrosis are the questions regarding accuracy of diagnosis, timing of intervention, safety of the procedure for both the fetus and mother, and, most importantly, the beneficial effects of interventions with regard to clinical outcomes, an issue which to date has not been properly evaluated. Furthermore, reliable echographic criteria of obstructive uropathy have not been well defined, especially early in pregnancy. A major dilemma, therefore, in the management of the fetus with bilateral hydronephrosis is selecting those fetuses who may benefit from early intervention (i.e., those fetuses with obstruction severe enough to compromise renal and pulmonary development, but not so severe that the renal damage is irreversible, even if relief of the obstructive process is accomplished. Several methods have been proposed to assess the functional capacity of the kidneys in a fetus suspected of having obstructive uropathy: evaluation of the sonographic appearance of the fetal kidneys, volume of amniotic fluid, and measurements of fetal urine electrolytes and proteins (Cendron et al., 1994b).

Renal dysplasia has been studied in various animal models (Beck, 1970; Berman and Maizels, 1982; Glick et al., 1983; Steinhardt et al., 1988). Its pathogenesis may be multifactorial, and several theories have been proposed: (1) early high grade obstruction; (2) lateral ectopia of the ureteral bud causing induction of the metanephric blastema in an abnormal area; (3) an abnormal metanephric blastema; or (4) abnormal induction of the metanephric blastema by the ureteral bud (Mackie and Stephens, 1975; Schwartz et al., 1981). The dysplastic fetal kidney is characterized by the presence of disorganized metanephric structures surrounded by fibrous tissue, which may harbor cortical cysts (Bernstein, 1976; Risdon, 1975). The sonographic detection of cortical cysts implies the presence of severe renal dysplasia and indicates irreversible renal damage. More than 90% of dysplastic kidneys with cortical cysts are associated with an obstructive process occurring early in nephrogenesis. Dysplastic kidneys display abundant fibrous tissue within the parenchyma which, on ultrasound, may appear more echogenic. As discussed earlier, increased renal echogenicity as seen on ultrasound in the fetus is less specific and of lower positive predictive value than the presence of cortical cysts (Mahoney et al., 1984). Furthermore, renal dysplasia may be associated with large cystic formations within the parenchyma. Multicystic renal dysplasia (MCDK) typically has cysts of varying size, interfaces between the cysts, nonmedial location of the largest cyst, and an absence of organized parenchyma (Fong et al., 1986). MCDK is usually unilateral and may be associated with contralateral urologic anomalies that warrant postnatal evaluation (Flack and Bellinger, 1993; Kleiner et al., 1986).

The amount of amniotic fluid is not a very useful prognostic indicator except at the extreme of oligohydramnios or anhydramnios (Bellinger et al., 1983; Crombleholme et al., 1990; Harrison et al., 1982b). Unfortunately, by the time the amniotic fluid volume has been reduced to pathologic levels, fetuses with obstructive uropathy already show features of renal dysplasia and pulmonary hypoplasia that may be incompatible with life (Bellinger et al., 1983; Crombleholme et al., 1988). In addition, genitourinary anomalies often are found in association with other congenital anomalies, especially chromosomal abnormalities (Glick et al., 1985; Morin et al., in press).

Two additional screening tools that have shown some promise in helping to determine fetal renal function and may provide some prognostic indicators are fetal urine production as measured by the amniotic fluid index (Doubilet and Benson, 1994) and fetal urine electrolyte sampling. As the fetal kidneys begin making urine at 13 weeks' gestation, an ultrafiltrate of fetal serum is produced, which is hypertonic because of selective tubular reabsorption of sodium and chloride in excess of free water (Hill and Lumbers, 1988; McCrory, 1972). Between 16 and 21 weeks' gestation, the fetal urine becomes progressively more hypotonic (McCance and Widdowson, 1953; Nicolini et al., 1993). Fetuses who display dilatation of the upper urinary tract and are found postnatally to have normal renal function produce hypotonic urine, whereas those with poor renal function have been shown to produce isotonic urine (Glick et al., 1985; Harvison et al., 1982a; McFayden et al., 1983; Weinstein et al., 1982). The reasons why the fetal kidney subjected to longstanding obstruction produces isotonic urine have not been clearly elucidated, but it has been suggested that intrinsic and parenchymal changes, such as dysplasia, may alter the reabsorption of sodium and chloride and thus cause varying degrees of salt wasting (Glick et al., 1985).

In an attempt to better ascertain fetal renal function, Glick and colleagues (1985) studied 20 fetuses with suspected obstructive uropathy using percutaneous aspiration of fetal urine via a 4 F balloon tip catheter inserted into the fetal bladder during gestation. In evaluating urine electrolytes, prognostic features for

good renal function were proposed. These urine electrolyte features of adequate renal function in a fetus with sonographic evidence of obstructive uropathy include a urinary sodium <100 mg, a chloride <90 mg, an osmolality <210 mOsm/L and a urine output >2 ml/hr. These criteria were considered in the context of normal renal echogenicity and in the face of normal to moderately decreased amniotic fluid. Despite use by some investigators (Oesch et al., 1982), urinary creatinine excretion has not been shown to be helpful in prognosticating the renal function in fetuses with obstructive uropathy. Since Glick and colleagues' initial report (1985), the prognostic criteria for renal function have been disputed. Wilkins and associates (1987) reviewed nine cases of fetal obstructive uropathy; the prognostic criteria were helpful in predicting poor outcome, whereas in the good prognostic criteria group of five fetuses, only one had a good outcome, but it happened to be the one who underwent in utero decompression using a vesicoamniotic shunt. Furthermore, Elder and co-workers (1990) reported several cases in which fetal urine electrolytes were felt to be misleading with regard to the ultimate renal function in fetuses with obstructive uropathy. Recently, in addition to fetal sodium, chloride, and osmolality, Nicolini and associates (1992) evaluated fetal urine creatinine, urea, electrolytes, calcium, and phosphate. Urinary calcium and sodium were found to be significantly higher in fetuses with renal dysplasia compared to those with lower urinary tract obstruction and normal clinical outcomes. Fetal urine calcium levels were felt to be the most sensitive indicator of renal dysplasia (100%), but only had a specificity of 60%. The sensitivity to urinary sodium was less sensitive (87), but was more specific (80%) than urinary calcium. β_2-Microglobulin, a urinary protein that can be measured in fetal urine, was reported by Muller and colleagues (1993) to be elevated in fetuses who had an elevated serum creatinine one year postnatally. More recently this group reported their experience with other urinary parameters using nuclear magentic resonance spectroscopy and found that fetuses with renal insufficiency excreted higher levels of certain amino acids, such as alanine, valine, and threonine (Eugene et al., 1994). However, to date, no reliable marker of renal damage that would allow early diagnosis of obstructive uropathy thus enabling early intervention prior to the onset of irrevocable renal dysfunction has been identified.

In utero intervention to relieve an obstructive process affecting the lower urinary tract is thought to improve neonatal outcome by restoring normal levels of amniotic fluid and thus avoiding pulmonary maldevelopment. When oligohydramnios occurs during the early stages of lung development (16 to 24 weeks' gestation) the fetus displays pulmonary hypoplasia, characterized by a delay in the structural development of the lungs (Nakayama et al., 1986; Wigglesworth et al., 1981). Pulmonary hypoplasia may occur in the fetus with oligohydramnios from (1) mechanical restriction of lung growth and thoracic development secondary to external compression and (2) insufficient amniotic fluid bathing developing airways, thus preventing stretching of the developing bronchi and bronchiole.

Several factors suggest that mechanical factors may prevent normal lung development. First, infants with bilateral renal agenesis and oligohydramnios have typical facial features and limb defects (flattened nose, recession of the chin, aberrant folding of the ears, spadelike hands, and talipes equinovarus) and hypoplastic lungs. However, in monoamniotic twin pregnancies in which one identical twin has bilateral renal agenesis, pulmonary hypoplasia is not present (Thomas and Smith, 1974). Similarly, newborn infants with bilateral renal agenesis and an alternate source of amniotic fluid such as esophagenal atresia (Thomas and Scott, 1974) or myelomeningocele (Bain and Scott, 1960) have more normal-appearing lungs histologically. Second, pulmonary hypoplasia results in the fetus with congenital diaphragmatic hernia. In this instance, the hypoplasia represents developmental arrest of both lungs secondary to direct compression by the herniated viscera (Inselman and Mellins, 1981).

If amniotic fluid levels are restored by relieving the obstruction early in gestation, survival rates are markedly improved, whereas untreated oligohydramnios has been associated with a near 100% neonatal mortality rate (Crombleholme et al., 1990). In utero decompression therefore would appear to prevent neonatal demise from pulmonary hypoplasia, but its effect on ultimate renal function is less clear. The severity of renal dysfunction in a fetus with obstructive uropathy depends on the timing and the severity of the obstruction. It has become clear that the pathophysiology of obstructive uropathy is quite variable with regard to its effect on the kidneys.

Fetal intervention for urologic anomalies detected prenatally by ultrasound has consisted primarily of methods that would allow improved drainage of the obstructed urinary tract. Indications for possible in utero intervention are listed in Table 44-7. As previously noted, although the primary objective of intervention is to restore normal fetal development, the primary cause of morbidity and mortality in the newborn is pulmonary hyperplasia (Landers and Hansen, 1991). Despite the introduction of new techniques, such as extracorporeal membrane oxygenation (ECMO), which has helped in the management of neonatal respiratory distress, in the long run the natural history of obstructive uropathy has been shown to be variable and in some cases extremely debilitating

TABLE 44-7
Prenatal Intervention for Hydronephrosis

Indications

Presumed obstructive hydronephrosis, persistent or progressive, bilateral or in a solitary unit
Oligohydramnios
Otherwise healthy fetus without severe structural or karyotypic abnormalities
Adequate fetal renal functional indices (urine output >2 ml/h, Na$^+$ <100 mmol/L, Cl$^-$ <90, osmolality <210 mOsm/kg H$_2$O)
Without overt renal dysplasia (minimal echogenicity, hydronephrosis proportional to lower tracts)
Adequate informed consent

Contradictions

Presence of associated severe anomalies
Chromosomal abnormalities
Unilateral hydronephrosis with an adequately functioning contralateral kidney
Bilateral hydronephrosis without oligohydramnios
Severely dysplastic kidneys
Evidence of urethral atresia
Presence of a normal twin

From Blyth B, Duckett JW: Neonatal obstructive uropathy. In Reed GB, Claireaux AE, Cockburn F (eds): *Diseases of the Fetus and Newborn*. London, Chapman and Hall, 1995.

(Churchill et al., 1990; Gibbons et al., 1993; Parkhouse et al., 1990).

A fetal surgery registry was established to determine the risk of fetal intervention and to evaluate the clinical outcomes with regard to survival and quality of life (Manning et al., 1986). To date, 90 patients have been entered from 20 centers (Crombleholme, 1994). In the initial report from the International Fetal Surgery Registry, 72 patients with suspected fetal obstructive uropathy were treated with a vesicoamniotic shunt. The most common diagnosis was posterior urethral valves (29%, 21 of 73 patients), whereas in 45% (33 of 73), the diagnosis was unknown or unreported. The overall survival rate was 41% (30/73). Eleven of the 43 deaths (26%) were from voluntary termination of pregnancy. Three deaths (7%) were thought to be related to intervention. Of the 29 patients that died in the perinatal period, 27 (93%) died from pulmonary hypoplasia, whereas only one (2%) died from renal failure. The clinical experience for fetal intervention clearly suffers from the lack of consistency and from the wide range of underlying diagnoses. The data have been collected from 20 centers with no apparent coherent approach to diagnoses and with no defined patient selection criteria. Some patients had oligohydramnios, whereas others were treated despite presence of normal amniotic fluid volumes.

Thus far, the efficacy of prenatal decompression of the urinary tract has not been evaluated clearly because of the lack of a prospective randomized trial. There are so few patients who may in fact benefit from

TABLE 44-8

Fetal Intervention in 57 Patients*

Procedure	Number of Cases
Vesicoamniotic or peritoneoamniotic shunt	21
Aspiration of bladder	
Single	11
Multiple	7
Aspiration of kidney	
Single	4
Multiple	3
Renoamniotic shunt	4
Attempted shunt	10
Radiographic study	6
External drainage, kidney or bladder	2
Ureterostomies	1
Vesicostomy	1

*Some fetuses underwent more than one procedure.

TABLE 44-9

Complications of Fetal Intervention in 57 Patients*

Complication	Number of Cases
Shunt migration or poor drainage	11
Onset of labor within 48 hr	7
Urinary ascites	4
Chorioamnionitis	3
Extrusion of shunt (laparotomy)	2
Amniotic fluid leak	2
Perforated jejunum	1
Periureteral scarring	1
Placental hemorrhage	1
No complications	32

*Some fetuses had more than one complication.

in utero intervention that such a trial may be difficult to accomplish. Furthermore, the indications for fetal intervention have not been clearly defined. The most critical factor in evaluating fetuses with obstructive uropathy is the amniotic fluid volume. If this volume is normal or slightly diminished, it is likely that the fetal renal function is satisfactory and that sufficient pulmonary development may take place obviating the need for intervention. Gestational age is important is determining whether drainage of the fetal urinary tract may result in a successful outcome or whether it may be more worthwhile delivering the child for early, immediate, definitive treatment of the urinary tract. Certainly early delivery of the child may provide the opportunity to decompress the urinary tract in a child who may already have some degree of pulmonary development.

The time of intervention procedures in the fetus is critical. If an obstruction is diagnosed before 20 weeks' gestation and there is associated anhydramnios, the probability of severe irreversible renal dysplasia is very high, and it is unlikely that fetal intervention will be effective in restoring any degree of renal function (Bellinger et al., 1983; Harris et al., 1982). Thus, in such cases, either voluntary termination of pregnancy is recommended or else the pregnancy is allowed to continue until term without fetal therapy. If oligohydramnios and hydronephrosis are detected at 32 weeks' gestation or later, early delivery of the fetus should be considered. In these cases, fetal lung maturity should be confirmed with a lecithin/sphingomyelin amniotic fluid ratio. Term delivery is usually recommended if the amniotic fluid volume is normal. There is, therefore, a critical window between 20 and 32 weeks' gestation during which fetal intervention might be considered in a small number of cases.

The simplest and safest method of intervention for fetal hydronephrosis is needle aspiration of the fetal bladder or kidney to assess renal function (Glick et al., 1985). The bladder can be drained and urine obtained for analysis. The fetal bladder may then be re-imaged after a few days (Manning et al., 1983) or alternatively, may be allowed to drain continuously for a few hours to determine urine output (Glick et al., 1985). The most common procedure for relief of an obstructed process in the fetus is vesicoamniotic or peritoneoamniotic shunt. The latter procedure has been reported in a few infants noted to have urinary ascites. Several interventional techniques have been reported and are listed in Table 44-8.

The complication rate for fetal intervention is high, and is usually 50% (Table 44-9). The most common problem is failure of the shunt to drain for an extended period, requiring shunt replacement. In most cases, the shunt drains for only 3 to 4 weeks. Although some of the shunts have migrated, in most patients the shunt appears to become inspissated with particulate matter from the amniotic fluid. In addition, there have been anecdotal reports of shunt induced–abdominal wall defects with herniation of the bowel through the trochar insertion site or maternal ascites from an amniotic fluid leak into the maternal peritoneal cavity (Mandell et al., 1991; Manning et al., 1986; Ronderos-Dumit et al., 1991). In the initial report from the fetal surgery registry in seven patients (12%), labor ensued within 2 days of the fetal intervention. Finally, cases of chorioamnionitis were noted to occur after a routine use of prophylactic antibiotics, and during a period of long-term (4 to 16 hours) bladder catheterization (Crombleholme et al., 1990). Therefore, it is clear that the use of vesicoamniotic shunts is limited by the relatively brief duration of decompression, risk of infection both for the mother and fetus, catheter obstruction or dislodgment, fetal injury during placement, and potential inadequate decompression of the fetal urinary tract.

Recently, open fetal surgical procedures and fetoscopic techniques have been devised to obviate the difficulties experienced with vesicoamniotic shunting, although these techniques are still in the experimental stages of development (Crombleholme et al., 1988a; Estes and Harrison, 1993; Estes et al., 1992). Anecdotal reports of endoscopic treatment also have appeared (Quintero et al., 1994).

In summary, fetal surgery for obstructive uropathy remains limited to a very small number of cases and is currently being investigated in various animal models. The procedure should only be carried out at a tertiary care center, and the interventional team should be experienced in the diagnosis, management, and follow-up of fetuses with congenital anomalies. The current trend is to support the fetus in utero without surgery and to let the pregnancy come to term (Marwick, 1993).

Other Forms of Prenatal Intervention with Urologic Application

Hydronephrosis is not the only urologic condition in which attempts have been made to modify postnatal outcome by prenatal methods. Meningomyelocele and congenital adrenal hyperplasia also have been detected prenatally and represent areas in which prenatal efforts may be beneficial.

Myelodysplasia occurs in approximately 1 per 1000 births in the United States, but over the last 50 years a steady decrease in the number of neural tube defects, including myelodysplasia, has been observed (Hobbins, 1991). Contributing to this decline is the prenatal recognition of defects by ultrasound or by elevations in α-feto protein (AFP) in the mother's serum. Maternal serum AFP concentrations greater than three standard deviations above mean are associated with a 70% rate of open neural tube defects (Scott et al., 1990). Ultrasonography can help in ascertaining the cause of an elevated serum AFP concentration by accurately determining the presence in the fetus of spina bifida. Prenatal counseling allows for management options to be reviewed with parents. Recent information suggests that cesarean delivery without labor resulted in a substantially better lower extremity motor function when compared prospectively to vaginal delivery (Luthy et al., 1991). The impact of the form of delivery on the function of the lower urinary tract is, however, unclear. Prenatal recognition of fetal hydrocephalus, which occurs in 80% to 90% of children with myelodysplasia, can allow earlier shunting and improved outcomes (Paidas and Cohen, 1994).

Congenital Adrenal Hyperplasia

Congenital adrenal hyperplasia (CAH) is an autosomal recessive disorder and the most common cause of ambiguous genitalia in the newborn. In girls, significantly elevated fetal adrenal androgen levels cause masculinization of the external genitalia. Masculinization is thought to occur between 10 and 16 weeks' gestation when the testes normally masculinize the genital tubercle. Prenatal diagnosis of CAH is based on the detection of elevated 17-hydroxyprogesterone and adrenal androgen concentrations in amniotic fluid and HLA typing of cultured amniotic fluid cells (Pollack et al., 1979; Warsos et al., 1980). However, these tests cannot be completed prior to 16 to 17 weeks' gestation, and if one waited until the diagnoses were made to institute therapy, it would be too late to prevent significant masculinization. Accordingly, suppression of the fetal pituitary-adrenal axis with a glucocorticoid during gestational weeks 10 to 16 has been performed in an attempt to prevent masculinization of the female fetus (David and Forest, 1984; Evans et al., 1985). This therapy has been used in pregnant women who have already delivered one child with CAH. If the testing determines that she has another girl with CAH, steroid therapy is continued. The purpose of the treatment is to prevent masculinization of the female external genitalia; it has no effect on the long-term need for steroid therapy following delivery.

David and Forest (1984) treated six mothers at risk with either hydrocortisone or dexamethasone in early pregnancy. In two mothers, it was determined that there was a female fetus with CAH. Steroid therapy was continued until term, and both were found to have a severe salt-wasting 21-hydroxylase deficiency. In one, the genitalia were essentially normal, and the other had mildly virilized genitalia, which probably would not need reconstructive surgery. Evans and co-workers (1985) reported one case of treatment of a fetus at risk for CAH. Fetal adrenal gland suppression was maintained by administering dexamethasone to the mother, but the infant was heterozygous for CAH.

In the future, prenatal diagnosis of CAH and other hereditary diseases may be facilitated using DNA probes (Matsumoto et al., 1988; Pang et al., 1990).

Important ethical and legal consideration also have evolved from the improvements in the prenatal diagnosis of congenital anomalies and, in particular, from attempts in treating these disorders (Colodny, 1986). The first and foremost ethical consideration is that invasive therapy for fetal hydronephrosis must be considered experimental. Much has yet to be learned with regard to the development of the lungs and urinary tract, as well as the pathophysiology of obstructive uropathy. Few of the reported efforts of therapeutic intervention have met with success or have been proved to alter the natural history of existing congenital anomaly, so as to provide objective improvements in clinical outcome.

Intimately related to the recognition that therapy for fetal hydronephrosis is experimental is the necessity of providing informed consent. Policies regarding informed consent for in utero surgery and fetal research were established by the District Council and Council on Scientific Affairs, the American Medical Association (1983). They state that (1) voluntary informed consent in writing should be given by the pregnant woman, acting in the best interest of the fetus; and (2) alternative treatments or methods of care, if any, should be reviewed carefully and explained fully. If safer and simpler treatment is known, it should be pursued. In addition, it has been recommended that an impartial physician, the mother's own physician, anesthetist, and other family members, particularly the father, be consulted to participate in the decision-making (Fletcher and Jonsen, 1984).

In conclusion, the management options for a fetus diagnosed early in gestation with bilateral hydronephrosis include the following:

1. Observation, which would involve monitoring of the amniotic fluid and its volume, evaluation of renal pelvic dilatation, evaluation of the renal parenchyma, size of the bladder, and emptying of the bladder. The ideal frequency of follow-up studies remains to be determined (Mandell et al., 1990). Serial ultrasounds are certainly recommended if the diagnosis is made prior to 30 weeks (Fugelseth et al., 1994).

2. Termination of the pregnancy if the urinary tract anomaly appears to be incompatible with postnatal life. These lesions include severe early obstructive uropathy with evidence of severe renal dysplasia and pulmonary hypoplasia with oligohydramnios or anhydramnios. In these cases, termination can be carried out before 24 weeks. Genetic counseling is certainly recommended in these conditions (Inati et al., 1994).

3. Early delivery can be carried out at gestational age 30 to 32 weeks or later. Evaluation of lung maturity is helpful to ascertain the risk for the fetus (Deppe et al., 1980). Delivery at a tertiary care facility is recommended in these cases.

4. Percutaneous shunting: indications for fetal intervention are listed in Table 44-7. Several catheter systems are available for use, but a versatile, reliable catheter has not yet been developed. Two experimental procedures, open fetal surgery and fetoscopic or endoscopic procedures, are on the horizon.

RADIOGRAPHIC EVALUATION OF THE URINARY TRACT IN THE NEWBORN

Prenatal Evaluation

Unilateral dilatation of the upper urinary tract of the fetus may be due to ureteropelvic obstruction (UPJ), unilateral vesicoureteral reflux (VUR), ureterovesical (UVJ) junction obstruction, renal duplication, nonrefluxing, nonobstructive megaureter, or idiopathic physiological dilatation of the urinary tract. However, the most common cause of unilateral hydronephrosis is UPJ obstruction (Harrison and Filly,

1991). All of these conditions can be seen with great variation in the degree of dilatation of the renal pelvis, calyces, and ureter. It should not be confused with dysplastic kidney or dilatation of the bowel. The long-term renal function in the affected renal unit is quite variable. In cases in which the degree of hydronephrosis is significant (>15 mm) with caliectasis and renal parenchymal thinning from a long-standing obstruction, renal function in the involved kidney may be severely compromised. If the obstruction has occurred before 24 weeks' gestation, dysplastic changes may be identifiable by an increase in the echogenicity of the kidney or the presence of cortical cysts (Mahoney et al., 1984).

The prenatal diagnosis of unilateral hydronephrosis may be suggestive of obstruction, but vesicoureteral reflux (VUR) also can be identified, especially during the cycles of filling and emptying of the fetal bladder. VUR is associated with changes in the degree of ureteral and pelvic dilatation (Helin and Persson, 1986; Najmaldin et al., 1990; Zerrin et al., 1993). Prenatal ultrasonographic identification of VUR requires follow-up in the postnatal period in the form of a postnatal ultrasound and voiding cystourethrogram (VCUG). Recent studies suggest that the natural history of prenatally diagnosed VUR differs from postnatally diagnosed VUR because it affects a higher percentage of males; it is more severe and is associated with a higher incidence of coexistent anomalies (Zerrin et al., 1993).

UVJ obstruction most commonly is found unilaterally. Dilatation of the ureter may be identified also with varying degrees, but massive renal pelvic dilatation is not usually seen. The dilated ureter can be confused with the bladder, pelvic cysts, or a dilated loop of bowel. Duplication of the upper urinary tract should be suspected when hydronephrosis is seen in conjunction with cystic dilatation of the upper pole of the kidney or the presence of a ureterocele in the bladder (Friedland et al., 1983).

If the amniotic fluid volume is normal and the fetus has no other anomalies before 30 weeks' gestation, one ultrasonographic evaluation will be necessary before birth to determine progression or regression of the hydronephrosis (Ghidini et al., 1990) (Fig. 44-12).

When bilateral hydronephrosis is identified early in gestation, of greatest concern is the possibility of a urinary tract obstruction. Bilateral hydronephrosis attributable to obstruction is most often infravesical, but also may occur at the level of the UVJ or UPJ. The most common cause of infravesical obstruction is posterior urethral valves, which occur in approximately 1 in 5000 to 1 in 8000 boys, with a wide spectrum of severity (Hendren, 1991).

It is thought that high intravesical pressure is transmitted to the upper urinary tracts, which contributes to the maldevelopment of the kidneys. The fetus may

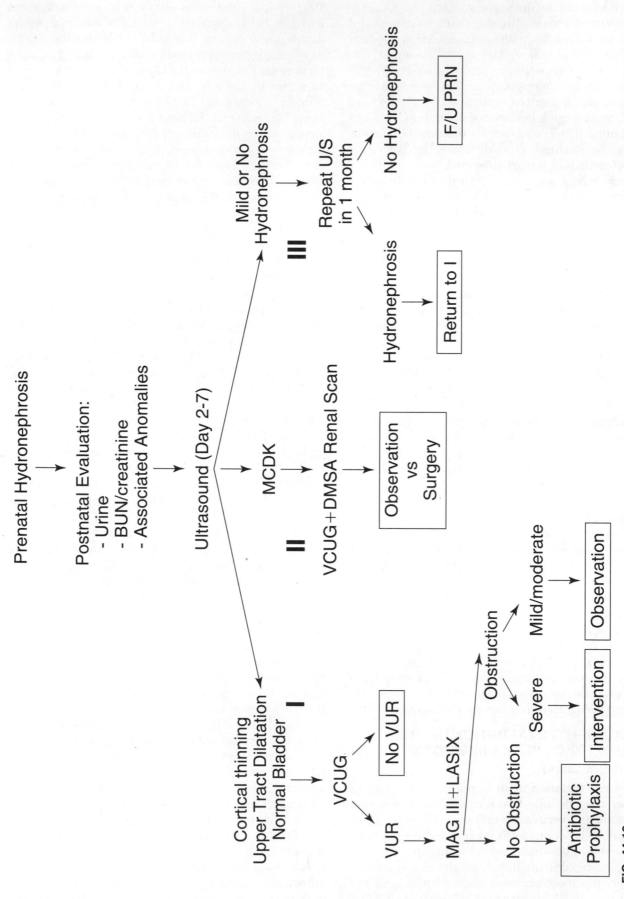

FIG. 44-12
Algorithm for the postnatal evaluation of fetal hydronephrosis. Abbreviations: MCDK. multicystic dysplastic kidney: VUR, vesicoureteral reflux. (From Cendron M, D'Alton ME, Crombleholme M: *Semin Perinatol* 1994; 18:163.)

respond to bladder outlet obstruction by several pop-off mechanisms including bladder diverticula, massive vesicoureteral reflux, or urinary ascites (Churchill et al., 1990; Wilson et al., 1988).

The fetus who presents with bilateral hydronephrosis should be evaluated for degree of dilatation and whether or not the criteria for minimal pyelectasis versus pathological hydronephrosis are met. The fetus with significant bilateral hydronephrosis and dilated bladder should undergo a complete diagnostic evaluation (Figs. 44-13, 44-14). This should include a complete ultrasound survey to identify any associated anomalies and a genetic amniocentesis because the incidence of associated chromosomal anomalies is approximately 10% (Manning et al., 1986; Wilson et al., 1988). The fetus with high-grade bladder outlet obstruction and decreasing amniotic fluid or oligohydramnios should undergo bladder tap for fetal urine Na, Cl, osmolality, Ca^{++}, PO_4, and β-$_2$-microglobulin (Glick et al., 1985; Muller et al., 1993). The fetal kidneys should be examined carefully to exclude cortical cysts or increased echogenicity (Mahoney et al., 1984). If the renal function is preserved as indicated by a favorable prognostic profile, fetal treatment should be considered. The treatment selected depends on the gestational age. Those at 32 weeks' gestation or later can be considered for early delivery and immediate postnatal decompression. Those fetuses at 28 to 32 weeks may be considered for short-term decompression in utero with vesicoamniotic shunts. The fetus diagnosed before 28 weeks' gestation should be considered for open vesicostomy or fetoscopic vesicocutaneous fistula to provide long-term decompression (Crombleholme et al., 1988a and b, 1991; Estes and Harrison, 1993; Harrison et al., 1987).

Postnatal Evaluation by Ultrasound

Over the past two decades, the radiologic evaluation of the newborn has changed because of technical improvements in ultrasonography. The presentation of the newborn with urologic anomalies also has changed, since a majority of cases are now detected in utero. Furthermore, because the newborn's GFR is low, in many cases nuclear medicine studies have replaced the intravenous urogram (IVU) in the workup of suspected obstructive processes within the urinary tract (Heyman and Duckett, 1988a).

Newborn ultrasonography is probably the most important initial step in the evaluation of the newborn urinary tract. It has even been proposed as a screening test that would complement prenatal ultrasound evaluation. Indeed, in a recent prospective study of 437 healthy infants between 2 and 10 months of age who underwent a screening ultrasound, six (1.4%) had a significant urologic anomaly (Steinhart et al., 1988). Such a percentage may be high and should be confirmed in a larger study. At the present time, its use

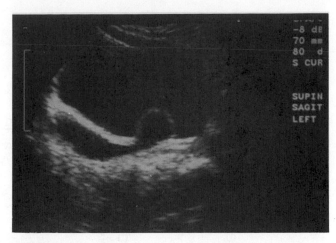

FIG. 44-13
Baby boy with bilateral hydroureteronephrosis and distended bladder requires prompt evaluation to diagnose ureteral valves.

is confined to the follow-up of fetuses diagnosed in utero with hydronephrosis and in the initial evaluation of newborns suspected of harboring congenital anomalies. These include babies with multiple congenital anomalies or chromosomal abnormalities, congenital heart disease, malformations of the ears, severe hypospadias, intersex conditions, myelodysplasia, single umbilical artery, family history of duplex systems or vesicoureteral reflux, and exposure to various teratogenes or cocaine (Greenfield et al., 1991; Leung et al., 1989; Selzman et al., 1993).

Ultrasonography of the abdomen in neonates and infants ideally should be performed in a warm, quiet room with adequate lighting. Most studies can be performed without sedation; feeding the infant or letting him/her suck on a pacifier often is comforting.

A urologic ultrasound examination in babies usually begins with the bladder, because the cold gel often stimulates a bladder contraction. Supine longitudinal views of the pelvis are performed to determine bladder volume and thickness, extravesical or intravesical masses, and to follow the course of a dilated ureter. A transverse scan is then performed to aid in determination of bladder volume. In females or in a newborn with ambiguous genitalia, the uterus may be visualized.

In a neonate with suspected posterior urethral valves, posterior urethral dilatation occasionally may be appreciated both in transvesical and perineal images (Cohen et al., 1994; Cremin and Aaronson, 1983).

Next, the kidneys are imaged. The kidneys are studied with longitudinal scans with particular attention to the upper poles (to detect the presence of duplication) and kidney size. Neonatal kidneys normally range from 3.3 to 5.0 cm in length, 2 to 3 cm in width, and 1.5 to 2.5 cm in diameter (McInnis et al., 1992). The best view of the right kidney is obtained through

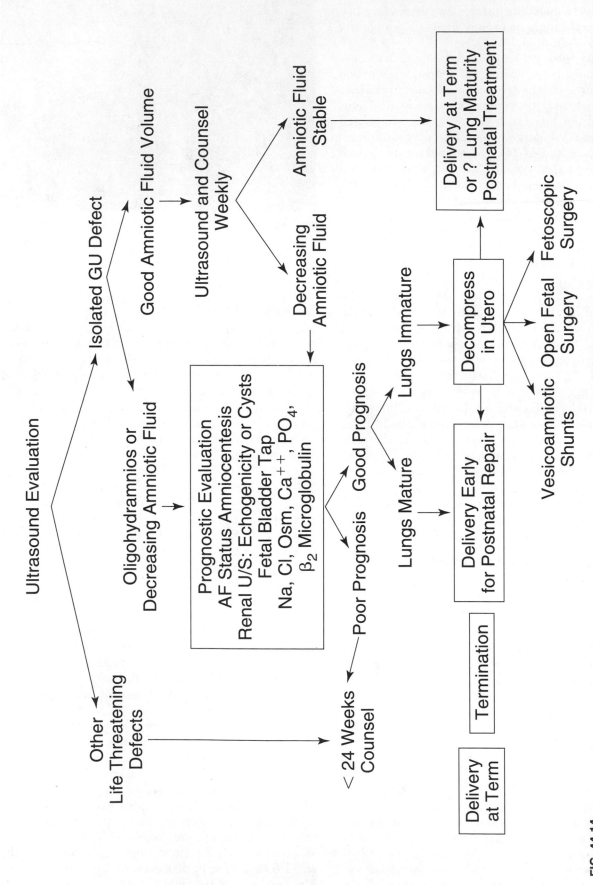

FIG. 44-14
Algorithm for the prenatal management of the fetus with bilateral hydronephrosis. (From Cendron M, D'Alton ME, Crombleholme M: *Semin Perinatol* 1994; 18:163.)

a supine longitudinal scan through the liver, whereas the left kidney is more likely to be visualized optimally by a prone longitudinal scan through the spleen. In infants with vesicoureteral reflux or infection, renal scarring may be detected, but calyceal morphology may not be distinct.

Attention also should be directed to identification of the adrenal glands. These structures are imaged optimally in the positions used to identify the upper poles of the kidneys. In the newborn, significant adrenal enlargement is suggestive of congenital adrenal hyperplasia. In such patients, the size of the adrenal glands may be compared with reported normal values (Oppenheimer et al., 1983).

The echogenicity of the kidneys should be assessed also. Organs with a uniform parenchymal composition, such as the liver and spleen, produce a homogeneous echo pattern that provides an excellent acoustic window for examining the adjacent kidney. In infants up to 6 months of age, cortical echogenicity may be equal to that of the liver. Another important feature is the prominent hypoechoic pyramids, which may be mistaken for dilated calyces or cysts (Haller et al., 1982).

Timing of the neonatal ultrasound is important to interpretation of its clinical relevance. The renal pelvis may be moderately dilated on antenatal sonography, yet appear normal in the first few days of life despite significant obstruction because oliguria during the first 24 to 48 hours of life may cause a distended renal pelvis to shrink transiently (Laing et al., 1984). If the neonatal ultrasound is normal, a voiding cystourethrogram should be obtained to determine whether reflux is present, and a renal ultrasound should be repeated in 3 weeks. Dejter and Gibbons (1989) reported on 49 dilated renal units detected antenatally, nine of which were normal on the postnatal evaluation done in the first few days of life. In follow-up, one had a UPJ obstruction, one had a ureterovesical junction obstruction, two had vesicoureteral reflux, and three had nonobstructive dilation of the collecting system necessitating continuing radiologic evaluation. Thus, 50% of neonates with antenatal hydronephrosis and a normal postnatal sonogram within 48 hours of birth required reconstructive surgery or had vesicoureteral reflux.

In order to standardize terminology, the grade of hydronephrosis has been standardized by the Society for Fetal Urology (Maizels et al., 1992) (Table 44-10). The hydronephrotic grade is based on the severity of renal pelvic and calyceal enlargement, as well as the presence of renal cortical atrophy. In general, only those kidneys with grade 3 or 4 (out of 4) hydronephrosis secondary to suspected obstruction require surgery (Maizels et al., 1994).

Further refinements in ultrasonographic technology, such as pulsed flow duplex doppler, have en-

TABLE 44-10

Society for Fetal Urology Grading of Hydronephrosis

Grade of Hydronephrosis	Central Renal Complex	Renal Parenchymal Thickness
0	Intact	Normal
1	Slight splitting	Normal
2*	Evident splitting, complex confined within renal border	
3	Wide-splitting pelvis dilated outside renal border and calices uniformly dilated	Normal
4	Further dilation of renal pelvis and calices (calices may appear convex)	Thin

From Maizels M, et al: *J Urol* 1992; 148:1609.
*An extrarenal pelvis extends outside the renal border, yet since the calices are not dilated hydronephrosis is grade 2. When the major calices are imaged but are not dilated, hydronephrosis is also grade 2.

hanced the ability to evaluate the newborn kidneys. This technique measures renal vascular resistance in the normal and dilated kidney and determines the resistive index, which estimates the renal vascular response to obstruction (Gilbert et al., 1993; Platt, 1992). The procedure is still experimental but has shown promising results in the clinical setting (Fung et al., 1994).

In summary, sonography is the least invasive method of evaluating and following infants with hydronephrosis. Although a urologic diagnosis may be suggested by sonography, other studies, such as VCUG, renal scan, and IVU are also necessary to establish the diagnosis. Subsequently, sonography is beneficial in observing the child by assessing renal growth and comparing degrees of calyceal dilation.

Intravenous Urography (IVU)

The indications and use of intravenous urography to assess the newborn urinary tract have decreased steadily over the last 20 years because of the increased availability of sonography and isotope imaging. The anatomic resolution of the IVU can be excellent but it should be remembered that, at birth, renal function may be too immature to allow for adequate concentration of the contrast material within the collecting system, thus preventing satisfactory visualization, which may be further obscured by copious bowel gas. However, 2 to 3 weeks after birth, visualization of the kidneys and collecting system can be obtained following administration of 2 to 3 ml/kg of contrast medium. The issue of whether to use ionic or nonionic contrast material is not resolved. The frequency of hypersensitivity reaction to ionic contrast media is lower in children than in adults, but is even less with the newer, nonionic (low osmolar) contrast. However, nonionic contrast is more expensive ($1/ml) than standard contrast media (14¢/ml).

The procedure used to carry out an IVU in a newborn is as follows: a scout film, a 1-minute film and a film at 7 to 10 minutes are obtained. Delayed films can be obtained to visualize a dilated renal pelvis and/or ureter. A urethral catheter in the bladder will prevent filling of a refluxing ureter. A dynamic interpretation of the IVU allows a functional assessment of renal function by evaluating the effects of an obstructive process on the appearance of the contrast material within the kidney and collecting system. This assessment is very operator dependent and does not offer the objective measurements provided by isotope imaging. Features of obstruction seen on IVU include calyceal dilatation, delayed appearance of contrast material in one renal unit compared to the normal kidney, and dilution of contrast material within the collecting system, either because of poor concentrating ability of the obstructed kidney or because of the mixing of contrast with urine accumulated within the obstructed system. A comparison with a normal contralateral kidney is necessary for this assessment. The interpretation of an IVU in the setting of a solitary kidney or bilateral hydronephrosis may be difficult.

The IVU provides excellent anatomic delineation of the upper urinary tract and can be used to identify specifically an area of obstruction, as well as whether the patient has a duplex collecting system. In addition, renal scarring from vesicoureteral reflux may be identified. However, its use for follow-up has diminished, since radionuclide imaging can fairly reliably provide quantitative estimation of relative renal function.

Retrograde Pyelography

With the radiologic studies currently available, retrograde pyelography rarely adds important diagnostic information in the evaluation of hydronephrosis in the newborn, even with a ureteropelvic junction obstruction (Rushton et al., 1994). In a neonate, urethral or ureteral injury may occur from the study. If ultrasound, IVP, and the renal scan do not provide sufficient visualization of the upper tract, antegrade pyelography usually is preferable to retrograde pyelography.

Voiding Cystourethrography

Any newborn with a prenatal diagnosis of hydronephrosis should undergo VCUG, even if the postnatal ultrasonogram is normal. Usually the study is obtained before the baby leaves the hospital because if vesicoureteral reflux is present, antimicrobial prophylaxis should be started. Furthermore, in male newborn infants infravesical obstruction must be excluded, even if sonography or isotope renography indicates probable upper tract obstruction.

In a boy with hydronephrosis, a radiographic VCUG always should be obtained to evaluate the lower urinary tract to exclude urethral and bladder disease. However, in girls, in whom these abnormalities are less common, it may not be so important to obtain a radiographic cystogram. A nuclear cystogram confers approximately 1% to 2% of the radiation exposure of a standard radiographic study, but the anatomic detail from the nuclear cystogram is considerably less than with the standard radiographic VCUG. Furthermore, the grading system for the nuclear cystogram has not been established, and the two studies are not always comparable. In addition, reflux associated with a duplication anomaly demonstrated on the radiographic VCUG might not be apparent on a nuclear study. Most children's hospitals have digital fluoroscopy units, which result in significantly less radiation exposure during a VCUG. Consequently, the clinician must decide which of the tests should be done.

Indications for VCUG in the newborn include the following conditions: prenatally diagnosed hydronephrosis, unilateral multicystic dysplastic kidney to rule out contralateral reflux, (Selzman and Edler, in press), suspected bladder outlet obstruction (posterior urethral valves, urethral anomalies), and suspected duplicated upper collecting system with or without ureterocele (Jee et al., 1993). If the neonate has ambiguous genitalia, contrast material should be injected into all genitourinary cavities, allowing the anatomic definition of the bladder and other genital cavities; this procedure is termed a genitogram.

Nuclear Medicine Studies

In the newborn with a suspected structural urologic anomaly, nuclear medicine studies play an important role in diagnosis, and in helping to direct treatment or assess results of therapy. Radionuclide studies of the kidneys (renograms) may be used to assess renal perfusion, glomerular function of each kidney, structural anomalies, and the presence or absence of obstruction. Although renograms complement ultrasonography and IVP by providing a quantitative assessment of perfusion and function, in certain instances the renal scan may be particularly advantageous over urography. For example, during the first 2 weeks when the neonatal GFR and concentrating ability of the kidneys are particularly low, the renal scan may provide an image of the urinary tract far superior to that obtained by IVP. In addition, in dehydrated infants or in a young infant with acute renal failure, the high solute load may cause further deterioration of renal function or have a deleterious effect on the child's fluid and electrolyte status.

Several radiopharmaceuticals are now available for renal imaging and functional analysis with technetium (Tc) 99m MAG-3 (mercaptoacetyltriglycerine) being the newest imaging agent. Tc 99m dimercaptosuccimic acid (DMSA) and Tc 99m diethylenetriaminepentaacetic acid (DTPA) have been available longer, as have TC 99m glucoheptonate (GHA): hippuran I-131 is seldom used. The advantages of radiopharmaceuticals include the absence of systemic pharmacologic effects or allergic reactions, lower radiation exposure than conventional urography and no need for fasting or special preparation of the bowel.

DTPA is cleared almost entirely by glomerular filtration (95%) without significant retention by the renal parenchyma. The remainder of the radionuclide is protein bound. The renal handling of DTPA can be divided into three phases that can be identified during the scan: (1) radionuclide uptake by the kidney, (2) transit through the renal parenchyma, and (3) washout into the collecting system. Estimation of glomerular filtration is determined by the activity recorded in the kidney between 1 and 3 minutes after injection of the radionuclide corresponding to parenchymal transit time. Differential renal function is computed by comparing diferential uptake from one to three minutes. Accumulation of radionuclide within the kidney is proportional to GFR. Gates (1982) described a method in which the renal uptake of radionuclide is expressed as a percentage of the injected dose and correlates with GFR in adults as determined by creatinine clearance (r = 0.95). Another method of estimating individual kidney clearance can be obtained by the determination of the extraction factor, which correlates well between initial renal uptake of DTPA without depth correction and GFR obtained by plasma clearance of DTPA (r = 0.92) in pediatric patients (Heyman and Duckett, 1988a). In the later phase of the study, the high urinary concentration of DTPA with normal or near normal renal function can provide excellent visualization of the upper urinary tract and bladder. Renal anomalies, such as pelvic kidney, crossed fused ectopia, horseshoe kidney, or urinary extravasation, can be detected using DTPA.

MAG-3 is secreted by the renal tubules and has a rate of excretion more than three times that of DTPA, with 73% normally excreted by 30 minutes (Eshima et al., 1990; Russell et al., 1988). The images obtained are similar to DTPA in older children, but in the neonate there is less background activity with MAG-3, making it a superior radiopharmaceutical. The disadvantage of MAG-3 is that its shelf life is much shorter, and it is more expensive than DTPA. Differential renal function is computed in an identical manner to DTPA (Pickworth et al., 1992).

[99m]DMSA is the most sensitive radiopharmaceutical for imaging the renal parenchyma in the absence of obstruction (Stoller and Kogan, 1986; Sty et al., 1987). In the neonate or premature infant, however, uptake of DMSA may be low due to renal functional immaturity, low plasma flow, and reduced bulk of tubular tissue (Gordon and Barratt, 1987). DMSA scanning provides functional information about the kidneys and demonstrates areas of decreased function, such as focal dysplasia, scarring, or acute infection (Bjorgvinsson et al., 1991; Risdon et al., 1994; Rushton et al., 1988). GHA provides similar images to DMSA. The disadvantage of DMSA and GHA is that renal cortical imaging is performed 4 hours after injection of the radiopharmaceutical. Consequently, these agents are used primarily for assessing renal cortical scarring.

Renal scanning usually is performed in the following situations (Taylor and Nally, 1995):

1. Assessing whether upper tract obstruction is present in a neonate or infant with hydronephrosis (diuretic renogram—MAG-3 or DTPA);
2. Confirming that a multicystic kidney has no function (MAG-3 or DTPA);
3. Determining whether the upper pole of an obstructed duplex system (ureterocele or ectopic ureter) functions (MAG-3, DTPA, DMSA, GHA);
4. Confirming that a kidney is absent in a neonate in whom the ultrasound demonstrates one kidney (MAG-3 or DTPA);
5. Demonstrating a fusion anomaly of the kidney (horseshoe kidney or crossed renal ectopia; MAG-3 or DTPA);
6. Determining whether a child has acute pyelonephritis (DMSA) or evidence of renal scarring from previous infection (DMSA, GHA, MAG-3).

Diuretic Renogram

Diuretic renography is a provocative method of evaluating patients found to have dilatation of the upper urinary tract in whom an obstructive process is suspected. The theoretical basis of this test is twofold: if an obstructive lesion is present, then (1) renal function, more specifically glomerular filtration, will be impaired; and (2) a dilated upper urinary tract will retain a larger amount of radionuclide that will not wash out if increased urine flow is generated by the administration of a diuretic (Conway and Maizels, 1992; Thrall et al., 1981). Two radionuclide tracers are available for diuretic renograms: DTPA and MAG-3. Imaging is superior with MAG-3 compared to DTPA because of a smaller volume of distribution and faster clearance (Heyman and Duckett, 1988b).

The technique for the diuretic renal scan is critical to its correct interpretation and requires attention to detail to assure reliability and reproducibility. In general, neonates and young infants are placed supine for the study; mechanical restraint usually is necessary. At some institutions infants are placed prone; however, because this may affect better upper tract drainage. Ideally the child should be well hydrated, because relative dehydration prolongs parenchymal transit and delays urinary excretion. MAG-3 or DTPA is injected intravenously as a bolus. Subsequently, 4-second posterior images are recorded with a high-resolution collimator. One minute after injection, images of the kidneys are obtained each minute. Normally the renal parenchyma is well visualized during the first minute, by 2 to 3 minutes activity is seen in the collecting system, and by 6 to 9 minutes the bladder is visualized.

The differential renal function of each kidney is calculated between 60 seconds and 180 seconds after injection of the radiopharmaceutical, which represents parenchymal transit. In the normal neonate, approximately 1.5% of DTPA is taken up by each kidney at 120 to 180 seconds, compared with 2.5% at 1 year of age (Heyman and Duckett, 1988a). This has been termed the "extraction factor" (Heyman and Duckett, 1988a) and reflects glomerular function. These figures have not been derived for MAG-3. On computer images, regions of interest are selected from each kidney and background activity is subtracted. The activity within each kidney is expressed as a percentage of the total renal counts, and this differential activity is used to compute differential renal function. In a kidney with a duplex system in which there is upper pole obstruction, the regions of interest of the affected kidney may be broken down further and used to determine relative function of the upper and lower segments.

To determine whether significant obstruction is present, furosemide is administered intravenously, with a recommended dosage of 1 mg/kg when the hydronephrotic system shows maximal accumulation of radionuclide, but not later than 30 to 60 minutes. It is important to distinguish hydronephrosis secondary to suspected UPJ obstruction from ureterovesical junction obstruction, in which the ureter should contain a large amount of radionuclide before furosemide is given (Barrett et al., 1983). The activity over each kidney is measured and the half-time clearance determined. The half-time (T ½) represents the number of minutes required for half of the radiopharmaceutical to drain from the collecting system after administration of furosemide. O'Reilly and colleagues (1979) have defined several types of responses to furosemide (Fig. 44-15). In the newborn, drainage typically is delayed, compared with drainage in the older child, primarily because the GFR is low. A nonobstructed system should have a T ½ less than 10 to 15 minutes, whereas a T ½ greater than 20 minutes is suggestive of obstruction. If T ½ is between 15 and 20 minutes, the results are indeterminate. The T ½ is computed from the peak of renal activity, not the actual time of diuretic administration, because if the hydronephrotic system is not completely filled when furosemide is administered, the radionuclide may continue to accumulate for several minutes in the collecting system

before it begins to drain. If a normal drainage pattern begins, then levels off, the slope of the drainage curve should be used to extrapolate T ½. If the collecting system does not fill completely within 1 hour after injection of MAG-3 or DTPA or if the kidney has less than 20% of total renal function, the diuretic washout curve may be prolonged, even if the system is not obstructed (Kass and Majd, 1985).

Technical Considerations Affecting Interpretation of Diuretic Renogram

Numerous variables may affect the interpretation of the diuretic renal scan, particularly in the newborn (Table 44-11) (Elder, 1992).

Renal Maturity.—In the newborn there is temporary but significant renal functional impairment that may confuse the diagnosis of obstruction by renography, because there is no readily available measurement to determine when renal function is too immature for diuretic renogram accuracy. Koff and associates (1988) studied the diuretic response of the normal kidney in 33 infants with unilateral hydronephrosis caused by either multicystic kidney or UPJ obstruction. These infants were not formally hydrated, nor was a bladder catheter used. In neonates younger than 1 month, 68% of the normal kidneys had a T ½

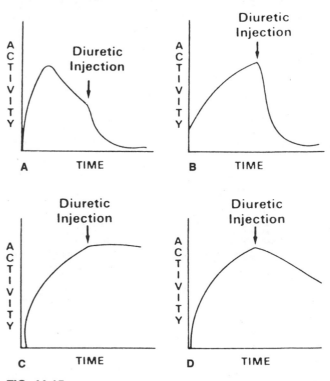

FIG. 44-15
Patterns of response to furosemide in DTPA renal scan. Normal response **(A),** dilated nonobstructed system **(B),** dilated obstructed collecting system **(C),** and equivocal response **(D).** (From Kelalis PP, King LR, Belman AB (eds): *Clinical Pediatric Urology,* ed 2 Philadelphia, WB Saunders Co, 1985.)

greater than 9 minutes; of the infants studied between 1 and 4 months, 33% had a prolonged T ½; and all infants older than 4 months had a normal T ½ in the normal kidney. Prematurity was a significant factor as well. Of nine full-term infants younger than 1 month, 5 (55%) had a T ½ less than 9 minutes in the normal kidney, whereas none of the eight premature infants had a T ½ less than 9 minutes. Consequently, when studying the neonate with a diuretic renal scan, drainage of the normal kidney must be assessed carefully. If the normal contralateral kidney shows impaired drainage, then the study is invalid and cannot be used to provide a satisfactory indication of whether obstruction is present. In these cases other clinical information must be used to assess the kidney with suspected obstruction. If the hydronephrotic kidney is functioning as well as the nonhydronephrotic kidney, then the renal scan should be repeated 6 to 12 weeks later.

Renal Function.—In a kidney with significantly reduced renal function secondary to a UPJ obstruction, posterior urethral valves, or with a primary renal functional abnormality, the diuretic renogram may be difficult or impossible to interpret. In general, if the differential renal function is less than 20% or if the kidney has not reached its peak intensity by 60 minutes after administration of MAG-3 or DTPA, the diuretic phase cannot be used to provide an indication of definite obstruction.

Hydration Effect.—State of hydration has an important effect on the diuretic response. Dehydration prolongs parenchymal transit and the diuretic response. In a study by Howmann-Giles and co-workers (1987), of 12 patients with prolonged T ½ in 10 the T ½ decreased to the normal range with infusion of 360 ml/m² normal saline solution over 30 minutes prior to the study. Although forced hydration is not physiologic, it reduces the likelihood that prolonged T ½ is secondary to prolonged parenchymal transit. In many centers the family is asked to feed the infant immediately before the study.

Dose and Timing of Diuretic Administration.—Although O'Reilly and colleagues (1978) recommended an administered dose of 0.5 mg/kg furosemide, in children, and in particular the newborn, 1 mg/kg provides a stronger and more reliable effect. If the infant is well hydrated, significant dehydration is unlikely to result. Children with renal insufficiency may require as much as 4 mg/kg furosemide to stimulate satisfactory diuresis. If a catheter is used to drain the bladder during the diuretic study, urine output can be measured to determine whether diuretic response is adequate.

The timing of diuretic administration is controversial. O'Reilly (1986) recommends administration at 20 minutes in all patients. However, in a nonobstructed hydronephrotic or poorly functioning kidney the radionuclide might not accumulate maximally in the collecting systems by 20 minutes. If furosemide is administered too soon, the radionuclide will continue to accumulate in the kidney for a variable period of time before drainage occurs, potentially simulating an obstructed kidney.

Bladder Effect.—Approximately 15% of children with UPJ obstruction have vesicoureteral reflux (Hollowell et al., 1989). Consequently, if the VCUG demonstrates reflux, bladder catheterization during the diuretic renogram is mandatory. Whether bladder catheterization should be done in all cases, however, is controversial. A full bladder impairs drainage of the upper tracts. Thus a nonobstructed kidney may begin to drain after furosemide is given, but the drainage response may be blunted as the bladder fills, spuriously prolonging the T ½. It can be argued that bladder catheterization is not a normal physiologic situation. Furthermore, infants often void during furosemide diuresis, and there may be some risk of causing iatrogenic urinary infection in the hydronephrotic kidney with placement of a urethral catheter. On the other hand, if the bladder is not catheterized it may be difficult to determine whether impaired upper-tract drainage is secondary to a distended bladder or to obstruction. The ideal diuretic renal scan should include a continuously drained bladder, although this is not routinely done by most pediatric nuclear medicine departments at present.

Outlined Regions of Interest.—Differential renal function is computed by comparing the differential uptake for 1 minute, between 1 and 3 minutes after injection of the radiopharmaceutical. The renal images that are analyzed, or "regions of interest," are extremely important to this analysis. Background activity from the liver or spleen may affect the number of counts, and this activity must be subtracted. In reality, the computed uptake of a kidney

TABLE 44-11

Factors Affecting Diuretic Renography in the Neonate

Renal maturity
Renal function
Hydration status
Type and dose of radiopharmaceutical
Dose of diuretic
Timing of diuretic administration
Vesicoureteral reflux
Volume of urine in bladder
Outlined regions of interest
Patient position
Patient movement
Capacity of upper tract
Severity of obstruction
Site of obstruction
Method of data interpretation

may be altered significantly by changing the region of interest. In some institutions, the regions are drawn outside the area of perceived renal activity; at other institutions the region of interest is drawn tightly to the edge of the kidney. Recognition of this variable is important because often the decision of whether to operate on a hydronephrotic kidney is based largely on whether the differential glomerular function is affected significantly. In some cases the hydronephrotic kidney may not seem to visualize significantly on IVP, yet the computed function on renal scan is good. The "extraction factor" (Heyman and Duckett, 1988a), on which the differential functions are based, allows computation of absolute renal function within each kidney and comparison of these values as the child grows.

Position of the Infant.—In some cases, drainage of urine from the kidney may be improved by placing the child in the prone or upright position rather than supine during the study because the bladder becomes more dependent.

Site of Obstruction.—If the neonate has a megaureter, ideally the renal pelvis and ureter should be filled with the radionuclide before furosemide is administered. If the diuretic is administered prematurely and renal pelvic drainage is impaired, the study probably should be repeated before deciding on a diagnosis of obstruction. If the diuretic is administered at the appropriate time, currently it is unresolved whether to assess drainage from the renal pelvis and ureter separately or as one entire system.

Interpretation of Diuretic Renogram

It should be remembered that the DTPA renal scan does not actually measure obstruction; rather, it monitors the ability of the kidney to respond to a volume challenge. Thus, accuracy of the study depends on a number of biologic factors that influence this response. The clinician should never rely on the written report to determine whether an obstructive lesion is present. The study should always be reviewed by the urologist to assess specifically which of these variables might have adversely affected the outcome of the test and whether it should be repeated under modified conditions or when renal function is better.

Another important aspect in evaluation of the study deals with the interpretation and comparison of follow-up examinations. For example, how does one assess stability or deterioration of renal function or obstruction? If the differential renal function remains stable but the T ½ becomes prolonged, is there deterioration of function, worsening obstruction, or is this simply a difference in technique between the two studies?

Recommended Protocol for Diuretic Renogram in the Neonate

Because the method of diuretic renography varies among nuclear medicine practitioners, and recognizing the limitations of the diuretic renogram in the neonate with hydronephrosis, the Society for Fetal Urology met recently with the Pediatric Nuclear Medicine Club to derive a standardized method for the diuretic renogram in the neonate (Conway and Maizels, 1992). Ideally, infants should be older than 1 month at renography to reduce the likelihood that renal function is immature, and premature infants should be even older before the initial renogram. Oral hydration is offered as desired, beginning 2 hours before the study. The bladder is catheterized to assure that it is empty, and the catheter is left to continuous open drainage or intermittent syringe evacuation of the bladder via the catheter. Urine output of 4 to 5 ml/min is expected during the active diuresis in a well-hydrated infant. Prophylactic antiseptic therapy is administered during the study and for 3 days afterwards. Prior to the study a dilute normal saline solution is administered at a rate of 10 ml/kg over 15 minutes, before infection of MAG-3 or DTPA, and is continued for 15 minutes after injection. The renogram should be recorded in the supine position. Following injection of MAG-3 or DTPA, the regions of interest encompass the entire kidney, including the dilated renal pelvis, with a region of interest for background subtraction defined as 2 pixels wide around the entire outer perimeter of the kidney. The percent differential renal function is determined by measuring the total counts of the renogram curve for each kidney minus background between the intervals of 90 and 150 seconds after the appearance of the abdominal aorta. Furosemide is administered at a dose of 1 mg/kg after 20 to 30 minutes or when the dilated pelvis or ureter is believed filled on the scintigram images. It may be necessary to place the patient in the prone position to allow the radioactive agent to be distributed evenly throughout the entire dilated pelvis and ureter. Methods used to monitor T ½ clearance include: (1) T ½ from the time of furosemide injection, (2) T ½ from the peak of the curve, and (3) T ½ of the extrapolated slope of the primary response to furosemide. Most probably one of the latter two will prove most accurate.

ANTEGRADE PERFUSION STUDIES OF UPPER URINARY TRACT

Another way to evaluate the hydronephrotic kidney is the Whitaker test, in which fluid is infused into the kidney at a constant rate and the differential increase in pressure in the kidney, compared with the pressure in the bladder, is measured. A variant of this, which is discussed briefly, is the constant-pressure perfusion test, in which fluid is infused at a constant pressure to assess the change in output.

Constant Volume Perfusion (Whitaker Test)

The Whitaker test generally is performed when other diagnostic tests, such as sonography, excretory urography, and diuresis renography, either do not agree or are inconclusive in establishing a diagnosis (Whitaker, 1979). The test is much more invasive than the other procedures because it requires insertion of a needle or small nephrostomy tube into the kidney, with the patient under general anesthesia.

After administration of general anesthesia, the child is placed in the prone position. Access to the hydronephrotic collecting system is obtained percutaneously, either using sonography or after injecting a bolus of contrast medium intravenously and imaging the kidney fluoroscopically. Spinal needles of 22 or 20 gauge are commonly used, although we have selectively used a pigtail nephrostomy tube. The needle resistance is subtracted from the renal pressure to determine intrapelvic pressure. If the kidney is extremely hydronephrotic, a second needle may be inserted into the kidney to measure the pressure continuously. A urethral catheter is inserted as well. A Harvard pump or similar apparatus is used to deliver a constant flow through the kidney at a set rate. Usually the bladder catheter is left open and allowed to drain during the procedure, except in situations of suspected secondary ureterovesical junction obstruction. Each institution has its own protocol for performing the study. In some centers the study is initiated by infusing 5 ml/min for 5 to 10 minutes and checking the renal pressure with a manometer or pressure transducer every 5 minutes. If the pressure remains within a physiologic range, the inflow is increased to 10 ml/min for another 5 to 10 minutes. In selected cases (generally older children) the fluid infusion is increased to 15 ml/min. This study also allows infusion of contrast medium to examine the upper urinary tract fluoroscopically, which often is as helpful as the pressure readings.

A maximum renal relative pressure (renal pelvic pressure minus needle resistance minus bladder pressure) less than 15 cm water indicates absence of obstruction; pressure greater than 22 cm water is indicative of resistance to urinary flow; and maximum pressure between 15 and 22 cm water is considered indeterminate.

The Whitaker test measures only drainage, not function. The clear implication is that the kidney that has impaired drainage by the Whitaker test is likely to develop renal functional impairment.

Numerous technical variables may influence the Whitaker test, including the concentration of contrast medium (if used), the gauge and length of the perfusion needle, temperature of the solution, and flow rate (Toguri and Fournier, 1982). For example, as the temperature of contrast increases, its viscosity decreases. Diminished viscosity of the infusate results in diminished resistance by viscous drag. Not surprisingly, viscous drag was greater using a 9-cm long needle, compared with a shorter needle. In these studies the greatest intrinsic resistance resulted with high rates of infusate flow using 25% contrast, with the maximum pressure difference 5.0 cm water at 11.5 ml/min.

Although the Whitaker test was developed in children, there are no reports of its use in large series in neonates and infants. Because the kidneys and ureters are smaller, we can speculate that the desired maximum rate of flow should be lower in an infant than in an older child or adult. However, no one is certain what the appropriate infusion rate should be. Is a dramatic rise in renal pressure at 10 ml/min significant? Assuming a two-kidney system, this infusion rate would be equivalent to 1200 ml/hr, which is a greater volume than the urinary output in most infants over 24 hours. Consequently, an infusate rate of 10 ml/hr is not physiologic. Furthermore, standards for abnormal renal pressure in neonates have not been established, although these should be similar to those in older children. In an unpublished report, Ransley noted that in neonates and infants with a UPJ obstruction, using a second needle to measure renal pressure, intrarenal pressures between 100 and 300 cm water have been obtained in some patients, even at infusate rates of only 5 ml/min (Ransley, 1992). More data are required to clarify this issue.

Constant Pressure Perfusion

The Whitaker, or constant volume perfusion test, assesses the compliance of the renal pelvis (and ureter in hydroureteronephrosis) with suspected upper tract obstruction. Upper tract obstruction is characterized by the necessity for increased renal pelvic pressure to cause urinary flow to the bladder. As a result of dissatisfaction with the Whitaker test, the study recently has been modified to use constant pressure perfusion rather than constant flow (Woodbury et al., 1989). Constant-pressure perfusion is independent of upper-tract compliance, uses low fixed pressures in the renal pelvis, and measures the rate of flow out of the upper tract into the bladder at various pressures. In a pig model, one kidney was isolated and a nephrostomy tube was inserted into the renal pelvis. A bag of saline solution served as the constant pressure reservoir, and the height of the bag was adjusted to achieve the desired intrarenal pelvic pressure. The contralateral ureter was clamped, and fluid outflow through the ureter was measured with a urethral catheter.

The authors found that in the normal pig, flow should always occur with renal pelvic pressures less than 5 cm water, with a flow rate of approximately 5 ml/min. At 10 cm water renal pelvic pressure, drainage was 12 ml/min. When partial obstruction was created, the flow rate from the kidney was more than 3 standard deviations below the normal curve. Using the Whitaker model of continuous flow in the same animals, an inflow of 5 ml/min yielded an equivocal pressure rise, and at a flow rate of 10 ml/min the system demonstrated obstruction.

In theory, the constant-pressure perfusion technique is advantageous over constant flow in that it measures flow out of the upper tract at various renal pelvic pressures. Furthermore, the results were more reproducible and had less overlap with normal or equivocal values. In the human, however, an obvious limitation in a patient with two kidneys is the difficulty in determining the outflow from the single obstructed kidney. The authors speculated that this might be accomplished by using radionuclide perfusion and assessing outflow by scintigraphy. Further work on this important model is under way.

MANAGEMENT OF THE NEWBORN WITH GENITOURINARY ANOMALIES

Parental Issues

Prenatal diagnosis of congenital anomalies not only has permitted counseling and early management but also has introduced a significant stressor during pregnancy, especially if invasive procedures are recommended (Harvard, 1992; Van Putte, 1988). This stress can be managed adequately by providing the parent(s) with adequate information and nondirective counseling (Inati et al., 1994). Difficult management decisions should be handled with a multidisciplinary approach coordinated by a genetic counselor who will act as the liaison between the parent(s), referring physician, and the perinatal team. The counseling should ensure comprehensive and compassionate care in cases where termination is considered or where the outcome of the pregnancy is poor.

Postnatally, the mother/child interactions are especially important in establishing bonding.

Bonding

Bonding refers to the strong emotional and affectional relationship that occurs between a mother and father and their newborn infant. Although bonding has been demonstrated to occur at the time of prenatal ultrasound (Fletcher and Evans, 1983), most important are the first few days or weeks of an infant's life (Marano, 1981). The classic references on this subject are by Klaus and Kennell (1976, 1982). The long-term significance of bonding is controversial, and there is extensive dialogue in the literature regarding the importance of the extensive early mother-newborn contact and its effect on the subsequent parent-child relationship and behavior (Klaus and Kennell, 1983; Korsch, 1983; Lamb, 1982; Lamb and Hwang, 1982). Early mother-infant contact has been associated with improved speech between mother and child at 2 years (Ringler et al., 1975), and at age 5, such offspring have been reported to have higher intelligence quotients and better scores on language comprehension tests than those with limited mother-infant contact in the neonatal period (Ringler et al., 1976). Furthermore, following neonatal illness and hospitalization, there is a significantly increased incidence of child abuse and neglect (Lynch and Roberts, 1977; O'Connor et al., 1980) and failure to thrive in the absence of organic causes (Shaheen et al., 1968).

Anesthesia

In general, neonatal surgery is quite safe from an anesthetic standpoint when the patient is healthy and a staff with extensive experience in pediatric anesthesia is available (Holzman, 1994). However, in the transition from fetus to neonate, there are important circulatory and hematologic considerations. In addition, newborn infants may be at risk for retrolental fibroplasia or postoperative apnea under certain circumstances.

Retrolental fibroplasia (RLF; retinopathy of prematurity) is a major cause of blindness or impaired vision in low-birth-weight infants on ventilators. When the retinal vasculature is immature, elevated inspired oxygen concentrations result in arterial oxygen tensions (PaO_2) higher than normal, with the potential for significant arterial narrowing and the destruction of newly formed capillary endothelium. A vasoproliferative process results, leading to RLF. There have been cases of RLF developing in infants in whom the only supplementary oxygen received was during anesthesia (Betts et al., 1977; Merritt et al., 1981). At a conceptional age of 40 weeks (i.e., term), approximately 40% of newborns have an immature retina. However, this incidence decreases to 0% at 45 weeks (Quinn et al., 1981). The risk of developing RLF in a child with an immature retina during anesthesia may be minimized by maintaining the PaO_2 less than 90 mm Hg (American Academy of Pediatrics [AAP]-American College of Obstetrics and Gynecologists [ACOG], 1983). At the Children's Hospital of Philadelphia, neonates under 45 weeks' conceptional age routinely undergo ophthalmologic examination to check for evidence of retinal immaturity, and at present, special efforts are made to adhere to the recommendations noted.

There is a subgroup of newborn infants that may develop an apneic episode following general anesthesia (Welborn and Greenspun, 1994). The primary group at risk consists of prematurely born infants who have had a previous episode of apnea, whether idiopathic or otherwise (Liu et al., 1983). Such infants less than 55 to 60 weeks' conceptional age (15 weeks after term) appear to be at particular risk (Kurth et al., 1987). Reasons for this higher risk are unclear. However, apneic episodes in prematurely born infants have been attributed to immaturity of the respiratory system (Shannon and Kelly, 1982a and b). In infants with a history of neonatal apnea, alveolar hypoventilation during sleep and an abnormal response to hypercapnia and hypoxia have been demonstrated (Hunt, 1981; Shannon et al., 1977). It is postulated that the anesthetics used (e.g., halothane), as well as narcotics, affect the ventilatory control mechanism and predispose to postoperative apnea for 48 hours (Liu et al., 1983). Infants born at term who have not experienced apnea do not appear to have an elevated risk for ventilatory complications following general anesthesia.

At birth, the ductus arteriosus constricts but has the potential to reopen during the first week of life under certain conditions. For example if PaO_2 falls to fetal levels within the first few days of life, the ductus arteriosus may reopen with right-to-left shunting of blood away from the lung, referred to as *persistent fetal circulation syndrome* (Crone, 1986). This phenomenon could be caused by a very brief episode of hypoxia, as potentially could occur during induction of anesthesia.

Finally, the red blood cells (RBCs) in the neonate are undergoing qualitative and quantitative changes. In the first few months of life, fetal hemoglobin predominates in RBCs and differs from adult hemoglobin in its inability to bind 2,3-diphosphoglycerate. This inability results in oxygen binding more efficiently to hemoglobin, making it more difficult to release oxygen to the tissues. Furthermore, during the first 3 to 4 months of life, the total hemoglobin concentration decreases to its lowest level. Thus, at 3 months of age, the infant's oxygen-carrying capacity may be compromised quantitatively and qualitatively (Crone, 1986). This effect is compensated for by an increase in cardiac output. However, the effects of many anesthetic agents include reduction of the cardiac output, increase of the intrapulmonary shunt (decreasing PaO_2), and decrease in peripheral oxygen consumption. The margin for error is reduced, and the risk of anesthesia may be increased in the first few weeks of life, particularly if hypovolemia, hypoxemia, or anemia is present and undetected.

The preceding discussion is not meant to exaggerate the anesthetic risks of neonatal surgery. With the skills

TABLE 44-12

Distribution of Abdominal Masses of 280 Patients in the Neonatal Period*

	Number
Kidney (65%)	
Hydronephrosis (UPJ obstruction, UVJ obstruction, ureterocele, etc.)	80 (28%)
Multicystic kidney	63 (22%)
Polycystic kidney disease	18
Renal vein thrombosis	5
Solid tumor	13
Ectopy	4
Total	183
Retroperitoneum (9%)	
Neuroblastoma	17
Teratoma	3
Hemangioma	1
Abscess	4
Total	25
Bladder (1%)	
Posterior urethral valves	2
Female genital system (10%)	
Hydrocolpos	16
Ovarian cyst	13
Total	31
Gastrointestinal (12%)	
Duplication	17
Giant cystic meconium ileus	4
Mesenteric cyst	3
Ileal atresia	2
Volvulus (ileum)	2
Teratoma (stomach)	1
Leiomyosarcoma (colon)	1
Meconium peritonitis with ascites	1
Ascites	1
Total	32
Hepatic or biliary (3%)	
Hemangioma (liver)	3
Solitary cyst (liver)	2
Hepatoma	1
Distended gallbladder	1
Choledochal cyst	1
Adenomatoid malformation of the lung	1
Total	9

Modified from Griscom NT: *AJR* 1965; 93:447; Raffensperger J, Abousleiman A: *Surgery* 1968; 63:514; Wedge JJ, Grosfeld JL, Smith JP: *J Urol* 1971; 106:770; Wilson DA: *Am J Dis Child* 1982; 136:147; Emanuel B, White H: *Clin Pediatr* 1968; 7:529.
*Distended bladder, hepatomegaly, and splenomegaly excluded in most series. UPJ = ureteropelvic junction; UVJ = ureterovesical junction.

of a pediatric anesthesiologist, general anesthesia may be administered safely to practically any infant, but the potential risks must be understood by the surgeon.

Abdominal Masses

An abdominal mass in the neonate demands urgent evaluation. Urologists working in institutions with newborn nurseries need to be familiar with the various causes of abdominal masses in the newborn and their evaluation because a large proportion of these are genitourinary in origin. Over the past few decades, the evaluation of such neonates has changed dramatically.

Table 44-12 shows the distribution of abdominal masses based on a collation of five large series. Excluded are babies with distended bladders without hydronephrosis, isolated splenomegaly, pyloric stenosis, pelvic tumors palpable only by rectal examination, and babies with hydrocolpos in whom the diagnosis was obvious because of a bulging imperforate hymen. Nearly two thirds of abdominal masses detected within the first month of life arise from the urinary tract, and 10% occur in the female genital system. One half are secondary to either hydronephrosis or multicystic kidney. It has been reported that during the first 2 days of life, an abdominal mass is more likely to be a multicystic kidney, whereas beyond 2 days of age, hydronephrosis is more common (Griscom, 1965).

Nearly all neonatal masses arising from the genitourinary tract may be diagnosed accurately based on history, physical examination, ultrasound, and nuclear renal scan.

The history may provide important clues to the source of the abdominal mass. One should inquire whether prenatal ultrasonography was performed, and if so, at which week of gestation. Ideally, these films should be obtained and reviewed. As has already been detailed, prenatal ultrasonography is extremely sensitive in identifying a variety of obstructive urologic lesions (Fig. 44-16). Normal prenatal ultrasound late in gestation in which the fetal urinary tract was visualized would tend to exclude hydronephrosis and multicystic kidney as etiologic factors (Fugelseth et al., 1994).

A history of fever developing in the neonatal period suggests an obstructive lesion, because febrile illnesses in the neonate are rare. Persistent vomiting in the first few days of life may be indicative of a gastrointestinal disorder. In a boy, the stream should be visualized, because the majority of boys with urethral valves have a weak urinary stream. Infants with severe dehydration and those with diabetic mothers have an increased incidence of renal vein thrombosis.

Family history is important as well. Infantile polycystic kidney disease is an autosomal recessive disorder, and infant deaths are often noted in the family history. Duplication of the urinary tract often is hereditary and has a polygenic mode of inheritance (O'Neill, 1990). Consequently, if there is a family history of duplication of the urinary tract, one might suspect an ectopic ureterocele or ureter as the diagnosis. Similarly, multicystic kidney disease has been noted to recur in family members.

Despite the variety of radiographic modalities available for urologic diagnosis, physical examination should not be forgotten as an important component of the evaluation. Several large clinical series performed prior to the widespread use of diagnostic ultrasound attest to the ability to detect a number of urogenital anomalies simply by abdominal palpation, including renal agenesis (kidney impalpable), horseshoe kidney (a midline bridge of tissue palpable), ectopic kidney (kidney lower than usual), and fused ectopia (altered renal shape associated with impalpable contralateral kidney) (Museles et al., 1971; Perlman and Williams, 1976; Sherwood et al., 1956). In these series, the incidence of renal anomalies detected at birth varied from 0.2% to 0.5%. In the first few days of life, the newborn is particularly easy to examine. The examination may be performed initially by carefully palpating the upper quadrants on either side. Supporting the right flank with the left hand, the examiner's right hand may be used to slide up subcostally to examine the upper quadrant. The kidney is almost always palpable in the newborn, is superior to the level of the umbilicus, and is situated in a vertical orientation. One should be able to palpate the upper pole. If the lower poles of the kidneys are positioned close to the midline, one should suspect a horseshoe kidney. In such circumstances, palpation along the anterior aspect of the spine may detect the isthmus. Lower quadrants are examined in the customary manner. Finally, by compressing the abdomen from both sides, one may detect a mobile abdominal mass, such as an intestinal duplication or ovarian cyst.

Another important aspect of examination is transillumination (Donn and Faix, 1985). This technique helps to distinguish between masses that are solid and those that are filled with fluid or air. In addition, in the neonate, it may aid in identifying the liver edge, stomach, bladder, and gallbladder. Bladder massage may be a helpful diagnostic aid. Rather than forcefully expressing the bladder (Credé method), one gently massages the bladder between the index finger and thumb. Within 1 to 2 minutes, if the bladder is moderately full, voiding will commence. One may judge the stream, assess residual urine, note bladder thickness, and obtain a clean urine specimen in this manner.

A complete examination also includes measurement of the blood pressure, assessment of the respiratory tract and genitalia, and a rectal examination. Hypertension may occur with neuroblastoma or infrequently with hydronephrosis. Respiratory distress in the newborn often is associated with bladder outlet obstruction and may be indicative of hypoplastic lungs. In a female infant, a bulging interlabial mass is suggestive of hydrometrocolpos. Rectal examination may help to

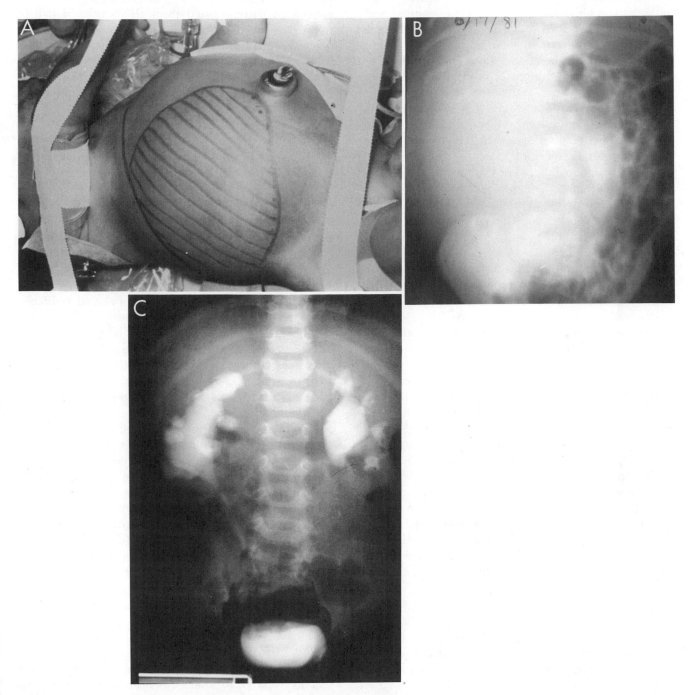

FIG. 44-16
Neonate with large abdominal mass discovered on prenatal ultrasonography and found to have bilateral hydronephrosis. **A,** Extent of palpable right abdominal mass is marked out. **B,** Preoperative intravenous pyelogram (IVP) showing large right abdominal mass and left hydronephrosis. The right kidney was found to be severely hydronephrotic secondary to a ureteropelvic junction obstruction, and a right pyeloplasty was performed. A left pyeloplasty was performed subsequently. **C,** Postoperative IVP demonstrating excellent function bilaterally.

disclose the origin of a solid lower abdominal tumor, such as a sacrococcygeal teratoma.

Following the physical examination, if the mass is thought to be renal, retroperitoneal, hepatic, or secondary to an abnormality of the female genital tract, ultrasonography is the next diagnostic step. In most cases, an experienced ultrasonographer is able to demonstrate the location of the mass and whether it is cystic or solid. In addition, a multicystic kidney has characteristic sonographic features that usually distinguish it from hydronephrosis. If it appears that the mass is either a hydronephrotic or multicystic kidney, a VCUG should be performed to assess whether there is vesicoureteral reflux and, in males, whether bladder outlet obstruction (i.e., posterior urethral valves) is present. If a tentative diagnosis of unilateral UPJ obstruction, ureterovesical junction obstruction, or multicystic kidney is made, the newborn may be discharged with its mother and allowed to return after 3 or 4 weeks for a renal scan. A scan should be performed urgently, as if the renal mass is a hydronephrotic kidney secondary to a ureteropelvic junction obstruction. Early pyeloplasty probably will be necessary.

If a solid tumor is suspected, an IVP or CT scan should be performed. It is likely that the mass represents a mesoblastic nephroma, and a nephrectomy should be performed before discharge from the hospital. Wilms' tumors rarely occur in the newborn period. The management of renal vein thrombosis is discussed later in the chapter. Other urologic problems that may require immediate treatment include posterior urethral valves, hydrocolpos, and an ovarian cyst.

The list in Table 44-12 should not be construed as a complete list of all neonatal abdominal masses. In our experience, other masses that have been encountered include focal renal dysplasia manifested as a unilateral solid renal mass (Elder et al., 1981) and oxalosis and neonatal leukemia (Gore and Shkolnik, 1982), both of which were diagnosed following the detection of bilateral renomegaly.

Multicystic Kidney

The multicystic kidney is the second most common cause of an abdominal mass in the neonate (see Table 44-12) and is the most common cause of an abdominal mass in the first 2 days of life (Griscom, 1965). It represents a severe form of renal dysplasia and is associated with ureteral atresia. The etiology is uncertain, although Stephens (1983) suggests that during migration of the developing kidney from the sacral to the lumbar level, the normal arterial cascade providing vascularity to the kidney may not occur, resulting in an ischemic insult, producing the multicystic kidney and associated ureteral atresia. In the past, nearly all multicystic kidneys were detected in the newborn fol-

lowing detection of an abdominal mass. However, the widespread use of antenatal ultrasound has resulted in the majority of multicystic kidneys being detected before birth. However, at times a multicystic kidney cannot be distinguished from an obstructed hydronephrotic kidney prenatally (Cooke et al., 1989). Therefore, prompt postnatal evaluation is necessary. The multicystic kidney is almost always unilateral, with the left side being more commonly involved (Filmer et al., 1974). Bilateral multicystic kidney is incompatible with life.

Diagnosis

Most multicystic kidneys detected by antenatal ultrasound are not palpable unless the cysts are quite large. In one recent series, only 13% were palpable (Gordon et al., 1988). When the kidney is palpable and enlarged, examination usually reveals a unilateral firm mass that has an irregular surface caused by the cysts and which may feel like a bunch of grapes. Transillumination demonstrates the mass to be lucent. Although the kidney usually is in a lumbar location, it may occur in a pelvic kidney (Pathak and Williams, 1964), crossed fused ectopia (Rosenberg et al., 1984), or a horseshoe kidney (Fig. 44-17). Ultrasound is usually diagnostic (Stuck et al., 1982), but occasionally strikingly resembles a kidney with a UPJ obstruction, termed the *hydronephrotic variant* (Sanders and Hartman, 1984). Thus, the diagnosis must be confirmed by DTPA or MAG-3 renal scan. A renal scan should demonstrate a photopenic area with less than 1% differential function. A few multicystic kidneys, however, have been reported to demonstrate significant function or renal scan in the neonate, leading to uncertainty about the diagnosis (Carey and Howards, 1988). Since the contralateral kidney has a 20% chance of being abnormal (Pathak and Williams, 1964; Vinocur et al., 1988), careful imaging of this kidney with an ultrasound is mandatory. In addition, a VCUG should be performed because there is a significant incidence of lower urinary tract anomalies and 15% have reflux (Selzman and Elder 1995a).

Management

Left untreated, most multicystic kidneys become smaller relative to total body size, and some regress completely (Avni et al., 1987; Gordon et al., 1988; Vinocur et al., 1988). In a registry of children with a multicystic kidney, 23% of those managed nonoperatively until 3 years of age showed complete regression (Wacksman and Phipps, 1993). Consequently, some feel that it is unnecessary to remove the incidentally detected multicystic kidney. Complications associated with multicystic kidneys include hypertension (Angermeier et al., 1992; Susskind et al., 1989), malig-

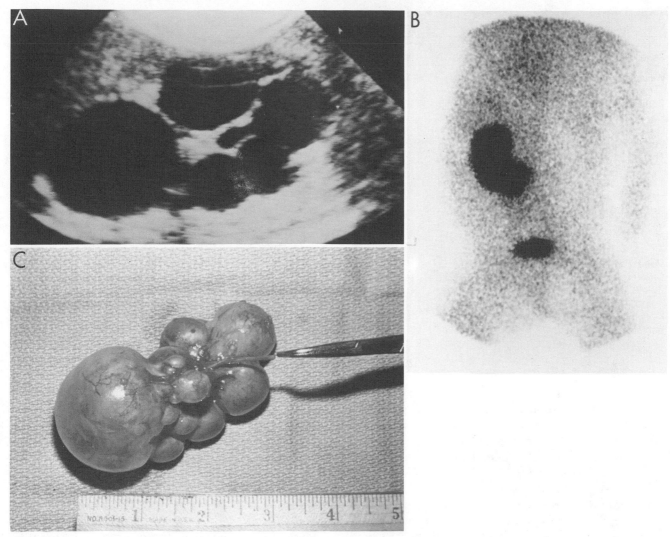

FIG. 44-17
Infant born with palpable right abdominal mass. **A,** Sonogram of right kidney demonstrating multiple echolucent cysts of varying sizes with no discernible cortex. **B,** DTPA renal scan demonstrating absence of flow and function on the right side. The infant also has a horseshoe kidney with a ureteropelvic junction obstruction of the left kidney on the left side of the image. **C,** Multicystic kidney, gross specimen.

nancy (Barrett and Wineland, 1980; Birken et al., 1985; Dimmick et al., 1989; Hartman et al., 1986; Oddone et al., 1994; Rackley et al., 1994), nodular renal blastema, which is a precursor to Wilms' tumor (Dimmick et al., 1989), and focal nephroblastomatosis (Vinocur et al., 1988). Because of the occult nature of these potential problems, annual follow-up with ultrasonography and blood pressure measurement is recommended. If any cysts enlarge, the stromal core increases in size, or hypertension develops, nephrectomy is recommended. Alternatively, in lieu of follow-up screening, nephrectomy may be performed as an outpatient through a 3-cm incision when the child is 3 to 12 months old (Elder et al., 1995b). The Section on Urology of the American Academy of Pediatrics has ongoing registry to determine the long-term "risks" of nonoperative management of multicystic kidneys.

Ureteropelvic Junction Obstruction

Congenital hydronephrosis secondary to UPJ obstruction is a common disorder of childhood, with an incidence approximating 1 in 1000. In the past, approximately 75% of children with this anomaly were diagnosed beyond 1 year of age (Snyder et al., 1980). However, with increasing use and improved sophistication of prenatal ultrasound, 30% to 50% of children with UPJ obstruction are diagnosed prenatally, before they become symptomatic. Currently less than 15% of neonates with a UPJ obstruction present with an abdominal mass. Other typical presentations include urinary tract infection, VATER (vertebral defects, anal

TABLE 44-13

Infant Pyeloplasties

Series	No. of Patients (Time Period)	Bilateral	M/F	L/R	Prenatal Diagnosis	Nephrostomy	Reoperation Rate
Williams and Karlaftis, 1966	26 (1951-1964)	10	17:9	?	0	All	Not reported
Robson et al, 1976	33	10	23:10	18:5	0	All, with stent	
Snyder et al, 1980	49 (1969-1978)	6	34:15	?	0	Almost all, with stent	9/49
Bejjani and Belman, 1872	11 (11/76-4/81)	2	5:6	6:3	?	3 (2 with stent)	1/11
Perlmutter et al, 1980	24 (1971-1978)	8	19:5	?	0	20/27 with stent	2/27
Thomas et al, 1982	16 (1964-1979)	4	?	?	0	"Advantageous"	7% of all patients had reoperation
Valayer and Adda, 1982	31 (1968-1980)	3	24:7	17:11	?	6	1/31
Roth and Gonzales, 1983	16 (1976-1982)	4	12:4	7:5	6	4 with stent	0/16
Murphy et al, 1984	21 (1973-1983)	4	10:11	9:8	6	All	1/21
King et al, 1984	11 (1982-1983)	0	?	?	?	Generally, no nephrostomy	
Mandell et al, 1984	6	0	?	2:4	6	?	0/6
Children's Hospital of Philadelphia (Sheldon et al, 1992)	28 (1973-1982)	5	21:7	13:10	5	17 nephrostomy and stent	2/31
Koyle and Ehrlich, 1988	17	3	?	?	17	6 (with stent)	0/20
Bernstein et al, 1988	67 (1981-1987)	6	?	?	52	45	1/67
Totals	356	65 (18.3%)	165:34 (2.2:1)	72:46 (1.6:1)			17/279 (6.1%)

atresia, *t*racheoesophageal fistula with *e*sophageal atresia, and *r*adial and *r*enal anomalies) screening, urinary ascites, and as an incidental finding during cardiac catheterization for congenital heart disease (Sheldon and Duckett, 1988).

In most series, the sex incidence and left-sided preponderance are similar to those described in older children (Table 44-13). Approximately two thirds of newborns with UPJ obstruction are boys, and in 60%, the obstruction is on the left side. Approximately 20% detected in the first year have a bilateral UPJ obstruction, whereas in children older than 1 year, bilateral involvement is less common (5%) (see Fig. 44-16). Approximately 15% have vesicoureteral reflux (Bernstein et al., 1988; Hollowell et al., 1989). In children with unilateral UPJ obstruction, contralateral renal anomalies have been described, including agenesis, duplication of the collecting system, malrotation, ectopia, and multicystic kidney. The etiology of UPJ obstruction is uncertain. The most attractive proposed theory is failure of recanalization of the metanephric cord between the fifth and sixth week of fetal development (Ruano-Gil et al., 1975).

Without ultrasound, the most common sign leading to diagnosis of UPJ obstruction in the newborn is the presence of an abdominal mass (Murphy et al., 1984; Robson et al., 1976). Other associated symptoms and signs include fever (secondary to UTI, most common in girls), hematuria, vomiting, and failure to thrive. In contrast, in older children, abdominal or flank pain

and UTI are the most common presentations (Elder et al., 1995a; Snyder et al., 1980). A spectrum of abnormalities is seen pathologically in UPJ obstruction (Hanna et al., 1976a and b). The UPJ may show reduced muscle bulk, muscular malorientation, thickened adventitia, and infiltration by inflammatory cells. Approximately 20% are normal by light microscopy (Hanna et al., 1976b). By electron microscopy, abundant collagen fiber is in the obstructed UPJ and between the muscle cells just proximal to the UPJ. In the renal pelvis, there is variable muscle cell damage with increased collagen and ground substance deposition and disrupted nexuses. An accessory lower pole renal artery is present in 10% to 20% of patients and usually is anterior to the obstructed UPJ (Rushton et al., 1994; Snyder et al., 1980; Uson et al., 1968). However, in most patients, the obstruction produced is due to a stenotic or dysfunctional UPJ that does not allow normal propulsion of urine from the renal pelvis to the ureter. When an accessory lower pole artery is present, a distended pelvis may pull the ureter up such that it drapes over the vessel and kinks the ureter, further obstructing the system. The vessel usually is an associated finding and not the primary cause of obstruction. There is a group of patients who appear to develop intermittent obstruction at the UPJ. In such patients, there appears to be a borderline functional obstruction, and during high rates of urine flow, the renal pelvis decompensates, resulting in severe abdominal pain and vomiting (Dietl's crisis). When the pelvis finally drains sufficiently, the pain resolves.

This situation exists more commonly in older children and adults and is rare in neonates.

Evaluation

In a newborn with hydronephrosis detected by prenatal sonography a UPJ obstruction often is suspected if the ureter is nondilated and the bladder is normal. In some cases there is an abdominal mass, but in most cases the exam is normal, and the perinatal finding is incidental (Figs. 44-18, 44-19, 44-20). If there is an abdominal mass, a solitary kidney or bilateral hydronephrosis, prompt evaluation is suggested. Otherwise, the workup does not need to be as urgent. Renal function should be assessed with serial serum creatinine levels, recognizing that it may not become normal (0.4 mg%) until 1 week of age. The radiologic evaluation consists of a renal ultrasound, VCUG, and diuretic renogram.

If the initial ultrasound is normal, the finding may be secondary to oliguria, which occurs immediately postnatally (Laing et al., 1984), and a repeat study should be performed in 3 weeks. Hydronephrosis should be graded according to the Society for Fetal Urology grading scale, from 0 to 4 (Maizels et al., 1992). If there is severe hydronephrosis with marked parenchymal thinning, generally seen in neonates with an abdominal mass secondary to a UPJ obstruction, or if there is bilateral hydronephrosis, a prompt VCUG and diuretic renogram should be done. In most cases the evaluation may be delayed until the infant is 4 to 6 weeks of age, to allow renal maturation with an increased GFR, which will enhance the accuracy of the diuretic renogram (Conway, 1992). In such cases the infant should be discharged on oral amoxicillin 50 mg daily. In addition, in boys with hydronephrosis circumcision is recommended to diminish the risk of urinary tract infection.

A VCUG is necessary to ascertain that the male urethra is normal and to determine whether there is vesicoureteral reflux, which is present in as many as 15% of children with a UPJ obstruction (Bernstein et al., 1988; Hollowell et al., 1989). At times the reflux may be high grade (Lebowitz and Blickman, 1983; Maizels et al., 1984) (Fig. 44-21). Performing a pyeloplasty in a child with reflux may subject the repair to high pressures and result in an anastomotic leak.

An IVP generally is not performed in neonates or infants less than 6 months of age with a suspected UPJ obstruction because the diuretic renogram provides much more information regarding function of the hydronephrotic kidney and severity of obstruction. Furthermore, visualization of the kidney is likely to be suboptimal because of insufficient concentration of the contrast media and overlying bowel gas. However, the study may provide important anatomic information if a duplication anomaly with obstruction of the lower pole UPJ is suspected. We tend to use the IVP as a follow-up study in older infants and toddlers with mild hydronephrosis secondary to an anomalous UPJ followed nonoperatively.

If an IVP is done, typical features include delay in visualization of the collecting system, variable hydronephrosis with a cut-off at the UPJ, and often there is parenchymal thinning. The *rim sign* is a reflection of the amount of parenchyma compressed by the hydronephrotic collecting system prior to contrast spilling into the pelvis. The *crescent sign* represents contrast media in the collecting ducts with a semicircular configuration caused by the stretched collecting ducts lying in a transverse fashion over the distended calyx. In general, the crescent sign is a more favorable indicator of good recoverability.

If an IVP is performed with a UPJ obstruction, delayed films should be obtained until the calyces and renal pelvis are seen. The timing of delayed films is important. One should double the length of time since the last film until the collecting system is seen (e.g., 1, 2, 4, 8, 16 hours, etc.). If there is vesicoureteral reflux, contrast excreted from the good kidney may reflux into the poorly functioning side and result in spurious renal function.

The most important diagnostic study is the "well-tempered" MAG-3 diuretic renogram. This study is covered in detail elsewhere in this chapter in the section on nuclear medicine studies. In general, extrapolating the drainage slope from the point of maximal activity, a T ½ greater than 20 minutes is consistent with obstruction. However, if the first study shows any drainage following diuretic administration and the differential renal function in the hydronephrotic kidney is at least 35% to 40%, we tend to follow the infant nonoperatively and repeat the "well-tempered" diuretic renogram 3 months later, because in some cases the obstruction reduces in severity or disappears with time. Exceptions to this approach include an infant with a solitary kidney, bilateral hydronephrosis, reduced renal function, an abdominal mass, or the rare infant with nearly constant abdominal pain, which has been attributed to colic.

With current methods of diagnosis, percutaneous nephrostomy and antegrade pyelography rarely are necessary. Antegrade pyelography may aid in distinguishing a UPJ obstruction from a multicystic kidney. However, the renal scan is likely to be as accurate, if not more accurate, since a congenital UPJ obstruction almost always demonstrates at least 5% function in the newborn, whereas a multicystic kidney demonstrates minimal or no flow or function. If the diagnosis is in doubt, an antegrade study of a multicystic kidney generally demonstrates that the cysts do not communicate.

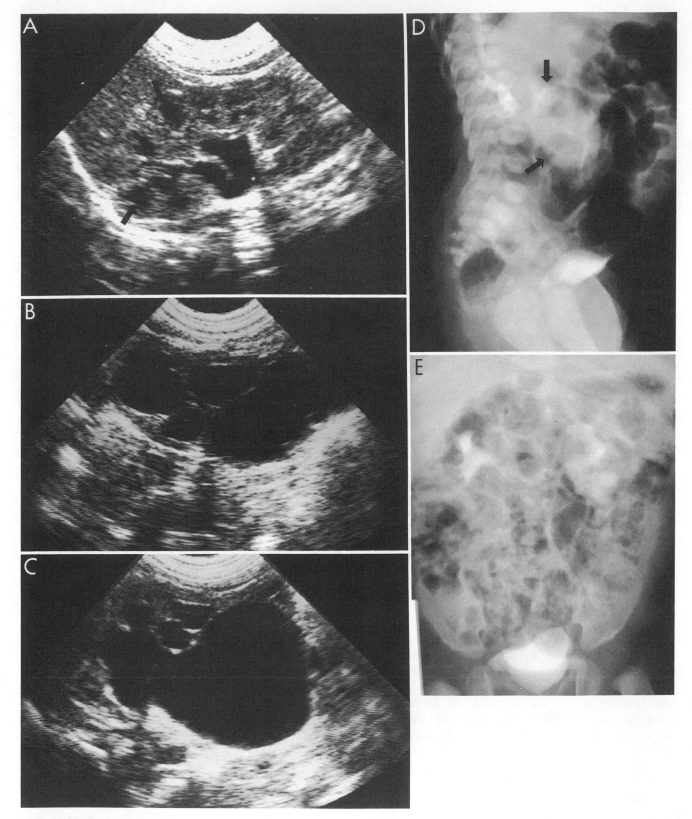

FIG. 44-18
A, Normal neonatal renal ultrasound. Note prominent intrarenal pelvis and corticomedullary junctions *(arrows)*. **B** and **C,** Renal ultrasounds in newborn with left ureteropelvic junction obstruction. Note large renal pelvis communicating with clubbed calyces. Cortex is quite thin. **D,** Intravenous pyelogram (IVP) performed at 1 week of age. Film was taken 1 hour, 45 minutes after injection. Note large left renal pelvis *(arrows)* of the left kidney. Patient underwent pyeloplasty in the neonatal period. **E,** IVP 2.5 months postpyeloplasty, a 15-minute film. Visualization of the left kidney was prompt. Note persistently clubbed calyces.

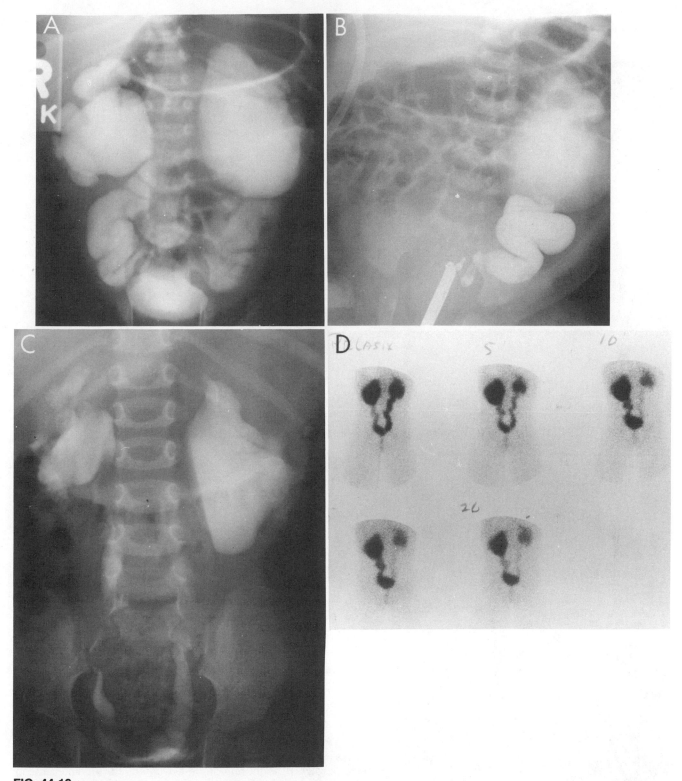

FIG. 44-19

Example of bilateral hydronephrosis that is apparently nonobstructive. As newborn, a large abdominal mass was palpable. Serum creatinine was 0.3 mg/dl. **A,** Intravenous pyelogram (IVP) performed at 3 days of age 5.5 hours after injection demonstrating marked bilateral hydroureteronephrosis with multiple transverse folds in the ureters. **B,** Left retrograde pyelogram performed at 2 months of age. Child was followed nonoperatively and maintained on antimicrobial prophylaxis. Serial IVPs and renal scans were obtained. **C,** IVP at 2½ years of age demonstrating nearly complete resolution of hydronephrosis. Renal units are dysmorphic. **D,** DTPA diuretic renogram at 3½ years of age. Left kidney is on left side of image. Percent uptake: left, 3.2%. Differential function: left, 46%; right, 54%. Cortical transit time: left, 3.5 minutes; right, 2.5 minutes. Following administration of furosemide, $T_{1/2}$; left kidney on left side of image, 9 minutes; right, less than 5 minutes.

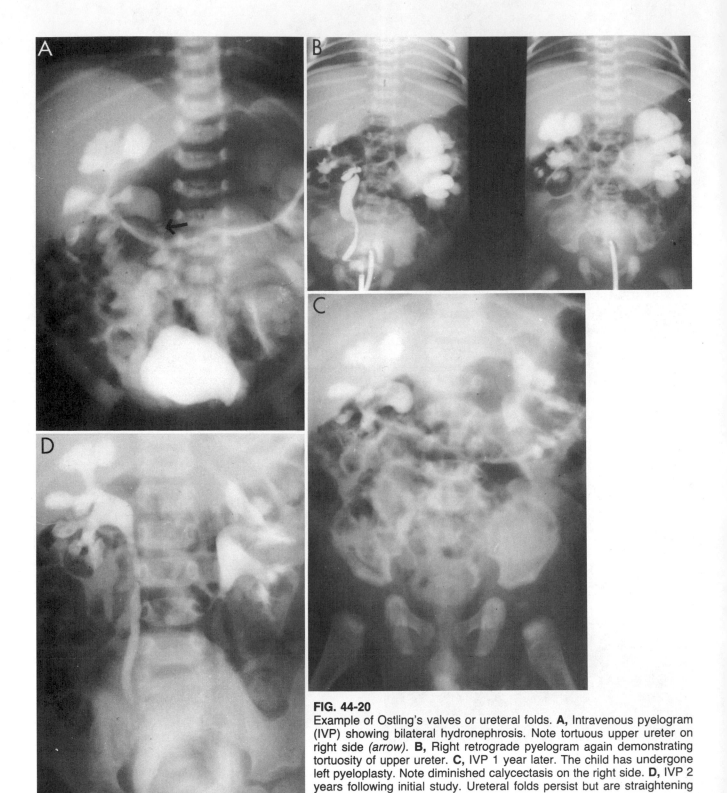

FIG. 44-20
Example of Ostling's valves or ureteral folds. **A,** Intravenous pyelogram (IVP) showing bilateral hydronephrosis. Note tortuous upper ureter on right side *(arrow).* **B,** Right retrograde pyelogram again demonstrating tortuosity of upper ureter. **C,** IVP 1 year later. The child has undergone left pyeloplasty. Note diminished calycectasis on the right side. **D,** IVP 2 years following initial study. Ureteral folds persist but are straightening out.

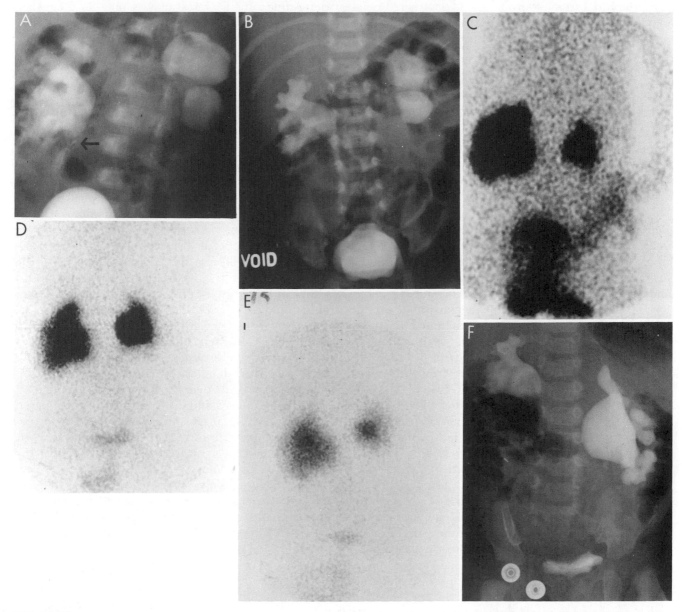

FIG. 44-21
Example of left ureteropelvic junction obstruction and bilateral vesicoureteral reflux. **A** and **B,** Voiding cystourethrogram demonstrating bilateral grade III-IV reflux. Note Ostling's valve or ureteral fold *(arrow)*. **B,** is postvoid film. **C,** Delayed image following DTPA renal scan performed at 3 weeks of age showing stasis in left kidney. $T_{1/2}$ normal on right, prolonged on left side. Percent uptake: left side, 1.2%; right side, 1.5%. Differential function, left, 45%; right, 55%. Because of excellent function in the left kidney on the left side of the image, it was decided not to perform a pyeloplasty at this time. **D** and **E,** DTPA diuretic renogram at 4 months of age. Left kidney is on the left side of the image. **D,** Prefurosemide image; **E,** image 15 minutes following administration of furosemide. $T_{1/2}$ on right side, 7 minutes; 40% washout of radionuclide at 20 minutes on the left side. Percent uptake: left, 2.7%; right, 2.1%. Differential function: left, 56%; right, 44%. **F,** Intravenous pyelogram performed at 5 months of age. Pyeloplasty has not yet been performed. Case demonstrates continued growth of left kidney despite obstruction on furosemide washout curve.

It may be worthwhile to place a percutaneous nephrostomy temporarily if the salvageability of an obstructed kidney is in doubt or in the presence of respiratory distress compounded by abdominal distention secondary to a tremendously dilated obstructed renal pelvis. Although percutaneous nephrostomy in the newborn is safe and generally successful (LiPuma et al., 1984), it may result in edema, inflammation, infection, or hemorrhage in the pelvis that can result in a very difficult pyeloplasty.

Immediate Versus Delayed Surgical Arrangement

In the human, nephrogenesis is completed by 36 weeks' gestation. At birth, blood flow is redistributed, with an increasing proportion directed to the peripheral nephrons. During the first 6 months of life, the GFR increases substantially, and the ability of the kidney to concentrate and acidify urine improves. The rate at which the GFR increases postnatally is dependent on glomerular permeability and glomerular perfusion pressure (Horster and Valtin, 1971). Chronic urinary tract obstruction results in decreasing GFR and renal blood flow, and impaired concentrating ability. These findings have been demonstrated experimentally in rats with hereditary congenital unilateral hydronephrosis (Friedman et al., 1979). Unfortunately, there is no reliable method to predict recovery of renal function following relief of obstruction (Walker et al., 1980).

In the newborn rat (corresponding to the human fetus in the last trimester), when partial ureteral obstruction is created, the GFR on the hydronephrotic side is variably affected, being 10% to 43% less than the contralateral side, with compensatory hypertrophy of the normal side (Josephson, 1983; Josephson et al., 1980, 1982, 1985). Furthermore, the single-nephron GFR may be elevated on the hydronephrotic side, with minimal redistribution of glomerular filtration (Josephson et al., 1985). The alterations in GFR appear to stabilize over time, as do the changes in renal morphology (Claesson et al., 1983; Josephson, 1983). Similar studies have been performed in the newborn guinea pig, which corresponds to the human in that nephron formation is complete at birth. In this model, neonatal ureteral obstruction results in variable hydroureteronephrosis, with the intraureteral pressure inversely proportional to a reduction in GFR (Chevalier, 1984). These studies suggest that although partial ureteral obstruction may cause diminished kidney function, the changes may not progress over time. In UPJ obstruction, there is partial obstruction that is variable in severity. Accordingly, one might infer from these studies that with a mild UPJ obstruction a mild diminution of renal function is likely to remain stable, whereas with high-grade obstruction, progressive deterioration of renal function is likely.

King and co-workers (1984) reported on a series of 11 infants who underwent pyeloplasty. Nearly all of the patients were 3 months of age or less, and the mean differential function of the involved kidney as determined by DTPA scan was only 17.6%. All of these children had follow-up renal scans, and the average percentage improvement in differential function was 107%. In contrast, in children more than 5 years of age undergoing pyeloplasty, the percentage improvement in differential function was only 16.4%. However, the mean preoperative function in the older patients was 27.9% (i.e., much higher than the infant group). Furthermore, the final percentage of differential function in the two groups was similar; 36.5% in the infants compared with 32.5% in the older group. These data do not infer that immediate neonatal pyeloplasty is necessary to provide optimal renal function. However, it is clear that the congenitally obstructed kidney can undergo substantial improvement in function following relief of obstruction. Mandell (1985) and co-workers (1984) also has advocated early postnatal reconstruction of UPJ obstruction. On the other hand, although relief of UPJ obstruction in infancy presumably would result in better improvement in renal function than if the pyeloplasty were performed later in childhood, Mikkelsen and colleagues (1982) found that patients who underwent pyeloplasty earlier than 30 *years* of age had significantly more functional improvement than patients over 30 years of age at operation.

To better understand the natural history of apparent UPJ obstruction in infants, Ransley and associates (1990) performed a study in which selected newborns with hydronephrosis and a suspected UPJ obstruction and satisfactory differential renal function were followed nonoperatively.

Their management plan separated patients into three groups based on the "function" of the "obstructed" kidney on DTPA diuretic renogram.

Group I   Normal function: normal uptake curve (parenchymal transit time) with greater that 40% of overall function

Group II   Moderately reduced function: delayed uptake curve with 10% to 40% of overall function

Group III Severely reduced function: flat uptake curve with less than 10% of overall function

Group I was managed expectantly. The concept was that if the kidney had good function despite a long period of antenatal obstruction, surgical intervention might not be necessary in an asymptomatic child. In those with moderately reduced function (Group II), it was assumed that the partial obstruction was severe enough to warrant early surgical therapy. If the renal function was severely affected, it was distinguished from a multicystic kidney either by antegrade pyelogram or temporary percutaneous nephrostomy.

Of a total of 142 kidneys, 106 were Group I, 27 were Group II, and nine were Group III (Ransley et al., 1990). Of the nine Group III patients, three (33%) underwent pyeloplasty and six (67%) had a nephrectomy because of poor function. Of the 27 Group II patients, 23 underwent early pyeloplasty. Of these, nine (39%) had marked improvement in differential function, five (22%) had moderate improvement, and nine (39%) had no change. Of the Group I patients, six underwent early pyeloplasty. Of the 100 patients who were followed nonoperatively, 23 (23%) eventually required a pyeloplasty, 19 (83%) by 3 years of age. Reasons given for pyeloplasty included deteriorating differential renal function in 14 (61%), UTI in three (13%), pain in one (4%), concentrating defect in 1 (4%), and "other" in 4 (18%). Of the 14 patients with deteriorating renal function, only five (36%) returned to the original level of differential function. Mean follow-up was less than 3 years. Of the 66 kidneys with renal pelvic diameter >12 mm, 23 (35%) eventually underwent pyeloplasty, whereas none of 34 with pelvic diameter <12 mm required surgical intervention.

This report was the first study of a large group of patients with suspected UPJ obstruction followed nonoperatively. In retrospect, there were significant problems with the methodology of the diuretic renograms used to diagnose obstruction. For example, only 0.2 mg/kg of furosemide was administered 20 minutes into the study, rather than 1 mg/kg at peak activity in the renal pelvis, as is currently recommended. Consequently, the diuretic stimulus was minimal. In addition, hydration prior to the diuretic renogram was not monitored. Furthermore, a catheter was not used to drain the bladder (Gordon et al., 1991). Finally, using a liberal definition of obstruction (decrease in activity to 75% within 10 minutes or to 50% of activity within 20 minutes), 27% of the Group I patients never showed an obstructive pattern. Therefore, this study is not ideal for documenting the natural history of suspected UPJ obstruction.

In a more recent report, Cartwright and associates (1992) studied 97 newborns with suspected UPJ obstruction. Of 39 with at least 35% differential renal function followed nonoperatively, only six (15%) underwent pyeloplasty, with average follow-up of 18 months (range 6 to 48). Of the three with differential renal function less than 40% who underwent pyeloplasty because of decreasing renal function, all returned to their initial levels. One might question whether early pyeloplasty in these three patients would have allowed renal function to improve to 50%, which would have been ideal. In those followed nonoperatively, all maintained differential functions greater than 40% with follow-up as late as 48 months.

In a provocative report, Koff and Campbell (1994) reported on 45 consecutive neonates with suspected UPJ obstruction followed nonoperatively, irrespective of severity of hydronephrosis, shape of the diuretic renogram curve or initial degree of functional impairment. Of the 30 with grade 2 or 3 hydronephrosis (Society for Fetal Urology grading scale) and at least 40% differential function, none required pyeloplasty, with maximum follow-up of 2.5 years. Of the 15 with grade 4 hydronephrosis and functional impairment (range 7.5% to 42%), follow-up showed complete disappearance of hydronephrosis in two, mild to marked improvement in five, and no change in eight. The washout curves became improved in all cases but became nonobstructed in only 4. Furthermore, the differential function improved in all of these kidneys.

Subsequently, Koff and Campbell (1994) reported 104 consecutive neonates with suspected unilateral UPJ obstruction managed nonoperatively, with follow-up as long as 5 years. In this study, only seven (7%) ultimately underwent pyeloplasty for reduction in differential renal function more than 10% or progression of hydronephrosis. Pyeloplasty returned renal function to prepyeloplasty levels in all cases. Of 16 with significantly reduced renal function on initial scan and grade 4 hydronephrosis, rapid improvement was noted on follow-up diuretic renograms in 15 and the washout curve became nonobstructive in six. In addition, hydronephrosis disappeared in six, improved in six, remained stable in three and deteriorated in one. Of interest is that none of their patients were reported to have an abdominal mass, whereas in our own experience, currently 10% of children undergoing pyeloplasty have an abdominal mass (Elder et al., 1995b).

These observations may be interpreted in several ways. First, it may be that some partially obstructed kidneys have significant functional impairment at birth, but that the capacity for renal maturation, with increasing GFR secondary to redistribution of blood flow to cortical nephrons, during the first year of life is maintained. Another explanation is that the early diuretic renogram is erroneous, and that during the period of transitional nephrology the differential renal function and capacity for washout in these kidneys is different than in older children. This position was vigorously disputed by Chung and co-workers (1993), who performed well-tempered diuretic renograms and found no significant differences in renal function or washout in neonatal and follow-up studies in patients managed nonoperatively. Finally, it must be remembered that all of these studies base "renal function" on the results of the differential renal function, which has significant potential for variability.

Elder and colleagues (in press[b]) reported the results of renal biopsies performed in 55 children undergoing pyeloplasty. Overall, 63% showed minimal or no obstructive histologic changes. However, of those with differential renal function greater than 40%, 21% showed significant histopathology (reduced glomerular number, glomerular hyalinization, interstitial inflammation). In contrast, of those with a differential function less than 40%, 33% showed minimal or no obstructive changes. Consequently, in 25% of the patients the findings on renal biopsy did not correspond to the computed differential renal function and suggest the need for more sensitive markers of obstruction.

The critical question in patients with suspected UPJ obstruction is what is obstruction? Koff and Campbell (1994) define obstruction as identifying "evidence of obstructive injury, such as a failure of expected improvement in renal function, compensatory hypertrophy in the contralateral kidney or progressive hydronephrosis." By this definition, no neonate with unilateral hydronephrosis would undergo pyeloplasty until follow-up studies confirmed evidence of obstructive injury. Allen (1992), on the other hand, has stated "it makes no more sense to wait for evidence of progressive renal damage before making diagnosis of obstruction than it does to wait for a tumor to metastasize before calling it a cancer." Peters defines obstruction as "a condition of impaired urinary drainage that if uncorrected will limit the ultimate functional potential of a developing kidney." Woodard (1993) states "to delay surgery . . . until measurable deterioration in renal function has occurred seems to deny the patient the benefit of state-of-the-art management." Unfortunately, no one knows how many of these children later will become symptomatic with abdominal or flank pain. Although there are many viewpoints on the indications for pyeloplasty and appropriate timing (Blyth, 1993; Flashner et al., 1993; King, 1993; Perez et al., 1991), the physician managing these infants nonoperatively must be able to provide assurance that no permanent injury will occur.

Our approach to neonates with a perinatal diagnosis of suspected UPJ obstruction is as follows (Blyth et al., 1993). In children with unilateral hydronephrosis, no abdominal mass, and a normal contralateral kidney, the hydronephrosis is graded (1 to 4). Those with grade 4 hydronephrosis are most likely to require pyeloplasty. We obtain a VCUG during the first few weeks of life, place the child on prophylactic penicillin or amoxacillin, and recommend circumcision for boys. At 6 week a well-tempered renogram is performed. If differential renal function is greater than 35% to 40% the child is managed nonoperatively, and kept on prophylaxis with trimethoprim-sulfamethoxazole, which is safe to administer after 2 months of age. Follow up– well tempered diuretic renography is performed 3 months later. If there is deterioration in differential

function, decrease in the extraction factor, or worsening of the diuretic washout curve, pyeloplasty is recommended. If these parameters remain stable or improved, follow-up of 3 to 6 months later with another diuretic renogram or IVP is performed, and management is individualized. If there is an abdominal mass, a solitary kidney, bilateral hydronephrosis, or impaired renal function, pyeloplasty is performed if there is any sign of obstruction. With this approach, approximately 40% of neonates with a suspected UPJ obstruction have been undergoing pyeloplasty at some point (Blyth et al., 1993).

On occasion, urography of the fetal or neonatal urinary tract may disclose mild to moderate hydronephrosis and a dilated ureter a few centimeters distal to the UPJ. In many of these patients, the apparent dilatation is secondary to *Ostling's valves*, which represent transverse folds of the upper ureter (Ostling, 1942). They are usually nonobstructive and resolve over time (see Fig. 44-20).

Pyeloplasty: Technical Points

The infant is admitted to the hospital on the day of surgery, and rooming in by one of the parents is encouraged. Preoperatively, the anterior or posterior location of the extrarenal pelvis is determined because it may help in determining the surgical approach. Lateral or oblique views on the urogram or ultrasound are helpful in this regard. The anterior muscle-splitting approach clearly is indicated if the pelvis is anterior (Duckett et al., 1980), but since the pelvis is posterior in the majority of infants, a lumbotomy incision may be preferred.

If a flank incision is used, the infant is placed with the appropriate flank elevated 30 degrees, with the opposite side flexed over a rolled towel. It is preferable not to enter the peritoneum, which should be mobilized widely and retracted medially. In general, the kidney does not need to be mobilized.

We have found the posterior lumbotomy to provide an excellent surgical approach to the kidney in the neonate (Gil-Vernet, 1965; Gonzalez and Aliabadi, 1987; Lurz, 1956; Pansadoro, 1983). The infant is placed in the supine position, and a towel is placed under the abdomen to push the kidneys further posteriorly. A 45-degree incision is made in the costovertebral angle. This approach is minimally traumatic because no muscles are cut. The exposure is optimal (except when the renal pelvis is anterior), and opening and closing the incision is rapid.

In general, a dismembered Anderson-Hynes pyeloplasty is performed. The pelvis is exposed completely by dissecting bluntly in the plane just superficial to its intrinsic blood supply. The dissection of the upper ureter should be minimal, just enough to permit resection of the narrow segment and spatulation. The ureter is not elevated or placed on traction with umbilical tape or vessel loop. Following these precautions results in the preservation of maximal blood supply to the anastomosis. When a large redundant pelvis is present, the pelvis is resected to 1 cm from the edge of the renal parenchyma. If a decompensated large-capacity floppy pelvis is left unresected, the likelihood of an unanticipated kink at the ureteropelvic anastomosis when filling occurs is increased.

Holding sutures are placed to help position the tissues for precise approximation and to avoid the need for handling the tissue with forceps. Optical magnification ($\times 2.0$ to 3.5) is beneficial in assuring precise suture placement and a watertight anastomosis. The pelvis is closed with a running 6-0 polyglycolic acid (PGA) suture. The ureteropelvic anastomosis is performed with 6-0 or 7-0 PGA sutures. Between three and five interrupted sutures are placed at the apex, allowing more precise alignment of this critical portion of the anastomosis. The remainder of the anastomosis is performed with a running stitch, allowing a watertight closure. The anastomosis is performed over a catheter passed a few centimeters down the ureter. Passage of a catheter into the bladder is avoided because it may cause edema of the ureterovesical junction, resulting in mild obstruction, increased intrapelvic pressure, and possible breakdown of the anastomosis. The renal pelvis should be irrigated well prior to closure to remove any blood clots.

There is no general consensus as to whether a nephrostomy or a ureteral stent should be used. Numerous series have demonstrated that a pyeloplasty in a neonate may be performed safely without proximal drainage (B jjani and Belman, 1982; Roth and Gonzales, 1983; Valayer and Adda, 1982). However, there are several points to be considered. It may be more difficult to produce a perfect anastomosis in a small ureter. Edema may make coaptation of the walls of the anastomosis more likely, leading to the postoperative synechiae, obstruction, or both. These considerations would encourage the use of a nephrostomy and possibly a stent. When a nephrostomy is not used, leakage of urine is common during the first few postoperative days. Although extravasation of urine without drainage induces an inflammatory tissue reaction, a minor amount of leakage is not problematic if the area is drained adequately. Therefore, proper management of the drain is essential.

Ipsilateral vesicoureteral reflux or a full bladder may subject the anastomosis to high intraluminal pressure and may result in excessive leakage from the fragile anastomosis. Cystoscopy or intraoperative urethral catheterization may cause sufficient irritation in a newborn to allow unwanted bladder distention and probably should be avoided, as should retrograde ureteral catheterization. If a nephrostomy is not used, the infant should be checked carefully during the first 24 hours and catheterized every 4 to 6 hours if the child does not void to prevent a significant increase in the intrapelvic pressure.

A nephrostomy tube generally is recommended with a solitary kidney, with a bilateral pyeloplasty, or if the ureter is unusually small or thin walled. In general, a 12 F Malecot catheter is used as a nephrostomy, with two of the wings excised. In a patient whose kidney has been demonstrated postoperatively to have little or no function, a nephrostomy provides a way of demonstrating postoperatively that no obstruction is present. The catheter is placed in a lower-pole calyx. Since there is a theoretical advantage in urine transversing the anastomosis immediately postoperatively, when a nephrostomy is used, an option is to clamp it immediately and use it as a backup only if there is significant drainage from the anastomosis, obstruction, or urinary infection. When the nephrostomy is left open, it may be allowed to drain into a double diaper. Such drainage eliminates twisting, kinking, and inadvertent removal of tubes that may occur when the infant moves about the crib with the nephrostomy tube attached to a drainage bag. The infant may be discharged with an indwelling nephrostomy as soon as feeding is progressing satisfactorily and the clinical situation is stable.

Delayed opening of the anastomosis protected by a nephrostomy is common in the infant pyeloplasty. Snyder and associates (1980) encountered this problem in 45% of their pyeloplasties performed in patients less than 1 year of age. Mandell and coworkers (1984) reported an average length of nephrostomy drainage of 51 days in six newborns undergoing early pyeloplasty. In delayed opening, the drainage tubing may be elevated (hump the tube) 30 cm to increase the intrapelvic pressure and encourage the anastomosis to open. Gravity drainage may be reinstituted if the baby is fussy and to check for residual urine.

A reoperation rate of 8% to 10% in infant pyeloplasties has been reported (see Table 44-13), similar to series of older patients, although with greater experience there have been lower complication rates. The technical failures may be secondary to traumatic dissection, devascularization of the ureter, excessive traction on the ureter resulting in ischemia or creation of an anastomosis that is too tight, or extravasation from an undrained anastomotic leak with subsequent fibrosis.

Follow-up studies may include an IVP, DTPA diuretic renal scan, or ultrasound. In general, we obtain an IVP 3 months postoperatively and a renal scan in 6 months. If an undrained urinoma is suspected, an ultrasound should be obtained.

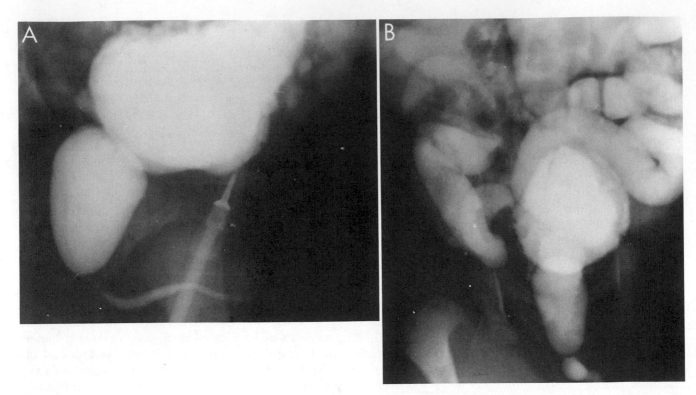

FIG. 44-22
A and **B**, Examples of voiding cystourethrogram demonstrating typical posterior urethral valves. Note dilated posterior urethra, hypertrophy of bladder neck, and trabeculated bladder. Bilateral vesicoureteral reflux demonstrated in **B**.

Posterior Urethral Valves

The most common cause of bladder outlet obstruction in the newborn is posterior urethral valves. The embryology, clinical features, and long-term management are described in Chapter 51. Although Young described three types of valves in 1919, presently only Type I and Type III valves are thought to be clinically significant. Type I valves are represented by leaflets or sails that extend distally from either side of the verumontanum to the anterior urethral wall at the level of the urogenital diaphragm. More than 90% of valves are Type I. A Type III valve is a diaphragm just distal to the verumontanum that has a small central perforation. Patients with Type III valves tend to have more severe bladder and upper urinary tract obstruction.

A recent study suggests that most congenital posterior urethral obstructions are similar. Dewan and co-workers (1992) performed antegrade voiding cystourethrography in boys with suspected valves. Subsequently, cystoscopy demonstrated that all had a "Type III" urethral membrane. After passing the cystoscope into the bladder and then withdrawing the cystoscope back into the urethra, all had the appearance of a Type I valve. This report suggests that the catheter used for VCUG disrupts the valve membrane, giving it a Type I appearance.

The incidence of posterior urethral valves is approximately 1 in 5000 to 8000 boys. At the Children's Hospital of Philadelphia, 120 boys with urethral valves have been treated between 1970 and 1985 (Hulbert and Duckett, 1986). Of these, half were less than 6 months of age and 30% less than 1 week of age at diagnosis.

There is a wide spectrum in the presenting symptomatology and long-term prognosis following treatment. Because of the high-grade bladder outlet obstruction throughout gestation, it is not uncommon for children with valves to have severely compromised renal function secondary to renal dysplasia.

Diagnosis

The newborn with urethral valves may have an abdominal mass (48%), failure to thrive (10%), urosepsis (8%), or urinary ascites (7%). When the bladder is empty, most will have a walnut-size firm mass in the pelvis which corresponds to the trabeculated bladder muscle. In as many as 48%, the diagnosis of valves has been suggested by prenatal ultrasonography (see Fig. 44-10). Prognosis is significantly better if ultrasound studies performed prior to 24 weeks' gestation were normal; more than half detected by 24 weeks died or were in chronic renal failure (Dinneen et al., 1993; Hutton et al., 1994). In addition, dyspnea at

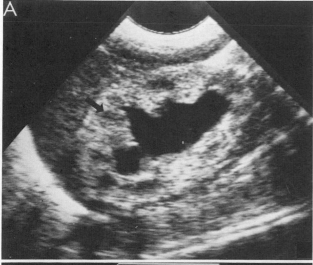

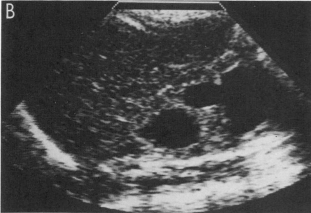

FIG. 44-23
Sonograms of kidneys from infants with posterior urethral valves. **A,** Corticomedullary junction is present *(arrow)*. At birth, creatinine rose to 2.8 mg/dl but fell to 0.6 mg/dl following valve ablation. **B,** Corticomedullary junction absent. The infant progressed to chronic renal failure.

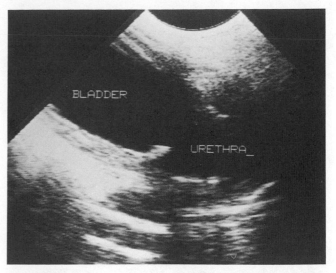

FIG. 44-24
Suprapubic ultrasound demonstrating dilated bladder and posterior urethra strongly suggestive of posterior urethral valves.

views of the renal collecting systems to assess pelvic and calyceal dilatation, as well as cortical echogenicity, which may be indicative of the presence of dysplasia. We have found that sonographic presence of the corticomedullary junction in newborns with urethral valves is an important prognostic indicator of good renal function following drainage of the urinary tract (Fig. 44-23). Conversely, if the corticomedullary junction is not visualized and does not appear on subsequent ultrasound examinations, most develop renal insufficiency (Hulbert et al., 1992). Suprapubic or perineal ultrasound may demonstrate the dilated posterior urethra, and thus one might establish the diagnosis of valves on the basis of an ultrasound before the VCUG is performed (Cohen et al., 1994) (Fig. 44-24).

Management

After the diagnosis of urethral valves is made, the bladder should be drained with either a urethral catheter or a suprapubic tube. Our preference is to use a 5 F or 8 F pediatric feeding tube. A Foley balloon catheter may not drain satisfactorily, because the balloon has a tendency to occlude the ureteral orifices (Jordan and Hoover, 1985). When passing the ureteral catheter, there is a tendency for the tip of the tube to bump on the bladder neck and coil in the dilated posterior urethra, compromising effective drainage. If there is a question, the appropriate position should be confirmed either by sonography or when the VCUG is done. Adjusting the tip of the catheter increases the likelihood of a secondary infection of the urinary tract.

birth associated with pneumothorax or pneumomediastinum may be the initial sign of severe urethral obstruction (Nakayama et al., 1986; Renert et al., 1972). A normal urinary stream is an infrequent finding.

When the diagnosis of urethral valves is suspected, a VCUG should be performed. A thick trabeculated bladder with a very distended posterior urethra and valve leaflets is seen. The VCUG should be performed with both anteroposterior and oblique views. Half of these patients have vesicoureteral reflux, and bladder neck hypertrophy or narrowing may be seen (Fig. 44-22). The radiographic appearance of urethral valves should not be confused with prune-belly syndrome, although both of these conditions can cause significant bladder and upper urinary tract dilatation.

The other important radiographic study is a renal and bladder ultrasound. It is critical to obtain baseline

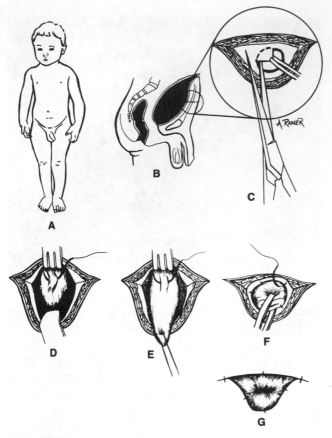

FIG. 44-25

A-G, Diagram of cutaneous vesicostomy. Incision is made halfway between the pubic symphysis and umbilicus. Holding sutures are placed through the bladder wall for traction, and the bladder is mobilized superiorly until the dome is reached. The dome of the bladder is then exteriorized.

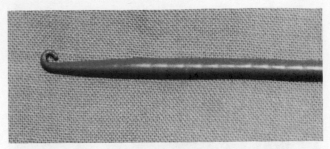

FIG. 44-26

Tip of insulated crochet hook developed by Whitaker and Sherwood (1986). Tip of hook engages only the valve leaflets. Crotch of hook is not insulated allowing diathermy ablation of valves.

Broad-spectrum antibiotics are given IV to minimize the chance of developing a nosocomial bacterial infection. Serum creatinine is monitored, and electrolyte abnormalities, including acidosis and hyperkalemia, need to be managed before surgical treatment of the lesion is undertaken.

Initial treatment of the valves is dependent on the age at presentation and the size and condition of the child. In the past, use of inappropriately large endoscopic instruments for valve ablation resulted in urethral strictures. With improvement in the optics of the 8 F pediatric cystoscope, fulguration may be done in many small infants with safety.

In more than 80% of patients, urethral valve ablation may be performed at diagnosis. In the 1970s, approximately half of these were performed through a perineal urethrostomy. More recently, nearly all have been performed in a standard transurethral manner (Hulbert and Duckett, 1986). In the newborn, the 8 F cystoscope is used to examine the bladder, with assessment of the degree of trabeculation, the presence of diverticula, and the position of the ureteral orifices, as well as examination of the valves. In many cases, the 10 F panendoscope or the 11.5 F resectoscope will traverse the newborn urethra for fulguration. Alternatively, the small Bugbee electrode (3 F) may be inserted beside the 8 F cystoscope and manipulated to fulgurate the valve cusps. The valve leaflets should be ablated at the 5 o'clock and 7 o'clock positions.

If the urethra is too small to accommodate the pediatric cystoscope and miniature Bugbee electrode, cutaneous vesicostomy is an alternative form of management (Duckett, 1974). The dome of the bladder should be brought to the skin at a level such that the posterior bladder wall will not prolapse into the stoma (Fig. 44-25). The vesicostomy should calibrate to 24 F.

A method of valve ablation prior to the availability of miniature endoscopic equipment was a modified crochet hook (Williams et al., 1973). However, because of complications and the development of better endoscopic equipment, that treatment has not enjoyed widespread use. More recently, Whitaker and Sherwood (1986) have redesigned the hook (Fig. 44-26) such that it engages only valves and not the bladder neck, verumontanum, or external sphincter. Except for the crotch of the hook, the entire instrument is insulated to prevent spread of diathermy current. It is important to use low cutting current with the device. It may be used under fluoroscopic guidance in the radiology suite without the necessity for general anesthesia. A cystogram in the operating room confirms adequate relief of obstruction. Experience with this technique over the past few years has confirmed its effectiveness in relieving bladder outlet obstruction, although some patients have required secondary valve ablation (Deane et al., 1988). Its most appropriate use may be in countries where miniature endoscopic equipment is unavailable.

Cromie and colleagues (1994) reported using a venous valvulotome to incise the valve leaflets at the 12 o'clock position under local anesthesia. Of the 10 pa-

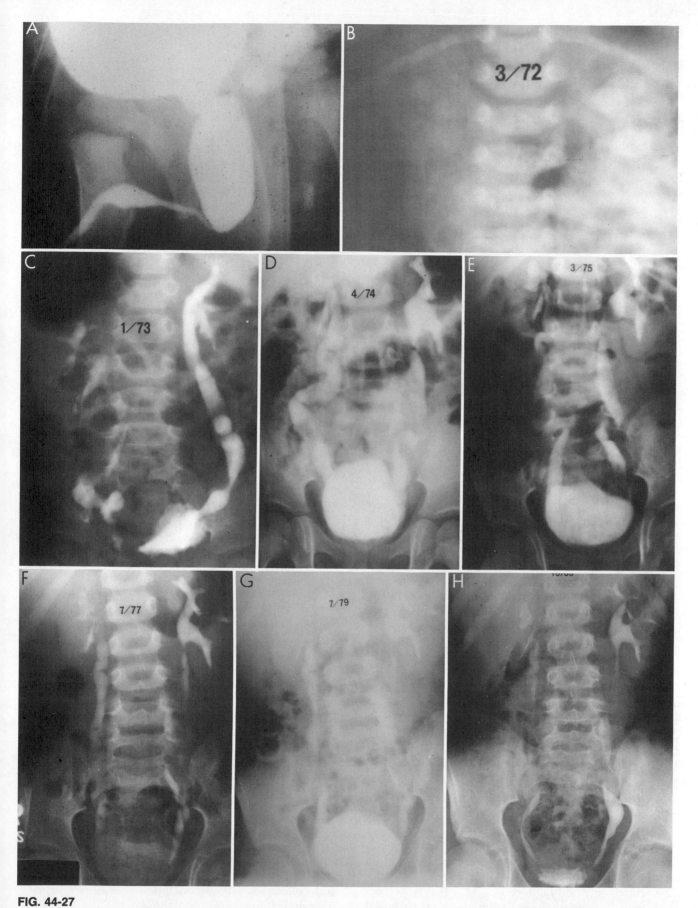

FIG. 44-27
Example of long-term follow-up in a patient with posterior urethral valves. Infant was born with urinary ascites. Child underwent primary resection of urethral valves. **A,** Voiding cystourethrogram with typical posterior urethral valves. **B,** Initial intravenous pyelogram demonstrating bilateral hydronephrosis. **C-H,** Initial improvement was observed, and long-term follow-up shows good results. Vesicoureteral reflux of the right kidney ceased within 3 years. Note the straightening of the ureters with time. (**A-G** from Duckett JW, Snow BW: Disorders of the urethra and penis. In Walsh PC, Gittes RF, Perlmutter AD, et al (eds): *Campbell's Urology,* ed 5. Philadelphia, WB Saunders Co, 1986.)

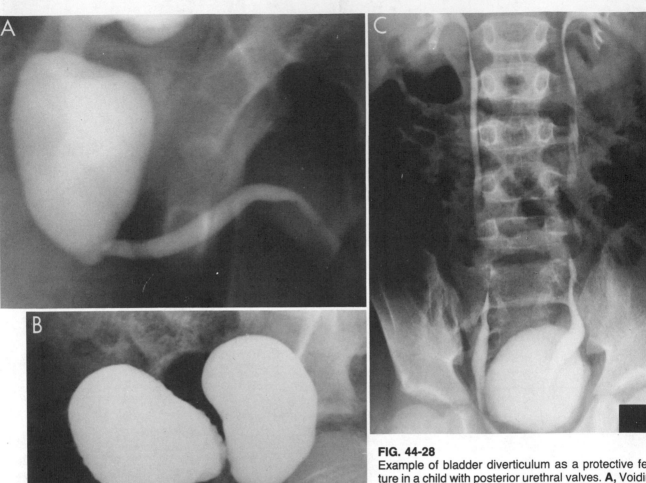

FIG. 44-28
Example of bladder diverticulum as a protective feature in a child with posterior urethral valves. **A,** Voiding cystourethrogram showing typical posterior urethral valves. **B,** Lateral image on cystogram showing large vesical diverticulum. **C,** IV urogram prior to valve ablation showing normal collecting systems and medial deviation of lower left ureter secondary to large diverticulum.

tients, two underwent later resection of small nonobstructive valve leaflet remnants.

Other techniques for valve ablation also have been described. Blind rupture of the valves using a small Fogarty catheter has been reported (Diamond and Ransley, 1987). Zaontz and Gibbons (1984) reported antegrade ablation of valves through an established vesicostomy. The technique also has been used percutaneously in neonates (Zaontz and Firlit, 1986). The technique involves distending the bladder and performing a percutaneous cystotomy with a 12 F trocar midway between the symphysis and umbilicus in the midline. The obturator may be removed, leaving the 12 F sheath in the bladder. The 11.5 F resectoscope then may be passed through the sheath with visualization of the valves through a 0-degree lens. Visualization has been reported to be quite good. Follow-

ing this procedure, neither a suprapubic tube nor a urethral catheter was necessary postoperatively.

Following definitive therapy, the child should be monitored closely by ultrasound to be certain that the upper urinary tracts are decompressed satisfactorily. A high serum creatinine should decrease gradually. In a newborn who has undergone only valve ablation, however, if the serum creatinine remains unchanged or does not decrease at least to 1.0 to 1.2 mg/dl, proximal diversion by vesicostomy or cutaneous pyelostomy may be necessary. We have not found that cutaneous ureterostomy or pyelostomy is more beneficial than cutaneous vesicostomy. Although Krueger and colleagues (1980) concluded that upper urinary tract diversion was optimal, these data have been challenged. Indeed, others have found, as we have, that cutaneous vesicostomy is as effective as upper urinary

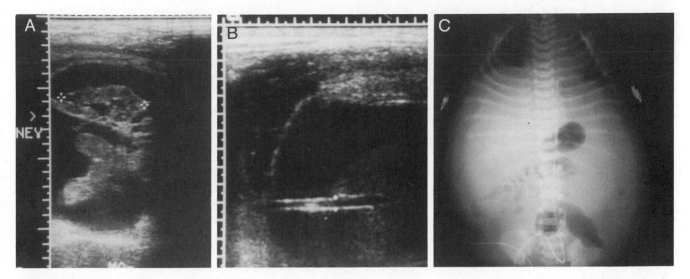

FIG. 44-29
Urinary ascites secondary to posterior urethral valves. **A,** Prenatal ultrasound, 38 weeks' gestation, showing right kidney and ascites. **B,** Massive ascites, resulting in stretching of umbilical vein *(arrow)* L = liver. **C,** Abdominal film at birth, showing characteristic appearance of ascites. Note umbilical artery catheter.

tract diversion (Fleisher et al., 1984). However, cutaneous pyelostomy may be necessary if a child has urosepsis secondary to pyonephrosis. If upper urinary tract diversion is performed, concurrent renal biopsy should be done to assess renal morphology.

The long-term prognosis for infants with posterior urethral valves is dependent on multiple factors (Rittenberg et al., 1988) (Fig. 44-27). Among the most important are the serum creatinine level 1 month following urinary drainage and whether vesicoureteral reflux or a large bladder diverticulum is present. In our experience, if the serum creatinine level falls below 1.0 mg/dl 1 month following treatment, renal function has remained sufficient to prevent the need for dialysis.

In patients with unilateral vesicoureteral reflux associated with nonfunction, the prognosis has been quite good. It has been called the VURD (valves, unilateral reflux, and dysplasia) syndrome (Hoover and Duckett, 1982). In a recent review of 12 patients, the nonfunctioning refluxing unit was on the left side in 92%, and in 83%, the kidney was dysplastic. The refluxing ureter acts as a pop-off valve, preventing the deleterious effects of high vesical pressure on the opposite kidney. A similar phenomenon occurs when a giant vesical diverticulum is present (Fig. 44-28). In five patients with this entity, all have good renal function, and some have surprisingly normal upper urinary tracts (Rittenberg et al., 1988). Finally, the presence of urinary ascites in newborns with posterior urethral valves has been recognized as another protective factor, with an upper or lower urinary tract leak allowing the kidneys to develop without the deleterious effects of high pressure (Adzick et al., 1985). In our experi-

ence, four (11%) of 36 infants with posterior urethral valves less than 1 week old had ascites (Rittenberg et al., 1988) (Fig. 44-29).

In our experience with 71 boys with valves and long-term follow-up, 20 (28%) had one of the protective mechanisms. Of these, only one (5%) had a serum creatinine greater than 1.0 mg/dl. In contrast, of the 51 boys without a pop-off mechanism, 20 (39%) had an elevated creatinine and seven (14%) were on dialysis or had undergone renal transplantation (Rittenberg et al., 1988).

More recently, the potentially devastating long-term consequences of urethral valves have become apparent. In a series of 98 boys with follow-up between 11 and 22 years, Parkhouse and colleagues (1988) reported that 31 (32%) had poor renal function; 10 (10%) had died of renal failure, 15 (15%) had end-stage renal failure, and six (6%) had chronic renal failure but were not yet on dialysis. Adverse prognostic factors included presentation under 1 year of age, bilateral vesicoureteral reflux, and diurnal incontinence beyond 5 years of age, the last being the most important factor. The association of diurnal incontinence and poor renal function in these patients most probably is related to detrusor instability and detrusor sphincter dyssynergia, which many of these boys develop, resulting in elevated upper urinary tract pressures and gradual deterioration in renal function.

The overall prognosis for these infants seems to be improving. For example, from 1973 to 1987 at the Children's Hospital of Philadelphia, only one child with urethral valves died, a 6-month-old with severe renal insufficiency and sepsis. In contrast, from 1971 to 1973, there were seven deaths. A number of other institutions have had a similar experience, which has been attributed to improved medical management of the renal and respiratory complications of valve disease. Nakayama and associates (1986), however, have suggested that many cases may be unreported because they are not recognized until autopsy. In addition, with the popularity of prenatal ultrasound, a number of pregnancies of fetuses with bilateral hydronephrosis with associated oligohydramnios may be terminated early.

When urethral valves are discovered in the newborn, it is likely that the infant will have high urine output resulting from a renal concentrating defect. Consequently, the parents of these infants should be advised that their child is much more likely than other infants to become severely dehydrated with viral gastroenteritis or other febrile infections that might increase the child's fluid requirements.

Anterior Urethral Valve

Another form of urethral obstruction that may be apparent in the newborn is the anterior urethral valve (Fig. 44-30). This anomaly is rare, and its embryologic origin is uncertain. Usually the valve is a filamentous cusp on the ventral aspect of the urethra, resulting in the development of a diverticulum that by virtue of its size may obstruct the distal urethra. Nearly all occur in the bulbous or pendulous urethra (Firlit and King, 1972). If the diverticulum is large, it may be visualized as a cystic mass on the ventral aspect of the penoscrotal junction, which increases in size when the infant voids. In addition, a prolonged dribbling stream is noted. If obstruction is severe, the neonate may develop renal insufficiency. Diagnosis is confirmed by VCUG. In addition, a renal ultrasound to assess the upper urinary tracts should be performed.

Treatment is based on the size of the diverticulum and renal function. If the diverticulum is small, the cusp may be ablated by transurethral resection. Another technique is incision with a venous valvotome (Cromie et al., 1994). However, in the majority of neonates, open surgical resection of the diverticulum and valve cusp is necessary. A 6 F silastic urethral stent may be left in place to drain continuously into the diaper for 10 to 14 days. If renal function is impaired, temporary catheter drainage of the bladder may be necessary to stabilize the infant and correct electrolyte abnormalities. If the serum creatinine fails to decrease to a satisfactory level, resection of the diverticulum and valve and perineal urethrostomy provide reliable drainage. Alternatively, cutaneous vesicostomy should be considered in these patients (Rushton et al., 1987).

Hematuria

Gross hematuria in the neonate is an uncommon event but requires emergency diagnosis (Brem, 1981).

The unusual nature of hematuria in this age group is exemplified by the report by Emanuel and Aronson (1974) in which only 35 cases were encountered at a busy children's hospital over a 27-year period. In that series, seven patients (20%) had renal vein thrombosis, seven (20%) had obstructive uropathy, and six (17%) had infantile polycystic kidney disease. In 11 (31%) of the patients, the cause of the hematuria was unknown.

Another cause of neonatal hematuria is stone disease, which occurs with some frequency in premature newborns receiving parenteral furosemide therapy and which is discussed later in this chapter.

Other potential causes of hematuria in the newborn include endocarditis (Oelberg et al., 1983), peripheral venous air embolus (Willis et al., 1981), and secondary to indomethacin therapy for patent ductus arteriosus (Corazza et al., 1984). Although renal disease is a common cause of hematuria in the older pediatric age groups, glomerulonephritis is rare in the newborn.

Renal Vein Thrombosis

As noted above, renal vein thrombosis (RVT) is a common cause of neonatal hematuria. In neonatal autopsy studies, the incidence of RVT varies from 1.9% (Cruikshanks, 1930) to 2.7% (Arneil et al., 1973), although among surviving neonates, the incidence clearly is much lower. There is a moderate male predominance.

The neonatal kidney seems to be particularly vulnerable to RVT because of low renal perfusion pressure. The condition occurs primarily in conditions associated with dehydration and polycythemic sludging. For example, infants of diabetic mothers experience an osmotic diuresis and have a substantially increased incidence of RVT. In addition, it may occur following diarrhea, perinatal stress, sepsis (fever with increased fluid requirements), cyanotic congenital heart disease (with resultant polycythemia), acute hypoxia, sickle cell disease, cytomegalovirus, hypotension and seizures, and is associated with polyhydramnios, toxemia and maternal diuretic use (Ricci and Lloyd, 1990; Vorlicky and Balfour, 1974). Sludging in the renal venules results from low perfusion pressure, whereas contracture of the extracellular volume leads to increased blood viscosity and further diminishes renal blood flow, with predisposition to thrombosis (Belman and King, 1972). RVT is thought to originate in the arcuate and interlobar veins at the corticomedullary junction. The thrombotic process extends along the venous tributaries to the cortex, as well as centrally along the interlobar veins to the main renal vein (Arneil et al., 1973; Lloyd, 1986). Following RVT, severe renal congestion occurs, leading to further impairment of arterial perfusion with thrombosis.

Among cases of RVT in childhood, almost 65% occur during the neonatal period, whereas 30% occur be-

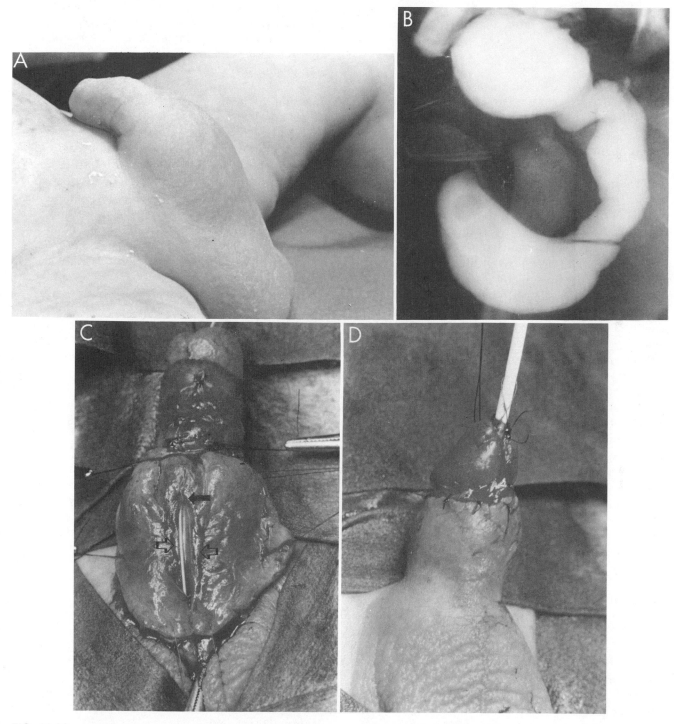

FIG. 44-30
Example of anterior urethral valve. **A,** Infant born with cystic firm mass at penoscrotal junction. **B,** Voiding cystourethrogram showing huge ventral diverticulum secondary to anterior urethral valve. Note distal anterior urethra. Infant also had bilateral vesicoureteral reflux. **C,** Neonate underwent primary open resection of valve and diverticulum. Intraoperative view demonstrates large diverticulum *(open arrows)* and anterior urethral valve *(solid arrow).* **D,** Postoperative photograph. A 6 F Silastic stent is used for bladder drainage.

yond the age of 1 year (Lloyd, 1986). In addition, it has been recognized prenatally (Evans et al., 1981). Evidence for the latter includes the finding of organized RVTs with calcification in the newborn period. An early postnatal renin-mediated hypertension may result.

Diagnosis

The classic features of neonatal RVT include (1) palpable renal mass (60%), (2) gross hematuria (70%), (3) thrombocytopenia (90%) less than $75,000/\mu L$, (4) consumptive coagulopathy (prolonged clotting time; elevated fibrin split products), (5) leukocytosis, (6) proteinuria, and (7) anemia (32%).

If there is edema of the lower extremities, one should suspect thrombosis of the inferior vena cava. In RVT, the blood pressure is usually normal or low. With bilateral RVT (20% of cases), the blood urea nitrogen (BUN) and serum creatinine levels usually are elevated. The prognosis of bilateral RVT is ominous compared with unilateral RVT.

As in the evaluation of other renal masses, ultrasonography is the initial procedure of choice for the diagnosis of RVT (Metreweli and Pearson, 1984; Ricci and Lloyd, 1990) and usually demonstrates an RVT with diffuse renal enlargement. Renal echo patterns are nonspecific. The associated clinical and laboratory features often provide confirmatory evidence to make the correct diagnosis.

An abdominal x-ray film is usually normal but may show calcified organized intrarenal thrombi, which usually have a lacelike pattern corresponding to the renal venous tree (Brill et al., 1977). An IVP is nearly always abnormal, with delayed opacification and renomegaly. Often there is nonvisualization of the involved kidney. In the newborn, a more effective method of assessing renal function is the DTPA scan (Nielander et al., 1983). Computed tomography or inferior vena cavography infrequently may be necessary to determine the extent of the thrombus.

Management

Because of the relative infrequency of cases of RVT, there is no general consensus as to optimal management. In the past, surgery often has been recommended, with either thrombectomy or nephrectomy performed. However, experience has demonstrated that operative management rarely is necessary on an emergency basis. Initial therapy is directed at correction of the fluid and electrolyte abnormalities and prevention of propagation of the venous thrombus. In the presence of acute renal failure, peritoneal dialysis may be necessary.

Careful attention must be paid to correcting dehydration and electrolyte abnormalities and to restoring acid-base balance. In addition, underlying conditions, such as cardiac disease, must be treated.

The extent of the venous thrombus must be assessed. If the ultrasound demonstrates unilateral involvement, no therapy may be necessary. A baseline renal scan should be obtained to assess function of the involved kidney, and CT may be used to provide a baseline for the extent of venous involvement (Greene et al., 1982). With bilateral RVT, the prognosis is much more ominous, particularly if the thrombus involves the vena cava as well (Gonzalez et al., 1982).

Definitive therapeutic options include prevention of propagation of the thrombus, thrombolysis, and formal thrombectomy. Systemic heparinization may be used to prevent thrombus propagation, although the risk of it occurring with restoration of fluid and electrolyte balance seems low. There is no consensus regarding the efficacy of heparin therapy for unilateral RVT (Lloyd, 1986).

The development of thrombolytic agents, such as urokinase (Gonzalez et al., 1982) and streptokinase (Burrow et al., 1984), provided the physician with a more definitive way of stimulating resolution of the thrombus, but they should be reserved for bilateral RVT. Whether to perform thrombectomy is controversial. With vena caval thrombosis, the vena cava may remain permanently occluded, but collateral venous channels generally develop and provide satisfactory drainage.

With improvement in the management of this condition, the overall survival rate has increased dramatically and has been reported to be 83% (Lloyd, 1986). Most deaths are related to the underlying disease, not renal infarction. Long-term sequelae include (1) a nonfunctioning, completely fibrosed, shrunken kidney; (2) a partially fibrosed kidney with impaired function; (3) renovascular hypertension; (4) nephrotic syndrome; (5) chronic renal infection; and (6) chronic renal tubular dysfunction (Stark and Geiger, 1973). Frequently, the prognosis may be inferred based on the DTPA scan performed during acute stages of the disease (Rasoulpour and McLean, 1980).

In unilateral RVT, the most serious complication is hypertension, which usually results from an atrophic kidney. In such cases, renin-mediated hypertension is present, and nephrectomy is curative (Smith et al., 1979). Jobin and co-workers (1982) reported that five of six patients followed 21 months to 12 years following neonatal RVT were hypertensive. However, only three had an atrophic kidney. Furthermore, not all patients with small scarred kidneys following RVT developed hypertension. If significant return of renal function is going to occur, visualization on the renal scan or IVP may be expected within 4 to 6 weeks (Belman, 1985). In some small kidneys labeled as "con-

TABLE 44-14

Major Causes of Renal Failure in the Neonate

Prerenal	Intrinsic	Postrenal
Hypotension secondary to:	Congenital anomalies	Posterior urethral valves
Sepsis	Cystic dysplasia	Anterior urethral valve
Maternal antepartum hemorrhage	Hypoplasia	Prune-belly syndrome
Twin-to-twin hemorrhage	Agenesis	Urethral atresia
Intrinsic neonatal hemorrhage	Polycystic kidney disease	Ectopic ureterocele
Cardiac surgery	Inflammatory	Ureteropelvic or ureterovesical obstruction
Congestive heart failure	Congenital syphilis or toxoplasmosis	Extrinsic tumor compressing bladder outlet
Asphyxia neonatorum	Pyelonephritis	
Dehydration	Metabolic	
? Intermittent positive pressure breathing	Oxalosis	
? Continuous positive airway pressure	Vascular	
	Renal vein thrombosis	
	Renal artery thrombosis	
	Hemolytic-uremic syndrome	
	Disseminated intravascular coagulation	
	Cortical necrosis	
	Perinatal asphyxia	
	Sepsis	
	Shock	
	Acute tubular necrosis	
	Nephrotoxins	
	Maternal use of nonsteroidal	
	antiinflammatory medication	
	Dehydration	
	Transient renal dysfunction	

genitally hypoplastic," unrecognized RVT is the probable underlying cause.

Renal Failure

With the development of intensive medical support for premature neonates, acute renal failure probably is occurring with increasing frequency. Acute renal failure should be suspected in any infant who has a sustained decrease in urine output to less than 1 ml/kg/hr, a persistent serum creatinine level greater than 1 mg/dl (in newborns beyond 34 weeks' gestation), or hematuria. Although renal failure may be associated with normal or even increased production of urine, most neonates with acute renal failure have oliguria or anuria.

Since 92% of term newborns pass urine within 24 hours of birth, and 99.4% within 48 hours (Sherry and Kramer, 1955), renal failure should be suspected in any infant who fails to void within 48 hours of birth.

In the neonate, as in the older child and adult, renal failure is characterized as prerenal, renal, or postrenal (Table 44-14). In prerenal and in many patients with intrinsic renal failure, the kidneys are basically normal, although the renal insult may result in permanent impairment of function (Wassner, 1985). In contrast, many patients with postrenal failure have irreversible renal damage, often from congenital abnormalities.

Renal development in the fetus whose mother is azotemic progresses normally. Often these infants are born prematurely. Interestingly, renal size at birth in these cases has been reported to be at the upper limits of normal (Brem et al., 1988), raising the possibility that compensatory growth might be occurring in utero.

Prerenal Failure

The most common cause of oliguria or anuria in the neonate is prerenal failure, secondary to underperfused kidneys that are intrinsically normal (Anand, 1982; Engle, 1986). In a review of 314 admissions to a neonatal intensive care unit, 72 infants were thought to have acute renal failure. Of these, 52 (72%) responded to a trial of volume expansion with an immediate and sustained increase in urine output and fall in creatinine clearance. Thus, they were classified as having prerenal failure (Norman and Asadi, 1979).

There are numerous causes of diminished renal perfusion that may cause renal failure in the neonate (see Table 44-14). Hypotension may result from sepsis, fetal-maternal hemorrhage, or abdominal bleeding, or may occur following surgical bleeding. Furthermore, renal blood flow may be compromised in patients with congestive heart failure or in those with a patent ductus arteriosus. In these patients, total blood volume may be normal or increased. Although continuous positive airway pressure or intermittent positive pressure breathing may diminish renal perfusion (Fewell and Norton, 1980; Furzan et al., 1981; Moore et al., 1974),

GFR usually is not affected if other predisposing factors are absent (Heijden et al., 1988). Finally, perinatal asphyxia or hypoxemia, which occurs in severe idiopathic RDS or secondary to complicated or traumatic deliveries, also may cause renal failure (Dauber et al., 1976; Torrado et al., 1974). The pathogenesis of hypoxemia-induced renal impairment is not entirely understood, but hypoxemia results in a diminished GFR and effective renal plasma flow (Guignard et al., 1976). It has been suggested that the low urinary water excretion may be secondary to a high serum concentration of ADH, because inappropriate ADH is a frequent complication of perinatal asphyxia (Guignard, 1982). However, newborn renal tubules are not known to be sensitive to ADH. Pathologic studies in perinatal hypoxia have not revealed any significant renal lesions. Nevertheless, the prognosis for these infants is variable, depending on the severity and duration of hypoxia. When it is severe, the prerenal failure may result in cortical necrosis.

Intrinsic Renal Failure

Intrinsic renal failure implies that inadequate kidney function is secondary to inherent kidney damage. All of the conditions that cause prerenal failure may result in intrinsic renal damage if the insult is severe.

A small proportion of these infants may have renal failure secondary to congenital renal anomalies. In most of these patients, the diagnosis can be made rapidly from a history of oligohydramnios, features of Potter's syndrome, or both.

Vascular complications are an important cause of neonatal renal failure. Renal vein thrombosis and renal artery thrombosis are covered elsewhere in this chapter. Disseminated intravascular coagulation may result from sepsis or necrotizing enterocolitis.

Hemolytic-uremic syndrome is characterized by a triad of microangiopathic hemolytic anemia, thrombocytopenia, and renal failure. Associated findings include fever and neurologic involvement. The disease predominantly affects infants and young children. A variety of agents has been implicated in its pathogenesis, including viruses and bacteria affecting erythrocytes, platelets, vascular endothelium, or the coagulation system (Levin and Barratt, 1984). Histologically, severe types of renal pathology are seen, although thrombotic microangiopathy involving the glomeruli is the most common pattern. The disease may occur in (1) a sporadic form with no seasonal variation in incidence and without a clear prodromal illness or respiratory symptoms or (2) in an epidemic form that usually occurs during the summer months and is associated with explosive diarrhea. The sporadic form carries a poor prognosis for ultimate renal function, whereas in the epidemic form, renal function usually is satisfactory ultimately (Trompeter et al.,

1983). Cortical necrosis occurs following renal insult, and is usually related to sepsis, hypoxia, or hypotension. Cortical necrosis represents an irreversible renal insult. One of the reasons that the newborn may be somewhat more susceptible to cortical necrosis is that blood flow in the neonatal kidney is directed more toward the juxtamedullary nephrons (Spitzer and Brandis, 1974).

Acute tubular necrosis (ATN) may result from the same insults as cortical necrosis but only if the insult is less severe. Often it is secondary to nephrotoxic medication. For example, aminoglycosides are potent nephrotoxic agents that have been studied much more in adults than in newborns. Since the GFR in the newborn is low, it is important to measure peak and trough drug levels when these agents are used. Although the blood flow distribution in the newborn kidney, which favors the juxtamedullary nephrons, might make aminoglycoside nephrotoxicity less common in the neonate (Cowan et al., 1980), toxicity has been demonstrated. Indomethacin, a prostaglandin synthesis inhibitor, is used in the pharmacologic closure of the ductus arteriosus in premature infants. Its major toxicity is renal, and Vert and associates (1980) reported transient oliguria in 16 of 18 infants treated with indomethacin. The toxic effect of indomethacin appears to be diminished considerably by the administration of concomitant furosemide (Yeh et al., 1982). Nonsteroidal antiinflammatory agents, such as indomethacin, also have been administered to diminish amniotic fluid volumes in women with polyhydramnios, presumably by diminishing fetal urine output. In a recent report, three premature infants with prenatal exposure to indomethacin developed renal failure, which was fatal in one case (Simeoni et al., 1989). Other agents that have been associated with oliguric renal failure include tolazoline, an α-sympatholytic agent used as a pulmonary vasodilator and angiotensin converting enzyme inhibitors (Cunniff et al., 1990; Guignard, 1982; Meeks and Sims, 1988).

Hypertonic angiographic contrast agents have been reported to cause RVT, medullary necrosis, ischemia, and renal insufficiency in the newborn and should be used carefully and only after adequate hydration of the infant (Gilbert et al., 1970).

Another recently described entity is transient oliguric renal failure with enlarged kidneys and echogenic medullary pyramids (Hijazi et al., 1988). In these patients, there was no apparent cause and all eventually had a normal serum creatinine; none required dialysis.

Postrenal Failure

There is a discussion of these entities elsewhere in this chapter, as well as other chapters in the text. In general, oligohydramnios is present if the obstruction is severe enough to cause renal failure in the newborn. Whether relief of obstruction may allow satisfactory renal function to occur depends on a number of factors, including the severity and duration of obstruction.

Pathophysiology

Although renovascular constriction and decrease in blood flow to nephrons is important in the development of renal failure, other factors may play a role as well. Siegel (1983) and co-workers (1984) have speculated that a disturbance of the adenine nucleotide system of the kidney may be important in the initiation and persistence of renal failure. Following tissue ischemia, there is cessation of cellular respiration and oxidative phosphorylation with depletion of adenosine triphosphate (ATP), adenosine diphosphate (ADP), and adenosine monophosphate (AMP) (Collins et al., 1977). As cellular energy production diminishes below a critical level, cell injury and death may occur. Experimentally, ATP–magnesium chloride has been used to preserve renal function following prolonged renal ischemia (Gaudio et al., 1982).

Diagnosis

The most important sign of acute renal failure in the neonate is oliguria, with a urine output of less than 1 ml/kg/hr. Measurement of urine output in premature infants may be inaccurate while they are in an incubator or isolette, because significant evaporation occurs within 15 minutes (Cooke et al., 1989). In infants, the newer highly absorbent diapers that contain a gel-based absorbent also may absorb ambient moisture, spuriously elevating recorded urine output.

Often, the history and physical examination provide important clues to the diagnosis. For example, as already discussed, RDS hypoxia, shock, congestive heart failure, and sepsis, as well as dehydration, may cause renal failure. Enlarged kidneys may be secondary to RVT, hydronephrosis, infantile polycystic kidney disease, or multicystic kidneys. Urinary ascites may be secondary to posterior urethral valves. The presence of edema usually indicates volume overload. In most of these conditions, treatment of the underlying condition will allow resolution of satisfactory renal function. However, until renal function does resolve, careful monitoring of electrolytes and volume status must be performed.

If the etiology of renal failure is not readily apparent from the initial clinical evaluation, a battery of studies is in order, including complete blood cell count with RBC morphology and platelet count; prothrombin time; partial thromboplastin time; serum electrolyte, BUN, creatinine, uric acid, calcium, phosphorus, glucose, total protein, and albumin concentrations; blood pH, oxygen (Po_2) and carbon dioxide (Pco_2) partial

TABLE 44-15

Diagnostic Indices in Neonatal Acute Renal Failure

	Prerenal	Intrinsic
Urine osmolality (mOsm/kg H_2O)	>400	<400
Urinalysis	Normal	>5 RBCs/HPF
Urine sodium (mEq/L)	31 ± 19	63 ± 35
Urinary (U)/plasma creatinine (P_{Cr})	29 ± 16	10 ± 4
Fe_{Na}%	<2.5 (x = 0.9)	>2.5 (x = 4.2)
RFI	<3.0 (x = 1.3)	>3.0 (x = 11.6)

Modified from Mathew OP, Jones AS, James E, et al: *Pediatrics* 1980; 65:57. HPF = high-power field: Fe_{Na}% = fractional sodium excretion; RFI = renal failure index [(U_{Na}/U_{Cr}) × P_{Cr}].

pressures, urinalysis; urine culture; urinary sodium concentration, creatinine clearance; osmolality; electrocardiogram (ECG); chest x-ray film; and renal ultrasound.

Postrenal causes of acute renal failure are apparent from the ultrasound examination. Using the studies shown in Table 44-15, Mathew and co-workers (1980) found that the fractional excretion of sodium and the renal failure index were of greatest value in distinguishing prerenal from intrinsic renal failure. Practically speaking, once volume overload and urinary obstructive causes are excluded, a fluid challenge may be given. In general, 20 ml/kg of normal saline or Ringer's lactate may be administered IV over 1 to 2 hours. If oliguria persists, furosemide in a dosage of 1 mg/kg of body weight is administered. If there is still no response, the dose of furosemide should be increased to 2 mg/kg. If no further increase of urine output is observed during the following hour, intrinsic renal failure should be suspected and fluid administration reduced. Although furosemide may protect the kidney during recovery from renal ischemia, after intrinsic renal failure has developed, repeated doses of furosemide may cause ototoxicity.

Management

After the cause of renal failure is determined, attention must be directed to the volume status and electrolytes of the infant while the underlying condition resolves.

Since acute renal failure is nearly always oliguric, fluid intake must be monitored carefully. Usually it is advisable to place a 5 F or 8 F pediatric feeding tube into the bladder to monitor urine output. Fluid intake should be restricted to insensible water loss plus other nonrenal losses, such as gastrointestinal. If the infant is normovolemic, urine losses should be measured and replaced with an equal volume each hour. In the presence of volume overload, the desired amount of weight loss should be subtracted from the total replacement fluids. In the newborn, daily insensible water loss is

40 ml/kg/24 hr, although it may be higher in low-birth-weight infants (Rahman et al., 1981). Insensible water loss is increased if the infant is under a radiant warmer or is febrile and is decreased if the neonate is on a respirator. Insensible water loss should be replaced as electrolyte-free water in a 10% dextrose solution. Urinary losses should be replaced with a solution containing the same concentration of sodium as is present in the urine. The neonate should be weighed at least every 12 hours to monitor fluid balance. A daily loss of 0.5% to 1.0% of body weight is to be expected (Rahman et al., 1981).

Hyponatremia may result from fluid overload with dilution of extracellular sodium. If the infant is asymptomatic, fluid and sodium restriction is adequate. If the infant is symptomatic or the sodium concentration is less than 120 mEq/L, 3% saline should be administered in a dose of 6 mL/kg over 1 to 2 hours (Engle, 1986), which should increase the serum sodium concentration by 5 mEq/L.

Hypertension is usually secondary to fluid overload and may be controlled by fluid restriction. If the blood pressure is above 120/80 mm Hg, hydralazine in a dose of 0.2 to 0.5 mg/kg intramuscularly or IV every 4 to 8 hours may be used. For extreme elevations in blood pressure, diazoxide (2 to 3 mg/kg IV) or sodium nitroprusside (0.5 μg/kg/min) may be used (Engle, 1986). Persistent hypertension requires investigation, because renal artery thrombosis is likely.

Hyperkalemia may be severe in the presence of acute renal failure and can be fatal if untreated. Accordingly, the potassium level should be monitored frequently and promptly treated if significantly elevated. However, before treatment, one must check to be certain that the specimen was not hemolyzed and that it was not drawn through a catheter containing a potassium-containing solution. If the potassium concentration is 7 mEq/L or less, it may be managed with cessation of potassium intake and administration of sodium polystyrene sulfonate (Kayexalate), which exchanges 1 mEq of potassium for 2 to 3 mEq of sodium (Rahman et al., 1981). Sodium polystyrene sulfonate, 1 g/kg body weight is mixed with 10% sorbitol or 10% dextrose in water (1 g/4 ml) and given rectally as a retention enema. It should be retained for 3 to 4 hours to have maximal effect. This dose of sodium polystyrene sulfonate should reduce serum potassium approximately by 1 mEq/L. Repeated doses of sodium polystyrene sulfonate may cause hypernatremia. If the serum potassium is greater than 7 mEq/L or ECG changes are present, more aggressive therapy is necessary. If only peaked T waves on the ECG are present, sodium bicarbonate, 2 mEq/kg IV, and sodium polystyrene sulfonate enemas may be used. If widening of the QRS complex is seen on ECG, 0.5 ml of 10% calcium gluconate should be given slowly IV, with constant ECG monitoring. It should be followed by sodium bicarbonate, 2 to 3 mEq/kg. The duration of effect of these agents is short, and dialysis should be instituted (Rahman et al., 1981). Another effective treatment is glucose, 2 g/kg, (administered as 25% dextrose) plus insulin, 0.5 unit/kg (Engle, 1986).

Metabolic acidosis usually is present in acute renal failure and may be managed with sodium bicarbonate, 1 to 3 mEq IV, to maintain the serum pH between 7.25 and 7.35.

Serum phosphorus and calcium may be abnormal in renal failure. The serum phosphorus concentration may be maintained within normal range by administering aluminum hydroxide, 20 mg/kg/day, three times daily orally to maintain a serum phosphorus level between 5 and 6 mg/dl. If hypocalcemia develops, 500 mg/day of calcium gluconate or carbonate should be started once the phosphorus concentration is normal and the gastrointestinal system allows normal intake. Intestinal absorption of calcium may be enhanced by using 0.1 to 0.4 mg/day of dihydrotachysterol (Rahman et al., 1981).

The nutritional status of infants with renal failure is important, because improved nutrition may diminish the metabolic complications of renal failure (Abel, 1983; Laouari and Kleinknecht, 1985). If the infant is able to tolerate feedings, breast milk is optimal, although PM 60/40 is satisfactory. If the infant is unable to tolerate enteral feedings, peripheral or central hyperalimentation should be used (Abel, 1983; Abitbol and Holliday, 1976).

Indications for dialysis include severe fluid overload, hyperkalemia, electrolyte abnormalities that cannot be corrected medically, or severe CNS depression secondary to uremia (Rahman et al., 1981). Peritoneal dialysis generally is performed, although hemodialysis has been reported (Sadowski et al., 1994).

Prognosis

The prognosis of infants with acute renal failure depends largely on the etiology. Chevalier and associates (1984) reviewed 16 neonates with acute renal failure and determined significant prognostic factors. Nine had renal failure secondary to perinatal asphyxia, and three were secondary to congenital heart disease. Half were oliguric. All of the nonoliguric infants survived, whereas half of the oliguric patients died, usually from renal failure. Of the eight oliguric patients, the three that were anuric 3 days or less and had demonstrable renal perfusion by renal scan survived. In contrast, all four infants who had anuria 4 days or longer and had no perfusion on renal scan died. Thus, anuria lasting 4 days or more and lack of visualization by renal scan are poor prognostic signs.

Another adverse prognostic sign is significant prematurity. For example, Meeks and Sims (1988) reported 30 neonates with a mean gestational age of 31 weeks; mortality was 90%.

Continuation of peritoneal dialysis in infants with renal failure is controversial. Wassner (1985) recommends that a renal biopsy be performed after 1 month. Stopping dialysis should be considered if it is determined that irreversible renal damage has occurred. The mortality rate for neonates requiring peritoneal dialysis is 60% (Matthews et al., 1990).

An alternative to dialysis in the newborn may be renal transplantation. With further experience in renal transplantation in the infant (Sheldon et al., 1985), renal transplantation in this age group may be efficacious.

Urinary Tract Infection

In the newborn, UTI often presents with symptoms and signs of sepsis, including fever (50%), weight loss (75%), and cyanosis (40%) (Winberg, 1986). Other findings include a distended abdomen, jaundice, and symptoms referable to the CNS, such as irritability and seizures. Thus, if a newborn is not growing satisfactorily and seems ill, a UTI should be suspected. In a series of infants less than 3 months of age with fever, 11% were secondary to UTI (Krober et al., 1985). In 75% of newborns, *Escherichia coli* is the etiologic agent, with *Klebsiella* accounting for approximately 10% (Ginsburg and McCracken, 1982).

In contrast to older age groups, between 70% and 80% of newborns with a UTI are boys (Ginsburg and McCracken, 1982). Beyond the neonatal period, the incidence of UTI in males drops considerably. The vast majority of newborn boys with symptomatic UTIs who do not have obstructive abnormalities are uncircumcised (Ginsburg and McCracken, 1982; Wiswell and Hachey, 1993; Wiswell et al., 1985). Pathogenic bacterial organisms colonize the newborn prepuce (Fussell et al., 1988), conferring a greater risk of UTI in uncircumcised boys until 3 to 6 months of age, when the foreskin usually begins to retract. In females, the highest incidence of UTI also is in the newborn period.

Diagnosis

The method of obtaining the urine specimen must be assessed before one decides that an infant has a UTI. For example, if a plastic bag is used to obtain the specimen, the genitalia must be washed thoroughly, the bag must be removed within a few minutes of voiding, and the urine either must be refrigerated or cultured immediately. Urine cultures obtained with a plastic bag are most informative if the culture is negative. If the culture from the plastic bag is a single organism with a colony count greater than 100,000/ ml and the infant is symptomatic, a UTI may be presumed, as long as the specimen was obtained by the previous guidelines. The presence of significant pyuria also provides confirmation that the neonate has a UTI.

On the other hand, in asymptomatic infants or uncircumcised boys, if the culture grows a mixed group of organisms or the colony count is less than 100,000/ ml, the urine specimen should be obtained in another manner. A catheterized specimen may be obtained by sterilely passing a 5 F or 8 F pediatric feeding tube into the bladder. If a urethral abnormality or preputial contamination is suspected, or if one has difficulty identifying the infant female urethra, a suprapubic aspirate (SPA) should be done (Fig. 44-31). Before an SPA is performed, the bladder should be palpable. In the newborn the bladder is an abdominal organ, and it is relatively easy to obtain a suitable specimen to culture. An SPA should not be attempted if the bladder is not palpable, because complications may result. The procedure is performed after cleaning the suprapubic area with an antiseptic solution. A 22-gauge needle then is inserted periappendicular to the lower abdominal wall in the midline one finger breadth above the pubic symphysis. A local anesthetic generally is not necessary.

Management

Since most neonates with a UTI have evidence of sepsis, and broad-spectrum parenteral antibiotics are necessary, these children should be hospitalized. Generally, IV gentamicin and ampicillin are given until the culture and sensitivities are available. Fever and vomiting may increase the infant's fluid requirements substantially, and urine output must be monitored closely. IV antibiotics should be continued until the infant has been afebrile for 48 hours, at which time a suitable oral agent may be used. However, if the child has a positive blood culture as well, parenteral antibiotics may need to be given for a longer period of time. Since the newborn's renal function is low, peak and trough aminoglycoside levels must be obtained on a regular basis.

Two antimicrobial agents that are used commonly in older children and adults should not be used in the newborn. Trimethoprim-sulfamethoxazole is a combination medication that interferes with bacterial folic acid metabolism and also in the newborn may interfere with bilirubin excretion and cause jaundice. Nitrofurantoin interferes with the bacterial Krebs' cycle but is contraindicated in the newborn because of potential hepatotoxicity and a risk of hemolytic anemia.

If a newborn has a symptomatic UTI, he or she should continue to be given oral antibiotics until a radiographic evaluation has been obtained. This evaluation should include a VCUG to study the lower urinary tract and either a renal ultrasound, IVP, or renal scan, depending on the age and findings of the

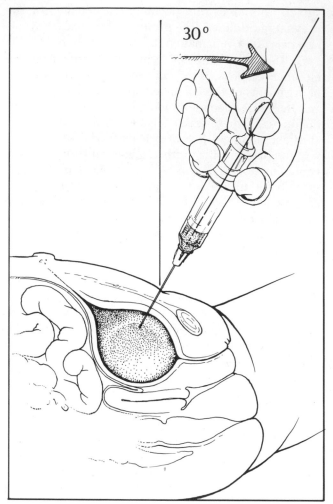

FIG. 44-31
Suprapubic aspiration for collection of bladder urine with a full bladder. The needle is inserted 2 cm cephalad to the pubic symphysis perpendicular to the axis of the child.

VCUG. The evaluation should be performed while the child is still in the hospital. An ultrasound does not provide sufficient visual evidence of the presence or absence of reflux (Zerin et al., 1993).

A renal ultrasound should be used to study the upper urinary tracts and the bladder. If either the ultrasound or VCUG is abnormal, a renal scan should be obtained. The specific type of scan to order depends on whether reflux, hydronephrosis, a duplex collecting system, or posterior urethral valves is identified (Taylor and Nally, 1995).

In a study of 100 patients less than 8 months of age with a UTI, 45% of the girls and 7% of the boys had a urinary tract abnormality. The most common finding was vesicoureteral reflux (Ginsburg and McCracken, 1982). In another study of newborns with UTIs, nearly half demonstrated varying degrees of reflux (Bergstrom et al., 1972). Thus, radiographic evaluation of these infants is important.

Even if reflux or an obstructive anomaly is not found, the child clearly is at risk for developing pyelonephritis. Since the kidneys are most likely to develop scarring secondary to reflux and infection during the first 2 years of life, a course of antimicrobial prophylaxis with nitrofurantoin or Trimethoprim-sulfamethoxazole should be used until the child is at least 1 year old. In addition, a follow up IVP or DMSA scan should be performed at 1 year of age to detect renal scarring.

Adrenal Hemorrhage

Because of its large size and hypervascularity in the newborn, the adrenal gland is susceptible to spontaneous hemorrhage or to trauma with subsequent hemorrhage. Small unilateral or bilateral adrenal hemorrhage is a common finding at postmortem examination of infants, but clinically significant neonatal adrenal hemorrhage is much less common. However, it is a condition that must be considered in the differential diagnosis of neonatal abdominal masses. In the past, it carried a high mortality rate (Black and Williams, 1973).

The pathogenesis of adrenal hemorrhage is not completely understood, but the relatively large size of the newborn adrenal glands, their hyperemia, and any condition that causes venous congestion or stasis within the adrenal tend to make the adrenal gland more susceptible to trauma (Smith and Middleton, 1979). Traumatic delivery seems to be an important factor (Smith and Middleton, 1979), but asphyxia, sepsis, hemorrhagic disorders, and hypoprothrombinemia also may be predisposing conditions (Khuri et al., 1980). Adrenal hemorrhage is reported to occur more commonly on the right side (Black and Williams, 1973), probably because venous engorgement caused by temporary vena caval occlusion or compression is dampened by the renal vein on the left side, whereas the right adrenal vein drains directly into the vena cava. In approximately 10% of patients, the condition is bilateral.

Diagnosis

A triad of findings is usually present with adrenal hemorrhage: (1) flank mass (more than 85%), (2) jaundice (more than 80%), and (3) mild anemia (approximately 50%) (Khuri et al., 1980; Smith and Middleton, 1979).

Jaundice is secondary to reabsorption of blood from the retroperitoneum and depends on the degree of hemorrhage and rapidity of reabsorption. Most clinically significant cases become apparent by the time the patient is 1 week of age.

As in the diagnosis of many adrenal masses, ultrasound is an extremely useful modality (Fig. 44-32). In general, a well defined–echo free area superior to an

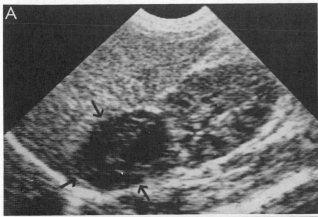

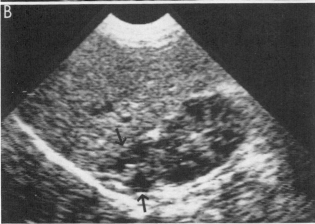

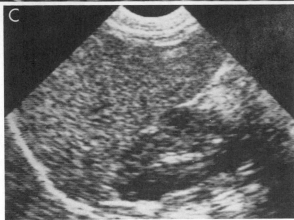

FIG. 44-32
Patient at 17 days of age, ultrasound of adrenal hemorrhage. **A,** 4.0- × 3.7- × 2.7-cm complex mass in region of right adrenal gland. Echolucent areas suggest liquefaction. **B,** Patient at 1 month of age. The mass has diminished in size, measuring 2.0 × 1.5 cm. **C,** Patient at 2 months of age. Adrenal gland is normal. Adrenal hemorrhage has resolved completely.

inferiorly displaced kidney is identified. In some cases, it may contain internal echoes, depending on the state of liquefaction within the adrenal gland. If clots and necrotic tissue are present in the hemorrhagic area, a mixed pattern is encountered. Following complete liquefaction, the mass becomes completely echo-free (Alanen and Kormano, 1984; Pery et al., 1981). Ultrasound is the best method to use to follow these infants, because it demonstrates the progressive decrease in size and resolution of the hemorrhagic area, as well as subsequent calcification (Pery et al., 1981).

In addition to serial hematocrits, serum bilirubin, and abdominal ultrasound, other studies should be performed. Measurement of the 24-hour urinary excretion of vanillylmandelic acid, homovanillic acid, and catecholamines is important because an increase in these substances, particularly vanillylmandelic acid, is virtually diagnostic of neuroblastoma. In addition, a CT scan may demonstrate the lesion, confirm that it is not a neoplasm and demonstrate that the ipsilateral kidney is functioning. Simultaneous renal vein thrombosis and idiopathic adrenal hemorrhage have a recognized association (Lebowitz and Belman, 1983) and probably explain reports of nonvisualization of the kidney on IVP in a small proportion of infants with adrenal hemorrhage (Khuri et al., 1980). An IVP is not necessary if a renal scan or CT scan is performed.

Management

In most patients, adrenal hemorrhage is a self-limited condition, particularly when the hematoma remains intracapsular. Rarely, with extensive hemorrhage, capsular rupture with retroperitoneal bleeding may occur. As discussed, ultrasonography is useful in following resolution of the hematoma. In addition, serial hematocrit and serum bilirubin levels are important. The adrenal typically calcifies following adrenal hemorrhage. Calcification may occur as early as 7 days and usually may be visualized radiographically about 2 weeks after the hemorrhage (Smith and Middleton, 1979). Initially, a thin rim of calcification is seen surrounding the mass. As reabsorption of the hematoma occurs, the calcified area condenses and takes the shape of the adrenal gland. In contrast, the calcification that frequently occurs in neuroblastoma typically is stippled throughout the mass.

Adrenal Abscess

An unusual complication of adrenal hemorrhage is adrenal abscess. Theories regarding the etiology of adrenal abscess have included (1) hematogenous bacterial seeding of a normal adrenal gland with subsequent abscess formation and (2) bacterial seeding of neonatal adrenal hemorrhage with formation of an abscess (Gibbons et al., 1978). In a review of reported cases of neonatal adrenal abscess, Atkinson and coworkers (1985) found that maternal infection at the time of delivery and forceps or breech delivery were common. Clinical findings included palpable mass, fever, leukocytosis, and jaundice. Most cases were diagnosed when the patient was between 1 and 4 weeks of age.

Ultrasound has been extremely useful in demonstrating the character and extent of the abscess. The mass is noted to be a suprarenal fluid-filled mass, and frequently layered debris is noted with changes in position. An IVP demonstrates an intense circumferential opacification of the margin of the abscess cavity related to the increased vascularity in the wall (Carty and Stanley, 1973; Gibbons et al., 1978). The differential diagnosis includes an obstructed upper pole duplication anomaly, adrenal hematoma or pseudocyst, upper pole hydrocalyx, neuroblastoma with hemorrhage and necrosis, and cystic Wilms' tumor (Atkinson et al., 1985). Failure of a suspected adrenal hemorrhage to resolve or evidence of a gradual increase in the size of the mass with evidence of systemic disease should raise suspicion.

Treatment of a neonatal adrenal abscess consists either of excision of the abscess or incision and drainage (Gibbons et al., 1978). Ideally, the diagnosis can be made before the suppurative process extends to adjacent organs; in almost one third of reported cases, the kidney has been removed (Atkinson et al., 1985). With improvements in neonatal sonographic imaging and percutaneous techniques, it is conceivable that needle aspiration under ultrasound guidance with abscess drainage and concomitant IV antibiotic therapy might be sufficient treatment.

Scrotal Mass

In most cases, a scrotal mass that is present at birth represents testicular torsion. Anatomically, testicular torsion in the newborn is extravaginal with twisting of the entire spermatic cord (Fig. 44-33). In contrast, in pubertal boys, testicular torsion is intravaginal. In the perinatal period, the cause of extravaginal torsion is speculated to be loose or absent connections between

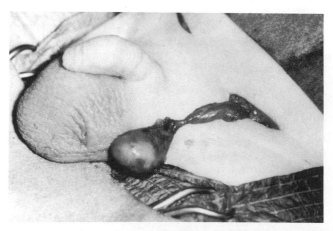

FIG. 44-33
Neonatal extravaginal testicular torsion, left side. Inguinal approach is preferable.

the testicular tunics and the scrotal wall. However, we are aware of a case of neonatal torsion that presented as a painless unilaterally enlarged firm testis at 1 week of age that was salvaged by detorsion.

In most neonates with testicular torsion, the event occurs in utero. Consequently, the mass is hard, painless, and does not transilluminate. The scrotal skin may be discolored and edematous.

Other diagnoses to consider include scrotal hematoma, incarcerated inguinal hernia, testis tumor (Levy et al., 1994), idiopathic testicular infarction, meconium peritonitis, and testicular strangulation secondary to an inguinal hernia. If the scrotal swelling transilluminates, it usually represents either a hydrocele or, less commonly, an inguinal hernia. Given these considerations, the diagnosis of testicular torsion in the newborn usually is straightforward. Scrotal ultrasound has demonstrated an inhomogeneously hypoechoic testis surrounded by a slightly echogenic rim (Zerin et al., 1990). Color Doppler sonography has not yielded higher diagnostic accuracy.

Whether to perform surgical exploration is controversial. In older boys with intravaginal testicular torsion, there is clearly a risk that the contralateral testis may undergo torsion as well. However, the long-term risk for contralateral intravaginal torsion seems low. In a survey of 67 pediatric surgeons and urologists in Great Britain, six cases of torsion of a solitary testis were identified. Overall, 89% sometimes or never performed a scrotal orchiopexy for a solitary testis (Mishriki et al., 1992). The newborn is at risk for developing testicular torsion until 4 to 8 weeks beyond term (Burge, 1987). However, Feins (1983) and LaQuaglia and associates (1987) reported on a 2 ½-month old boy with a large acute hydrocele secondary to torsion of the spermatic cord. On the contralateral side was a small fibrotic calcified testis, which presumably resulted from in utero torsion, and apparently was unrecognized at birth. Kay and co-workers (1980) reported on a newborn with testicular torsion diagnosed when he was 22 hours old. The contralateral testis apparently was small and nonviable secondary to previous intrauterine torsion. Bilateral testicular torsion has been reported to occur synchronous at 24 hours of age (Jerkins et al., 1983). Neonatal testicular torsion has occurred as late as 2 to 10 weeks of age in term infants and in some patients has been intravaginal rather than extravaginal (Guiney and McGlinchey, 1981; Jerkins et al., 1983).

We are not aware of any cases of testicular torsion discovered at delivery that have been salvaged. Consequently, we do not advocate routine immediate surgical exploration in which unilateral testicular torsion is suspected at the time of delivery. There is little possibility that the involved testis may be saved by an immediate exploration, and there appears to be only a small chance that the opposite testis may twist. In a newborn male with suspected bilateral torsion, prompt exploration is necessary on the remote chance that one of the testes might be salvaged.

Testicular exploration should be performed through an inguinal incision to identify accurately the abnormality and to be certain that an inguinal hernia, patent processus vaginalis, or abdominal abnormality may be recognized and managed appropriately.

The other diagnosis of concern in the newborn is testicular tumor (Levy et al., 1995). However, testicular neoplasms are extremely rare in the neonate and almost always are teratomas, which are benign. Consequently, prompt exploration to rule out a tumor does not seem warranted.

Ascites

Ascites refers to an abnormal accumulation of fluid in the peritoneal cavity. In the neonate, ascites are uncommon and most commonly are secondary to extravasation from the urinary tract, accounting for 25% of cases. Other causes of neonatal ascites include gastrointestinal disorders (bowel obstruction), cardiac disease, liver disease, toxoplasmosis, ovarian cyst, and chylous ascites. In 15% of patients, the diagnosis is unknown (Griscom et al., 1977).

As many as 70% of newborns with urinary ascites have posterior urethral valves (Scott, 1976) (see Fig. 44-29). Other etiologies include urethral atresia, vesicoureteral reflux, neurogenic bladder, ureterocele, ureteral stenosis, and bladder perforation (Griscom et al., 1977; Trulock et al., 1985). In most patients with urinary ascites, the site of extravasation is unknown. When extravasation from a fornix or the renal pelvis occurs, urine may accumulate within the retroperitoneum with subsequent rupture into the peritoneum. In other patients, there may be rupture of the distended pelvis directly into the peritoneal cavity. In cases of bladder perforation, the dome of the bladder ruptures into the peritoneal cavity.

Earlier reviews emphasized the significant mortality associated with urinary ascites, as high as 70% (Griscom et al., 1977; Scott, 1976). More recently, with improved neonatal care, mortality has been considerably lower, approximately 12% (Greenfield et al., 1982).

In some neonates with ascites, the condition may not be evident until 1 or 2 weeks of age. In such patients, poor feeding, vomiting, and progressive abdominal distention are reported.

In most cases, neonates with ascites should be evaluated initially by abdominal ultrasound, which confirms the presence of ascitic fluid and may demonstrate dilation of the upper urinary tracts or a distended, thick-walled bladder in the presence of obstructive uropathy. However, if the kidneys are decompressed because of forniceal rupture, the dilation may be minimal. A VCUG should be performed to determine whether posterior urethral valves are present, to aid in detecting whether the site of extravasation is the bladder, and to detect reflux. A peritoneal tap may be necessary, particularly if severe abdominal distention is present or if respiratory function is compromised. In other cases, it is performed for diagnostic purposes. In patients with urinary ascites, one would expect to find an elevated BUN concentration and creatinine in the ascitic fluid. However, since the ascites equilibrate with serum rapidly, it is not a valid study. Because of their ineffective excretion, serum BUN concentration and creatinine usually are elevated.

Management

Parenteral antibiotics should be instituted. Following stabilization of the infant, adequate urinary diversion should lead to resolution of the ascites, since the reduced pressure on the upper urinary tracts will allow the leak to close. An 8 F pediatric feeding tube placed into the bladder should achieve this. If it does not, cutaneous vesicostomy or possibly even cutaneous pyelostomy may be necessary. Once the child has been stabilized sufficiently, operative ablation of the valves may proceed.

Urinary ascites may be secondary to a problem other than urethral valves. For example, a ruptured bladder is present in 25% of newborns with urinary ascites. Although the most common cause is urethral valves, it also may be secondary to neurogenic bladder (Mann et al., 1974) or iatrogenic during umbilical artery cutdown (Hepworth and Milstein, 1984; Redman et al., 1979). In nearly all patients, it has been discovered within the first day or two of life. Management has consisted of suprapubic cystostomy or cutaneous vesicostomy, with a survival rate of 94% (Trulock et al., 1985).

Ultimately, many have surprisingly normal-appearing upper urinary tracts (Adzick et al., 1985; Greenfield et al., 1982; Parker, 1974). The upper or lower leak from the urinary tract seems to act as a pop-off valve and allows renal development to proceed more normally (Rittenberg et al., 1988).

Related to urinary ascites is the *isolated perirenal urinoma* (Adzick et al., 1985) (Fig. 44-34). In some patients, it is secondary to urethral valves, and in others it is secondary to UPJ obstruction. Interestingly, when the urinoma is contained within Gerota's fascia, the kidney usually is severely dysplastic (Adzick et al., 1985). Presumably, severe obstruction has occurred, and if the leaking urine is contained within Gerota's fascia, there is insufficient decompression of the urinary tract to allow satisfactory renal development. When this condition occurs bilaterally in the

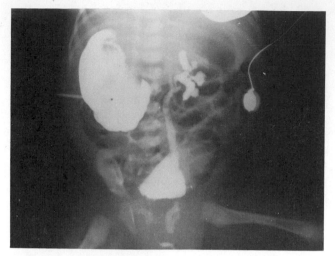

FIG. 44-34
Neonate with right perirenal urinoma secondary to posterior urethral valves. Simultaneous cystogram shows left vesicoureteral reflux.

absence of ascites, the outcome is always fatal (Adzick et al., 1985).

Other Neonatal Conditions of Urologic Conditions

The foregoing discussion has not been exhaustive in describing all urologic conditions that may affect the neonate. However, anomalies not mentioned are covered extensively in other chapters.

Vesicoureteral reflux may be discovered in the newborn in a variety of settings. Prenatal ultrasonography may disclose a variably dilated renal pelvis that is found to be secondary to reflux on postnatal evaluation (Scott, 1987). Approximately half of newborns with a febrile UTI have reflux (Ginsburg and McCracken, 1982). In most cases, these infants may be followed with an annual nuclear cystogram and IV urogram or renal scan, and maintained on prophylactic antimicrobials until the reflux resolves. If the reflux is massive, resulting in a *megaureter*, more careful evaluation is mandatory.

In a child with a megaureter, the condition may be obstructive or nonobstructive and refluxing or nonrefluxing (Elder, 1988). The dilated upper urinary tract may be evaluated with a MAG-3 diuretic renogram to assess whether there is obstruction or diminished renal function. False-negative and false-positive scans may occur; thus, follow-up evaluation should be planned in 3 to 6 months. We have found that the majority of neonates with a primary obstructive megaureter can be managed safely nonoperatively (Keating et al., 1989). However, if the differential renal function in the affected kidney is reduced significantly, tailored ureteral reimplantation should be performed in the first few months of life by a surgeon familiar with operating on the neonatal urinary tract (Green-

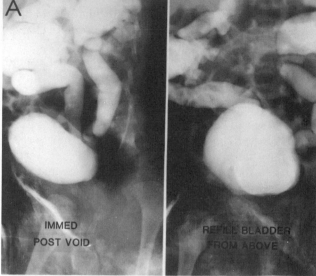

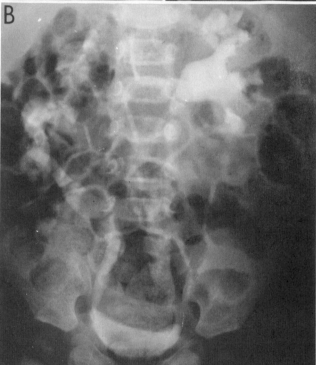

FIG. 44-35
Newborn with bilateral grade V reflux and congenital heart disease. **A,** Voiding cystourethrogram demonstrating severe reflux. The infant was placed on a program of clean intermittent catheterization to decompress the upper urinary tracts during recovery from corrective heart surgery. **B,** Intravenous pyelogram 6 weeks after bilateral transtrigonal ureteral reimplantation. Tapering was not necessary.

field et al., 1993). One must be certain to remove the narrowed distal ureteral segment and part of the redundant ureter. Although Hendren's (1969) technique of extensive ureteral excisional tapering has been popular in the past, more recently, ureteral plication has been demonstrated to be a very reliable method of repair, with a lower incidence of postoperative obstruction and shortened hospitalization (Ehrlich, 1985). Two techniques have been used; ureteral plication (Starr, 1979) and ureteral folding (Ehrlich, 1985; Kalicinsky et al., 1977). The tailoring needs to be performed only up to a few centimeters proximal to the intramural segment. In general, we have stented these tailored ureters for 3 or 4 days.

If bilateral Grade IV to V reflux is present with resultant massive dilatation of the urinary tract, early intervention should be considered. Options include ureteral reimplantation, cutaneous vesicostomy, intermittent catheterization, or a combination of these (Fig. 44-35).

Most of these patients are male and will present with an elevated creatinine, which will trend downward during the first year of life.

A complication of bilateral high-grade reflux is the *megacystis-megaureter* syndrome (Williams, 1954; Burbige et al., 1984) (Fig. 44-36). This syndrome affects primarily boys. Most of the voided urine refluxes into the upper urinary tracts, resulting in a weak urinary stream, a large bladder, and significant residual urine mimicking bladder outlet obstruction. However, the bladder is smooth-walled, and no obstructive component is delineated on VCUG. This pattern of constant recycling of large volumes of refluxing urine has been termed *aberrant micturition* (Hutch, 1966). Ureteral reimplantation with tapering is necessary to correct the condition, although cutaneous vesicostomy is a temporizing procedure that allows the ureters to diminish in caliber, which may facilitate later ureteral reimplantation (see Fig. 44-36). Reduction cystoplasty is not necessary or effective.

The *megacystis-microcolon-intestinal hypoperistalsis syndrome* was described in 1976 (Berdon et al., 1976) and is characterized by abdominal distention, lax abdominal musculature, a huge bladder, incomplete intestinal rotation, bilious vomiting, and diminished or absent intestinal peristalsis. Approximately 80% of patients are female, and nearly 30 cases have been reported (Redman et al., 1984). All patients have microcolon and small bowel dilatation. The etiology of this condition is unknown. Unfortunately, most infants die within 1 or 2 years of life because of an inability to obtain sufficient nutrition through their abnormal gastrointestinal tracts. Vesicoureteral reflux usually is present, but generally is low or moderate in grade. Bladder emptying may be ineffective, and clean intermittent catheterization may be necessary to assure vesical drainage. A nonlethal variant of this syndrome is pseudo-Hirschsprung's disease, in which there is megacystis and colonic dilatation without aganglionosis.

The *prune-belly syndrome* probably represents a transient congenital urethral membrane obstruction at 8 to 10 weeks gestation, resulting i[n] [obstruc]tion of the upper urinary tract. Th[e urethra] canalizes and decompresses the syst[em. The] stigmata of prune-belly syndrome, w[ith a] dilated bladder and upper urinary tract, [bilateral] cryptorchism, and the characteristic wrinkled a[b]domen. Some of these neonates have severe renal dysplasia and associated pulmonary hypoplasia. The prognosis probably depends on how soon the urethra recanalizes.

The newborn with *classic bladder exstrophy* usually is otherwise healthy and has normal renal function. Associated anomalies of other organ systems are infrequent. We believe that primary closure within 48 hours of birth is ideal in nearly all cases, because the bony pelvis usually can be brought together anteriorly without the need for iliac osteotomies because of residual circulating maternal relaxin. Early closure is recommended even if the bladder is small.

In contrast, *cloacal exstrophy* represents the most devastating urologic congenital anomaly. These infants are likely to have anomalous upper urinary tracts and defects in the spine and gastrointestinal tract.

Hypertension is usually related to a vascular abnormality in the neonate (Guignard et al., 1989). In the normal full-term newborn, blood pressure is 72 mm Hg systolic and 47 mm Hg diastolic. The most common etiologies are coarctation of the aorta and *renal artery thrombosis* secondary to umbilical artery catheter complication. In the latter condition, if aggressive antihypertensive management is ineffective, a nephrectomy should be performed.

Micropenis is a small penis that is structurally normal but more than 2.5 SD below the mean in stretched penile length (Aaronson, 1994). In a full-term newborn, the critical length is 2.5 cm. Many of these patients have a cerebral abnormality involving the hypothalamic-pituitary axis. Early evaluation of the etiology followed by testosterone stimulation should be performed. If penile growth does not occur with androgen stimulation, gender reassignment should be considered.

Circumcision   Ethical

In pediatrics, few topics generate as much controversy as whether a newborn male should undergo circumcision, mostly because indications for neonatal circumcision have been obscured by factors, such as cultural prejudices, parental preferences, presumption about medical necessity and health benefits, physicians' biases, and aesthetic choices of the family, physician and society (Ross and Elder, 1991). It remains the most common surgical operation carried out in the United States. Conversely, it is seldom performed in European countries, China, and South America. The National Center for Health Statistics

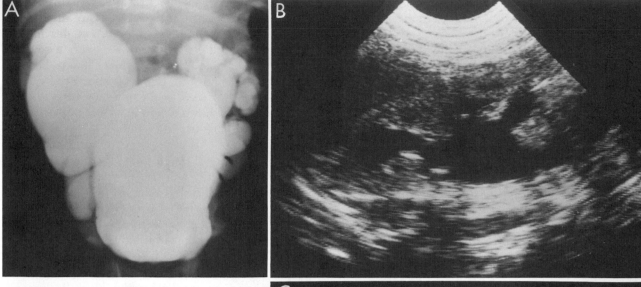

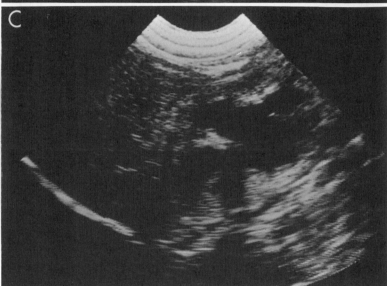

FIG. 44-36
Newborn with distended abdomen and renal insufficiency. **A,** Voiding cystourethrogram shows huge smooth-walled bladder with bilateral grade V reflux, the typical picture of megacystis-megaureter syndrome. **B,** and **C,** Following cutaneous vesicostomy, renal function improved, with serum creatinine clearance dropping to 0.7 mg/dl. Ultrasound at 9 months of age shows nicely decompressed upper urinary tracts. Cortex is quite thin. **B,** Left kidney. **C,** Right kidney.

reports that 61% (or 1,190,000) American boys were circumcised during 1981 (Poland, 1990).

It has been estimated that approximately one sixth of the world's population practices circumcision for religious reasons (Chebel, 1992; Nesbitt et al., 1986). The practice goes back to as early as 2300 B.C. in Egypt and it has been suggested that it may have derived from the practice of mutilating prisoners of war while retaining them capable of laboring as slaves (Burger and Guthrie, 1974). This may have translated to the ritual circumcision imbued with great moral significance that has been carried out in the Jewish and Moslem cultures.

Circumcision as a means of preventing disease was strengthened by the two World Wars and the increased belief in the United States, Canada, and Australia that circumcision provided an additional measure of hygiene (Gellis, 1978). By the 1960s, the indications for neonatal circumcision came under in-

creased scrutiny and two reports by the Task Force of Neonatal Circumcision from the American Academy of Pediatrics (AAP) have tried to define guidelines for the procedure (Schoen et al., 1989; Thompson et al., 1975). In 1975, the conclusion was that routine neonatal circumcision had no valid medical indications. However, in 1989, as several published reports had suggested that uncircumcised infants were at increased risk for urinary tract infection (UTI), the AAP concluded that "newborn circumcision has potential medical advantages, as well as disadvantages and risks." But this report stops short of recommending routine circumcision and there is no general consensus (Devine et al., 1995). The urologist is on occasion called upon to render an opinion or carry out neonatal circumcision and must be cognizant of the facts to enable him to make an objective recommendation which will allow the parents to make an informed decision for a child who is unable to give consent.

More often, the urologist is consulted for an injury sustained after neonatal circumcision.

The complication rate after circumcision ranges between 0.2% and 5% (Gee and Answell, 1976; Kaplan, 1983; Schoen et al., 1989). Immediate complications include pain, hemorrhage, removal of insufficient or excessive penile skin, entrapped penis from scarring of the skin edges over the glans, infection, meatiness, and urinary retention from a tight bandage. Often, early morbidity can be attributed to inexperience by the person performing the procedure (junior house officer). In addition, the megameatal form of hypospadias, the scaphoid variant of megalourethra or torsion of the penis may not be recognized until after the circumcision is performed (Redman, 1988). Late complications include: meatal stenosis, which may require meatoplasty; formation of a synechium, or skin bridge between residual prepuce and glans; chordee; inclusion cyst at the circumcision line; urethrocutaneous fistula; removal of a portion of the glans; and slough of a portion or the entire penis from excessive use of cautery. Such complications must be managed by the urologist with the potential medicolegal implications. The cost of these complications and of the potential lawsuits has not been, to our knowledge, estimated.

In addition to the cost of circumcision is the overall cost of routine circumcision on health care, which currently is being borne mostly by insurance companies and has been estimated to be about $140 million per year (Poland, 1990). An accurate cost benefit analysis of neonatal circumcision is nearly impossible. Several reports have attempted to justify neonatal circumcision by balancing its cost against the risk of penile cancer or UTI in uncircumcised males (Cadman et al., 1984; Warner and Strachin, 1981; Wiswell and Geschke, 1989). Economic issues aside, entrenchment of circumcision in American society remains strong as reflected that even extensive counseling in prepared childbirth classes regarding the risks of circumcision and the 1975 recommendations of the AAP Committee have failed to alter significantly the incidence of circumcision (Herrera et al., 1983; Land and Policastro, 1983). Nevertheless, a debate in the lay press has been ongoing and several anticircumcision groups have developed, including INTACT (Everson, Wash.) (Romberg, 1985) and the Newborn Rights Society (St. Peters, Pa.).

There are several nonreligious justifications supporting neonatal circumcision to assure good hygiene. These include the prevention of UTI, penile cancer, venereal diseases, cervical cancer, and phimosis, as well as lessening the risk of balanoposthitis. Recent reports linking the presence of an intact foreskin and UTIs in the first 6 months of life have been responsible for the resurgence of the sentiment in favor of neonatal circumcision. In 1986, Roberts theorized that circum-

cision prevented colonization of the prepuce by uropathogens, which would then enter the urethra and cause an ascending UTI. Subsequently, epidemiologic studies have shown a ten-fold increase in the incidence of UTIs among uncircumcised male infants with a higher risk of serious sequelae, such as bacteriemia and meningitis (Ginsburg and McCracken, 1982; Herzog, 1989; Wiswell and Geschke, 1989; Wiswell et al., 1985). There was also an increased risk for UTIs in young uncircumcised males (median age 30) in a recent retrospective study by Spaeh and associates (1992). These studies have been criticized because of their retrospective nature. Furthermore, despite findings that, uncircumcised infants harbor uropathogens under the prepuce, (Wiswell et al., 1988), these organisms have not been directly implicated as the cause of UTIs. Nonetheless, circumstantial evidence and demographics show that uncircumcised boys are at increased risk for UTIs but routine neonatal circumcision may in fact only prevent UTIs in only 1% to 2% of all newborn males.

Squamous cell carcinoma of the penis is extremely rare in males circumcised at birth (Schoen, 1991). Penile cancer occurs much more frequently in areas where circumcision is not practiced and poor hygiene is prevalent. For example, in Brazil, the rate of penile cancer is 10 times higher in poor regions as compared to the more developed parts of the country. The incidence of penile cancer in the United States is reported to be between 0 and 2.1 per 100,000, representing less than 1% of all cancers in men (Waterhouse et al., 1982). This incidence is similar to that of Denmark (1.1 per 100,000) and Japan (0.3 per 100,000), countries where neonatal circumcision is not practiced routinely.

An association between cervical cancer and a sex partner who is uncircumcised has been postulated on the basis of a low rate of cervical cancer observed in Jewish women (Herbst, 1987). However, subsequent studies have not been able to corroborate this cause-and-effect relationship. Instead, several other factors have been implicated for cervical cancer, such as age of first intercourse, multiple sexual partners, and age of childbearing (Kessler, 1991). Finally, it has been suggested that the foreskin may serve as a reservoir for sexually transmitted diseases, and, more recently, an association between immunodeficiency virus (HIV) infection and the presence of the prepuce was postulated (Marx, 1989). However, these studies have been disputed and the protective effect of circumcision is unproven (Ross and Elder, 1991).

Since circumcision is so prevalent in the United States, education regarding hygiene of the uncircumcised penis has lapsed, and benign neglect may have contributed to an increased rate of balanoposthitis and phimosis in boys who have not been properly in-

retract their foreskin and wash their penis. understanding of the relationship between prepuce can help illustrate the care of the cised penis. In the newborn, physiologic s of the inner aspect of the prepuce to the glans prevent retraction and serve to protect the glans. Desquamated cells may accumulate and form smegma beads, which are benign. Over the first year or two of life, separation of the glans from the prepuce occurs progressively such that by 1 year of age, 50% of boys can have their foreskin retracted, and by 5 years of age, 90% (Herzog and Alvarez, 1986). It is, therefore, imperative to start teaching boys at 1 to 2 years of age to gently retract their foreskin themselves.

If circumcision is carried out, a careful review of the potential complications should be given to the parents and informed consent obtained. Various instruments and procedures can be used including Gomco clamp, Bronstein or Mogen clamp, and Plastibell (Ross and Elder, 1991). None have a significant advantage over the other, and use of one over the other has been a matter of personal preference. Prior to circumcision, in a neonate, a check of the patient's identification is crucial. Administration of Vitamin K in advance of the procedure and a check for a family history of bleeding diseases may help prevent hemorrhage. Recently, a trend has emerged encouraging the use of local anesthesia for circumcision in the newborn. This trend has been supported by the AAP. Physiologic response and behavioral changes have been demonstrated to decrease with the use of local anesthesia (Benini et al., 1993; Masciello, 1990; Weatherstone et al., 1993). Postsurgical care of the penis involves placement of a nonconstricting Vaseline or xeroform bandage which stays on for 24 hours and subsequent gentle cleansing. Application of Vaseline or any petroleum based ointment prevents sticking of the glans to the remaining preputial skin or to the diaper. Parents must be made aware of the potential for slight bleeding.

UROLOGIC PROBLEMS IN THE NEONATAL INTENSIVE CARE UNIT

Candidiasis

With improvement in the respiratory, nutritional, and antimicrobial management of preterm infants, increasing numbers of extremely premature neonates are surviving. However, these neonates often are intubated for weeks and receive long-term IV hyperalimentation with the resultant risk of bacterial superinfection. A significant number develop systemic candidiasis, with an incidence ranging from 4% in those weighing 1500 g to 10% in those with a birth weight less than 1000 g (Baley et al., 1981).

In the past, primary renal candidiasis in 18 preterm infants had a mortality rate of 60% (Pappu et al., 1984).

Nearly all infants that develop renal candidiasis have a variety of predisposing features, including treatment with broad-spectrum antibiotics and prolonged fluid therapy with central or peripheral (or both) intravascular catheters or needles. Approximately half weigh less than 1500 g at birth. The most common clinical manifestation is the development of oliguria or anuria, which occurs in 85% of patients. Physical findings also may include hypertension, a palpable flank mass or abdominal distention, and subcutaneous abscesses. The serum creatinine often is elevated.

The diagnosis is made by urine culture obtained by suprapubic bladder tap or percutaneous renal aspiration. Renal candidiasis is confirmed by the presence of more than 10,000 colonies of *Candida albicans*/per milliliter of urine, isolating *Candida* in the sediment obtained from 10 ml of suprapubic urine centrifuged for 3 minutes at 3000 rpm (Kozinn et al., 1978), or growth of *Candida* in urine obtained from the kidney.

Early in the disease course of *systemic* candidiasis, the urine culture may be positive, although the blood cultures may be negative. In such cases, primary renal candidiasis is excluded by the absence of pathologic changes on renal ultrasonography and by the presence of *Candida* from other sources, such as the endotracheal tube or IV catheter. A positive urine culture for *Candida* should prompt an arterial (not venous) blood culture, followed by antifungal therapy (Smith and Congdon, 1985). Systemic candidiasis can be detected early and possibly avoided by routine urine cultures by suprapubic bladder aspiration in the neonatal intensive care unit (ICU) (Smith and Congdon, 1985). With current antifungal therapy, few infants die from either systemic candidiasis or its treatment, but rather from complications of its predisposing factors.

Radiographic evaluation may demonstrate unilateral or bilateral hydronephrosis associated with an intrapelvic filling defect that represents a fungal ball. Renal scan or IV urogram generally demonstrates that the involved kidney or kidneys exhibit poor function.

The treatment of renal candidiasis involves IV antifungal therapy in conjunction with local instillation of antifungal agents, surgical removal of the fungal balls, or both. At present, 5-flucytosine and amphotericin B are the drugs of choice for primary IV therapy. When used in combination, these drugs are synergistic (Rabinovich et al., 1974) and prevent the emergence of a resistant strain. An adverse effect of 5-flucytosine is bone marrow suppression, and amphotericin B may cause nephrotoxicity, hypotension, and thrombocytopenia. The latter drug has been well tolerated in infants by gradually increasing the dose of 0.25 to 1.0 mg/kg/day. Furthermore, by combining these two agents, the therapeutic doses of the individual drugs are smaller, diminishing the risk of toxic effect (Hermans and Keys, 1983). The imidazole derivatives, miconazole and ketoconazole, which have been used to treat fungal infections in adults, have not been used widely in the treatment of infant renal candidiasis.

IV antifungal therapy may be necessary for 4 to 6 weeks. In general, the end point of therapy is the inability to isolate *C. albicans* from specimens of urine sediment obtained 1 week apart (Michigan, 1976). Alternatively, the *Candida* antigen mannin may be found in the sera of patients with disseminated candidiasis (Schreiber et al., 1984). If mannin is detected, antifungal therapy should be continued until the antigen is no longer detected.

When a large fungal ball is present, medical management often is not sufficient. Most cases will require a percutaneous nephrostomy to be placed in the involved kidney so that irrigation with a solution of amphotericin B (1 mg in 100 ml of normal saline daily) may be performed. The irrigant provides a high concentration of antifungal agent, allows the bezoar to dissolve gradually, and provides a flushing effect (Bartone et al., 1988; Mazer and Bartone, 1982). Percutaneous removal of the fungal ball may be achieved under anesthesia. Alternatively, open surgical removal of the bezoar or nephrectomy may be necessary.

Nephrolithiasis

One of the more common urologic problems encountered now with the improved care of the premature neonate is the development of renal calcifications secondary to furosemide administration (Gilsanz et al., 1985; Hufnagle et al., 1982; Noe et al., 1984). The overall incidence of nephrolithiasis in infants treated in the neonatal ICU is approximately 2.5% (Gilsanz et al., 1985; Hufnagle et al., 1982) and was 11% in those weighing 1250 g or less (Gilsanz et al., 1985). Furosemide is used extensively in the management of infants with patent ductus arteriosus and to mobilize interstitial water in RDS secondary to bronchopulmonary dysplasia, and results in substantial hypercalciuria. Filtered calcium, in large part, is resorbed in the proximal tubule in the loop of Henle. Furosemide further increases the excretion of calcium, as well as sodium and potassium.

The development of urolithiasis in these preterm infants appears to be multifactorial: (1) high doses of furosemide necessary to control the bronchopulmonary dysplasia, (2) prolonged half-life of furosemide in premature infants, and (3) development of secondary hyperparathyroidism. Other contributing factors include excessive calcium intake, phosphate depletion, chronic corticosteroid therapy, distal renal tubular acidosis, excessive glucose intake, and immobilization. Furthermore, nephrocalcinosis is more common in low-birth-weight neonates with a family history of

stone disease and in white neonates (Karlowicz et al., 1993).

Essentially all of the reported infants developing renal calcifications or calculi have received furosemide 2 mg/kg/day or more for at least 2 weeks, with a mean duration of therapy of approximately 4 weeks before calcification was noted (Hufnagle et al., 1982). Many of the affected infants have received furosemide in doses substantially higher than 2 mg/kg/day. Importantly, long-term use of furosemide in the premature infant is associated with ototoxicity (Peterson et al., 1980) and secondary hyperparathyroidism (Gilsanz et al., 1985; Venkataraman et al., 1983).

The half-life of furosemide in the premature infant is prolonged. In the normal adult, the plasma half-life of the drug is between 33 and 100 minutes (Beermann et al., 1977) compared with values between 4 and 44 hours in neonates (Aranda et al., 1978; Peterson et al., 1980). In adults, slightly more than half of total plasma clearance of furosemide is accounted for by renal clearance (Beermann et al., 1975, 1977), with the remainder excreted through the biliary and intestinal tracts. However, in the premature infant, the GFR is low, hepatic function is immature, and furosemide is excreted unchanged almost entirely in the urine (Tuck et al., 1983). Thus, the prolonged half-life of furosemide also contributes to the development of hypercalciuria.

All of the infants who developed nephrolithiasis had a gestational age of 34 weeks or less at birth. Interestingly, in a 20-year review of pediatric stone disease at the Mayo Clinic, no child less than 1 year of age was reported (Malek and Kelalis, 1975). In these preterm infants with stone disease, the spot urine calcium–urine creatinine concentration ratio (mg/mg) has been significantly elevated, greater than 3.0 (normal less than 1.24) (Noe et al., 1984). The total urinary excretion of calcium has varied from 15 to 30 mg/kg/day of calcium compared with a normal level of less than 4 mg/kg/day of calcium (Hufnagle et al., 1982).

Most of the infants developing nephrolithiasis have been asymptomatic, although in one series six of ten had a UTI, and three had associated sepsis (Hufnagle et al., 1982). It is likely that the infections were related to colonization of the catheterized urinary tract.

Preterm infants in ICUs often have frequent radiographic evaluation, and the renal calculi may be detected by a careful radiologist. At times, the stones may continue to grow undetected, and a few staghorn calculi have been reported. In patients with suspected renal calculi, ultrasonography will provide confirmation of the suspected diagnosis and may demonstrate other areas of nephrocalcinosis.

The treatment of renal calculi in these infants generally is nonoperative. Administration of 20 mg/kg/day, of chlorothiazide, concurrently with furosemide has resulted in radiographic diminution or disappearance of most calculi. A few infants have undergone early surgical removal of the calculus. Extracorporeal shock wave lithotripsy has been used in only a few of these patients.

The mortality rate has been high because of the severity of the bronchopulmonary dysplasia. Postmortem examination of affected kidneys has demonstrated the calculi to be composed of calcium oxalate and calcium phosphate. In general, the microscopic renal involvement is bilateral, even if only one side is involved on x-ray film. Calcium deposits have been found in the collecting tubules and interstitial areas of the renal papillae. Ezzedeen and co-workers (1988) reported on the follow-up between 9 and 56 months of nine neonates with renal calcification. Total resolution was noted in four patients and improvement in one with medical management. Renal length was normal in 17 of 18 kidneys, but GFR was reduced in four patients. The need for continued urologic management in such patients is apparent.

The differential diagnosis of intrarenal calcification in the premature infant is limited. In addition to renal calculi, renal calcification following renal cortical necrosis (Leonidas et al., 1971) and RVT (Sutton et al., 1977) has been reported. In renal cortical necrosis, peripheral linear calcifications are found, whereas following RVT, lacelike and reticular calcifications are suggestive of an intravascular location (Gilsanz et al., 1985). Nephrocalcinosis in association with metabolic disorders, such as primary hyperoxaluria, has not been reported in infants less than 2 months of age.

In summary, the urologist should recognize that preterm infants are at risk for the development of renal calculi when they are receiving high doses of furosemide and that, in most cases, the problem may be managed by administration of concurrent chlorothiazide.

Umbilical Artery Catheter Complications

Another condition of urologic significance related to improved intensive care management of premature neonates is complications of umbilical artery catheterization. These catheters have been used for more than 20 years and have become standard in the treatment of sick newborn infants. Usual indications include the need to gain arterial access for reliable monitoring and blood pressure, frequent blood sampling for blood gas and pH values, exchange transfusion, cardiac catheterization, and infusion of fluid and nutrients. It is estimated that approximately 2% of all infants have an umbilical artery catheter (Caeton and Goetzman, 1985). Until recently, polyvinyl chloride catheters impregnated with barium in sizes 3.5 F and 5 F have been used. The most serious complication of these catheters has been thrombosis, which occurs in as many as 30% of such newborns (Goetzman et al., 1975; Marsh et al., 1975; O'Neill et al., 1981). However, the overall incidence of major complications is approximately 3% (Stringel et al., 1985).

Small infants appear to be at greater risk for the development of thrombotic complications from an umbilical artery than larger infants, but the size of the catheter does not appear to play a role. The level of catheter placement is quite controversial. Although catheters placed at the level of the thoracic aorta have a significantly lower incidence of complications, when complications do occur, they tend to be much more devastating.

One of the most serious complications associated with the use of such catheters is occlusion of the distal aorta secondary to thrombosis. The diagnosis is suggested by the development of congestive heart failure, hypertension, and lower limb ischemia. Involvement of one or both renal arteries is suggested by the development of anuria. Often, patients have had demonstrable low-flow states, hypoxia, hypercoagulable states, and sepsis (Wigger et al., 1970). Placement of the umbilical artery catheter below the thoracic aorta and frequent replacement or manipulation predispose to thrombosis (Marsh et al., 1975).

Clinically, manifestations of renal-aortic thrombosis include blanching or mottling of the lower extremities, difficulty in maintaining catheter patency, narrowing of the pulse pressure obtained through the catheter, hypertension, and metabolic acidosis (Krueger et al., 1985). Usually the diagnosis can be made by noninvasive means. Ultrasound and technetium aortic flow scans are quite helpful. In general, aortography is not necessary to confirm the diagnosis, although at times it is performed because of suspected congenital heart disease or coarctation.

Aortic thrombosis is considered by most to require immediate surgical management (Krueger et al., 1985; Lofland et al., 1988) and can result in a high rate of infant salvage if associated medical problems are reasonably well controlled. Recently, Malin and associates (1985) presented a series of three patients with obstructive aortic thrombosis and renovascular hypertension who did not undergo surgery but instead received aggressive supportive medical therapy, with demonstrable resolution of the thrombosis over a 4-week period. Medical treatment included peritoneal dialysis for acute renal failure and use of as many as five different antihypertensive medications. At late follow-up, all three of these infants were free of hypertension, and one had moderate renal insufficiency. The use of heparin or thrombolytic agents may be contraindicated because of the risk of developing intracranial hemorrhage, particularly in the hypertensive neonate (Malin et al., 1985). Clearly, the optimal management of such infants has not been resolved.

Persistent hypertension in infants with aortic thrombosis strongly suggests renal involvement and must be managed aggressively with diuretics and fluid restriction to deplete the extracellular fluid overload. β-Blockers are an important mainstay of antihypertensive therapy. Captopril may be beneficial because the hypertension is renin-mediated (Bifano et al., 1982; Plummer et al., 1976).

Because of the potential risks with the use of catheters for vascular access, there has been a recent reexamination of the necessity for their use (Caeton and Goetzman, 1985; Tooley and Myerberg, 1978). Catheters that are less thrombogenic are now becoming available (Caeton and Goetzman, 1985). Other umbilical artery catheter complications of urologic significance include vesicoumbilical fistula (Waffarn et al., 1980) and urinary ascites (Dmochowski et al., 1986; Vordermark et al., 1980).

REFERENCES

Aaronson IA: Micropenis: medical and surgical implications. *J Urol* 1994; 152:4.

Aaronson IA, Cremin BJ: *Clinical Paediatric Uroradiology*. New York, Churchill Livingstone Inc, 1984, p 29.

Abel RM: Nutritional support in the patient with acute renal failure. *J Am Coll Nutr* 1983; 2:33.

Abitbol CL, Holliday MA: Total parenteral nutrition in anuric children. *Clin Nephrol* 1976; 5:153.

Abramovich DR, Heaton B, Page KR: Transfer of labelled urea creatinine and electrolytes between liquor amnii and the feto-placental unit in midpregnancy. *Eur J Obstet Gynaecol Reprod Biol* 1974; 4/4:143.

Adzick NS, Harrison MR, Flake AW, et al: Urinary extravasation in the fetus with obstructive uropathy. *J Pediatr Surg* 1985; 20:608.

Alanen A, Kormano M: Real time sonographic diagnosis of adrenal haemorrhage. *Eur J Radiol* 1984; 4:210.

Alcaraz A, Vinaixa F, Tejedo-Mateau A, et al: Obstruction and recanalization of the ureter during embryonic development. *J Urol* 1991; 145:410.

Alexander DP, Nixon DA: The foetal kidney. *Br Med Bull* 1961; 17:112.

Alexander DP, Nixon DA: Plasma clearance of p. amino hippuric acid by the kidneys of fetal, neonatal, and adult sheep. *Nature* 1962; 194:483.

Allen KS, Arger PH, Mennuti M: Effect of maternal hydration on fetal pyelectasis. *Radiology* 1987; 163:807.

Allen TD: The swing of the pendulum. *J Urol* 1992; 148:534.

American Academy of Pediatrics (AAP)–American College of Obstetricians and Gynecologists (ACOG): *Guidelines for Perinatal Care*. Chicago, American Academy of Pediatrics, 1983, p 212.

American College of Obstetrics and Gynecologists. Practice guidelines, 1993.

American Institute for Ultrasound in Medicine: AIUM official statements. Rockville, MD, AIUM reported, Nov 1993, p 6.

Ames RG: Urinary water excretion and neurohypophysical function in full-term and premature infants shortly after birth. *Pediatrics* 1953; 12:272.

Anand SK: Acute renal failure in the neonate. *Pediatr Clin North Am* 1982; 29:791.

Angermeier KW, Kay R, Levin R: Hypertension as a complication of multicystic kidney. *Urology* 1992; 39:55.

Aperia A, Broberger O, Thodenius K, et al: Developmental study of the renal response to an oral salt load in preterm infants. *Acta Paediatr Scand* 1974; 63:517.

Aranda JV, Perez J, Sitar DS, et al: Pharmacokinetic disposition and protein binding of furosemide in newborn infants. *J Pediatr* 1978; 93:507.

Arant BS Jr: Developmental patterns of renal functional maturation compared in the human neonate. *J Pediatr* 1978; 92:705.

Arant BS Jr: Non-renal factors influencing renal function during the perinatal period. *Clin Perinatol* 1981; 8:225.

Arant BS Jr: Estimating glomerular filtration rate in infants. *J Pediatr* 1984a; 104:890.

Arant BS Jr: Renal disorders of the newborn infant. *Contemp Issues Nephrol* 1984b; 12:111.

Arger PH, Coleman BG, Mintz MC, et al: Routine fetal genitourinary tract screening. *Radiology* 1985; 156:485.

Arneil GC, MacDonald AM, Murphy AV, et al: Renal venous thrombosis. *Clin Nephrol* 1973; 1:119.

Atkinson GO Jr, Kodroff MB, Gay BB Jr, et al: Adrenal abscess in the neonate. *Radiology* 1985; 155:101.

Avni EF, Rodesh F, Schulman CC: Fetal uropathies: diagnostic pitfalls and management. *J Urol* 1985; 134:921.

Avni EF, Thoua Y, Lalmand B, et al: Multicystic dysplastic kidney: natural history from in utero diagnosis and postnatal follow-up. *J Urol* 987; 138:1420.

Bain AD, Scott JS: Renal agenesis and severe urinary tract dysplasia: a review of 50 cases with particular reference to the associated anomalies. *Br Med J* 1960; 1:841.

Baley JE, Annable WL, Kliegman RM: Candida endophthalmitis in the premature infant. *J Pediatr* 1981; 98:458.

Barnett H, Vesterdal J, McNamara H, et al: Renal water excretion in premature infants. *J Clin Invest* 1952; 31:1069.

Barratt TM: The nephrological background to urology. In Williams DI (ed): *Urology in Childhood*. New York, Springer-Verlag, 1974, p 1.

Barrett DM, Wineland RE: Renal cell carcinoma in multicystic dysplastic kidney. *Urology* 1980; 15:152.

Barrett RJ, Rayburn WF, Barr M Jr: Furosemide (Lasix) challenge test in assessing bilateral fetal hydronephrosis. *Am J Obstet Gynecol* 1983; 147:846.

Bartone FF, Hurwitz RS, Rojas EL, et al: The role of percutaneous nephrostomy in the management of obstructing candidiasis of the urinary tract in infants. *J Urol* 1988; 140:338.

Beck D: Intrauterine renal surgery: techniques for exposing the fetal kidney during the last two-thirds of gestation. *Invest Urol* 1970; 8:182.

Beermann B, Dalen E, Lindstrom B: Elimination of furosemide in healthy subjects and in those with renal failure. *Clin Pharmacol Ther* 1977; 22:70.

Beermann B, Dalen E, Lindstrom B, et al: On the fate of furosemide in man. *Eur J Clin Pharmacol* 1975; 9:57.

Behrman RE, Kliegman RM: High-risk pregnancies. In Behrman RD, Vaughn VC (eds): *Nelson Textbook of Pediatrics*. Philadelphia, WB Saunders Co, 1983, p 329.

Bejjani B, Belman AB: Ureteropelvic junction obstruction in newborns and infants. *J Urol* 1982; 128:770.

Bell EF, Warburton D, Stonestreet BS, et al: High-volume fluid intake predisposes premature infants to necrotising enterocolitis. *Lancet* 1979; 2:90.

Bell EF, Warburton D, Stonestreet BS, et al: Effect of fluid administration on the development of symptomatic patent ductus arteriosus and congestive heart failure in premature infants. *N Engl J Med* 1980; 302:598.

Bellinger MF, Comstock CH, Grosso D, et al: Fetal posterior urethral valves in renal dysplasia at 15 weeks gestational age. *J Urol* 1983; 129:1238.

Belman AB: Renal vascular thrombosis and adrenal hemorrhage. In PP Kelalis, LR King, AB Belman (eds): *Clinical Pediatric Urology*, ed 2. Philadelphia, WB Saunders Co, 1985, p 1079.

Belman AB, King LR: The pathology and treatment of renal vein thrombosis in the newborn. *J Urol* 1972; 107:852.

Benini F, Johnston C, Paucher D, et al: Topical anesthesia during circumcision in newborn infants. *JAMA* 1993; 270(7):850.

Berdon WE, Baker DH, Blanc WA, et al: Megacystismicrocolon-intestinal hypoperistalsis syndrome: a new cause of intestinal obstruction in the newborn: report of radiologic findings in five newborn girls. *AJR* 1976; 126:957.

Bergstrom T, Larson H, Lincoln K, et al: Studies of urinary tract infections in infancy and childhood: XII. Eighty consecutive patients with neonatal infection. *J Pediatr* 1972; 80:858.

Berman DJ, Maizels M: The role of urinary obstruction in the genesis of renal dysplasia. A model in the chick embryo. *J Urol* 1982; 128:1091.

Berstein J: A classification of renal cysts. In Gardner KD (ed): *Cystic Disease of the Kidney*. New York, John Wiley and Sons, 1976; pp 7-30.

Bernstein GT, Mandell J, Lebowitz RL, et al: Ureteropelvic junction obstruction in the neonate. *J Urol* 1988; 140:1216.

Betts EK, Downes JJ, Schaffer DB, et al: Retrolental fibroplasia and oxygen administration during general anesthesia. *Anesthesiology* 1977; 47:518.

Bifano E, Post EM, Springer J, et al: Treatment of neonatal hypertension with captopril. *J Pediatr* 1982; 100:143.

Birken G, King D, Vane D, et al: Renal cell carcinoma arising in a multicystic dysplastic kidney. *J Pediatr Surg* 1985; 20:619.

Birnholz JC: Determination of fetal sex. *N Engl J Med* 1983; 309:942.

Bjorgvinsson E, Majd M, Eggli KD: Diagnosis of acute pyelonephritis in children: comparison of sonography and 99mTc-DMSA scintigraphy. *Am J Roentgenol* 1991; 157:539.

Blachar A, Blachar Y, Livne P, et al: Clinical outcome and follow-up of prenatal hydronephrosis. *Pediatr Nephrol* 1994; 8:30.

Black J, Williams DI: Natural history of adrenal hemorrhage in the newborn. *Arch Dis Child* 1973; 48:183.

Blane CE, Koff SA, Bowerman RA, et al: Nonobstructive fetal hydronephrosis: sonographic recognition and therapeutic implications. *Radiology* 1983; 147:95.

Blythe B, Duckett JW: Neonatal obstructive uropathy. In Reed GB, Claireaux AE, Cockburn F (eds): *Diseases of the Fetus and Newborn*. London, Chapman and Hall, 1995.

Blyth B, Snyder HM, Duckett JW: Antenatal diagnosis and subsequent management of hydronephrosis. *J Urol* 1993; 149:693.

Bourke WG, Clarke TA, Mathews TA, et al: Isolated single umbilical artery — the case for routine renal screening. *Arch Dis Child* 1993; 68:600.

Brace RA: Fetal fluid balance. In *Textbook of Fetal Physiology*. Thornburn GD, Harding R (eds): Oxford, England, Oxford University Press, 1994, pp 205-208.

Brace RA, Wolf EJ: Normal amniotic fluid volume changes throughout pregnancy. *Am J Obstet Gynecol* 1989; 161:382.

Brem AS: Neonatal hematuria and proteinuria. *Clin Perinatol* 1981; 8:321.

Brem AS, Singer D, Anderson L, et al: Infants of azotemic mothers: a report of three live births. *Am J Kidney Dis* 1988; 12:299.

Brill PW, Mitty HA, Strauss L: Renal vein thrombosis: a cause of intrarenal calcification in the newborn. *Pediatr Radiol* 1977; 6:172.

Brocklebank JT: Kidney function in the very low birthweight infant. *Arch Dis Child* 1992; 64:1140.

Bronshtein M, Bar-Hava T, Blumenfel Z: Differential diagnosis of the non-visualized fetal urinary bladder by transvaginal sonography in the early second trimester. *Obstet Gynecol* 1993; 82:490.

Bronshtein M, Yotte JM, Brandes JM, et al: First and early second-trimester diagnosis of fetal urinary tract anomalies using transvaginal sonography. *Prenat Diag* 1990; 10:653.

Burbige DM, Griffiths MD, Malone PS, et al: Fetal vesicoureteral reflux: outcome following conservative postnatal management. *J Urol* 1992; 148:1743.

Burbige KA, Lebowitz RL, Colodny AH, et al: The megacystis-megaureter syndrome. *J Urol* 1984; 131:1133.

Burge DM: Neonatal testicular torsion and infarction: aetiology and management. *Br J Urol* 1987; 59:70.

Burger R, Guthrie TH: Why circumcision? *Pediatrics* 1974; 54:362.

Burrow CR, Walker WG, Bell WR, et al: Streptokinase salvage of renal function after renal vein thrombosis. *Ann Intern Med* 1984; 100:237.

Cadman D, Gafini A, McNamee J: Newborn circumcision, an economic perspective. *Canadian Med Assoc J* 1984; B1:1353.

Caeton AJ, Goetzman BW: Risky business: umbilical artery catheterization. *Am J Dis Child* 1985; 139:120.

Caldamone AA, Snyder HM, Duckett J: Ureteroceles in children: follow-up of management with upper-tract approach. *J Urol* 1984; 136:1130.

Cameron G, Chambers R: Direct evidence of function in kidney of an early human fetus. *Am J Physiol* 1983; 123:482.

Campbell S, Wladimiroff JW, Dewurst CJ: The antenatal measurement of fetal urine production. *J Obstet Gynecol Proc Common* 1973; 80:680.

Carey PO, Howards SS: Multicystic dysplastic kidneys and diagnostic confusion on renal scan. *J Urol* 1988; 139:83.

Carter BB, Moores RR, Battaglia FC: Placental transport and fetal and placental metabolism of amino acids. *J Nutr Biochem* 1991; 2:4.

Cartwright PC, Duckett JW, Keating MA, et al: Managing apparent ureteropelvic junction obstruction in the newborn. *J Urol* 1992; 148:1224.

Carty A, Stanley P: Bilateral adrenal abscesses in a neonate. *Pediatr Radiol* 1973; 1:63.

Celio MR, Groscurth P, Imagam T: Ontogeny of renin immunoreactive cells in the human kidney. *Anat Embryol* 1985; 173:143.

Cendron M, D'Alton ME, Crombleholme M: Prenatal diagnosis and management of the fetus with hydronephrosis. *Semin Perinatol* 1994a; 18-3:163.

Cendron M, Morin L, Crombleholme TM, et al: Early minimal fetal hydronephrosis: clinical outcomes and implications for management. Abstract 3, Section on Urology. American Academy of Pediatrics, Dallas, 1994b.

Chandhoke PS, Kogan BA, Al-Dahwi A, et al: Monitoring renal function in children with urological abnormalities. *J Urol* 1990; 144:601.

Chebel M: Histoire de la circoncision, des origines a nos jours. In Bolland (ed): Paris, France, 1992.

Chevalier RL: Chronic partial ureteral obstruction in the neonatal guinea pig. II. Pressure gradients affecting glomerular filtration rate. *Pediatr Res* 1984; 18:1271.

Chevalier RL, Campbell F, Brenbridge ANAG: Prognostic factors in neonatal acute renal failure. *Pediatrics* 1984; 74:265.

Chez RA, Smith FG, Hutchinson DL: Renal function in the intrauterine primate fetus. *Am J Obstet Gynecol* 1964; 90:128.

Chung S, Majd M, Rushton HG: Diuretic renography in the evaluation of neonatal hydronephrosis: is it reliable? *J Urol* 1993; 150:765.

Churchill BM, McLorie GA, Khoury AE, et al: Emergency treatment and long-term follow-up of posterior urethral valves. *Urol Clin North Am* 1990; 17:343.

Claesson G, Josephson S, Robertson B: Experimental partial ureteric obstruction in newborn rats: IV. Do the morphological effects progress continuously? *J Urol* 1983; 130:1217.

Cohen HL, Susman M, Haller JO, et al: Posterior urethral valve: transperineal US for imaging and diagnosis in male infants. *Radiology* 1994; 192:261.

Collins GM, Taft P, Green RD, et al: Adenine nucleotide levels in preserved and ischemically injured canine kidneys. *World J Surg* 1977; 1:237.

Colodny AH: Fetal diagnosis and therapy: legal, ethical, religious, moral issues. *Dial Pediatr Urol* 1986; 9:1.

Conley AJ, Masson JI: Endocrine function of the placenta. In Thornburn GD, Harding R (eds): *Textbook of Fetal Physiology*. Oxford Medical Publications, 1994, pp 16-29.

Conway JJ, Maizels M: The "well-tempered" diuretic renogram: a standard method to examine the asymptomatic neonate with hydronephrosis or hydroureteronephrosis. *J Nucl Med* 1992; 33:2047.

Cooke RJ, Werkman S, Watson D: Urine output measurement in premature infants. *Pediatrics* 1989; 83:116.

Coplen DE, Hare JY, Zderic SA, et al: Ten-year experience with antenatal in utero intervention. *J Urol* (in press).

Corazza MS, Davis RF, Merritt TA, et al: Prolonged bleeding time in preterm infants receiving indomethacin for patent ductus arteriosus. *J Pediatr* 1984; 105:292.

Corey HE, Spitzer A: Renal blood flow and glomerular filtration rate during development. In Edleman CM (ed): *Pediatric Kidney Diseases*, ed 2. Boston, Little Brown Company, 1992, pp 49-77.

Corteville JE, Gray DL, Crane JP: Congenital hydronephrosis: correlation of fetal ultrasonographic findings with fetal outcome. *Am J Obstet Gynecol* 1991; 165:384.

Coulthard G: Comparison of methods of measuring renal function in pre-term babies using insulin. *J Pediatr* 1983; 102:923.

Coulthard MG: Maturation of glomerular filtration in pre-term and mature babies. *Early Human Develop* 1985; 11:281.

Council on Scientific Affairs, American Medical Association: In utero fetal surgery. *JAMA* 1983; 250:1443.

Courteville J, Gray DL, Crane JP: Congenital hydronephrosis: correlation of fetal ultrasound findings with infant outcomes. *Am J Obstet Gynecol* 1991; 165:384.

Cowan RH, Jukkola AF, Arant BS Jr: Pathophysiologic evidence of gentamicin nephrotoxicity in neonatal puppies. *Pediatr Res* 1980; 14:1204.

Cremin BJ, Aaronson IA: Ultrasonic diagnosis of posterior urethral valve in neonates. *Brit J Radiol* 1983; 56:435.

Crombleholme TM: Invasive fetal therapy: current status and future directions. *Semin Perinatol* 1994; 18(IV):385.

Crombleholme TM, Harris MR, Langer JC, et al: Early experience with open fetal surgery for congenital hydronephrosis. *J Pediatr Surg* 1988a; 23:1114.

Crombleholme TM, Harrison MR, Golbus MS, et al: Fetal intervention in obstructive uropathy: prognostic indicators and efficacy of intervention. *Am J Obstet Gynecol* 1990; 162:1239.

Crombleholme TM, Harrison MR, Longaker MT, et al: Prenatal diagnosis and management of bilateral hydronephrosis. *Pediatr Nephrol* 1988b; 2:334.

Cromie WJ, Cain MP, Bellinger MF, et al: Urethral valve incision using a modified venous valvulotome. *J Urol* 1994; 151:1053.

Crone RK: Postnatal urinary tract dilatation: diagnosis/management dilemmas. *Dial Pediatr Urol* 1986; 9(2):5.

Cruikshanks JN: Causes of 800 neonatal deaths. In *Special Report Series*. Medical Research Council, 1930, p 145.

Cuniff C, Jones KL, Phillipson J, et al: Oligohydramnios sequence and renal tubular malformation associated with maternal enalapril use. *Am J Obstet Gynecol* 1990; 162:187.

Dauber IM, Krauss AN, Symchych MD, et al: Renal failure following perinatal anoxia. *J Pediatr* 1976; 88:851.

David M, Forest MG: Prenatal treatment of congenital adrenal hyperplasia resulting from 21-hydroxylase deficiency. *J Pediatr* 1984; 105:799.

Deane AM, Whitaker RH, Sherwood T: Diathermy hook ablation of posterior urethral valves in neonates and infants. *Br J Urol* 1988; 62:593.

Dejter SW Jr, Gibbons MD: The fate of infant kidneys with fetal hydronephrosis but initially normal postnatal sonography. *J Urol* 1989; 142:661.

DeKlerk DP, Marshall FF, Jeffs RD: Multicystic dysplastic kidney. *J Urol* 1977; 118:306.

Deppe R, Boehm JJ, Nosekja JA, et al: Antenatal corticosteroids to prevent neonatal respiratory distress syndrome. Risk versus benefit considerations. *Am J Obstet Gynecol* 1980; 137:338.

Devine, et al: The circumcision controversy. *AUA Update* 1995; lesson 14.

Dewan PA, Zappala SM, Ransley PG, et al: Endoscopic reappraisal of the morphology of congenital obstruction of the posterior urethra. *Br J Urol* 1992; 70:439.

Diamond DA, Ransley PG: Fogarty balloon catheter ablation of neonatal posterior urethral valves. *J Urol* 1987; 137:1209.

Diamond DA, Saunders R, Jeff RD: Fetal hydronephrosis: considerations regarding urologic intervention. *J Urol* 1984; 131:1155.

Dimmick JE, Johnson HW, Coleman GV, et al: Wilms' tumorlet, nodular renal blastema, and multicystic renal dysplasia. *J Urol* 1989; 142:484.

Dinneen MD, Dhillon HK, Ward HC, et al: Antenatal diagnosis of posterior urethral valves. *Br J Urol* 1993; 72:364.

Dmochowski RR, Crandell SS, Corriere JN: Bladder injury and uroascites from umbilical artery catheterization. *Pediatrics* 1986; 77:421.

Donald I, MacVicar J, Brown TG: Investigation of abdominal masses by pulsed ultrasound. *Lancet* 1958; 1:1188.

Donn SM, Faix RG: Transillumination in neonatal diagnosis. *Clin Perinatol* 1985; 12:3.

Doubilet PM, Benson CB: Ultrasound evaluation of amniotic fluid. In Callen PW (ed): *Ultrasonography and Obstetrics and Gynecology*. Philadelphia, WB Saunders, 1994, pp 475-476.

Duckett JW Jr: Cutaneous vesicostomy in childhood: the Blocksom technique. *Urol Clin North Am* 1974; 1:485.

Duckett JW Jr, Gibbons MD, Cromie WJ: An anterior extraperitoneal muscle-splitting approach for pediatric renal surgery. *J Urol* 1980; 123:79.

Edelmann CM Jr: Maturation of the neonatal kidney. In Becker EL (ed): *Proceedings of the Third International Congress of Nephrology*, vol 3. Basel, Karger, 1967, p 1.

Edelmann CM Jr, Barnett HL, Troupkou V: Renal concentrating mechanisms in newborn infants. Effect of dietary protein and water content, role of urea, and responsiveness to antidiuretic hormone. *J Clin Invest* 1960; 39:1062.

Ehrlich RM: The ureteral folding technique for megaureter surgery. *J Urol* 1985; 134:668.

Elder JS: Megaureter in children. *AUA Update Series* 1988; 7:185.

Elder JS: In utero ultrasonography: impact on urology. *J Endourol* 1992; 6:279.

Elder JS, Duckett JW, Snyder HM: Intervention for fetal obstructive uropathy: has it been effective? *Lancet* 1987; b-2:1007.

Elder JS, Hladky D, Selzman AA: Outpatient nephrectomy for non-functioning kidneys. *J Urol* 1995; 154:712.

Elder JS, Klacsmann PG, Sanders RC, et al: Clinicopathological conference: flank mass in a neonate. *J Urol* 1981; 126:94.

Elder JS, O'Grady JP, Ashmead G, et al: Evaluation of fetal renal function: unreliability of urinary electrolytes. *J Urol* 1990; 144:574.

Elder JS, Stansbrey R, Dahms BB, et al: Renal histologic changes secondary to ureteropelvic junction obstruction. *J Urol* 1995; 154:719.

Elinder G, Aperia A: Effect of aldosterone blocking on distal sodium reabsorption during development. *Eur J Pediatr* 1983; 140:166.

Ellis CEG, Bennett MJ: Routine ultrasound screening in pregnancy. In Bennett MJ (ed): *Ultrasound in Perinatal Care*. New York, John Wiley and Sons, Inc, 1984, p 49.

Emanuel B, Aronson N: Neonatal hematuria. *Am J Dis Child* 1974; 128:204.

Emanuel B, White H: Intravenous pyelography in the differential diagnosis of renal masses in the neonatal period. *Clin Pediatr* 1968; 7:529.

Engle WD: Evaluation of renal function and acute renal failure in the neonate. *Pediatr Clin North Am* 1986; 33:129.

Eshima D, Fritzberg AR, Taylor A Jr: ^{99m}Tc Renal tubular function agents: current status. *Semin Nucl Med* 1990; 20:28.

Estes JM, Harrison MR: Fetal obstructive uropathy. *Semin Pediatr Surg* 1993; 2:129.

Estes JM, MacGillivray TE, Hedrick M, et al: Fetoscopic surgery for the treatment of congenital anomalies. *J Pediatr Surg* 1992; 27:950.

Evans DJ, Silverman M, Bowley NB: Congenital hypertension due to unilateral renal vein thrombosis. *Arch Dis Child* 1981; 56:306.

Evans MI, Chrousos GP, Mann DW, et al: Pharmacologic suppression of the fetal adrenal gland in utero. Attempted prevention of abnormal external genital masculinization and suspected congenital adrenal hyperplasia. *JAMA* 1985; 253:1015.

Ewigman BG, Crane JP, Frigoletto FD, et al and The RADIUS Study Group: Effect of prenatal screening on perinatal outcome. *N Engl J Med* 1993; 329:821.

Ezzedeen F, Adelman RD, Ahlfors CE: Renal calcification in preterm infants: pathophysiology and long-term sequelae. *J Pediatr* 1988; 113:532.

Feins NR: To pex or not to pex. *J Pediatr Surg* 1983; 18:697.

Fernbach SK, Maizels M, Conway JJ: Ultrasound grading of hydronephrosis: introduction of the system used by the Society for Fetal Urology. *Pediatr Radiol* 1993; 23:478.

Fetterman GH, Shuplock NA, Philipp FJ, et al: The

growth and maturation of human glomeruli and proximal convolutions from term to adulthood: studies by microdissection. *Pediatrics* 1965; 35:601.

Fewell JE, Norton JB: Continuous positive airway pressure impairs renal function in newborn goats. *Pediatr Res* 1980; 14:1132.

Filmer RB, Taxy JB, King LR: Renal dysplasia: clinicopathological study. *Trans Am Assoc Genitourin Surg* 1974; 66:18.

Finberg H: Renal ultrasound: anatomy and technique. *Semin Ultrasound* 1981; 2:7.

Firlit CF, King LR: Anterior urethral valves in children. *J Urol* 1972; 108:972.

Flack CE, Bellinger MF: The multicystic dysplastic kidney and contralateral vesicoureteral reflux: protection of the solitary kidney. *J Urol* 1993; 150:1873.

Flake AW, Adzick NS, Harrison TR, et al: Ureteropelvic junction obstruction. *J Pediatr Surg* 1986; 21:1058.

Flashner SC, Mesrobian HG, Flatt JA, et al: Nonobstructive dilatation of upper urinary tract may later convert to obstruction. *Urology* 1993; 42:569.

Fleisher MH, Churchill BM, McLorie GA, et al: Posterior urethral valves—a role for temporary cutaneous vesicostomy. *J Urol* 1984; 131:150A.

Fletcher JC, Evans MI: Maternal bonding in early fetal ultrasound examinations. *N Engl J Med* 1983; 308:392.

Fletcher JC, Jonsen AR: Ethical considerations. In Harrison MR, Golbus MS, Filly RA (eds): *The Unborn Patient: Prenatal Diagnosis and Treatment*. Orlando, Fla, Grune & Stratton, 1984, p 159.

Fong EF, Rahman MR, Rose T, et al: Fetal renal cystic disease: sonographic-pathologic correlation. *Am J Roentgenol* 1986; 146:767.

Fouser L, Avner ED: Normal and abnormal nephrogenesis. *Am J Kidney Diseases* 1993; 21:64.

Friedland G, Filly RA, Goris M, et al: Uroradiology: an integrated approach. New York, Churchill-Livingstone, 1983.

Friedman J, Hoyer JR, McCormick B, et al: Congenital unilateral hydronephrosis in the rat. *Kidney Int* 1979; 15:567.

Fugelseth D, Lidemann R, Sande HA, et al: Prenatal diagnosis of urinary tract anomalies. The value of two ultrasound examinations. *Acta Obstet Gynecol Scand* 1994; 73:290.

Fung LCT, Steckler RE, Khoury AE, et al: Intrarenal resistive index correlates with renal pelvis pressures. *J Urol* 1994; 152:607.

Furzan JA, Gabriele G, Wheeler JM, et al: Regional blood flows in newborn lambs during endotracheal continuous airway pressure and continuous negative pressure breathing. *Pediatr Res* 1981; 15:874.

Fussell EN, Kaack MB, Cherry R, et al: Adherence of bacteria to human foreskins. *J Urol* 1988; 140:997.

Garmel SH, D'Alton ME: Diagnostic ultrasound in pregnancy: an overview. *Semin Perinatol* 1994; 18(3):117.

Garrett WJ, Grunwald G, Robinson DE: Prenatal diagnosis of fetal polycystic kidney by ultrasound. *J Obstet Gynecol* 1970; 10:7.

Gates GF: Glomerular filtration rate: estimation from fractional renal accumulation of ^{99m}Tc DTPA. *Am J Radiol* 1982; 138:565.

Gaudio KM, Taylor MR, Chaudry IH, et al: Accelerated recovery of single nephron function by the postischemic infusion of ATP-MgC12. *Kidney Int* 1982; 22:13.

Gee WF, Ansell JS: Neonatal circumcision: a ten-year overview with comparison of the Gomco clamp and plastibell device. *Pediatrics* 1976; 58:824.

Gellis SS: Circumcision. *Am J Dis Child* 1978; 132:1168.

Ghidini A, Sirtori M, Vergani P, et al: Ureteropelvic obstruction in utero and ex utero. *Obstet Gynecol* 1990; 75:805.

Gibbons MD, Duckett JW Jr, Cromie WJ, et al: Abdominal flank mass in the neonate. *J Urol* 1978; 119:671.

Gibbons MD, Horan HA, Dejter SW, et al: Extracorporeal membrane oxygenation: an adjunct in the management of the neonate with severe respiratory distress and congenital urinary tract anomalies. *J Urol* 1993; 150:434.

Gilbert EF, Khoury GH, Hogan GR, et al: Hemorrhagic renal necrosis in infancy: relationship to radiopaque compounds. *J Pediatr* 1970; 76:49.

Gilbert RD: Control of fetal cardiac output during changes in blood volume. *Am J Phys* 1980; 238:1180.

Gilbert R, Garra B, Gibbons MD: Renal duplex doppler ultrasound: an adjunct in the evaluation of hydronephrosis in the child. *J Urol* 1993; 150:1192.

Gilsanz V, Fernal W, Reid BS, et al: Nephrolithiasis in premature infants. *Radiology* 1985; 154:107.

Gil-Vernet J: New surgical concepts in removing renal calculi. *Urol Int* 1965; 20:255.

Ginsburg CM, McCracken GH Jr: Urinary tract infections in young infants. *Pediatrics* 1982; 69:409.

Gleason CA: Prostaglandins and the developing kidney. *Semin Perinatol* 1987; 11:12.

Glick PL, Harrison MR, Golbus MS, et al: Management of the fetus with congenital hydronephrosis: II. Prognostic criteria and selection for treatment. *J Pediatr Surg* 1985; 20:376.

Glick PL, Harrison MR, Noall RA, et al: Correction of congenital hydronephrosis in utero: III. Early midtrimester ureteral obstruction produces renal dysplasia. *J Pediatr Surg* 1983; 18:681.

Goetzman BW, Stadalnik RC, Bogren HC, et al: Thrombotic complications of umbilical artery catheters: a clinical and radiographic study. *Pediatrics* 1975; 56:374.

Goldsmith DI, Drukker A, Blaufox MD, et al: Hemodynamic and excretory response of the neonatal canine kidney to acute volume expansion. *Am J Physiol* 1979; 237(5):F-392.

Gomez RA, Lynch KR, Chevalier RL, et al: Renin and angiotensin gene expression and intrarenal renin distribution during ACE inhibition. *Am J Physiol* 1988; 254:F582.

Gonzalez R, Aliabadi H: Posterior lumbotomy in pediatric pyeloplasty. *J Urol* 1987; 137:468.

Gonzalez R, Reimberg Y, Burke B, et al: Early bladder outlet obstruction in fetal lambs induces renal dysplasia and prune belly syndrome. *J Pediatr Surg* 1990; 25(3):342.

Gonzalez R, Schwartz S, Sheldon CA, et al: Bilateral renal vein thrombosis in infancy and childhood. *Urol Clin North Am* 1982; 9:279.

Gordon I, Barratt TM: Imaging the kidneys and urinary tract in the neonate with acute renal failure. *Pediatr Nephrol* 1987; 1:321.

Gordon I, Dhillon HK, Gatanash H, et al: Antenatal diagnosis of pelvic hydronephrosis: assessment of renal function and drainage as a guide to management. *J Nucl Med* 1991; 32:1649.

Gordon AC, Thomas DFM, Arthur RJ, et al: Multicystic dysplastic kidney: is nephrectomy still appropriate? *J Urol* 1988; 140:1231.

Gore RM, Shkolnik A: Abdominal manifestations of pediatric leukemias: sonographic assessment. *Radiology* 1982; 143:207.

Grannum P, Bracker M, Silverman R, et al: Assessment of fetal kidney size in normal gestation by comparison of ratio of kidney circumference to abdominal circumference. *Am J Obstet Gynecol* 1980; 136:249.

Gray SW, Skandalakis JE: *Embryology for Surgeons*. Philadelphia, WB Saunders Co, 1972, p 31.

Greene A, Cromie WJ, Goldman M: Computerized body tomography in neonatal renal vein thrombosis. *Urology* 1982; 20:213.

Greenfield SP, Griswold JJ, Wan J: Ureteral reimplantation in infants. *J Urol* 1993; 150:1460.

Greenfield SP, Hensle TW, Berdon WE, et al: Urinary extravasation in the newborn male with posterior urethral valves. *J Pediatr Surg* 1982; 17:751.

Greenfield SP, Rutigliano E, Steinhardt A, et al: Genitourinary malformations and maternal cocaine abuse. *Urology* 1991; 37:455.

Grignon A, Giljon R, Filiatrault D, et al: Urinary tract dilatation in utero: classification and clinical applications. *Radiology* 1986; 160:645.

Griscom NT: The roentgenology of neonatal abdominal masses. *Am J Radiol* 1965; 93:447.

Griscom NT, Colodny AH, Rosenberg HK, et al: Diagnostic aspects of neonatal ascites: report of 27 cases. *Am J Roentg* 1977; 128:961.

Gruppe WE: The dilemma of intrauterine diagnosis of congenital renal disease. *Pediatr Clin North Am* 1987; 34(3):629.

Guignard J-P: Renal function in the newborn infant. *Pediatr Clin North Am* 1982; 29:777.

Guignard J-P, Gouyon JB, Adelman RD: Arterial hypertension in the newborn infant. *Biol Neonate* 1989; 55:77.

Guignard J-P, John EG: Renal function in the tiny, premature infant. *Clin Perinatol* 1986; 13:377.

Guignard J-P, Torrado A, Mazouni SM, et al: Renal function in respiratory distress syndrome. *J Pediatr* 1976; 88:845.

Guiney EJ, McGlinchey J: Torsion of the testes and the spermatic cord in the newborn. *Surg Gynecol Obstet* 1981; 152:273.

Haller JO, Berdon WE, Friedman AP: Increased renal cortical echogenicity: a normal finding in neonates and infants. *Radiology* 1982; 142:173.

Hanna MK, Jeffs RD, Sturgess JM, et al: Ureteral structure and ultrastructure: I. The normal human ureter. *J Urol* 1976a; 116:718.

Hanna MK, Jeffs RD, Sturgess JM, et al: Ureteral structure and ultrastructure: II. Congenital ureteropelvic junction obstruction and primary obstructive megaureter. *J Urol* 1976b; 116:725.

Harrison MR, Filly RA: The fetus with obstructive uropathy: pathophysiology, natural history, selection and treatment. In Harrison MR, Golbus MS, Filly RA (eds): *Fetal Diseases and Their Management*. Philadelphia, WB Saunders, 1991, pp 328-393.

Harrison MR, Filly RA, Parer JT: Management of the fetus with urinary tract malformation. *JAMA* 1982a; 246:635.

Harrison MR, Golbus MS, Filly RA, et al: Fetal surgery for congenital hydronephrosis. *N Engl J Med* 1982b; 306:591.

Harrison RM, Golbus MS, Filly RA, et al: In utero treatment of urinary tract obstruction. *Am J Obstet Gynecol* 1982c; 142:383.

Harrison MR, Golbus MS, Filly RA: Ultrasonography. In Harrison MR, Golbus MS, Filly RA (eds): *The Unborn Patient: Prenatal Diagnosis and Treatment*. Orlando, Fla, Grune & Stratton, Inc, 1984, pp 33-123.

Harrison MR, Golbus MS, Filly RA, et al: Fetal hydronephrosis: selection and surgical repair. *J Pediatr Surg* 1987; 22:556.

Harrison MR, Nakayama DK, Noall R, et al: Correction of congenital hydronephrosis in utero II. Decompression reverses the effect of obstruction in the fetal lung and urinary tract. *J Pediatr Surg* 1982c; 17:965.

Hartman GE, Surolik LM, Shochat SJ: The dilemma of the multicystic dysplastic kidney. *Am J Dis Child* 1986; 140:925.

Harvard JR: Emotion in women undergoing amniocentesis in the second trimester of pregnancy. *J Perinatal* 1992; 12:257.

Haswell GL, Morris JA: Amniotic fluid volume studies. *Obstet Gynecol* 1973; 42:725.

Heijden AJ, Grose WFA, Ambagtsheer JJ, et al: Glomerular filtration rate in the preterm infant: the relation to gestational and postnatal age. *Eur J Pediatr* 1988; 148:24.

Helin I, Persson PH: Prenatal diagnosis of urinary tract abnormalities by ultrasound. *Pediatrics* 1986; 78:879.

Hendren WH: Operative repair of megaureter in children. *J Urol* 1969; 101:491.

Hendren WH: Posterior urethral valves in boys: a broad clinical spectrum. *J Urol* 1991; 106:298.

Hepworth RC, Milstein JM: The transected urachus: an unusual cause of neonatal ascites. *Pediatrics* 1984; 73:397.

Herbst AL: Intraepithelial neoplasia of the cervix. In Droegemueller W, Herbst AL, Mishell DR, et al (eds): *Comprehensive Gynecology*. St Louis, Mosby, 1987, pp 729-766.

Hermans PE, Keys TF: Antifungal agents used for deep-seated mycotic infections. *Mayo Clin Proc* 1983; 58:223.

Herrera AJA, Cochran B, Herrera A, et al: Parental information and circumcision in highly motivated couples with higher education. *Pediatrics* 1983; 71:233.

Herzog LW: Urinary tract infections and circumcision: A case control study. *Am J Dis Child* 1989; 143:348.

Herzog LW, Alvarez SR: The frequency of foreskin problems in uncircumcised children. *Am J Dis Child* 1986; 140:254.

Heyman S, Duckett JW: The extraction factor: an estimate of single kidney function in children during routine radionuclide renography with ^{99m}Tc DTPA. *J Urol* 1988a; 140:780.

Heyman S, Duckett JW: Radionuclide studies of the urinary tract in children. *AUA Update Series* 1988b; Lesson 24, vol XI, p 1.

Hijazi Z, Keller MS, Gaudio KM, et al: Transient renal dysfunction of the neonate. *Pediatrics* 1988; 82:929.

Hill KJ, Lumbers ER: Renal function in adult and fetal sheep. *J Dev Physiol* 1988; 10:249.

Hoddick WK, Filly RA, Mahony BS, et al: Minimal fetal renal pyelectasis. *J Ultrasound Med* 1985; 4:85.

Hollowell JA, Altman HA, Snyder HM, et al: Coexisting ureteropelvic junction obstruction and vesicoureteral reflux: diagnostic and therapeutic implications. *J Urol* 1989; 142:490.

Holzman RS: Morbidity and mortality in pediatric anesthesia. *Pediatr Clin North Am* 1994; 41:239.

Homsy YL, Williot P, Danais S: Transient-ional neonatal hydronephrosis: facts of fantasy. *J Urol* 1986; 136:339.

Hoover DL, Duckett JW Jr: Posterior urethral valves, unilateral reflux and renal dysplasia: a syndrome. *J Urol* 1982; 128:994.

Horster M, Valtin H: Postnatal development of renal function: micropuncture and clearance studies in the dog. *J Clin Invest* 1971; 50:779.

Howman-Giles R, Uren R, Roy LP, et al: Volume expansion diuretic renal scan in urinary tract obstruction. *J Nucl Med* 1987; 28:824.

Hufnagle KG, Khan SN, Penn D, et al: Renal calcifications: a complication of long-term furosemide therapy in preterm infants. *Pediatrics* 1982; 70:360.

Hulbert WC, Duckett JW: Prognostic factors in infants with posterior urethral valves. *J Urol* 1986; 135:121.

Hulbert WC, Rosenberg HK, Cartwright PC, et al: The predictive value of ultrasonography in evaluation of infants with posterior urethral valves. *J Urol* 1992; 148:122.

Hunt CE: Abnormal hypercarbic and hypoxic sleep arousal responses in near-miss SIDS infants. *Pediatr Res* 1981; 15:1462.

Hutch JA: Aberrant micturition. *J Urol* 1966; 96:743.

Hutchinson DL, Gray MJ, Plentl AA, et al: The role of the fetus in the water exchange of the amniotic fluid of normal and hydramniotic patients. *J Clin Invest* 1959; 38:971.

Hutton KAR, Thomas DFM, Arthur RJ, et al: Prenatally detected posterior urethral valves: is gestational age at detection a predictor of outcome. *J Urol* 1994; 152:698.

Inati MN, Lazar EC, Haskin-Leahy L: The role of the genetic counselor in a perinatal unit. *Semin Perinatol* 1994; 18:133.

Inselman LS, Mellins RB: Growth and development of the lung. *J Pediatr* 1981; 98:1.

Janovsky M, Martinek J, Stanincova V: Antidiuretic activity in the plasma of human infants after a load of sodium chloride. *Acta Paediatr Scand* 1965; 54:543.

Jeanty P, Dramaix-Wilmet M, Elkhazen N, et al: Measurement of fetal kidney growth on ultrasound. *Radiology* 1982; 144:159.

Jee LD, Rickwood AMK, Williams MPL, et al: Experience with duplex system anomalies detected by prenatal ultrasonography. *J Urol* 1993; 149:808.

Jerkins GR, Noe HN, Hollabaugh RS, et al: Spermatic cord torsion in the neonate. *J Urol* 1983; 129:121.

Jobin J, O'Regan S, Demay G, et al: Neonatal renal vein thrombosis: long-term follow-up after conservative management. *Clin Nephrol* 1982; 17:36.

John E, Goldsmith DI, Spitzer A: Developmental changes in glomerular vasculature: physiologic implications. *Clin Res* 1980; 28:450A.

Johnson CE, Elder JS, Judge NE, et al: The accuracy of antenatal ultrasonography in identifying renal abnormalities. *Am J Dis Child* 1992; 146:1181.

Jones CT: Endocrine function of the placenta. *Baillieres Clin Endocrinol Metab* 1988; 3:755.

Jones C, Millan MA, Naftolin F, et al: Characterization of angiotensin II receptors in the rat fetus. *Peptides* 1989; 10:459.

Jordan GH, Hoover DL: Inadequate decompression of the upper tracts using a Foley catheter in the valve bladder. *J Urol* 1985; 134:137.

Josephson S: Experimental obstructive hydronephrosis in newborn rats: III. Long-term effects on renal function. *J Urol* 1983; 129:396.

Josephson S, Ericson AC, Sjoquist M: Experimental obstructive hydronephrosis in newborn rats: VI. Long-term effects on glomerular filtration and distribution. *J Urol* 1985; 134:391.

Josephson S, Robertson B, Claesson G, et al: Experimental obstructive hydronephrosis in newborn rats: I. Surgical technique and long-term morphologic effects. *Invest Urol* 1980; 17:478.

Josephson S, Wolgast M, Ojteg G: Experimental obstructive hydronephrosis in newborn rats: II. Long-term effects on renal blood flow distribution. *Scand J Urol Nephrol* 1982; 16:179.

Kalicinsky ZH, Kansy J, Kotarbinska B, et al: Surgery of megaureters-modification of Hendren's operation. *J Pediatr Surg* 1977; 12:183.

Kaplan GW: Complications of circumcision. *Urol Clin North Am* 1983; 10:543.

Karlowicz MG, Katz ME, Adelman RD, et al: Nephrocalcinosis in very low birth weight neonates: family history of kidney stones and ethnicity as independent risk factors. *J Urol* 1993; 122:635.

Kass EJ, Majd M: Evaluation and management of upper urinary tract obstruction in infancy and childhood. *Urol Clin North Am* 1985; 12:133.

Kay R, Strong DW, Tank ES: Bilateral spermatic cord torsion in the neonate. *J Urol* 1980; 123:293.

Keating MA, Escala J, Snyder H, et al: Changing concepts in management of primary obstructive megaureter. *J Urol* 1989; 142:636.

Kessler II: Etiological concepts in cervical carcinogenesis. *Gynecol Oncol* 1991; 12:S7.

Khuri FJ, Alton DJ, Hardy BE, et al: Adrenal hemorrhage in neonates: report of 5 cases and review of the literature. *J Urol* 1980; 124:684.

King LR: Fetal hydronephrosis: what is the urologist to do? *Urology* 1993; 42:229.

King LR, Coughlin PWF, Bloch EC, et al: The case for immediate pyeloplasty in the neonate with ureteropelvic junction obstruction. *J Urol* 1984; 132:725.

Kirya C, Werthman M: Neonatal circumcision and dorsal penile nerve block: a painless procedure. *J Pediatr* 1978; 92:998.

Klaus MH, Kennell JH: *Maternal-Infant Bonding*. St Louis, Mosby, 1976.

Klaus MH, Kennell JH: Parent-infant bonding, ed 2, St Louis, Mosby, 1982.

Klaus MH, Kennell JH: Parent-to-infant bonding: Setting the record straight. *J Pediatr* 1983; 102:575.

Klein DJ, et al: Chondroitin sulfate proteoglycan synthesis and reutilization by B-D Xyloside-initiated chondroitin/dermatan sulfate glycosaminoglycans in the fetal kidney branching morphogenesis. *Dev Biol* 1989; 133:515.

Kleiner B, Callen PW, Filly RA: Sonographic analysis of the fetus with ureteropelvic junction obstruction. *Am J Radiol* 1987; 148:359.

Kleiner B, Filly RA, Mack L, et al: Multicystic dysplastic kidney: observations of contralateral disease in the fetal population. *Radiology* 1986; 161:27.

Koff SA, Campbell KD: Non-operative management of unilateral neonatal hydronephrosis: natural history of poorly functioning kidneys. *J Urol* 1994; 152:593.

Koff SA, McDowell GC, Byard M: Diuretic radionuclide assessment of obstruction in the infant: guidelines for successful interpretation. *J Urol* 1988; 140;1167.

Korsch BM: More on parent-infant bonding. *J Pediatr* 1983; 102:249.

Kotchen TA, Strickland AL, Rice TW, et al: A study of the renin-angiotensin system in newborn infants. *J Pediatr* 1972; 80:938.

Koyle MA, Ehrlich RM: Management of ureteropelvic junction obstruction in neonate. *Urology* 1988; 31:496.

Kozinn PJ, Taschdjian CL, Goldberg PK, et al: Advances in the diagnosis of renal candidiasis. *J Urol* 1978; 119:184.

Krober MS, Bass JW, Powell JM, et al: Bacterial and viral pathogens causing fever in infants less than 3 months old. *Am Dis Child* 1985; 139:889.

Krueger RP, Hardy BE, Churchill BM: Growth in boys with posterior urethral valves. Primary valve resection vs upper tract diversion. *Urol Clin North Am* 1980; 7:265.

Krueger TC, Neblett WW, O'Neill JA, et al: Management of aortic thrombosis secondary to umbilical artery catheters in neonates. *J Pediatr Surg* 1985; 20:328.

Kurjak A, Kirkinen P, Latin V, et al: Ultrasonic assessment of fetal kidney function in normal and complicated pregnancies. *Am J Obstet Gynecol* 1981; 141:266.

Kurjak A, Latin V, Mandruzzato G, et al: Ultrasound diagnosis and perinatal management of fetal genitourinary abnormalities. *J Perinatol Med* 1984; 12:291.

Kurth CD, Spitzer AR, Broennle AM, et al: Postoperative apnea in preterm infants. *Anesthesiology* 1987; 66:483.

Laing FC, Burke VD, Wing VW, et al: Postpartum evaluation of fetal hydronephrosis: optimal timing for follow-up sonography. *Radiology* 1984; 152:423.

Lamb ME: Early contact and maternal-infant bonding: one decade later. *Pediatrics* 1982; 70:763.

Lamb ME, Hwang CP: Maternal attachment and mother-neonate bonding: a critical review. In Lamb ME, Brown AL (eds): *Advances in Developmental Psychology*, vol 2, Hillsdale, NJ, Erlbaum, 1982.

Land JA Jr, Policastro AM: Parental information and circumcision: another look (letter). *Pediatrics* 1983; 72:142.

Landers C, Hansen TM: Pulmonary problems associated with congenital renal malformation. In Gonzales ET Jr, Roth D (eds): *Common Problems in Pediatric Urology*. St Louis, Mosby, 1991, ch 9, pp 85-98.

Laouari D, Kleinknecht C: The role of nutritional factors in the course of experimental renal failure. *Am J Kidney Dis* 1985; 5:147.

LaQuaglia MP, Bauer SB, Eraklis A, et al: Bilateral neonatal torsion. *J Urol* 1987; 138:1051.

Lawson TL, Fowley WD, Berland LL, et al: Ultrasonic evaluation of fetal kidneys: analysis of normal size and frequency of visualization related to stage of pregnancy. *Radiology* 1981; 138:153.

Lebowitz JM, Belman AB: Simultaneous idiopathic adrenal hemorrhage and renal vein thrombosis in the newborn. *J Urol* 1983; 129:574.

Lebowitz RL, Blickman JG: The coexistence of ureteropelvic junction obstruction and reflux. *Am J Radiol* 1983; 140:231.

Lebowitz RL, Griscom NT: Neonatal hydronephrosis: 146 cases. *Radiol Clin North Am* 1977; 15:49.

Leonidas JC, Berdon WE, Gribetz D: Bilateral renal cortical necrosis in the newborn infant: roentgenographic diagnosis. *J Pediatr* 1971; 79:623.

Leung AKC, Robson WLM: Single umbilical artery. A report of 159 cases. *Am J Dis Child* 1989; 143:108.

Levin M, Barratt TM: Haemolytic uraemic syndrome. *Arch Dis Child* 1984; 59:397.

Levy DA, Abdul-Karim FW, Miraldi FS, Elder JS: Effect of human chorionic gonadotropin before spermatic vessel ligation in prepubertal rat testis. *J Urol* 1995; 154:738.

LiPuma JP, Haaga JR, Bryan PJ, et al: Percutaneous nephrostomy in neonates and infants. *J Urol* 1984; 132:722.

Liu LMP, Cote CJ, Goudsouzian NG, et al: Life-threatening apnea in infants recovering from anesthesia. *Anesthesiology* 1983; 59:506.

Lloyd DA: Renal vein thrombosis. In Welch KJ, Randolph JG, Ravitch MM, et al (eds): *Pediatric Surgery*, ed 4. Chicago, Year Book Medical Publishers, 1986, vol 2, p 1146.

Lofland GK, Russo P, Sethia B, et al: Aortic thrombosis in neonates and infants. *Am Surg* 1988; 208:743.

Lorenz R and Kuhn M: Multidisciplinary team counseling for fetal anomalies. *Am J Obstet Gynecol* 1989; 161:263.

Lotgering FK, Wallenburg HCS: Mechanisms of production and clearance of amniotic fluid. *Semin Perinatal* 1986; 10:94.

Lurz H: Ein muskelschonender Lumbalschnitt zur Freilegung der Nieren. *Chirurgie* 1956; 27:125.

Lynch MA, Roberts J: Predicting child abuse: signs of bonding failure in the maternity hospital. *Br Med J* 1977; 1:624.

Mackie GG, Stephens FD: Duplex kidneys: a correlation of renal dysplasia with position of the ureteral orifice. *J Urol* 1975; 114:274.

Mahoney BS, Filly RA, Callen PW, et al: Sonographic evaluation of fetal renal dysplasia. *Radiology* 1984; 152:143.

Maisels MJ, Hayes B, Conrad S, et al: Circumcision: the effect of information on parental decision-making. *Pediatrics* 1983; 71:453.

Maizels M, Mitchell B, Kass E, et al: Outcome of nonspecific hydronephrosis in the infant: a report from the registry of the Society for Fetal Urology. *J Urol* 1994; 152:2324.

Maizels M, Reisman ME, Flom ES, et al: Grading nephroureteral dilatation detected in the first year of life: correlation with obstruction. *J Urol* 1992; 148:609.

Maizels M, Smith CK, Firlit CF: The management of children with vesicoureteral reflux and ureteropelvic junction obstruction. *J Urol* 1984; 131:722.

Malek RS, Kelalis PP: Pediatric nephrolithiasis. *J Urol* 1975; 113:545.

Malin SW, Baumgart S, Rosenberg HK, et al: Nonsurgical management of obstructive aortic thrombosis complicated by renovascular hypertension in the neonate. *J Pediatr* 1985; 106:630.

Mandell J: Early postnatal reconstruction of UPJ obstruction diagnosed in utero. *Dial Pediatr Urol* 1985; 8:3.

Mandell J, Blyth B, Peter CA, et al: The natural history of structural genitourinary defects detected in utero. *Radiology* 1991; 178:194.

Mandell J, Greene MF, et al: Fetal abdominal wall defect: a new complication of vesicoamniotic shunting. *Fetal Diagn Ther* 1991; VI:111.

Mandell J, Kinard HW, Mittelstaedt CA, et al: Prenatal diagnosis of unilateral hydronephrosis with early postnatal reconstruction. *J Urol* 1984; 132:303.

Mandell J, Lebowitz RL, Peters CA, et al: Prenatal diagnosis of the megacystis-megaureter association. *J Urol* 1992a; 148:1487.

Mandell J, Peters CA, Estroff JA, et al: Late onset severe oligohydramnios associated with genitourinary anomalies. *J Urol* 1992b; 148:515.

Mandell G, Peters CA, Retik AB: Current concepts in the prenatal diagnosis and management of hydronephrosis. *Urol Clin North Am* 1990; 17:247.

Mann CM, Leape LL, Holder TM: Neonatal urinary ascites: report of 2 cases of unusual etiology and a review of the literature. *J Urol* 1974; 111:124.

Manning FA, Harman CR, Lange IR, et al: Antepartum chronic fetal vesicoamniotic shunts for obstructive uropathy: a report of two cases. *Am J Obstet Gynecol* 1983; 145:819.

Manning FA, Harrison MR, Rodeck CH, et al: Catheter shunts for fetal hydronephrosis and hydrocephalus. Report of the International Fetal Surgery Registry. *N Engl J Med* 1986; 315:336.

Marano HE: Biology is one key to the bonding of mothers and babies. *Smithsonian*, Feb 1981, p 63.

Marras A, Mereu G, Dessi C, et al: Oligohydramnios and extrarenal abnormalities in Potter's syndrome. *J Pediatr* 1983; 102:597.

Marsh JL, King W, Barrett C, et al: Serious complications after umbilical artery catheterization for neonatal monitoring. *Arch Surg* 1975; 110:1203.

Marwick C: Coming to terms with indications for fetal surgery. *JAMA* 1993; 270(17):2025.

Marx JL: Circumcision may protect against the AIDS virus. *Science* 1989; 245:470.

Masciello A: Anesthesia for neonatal circumcision: local anesthesia is better than dorsal penile nerve block. *Obstet Gynecol* 1990; 75:834.

Mathew OP, Jones AS, James E, et al: Neonatal renal failure: usefulness of diagnostic indices. *Pediatrics* 1980; 65:57.

Matsumoto T, Kondoh T, Kamei T, et al: Prenatal DNA analysis in four embryos/fetuses at risk of 21-hydroxylase deficiency. *Eur J Pediatr* 1988; 148:288.

Matthews DE, West KW, Rescorla FJ: Peritoneal dialysis in the first 60 days of life. *J Pediatr Surg* 1990; 25:110.

Mazer MJ, Bartone FF: Percutaneous antegrade diagnosis and management of candidiasis of the upper urinary tract. *Urol Clin North Am* 1982; 9:157.

McCance RA, Naylor NJB, Widdowson EM: The response of infants to a large dose of water. *Arch Dis Child* 1954; 29:104.

McCance RA, Widdowson EM: Renal function before birth. *Proc R Soc Lond* 1953; 141:488.

McCrory WW: *Developmental Renal Function in Utero.* Cambridge, Harvard University Press, 1972, pp 51-78.

McCrory WW: Regulation of renal functional development. *Urol Clin North Am* 1980; 7:243.

McCurdy FA: Renal functional development with an approach to the evaluation of the obstructed urinary tract. *AUA Update Series* 1983; 3:1.

McFayden IR, Wigglesworth GS, Dillon MG: Fetal urinary tract obstruction: is active intervention before delivery indicated? *J Obstet Gynecol* 1983; 90:342.

McHugo Jm, Shafi MI, Rowlands D, et al: Pre-natal diagnosis of adult polycystic kidney disease. *Br J Radiol* 1988; 61:1072.

McInnis AN, Felman AH, Kaude JV, et al: Renal ultrasound in the neonatal period. *Pediatr Radiol* 1982; 12:15.

Meeks ACG, Sims DG: Treatment of renal failure in neonates. *Arch Dis Child* 1988; 63:1372.

Mercer LJ, Brown LG, Petres RE, et al: A survey of pregnancies complicated by decreased amniotic fluid. *Am J Obstet Gynecol* 1984; 149:355.

Merritt JC, Sprague DH, Merritt WE, et al: Retrolental fibroplasia: a multifactorial disease. *Anesth Analg* 1981; 60:109.

Metreweli C, Pearson R: Echographic diagnosis of neonatal renal venous thrombosis. *Pediatr Radiol* 1984; 14:105.

Michigan S: Genitourinary fungal infections. *J Urol* 1976; 116:390.

Mikkelsen SS, Rasmussen BS, Jensen TM, et al: Long-term follow-up of patients with hydronephrosis treated by Anderson-Hynes pyeloplasty. *Br J Urol* 1992; 79:121.

Miller ME, Higginbottom M, Smith DW: Short umbilical cord: its origin and relevance. *Pediatrics* 1981; 67:618.

Mishriki SF, Winkle AC, Frank JD: Fixation of a single testis: always, sometimes, or never. *Br J Urol* 1992; 69:311.

Molteni RA, Stys SJ, Battaglice FC: Relationship of fetal and placental weight in human beings: fetal/placental weight ratios at various gestational ages and birth weight distributions. *J Reprod Med* 1978; 21:327.

Moore ES, Galvez MB, Paton JB, et al: Effects of positive pressure ventilation on intrarenal blood flow in infant primates. *Pediatr Res* 1974; 8:792.

Moore KL: *The Developing Human. Clinically Oriented Embryology*, ed 3. Philadelphia, WB Saunders Co, 1982.

Moore TR, Coyle GA: The amniotic fluid index normal human pregnancy. *Am J Obstet Gynecol* 1990; 162:168.

Morin L, Cendrom M, Crombleholm TM, et al: Minimal hydronephrosis in the fetus: clinical significance and implication for management. *J Urol* (in press).

Muller F, Dommergues M, Mandelbrot L, et al: Fetal urinary biochemistry predicts postnatal renal function in children with bilateral obstructive uropathy. *Obstet Gynecol* 1993; 82:813.

Murphy JP, Holder TM, Ashcraft KE, et al: Ureteropelvic junction obstruction in the newborn. *J Pediatr Surg* 1984; 19:642.

Museles M, Gaudry CL Jr, Bason WM: Renal anomalies in the newborn found by deep palpation. *Pediatrics* 1971; 47:97.

Naeye RL: Umbilical cord length: clinical significance. *J Pediatr* 1985; 107:278.

Najmaldin A, Burge DM, Atwell JD: Fetal vesicoureteral reflux. *Br J Urol* 1990; 65:403.

Nakamura KT, Matherne GP, McWeeny OS, et al: Renal hemodynamics and functional changes during the transition from fetal to postnatal life in conscious sheep. *Pediatr Res* 1986; 20:452A.

Nakayama DK, Harrison MR, deLorimer AA: Prognosis of posterior urethral valves presenting at birth. *J Pediatr Surg* 1986; 21:43.

Nesbitt TE, King LR: Zirkumzision. In Hohenfellner R, Thuroff JW, Schulte-Wisserman M (eds): *Kinderurologie in Klinik und Praxis*. Stuttgart, New York, Thieme, 1986, p 522.

Nicolini U, Fisk NM, Rodeck CM, et al: Fetal urine biochemistry: an index of renal maturation and dysfunction. *Am J Obstet Gynecol* 1992a; 99:46.

Nicolini U, Fisk NM, Rodeck CH, et al: Fetal urine biochemistry: an index of renal maturation and dysfunction. *Obstet Gynecol* 1993; 82:813.

Nielander AJM, Bode WA, Heidendal GAK: Renography in diagnosis and follow-up of renal vein thrombosis. *Clin Nucl Med* 1983; 8:56.

Nimrod C, Varela-Gittings F, Machin G, et al: The effect of very prolonged membrane rupture on fetal development. *Am J Obstet Gynecol* 1984; 148:540.

Noe HN, Bryant JF, Roy S III, et al: Urolithiasis in preterm neonates associated with furosemide therapy. *J Urol* 1984; 132:93.

Noe NH, Magill HL: Progression of mild ureteropelvic junction obstruction in infancy. *Urology* 1987; 30:348.

Norman ME, Asadi FK: A prospective study of acute renal failure in the newborn infant. *Pediatrics* 1979; 63:475.

O'Connor S, Vietze PM, Sherrod KB, et al: Reduced incidence of parenting inadequacy following rooming-in. *Pediatrics* 1980; 66:176.

Oddone M, Marino C, Sergi C, et al: Wilms' tumor arising in a multicystic kidney. *Pediatr Radiol* 1994; 24:236.

Oelberg DG, Fisher DJ, Gross DM, et al: Endocarditis in high-risk neonates. *Pediatrics* 1983; 71:392.

Oesch I, Jann X, Bettex M: Ultrasonographic antenatal detection of obstructed bladder: diagnosis and management. *Eur Urol* 1982; 8:78.

Ohlsson R: Growth factors, protooncogenes and human placental development. *Cell Differ Dev* 1989; 28:1.

Olbing H, Blaufox MD, Aschinberg LC, et al: Postnatal changes in renal glomerular blood flow distribution in puppies. *J Clin Invest* 1973; 52:2885.

Oliver J: *Nephrons and Kidneys*. New York, Harper & Row, 1968.

O'Neill JA Jr, Neblett WW III, Born ML: Management of major thromboembolic complications of umbilical artery catheters. *J Pediatr Surg* 1981; 16:972.

Oppenheimer DA, Carroll BA, Yousem S: Sonography of the normal neonatal adrenal gland. *Radiology* 1983; 146:157.

O'Reilly PH: Diuresis renography eight years later: update. *J Urol* 1986; 136:993.

O'Reilly PH, Lawson RS, Shields RA, et al: Idiopathic hydronephrosis—the diuresis renogram: a new noninvasive method of assessing equivocal pelvioureteral junction obstruction. *J Urol* 1979; 121:153.

O'Reilly PH, Testa HJ, Lawson RS, et al: Diuresis renography in equivocal urinary tract obstruction. *Br J Urol* 1978; 50:76.

Osathanondh V, Potter EL: Development of human kidneys as shown by microdissection: I. Preparation of tissue with reasons for possible misinterpretations of observations. II. Renal pelvis, calyces, and papillae. III. Formation and interrelationship of collecting tubules and nephrons. *Arch Pathol* 1963; 76:1271.

Ostling K: The genesis of hydronephrosis particularly with regard to the changes at the ureteropelvic junction. *Acta Chir Scand (Suppl)* 1942; 86:72.

Pang S, Pollack MS, Marshall RN, et al: Prenatal treatment of congenital adrenal hyperplasia due to 21-hydroxylase deficiency. *N Engl J Med* 1990; 322:111.

Pansadoro V: The posterior lumbotomy. *Urol Clin North Am* 1983; 10:573.

Pappu LD, Purohit DM, Bradford BF, et al: Primary renal candidiasis in two preterm neonates. Report of cases and review of literature on renal candidiasis in infancy. *Am J Dis Child* 1984; 138:934.

Parker RM: Neonatal urinary ascites: a potentially favorable sign in bladder outlet obstruction. *Urology* 1974; 3:589.

Parkhouse HF, Barratt TM, Dillon MJ, et al: Long-term outcome of boys with posterior urethral valves. *Br J Urol* 1988; 62:59.

Parkhouse HF, Barratt TM, Dillon MJ, et al: Long-term status of patients with posterior urethral valves. *Urol Clin North Am* 1990; 17:373.

Parmley TH. Seeds AE: Fetal skin permeability to isotopic water (THO) in early pregnancy. *Am J Obstet Gynecol* 1970; 108:128.

Pathak IG, Williams DI: Multicystic and cystic dysplastic kidneys. *Br J Urol* 1964; 36:318.

Patten RM, Mack LA, Wang KY, et al: The fetal genitourinary tract. *Radiol Clin North Am* 1990; 28:115.

Perez LM, Friedman RM, King LR: The case for relief of ureteropelvic junction obstruction in neonates and young children at time of diagnosis. *Urology* 1991; 38:195.

Perlman M, Williams J: Detection of renal anomalies by abdominal palpation in newborn infants. *Br Med J* 1976; 2:347.

Perlmutter AD, Kroovand RL, Lai YW: Management of ureteropelvic obstruction in the first year of life. *J Urol* 1980; 123:535.

Pery M, Kaftori JK, Bar-Maor JA: Sonography for diagnosis and follow-up of neonatal adrenal hemorrhage. *J Clin Ultrasound* 1981; 9:397.

Peterson RG, Simmons MA, Rumack BH, et al: Pharmacology of furosemide in the premature newborn infant. *J Pediatr* 1980; 97:139.

Pickworth FE, Vivian GC, Franklin K, et al: ^{99m}Tc-mercapto acetyl triglycine in paediatric renal tract disease. *Br J Rad* 1992; 65:21.

Philipson EH, Sokal RJ, Williams T: Oligohydramnios: clinical associations and pediatric value for intrauterine growth retardation. *Am J Obstet Gynecol* 1983; 146:271.

Platt JF: Duplex doppler evaluation of native kidney dysfunction: obstruction and non-obstructive disease. *Am J Radiol* 1992; 158:1035.

Plummer LB, Kaplan GW, Mendoza SA: Hypertension in infants—a complication of umbilical artery catheterization. *J Pediatr* 1976; 89:802.

Poland RL: The question of routine neonatal circumcision. *N Engl J Med* 1990; 322:1312.

Pollack MS, Levine LS, Pang S, et al: Prenatal diagnosis of congenital adrenal hyperplasia (21-hydroxylase deficiency) by HLA typing. *Lancet* 1979; 1:1107.

Potter EL: Bilateral absence of ureters and kidneys. *Obstet Gynecol* 1965; 25:3.

Potter EL: *Normal and Abnormal Development of the Kidney*. Chicago, Year Book Medical Publishers, 1972.

Queenan JT: Polyhydramnios and oligohydramnios. In Fanaroff AA, Martin RJ (eds): *Behrman's Neonatal-Perinatal Medicine: Diseases of the Fetus and Infant*. St Louis, Mosby, 1983, p 44.

Queenan JT, Gadow EC: Polyhydramnios: chronic versus acute. *Am J Obstet Gynecol* 1970; 108:349.

Queenan JT, Thompson W, Whitfield CR, et al: Amniotic fluid volume in normal pregnancies. *Am J Obstet Gynecol* 1972; 114:34.

Quinn GE, Betts EK, Diamond GR, et al: Neonatal age (human) at retinal maturation. *Anesthesiology* 1981; 55:A326.

Quintero RA, Hume R, Smith C, et al: In utero endoscopic treatment of posterior urethral valves. Presented 13th International Fetal Medicine and Surgery Society, May 1994, Antwerp, Belgium.

Rabinovich S, Shaw BD, Bryant T, et al: Effect of 5-flurocytosine and emphotericin B on *Candida albicans* infection in mice. *J Infect Dis* 1974; 130:28.

Rabinowitz R, Peters MT, Vyas S, et al: Measurement of fetal urine production in normal pregnancy by real-time ultrasonography. *Am J Obstet Gynecol* 1989; 161:1264.

Rackley R, Angermeier KW, Levin H, et al: Renal cell carcinoma arising in a regressed multicystic dysplastic kidney. *J Urol* 1994; 152:1543.

Raffensperger J, Abousleiman A: Abdominal masses in children under one year of age. *Surgery* 1968; 63:514.

Rahman N, Boineau FG, Lewy JE: Renal failure in the perinatal period. *Clin Perinatol* 1981; 8:241.

Ransley P: Personal communication, 1992.

Ransley PG, Dhillon HK, Gordon I, et al: The postnatal management of hydronephrosis diagnosed by prenatal ultrasound. *J Urol* 1990; 144:584.

Rasoulpour M, McLean RH: Renal venous thrombosis in neonates. initial and follow-up abnormalities. *Am J Dis Child* 1980; 134:276.

Redman HF, Jimenez JF, Golladay ES, et al: Megacystis-microcolon-intestinal hypoperistalsis syndrome: case report and review of the literature. *J Urol* 1984; 131:981.

Redman JF: Rare penile anomalies presenting with complication of circumcision. *Urology* 1988; 32:130.

Redman JF, Seibert JJ, Arnold W: Urinary ascites in children owing to extravasation of urine from the bladder. *J Urol* 1979; 122:409.

Reitelman C, Perlmutter AD: Management of obstructing ectopic ureteroceles. *Urol Clin North Am* 1990; 17(2):317.

Renert WA, Berdon WE, Baker DH, et al: Obstructive urologic malformations of the fetus and infant—relation to neonatal pneumomediastinum and pneumothorax (air block). *Radiology* 1972; 105:97.

Reznick VM, Kaplan GW, Murphy G, et al: Follow up of infants with bilateral renal disease detected in utero. *Am J Dis Child* 1988; 142:453.

Ricci MA, Lloyd DA: Renal venous thrombosis in infants and children. *Arch Surg* 1990; 125:1195.

Ringler NM, Kennell JH, Jarnella R, et al: Mother-to-child speech at 2 years—effects of early postnatal contact. *J Pediatr* 1975; 86:141.

Ringler N, Trause MA, Klaus M: Mother's speech to her two-year old: its effect on speech and language comprehension at 5 years. *Pediatr Res* 1976; 10:307.

Risaun W and Ekblom P: Production of a heparin-binding angiogenesis factor by the embryonic kidney. *J Cell Biol* 1986; 103:1101.

Risdon RA: Renal dysplasia: a clinico-pathological study of 76 cases. *J Clin Path* 1975; 24:57.

Risdon RA: Renal dysplasia: a clinico-pathological study of 76 cases. *J Clin Path* 1975; 24:57.

Risdon RA, Godley ML, Gordon I, Ransley PG: Renal pathology and ⁹⁹ᵐTc-DMSA image before and after treatment of evolving pyelonephritic scar: experimental study. *J Urol* 1994; 152:1260.

Rittenberg MH, Hulbert WC, Snyder HM, et al: Protective factors in posterior urethral valves. *J Urol* 1988; 140:993.

Roberts JA: Does circumcision prevent urinary tract infections? *J Urol* 1986; 135:991.

Robichaux AG, Mandell J, Greene MF, et al: Fetal abdominal wall defect: a new complication of vesical amniotic shunting. *Fetal Diagn Ther* 1991; VI:11.

Robillard JE, Sessions C, Burmeister L, et al: Influence of fetal extracellular volume contraction on renal reabsorption of bicarbonate in fetal lambs. *Pediatr Res* 1977; 11:649.

Robillard JE, Smith FG, Segar JL, et al: Renal function in the fetus. In Thronburn GD, Harding R (eds): *Textbook of Fetal Physiology*. Oxford, England, Oxford University Press, 1994, pp 196-204.

Robillard JE, Weissman DN, Herin P: Ontogeny of single glomerular perfusion rate in fetal and newborn lambs. *Pediatr Res* 1981; 15:1248.

Robson WJ, Rudy SM, Johnston JH: Pelviureteric obstruction in infancy. *J Pediatr Surg* 1976; 11:57.

Rodriguez-Soriano J, Vallo A, Castillo G, et al: Renal handling of water and sodium in infancy and childhood: a study using clearance methods during hypotonic saline diuresis. *Kidney Int* 1981; 20:700.

Romberg R: *Circumcision: The Painful Dilemma*. South Hadley, Mass, Bergin & Garvey Publishers, 1985.

Romero R, Cullen M, Grannum P, et al: Antenatal diagnosis of renal anomalies with ultrasound: III. Bilateral renal agenesis. *Am J Obstet Gynecol* 1985; 151:38.

Romero R, Cullen M, Jeanty P, et al: The diagnosis of congenital renal anomalies with ultrasound: II. Infantile polycystic kidney disease. *Am J Obstet Gynecol* 1984; 150:259.

Ronderos-Dumit D, Nicolini U, Vaughan J, et al: Uterine-peritoneal amniotic fluid leakage: an unusual complication of intrauterine shunting. *Obstet Gynecol* 1991; 78:1913.

Roodhooft AM, Birnholz JC, Holmes LB: Familial nature of congenital absence and severe dysgenesis of both kidneys. *N Engl J Med* 1984; 310:1341.

Rosenberg HK, Snyder HM III, Duckett J: Abdominal mass in a newborn: multicystic dysplasia of crossed fused renal ectopia—ultrasonic demonstration. *J Urol* 1984; 131:1160.

Rosenfield AT, Taylor KJW, Jaffe CC: Clinical applications of ultrasound tissue characterization. *Radiol Clin North Am* 1980; 18:31.

Ross J, Elder JS: Much said, little settled about circumcision. *Contemp Urol* Nov 1991, pp 32-45.

Roth DR, Gonzales ET Jr: Management of ureteropelvic junction obstruction in infants. *J Urol* 1983; 129:108.

Royer P: The kidney in the newborn. In Royer P, Habib R, Mathieu H, et al (eds): *Pediatric Nephrology*. Philadelphia, WB Saunders Co, 1974, pp 116-127.

Ruano-Gil D, Coca-Payeras A, Tejedo-Mateu A: Obstruction and normal recanalization of the ureter in the human embryo. Its relation to congenital ureteric obstruction. *Eur Urol* 1975; 1:287.

Rubin MI, Bruck E, Rappoport M: Maturation of renal function in childhood: clearance studies. *J Clin Invest* 1949; 28:1144.

Rudolph AM, Heyman MA: Fetal and neonatal circulation and respiration. *Ann Rev Physiol* 1974; 36:187.

Rushton HG, Majd M, Chandra R, et al: Evaluation of ⁹⁹ᵐDMSA renal scans in experimental acute pyelonephritis in piglets. *J Urol* 1988; 140:1169.

Rushton HG, Parrott TS, Woodard JR, et al: The role of vesicostomy in the management of anterior urethral valves in neonates and infants. *J Urol* 1987; 138:107.

Rushton HG, Salem Y, Belman AB, et al: Pediatric pyeloplasty: is routine retrograde pyelography necessary? *J Urol* 1994; 152:604.

Russell CD, Thorstad B, Yester MV, et al: Comparison of technetium ⁹⁹ᵐMAG-3 with iodine-131 hippuran by a simultaneous dual channel technique. *J Nucl Med* 1988; 29:1189.

Sadowski RH, Harmon WE, Jalse K: Acute hemodialysis of infants weighing less than five kilograms. *Kidney Int* 1994; 45:903.

Samparo FJB, Aragao AHM: Study of the fetal kidney length growth during the second and third trimesters of gestation. *Eur Urol* 1989; 25:4.

Sanders RC, Hartman DS: The sonographic distinction between neonatal multicystic kidney and hydronephrosis. *Radiology* 1984; 151:621.

Saunders P, Rhodes P: The origin and circulation of the amniotic fluid. In Fairweather DVI, Eskes TKAB (eds): *Amniotic Fluid. Research and Clinical Application*. Amsterdam, Excerpta Medic, 1975; pp 1-18.

Savin VJ: Ultrafiltration in single isolated human glomeruli. *Kidney Int* 1983; 24:748.

Saxen L, Sariola H: Early organogenesis of the kidney. *Pediatr Nephrol* 1987; 1:385.

Schlondorff D, Weber H, Trizna W, et al: Vasopressin responsiveness of renal adenylate cyclase in newborn rats and rabbits. *Am J Physiol* 1978; 234:F16.

Schmitmeijer RT, Van der Harten JJ: Unilateral multicystic kidney and contralateral hydronephrosis in the newborn. *Br J Urol* 1975; 47:176.

Schoen EJ: The relationship between circumcision and cancer of the penis. *Cancer J Clinicians* 1991; 41:306.

Schoen EJ, Anderson G, Bohon C, et al: Report on the Task Force on Circumcision. *Pediatrics* 1989; 84:388.

Schreiber JR, Maynard E, Lew MA: *Candida* antigen detection in two premature neonates with disseminated candidiasis. *Pediatrics* 1984; 74:838.

Schwartz GJ, Feld LG, Langford DJ: A simple estimate of glomerular filtration rate in full-term infants during the first year of life. *J Pediatr* 1984; 104:849.

Schwartz GJ, Gauthier B: A simple estimate of glomerular filtration rate in adolescent boys. *J Pediatr* 1985; 106:522.

Schwartz GJ, Haycock GB, Edelmann CM Jr, et al: A simple estimate of glomerular filtration rate in children derived from body length and plasma creatinine. *Pediatrics* 1976; 58:259.

Schwartz RD, Stephens FD, Cussen LJ: The pathogenesis of renal dysplasia: II. The significance of lateral and medial ectopy of the ureteral orifice. *Invest Urol* 1981; 19:97.

Scott JES: Fetal ureteric reflux. *Br J Urol* 1987; 59:291.

Scott JE, Lee REJ, Hunter EW, et al: Ultrasound screening of newborn urinary tract. *Lancet* 1991; 338:1571.

Scott TW: Urinary ascites secondary to posterior urethral valves. *J Urol* 1976; 116:87.

Seeds AE: Current concepts of amniotic fluid dynamics. *Am J Obstet Gynecol* 1985; 138:575.

Selzman AA, Elder JS: Vesicoureteral reflux in children with a multicystic kidney. *J Urol* 1995; 153:1252.

Selzman AR, Elder JS, Magstone TB: Urologic consequences of myelodysplasia and other congenital abnormalities of the spinal cord. *Urol Clin North Am* 1993; 42:620.

Sariola H, Peault B, LeDouarin et al: Extra-cellular matrix and capillary ingrowth in interspecies chimeric kidneys. *Cell Differ* 1984; 15:43.

Shaheen E, Alexander D, Truskowsky M, et al: Failure to thrive—a retrospective profile. *Clin Pediatr* 1968; 7:255.

Shannon DC, Kelly DH: SIDS and near-SIDS (first of two parts). *N Engl J Med* 1982a; 306:959.

Shannon DC, Kelly DH: SIDS and near-SIDS (second of two parts). *N Engl J Med* 1982b; 306:1022.

Shannon DC, Kelly DH, O'Connell K: Abnormal regulation of ventilation in infants at risk for sudden-infant-death syndrome. *N Engl J Med* 1977; 297:747.

Sheldon CA, Duckett JW: Infant pyeloplasty. *AUA Update Series* 1988; 7:289.

Sheldon CA, Duckett JW, Snyder HM: Evolution in the management of infant pyeloplasty. *J Ped Urol* 1992; 27:501.

Sheldon CA, Elick B, Najarian JS, et al: Improving survival in the very young renal transplant recipient. *J Pediatr Surg* 1985; 20:622.

Sherry SN, Kramer I: The time of passage of the first stool and the first urine by the newborn infant. *J Pediatr* 1955; 46:158.

Sherwood DW, Smith RC, Lemmon RH, et al: Abnormalities of the genitourinary tract discovered by palpation of the abdomen of the newborn. *Pediatrics* 1956; 18:782.

Sholder AJ, Maizels M, Depp R: Cautious antenatal intervention. *J Urol* 1988; 139:1026.

Siegel NJ: Amino acids and adenine nucleotides in acute renal failure. In Brenner BM, Lazarus JN, Myers BD (eds): *Acute Renal Failure*. Philadelphia, WB Saunders Co, 1983, pp 741-752.

Siegel SR, Oh W: Renal function as a marker of human fetal maturation. *Acta Paediatr Scand* 1976; 65:481.

Simeoni U, Messer J, Weisburd P, et al: Neonatal renal dysfunction and intrauterine exposure to prostaglandin synthesis inhibitors. *Eur J Pediatr* 1989; 148:371.

Sivit CJ, Hill MC, Larsen JW, et al: The sonographic evaluation of fetal anomalies in oligohydramnios between 16 and 30 weeks' gestation. *AJR* 1986; 146:1277.

Smith FG, Nakamura KT, Segar JL, et al: Renal function in utero. In Polin RA, Fox WW (eds): *Fetal and Neo-*

natal Physiology. Philadelphia, WB Saunders, 1993, pp 1187-1195.

Smith FG, Robillard JE: Pathophysiology of fetal renal disease. *Semin Perinatol* 1989; 13:305.

Smith H, Congdon P: Neonatal systemic candidiasis. *Arch Dis Child* 1985; 60:365.

Smith JA Jr, Lee RE, Middleton RG: Hypertension in childhood from renal vein thrombosis. *J Urol* 1979; 122:389.

Smith JA, Middleton RG: Neonatal adrenal hemorrhage. *J Urol* 1979; 122:674.

Snyder HM III, Lebowitz RL, Colodny AG, et al: Ureteropelvic junction obstruction in children. *Urol Clin North Am* 1980; 7:273.

Solomon S, Hathaway S, Curb D: Evidence that the renal response to volume expansion involves a blood-borne factor. *Biol Neonate* 1979; 35:113.

Spaeh DH, Stapleton AE, Stamm WE: Lack of circumcision increases the risk of urinary tract infection in young men. *JAMA* 1992; 267:679.

Spitzer A: The role of the kidney in sodium homeostasis during maturation. *Kidney Int* 1982; 21:539.

Spitzer A: *Factors Underlying the Increase in Glomerular Filtration Rate During Development Morphology and Function*. New York, Mason Publishing Co, 1992, ch 16.

Spitzer A, Brandis M: Functional and morphologic maturation of the superficial nephrons. Relationship to total kidney function. *J Clin Invest* 1974; 53:279.

Spitzer A, Edelmann CM Jr: Maturational changes in pressure gradients for glomerular filtration. *Am J Physiol* 1971; 221:1431.

Stark H, Geiger R: Renal tubular dysfunction following vascular accidents of the kidneys in the newborn period. *J Pediatr* 1973; 83:933.

Starr A: Ureteral plication: a new concept in ureteral tailoring for megaureter. *Invest Urol* 1979.

Stein SC, Feldman JG, Friedlander M, et al: Is myelomeningocele a disappearing disease? *Pediatrics* 1982; 69:511.

Steinhardt GF, Vogler G, Salinas-Madrigal L, et al: Induced renal dysplasia in the young pouch opossum. *J Pediatr Surg* 1988; 23:1127.

Steinhart JM, Kuhn JP, Eisenberg B, et al: Ultrasound screening of healthy infants for urinary tract abnormalities. *Pediatrics* 1988; 82:609.

Stephens FD: *Congenital Malformations of the Urinary Tract*. New York, Praeger Scientific Co, 1983, p 195.

Stephens JD, Sherman S: Determination of fetal sex by ultrasound. *N Engl J Med* 1983; 309:984.

Stestes JM, MacGillivray TE, Hedrick M, et al: Fetoscopic surgery for the treatment of congenital anomalies. *J Pediatr Surg* 1992; 27:950.

Stewart CL, Jose PA: Transitional nephrology. *Urol Clin North Am* 1985; 12:143.

Stoller ML, Kogan BA: Sensitivity of ^{99m}DMSA for the diagnosis of chronic pyelonephritis: clinical and theoretical considerations. *J Urol* 1986; 135:977.

Stringel G, Mercer S, Richler M, et al: Catheterization of the umbilical artery in neonates: surgical implications. *Can J Surg* 1985; 28:143.

Stuck KJ, Koff SA, Silver TM: Ultrasonic features of multicystic dysplastic kidney: expanded diagnostic criteria. *Radiology* 1982; 143:217.

Sty Jr, Wells RG, Starkshak RJ, et al: Imaging in acute renal infections in children. *Am J Radiol* 1987; 148:471.

Sulyok E: The relationship between electrolyte and acid-base balance in the premature infant during early postnatal life. *Biol Neonate* 1976; 17:227.

Sulyok E, Heim T, Soltesz G, et al: The influence of maturity on renal control of acidosis in newborn infants. *Biol Neonate* 1972; 21:418.

Sulyok E, Nemeth M, Tenyi I, et al: Postnatal development of renin-angiotensin-aldosterone system, RAAS, in relation to electrolyte balance in premature infants. *Pediatr Res* 1979; 13:817.

Susskind MR, Kim KS, King LR: Hypertension and multicystic kidney. *Urology* 1989; 34:362.

Sutton TJ, Leblanc A, Gauthier N, et al: Radiological manifestations of neonatal renal vein thrombosis on follow-up examinations. *Radiology* 1977; 122:435.

Tavani N Jr, Calcagno P, Zimmet S, et al: Ontogeny of single nephron filtration distribution in canine puppies. *Pediatr Res* 1980; 14:799.

Taylor A Jr, Nally JV: Clinical applications of renal scintigraphy. *AJR* 1995; 164:31.

Thomas DFM: Fetal uropathy. *Br J Urol* 1990; 66:225.

Thomas DFM, Agrawal N, Laidin AZ, et al: Pelviureteric obstruction in infancy and childhood. A review of 117 patients. *Br J Urol* 1982; 54:204.

Thomas IT, Smith DW: Oligohydramnios, cause of the nonrenal features of Potter's syndrome, including pulmonary hypoplasia. *J Pediatr* 1974; 84:811.

Thompson HC, King LR, Knox E, et al: Ad Hoc Task Force on Circumcision—report. *Pediatrics* 1975; 56:610.

Thrall JM, Koff SA, Keyes JW Jr: Diuretic radionuclide urography and scintigraphy in the differential diagnosis of hydronephrosis. *Semin Nucl Med* 1981; 11:85.

Toguri AG, Fournier G: Factors involving the pressure-flow perfusion system. *J Urol* 1982; 127:1021.

Tomoda S, Brace R, Longo LD: Amniotic fluid volumes and fetal swallowing rate in sheep. *Am J Physiol* 1985; 249:R133.

Tooley WH, Myerberg DZ: Should we put catheters in the umbilical artery? *Pediatrics* 1978; 62:853.

Torrado A, Guignard JP, Prod'hom LS, et al: Hypoxaemia and renal function in newborns with respiratory distress syndrome (RDS). *Helv Paediatr Acta* 1974; 29:399.

Trompeter RS, Schwartz R, Chantler C, et al: Haemolyticuraemic syndrome: an analysis of prognostic features. *Arch Dis Child* 1983; 58:101.

Trulock TS, Finnerty DP, Woodard JR: Neonatal bladder rupture: case report and review of literature. *J Urol* 1985; 133:271.

Tuchmann-Duplessis H: *Illustrated Human Embryology*. New York, Springer-Verlag, 1972.

Tuck S, Morselli P, Broquaire M, et al: Plasma and urinary kinetics of furosemide in newborn infants. *J Pediatr* 1983; 103:481.

Tulassay T, Machay T, Kiszel J, et al: Effects of continuous positive airway pressure on renal function in prematures. *Biol Neonate* 1983; 43:152.

Uson AC, Cox LA, Lattimer JK: Hydronephrosis in infants and children. *JAMA* 1968; 205:323.

Valayer J, Adda G: Hydronephrosis due to pelviureteric obstruction in infancy. *Br J Urol* 1982; 54:451.

Van Putte A: Perinatal bereavement crisis: coping with negative outcomes from prenatal diagnosis. *J Perinat Neonat Nurs* 1988; 2:12.

Venkataraman PS, Hahn BK, Tsang RC, et al: Secondary hyperparathyroidism and bone disease in infants receiving long-term furosemide therapy. *Am J Dis Child* 1983; 137:1157.

Vert P, Bianchetti G, Marchal F, et al: Effectiveness and pharmacokinetics of indomethacin in premature newborns with patent ductus arteriosus. *Eur J Clin Pharmacol* 1980; 18:83.

Vinocur L, Slovis TL, Perlmutter AD, et al: Follow-up studies of multicystic dysplastic kidneys. *Radiology* 1988; 167:311.

Vordermark JS II, Buck AS, Dresner ML: Urinary ascites resulting from umbilical artery catheterization. *J Urol* 1980; 124:751.

Vorlicky LN, Balfour HH Jr: Cytomegalovirus and renal vein thrombosis in a newborn infant. *Am J Dis Child* 1974; 127:742.

Wacksman J, Phipps L: Report of the multicystic kidney registry: preliminary findings. *J Urol* 1993; 150:1870.

Waffarn F, Devaskar UP, Hodgman JE: Vesico-umbilical fistula: a complication of umbilical artery cutdown. *J Pediatr Surg* 1980; 15:211.

Walker RD, Richard GA, Bueschen AJ, et al: Pathophysiology and recoverability of function and structure in obstructed kidneys. *Urol Clin North Am* 1980; 7:291.

Wallenburg HCS: The amniotic fluid: I. Water and electrolyte homeostasis. *J Perinatal Med* 1977; 5:193.

Warner E, Strachin E: Benefits and risks of circumcision. *Can Med Assoc J* 1981; 125:967.

Warsos SL, Larsen JW, Kent SG, et al: Prenatal diagnosis of congenital adrenal hyperplasia. *Obstet Gynecol* 1980; 55:751.

Wassner SJ: Acute renal failure. In Nelson NM (ed): *Current Therapy in Neonatal/Perinatal Medicine, 1985-1986*. Toronto, Marcel Decker, 1985, p 137.

Waterhouse J, Shanmuguratnam K, Muir C, et al: Cancer incidence in five continents. *JARC Sci Pub* 1982; 4:750.

Watson AR, Readett D, Nelson CS, et al: Dilemmas associated with antenatally detected urinary tract abnormalities. *Arch Dis Child* 1988; 63:719.

Weatherstone KB, Rasmussen LB, Evenberg A, et al: Safety and efficacy of a topical anesthetic for neonatal circumcision. *Pediatrics* 1993; 92(5):710.

Wedge JJ, Grosfeld JL, Smith JP: Abdominal masses in the newborn: 63 cases. *J Urol* 1971; 106:770.

Weinstein L, Anderson CF, Finley PR, et al: The in utero management of urinary outflow obstruction. *J Clin Ultrasound* 1982; 10:465.

Welborn LG, Greenspun JC: Anesthesia and apnea: perioperative considerations in the former preterm infant. *Ped Clin North Am* 1994; 41:181.

Whitaker RH: The Whitaker test. *Urol Clin North Am* 1979; 6:529.

Whitaker RH, Sherwood T: An improved hook for destroying posterior urethral valves. *J Urol* 1986; 135:531.

Wigger HJ, Bransilver BR, Blanc WA: Thromboses due to catheterization in infants and children. *J Pediatr* 1970; 76:1.

Wigglesworth JS, Desai R, Guerrini P: Fetal lung hypoplasia: biochemical and structural variations and their possible significance. *Arch Dis Child* 1981; 56:606.

Wilkins BH: Renal function in sick, very low birthweight infants: glomerular filtration rate. *Arch Dis Child* 1992; 67:1124.

Wilkins IA, Chitkara U, Lynch L, et al: The non-predictive value of fetal urine electrolytes: preliminary report of outcomes and correlation with pathologic diagnosis. *Am J Obstet Gynecol* 1987; 157:694.

Williams DI: The chronically dilated ureter. Hunterian lecture. *Ann R Coll Surg Engl* 1954; 14:107.

Williams DI, Karlaftis CM: Hydronephrosis due to pelviureteric obstruction in the newborn. *Br J Urol* 1966; 38:138.

Williams DI, Whitaker RH, Barratt TM, et al: Urethral valves. *Br J Urol* 1973; 45:200.

Willis J, Duncan C, Gottschalk S: Paraplegia due to peripheral venous air embolus in a neonate: a case report. *Pediatrics* 1981; 67:472.

Wilson DA: Ultrasound screening for abdominal masses in the neonatal period. *Am J Dis Child* 1982; 136:1147.

Wilson RD, Morrison MG, Wittmann BK, et al: Clinical follow up of fetal urinary tract anomalies diagnosed prenatally by ultrasound. *Fetal Ther* 1988; 3:141.

Winberg J: Urinary tract infections in infants and children. In Walsh PC, Gittes RF, Perlmutter AD, et al: (eds): *Campbell's Urology*, ed 5. Philadelphia, WB Saunders Co, 1986, p 831.

Wiswell TE, Geschke DW: Risks from circumcision during the first month of life compared to those for uncircumcised boys. *Pediatrics* 1989; 83:1011.

Wiswell TE, Hachey WE: Urinary tract infection and the uncircumcised state: an update. *Clin Ped* 1993; 32:130.

Wiswell TE, Miller GM, Gelston HM Jr, et al: Effect of circumcision status on periurethral bacterial flora during the first year of life. *J Pediatr* 1988; 113:442.

Wiswell TE, Smith TR, Bass JW: Decreased incidence of urinary tract infections in circumcised male infants. *Pediatrics* 1985; 75:901.

Wladimiroff JW: Effect of furosemide on fetal urine production. *Br J Obstet Gynaecol* 1975; 82:221.

Wladimiroff JW, Campbell S: Fetal urine–production rates in normal and complicated pregnancy. *Lancet* 1974; 1:151.

Wladimiroff JW, van Otterlo LC, Wallenburg HC, et al: A combined ultrasonic and biochemical study of fetal renal function in the term fetus. *Eur J Obstet Gynaecol Reprod Biol* 1976; 6:103.

Wolpert JJ, Woodard JR, Parrott TS: Pyeloplasty in the young infant. *J Urol* 1989; 142:573.

Woodard JR: Hydronephrosis in the neonate. *Urology* 1993; 42:620.

Woodbury PW, Mitchell ME, Scheidler DM, et al: Constant pressure perfusion: a method to determine obstruction in the upper urinary tract. *J Urol* 1989; 142:632.

Yared A, Lon V, Ichikawa I: Functional development of the kidney. *Contemp Issues Nephrol* 1984; 12:61.

Yeh TF, Wilks A, Singh J, et al: Furosemide prevents the renal side effects of indomethacin therapy in premature infants with patent ductus arteriosus. *J Pediatr* 1982; 101:433.

Young HH, Frontz WA, Baldwin JC: Congenital obstruction of the posterior urethra. *J Urol* 1919; 3:289.

Zaontz MR, Firlit CF: Percutaneous antegrade ablation of posterior urethral valves in infants with small-caliber urethras: an alternative to urinary diversion. *J Urol* 1986; 136:247.

Zaontz MR, Gibbons MD: An antegrade technique for ablation of posterior urethral valves. *J Urol* 1984; 132:982.

Zerrin JM, DiPietro MA, Grignon A, et al: Testicular infarction in the newborn: ultrasound findings. *Ped Rad* 1990; 20:329.

Zerrin JM, Ritchey ML, Chang ACH: Incidental vesicoureteral reflux in neonates with antenatally detected hydronephrosis and other renal abnormalities. *Pediatr Radiol* 1993; 187:157.

CHAPTER 45

Anomalies of the Kidney

Stephen A. Koff
Henry A. Wise II

ANOMALIES OF NUMBER
Renal Agenesis
Embryologic Considerations

For the kidney to develop properly, a normal ureteral bud must penetrate a normal metanephric blastema at the proper time. These events typically occur between the fifth and the seventh week of gestation. Major factors that alter the morphology or sequence of these events, such as absence of the nephrogenic ridge or failure of ureteral bud formation, will prevent the kidney from developing. Although the kidney will obviously not form in the absence of metanephric tissue, it is genuinely unclear in renal agenesis which is the primary developmental abnormality, the nephrogenic ridge or the ureteral bud. Studies by Potter (1965) on the fetus and infant suggest that the primary abnormality rests in failure to develop a normal ureteral bud; she observed that if any portion of the ureter was present, some identifiable renal tissue usually existed. In contrast, an extensive review of autopsy material by Ashley and Mostofi (1960) disclosed that in many cases of renal agenesis there was partial or complete formation of the ureteral and wolffian duct structures. They also observed examples of renal dysgenesis occurring without a formed ureter. Although these findings are to some extent conflicting, they do support a theory that the ureteral bud directly stimulates the differentiation of the renal parenchyma and they also indicate that the potential for renal differentiation rests in the nephrogenic ridge itself. This potential suggests that the stimulus for ureteral bud formation resides, at least partly, in the developing metanephros.

The embryologic basis for renal agenesis appears to be an early insult to the developing ureteral bud, which prevents normal renal organogenesis from progressing. The ultimate clinical expression of this teratogenic event depends on its severity and extent (unilateral or bilateral renal agenesis) and on the sex of the fetus since wolffian duct derivatives are much less commonly affected than Müllerian duct structures. Also, even though there is close proximity between the renal and gonadal anlage on the nephrogenic ridge, injuries to the developing gonads are exceedingly rare in this condition.

Bilateral Renal Agenesis

Bilateral renal agenesis anomaly is rare, with an incidence of approximately 1 in 4000 births. It occurs much more frequently in males than in females (72%), and most affected infants are of low birth weight (less than 2.5 kg). Amniotic fluid is characteristically absent in all cases, although no other feature of pregnancy or maternal state is abnormal. About one third of births are stillborn; the survivors usually succumb to the effects of severe pulmonary hypoplasia within a short time.

The kidneys and renal arteries are usually completely absent, although dysgenetic vestiges may be noted at times. The ureters are completely absent in about one half of the infants, as is the bladder, which often is absent or hypoplastic. The adrenal glands are usually present but typically ovoid since they are not compressed by the kidneys and fail to assume their characteristic shape (Ashley and Mostofi, 1960). The infant with bilateral renal agenesis is characteristically deformed. The face is prematurely senile, with a flat nose, large flattened and lowered ears, and a depression below the lower lip. A prominent skin fold covers the inner canthus of each eye. In addition, the legs are often bowed and clubbed. This constellation of features, along with pulmonary hypoplasia, has been termed *Potter's syndrome* (Figs. 45-1 and 45-2). However, these features are not pathognomonic or specific for bilateral renal agenesis. Elegant experimental studies on the fetal rat subjected to repeated amniocentesis (DeMyer and Baird, 1969), observations by

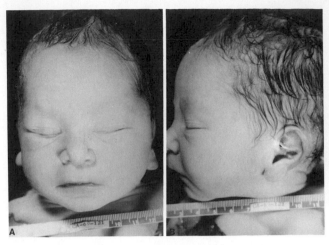

FIG. 45-1
A and **B,** Characteristic Potter's facies in an anephric child who survived only hours. Note flat nose, large flattened and lowered ears, depression below lower lip, and inner canthal skin folds.

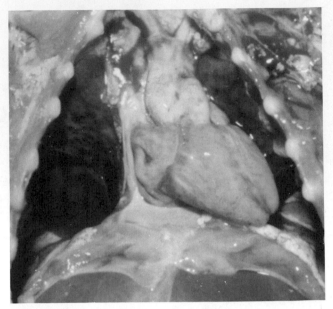

FIG. 45-2
Bell-shaped chest and pulmonary hypoplasia in stillborn child with bilateral renal agenesis.

Bain and associates (1964) on infants with leakage of amniotic fluid, and documentation of Potter's syndrome in babies with polycystic kidney disease, bilateral renal dysplasia, and urethral atresia or obstruction indicate that all of the features of Potter's syndrome are attributable to the mechanical effects of insufficient amniotic fluid volume.

Bilateral renal agenesis is incompatible with life, and thus its clinical significance is limited. With characteristic body features and associated oligohydramnios, the diagnosis should be readily apparent and can be confirmed easily by ultrasonography, renal scintigraphy, and if necessary, umbilical artery catheterization with aortography. In addition, improved technology has permitted ultrasonographic diagnosis of Potter's syndrome prenatally, which raises important controversies and implications in fetal therapeutics (Heliln et al., 1983).

Unilateral Renal Agenesis

Because of the potentially asymptomatic nature of unilateral renal agenesis, its reported incidence varies according to the population surveyed. Necropsy studies suggest an occurrence of about 1 in 1000, whereas clinical presentation may be 1 in 1500 (Emanuel et al., 1974; Longo, 1952; Thompson and Lynn, 1966). Males dominate in a ratio of 1.8:1 (Doroshow and Abeshouse, 1961).

The clinical significance of solitary kidney relates to associated genital abnormalities and cystic dilations within the pelvis and to its potential for pathologic complications. Genital anomalies occur commonly and are three to four times more frequent in females than in males. In girls, partial or complete nonunion of the Müllerian ducts is the most commonly occurring em-

bryologic defect. This defect may be expressed clinically as an obstructed hemivagina and uterus didelphis to produce a pelvic mass with menstrual irregularities and discomfort. These signs and symptoms often are diagnosed incorrectly as an ovarian mass because hematocolpometra is seldom considered as a likely diagnostic possibility in otherwise healthy, menstruating young women (Stassart et al., 1992; Yoder and Pfister, 1976) (Fig. 45-3). A spectrum of renal anomalies, including unilateral agenesis, may occur in certain patients with the *Mayer-Rokitansky-Kuster-Hauser Syndrome*, which is defined by congenital absence of the vagina and uterus. Two forms of this condition occur in otherwise normal genotypic and phenotypic females who have a shallow pouch replacing the vagina. In the typical form, there is complete absence of the vagina, associated with bilateral symmetrical rudimentary uterine anlagen (noncanalized muscular buds) and normal ovaries and fallopian tubes. In the atypical form, the uterine remnants are asymmetric (aplastic or enlarged), the fallopian tubes are abnormal (aplastic or hypoplastic), and the ovaries may be cystic and anomalous. Interestingly, the ovarian and renal anomalies occur almost exclusively in the atypical form of this syndrome (Pinsonneault and Goldstein, 1985; Strubbe et al., 1992; Tarry et al., 1986).

Genital anomalies are much less frequent in males, although hypospadias, undescended testes, hypoplastic or absent vas deferens, and seminal vesicle and prostatic cysts have been reported (Kaneti et al., 1988). In both sexes patients with ipsilateral renal agenesis (or severe dysplasia) may develop cystic di-

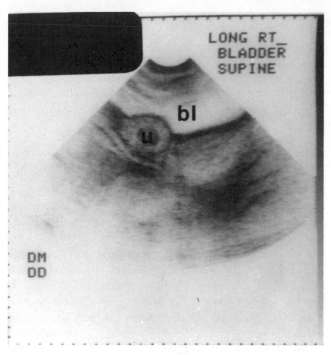

FIG. 45-3
Pelvic ultrasonogram demonstrates right-sided partially fluid-filled pelvic mass in a 15-year-old girl with solitary left kidney and menstrual irregularity. The mass proved to be an obstructed duplication of the uterus and vagina with hematometrocolpos. *u* uterus; *bl* bladder.

lations within the pelvis. In males these typically represent seminal vesicle cysts, whereas in females, Gartner's cysts occur. Sheih and co-workers (1990) performed screening renal ultrasound studies on 280,000 children and found 235 with a congenital solitary kidney. Of these, 13 had seminal vesicle or Gartner's cysts, an incidence of 0.005%. The embryologic connection between renal agenesis and pelvic cystic disease was made more obvious in those cases where dilated ureters were identified entering the cysts (see below).

Except as noted above the gonads and the remaining kidney are usually normal, and the ipsilateral adrenal gland would be expected to be normal because of its separate embryologic development. Interestingly, the adrenal has been reported to be absent in about 10% of cases of renal agenesis (Nakada et al., 1988). Associated nongenitourinary tract anomalies occur in up to 25% of affected individuals and commonly involve the cardiovascular, gastrointestinal, and skeletal systems.

The diagnosis of unilateral renal agenesis is often made during an evaluation for urinary symptoms or as part of an investigation in patients with abnormalities of the external genitalia or other organ systems. Females often are identified at puberty during an evaluation for menstrual irregularities or a mass. In males, the external genitalia may give a clue to diagnosis, but

finding an absent vas deferens or hypoplastic epididymis does not necessarily indicate that there will be an absence of the kidney (Charny and Gillenwater, 1965; Trigaux et al., 1991). Likewise, absence of the kidney does not signify absence of the testis in those instances in which the testis is undescended and impalpable. The clinical diagnosis of unilateral renal agenesis and its relationship to multicystic renal dysplasia become confusing and even more significant when fetal ultrasound studies are considered. Mesrobian (1993) reported on the occurrence of unequivocal unilateral multicystic renal dysplasia in three fetuses detected during maternal ultrasound examination, which completely disappeared during fetal development so that no trace of a kidney or cystic structure was seen on subsequent ultrasonograms performed after birth. Thus it is apparent that some solitary kidneys may not result from a lack of induction of the metanephric blastema, but rather their occurrence reflects an acquired insult to the developing kidney. The incidence and significance of this finding require further classification, but the study does help to explain certain embryologic findings, such as cystic dilations of the seminal vesicle or Gartner's duct associated with renal agenesis. Some of these cases may represent ureteral ectopia with early and total obstructive renal injury.

Investigations used to make the diagnosis of unilateral renal agenesis can include excretory urography, ultrasonography, radionuclide imaging, computed tomography, and magnetic resonance imaging. These tests make it virtually unnecessary to perform arteriography for diagnosis. Cystoscopy is usually not helpful even though it may reveal an asymmetric or absent hemitrigone typically without visualization of a ureteral orifice. However, these cystoscopic findings are not pathognomonic of renal agenesis. They merely indicate that the ureter does not enter the bladder normally; it may be ectopic. Consequently, cystoscopy is no longer recommended to confirm the diagnosis of renal agenesis.

Although the susceptibility of a solitary kidney to pathologic complications is now recognized to be no greater than that of a normal kidney, early studies suggested that solitary kidneys were predisposed to disease and carried an increased mortality. In recent times, such a potential has not been observed, and unilateral renal agenesis is compatible with normal longevity. However, in following the clinical course of 157 patients with unilateral renal agenesis, Argueso and associates (1992) found that although survival data was the same as for age-matched controls, there was an increased risk of developing proteinuria, hypertension, and renal insufficiency. Prolonged follow-up of these patients thus appears warranted.

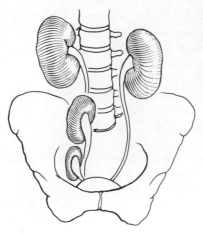

FIG. 45-4
Ascent of kidney is associated with medial rotation.

Hereditary Renal Adysplasia

Most cases of renal agenesis and renal dysplasia generally have been considered as isolated findings, occurring sporadically and not as part of any inherited syndromes. Alternatively, recent reports suggest that because of a common pathogenesis, renal agenesis, small kidneys with solid dysplasia, and large kidneys with solid or cystic dysplasia should be viewed as a spectrum of diseases that includes multicystic renal dysplasia. In addition, familial renal agenesis and dysplasia have been shown to occur together and to be inherited along autosomal dominant lines with variable inheritance (Bernstein, 1991; Murugasu et al., 1991; Roodhooft, 1984; Squires, 1987).

Hereditary renal adysplasia was first described by Buchta and associates in 1973 as the occurrence of renal agenesis and hypoplasia/dysplasia in two kindreds in which a predominantly autosomal dominant inheritance pattern with variable penetrance was suggested. Roodhooft (1984) clarified the familial nature of bilateral renal adysplasia and found that 9% of parents and siblings of afflicted individuals had asymptomatic renal abnormalities. Recent evidence by Murugasu and colleagues (1991), who studied three kindreds with hereditary renal adysplasia where two or more children in each family were affected, indicated that (1) at least one family member had a clinically silent anomaly, (2) normal kidneys in parents did not protect offspring from developing anomalies, and (3) empiric risks for offspring and first-degree relatives were 50% and 25%, respectively. These findings suggest that the strong genetic predisposition is along the lines of a dominant gene with variable expression. Because of this higher-than-expected incidence of silent genitourinary tract abnormalities and the increased risk to parents of having another infant so affected, there is a strong need for careful and complete genetic screening of the proband's family, pregnancies, and subsequent children. Although the risks of recurrence of the different forms of hereditary renal adysplasia have generally applied only to the renal components, Battin (1993) has identified a kindred in which Müllerian duct abnormalities (vaginal atresia or anomaly) were inherited in an autosomal dominant pattern.

Supernumerary Kidney

The supernumerary kidney is a rare condition in which a free accessory renal organ exists as a distinctly separate parenchymatous mass and blood supply associated with two usually normal kidneys. It is generally distinguishable from the normal ipsilateral kidney by its smaller size and abnormal position. Typically, the supernumerary kidney is located caudal to the normal kidney. When in this position, the supernumerary ureter is usually a bifid branch of the normal ureter. This contrasts with the cranially placed supernumerary kidney, whose ureter is characteristically completely duplicated and separate from the normal ureter and may empty ectopically (N'Guessan and Stephens, 1983). Pathologic conditions, such as calculus disease and hydronephrosis, have been reported in more than 50% of patients. However, it may not indicate a true increased susceptibility but may merely be an indication for their recognition (Carlson, 1950; Sasidharan et al., 1976). When it is diagnosed, therapy for supernumerary kidney should be directed toward and reserved for pathologic processes affecting the kidney rather than simply its abnormal position or apparent redundancy.

ANOMALIES OF POSITION
Embryologic Considerations

During normal embryologic development, the permanent kidneys are positioned initially in the pelvis opposite the sacral somites, with their pelves facing anteriorly. Through a combination of axial trunk lengthening, elongation of the ureter, intrinsic renal growth, and rotation, the metanephros ascends to a higher position (Fig. 45-4). By the eighth week of gestational life, migration has been completed, and the kidney resides in the upper retroperitoneum opposite the second lumbar vertebra with the hilum facing medially. During ascent, the vascular supply to the kidney is locally derived until it reaches its final position, where the main renal arteries and veins develop. Because of the interdependence of renal ascent, rotation, and vascular supply, anomalies of renal position are often associated with bizarre and at times puzzling alterations in morphology and function that become interpretable and subject to classification only on the basis of these embryologic processes.

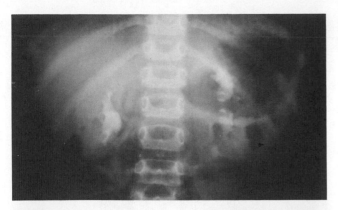

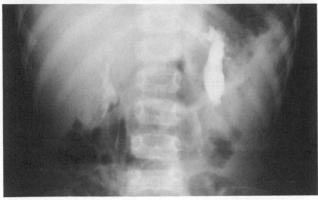

FIG. 45-5
Excretory urogram of malrotated left kidney with pelvis pointed anteriorly demonstrates normal calyces *(top)* and slightly dilated pelvis *(bottom)*.

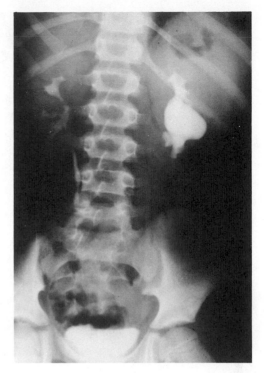

FIG. 45-6
Excretory urogram of malrotated left kidney demonstrates dysmorphic renal pelvis and hydronephrosis proved to be nonobstructive by diuretic radionuclide studies.

Malrotation

Malrotation may be unilateral or bilateral and may affect a normally positioned or ectopic kidney. The kidney is commonly rotated around its vertical axis, and in most cases the pelvis is aimed somewhat anteriorly somewhere between the fetal and normal adult positions (Fig. 45-5). Rarely, this situation can be reversed, with the pelvis pointing posteriorly. The renal vessels are usually normal when the kidney is malrotated but in its normal retroperitoneal position, which excludes a vascular cause for the anomaly.

Although the malrotated kidney is generally no more predisposed to pathologic conditions than is the normal kidney, malrotation is often accompanied by dysmorphism of the pelvis and calyces, especially in the presence of renal ectopy and fusion. Consequently, the malrotated kidney and pelvis may look hydronephrotic or deformed or may have a bizarre shape that suggests extrinsic compression or the presence of tumor (Fig. 45-6). In most instances, these appearances are illusory and are due as well to abnormal planes of projection on the excretory urogram. However, at times, special diagnostic studies may be needed to exclude obstruction and to establish a correct diagnosis.

Renal Ectopy

When the kidney occupies a position outside of its normal retroperitoneal location, it is termed ectopic. Ectopy may be acquired, as in ptosis, where the renal vasculature and ureteral length are normal. In contrast, congenital renal ectopia usually represents a developmental arrest during renal ascent so that the kidney occupies a pelvic, iliac, or abdominal location (see Fig. 45-4), having a shorter-than-normal ureter and an abnormal vascular supply. Malrotation is a usual accompaniment, with the pelvis typically directed anteriorly (Fig. 45-7).

Pelvic Kidney

In most cases of simple (ipsilateral) renal ectopy, the kidney is located within the confines of the bony pelvis and often is termed a *pelvic kidney* (Fig. 45-8). In this position, it overlies the pelvic bones and lumbosacral vertebrae, which makes its visualization on urography difficult even when renal function is well preserved. Diagnostic difficulty is further compounded by poor renal function and by the renal pelvis and calyces assuming an abnormal and often unex-

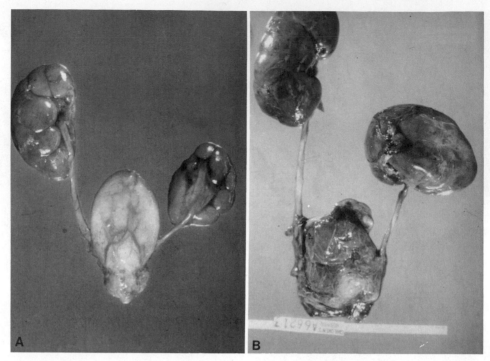

FIG. 45-7
A, Ectopic left kidney shows incomplete rotation with renal pelvis aiming anteriorly. **B,** Ectopic left kidney, which has ascended higher than **A,** has completed normal medial rotation but has an abnormal axis.

pected attitude that markedly impairs recognition (Fig. 45-9).

Pelvic kidneys are more susceptible to calculous formation than normal ones. They also are more frequently observed to be hydronephrotic, the cause of which may be true obstruction or nonobstructive dilation caused by vesicoureteral reflux, dysmorphism, malrotation. Because nonobstructive dilation occurs in over 50% of cases (Gleason et al., 1994) careful assessment must be made before the dilated kidney is assumed to be obstructed and treatment initiated. If reconstructive surgery is necessary, angiography may be required to characterize an unpredictable renal vasculature (Fig. 45-10). Also, the presence and status of the opposite kidney must be determined in case nephrectomy is required (Anderson and Harrison, 1965). In general, the prognosis in renal ectopia is primarily related to the presence of any associated urological disease and not directly related to ectopia alone (Gleason et al., 1994).

In clinical series, ectopic kidneys are frequently symptomatic in up to 40% to 50% of patients (Downs et al., 1973). Symptoms are generally on the basis of urinary infection, abdominal mass, or pain stimulating gastrointestinal disease. The autopsy incidence of this condition, 0.14% (Campbell, 1951), is much greater than is the clinical expression, 0.008%, based on hospital admissions (Kelalis et al., 1973). This finding suggests that in many cases the anomaly is asymptomatic and remains unrecognized. Prognosis ultimately de-

pends on whether the pelvic kidney is solitary and whether the contralateral kidney is normal, as reflected in the Downs and associates (1973) series, where renal disease developed in 40% of patients with a solitary ectopic kidney (representing about 10% of patients with pelvic kidney), and 15% did not survive early adulthood. The clinical significance of ectopic kidney is reinforced by the fact that in up to 50% of patients the contralateral kidney may be abnormal (Malek et al., 1971).

Prognosis also depends on the severity of associated anomalies, which are particularly common with renal ectopy, and may coexist in up to 85% of patients (Malek et al., 1971). In addition to the high incidence (15% to 45%) of genitourinary tract anomalies, such as hypospadias, undescended testis, and vaginal agenesis, associated anomalies typically include the skeletal, cardiovascular, and gastrointestinal systems. This high incidence of associated abnormalities requires thorough investigation, particularly in children found to have renal ectopy. Similarly, the presence of skeletal and especially vertebral anomalies should raise high the level of suspicion for coexisting renal abnormality (Donahoe and Hendren, 1980). Maizels and Stephens (1979) have identified and defined an embryologic explanation for this close relationship between renal ectopy and vertebral anomalies in a series of elegant experiments. By deforming the developing caudal trunk of the chick embryo, they could regularly induce scoliosis, which, when present, was associated

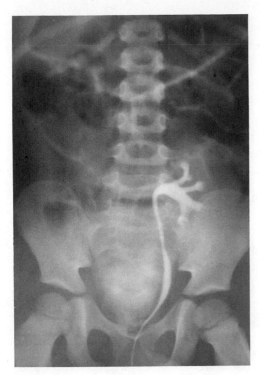

FIG. 45-8
Retrograde study of normally rotated and formed pelvic kidney with short ureter.

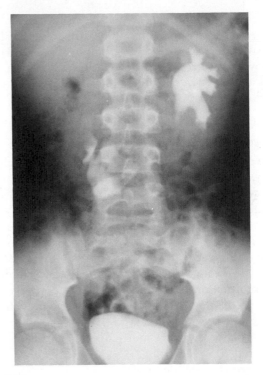

FIG. 45-9
Right pelvic kidney overlies the lumbosacral spine and is difficult to visualize on excretory urogram.

with a 62% incidence of renal ectopia. Equally important was the relatively high incidence of associated anomalies of the mesonephros, mesonephric duct, and Müllerian duct comparable with that reported in the clinical literature. As a result of these studies, they have proposed that an environmental teratogen affecting the hind end of the embryo at a critical period of about 5 to 7 weeks' gestation may lead to abnormal growth of the spine. This abnormal growth of the spine, in turn, would limit renal ascent to produce ectopia and deflect the mesonephric duct away from the cloaca, leading to abnormalities of these structures or of the Müllerian duct system. Such studies and their clinical correlates clearly indicate that the development of the lower end of the embryo is a highly complex process with multisystem interdependence. The clinician, therefore, must keenly recognize the interrelationships between renal anomalies and other genitourinary and somatic abnormalities to provide the thorough investigation necessary to uncover their presence and to interpret their significance.

Thoracic Kidney

Thoracic kidney is a rare form of renal ectopy where the kidney protrudes or projects at least in part above the diaphragm. It is distinguishable from diaphragmatic hernia in which other abdominal viscera occupy the chest cavity as well. Embryologically, it is uncertain whether the kidney ascends before the diaphrag-

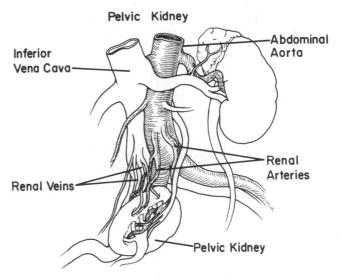

FIG. 45-10
Unpredictable renal vasculature to pelvic kidney is derived from surrounding major vascular trunks.

matic leaflets close normally or whether delayed diaphragmatic formation enhances the exaggerated renal ascent (Burke et al., 1967).

Because the thoracic kidney is typically asymptomatic and otherwise normal except for position, the diagnosis is usually made on routine chest roentgenogram. The ureter is longer than normal to reach the bladder, but unlike the pelvic kidney, the renal vasculature is not anomalous and typically arises as a single renal artery and vein. Once a diagnosis has been confirmed by excretory urography (Fig. 45-11), no therapy is required because neither the ectopic thoracic kidney nor its contralateral mate are predisposed to pathologic disturbances.

ANOMALIES OF POSITION AND FUSION
Embryologic Considerations

The classification of embryologic anomalies includes kidneys that have migrated to become contiguous or fused with their contralateral mate; it is subdivided clinically on the basis of whether both or only one kidney moves toward or crosses the midline. In horseshoe kidney, the most common fusion abnormality, both kidneys have migrated, whereas in crossed ectopia, usually only one kidney has crossed the midline. In both situations the blood supply is unpredictably abnormal, arising from multiple sources; in addition, the kidneys are malrotated to some degree because fusion usually prevents normal rotation from being completed.

Numerous eclectic embryologic theories have sought to provide an explanation for these different events, which occur very early in gestation. These explanations include faulty ureteral bud development, abnormalities of renal vasculature limiting ascent, and other teratogenic factors (Kelalis et al., 1973; McDonald and McClellan, 1957). More recently, Cook and Stephens (1977) have proposed a more unified theory that relates the position and fusion anomalies to abnormal variations in growth or flexion of the hind end of the developing embryo and to the subsequent induction of one or two nephrogenic cords. They propose that horseshoe kidney and its variants may be due to midline fusion of the two renal blastemata while they are still confined to the true pelvis. This fusion results from excessive ventral flexion of the hind end of the embryo, which pushes the kidneys together (Fig. 45-12). Alternatively, a combination of exaggerated ventral and lateral flexion with rotation of the tail might carry the cloaca and its attached ducts across the midline to allow the development of a fused kidney from a single nephrogenic cord that has been intercepted by ureteral buds from both wolffian ducts.

Crossed Renal Ectopy

Crossed renal ectopy is an uncommon condition with an autopsy incidence of about 1 in 2000 and a slight male predominance (Abeshouse and Bhisitkul, 1959; McDonald and McClellan, 1957). It occurs when the ureter occupies its normal position in the bladder but crosses the midline to join an ectopic kidney, which, in 90% of patients, is fused to its mate. In their comprehensive study, McDonald and McClellan (1957) subdivided this condition into four groups: (1)

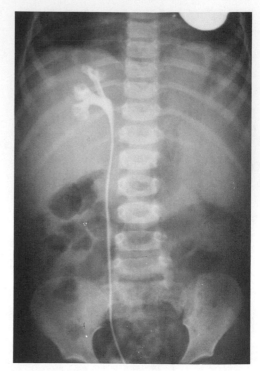

FIG. 45-11
Thoracic kidney, evaluated by retrograde pyelography, is entirely normal but abnormally positioned.

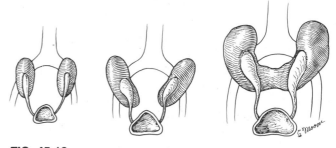

FIG. 45-12
Presumed embryologic sequence in the formation of horseshoe kidney.

crossed ectopia with fusion, (2) crossed ectopia without fusion, (3) solitary crossed ectopia, and (4) bilateral crossed ectopia (Fig. 45-13). Crossed renal ectopia with fusion, the most common of these entities, was further classified into six categories based on morphologic appearance (Fig. 45-14). Of these, the most common form appears to be fusion with the ectopic kidney placed inferiorly.

Although both urinary and nonurinary anomalies can be associated with this condition, their incidence is low, and they are not seen as frequently as in unilateral agenesis or pelvic kidney. However, a variety of abnormalities, including sacral agenesis, scoliosis, and cardiovascular and gastrointestinal anomalies,

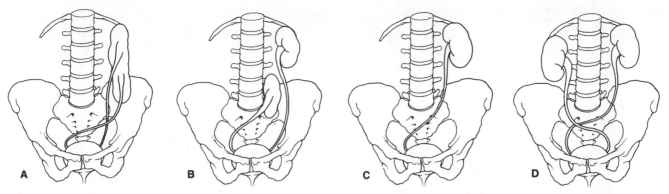

FIG. 45-13
Types of crossed renal ectopia: **A,** fused; **B,** nonfused; **C,** solitary; **D,** bilateral. (Modified from McDonald JH, McClellan DS: *Am J Surg* 1957; 93:995.)

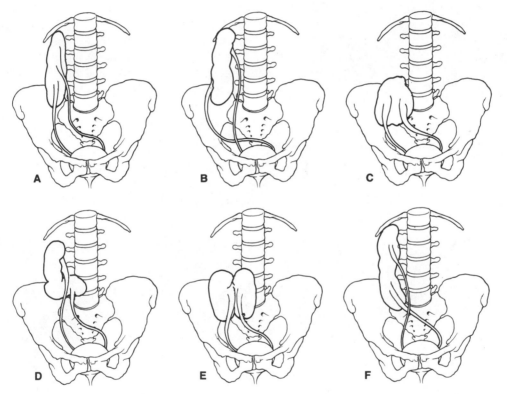

FIG. 45-14
Six types of crossed renal ectopia with fusion: **A,** ectopic kidney superior; **B,** sigmoid or S-shaped kidney; **C,** lump kidney; **D,** L-shaped kidney; **E,** disk kidney; **F,** ectopic kidney inferior. (Modified from McDonald JH, McClellan DS: *Am J Surg* 1957; 93:995.)

have been reported (Kelalis et al., 1973; McDonald and McClellan, 1957).

Many patients with crossed renal ectopia remain entirely asymptomatic. However, because of associated malrotation, a significant proportion of these kidneys display pelvocalyceal dysmorphism that simulates hydronephrosis. In some instances, an abnormal ureteropelvic junction position and aberrant blood vessels may actually interfere with pelvic emptying to produce obstruction and predispose to uri-

nary infection and calculous formation. Also, reflux commonly is observed to be associated with this anomaly.

Excretory urography is usually adequate to outline the anatomy of normally functioning crossed ectopic moieties (Figs. 45-15 and 45-16). However, because of the high incidence of reflux, voiding cystography and radionuclide studies that evaluate the functional significance of collecting system dilation are recommended. If surgery is required, angiography may be

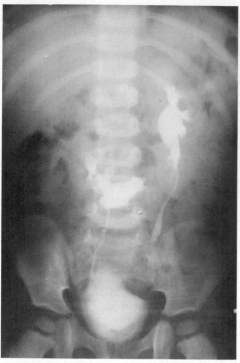

FIG. 45-15
L-shaped crossed fused renal ectopia with renal pelvis over-lying spine is visualized by excretory urography. Note mal-rotation of left kidney.

particularly useful because Rubinstein and associates (1976) have shown that the vascular supply to both the ectopic and nonectopic kidney may be anomalous.

Horseshoe Kidney

Horseshoe kidney is the most common fusion anomaly, with an incidence of approximately 1 in 400 births and a male predominance (Glenn, 1959; Segura et al., 1972). It presents great variability in morphology, position, and vascular supply. In more than 90%, there is true fusion of the lower poles, which form an isthmus and become medially directed (Fig. 45-17). The site of fusion may lie over the midline or may be asymmetrically positioned to one side. Depending on the degree of fusion, the isthmus may be composed of thick functioning parenchyma or merely a fibrous band that serves to tether the lower poles of anatomically independent renal masses. In most instances, the kidneys are located in their proper retroperitoneal positions, with the isthmus placed anterior to the great vessels at about the level of L4 or L5. The ureters typically course in front of the isthmus, descending from anteriorly facing renal pelves. Blood supply to the horseshoe kidney is variable, with the fused segment receiving a particularly unpredictable blood supply from branches of the common iliac, aorta, and at times the hypogastric and middle sacral arteries (Boatman et al., 1971). If large portions of the renal parenchyma fuse, the resulting kidney may lose its

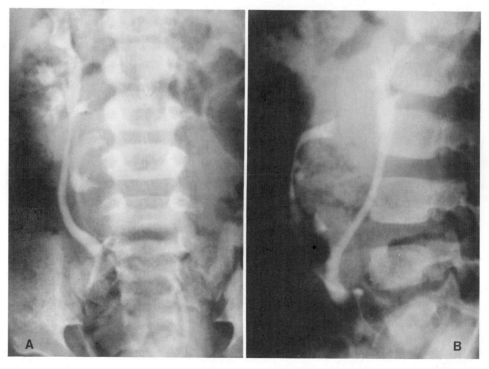

FIG. 45-16
A, Crossed renal ectopia with crossed kidney fused inferiorly is demonstrated on excretory urogram. **B,** Lateral film shows orientation of collecting systems to be anterior for inferior ectopic kidney and posterior for superior kidney.

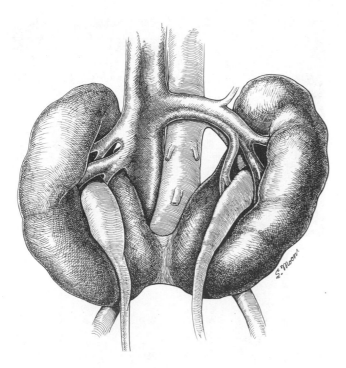

FIG. 45-17
Classic features of horseshoe kidney. Fusion of lower poles produces an isthmus and shifts the axis of the kidneys toward the lumbosacral vertebrae.

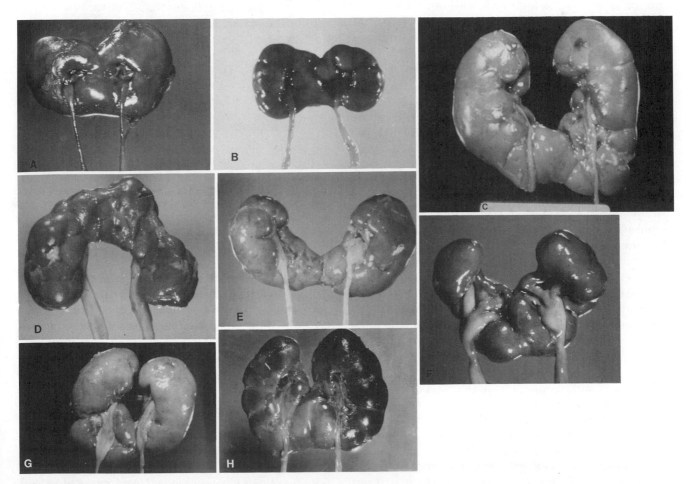

FIG. 45-18
Horseshoe kidney. **A-H,** Specimens show wide variation in degree of fusion, thickness of the isthmus, ureteral morphology, renal axis, and horseshoe appearance. Note fusion of upper poles in **D.**

horseshoe shape and become a flattened disc or lump kidney, which often has a pelvic location (Fig. 45-18).

Associated anomalies occur in at least one third of patients regardless of whether the horseshoe kidney is itself symptomatic. These anomalies include multisystem disturbances of the skeletal and cardiovascular systems and gastrointestinal tract, as well as genitourinary abnormalities. It appears that horseshoe kidneys are more common in infants succumbing to multiple congenital anomalies, but the kidney itself is rarely the cause for their deterioration (Zondek and Zondek, 1964). Boatman and colleagues (1971) documented an increased incidence of male and female genital anomalies with this condition. Also, an increased frequency of ureteral duplication with obstructive sequelae (e.g., ureterocele) and reflux has been reported (Pitts and Muecke, 1975; Segura et al., 1972).

At least one third and perhaps an even greater proportion of patients with horseshoe kidney remain entirely asymptomatic. When symptoms are present, they typically relate to calculi, hydronephrosis, infection, or hematuria. A high incidence of calculous disease has been attributed to a combination of partial obstruction and stasis; however, a review of this problem by Evans and Resnick (1981) disclosed that metabolic causes for kidney stone disease were no less frequent in patients with horseshoe kidney than in the general population. The treatment of calculi in a horseshoe kidney requires special consideration with regard to extracorporeal shock wave lithotripsy (ESWL) therapy and endourological techniques (Cussenot, 1992; Esuvaranthan, 1991; Serrate, 1991).

Hydronephrosis was present in 80% of the children reviewed by Segura and associates (1972) and a comparable figure was reported by Odiase (1983). Hydronephrosis may be due to ureteropelvic junction obstruction, which reflects the usual high insertion of the ureter into the pelvis, as well as displacement by the fused isthmus. However, hydronephrosis also may be consequent to vesicoureteral reflux or to pelvocalyceal dysmorphism consequent to malrotation, ectopy, and parenchymal distortion. Differentiation between obstructive and nonobstructive conditions is obviously essential for precise diagnosis and effective therapy (Fig. 45-19).

Dysplasia and neoplasia have been reported to occur in horseshoe kidney. Wilms' tumor, angiomyolipoma, teratoma, and transitional cell carcinoma have all been documented (Castro and Green, 1975; Feldman and Lome, 1982; Gay et al., 1983; Schacht et al., 1983). Reed and Robinson (1984) have suggested that the incidence of transitional cell carcinoma is three times that of normal kidneys, perhaps related to the stasis of carcinogens.

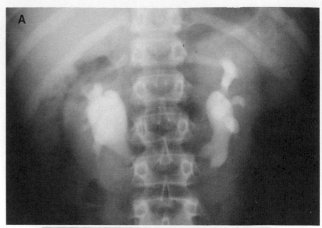

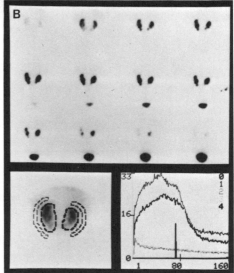

FIG. 45-19

A, Excretory urogram shows horseshoe kidney with bilateral hydronephrosis greater on the right side. **B,** Diuretic radionuclide study indicates that isthmus has no appreciable blood flow *(bottom left).* Also, scintiscans *(above)* and histogram curves *(bottom right)* illustrate rapid nonobstructed tracer transit and exclude mechanical obstruction.

The radiographic diagnosis of horseshoe kidney, although difficult with ultrasonography if the isthmus is not detected, is usually easily made with excretory urogathy if the renal segments function well; the vertical line of axis through the kidneys will point toward the lumbosacral spine, and there will be ureteral deviation by the isthmus. However, in children with spina bifida and a thoracolumbar gibbus deformity, the axis of the kidneys may be distorted to simulate a horseshoe kidney (Fernbach and Davis, 1986).

The addition of diuretic radionuclide imaging has been helpful in patients with horseshoe kidney because it reliably establishes whether the isthmus contains functioning parenchyma (Hosokawa et al., 1983), and it distinguishes true obstructive hydronephrosis from nonobstructive dilation (Thrall et al., 1981) (see

Fig. 45-19). To these studies, voiding cystography should be added because of the predictably high incidence of vesicoureteral reflux. If surgery for a diseased horseshoe kidney is contemplated, angiographic study may be required to characterize the variable arterial supply to the kidney.

Treatment and prognosis for horseshoe kidney, particularly for associated hydronephrosis, have changed considerably over the years, reflecting both conceptual evolution and technologic advance. In early series, Smith and Orkin (1945) believed that horseshoe kidney was almost always diseased and in need of surgical therapy, especially division of the isthmus. Later, Glenn in 1959 observed instead that nonoperative follow-up of horseshoe kidneys was compatible with a symptom-free course; less than 25% of patients required surgery for calculus or obstruction. Also, none of Glenn's patients required division of the isthmus for pain relief, a practice that since has no longer been popular. Division of the isthmus, however, was often believed to be necessary in conjunction with pyeloplastic surgery for obstruction or alone to improve drainage. However, symphysiotomy as an isolated procedure is not frequently performed today because the position of the kidneys, the course of the ureters, and the effect on drainage are not significantly altered; thus, the benefits of surgery do not appear to outweigh the associated risks (Pitts and Muecke, 1975). With attention directed toward eliminating proven obstruction by pyeloplasty and correcting reflux-induced pelvic overdistention by ureteral reimplantation when necessary, many have reported a very favorable prognosis for these patients in several large series (Culp and Winterringer, 1955; Glenn, 1959; Pitts and Muecke, 1975). The presence of a horseshoe kidney can significantly affect the management of other disease conditions involving the kidney and retroperitoneum, such as renal and testicular neoplasm, aortic aneurysm and renal transplantation. Special considerations and alterations in therapy may be required (Hohenfellner et al., 1992; O'Hara, 1993; Ratner and Zibari, 1993).

ANOMALIES OF THE RENAL COLLECTING SYSTEM

Calyx

Calyceal Diverticulum

A calyceal diverticulum is a cystic cavity located peripheral to an otherwise normal minor calyx with which it communicates through a narrow channel. It is lined by transitional epithelium, may be multiple, and can occur anywhere in the kidney, although the upper calyx is affected most frequently. Because the incidence in children and adults is approximately the same, it is considered to be a defect in embryo-

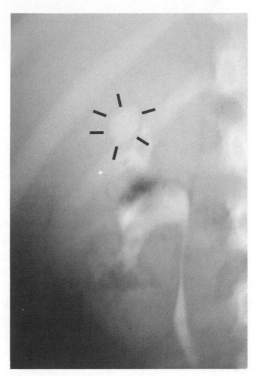

FIG. 45-20
Excretory urographic demonstration of a calyceal diverticulum.

genesis, although the embryology is unclear. One plausible explanation is based on persistence of later generations of the dividing ureteral bud that fail to degenerate and persist as calyceal diverticula, enlarging because of the backflow of urine (Middleton and Pfister, 1974; Timmons et al., 1975).

Diagnosis usually is made on excretory urography, although the neck of the diverticulum is best outlined on retrograde study (Fig. 45-20). In the evaluation, they must be distinguished from other acquired abnormalities, such as cortical abscess, papillary necrosis, and tuberculosis. Calyceal diverticula may be entirely asymptomatic, but there is an increased incidence of milk of calcium and stone formation within the poorly draining cavity, which in turn may cause secondary complications of pain, infection, and hematuria (Yeh et al., 1992). Surgery is rarely necessary, but if required, eradication can be accomplished by dividing the calyceal neck and marsupializing the cyst (Williams et al., 1969).

Megacalycosis

Megacalycosis is a nonobstructive condition in which the calyces are dilated, malformed, and often increased in number in the absence of ureteropelvic junction obstruction or enlargement of the renal pelvis. Megacalycosis or megacalyces are much more common in males, and the usual presenting symptoms in children are urinary tract infections, which are not necessarily related. In adults, megaureter is associated in 10% to 20% of patients and must be proved to be nonobstructive before a diagnosis of megacalycosis can be made with certainty (Gittes, 1984). Histologically, the renal cortex is normal, but the medulla is underdeveloped, which correlates with malformation of the renal papillae and an almost universally present defect in tubular concentrating ability.

The diagnosis of megacalycosis can be made only when there is no anatomically or functionally definable site of obstruction in the urinary tract. However, the etiology may involve a transient obstruction in fetal life during the period of early parenchymal development (Gittes, 1984; Johnston, 1973). The observations on transient fetal hydronephrosis and the similarity between megacalycosis and postoperative appearance of successfully corrected ureteropelvic junction obstruction give credence to this theory. Occasionally, the clinical features and radiographic findings of these two conditions appear to overlap, which leads to diagnostic confusion (O'Reilly, 1989).

Megacalycosis must be differentiated from true obstructive uropathy and from acquired conditions that produce infundibular scarring and calyceal dilation. As a nonobstructive anatomic deformity, the overall prognosis is excellent.

Infundibulopelvic Stenosis

Infundibulopelvic stenosis is a rare form of congenital hydrocalycosis in which the narrowed and obstructive infundibula drain variably dilated calyces into a small, nonobstructed renal pelvis (Fig. 45-21). Although the etiology of this condition is unknown, it may have embryologic significance as a link in the spectrum of congenital upper urinary tract obstructive anomalies, which ranges from infundibulopelvic dysgenesis, hydrocalycosis, and calyceal diverticulum through ureteropelvic junction obstruction to severe multicystic renal dysplasia (Kelalis and Malek, 1983; Uhlenhuth, 1990). Clinically, infundibulopelvic stenosis must be differentiated from renal malignancy, as well as from the more recognizable and correctable forms of hydronephrosis. Unless it is associated with significant renal parenchymal dysplasia, this abnormality rarely progresses (Lucaya et al., 1984; Schneider et al., 1988).

Ureteropelvic Junction Obstruction

Prior to the era of ultrasonography, hydronephrosis caused by obstruction at the ureteropelvic junction was considered a common cause of hydronephrosis in children and adolescents. Although its overall incidence was difficult to estimate, presentation was frequently in younger children; 25% of cases were diagnosed within the first year of life, and 50% were recognized before the age of 5 years (Johnston et al.,

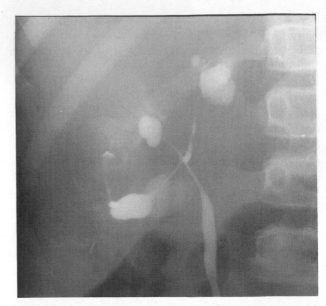

FIG. 45-21
Infundibulopelvic stenosis. Excretory urogram demonstrates dilated calyces and narrowed, elongated infundibula, which fuse to form narrowed upper ureter; renal pelvis, although almost nonexistent, is not obstructed.

1977; Williams and Karlaftis, 1966; Williams and Kenawi, 1976). With the use of routine perinatal ultrasonography, hydronephrosis suspected of being caused by ureteropelvic junction (UPJ) obstruction is now recognized in nearly 1 in 500 live births (Arger et al., 1985; Grignon, 1986). This condition occurs more commonly in males, especially neonates, with left-sided lesions predominating. Bilateral obstruction has been reported to occur in 10% to 40% of patients and, again, is more common in infants (Lebowitz and Griscom, 1977; Uson et al., 1968; Williams and Kenawi, 1976). Occasionally, UPJ obstruction occurs in a duplicated kidney and usually affects the lower pole moiety (Fig. 45-22).

Pathophysiology

Hydronephrosis may be caused by a variety of anatomical lesions or functional disturbances of the UPJ that restrict urinary flow across this region either by compression of the UPJ and/or by interference with peristalsis. Since complete obstruction to the UPJ causes relatively rapid renal destruction, most clinical cases of hydronephrosis are thus suspected of being caused by a partial rather than a total obstruction. Although hydronephrosis associated with partial UPJ obstruction has a potential to cause progressive dilation and renal deterioration, such does not necessarily occur. In some instances a state of equilibrium will occur, whereas in others there may even be spontaneous improvement. These phenomena are recognized clinically in patients with lifelong UPJ-type hydronephrosis who have no measurable reduction in renal function (Fig. 45-23) and in those followed non-

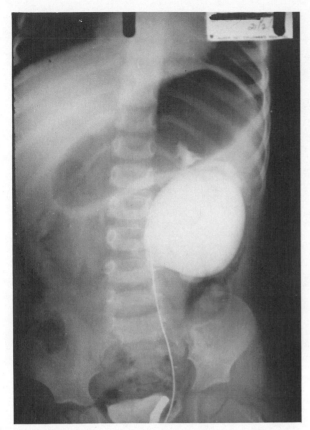

FIG. 45-22
Sequential retrograde pyelograms of each moiety of a duplicated kidney demonstrates UPJ obstruction affecting the lower pole.

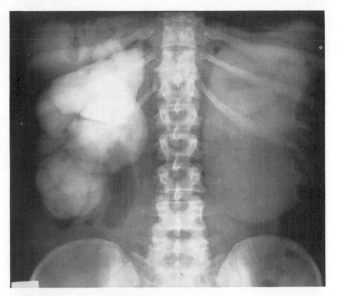

FIG. 45-23
Incidentally discovered bilateral congenital UPJ-type hydronephrosis in a 72-year-old woman who had normal renal function and no symptoms attributable to the urinary tract.

operatively who develop neither loss of renal function nor progressive urinary tract dilatation (Bratt 1977; Nilsson, 1979). Also, the clinical observations that as many as 40% of patients show no measurable radiographic improvement after pyeloplasty for UPJ obstruction suggest that partial obstruction is not functionally significant (Drake, 1978; Hendren, 1980; Johnston, 1977; Williams and Kenawi, 1976). Experimental studies support these clinical observations. Application of a ligature to the UPJ or burying the ureter in the psoas muscle in dogs produces initial hydronephrosis but thereafter not all kidneys progressively dilated; some reached an equilibrium, dilated no further, and maintained stable renal function (Koff, 1983; Olesen and Madsen, 1968).

The potential for progression or equilibration in hydronephrosis appears to be determined by several physiologic factors. These include: (1) urinary output and flow rates during diuresis, (2) the anatomy and function of the ureteropelvic junction, (3) glomerular and tubular renal function, and (4) pelvic compliance. Experimental pelvimetric studies have helped to clarify the relative importance and interrelationship between these factors. Pelvimetric study of the renal pelvis involves temporarily occluding the ureteropelvic junction while infusing saline into the pelvis and

simultaneously measuring renal pelvic pressure and volume (Koff, 1981,1983; Olsen, 1979). This is analogous to a cystometric examination in which a pressure volume curve is generated that describes the visceroelastic properties of the renal pelvis. The results of numerous pelvimetric studies have shown that all kidneys, whether normal, obstructed, dilated but nonobstructed, or previously obstructed, are characterized by a similar shaped pelvimetric curve: low-pressure filling or accommodation occurs until a critical pelvic volume that is unique for each pelvis is reached, the "capacity volume" of the renal pelvis. This capacity volume is analogous to bladder capacity and represents the volume above which low-pressure accommodation is no longer possible and overstretching of pelvic smooth muscle, elastic and connective tissue components occurs. Above this volume, pressures rise rapidly as volume expands further (Fig. 45-24). As the size of the pelvis increases, two important pelvimetric changes take place that determine the likelihood for progressive hydronephrotic dilation and renal damage: (1) the pelvis stretches and its capacity volume and compliance increase and this causes (2) the slope of the pelvimetric curve above the capacity volume to flatten (Fig. 45-25). As a result, large hydronephrotic kidneys require proportionately greater volumes of urine to overdistend their pelves and to develop high intrapelvic pressures; and once the pelvis is overdistended, intrapelvic pressures rise at a much slower rate in kidneys with large pelves than in those with small pelves. These findings explain (1) why kidneys with a small intrarenal pelvis are more vulnerable to renal damage from obstruction: they will rapidly develop high intrapelvic pressures; and (2) why kidneys

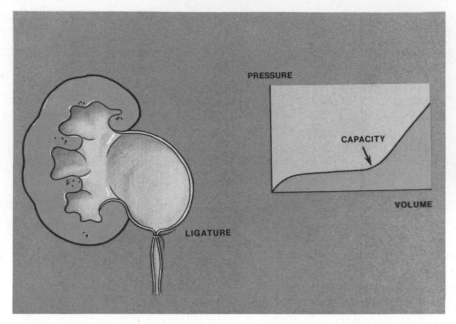

FIG. 45-24
Pelvimetric study of the renal pelvis displays characteristic pelvimetric tracing that defines the capacity of the renal pelvis and the slopes of the accommodation and filling phases below and above capacity.

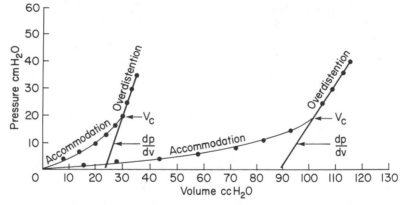

FIG. 45-25
During progression of hydronephrosis, pelvimetric studies demonstrate an increase in pelvic capacity (V_c) and a decrease in the slope of the overdistention portion of the curve (dp/dv) (From Koff SA: *Invest Urol* 1981; 19:85. Used by permission.)

with large pelves are seemingly protected from obstructive injury: they can accept larger volumes of urine before pressures begin to rise and once overdistended, pressures rise at a much more gradual rate. Consequently, once kidneys develop a large extrarenal pelvis with relatively increased compliance as a result of partial obstruction, they may reach a state of hydronephrotic equilibrium and deteriorate no further (Bullock, 1984; Koff, 1983).

Experimental studies also have shown that a partial UPJ obstruction that is capable of causing a normal kidney to initially dilate and become significantly hydronephrotic may not be significant enough to cause the now dilated kidney to develop progressive hydronephrosis or renal injury. The kidney may no longer be able to induce a diuresis sufficient to overfill the

renal pelvis and to cause intrarenal pressures to rise. In this setting because of acquired changes in pelvic size, compliance, renal function and nephron mass, hydronephrosis may have become a beneficial compensatory mechanism that protects the kidney from further injury (Koff, 1983; Koff and Whitaker, 1985). These interrelationships and observations have special importance in neonatal hydronephrosis, where the combination of a disproportionately large, stretchy, highly compliant renal pelvis, immature renal function, and reduced urinary output tend to minimize or eliminate completely the potentially harmful effects of partial UPJ obstruction and in some cases allow hydronephrosis to spontaneously improve. Witness the fact that reviews of the natural history of unoperated UPJ-type neonatal hydronephrosis indicate

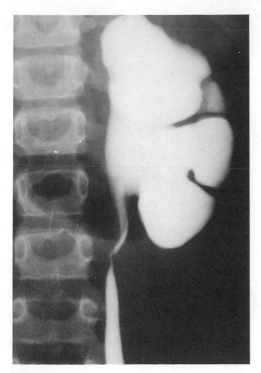

FIG. 45-26
Ureteropelvic junction obstruction caused by narrowed segment of upper ureter.

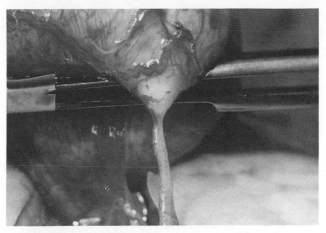

FIG. 45-27
Anatomic appearance of intrinsic UPJ obstruction caused by narrowed upper ureteral segment.

that only approximately 20% of affected infants will demonstrate deterioration of renal function or progression of hydronephrosis and require pyeloplasty (Chung et al., 1992; Koff and Campbell, 1992, 1994).

Ureteropelvic Junction Anatomy

A variety of anatomic abnormalities can affect the ureteropelvic junction to cause restriction of flow and obstruction. *Intrinsic* lesions are recognized easily during radiographic evaluation and at the time of surgery. Although true strictures at the ureteropelvic junction are rare findings, the upper segment of the ureter is often visibly narrowed and thinned but probe-patent (Figs. 45-26 and 45-27). This narrowing may represent an arrest in development (Allen, 1970) that can be explained embryologically by the fact that during fetal life the ureter undergoes a continuous process of obstruction and recanalization, which, if incomplete, may produce narrowing and obstruction (Ruano-Gil et al., 1975). The fetal ureter also may show intraluminal muscular invaginations, folds or valvelike structures, which can persist postnatally; ordinarily these are nonobstructive and disappear with time. However, if these folds become overdeveloped, they may produce obstruction to the upper ureter or ureteropelvic junction (Johnston, 1969) (Fig. 45-28).

Although there is no histologic difference between the normal ureteropelvic junction and the remainder of the upper urinary collecting system (Kinch, 1982), histologic differences have been identified in cases of obstruction by several authors, but their findings and interpretations have differed. Abnormalities include a preponderance of longitudinal muscle fibers, excessive collagen fibers in and around muscle bundles, and compromised or attentuated muscle bundles (English et al., 1982; Hanna et al., 1976; Kaneto et al., 1991; Murnaghan, 1958; Notley, 1968; Starr, 1992). All of these changes can, to some extent, interfere with normal ureteral peristalsis and urine transport, but it remains genuinely unresolved as to whether these changes better represent the cause or are merely a histologic effect of the obstruction.

Extrinsic mechanical abnormalities at or below the ureteropelvic junction may produce morphologic alterations and functional disturbances that impair pelvic emptying. This type of obstruction is commonly caused by an aberrant or accessory renal artery or early branching vessel to the lower pole of the kidney or a similarly positioned fibrous band that typically passes anterior to the pelvis and ureter to produce kinking, compression, or both. Although this type of ureterovascular hydronephrosis has been reported to occur in up to 40% of patients not all observers are convinced that the crossing vessel or band is the sole or inciting cause of the obstruction. (Ericsson et al., 1961; Johnston et al., 1977; Nixon, 1953). In many instances, an underlying primary intrinsic disturbance of the UPJ may exist or coexist to produce obstruction that results in pelvic overdistention and rotation. This rotation may then distort the normal anatomy and give the illusion that vessels or bands are the primary cause of obstruction. Stephens' (1982) observations on ureterovascular hydronephrosis support this view by indicating that transient or permanent defects in medial rotation of the renal pelvis predispose the uretero-

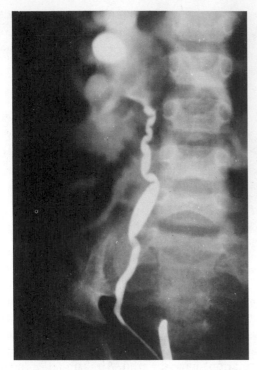

FIG. 45-28
Ureteropelvic junction obstruction associated with prominent ureteral folds.

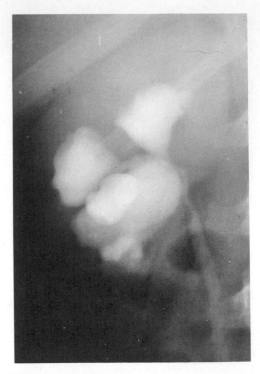

FIG. 45-29
Ureteropelvic junction obstruction associated with high insertion of the ureter into the pelvis.

pelvic junction to vascular obstruction. Insertion of the ureter high onto the pelvis instead of in a dependent position may produce a similar type of mechanical obstruction that combines a deficiency in ureteropelvic junction funneling with pelviureteral adhesions that can angulate and/or compress the ureter against the expanding pelvis (Figs. 45-29 and 45-30). Extrinsic obstructions of this type have important clinical implications, especially at the time of surgical repair. It must not be assumed that apparent extrinsic compressions or mechanical disturbances are the sole cause of impaired pelvic emptying and that their correction will relieve obstruction. The possibility that a coexisting intrinsic disturbance at the ureteropelvic junction also exists must be considered, assessed intraoperatively, and, if present, treated appropriately. In addition, it has been hypothesized that in some cases ureteropelvic junction obstruction may be caused entirely by a functional disturbance in the ability of the pelvis and upper ureter to function synchronously to initiate, form, or conduct peristaltic waves across the ureteropelvic junction (Constantinou and Djurhuus, 1982; Whitaker, 1973). This concept is obvious in those cases where there is no other cause apparent for the obstruction, but it also may be operative in certain cases where after release of an obvious extrinsic obstruction, the now normally appearing ureteropelvic junction does not function properly and resection

of an adynamic UPJ segment is required for complete relief of obstruction.

Ureteropelvic Junction Function

The different forms of pathologic anatomy of the UPJ, intrinsic and extrinsic, not only produce dissimilar degrees of static compression and obstruction at the UPJ, they also produce altogether different patterns of urinary flow across the UPJ that have important clinical implications. These distinctive flow patterns determine to a great extent the potential for progression or equilibration of hydronephrosis, and they influence the accuracy of diagnostic tests that aim to assess obstruction in hydronephrosis (Koff et al., 1986). Intrinsic obstructions, such as ureteral narrowing or an adynamic segment, tend to be fixed in severity, to produce a constant degree of obstruction, and are characterized by a linear pressure-flow curve in which the rate of flow across the UPJ is determined and driven primarily by increases in intrapelvic pressure. This flow pattern has been termed *pressure dependent*. In contrast, extrinsic UPJ obstructions, such as kinks, angulations, or compressing bands or vessels, tend to vary in severity, to produce a changing degree of resistance, and are characterized by a nonlinear pressure-flow curve in which flow rate depends primarily on renal pelvic volume and is determined by how tightly the ureter is kinked by or compressed

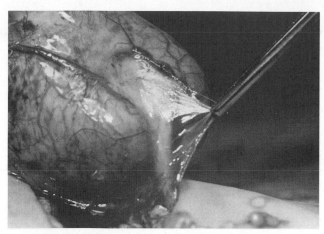

FIG. 45-30
Anatomy of extrinsic UPJ obstruction demonstrates adventitial tissue compressing the upper ureter against the overdistended renal pelvis.

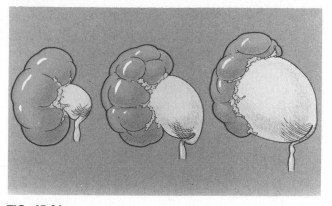

FIG. 45-31
Representation of the sequence of events involved in activation of an extrinsic volume-dependent obstruction by diuresis that causes renal pelvic volume expansion and overdistention. This allows adventitial bands to tightly compress the ureter against the dilating renal pelvis.

against the overdistended renal pelvis. This flow pattern has been termed *volume dependent*, because even at high pressures, flow may be low or absent. With this pattern, when pelvic volumes are small, resistance is usually low, and obstruction may be absent altogether. However, during a diuresis when the pelvis enlarges to a sufficient volume, obstruction may be activated, produce ureteral compression, and thereby induce self-perpetuating progression of obstruction by causing further pelvic enlargement, which increases obstructive compression. This sequence of events may be recognized clinically and at surgery in cases where adventitial bands bind the pelvis and ureter together and become more compressive as the pelvis overfills and the bands are drawn taut (Fig. 45-31).

In trying to relate the anatomy and function of the UPJ to its clinical behavior, it appears that intrinsic or extrinsic obstructions with pressure and volume-dependent flow patterns can explain many of the differences observed in the way kidneys respond to partial obstruction and the difficulties encountered in trying to diagnose obstruction. These discrepancies are related primarily to the intermittency of the obstruction. Intrinsic obstructions are almost always continuously present, whereas extrinsic obstructions are not active at all times but instead fluctuate, depending on the renal pelvic volume. Renal function and the ability of the kidney to initiate and sustain a diuresis are thus major factors in determining the timing and extent of pelvic overdistention and if obstruction becomes activated.

The diagnosis of obstruction can be particularly difficult in cases of intermittent obstruction, especially if the pelvis is minimally or not dilated between episodes of overdistention, because diagnostic tests may simply report that urine flows freely across the UPJ. In this setting, successful diagnosis often requires provocative testing during ultrasound or excretory urography with fluid loading to induce a diuresis; dynamic studies, such as diuretic renography or Whitaker's pressure-perfusion test, also may be particularly helpful in provoking or sustaining pelvic overdistention (Koff et al., 1986). Occasionally, testing must be performed during an episode of pain because this will be the only way to actually prove the diagnosis (Malek, 1983).

Presentation

In cases of symptomatic ureteropelvic junction obstruction, the presenting signs and symptoms depend on the age of the patient. Pain, hematuria, or urinary infection are more common in older children, whereas infants usually present with a palpable abdominal mass (Johnston et al., 1977; Snyder et al., 1980; Williams and Karlaftis, 1966). The pain often simulates gastrointestinal disease, especially if it is intermittent and associated with vomiting. Hematuria, which often occurs after mild abdominal trauma, is particularly significant because it reflects an increased susceptibility of the already dilated kidney to injury. Episodic intermittent flank pain associated with increased fluid intake is another recognizable presentation pattern that indicates sudden overdistention of the renal pelvis associated with diuresis.

Congenital anomalies commonly are associated with ureteropelvic junction obstruction and may occur in up to 50% of patients (Lebowitz and Griscom, 1977; Robson et al., 1976; Uson et al., 1968); however, genitourinary tract abnormalities usually are seen in only

10% of patients (Johnston et al., 1977; Snyder et al., 1980).

Diagnostic Evaluation

Most cases of perinatal hydronephrosis are detected initially by ultrasonography. UPJ obstruction is suspected when the pelvis is enlarged and the ureter is not dilated. In this age group, a voiding cystogram is required to exclude vesicoureteral reflux, which can produce renal pelvic and calyceal dilation indistinguishable from obstruction. In older patients, an excretory urogram is often the first study to identify hydronephrosis. The pattern of hydronephrosis caused by ureteropelvic junction obstruction has a characteristic radiographic appearance; the pelvicalyceal system is dilated, contrast transitions abruptly at the ureteropelvic junction, and the ureter is either nonvisualized or of normal caliber (Fig. 45-32). These diagnostic findings also may be produced by (1) obstruction at the ureterovesical junction with incomplete visualization of a dilated ureter, (2) lower urinary tract obstruction, or (3) vesicoureteral reflux. To exclude these other causes, one should obtain delayed filming (during excretory urography) and perform voiding cystography. However, visualization of a normal ureter on delayed films does not exclude significant UPJ obstruction, nor does identification of reflux or a dilated ureter exclude coexisting obstruction at the ureteropelvic junction. Reflux associated with hydronephrosis may present particular diagnostic difficulty (Fig. 45-33). If there is trapping of urine in the pelvis following voiding, and pelvic dilation persists, UPJ obstruction may coexist. In this setting, a diuretic renogram may be required to determine if primary UPJ obstruction exists, but it must be performed using a continuously draining bladder catheter to allow the UPJ to be analyzed independently by eliminating reflux-induced pelvic overdistention. The use of diuretic renography and constant perfusion pressure flow testing also are required whenever the diagnosis of UPJ obstruction is equivocal (Koff, 1982; O'Reilly et al., 1978; Whitaker, 1973). A more detailed discussion of the application of diagnostic tests in the diagnosis of hydronephrosis is presented in Chapter 21.

Prior to surgical treatment of UPJ obstruction it is necessary to prove that the ureter is normal in caliber and not obstructed. In some cases this information can be obtained by visualization of a normal ureter on excretory urography or noting normal ureteral transport and size at renography. When required, precise anatomic delineation of the ureter, pelvis, and UPJ may be obtained prior to surgery by retrograde or antegrade pyelography.

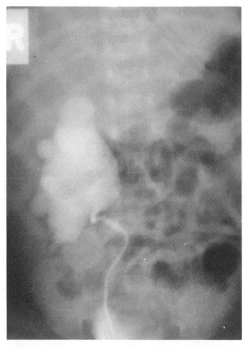

FIG. 45-32
Ureteropelvic junction obstruction demonstrated by retrograde pyelogram illustrates characteristic features. Pelvicalyceal dilation and abrupt transition at ureteropelvic junction to normal-caliber ureter are noted.

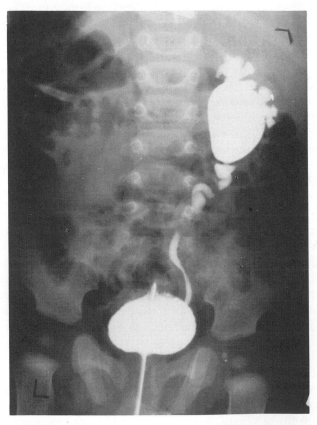

FIG. 45-33
When mild reflux is associated with pelvic hydronephrosis UPJ obstruction may coexist even though refluxed urine crosses the UPJ. A postvoiding study is required. If hydronephrosis persists, diuretic renography performed with a continuously draining bladder catheter is required.

Prognosis

The prognosis for kidneys obstructed at the ureteropelvic junction is generally good when surgery is performed in childhood. Anticipated renal recoverability generally correlates inversely with the age of the patient and with the duration and severity of obstruction and the extent of renal injury. Because of the unpredictably great potential for renal recoverability in young children, reconstructive surgery is almost always performed in childhood with nephrectomy reserved for only the most hopelessly damaged and dysplastic specimens.

RENAL VASCULAR ANOMALIES
Aberrant and Accessory Vessels

Normal vascular anatomy of the kidney and its variations are described and discussed in Chapter 14. In addition to normal variations, two anomalies of blood supply must be recognized: aberrant and accessory renal vessels. The term *aberrant* should be reserved for arteries that originate from vessels other than the aorta or main renal artery (Graves, 1954). True aberrant vessels are rare except in association with anomalies of renal position and fusion, such as renal ectopia and horseshoe kidney, where they may arise from a number of nearby major arterial trunks.

Accessory renal arteries are multiple arterial branches supplying the same renal segment. They occur rather frequently (23%) and are more common on the left side (Fig. 45-34). Accessory arteries enter the lower pole twice as frequently as the upper pole and typically pass caudal to the main renal artery (Anson and Kurth, 1955).

Vascular anomalies typically become clinically significant only when they interfere with urinary drainage to produce symptoms or to create unexplained filling defects on the excretory urogram. Characteristic vascular-induced patterns include ureteropelvic junction obstruction caused by an aberrant or accessory vessel to the lower pole and superior infundibular compression producing calyceal enlargement and pain (Fraley, 1966).

Renal Arteriovenous Fistula

Congenital arteriovenous fistula is a rare condition characterized by multiple communications between the main or segmental renal arteries and veins. It has a cirsoid shape that resembles varices and often does not present clinically until the third or fourth decade, with females being affected three times as often as males, and the right kidney more commonly is involved (Kopchick et al., 1981; Takaha et al., 1980; Yazaki et al., 1976). This type of congenital arteriovenous fistula accounts for less than 30% of all such fistulas; it is etiologically distinguishable from the aneurysmal type that is presumed to develop from a congenital aneurysm that erodes into a contiguous vein and slowly enlarges. The remaining types of arteriovenous fistulas are acquired and reflect traumatic or spontaneous causes, such as fibrodysplasia, arteriosclerosis, neoplasia, trauma, and especially renal biopsy, where a 15% incidence of often transient fistualization is observed (Bron and Redman, 1968; Oxman et al., 1973; Stanley et al., 1975).

Symptoms and signs of arteriovenous fistula reflect local or systemic disturbances and depend on size. A loud bruit is often heard in the abdomen. Hematuria occurs frequently and is probably related to the superficial location just below the pelvicalyceal walls. As the lesion enlarges, major shunting with rapid blood passage into the venous system will deprive the renal parenchyma of perfusion and may produce renin-mediated hypertension (Maldonado et al., 1964; McAlhany et al., 1971). With a large fistula, high output cardiac failure may be induced because of the combined effects of increased venous return and lowered peripheral resistance (Messing et al., 1976).

Despite significant signs and symptoms, excretory urography may be normal in about 50% of patients. Characteristic urographic signs when present include segmental reduction in renal function, distortion of calyces or pelvis by an enlarging mass, and filling defects caused by clot (DeSai and DeSautels, 1973). Diagnosis is best proved by renal arteriography where the tortuous vascular channels, shunting with early filling of venous vessels, and an enlarged renal vein are virtually pathognomonic (Fig. 45-35). However, the color doppler may provide simple noninvasive followup especially after therapy (Yura et al., 1991). Specific treatment depends on the etiology, size, and location of the arteriovenous fistula. Small lesions may be managed conservatively and nonoperatively, because when traumatically induced they are often sub-

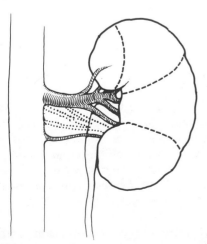

FIG. 45-34
Accessory renal arteries more commonly supply lower pole of left kidney.

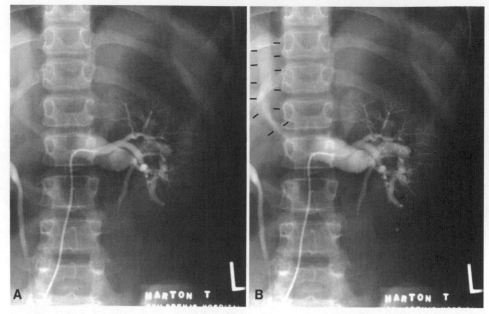

FIG. 45-35
Arteriovenous fistula involving lower pole of left kidney visualized by selective arteriography. **A,** Early injection film shows tortuous vascular channels and early filling of enlarged renal vein. **B,** Later film shows prominent, dilated renal vein and contrast in inferior vena cava.

ject to spontaneous cure. Medium-sized symptomatic fistulas have been treated effectively by transcatheter embolization (Bookstein and Goldstein, 1973). Large lesions, especially when accompanied by renal artery disease, are best managed by extirpation, which often requires partial or total nephrectomy.

Renal Artery Aneurysm

As with arteriovenous fistula, renal artery aneurysm is being discovered more commonly, perhaps because of the increased use of abdominal aortography and selective renal angiography to investigate patients with suspected renovascular hypertension. These studies have facilitated a more representative clinical profile of this rare condition. Aneurysms of the renal artery are found with equal frequency in both sexes and have been reported in patients ranging in age from 1 month to 82 years. Reflecting the often associated hypertension, about 50% of lesions are discovered in the fifth decade. Renal artery aneurysms constitute about 19% of all aneurysms; 80% are unilateral, 17% are intrarenal, and in 30% of patients the lesions are multiple (Abeshouse, 1951; Glass and Uson, 1967; Leary and Utz, 1971; Love et al., 1981; McLelland, 1957; Poutasse, 1975; Smith and Hinman, 1967).

Renal artery aneurysms are classified as either true or false. A false aneurysm is usually traumatic in origin, with walls that are derived from tissues other than the artery. In contrast, true aneurysms must contain at least one normal arterial wall component in

their walls and may be congenital or acquired. They are subdivided according to their appearance, which includes saccular, fusiform, or dissecting aneurysms (Altebarmakian et al., 1979; Cerny et al., 1968).

Saccular aneurysms are the most common form of true renal artery aneurysms in adults. They communicate with the arterial lumen through a channel that may be wide or narrow and characteristically occur at a point of bifurcation of the renal artery unassociated with renal artery stenosis. They are presumed to be due to a weakness in the elastic tissue layer that may be congenital or due to arteriosclerosis or medial arterial degenerative disease. In children, most renal artery aneurysms are associated with neurofibromatosis or medial fibrodysplasia accompanied by renal artery stenosis. They occur distal to the points of bifurcation and are thought to result from poststenotic flow disturbances (Slawin et al., 1991; Stanley and Fry, 1981).

Generally, the clinical signs and presentation of renal artery aneurysms are nonspecific and varied and depend on the size of the aneurysm. Most small aneurysms, especially in children, are silent, but because of altered hemodynamics within, they are prone to enlarge and calcify. Typical symptoms include pain, hematuria, and hypertension, which is usually renin-mediated.

These symptoms may be associated with a bruit heard in the abdomen (Glass and Uson, 1967). In addition to potential cure of hypertension, the most important reason for surgical treatment of renal artery aneurysms is the danger of spontaneous rupture. Asymptomatic aneurysms, less than 1.5 cm in diameter and fully calcified, are generally unlikely to rupture and may be followed conservatively. However, when aneurysms are larger than 2.5 cm, incompletely calcified, or associated with uncontrolled hypertension, surgical therapy is recommended (Martin et al., 1989; Poutasse, 1975). In cases of medial fibrodysplasia producing arterial stenosis and hypertension, nephrectomy has been the preferred therapy, especially for the small kidney. However, aortofemoral bypass grafts, transcatheter renal artery embolization and percutaneous transluminal angioplasty may soon eclipse nephrectomy as the therapeutic option of choice (Slawin et al., 1991).

REFERENCES

Abeshouse BS: Renal aneurysms, report of 2 cases and review of the literature. *Urol Cutan Rev* 1951; 55:451.

Abeshouse BS, Bhisitkul I: Crossed renal ectopia with and without fusion. *Urol Int* 1959; 9:63.

Allen TD: Congenital ureteral stricture. *J Urol* 1970; 104:196.

Altebarmakian VR, Caldamone AA, Dachelet RJ, et al: Renal artery aneurysm. *Urology* 1979; 13:257.

Anderson EE, Harrison JH: Surgical importance of the solitary kidney. *N Engl J Med* 1965; 273:683.

Anson BJ, Kurth LE: Common variations in the renal blood supply. *Surg Gynecol Obstet* 1955; 100:157.

Arger PH, Coleman BG, Mintz MC, et al: Routine fetal genitourinary tract screening. *Radiology* 1985; 156:485.

Argueso LR, Ritchey ML, Boyle ET, et al: Prognosis of patients with unilateral renal agenesis. *Ped Nephrol* 1992; 6:412.

Ashley DJB, Mostofi FK: Renal agenesis and dysgenesis. *J Urol* 1960; 83:211.

Bain A, Smith I, Gault I: Newborn after prolonged leakage of liquor amnii. *Br Med J* 1964; 2:598.

Battin J, Lacombe D, Leng JJ: Familial occurrence of hereditary renal adysplasia with Müllerian anomalies. *Clin Genet* 1993; 43:23.

Bernstein J: The multicystic kidney and hereditary renal adysplasia. *Am J Kidney Diseases* 1991; 18:495.

Boatman DL, Cornell SH, Kolln CP: The arterial supply of horseshoe kidneys. *AJR* 1971; 113:447.

Bookstein JJ, Goldstein HM: Successful management of post biopsy arteriovenous fistula with selective arterial embolization. *Radiology* 1973; 109:535.

Bratt CG, Aurell M, Nilsson S: Renal function in patients with hydronephrosis. *Brit J Urol* 1977; 49:249.

Bron KM, Redman H: Renal arteriovenous fistula and fibromuscular hyperplasia, a new association. *Ann Intern Med* 1968; 68:1039.

Buchta RM, Viseskul C, Gilbert EF, et al: Familial bilateral renal agenesis and hereditary renal adysplasia. *Z Kinderheilkunde* 1973; 115:111.

Bullock KN, Whitaker RH: Does good upper tract compliance preserve renal function? *J Urol* 1984; 131:914.

Burke EC, Wenzl JE, Utz DC: The intrathoracic kidney. Report of a case. *Am J Dis Child* 1967; 113:487.

Campbell MF: Embryology and anomalies of the urogenital tract. In Walsh PC, Gittes RF, Perlmutter AD, et al (eds): *Clinical Pediatric Urology*. Philadelphia, WB Saunders, 1951, pp 159-353.

Carlson H: Supernumerary kidney: a summary of fifty-one reported cases. *J Urol* 1950; 64:224.

Castro JE, Green NA: Complications of horseshoe kidney. *Urology* 1975; 6:344.

Cerny JC, Chang LY, Fry WJ: Renal artery aneurysms. *Arch Surg* 1968; 96:653.

Charny CW, Gillenwater JY: Congenital absence of the vas deferens. *J Urol* 1965; 93:399.

Chung YK, Chang PY, Lin CJ, et al: Conservative treatment of neonatal hydronephrosis. *J Formosan Med Assoc* 1992; 91:77.

Constantinou CE, Djurhuus JC: Urodynamics of the multicalyceal upper urinary tract. In O'Reilly PN, Gosling JA (eds): *Idiopathic Hydronephrosis*. New York, Springer-Verlag, 1982, pp 16-43.

Cook WA, Stephens FD: Fused kidneys: morphologic study and theory of embryogenesis. *Birth Defects* 1977; 13:327.

Culp OS, Winterringer JR: Surgical treatment of horseshoe kidney: Comparison of results after various types of operations. *J Urol* 1955; 73:747.

Cussenot O, Desgrandchamps F, Ollier P, et al: Anatomical basis of percutaneous surgery for calculi in horseshoe kidney. *Surg Radiol Anat* 1992; 14:209.

DeMyer W, Baird I: Mortality and skeletal malformations from amniocentesis and oligohydramnios in rats: cleft palate, club foot, microstomia, adactyly. *Teratology* 1969; 2:33.

DeSai SG, DeSautels RE: Congenital arteriovenous malformation of the kidney. *J Urol* 1973; 110:17.

Donahoe PK, Hendren WH: Pelvic kidney in infants and children: experience with 16 cases. *J Pediatr Surg* 1980; 115:486.

Doroshow L, Abeshouse BS: Congenital unilateral solitary kidney: report of 37 cases and a review of the literature. *Urol Surv* 1961; 11:219.

Downs RA, Lane JW, Burns E: Solitary pelvic kidney. Its clinical implications. *Urology* 1973; 1:51.

Drake DP, Stevens PS, Eckstein HB: Hydronephrosis secondary to ureteropelvic obstruction in children: a review of 14 years of experience. *J Urol* 1978; 119:649.

Emanuel B, Nachman R, Aronson N, et al: Congenital solitary kidney. *Am J Dis Child* 1974; 127:17.

English PJ, Testa HJ, Gosling JA, et al: Idiopathic hydronephrosis in childhood—a comparison between diuresis renography and upper urinary tract morphology. *Br J Urol* 1982; 54:603.

Ericsson NO, Rudhe U, Livaditis A: Hydronephrosis associated with aberrant renal vessels in infants and children. *Pediatr Surg* 1961; 50:687.

Esuvaranathan K, Tan EC, Tung KH, et al: Stones in horseshoe kidneys: results of treatment by ESWL and endourology. *J Urol* 1991; 146:1213.

Evans WP, Resnick MI: Horseshoe kidney and urolithiasis. *J Urol* 1981; 121:620.

Feldman SL, Lome LG: Renal dysplasia in horseshoe kidney. *Urology* 1982; 20:74.

Fernbach SK, Davis TM: The abnormal renal axis in children with spina bifida and gibbus deformity—the pseudohorseshoe kidney. *J Urol* 1986; 136:1258.

Fraley EE: Vascular obstruction of superior infundibulum causing nephralgia. A new syndrome. *N Engl J Med* 1966; 275:1403.

Gay BB, Dawes RK, Atkinson GO, et al: Wilms' tumor in horseshoe kidneys: radiologic diagnosis. *Radiology* 1983; 146:693.

Gittes RF: Congenital megacalices. In Stamey TA (ed): *1984 Monographs in Urology*. Princeton, NJ, Custom Publishing Services, 1984, pp 1-19.

Glass PM, Uson AC: Aneurysms of the renal artery, a study of 20 cases. *J Urol* 1967; 98:285.

Gleason PE, Kelalis PP, Husman DA, et al: Hydronephrosis in renal ectopia: incidence, etiology and significance. *J Urol* 1994; 151:1660.

Glenn JF: Analysis of 51 patients with horseshoe kidney. *N Engl J Med* 1959; 261:684.

Graves FT: The anatomy of the intrarenal arteries and its application to segmental resection of the kidney. *Br J Surg* 1954; 42:132.

Grignon A, Filiatrault D, Homsy Y, et al: Ureteropelvic junction stenosis: antenatal ultrasonographic diagnosis, postnatal investigation and follow-up. *Radiology* 1986; 160:649.

Hanna MK, Jeffs RD, Sturgess JM, et al: Ureteral structure and ultrastructure, part II: Congenital ureteropelvic junction obstruction and primary obstructive megaureter. *J Urol* 1976; 116:725.

Heliln I, Axelsson I, Persson PH: Prenatal diagnosis of Potter's syndrome by ultrasound. *Acta Paediatr Scand* 1983; 72:939.

Hendren WH, Radhakrishman J, Middleton AW Jr: Pediatric pyeloplasty. *J Ped Surg* 1980; 15:133.

Hohenfellner R, Schultz-Lampel D, Lampel A, et al: Tumor in the horseshoe kidney: clinical implications and review of embryogenesis. *J Urol* 1992; 147:1098.

Hosokawa S, Kawamura J, Tomoyoshi T, et al: Congenital renal anomaly evaluation with technetium-dimercaptosuccinic acid renal scintigraphy. *Am J Kidney Dis* 1983; 2:655.

Johnston JH: The pathogenesis of hydronephrosis in children. *Br J Urol* 1969; 41:724.

Johnston JH: Megacalycosis: A burnt out obstruction? *J Urol* 1973; 110:344.

Johnston JH, Evans JP, Glassberg KI, et al: Pelvic hydronephrosis in children: a review of 219 personal cases. *J Urol* 1977; 117:97.

Kaneti J, Lissmer L, Smailowitz Z, et al: Agenesis of kidney associated with malformations of the seminal vesicle. Various clinical presentations. *Int Urol Nephrol* 1988; 20:29.

Kaneto H, Orikasa S, Chiba T, et al: Three-D muscular arrangement at the ureteropelvic junction and its changes in congenital hydronephrosis: a stereo-morphometric study. *J Urol* 1991; 146:909.

Kelalis PP, Malek RS: Infundibulopelvic stenosis. *J Urol* 1983; 125:568.

Kelalis PP, Malek RS, Segura FW: Observations on renal ectopia and fusion in children. *J Urol* 1973; 110:588.

Kinch P: A morphometric study of the pelvi-ureteric junction and review of the pathogenesis of upper ureteric obstruction. *Pathology* 1982; 14:309.

Koff SA: The diagnosis of obstruction in experimental hydronephrosis; mechanisms for progressive urinary tract dilation. *Invest Urol* 1981; 19:85.

Koff SA: Ureteropelvic junction obstruction: role of newer diagnostic methods. *J Urol* 1982; 127:898.

Koff SA: Determinants of progression and equilibrium in hydronephrosis. *Urology* 1983; 21:496.

Koff SA, Campbell K: Nonoperative management of unilateral newborn hydronephrosis. *J Urol* 1992; 148:525.

Koff SA, Campbell K: Nonoperative management of unilateral neonatal hydronephrosis: natural history of poorly functioning kidneys. *J Urol* 1994; 152:593.

Koff SA, Hayden LJ, Cirulli C, et al: Pathophysiology of ureteropelvic junction obstruction: experimental and clinical observations. *J Urol* 1986; 136:336.

Koff SA, Whitaker RH: Recent advances in the diagnosis of upper urinary tract obstruction. In Whitaker RH and Woodard JR (eds): *Pediatric Urology*. London, Butterworths, 1985.

Kopchick JH, Bourne NK, Fine SW, et al: Congenital renal arteriovenous malformations. *Urology* 1981; 17:13.

Leary FJ, Utz DC: Miscellaneous vascular lesions affecting the urinary tract (aneurysms of the renal artery). In Emmett JL, Witten DM (eds): *Clinic Urography* vol 3. Philadelphia, WB Saunders Co, 1971, p 1639.

Lebowitz RL, Griscom NT: Neonatal hydronephrosis: 146 cases. *Radiol Clin North Am* 1977; 15:49.

Longo VJ: Congenital solitary kidney. *J Urol* 1952; 68:63.

Love WK, Robinette MA, Vernon CP: Renal artery aneurysm rupture in pregnancy. *J Urol* 1981; 126:809.

Lucaya J, Enriquez G, Delgado R, et al: Infundibulopelvic stenosis in children. *Am J Radiol* 1984; 142:471.

Maizels M, Stephens FD: The induction of urologic malformations. Understanding the relationship of renal ectopia and congenital scoliosis. *Invest Urol* 1979; 17:209.

Maldonado JE, Sheps SG, Bernatz PE, et al: Renal arteriovenous fistula. *Am J Med* 1964; 37:499.

Malek RS: Intermittent hydronephrosis: the occult ureteropelvic obstruction. *J Urol* 1983; 130:863.

Malek RS, Kelalis PP, Burke EC: Ectopic kidney in children and frequency of association with other malformations. *Mayo Clin Proc* 1971; 46:461.

Martin RS, Meacham PW, Ditesheim JA, et al: Renal artery aneurysm: Selective treatment for hypertension and prevention of rupture. *J Vasc Surg* 1989; 9:26.

McAlhany JC Jr, Black HC Jr, Hanback LD Jr, et al: Renal arteriovenous fistula as a cause of hypertension. *Am J Surg* 1971; 122:117.

McDonald JH, McClellan DS: Crossed renal ectopia. *Am J Surg* 1957; 93:995.

McLelland R: Renal artery aneurysm. *AJR* 1957; 78:256.

Mesrobian HG, Rushton HG, Bulas D: Unilateral renal agenesis may result from in utero regression of multicystic renal dysplasia. *J Urol* 1993; 150:793.

Messing E, Kessler R, Kaveney PB: Renal arteriovenous fistulas. *Urology* 1976; 8:101.

Middleton AW, Pfister RD: Stone-containing pyelocaliceal diverticulum: embryogenic anatomic, radiologic and clinical characteristics. *J Urol* 1974; 111:2.

Murnaghan GF: The dynamics of the renal pelvis and ureter with reference to congenital hydronephrosis. *Br J Urol* 1958; 30:321.

Murugasu BF, Cole BR, Hawkins EP, et al: Familial renal dysplasia. *Am J Kidney Dis* 1991; 18:490.

Nakada T, Furuta H, Kazama T, et al: Unilateral renal agenesis with or without ipsilateral adrenal agenesis. *J Urol* 1988; 140:933.

N'Guessan G, Stephens FD: Supernumerary kidney. *J Urol* 1983; 130:649.

Nilsson S, Aurell M, Bratt CG: Maximum urinary concentration ability in patients with idiopathic hydronephrosis. *Br J Urol* 1979; 51:432.

Nixon HH: Hydronephrosis in children: a clinical study of 78 cases with special reference to the role of aberrant renal vessels and the results of conservative operations. *Br J Surg* 1953; 40:601.

Notley RG: Electron microscopy of the upper ureter and the pelvi-ureteric junction. *Br J Urol* 1968; 40:37.

Odiase VON: Horseshoe kidney. A review of 25 cases. *J R Coll Surg* 1983; 28:41.

O'Hara PJ, Hakaim AG, Hertzer NR, et al: Surgical management of aortic aneurysm and coexistent horseshoe kidney: review of 31 year experience. *J Vasc Surg* 1993; 17:940.

Olesen S, Madsen PO: Function during partial obstruction following contralateral nephrectomy in the dog. *J Urol* 1968; 99:692.

Olsen PR: The renal pelvis and ureteral peristalsis. I. Pelvometry. *Scand J Urol Nephrol* 1979; 13:269.

O'Reilly PH: Relationship between intermittent hydronephrosis and megacalycosis. *Brit J Urol* 1989; 64:125.

O'Reilly PH, Testa HJ, Lawson RS, et al: Diuresis renography in equivocal urinary tract obstruction. *Br J Urol* 1978; 50:76.

Oxman HA, Sheps SG, Bernatz PE, et al: An unusual cause of renal arteriovenous fistula—fibromuscular dysplasia of the renal arteries. Report of a case. *Mayo Clin Proc* 1973; 48:207.

Pinsonneault O, Goldstein DP: Obstructing malformations of the uterus and vagina. *Fertil Steril* 1985; 44:241.

Pitts WR, Muecke EC: Horseshoe kidneys: a 40 year experience. *J Urol* 1975; 113:743.

Potter EL: Bilateral absence of ureters and kidneys. *Obstet Gynecol* 1965; 25:3.

Poutasse EF: Renal artery aneurysms. *J Urol* 1975; 113:443.

Ratner LE, Zibari G: Strategies for successful transplantation of the horseshoe kidney. *J Urol* 1993; 150:958.

Reed HM, Robinson ND: Horseshoe kidney with simultaneous occurrence of calculi, transitional cell and squamous cell carcinoma. *Urology* 1984; 23:62.

Robson WJ, Rudy SM, Johnston JH: Pelviureteric obstruction in infancy. *J Pediatr Surg* 1976; 11:57.

Roodhooft AM, Birnholz JC, Holmes LB: Familial nature of congenital absence and severe dysgenesis of both kidneys. *N Engl J Med* 1984; 310:1341.

Ruano-Gil D, Coca-Payeras, Tejedo-Mateu A: Obstruction and normal recanalization of the ureter in the human embryo. Its relation to congenital ureteric obstruction. *Eur Urol J* 1975; 1:287.

Rubinstein ZJ, Hertz M, Shahin N, et al: Crossed renal ectopia: angiographic findings in six cases. *AJR* 1976; 126:1035.

Sasidharan K, Babu AS, Rao MM, et al: Free supernumerary kidney. *Br J Urol* 1976; 48:388.

Schacht MJ, Sakowica B, Rao MS, et al: Intermittent abdominal pain in a patient with horseshoe kidney. *J Urol* 1983; 130:749.

Schneider K, Martin W, Helmig FJ, et al: Infundibulopelvic stenosis—evaluation of diagnostic imaging. *Eur J Radiol* 1988; 8:172.

Segura JW, Kelalis PP, Burke EC: Horseshoe kidney in children. *J Urol* 1972; 108:333.

Serrate R, Regue R, Prats J, et al: ESWL as treatment for lithiasis in horseshoe kidney. *Eur Urol* 1991; 20:122.

Sheih CP, Hung CS, Wei CF, et al: Cystic dilations within the pelvis in patients with ipsilateral renal agenesis or dysplasia. *J Urol* 1990; 144:324.

Slawin KM, Reilley EA, Baise J, et al: Renal artery aneurysm in the pediatric patient. *NY State J Med* 1991; 91:547.

Smith EC, Orkin LA: A clinical and statistical study of 471 congenital anomalies of the kidney and ureter. *J Urol* 1945; 53:11.

Smith JN, Hinman F Jr: Intrarenal arterial aneurysms. *J Urol* 1967; 97:990.

Snyder HM, Lebowitz RL, Colodny AH, et al: Ureteropelvic junction obstruction in children. *Urol Clin North Am* 1980; 7:273.

Squires EC, Morden RS, Bernstein J: Renal multicystic dysplasia: an occasional manifestation of the hereditary renal adysplasia syndrome. *Am J Med Genetics* 1987; 3:279.

Stanley JC, Fry WJ: Pediatric renal artery occlusive disease and renovascular hypertension. Etiology, diagnosis and operative treatment. *Arch Surg* 1981; 116:669.

Stanley JC, Rhodes EL, Gwertz BL, et al: Renal artery aneurysms. Significance of macroaneurysms exclusive of dissections and fibrodysplastic mural dilations. *Arch Surg* 1975; 110:1327.

Starr NT, Maizels M, Chou P: Microanatomy and morphometry of the hydronephrotic "obstructed" renal pelvis in asymptomatic infants. *J Urol* 1992; 148:519.

Stassart JP, Nagel TC, Prem KA, et al: Uterus didelphys, obstructed hemivagina, and ipsilateral renal agenesis: the University of Minnesota experience. *Fertil Steril* 1992; 57:756.

Stephens FD: Ureterovascular hydronephrosis and the "aberrant" renal vessels. *J Urol* 1982; 128:984.

Strubbe EH, Willemsen WNP, Lemmens JAM, et al: Mayer-Rokitansky-Kuster-Hauser Syndrome: distinction between two forms based on excretory urographic, sonographic, and laparoscopic findings. *AJR* 1992; 160:331.

Takaha M, Matsumoto A, Ochi K, et al: Intrarenal arteriovenous malformation. *J Urol* 1980; 124:315.

Tarry WF, Duckett JW, Stephens FD: The Mayer-Rokitansky syndrome: pathogenesis, classification and management. *J Urol* 1986; 136:648.

Thompson DP, Lynn HB: Genital anomalies associated with solitary kidney. *Mayo Clin Proc* 1966; 41:538.

Thrall J, Koff SA, Keyes JW Jr: Diuretic radionuclide renography and scintigraphy in the differential diagnosis of hydroureteronephrosis. *Semin Nucl Med* 1981; 11:89.

Timmons JW, Malek RS, Hattery RR, et al: Caliceal diverticulum. *J Urol* 1975; 114:6.

Trigaux JP, Van Beers B, Delchambre F: Male genital tract malformations associated with ipsilateral renal agenesis: sonographic findings. *J Clin Ultrasound* 1991; 19:3.

Uhlenhuth E, Amin M, Harty JI, et al: Infundibular pelvic dysgenesis. A spectrum of obstructive renal disease. *Urology* 1990; 35:334.

Uson AC, Cox LA, Lattimer JK: Hydronephrosis in infants and children. *JAMA* 1968; 205:323.

Whitaker RH: Diagnosis of obstruction in dilated ureters. *Ann R Coll Surg Engl* 1973; 53:153.

Williams DI, Karlaftis CM: Hydronephrosis due to pelviureteric obstruction in the newborn. *Br J Urol* 1966; 38:138.

Williams DI, Kenawi MM: The prognosis of pelviureteric obstruction in childhood. A review of 190 cases. *Eur Urol* 1976; 2:57.

Williams G, Blandy JP, Tresidder GC: Communicating cysts and diverticula of the renal pelvis. *Br J Urol* 1969; 41:163.

Yazaki T, Tomita M, Akimoto M, et al: Congenital renal arteriovenous fistula; case report, review of Japanese literature and description of non-radical treatment. *J Urol* 1976; 116:415.

Yeh HC, Mitty HA, Halton K, et al: Milk of calcium in renal cysts: new sonographic features. *J Ultrasound Med* 1992; 11:195.

Yoder IC, Pfister RD: Unilateral hematocolpos and ipsilateral renal agenesis: report of two cases and review of the literature. *AJR* 1976; 127:303.

Yura T, Yuasa S, Ohkawa M, et al: Noninvasive detection and monitoring of renal arteriovenous fistula by color doppler. *Am J Nephrol* 1991; 11:250.

Zondek LH, Zondek T: Horseshoe kidney and associated congenital malformations. *Urol Int* 1964; 18:347.

CHAPTER 46

Anomalies of the Ureter

Howard M. Snyder III

NEW TERMINOLOGY

Literature on anomalies of the ureter has been often confusing because of the multitude of terms used. For example, *orthotopic* has been used to describe an intravesical upper pole ureterocele associated with a duplex system or a ureterocele associated with a single system or even the orifice of a lower pole duplicated ureter that is lateral to the normal point of entry into the bladder at the corner of the trigone. The term *ectopic* has also been confusing. Some have used it to characterize a ureter or ureterocele that is located at the bladder neck or more distally, whereas others have used this term to simply describe the ureter draining the upper pole of a duplex kidney even when that orifice is in a normal position in the bladder. There have been a plethora of terms used to characterize ureteroceles, such as *childhood, adult, giant, orthotopic, simple, and ectopic*. Simple and orthotopic have been most frequently used to describe a small ureterocele located proximal to the bladder neck. However, some authors use simple to imply a single system ureterocele.

In an effort to clarify the confusion produced by this varied terminology, the Urologic Section of the American Academy of Pediatrics Committee on Terminology, Nomenclature, and Classification has suggested a simplified terminology for duplex systems, ectopic ureters, and ureteroceles (Glassberg et al., 1984). It is hoped that if a general usage of these terms is achieved, future confusion in the literature will be reduced. The recommendation of the terminology committee is that the term *duplex kidney* be used instead of double kidney. Ectopic and orthotopic should not be used as synonyms corresponding to upper and lower pole ureters or orifices. It is recommended that *upper* or *lower pole ureter* or *ureteral orifice* be used instead. The term ectopic is best restricted to describing a ureter and its orifice that drains at a site on the proximal lip of the bladder neck or more caudally, whether the ureter is part of a duplex or single renal system. *Ectopic ureterocele* is a useful term to describe a ureterocele that has a portion situated at the bladder neck or in the urethra. Orthotopic is a confusing term that is best avoided; it is better to use the term *intravesical ureterocele* to describe a ureterocele proximal to the bladder neck. The term simple should be dropped to describe an intravesical ureterocele, because it does not clarify whether the ureterocele is part of a single or duplex system.

The following glossary of terms has been recommended by the Committee on Terminology and will be used in this chapter.

Glossary of Terms

Duplex kidney—A kidney in which two pelvicalyceal systems are present.

Upper (lower) pole—One of the components of a duplex system.

Duplex (duplicated) system—A renal unit in which the kidney has two pelvicalyceal systems and is associated with a single ureter or bifid ureters (partial or incomplete duplication) or two ureters (double ureters) that empty separately into the bladder (complete duplication).

Bifid system—A form of duplication in which two pelvicalyceal systems join at the ureteropelvic junction (bifid pelvis) or in which two ureters join before emptying into the bladder (bifid ureters).

Double ureters—The two ureters associated with complete duplication. Each independent ureter drains a separate pelvicalyceal system and opens separately into the urinary or genital tract.

Upper (lower) pole ureter—The ureter that drains the upper (lower) pole of a duplex system.

Upper (lower) pole orifice—The orifice associated with the ureter that drains the upper (lower) pole of a duplex kidney; the orifice of an upper (lower) pole ureter.

Lateral ectopia (of ureteral orifice)—An orifice situated lateral to the normal position.

Caudal or medial ectopia (of ureteral orifice)—An

orifice situated at the proximal lip of the bladder neck or beyond.

Ectopic ureter—A ureter that drains to an abnormal site. However, since the term has been used so widely to mean a ureter whose orifice is ectopic caudally, this latter definition still is acceptable.

Intravesical ureterocele—A type of ureterocele that is located entirely within the bladder. An intravesical ureterocele may be associated with a single system but also may be associated with the upper pole ureter of a completely duplicated system; only rarely is it associated with a lower pole ureter.

Ectopic ureterocele—A type of ureterocele in which some portion of the ureterocele is situated permanently at the bladder neck or in the urethra. The orifice may be situated in the bladder, at the bladder neck, or in the urethra. Ureteroceles can be characterized further as stenotic, sphincteric, sphincterostenotic, cecoureteroceles, blind, and nonobstructive, as suggested by Stephens (1971).

Embryology of the Ureteral Bud

The spectrum of ureteral anomalies to be presented in this chapter is better understood in light of the embryology of the ureteral bud. Associated renal abnormalities can be understood in terms of differences in induction of renal tissue from the metanephric ridge produced by ureteral buds arising at various levels from the mesonephric duct. Normally, the ureter begins development at approximately the end of the fourth week of embryonic life as a bud taking its origin from the mesonephric (wolffian) duct at the point at which the duct bends sharply ventrally (the elbow) (Fig. 46-1). The ureteral bud grows rapidly to penetrate the metanephric blastemal ridge. By 5 weeks of gestation, the renal pelvis can be discerned. As subsequent renal differentiation takes place, the ureteral bud will produce the entire renal collecting system: ureter, renal pelvis, calyces, papillary ducts, and collecting tubules.

The "elbow" of the mesonephric duct is the point where the ureteral bud normally joins the duct and is the point at which the mesonephric duct bends forward and medially to join the ventral aspect of the cloaca. The portion of the mesonephric duct distal to the point of origin of the ureteral bud is referred to as the *common excretory duct*. The mesonephric duct is progressively absorbed into the portion of the cloaca that will become the urogenital sinus. The common excretory duct has been absorbed into the urogenital sinus by the eighth week of development, and the ureter and mesonephric duct are then independently joined to the urogenital sinus. Initially, the ureteral bud is below and medial to the mesonephric duct, and

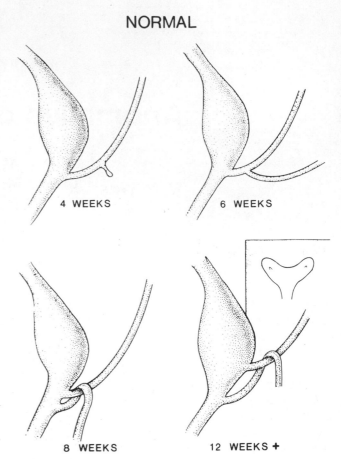

NORMAL

4 WEEKS

6 WEEKS

8 WEEKS

12 WEEKS +

FIG. 46-1
Normal embryology of ureteral bud from the mesonephric duct.

they are closely approximated. As development proceeds the ureteral orifice migrates cephalad and laterally while the mesonephric duct moves distally and medially to finally achieve its normal entry position in the posterior urethra at the verumontanum. The mesonephric duct will become the epididymis, seminal vesical, and vas deferens. By the twelfth week of development, the ureteral orifice and mesonephric duct have achieved their final position. It is the migration of the ureteral bud and mesonephric duct that causes the mesonephric duct and thus the vas to cross over the ureter ventrally.

In normal embryology the point at which the distal mesonephric duct joins the urogenital sinus indicates the eventual location of the bladder neck. As the common excretory duct (mesonephric duct below the point of origin of the ureteral bud) is incorporated into the expanding urogenital sinus, it forms the tissue of the bladder trigone. After ureteral bud and mesonephric duct migration is complete, the final positions of the ejaculatory duct and the ureteral orifice are usually roughly equidistant from the bladder neck.

NORMAL SITE

BIFID BUD

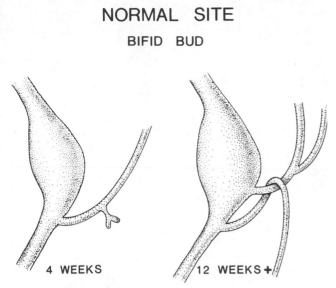

4 WEEKS

12 WEEKS +

FIG. 46-2
Bifid ureteral bud at normal site leading to incomplete duplication of ureter.

If this brief outline of normal embryology is borne in mind, it becomes much simpler to understand the pathologic conditions to be presented in this chapter. These anomalies are best understood as abnormalities of origin or division of the ureteral bud.

If the origin of the ureteral bud is at a normal site on the mesonephric duct but the bud bifurcates shortly after its origin, an incomplete duplication of the ureter will be seen (Fig. 46-2). If this division of the ureteral bud occurs late (fifth week), when the ureter is growing into the metanephric blastema, a bifid pelvis will be all that is seen. Before the fifth week, bifurcation of the ureteral bud will lead to varying degrees of ureteral duplication but with fusion distally to form a single ureter entering the bladder.

Primary vesicoureteral reflux can be understood to result from a ureteral bud that takes origin at a lower-than-normal position on the mesonephric duct (Fig. 46-3). As this low ureteral bud is incorporated into the urogenital sinus, a standard period of ureteral migration would lead it to be carried more laterally and cranially than normal. In this position less trigonal support for the ureter might be expected. This embryologic explanation would account for what is found clinically in primary reflux: a lateral ureteral orifice with a shortened submucosal tunnel permitting vesicoureteral reflux (Ambrose and Nicolson, 1962; Stephens and Lenaghan, 1962; Tanagho and Hutch, 1965).

If the ureteral bud were to have its origin marginally higher than normal on the mesonephric duct, a minor and nonpathologic degree of displacement of the ureteral orifice toward the bladder neck might result (Fig.

LOW BUD

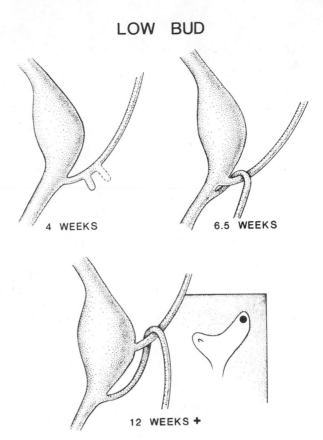

4 WEEKS

6.5 WEEKS

12 WEEKS +

FIG. 46-3
Low origin of the ureteral bud from the mesonephric duct leading to laterally ectopic ureteral orifice and vesicoureteral reflux.

46-4). However, if the ureteral bud were to originate very high on the mesonephric duct, it might fail to be incorporated into the bladder altogether and end in the urethra or mesonephric remnants (Fig. 46-5). In the male human these remnants constitute the epididymis, vas, and seminal vesical. In the female human Gartner's duct is the distal remnant of the mesonephric duct. It runs from the broad ligament of the uterus along the lateral wall of the vagina to end at the hymen. A very high origin of the ureteral bud in the female could end anywhere along this duct and with secondary rupture of the duct into the vagina resulting in a vaginally ectopic ureter. This discussion, then, provides the explanation for the main sites of ectopic ureters in males and females. The important difference between the two sexes is attributed to the fact that in the male, all ectopic ureters terminate above the level of the external urethral sphincter so that urinary incontinence is uncommon. In the female, by contrast, ectopic ureters commonly exit below sphincteric control, which accounts for the history of constant wetting from the ectopic ureter in spite of normal voiding of urine from ureters terminating in the bladder.

HIGH BUD

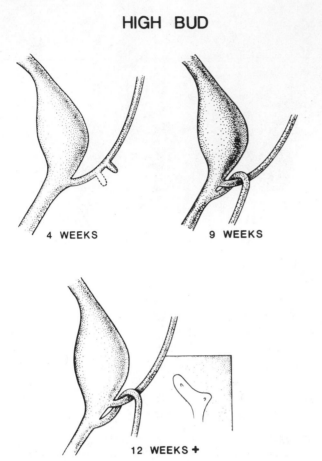

4 WEEKS   9 WEEKS

12 WEEKS +

FIG. 46-4
High origin of the ureteral bud from mesonephric duct leading to mild degree of ureteral ectopia toward the bladder neck but still on trigone.

VERY HIGH BUD

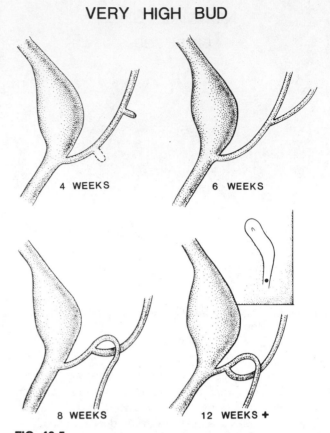

4 WEEKS   6 WEEKS

8 WEEKS   12 WEEKS +

FIG. 46-5
Very high origin of ureteral bud from mesonephric duct leading ectopic ureter to maintain contact with mesonephric remnants (vas, epididymis, or seminal vesicle).

The presence of two ureteral buds having independent origin from the mesonephric duct accounts for some of the most fascinating of ureteral anomalies. If the two buds arise close to the normal point of ureteral origin from the mesonephric duct, a complete ureteral duplication may result without any significant consequence (Fig. 46-6). By contrast, if two buds are present, with one located normally and one low, the result would be complete duplication with vesicoureteral reflux into the ureter, which during migration was carried most cranially and laterally, that is, the lower pole ureter (Fig. 46-7). This anomaly is a frequent clinical finding (Ambrose and Nicolson, 1964). With a duplication of the ureteral bud with one in a normal location and one high, the high ureter would be formed to end more caudally and medially than normal (Fig. 46-8). Thus the upper pole ureter is the one that ends ectopically. This embryologic review explains the Meyer-Weigert law: When complete ureteral duplication exists, the medial and distal ureteral orifice is that of the ureter to the upper pole of the kidney

(Meyer, 1907; Weigert, 1877). Occasional exceptions to this law have been reported (Lund, 1949).

To complete a presentation of the caudal embryology of the ureter, one must include a discussion of the origin of ureteroceles. Ureteroceles can be defined as a cystic dilatation of the terminal portion of the ureter. Ureteroceles associated with a single ureter are seen in children, usually as intravesical ureteroceles; however, ureteroceles associated with complete ureteral duplication are more common. In this situation they are at the distal end of the ureter. They drain the upper pole collecting system and are most commonly ectopic ureteroceles, that is, a ureterocele with some portion situated permanently at the bladder neck or in the urethra.

Chwalla (1927) suggested that ureteroceles have an obstructive etiology. Chwalla pointed out a two-cell-layer ureteral membrane that is present in the embryo at the time the ureteral bud arises from the mesonephric duct. If this membrane did not completely break down, an obstructed ureteral-meatal orifice would result, leading to the formation of a ureterocele. The ureteroceles seen with stenotic orifices or asso-

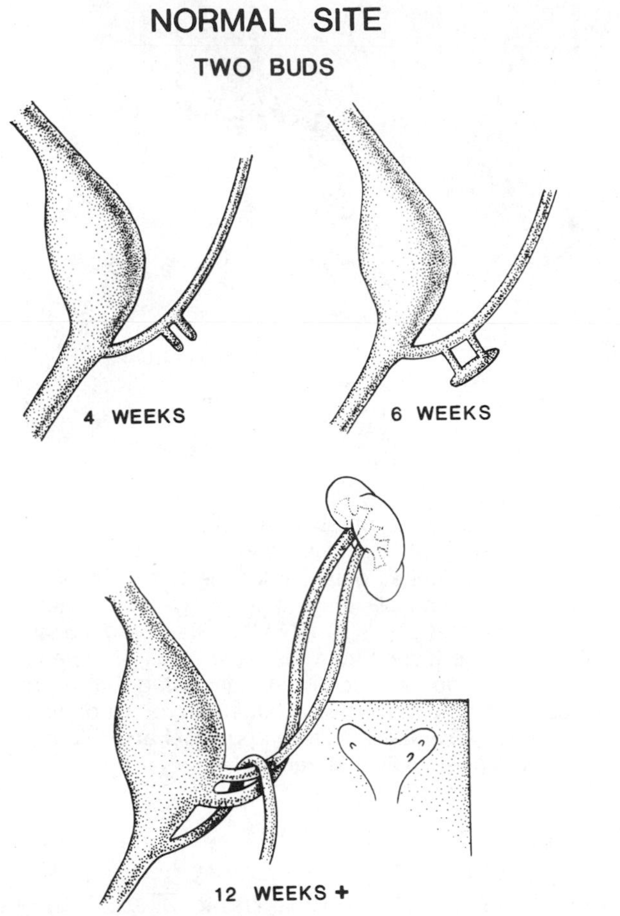

NORMAL SITE
TWO BUDS

4 WEEKS

6 WEEKS

12 WEEKS +

FIG. 46-6
Two ureteral buds at normal site on mesonephric duct leading to complete duplication of the ureter without pathologic sequelae.

TWO BUDS
ONE NORMAL, ONE LOW

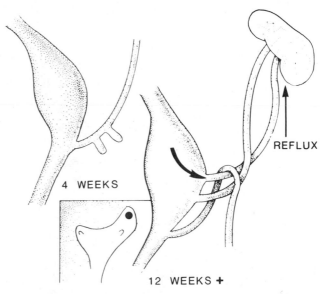

4 WEEKS

12 WEEKS +

REFLUX

FIG. 46-7
Two ureteral buds, one normal and one low on the mesonephric duct, leading to complete ureteral duplication with lower pole vesicoureteral reflux.

TWO BUDS
ONE NORMAL, ONE HIGH

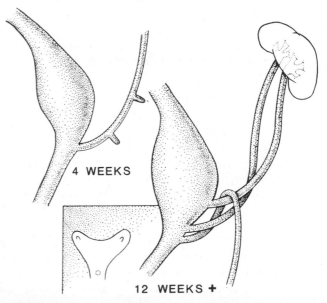

4 WEEKS

12 WEEKS +

FIG. 46-8
Two ureteral buds, one normal and one high on the mesonephric duct, leading to complete ureteral duplication with ectopic upper pole ureter.

ciated with muscular hypertrophy of the ureteral wall (or both) fit into this postulated origin well. But Stephens (1963) and others have described cases in which ureteroceles are found to have large ureteral orifices or, rarely, to be associated with a blind-ending ureter. Such cases make obstruction unsatisfactory as a total explanation for ureteroceles.

Alternatively, it has been suggested that the distal ureteral segment may be acted on by the same force that causes the expansion of the urogenital sinus to form the bladder (Stephens, 1971; Tanagho, 1976, 1979). If this theory were an adequate explanation for ureterocele formation, all caudal ectopic ureters should be associated with a ureterocele, which is not the case. Perhaps an explanation lies in Tanagho's (1976, 1979) postulation of an additional factor: delay in establishment of the lumen of the ureteral bud with that of the mesonephric duct. Perhaps this delay could be the triggering factor that produces ureteral expansion (Fig. 46-9). It is clear that our understanding of ureterocele embryology remains incomplete.

TWO BUDS
UPPER DELAYED LUMEN

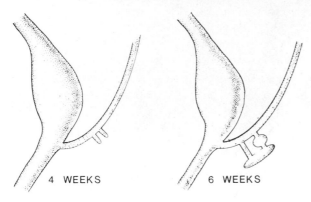

4 WEEKS   6 WEEKS

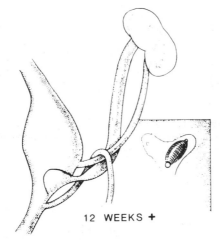

12 WEEKS +

FIG. 46-9
Two ureteral buds with delay in establishment of lumen of upper ureteral bud leading to development of upper pole ureterocele.

Relation of Ureteral Bud Position to Renal Morphology

Renal tissue associated with ectopic ureters and ureters joining ureteroceles is frequently dysplastic or hypoplastic and has minimal, if any, function. In 1975 Mackie and Stephens suggested that this finding could be associated with an abnormal origin of the ureteral bud from the mesonephric duct, which, as we have seen, may account for the caudal embryologic explanation for ectopic ureters and ureteroceles (Fig. 46-10). According to this theory, the metanephric ridge is made up of blastema with variable potential for the formation of normal renal tissue. The best potential exists in the central zone of the ridge, which would be the area normally penetrated by a ureteral bud having origin from a normal location on the mesonephric duct. This normal ureteral bud would thus be expected to induce a kidney from the metanephric blastema with the best potential to form a normal

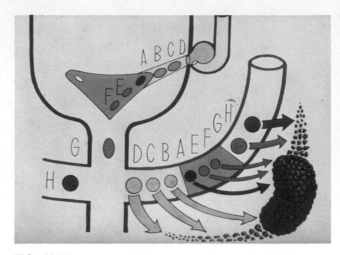

FIG. 46-10
Stephens' theory that an abnormal origin of the ureteral bud from the mesonephric duct leads to induction of metanephric blastema with limited potential for the formation of normal renal tissue. Composite diagram showing how a ureteral bud with near-normal origin **(A, E, F)** from the mesonephric duct will induce the kidney from the main mass of metanephric blastema and for a good kidney associated with a ureteral orifice on the trigone. Ureteral buds with an abnormal origin will induce blastema with limited potential and will be associated with an ectopic ureteral orifice.

kidney. On either side of the central zone of the metanephric ridge, the blastema may have a lesser potential to form normal renal tissue. Thus, if the ureteral bud is located above or below the normal point of origin, it may grow to induce renal tissue from blastema with an increased propensity for dysplasia or hypoplasia. This theory appears to hold best for the upper pole ureters seen in complete duplications associated with ectopic ureters or ureteroceles. Less commonly, occasional lateral ectopic ureteral orifices associated with vesicoureteral reflux may also be found attached to ureters draining dysplastic or hypoplastic renal tissue. Thus the Mackie and Stephens theory provides an attractive explanation for abnormal renal tissue associated with a ureteral orifice either cranial or caudal from the location of a normal ureteral orifice at the corner of the trigone.

Occasionally, quite normal renal tissue is found associated with ectopic ureteral orifices (Kesavan et al., 1977; Schlecker et al., 1986) or ureteroceles. An explanation might lie in growth of a ureteral bud that is not perfectly straight toward the metanephric ridge. If the bud were to stray a bit, it might come to induce metanephric blastema with good potential for the formation of normal renal tissue. Thus we might explain the normal renal tissue that is occasionally associated with an abnormally located ureteral orifice as well as the occasional converse association of a normal ureteral orifice with dysplastic or hypoplastic renal parenchyma.

Ureteral Duplication

Incidence, Genetics, and Associated Anomalies

Ureteral duplication constitutes the most frequently seen ureteral anomaly. In an autopsy population, ureteral duplication appears to occur in approximately 1 in 125 patients, or 0.8% (Campbell, 1970; Nation, 1944). Bilateral duplication is seen in approximately 40% of cases (Timothy et al., 1971). The right and left kidneys are affected equally. In clinical series, there are twice as many females with duplications as males. In series where urography has been done for urinary symptoms, there is a much higher incidence of duplication: 2% to 4% (Hartman and Hodson, 1969). Urinary infection is the most common associated finding. From the previous embryologic discussion, it is clear why a duplication might be associated with upper tract stasis from obstruction or reflux.

A genetic analysis of duplication indicates this anomaly may be transmitted as an autosomal dominant trait with incomplete penetrance (Cohen and Berant, 1976). When an index child with a duplication is found in a family, the frequency of a sibling being found with a duplication rises from 1 in 25 to 1 in 8 or 9 (Atwell et al., 1974; Babcock et al., 1977; Whitaker and Danks, 1966).

Patients with ureteral duplication are also found to have an increased incidence of other urinary tract anomalies. In the radiographic review of Privett and colleagues (1976), 29% of the duplex units reviewed exhibited scarring, hydronephrosis, or both. Histologically, renal hypoplasia or dysplasia and pyelonephritic scarring have an increased incidence. None of these findings is surprising in light of the previous embryologic discussion. Clinically, one would expect to see an increased incidence of childhood urinary tract infections when duplications are present because of associated reflux or obstruction, and indeed, this increase is what has been found (Campbell, 1970; Kretschmer, 1937).

Incomplete Ureteral Duplication: Y Ureter

An incomplete ureteral duplication with a common ureteral stem entering the bladder is the result of a bifurcation of the ureteral bud after it has taken its origin from the mesonephric duct. The degree of duplication is determined by the level of the bifurcation. A bifid renal pelvis is the result of the highest level of bifurcation and is seen in approximately 10% of the population. It is best viewed as a variant of normal. Of the other incomplete duplications, approximately 25% are found to divide in the distal or proximal third of the ureter, whereas the remaining 50% divide in the middle section. In most instances this form of ureteral duplication presents as an incidental finding. However, with a Y junction in the ureter, it is possible for urine to be passed down to the junction and then,

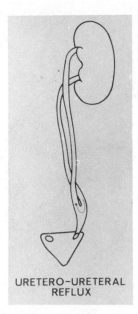

URETERO-URETERAL
REFLUX

FIG. 46-11

Yo-yo reflux: incomplete ureteral duplication and ureteroureteral reflux.

in a retrograde fashion, up the other side of the Y (Campbell, 1967; Tresidder et al., 1970). This ureteral reflux, or yo-yo, can rarely lead to stasis and ureteral dilatation (Fig. 46-11). It is most common when the bifurcation is at a low position but is rare if the duplication ends in the intramural portion of the ureter (Lenaghan, 1962). It has been reported in a blindending bifid ureter (Kontturi and Kaska, 1972). When yo-yo is present, there may be associated infection or flank discomfort.

Diagnosis is established by intravenous pyelography (IVP), particularly if fluoroscopic observation is used to observe the ureteral reflux (Kaplan and Elkin, 1968). A voiding cystourethrogram (VCUG) is essential to eliminate ureteral dilatation due to simple vesicoureteral reflux, which is much more common.

When surgical treatment is warranted, the operation will depend on the level of the duplication. If the duplication is very low, a reimplantation of the ureters into the bladder with separate ureteral orifices may be possible (Amar, 1972). When the duplication is higher, ureteropyelostomy or ureteroureterostomy at renal level with excision of most of the distal duplicated ureter is curative (Amar, 1970).

On occasion, ureteropelvic junction obstruction may be found in association with incomplete duplex systems and may pose interesting reconstructive problems (Ossandon et al., 1981). Usually the lower pole ureter is short (Fig. 46-12), and a side-to-side anastomosis of the obstructed lower pole pelvis to the upper pole ureter is required to deal effectively with the problem.

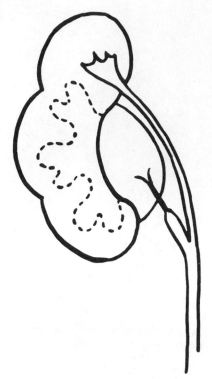

FIG. 46-12
Ureteropelvic junction obstruction in lower pole of duplex kidney. Usually the lower pole ureter is too short for a ureteropyelostomy and, accordingly, a side-to-side anastomosis of the pelvis to the upper pole ureter is performed.

Incomplete Ureteral Duplication: Blind-Ending Ureter

A very rare form of incomplete duplication has a blind-ending ureteral stump proximally (Albers et al., 1971; Peterson et al., 1975; Schultze, 1967). The embryologic explanation lies in a ureteral bud that bifurcates but has only one limb succeed in inducing associated renal parenchyma. Most of these duplications are in the middle or distal ureter. Women are three times more likely to exhibit this, and it is seen most frequently on the right side. A ureteral diverticulum may be confused with this entity (Rank et al., 1960). Culp's (1947) somewhat arbitrary criteria help to better define the true blind-ending bifid ureter: those blind-ending structures whose lumen joins that of the ureter at a clear angle, whose length is at least twice the width, and whose histologic characteristics resemble the ureter. Occasionally a blind-ending ureteral duplication may end in the bladder and be confused with a periureteral diverticulum because of the frequent association of vesicoureteral reflux in this situation (Marshall and McLoughlin, 1978).

The rare patient with a blind-ending duplication who has symptoms generally has them in the third or fourth decade. Flank pain associated with infection or calculi constitutes the most frequent presentation. A retrograde ureterogram may be required for diagnosis, because the blind duplication may not fill on IVP. Treatment consists of surgical excision of the duplication.

Incomplete Ureteral Duplication: Inverted Y Ureter

The inverted Y ureter is the rarest of all anomalies of ureteral branching. The embryologic explanation presumably lies in two separate ureteral buds arising from the mesonephric duct but fusing prior to penetrating the metanephric ridge. This anomaly has been seen almost exclusively in females (Klauber and Reid, 1972). If one limb is distally ectopic, urinary incontinence may result. Treatment is directed at problems caused by the ectopic limb. Usually resection of this limb is required. An inverted Y ureteral duplication with one blind-ending ureter has been reported (Britt et al., 1972).

Complete Ureteral Duplication and Vesicoureteral Reflux

When a complete ureteral duplication is present, vesicoureteral reflux is the most common cause of acquired renal disease. Reflux typically occurs into the lower moiety of a duplicated kidney drained by a ureter that had an abnormally caudal origin on the mesonephric duct, leading to a laterally ectopic ureteral orifice with shortened submucosal tunnel and vesicoureteral reflux (Ambrose and Nicolson, 1964). The upper pole ureter with its orifice medial and more distal (Meyer-Weigert law) has a longer submucosal tunnel and usually does not reflux. When reflux into both upper and lower pole ureteral orifices is seen, cystoscopy usually reveals that both orifices are side by side in a laterally ectopic position. This anomaly is embryologically explained by two ureteral buds close to one another, having an origin in a position caudal to normal on the mesonephric duct. Reflux into the upper pole ureter also may occur if its orifice is ectopic in the bladder neck or urethra, because the ureter reaches this point separately without trigonal support for an adequate submucosal tunnel. The child with duplication and reflux presents most commonly with urinary tract infection, as does the child with single-system reflux. The presence of complete ureteral duplication appears to increase the likelihood that reflux will be found. Fehrenbaker and co-authors (1972) found reflux in more than two thirds of children with duplex systems who presented with a urinary tract infection. The IVP and the VCUG establish the diagnosis by showing a duplex renal system with vesicoureteral reflux usually only into the lower pole collecting system (Fig. 46-13).

The treatment of duplicated ureters with reflux adheres to the same principles that govern the single-system ureter with reflux. When the grade of reflux

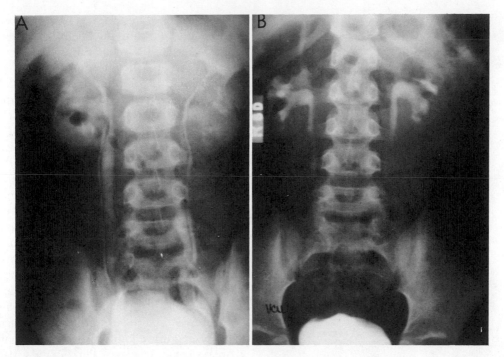

FIG. 46-13
Complete ureteral duplication and vesicoureteral reflux. **A,** Intravenous pyelogram showing completed duplication of ureters. **B,** Voiding cystourethrogram showing bilateral lower pole vesicoureteral reflux.

is low, spontaneous resolution with linear growth of the child accompanied by lengthening of the submucosal tunnel of the ureter usually avoids the need for surgery. Antibiotic prophylaxis and radiographic monitoring intermittently suffice for treatment. Surgical management may be more appropriate when the grade of reflux is high and the likelihood of spontaneous resolution is small. In a complete duplication, the distal 2 to 3 cm of the two ureters usually are bound in a common muscular sheath, making their separation dangerous to one or both ureters. Surgical correction of reflux thus involves mobilization of the common sheath and reimplantation of the common sheath, even though reflux has been observed in only one ureter (Barrett et al., 1975; Johnston and Heal, 1971). When the lower pole parenchyma is very diminutive, a common sheath reimplant generally still suffices unless there is major ureteral dilatation. This approach avoids the need for a renal operation, although the possible rare later development of hypertension secondary to the retained nubbin will have to be borne in mind.

Ureteral Triplication

Ureteral triplication is one of the rarest anomalies of the upper urinary tract. In their review of the literature in 1978, Kohri and colleagues could find only 75 cases. The embryologic explanation for ureteral triplication would be the presence of three ureteral buds taking origin separately on the mesonephric

duct. If there is early division of the ducts, partial triplication would result, as has been reported. In most cases all three ureters drain through a single orifice (Kohri et al., 1978). The left side appears to be affected most commonly, and trifid ureters are seen most frequently in females (Perkins et al., 1973). Symptoms may be infection, incontinence, or pain (Livaditis et al., 1964). Ureteral triplication in association with an ectopic ureter (Youngson, 1985; Zaontz and Maizels, 1985) and ureterocele (Finkel et al., 1983) has been reported. Surgical treatment must be individualized.

Ureteral quadruplication is most rare but has been described by Soderdahl and colleagues (1976).

Ureterocele

Terminology and Definitions

A ureterocele is defined as a cystic dilatation of the intravesical submucosal ureter. As previously mentioned, according to the guidelines of the Committee on Terminology of the Urologic Section of the American Academy of Pediatrics, ureteroceles contained entirely within the bladder are referred to as intravesical ureteroceles, and a ureterocele that has some portion of it situated permanently at the bladder neck or urethra regardless of the position of the orifice is termed an ectopic ureterocele. A *single-system ureterocele* is associated with a kidney with only one ureter, whereas a *duplex-system ureterocele* refers to one associated with the upper pole of a kidney with

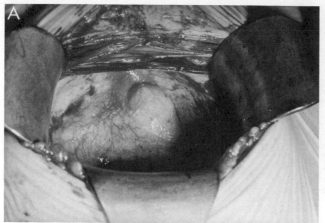

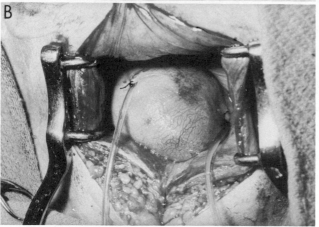

FIG. 46-14
A, Small ureterocele. Lower pole ureteral orifice can be seen to be elevated by the ureterocele. **B,** Large ureterocele. Catheters are in the orifice of the ureterocele and ipsilateral lower pole ureteral orifice.

a complete ureteral duplication. The embryology of ureteroceles has been much debated (see previous discussion), and it is clear that we are unable to account for all ureteroceles by one explanation. Usually the wall of a ureterocele exhibits attenuated muscle and collagen (Subbiah and Stephens, 1972; Tokunaka et al., 1981). Ureteroceles vary greatly in size from ones that may be difficult to visualize to ones that are so large as to fill virtually the entire bladder (Fig. 46-14). The orifice of a ureterocele may be stenotic, normal in size, or occasionally even patulous. They may be located intravesically or extravesically.

Incidence and Diagnosis

The incidence of ureteroceles was reported in 1951 by Campbell to be 1 in 4000 autopsies in children. Malek and co-authors (1972b) report an incidence between 1 in 5000 and 1 in 12,000 general pediatric admissions. Both of these estimates are probably low, suggesting that small ureteroceles were missed. Uson and colleagues (1961) reported an incidence of 1 in

500 autopsies. Ureteroceles occur most commonly in whites and are unusual in blacks. Although females are affected four to seven times as commonly as males, the malformation is often more complex in the male (Eklof et al., 1978). Some series have demonstrated a slight left-sided predominance; approximately 10% are bilateral (Royle and Goodwin, 1971). Ectopic ureteroceles, as opposed to intravesical ones, make up approximately 60% to 80% of most series (Ericsson, 1954; Mandell et al., 1980; Stephens, 1963). In approximately 80%, ureteroceles are associated with the upper pole ureter of a duplex kidney (Brock and Kaplan, 1978). Single-system ectopic ureteroceles are rare, usually occur in males, and may be associated with cardiac and genital anomalies (Johnson and Perlmutter, 1980). Very rarely, a ureterocele may be associated with a blind-ending ureter (Amar, 1971). Associated urologic anomalies, especially renal anomalies of fusion and ectopia, are frequently seen with ureteroceles. When the ureterocele arises from the upper pole of a duplex kidney, the upper pole frequently displays renal dysplasia (Perrin et al., 1974; Snyder et al., 1983). Lesions of the nephroblastomatosis complex have also been identified with upper pole parenchyma associated with ureteroceles (Snyder et al., 1983).

Ericsson (1954) was the first to make an effort at classifying ureteroceles. *Simple ureteroceles* were defined as ones contained entirely within the bladder, and ectopic ureteroceles were defined as ones that extended to the bladder neck or urethra. The clearer classification given earlier in the chapter eliminates the confusing term "simple." Stephens (1963) provided a more complex classification that was intended to more completely describe the pathologic anatomy of ureteroceles. He described *stenotic ureteroceles* (approximately 40%) as being located entirely within the bladder and having a small ureteral orifice. The orifice could vary from pinpoint with a constantly tense ureterocele to larger orifices that permit some decompression of the ureterocele, with the ureterocele being visible only when a peristaltic wave fills it. Stenotic ureteroceles tend to show more musculature in the wall of the ureterocele than other varieties of ureteroceles. The muscle is predominantly longitudinal in orientation. Stephens (1963) classified *sphincteric ureteroceles* (approximately 40%) as ones with an orifice confined within the internal sphincter. Thus they are a form of ectopic ureterocele. Compression by the internal sphincter obstructs drainage from the ureterocele, and thus emptying occurs only during voiding. The size of the meatus may be normal or even large. This type of ureterocele may be shown to exhibit vesicoureteral reflux (9%) (Sen et al., 1990). The wall of sphincteric and sphincterostenotic ureteroceles shows musculature that is deficient and oriented in a helical rather than longitudinal pattern.

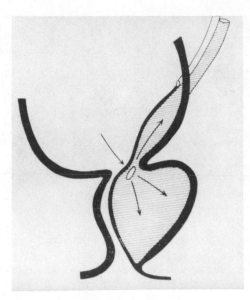

FIG. 46-15
Cecoureterocele: ureterocele with tonguelike projection extending down urethra submucosally.

Stephens' *sphincterostenotic ureteroceles* (approximately 5%) have a stenotic meatus located at the bladder neck or more distally and thus are again a form of an ectopic ureterocele. These ureteroceles tend to be large and tense. Because they do not decompress during voiding as sphincteric ones do, the tense ureterocele may act as a ball valve in the bladder outlet, producing urethral obstruction. In the female it may prolapse through the urethral meatus. Stephens' fourth type of ureterocele is referred to as a *cecoureterocele* (Fig. 46-15). Here, although the meatus of the ureterocele is in the bladder, a tongue of the ureterocele extends down the urethra. At the time of ureterocele excision, if this tonguelike projection is not carefully excised, a mucosal flap may be left capable of producing a valvelike obstruction of the urethra (Ashcraft and Hendren, 1979).

Although today more frequently ureteroceles are being detected before birth by antenatal maternal ultrasound, infection continues to be a common presentation for ureteroceles (Caldamone et al., 1984; Johnston and Johnson, 1969; Malek et al., 1972a). This infected obstructed system may lead to the picture of full gram-negative sepsis. At other times infants may simply exhibit failure to thrive or nonspecific gastrointestinal symptoms as seen with other obstructive uropathies in infancy. On occasion, an infant will present with a palpable abdominal mass representing the bladder or the obstructed renal unit. Prolapse of a ureterocele in the female leads to bladder outlet obstruction, which constitutes the most common urethral obstruction seen in girls (Klauber and Crawford, 1980). Prolapsing ureteroceles can also occasionally

obstruct the urethra in boys (Diard et al., 1981; Noe, 1978). Usually this obstruction occurs with a duplex system ureterocele but can rarely occur with a single-system intravesical ureterocele as well. The "ball-valving" obstructive ureteroceles tend to be tense large ones that Stephens would classify as stenotic. However, most ureteroceles are not obstructive because they are compressible during voiding. Hematuria may occur from minor trauma to the dilated system or rarely from the presence of a stone. At times the only symptom is abdominal or flank pain. When incontinence is a presenting symptom, it is usually secondary to infection. Occasionally, a large ureterocele with an abnormal lax bladder neck may lead to incontinence before or after the ureterocele is surgically treated (Husmann et al., 1994; Leadbetter, 1970). Although, historically, in the diagnosis of a ureterocele, the most useful study has been the IVP (Berdon et al., 1968; Sherwood and Stevenson, 1969; Williams et al., 1972), today there is increasing importance for ultrasound, which often can clearly identify a ureterocele (Fig. 46-16). When the associated renal unit exhibits good function, the IVP demonstrates a characteristic "cobra head" or "spring onion" deformity of the distal ureter that is produced when opacified urine in the ureterocele is surrounded by a radiolucent halo that represents the wall of the ureterocele (Fig. 46-17). Renal function adequate to produce this characteristic image is most frequently seen with single-system intravesical ureteroceles. Most ectopic ureteroceles are associated with the upper pole of a duplex kidney that exhibits minimal or no function (90%, Caldamone et al., 1984; 74%, Sen et al., 1992). In these cases the radiographic signs of a ureterocele are primarily negative, reflecting the displacement of the functioning lower pole renal unit and ureter by the hydronephrotic upper pole segment. The lower pole renal unit is often downward and laterally displaced, producing the characteristic "drooping lily" sign (Fig. 46-18). The lower pole ureter may be tortuous and displaced away from the spine as it wraps around the dilated upper pole ureter. At the bladder level, a negative shadow may be seen, suggesting the presence of a ureterocele (Fig. 46-18). The negative shadow can vary from a large, tense, round shadow occupying much of the bladder volume to a minor irregularity along the floor of the bladder. This negative shadow has to be differentiated from a bladder calculus, blood clot, bladder tumor, or gas in the rectum. In single-system ureteroceles the absence of function or associated hydroureteronephrosis may help clarify the issue, but in a ureterocele associated with a duplex unit, especially if there is little hydroureteronephrosis, the diagnosis may be more difficult. The early films and the postvoid films from a urogram should be examined closely for the ureterocele, because once the bladder is filled with contrast,

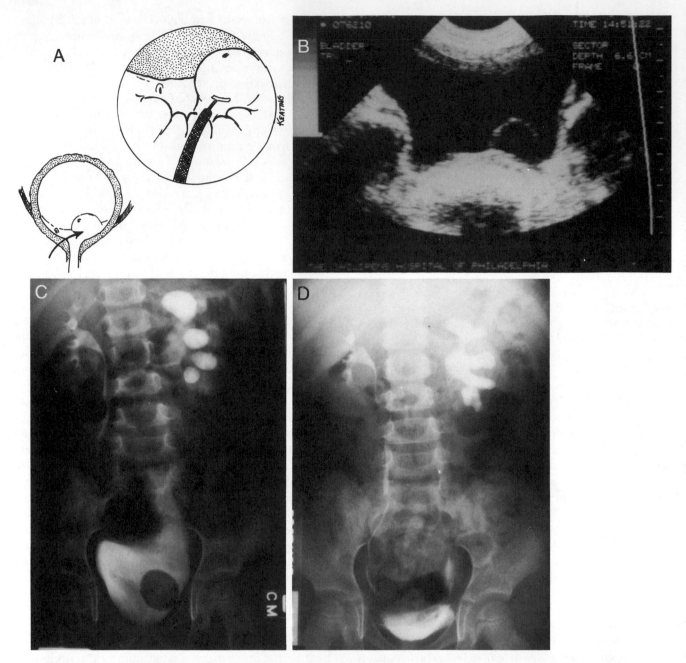

FIG. 46-16
A, Low transverse ureterocele incision. A short (2 to 3 mm) low incision just above the bladder wall is made by an initial puncture and then a sidewise movement of the Bugbee. The incision includes the ureteral orifice only if it is low. **B,** Single-system intravesical ureterocele: ultrasound clearly shows the ureterocele. **C,** Single-system intravesical ureterocele: intra-venous pyelogram (IVP) shows hydronephrotic left kidney with intravesical negative filling defect produced by ureterocele. **D,** Same case as **B** and **C:** IVP 3 months after a low transverse incision. Voiding cystourethrogram shows no reflux.

the ureterocele may be obscured. Intravesical ureteroceles tend to be defined by contrast that nearly surrounds them as opposed to ectopic ureteroceles, which are poorly separated by contrast from the floor of the bladder.

A VCUG is an integral part of the urographic evaluation of a ureterocele (Fig. 46-19). With duplex ure-

teroceles, reflux is seen to the ipsilateral lower pole in approximately 50% of cases (Fig. 46-19) (Brock and Kaplan, 1978; Caldamone et al., 1984; Sen et al., 1992). Most often they are compressible ureteroceles that provide poor support for the submucosal course of the lower pole ureter. In between 10% and 20% of cases (Kelalis, 1976; Leong et al., 1980; Sen et al.,

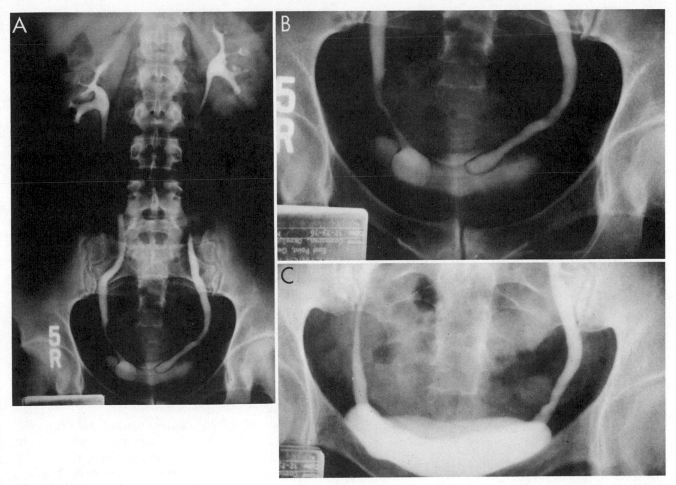

FIG. 46-17
Bilateral single-system simple ureteroceles. **A,** Intravenous pyelogram (IVP) showing normal kidneys and minimal obstruction. **B,** Bladder showing typical cobra head deformity of distal ureter with small ureterocele and good renal function. **C,** Bladder later in IVP showing how accumulation of contrast may obscure ureterocele.

1992), there is reflux into the ureterocele when it is part of a duplex kidney. Reflux is less frequent but can also occur into single-system ureteroceles (Bordon and Martinez, 1977; Sen et al., 1992). Reflux usually occurs into a wide-mouth (often sphincteric) ureterocele or cecoureterocele or a ruptured one.

When ruptured, a ureterocele typically is seen as an irregular cavity filling beyond the bladder outline with an edge that constitutes a filling defect within the bladder shadow. The VCUG is also useful to ascertain the degree of detrusor backing present for the ureterocele. If detrusor support is poor and the ureterocele prolapses through the detrusor with voiding, the ureterocele may mimic a bladder diverticulum (Fig. 46-20) (Cremin et al., 1974; Weiss and Spackman, 1974). Prolapse may occur either into the dilated ureter associated with the ureterocele or through the hiatus paraureterally (Koyanagi et al., 1980). Occasionally following decompression of a ureterocele, detrusor backing may appear to improve. When tense,

a ureterocele may obstruct the ipsilateral lower pole ureter or contralateral ureter as well as the bladder outlet. Occasionally in males, an ectopic ureterocele can prolapse and produce an image that may be confused with posterior urethral valves (Fenelon and Alton, 1981).

Ureteroceles often present some of the most challenging diagnostic dilemmas seen in uroradiology. Not only can the bladder outlet be obstructed, but there may be ipsilateral or contralateral obstruction or reflux produced.

The advent of ultrasonography has greatly assisted in sorting out these diagnostic dilemmas (Athey et al., 1983; Nussbaum et al., 1986; Summer et al., 1980) and with the advent of antenatal ultrasound has become an increasingly common way for ureteroceles to be discovered. The ultrasound appearance of a ureterocele can be deceiving, however, and accurate diagnosis requires an experienced radiologist. As many ureteroceles are compressible with bladder filling, ob-

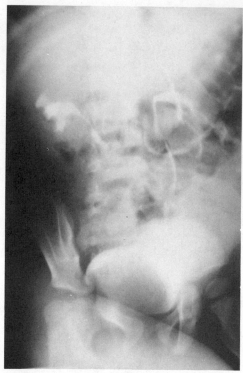

FIG. 46-18
Large ureterocele associated with nonfunctioning upper pole of duplicated right kidney. Intravenous pyelogram shows right lower pole is pushed down and outward (the drooping lily sign). A paucity of calyces is evident, and the upper pole infundibulum is absent.

servation when the bladder is very full may miss the mucosal irregularity of the bladder base, and the dilated ureter behind the bladder may be confused with an ectopic ureter or primary obstructive megaureter.

Computed tomography usually plays little role in the diagnosis of children with ureteroceles. Occasionally a diethylenetriamine pentaacetic acid (DTPA) renal scan may help to evaluate function in an upper pole renal unit, but it should be emphasized that neither the scan nor the IVP is able to predict the degree of recovery of function. In general, I agree with King and colleagues (1983) that if there is no function on delayed films from an IVP, it is unlikely that the associated renal unit with a ureterocele merits salvaging.

Cystoscopy is most useful in detection of ureteroceles, but the findings can be highly variable and, at times, confusing. When a ureterocele is small, it may not be evident until a peristaltic wave or flank compression fills it. Then a fine jet of urine from the meatus may be seen. Very large ureteroceles may make identification of any ureteral orifice in the bladder impossible. When bilateral obstruction is produced by a ureterocele, it is occasionally difficult to tell which system gave origin to the ureterocele. Injection of the ureterocele with contrast medium and

an intraoperative radiograph may sort out the anatomy. A small needle wedged into the end of a fine ureteral catheter can be used to puncture the ureterocele under direct vision at cystoscopy. Alternatively, a spinal needle passed transabdominally into the bladder and thus into the ureterocele with cystoscopic control may also be successful. With bladder filling, compressible ureteroceles may come to resemble only a minor mucosal fold; therefore, the bladder should be inspected when nearly empty as well as when full. Compression of the flank may push fluid into the ureterocele, making it more easily seen. When the kidney is infected, flank massage also can demonstrate the orifice of a ureterocele as pus jets from it. When the ureterocele has poor detrusor support and prolapses, at cystoscopy one may misdiagnose a bladder diverticulum (Snyder and Johnston, 1978). As the bladder is emptied and the flank compressed, the ureterocele may fill again, permitting the correct diagnosis to be made. Conversely, when the bladder is empty, the redundant mucosa of a periureteral diverticulum may be mistaken for a collapsed ureterocele. Once again, examination of the area in question when the bladder is full should permit recognition of a true diverticulum. Trigonal cysts are very rare but when present can be confused with a ureterocele at cystoscopy (Tacciuoli et al., 1976). Injection of contrast into the cyst, as previously described, or ultrasound should help to diagnose these rare cases. Occasionally the dilated lower end of an ectopic ureter may elevate the trigone, causing a "pseudoureterocele" by ultrasound, VCUG, or cystoscopy (Fig. 46-21) (Gill, 1980).

Because contralateral duplications are common with ureteroceles, it is worth every effort to assess the contralateral anatomy at cystoscopy. In this way possible damage to an inapparent ureteral orifice may be avoided.

The Choice of Strategy for Ureterocele Treatment

With the advent of successful ureterocele treatment by endoscopic incision (Fig. 46-16), the algorithm for the management of ureteroceles has become more complex. This is truly an area of great sophistication in pediatric urologic management. There are a number of factors that must be borne in mind in determining which approach to take. *The age of the patient* is a first consideration. In the infant requiring decompression of an obstructive uropathy detected before birth, endoscopic incision has the advantage of providing a simple and direct decompression of the obstructive uropathy. It is impressive in the series reported from Great Ormond Street (Etker et al., 1994) that there were no cases of urosepsis following decompression. That would appear to be a major advantage in treatment of the infant. After toilet training, bladder neck surgery is as highly symptomatic for the

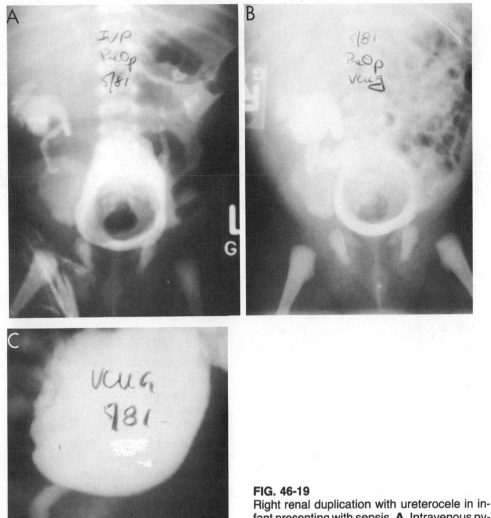

FIG. 46-19
Right renal duplication with ureterocele in infant presenting with sepsis. **A,** Intravenous pyelogram showing large ureterocele associated with nonfunctioning upper pole of right kidney. Lower pole shows drooping lily sign, and right lower pole ureter is tortuous as it wraps around the dilated upper pole ureter. **B,** Voiding cystourethrogram showing right lower pole vesicoureteral reflux. **C,** Voiding cystourethrogram showing that despite its size, the ureterocele does not obstruct the bladder outlet. Bladder full of contrast obscures the ureterocele.

child as any that is carried out on the bladder. Excision of a ureterocele and trigonal and possibly bladder neck reconstruction thus is preferable to avoid, if possible. Here the attractiveness of a "simplifed" approach with an upper pole partial nephrectomy and decompression of the ureterocele becomes evident.

The amount of functioning parenchyma is another issue. There is clearly greater salvage of parenchyma that has never been infected and, accordingly, our approach to asymptomatic infants who have never experienced pyelonephritis may permit better salvage of renal parenchyma. It is important to remember that usually the upper pole system serving the ureterocele typically makes up only the parenchyma subserved by the upper pole infundibulum (Privett et al., 1976), so in most cases, one should not let preservation of function be a paramount part of decision-making. On the other hand, a poorly functioning renal unit that is serving a decompressed ureterocele with no reflux has little or no indication to be removed.

A more important issue is whether *the kidney is single or duplex.* In a single-system ureterocele, it

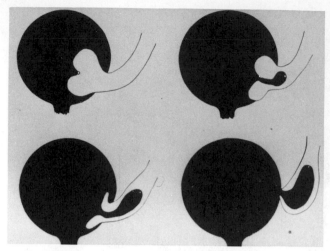

FIG. 46-20
Illustration of how prolapse of a ureterocele through the ureteral hiatus may mimic a bladder diverticulum.

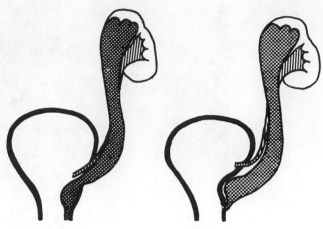

FIG. 46-21
Ureterocele *(left)* and "pseudo-ureterocele" *(right)*: an ectopic ureter can occasionally elevate the floor of the bladder sufficiently to mimic a ureterocele *(right)*, (From Gill, B.: *Br J Urol* Ureteric ectopy in children. 1980; 52:257. Used by permission.)

would appear that a primary endoscopic approach would be almost always rational as definitive therapy through open surgery is directed at the bladder level and, after endoscopic incision, one would have the advantage of reimplanting a smaller decompressed ureter should postendoscopic incision vesicoureteral reflux lead to an open operation. When the renal unit is duplex, then the decision is more complex. Some of the issues to be subsequently mentioned may be more critical in this setting.

Whether *the ureterocele is intravesical or extravesical* would be an important issue, because both the endoscopic and open surgical reconstructions vary. While Blyth and colleagues (1993) found that better than 90% of intravesical ureteroceles could be definitively decompressed by endoscopic incision without a need for subsequent surgery for reflux, their experience with extravesical ureteroceles was much less satisfactory. With extravesical ureteroceles, 50% of the cases came to secondary surgery. There may be a technical issue in this high incidence, as a recent paper by Schlussel and co-authors (1994) reported no real difference in secondary procedures between intravesical and extravesical ureteroceles in a small series.

Detrusor backing is also an important consideration in that a poorly supported ureterocele that everts during voiding and becomes a bladder diverticulum may be more likely to require secondary reconstruction of the trigone than one that is well supported. However, occasionally after ureterocele decompression, the support appears to improve, making it impossible to say that poor detrusor backing of the ureterocele is a firm predictor of the need for open bladder surgery.

The degree of ureteral dilation is another factor. When there is a small ureter running to a small intravesical ureterocele that is detected when one is operating for what is felt to be primary reflux, the reimplantation of the ureter from the poorly functioning upper pole serves as very good definitive treatment (Bauer and Retik, 1978). If, on the other hand, the ureter associated with the ureterocele is massively dilated, as is so often the case, attempts at reimplantation of such a system will be frought with a greater complication rate than an ablative operation aimed at the upper pole of the kidney.

What is emerging as the single important predictor of the need for open surgery is *associated vesicoureteral reflux*. The review by Sen and colleagues (1992) indicated that one can expect to see approximately 50% of ipsilateral lower pole ureters exhibit reflux. Approximately 25% of contralateral ureters reflux, and in about 10% of cases, reflux was seen into the ureterocele bearing unit. If high-grade reflux is associated with a ureterocele, it would appear that a primary endoscopic incision would be logical because subsequent surgery at the bladder level, while likely, will be facilitated by decompression of the ureterocele. If there is no vesicoureteral reflux, when the attractiveness of a "simplified" approach by an upper pole partial nephrectomy for a duplex ureterocele rises. In a review by Husmann and colleagues (1994), it is readily evident that reflux was the major factor leading to the need for subsequent surgery after an upper pole partial nephrectomy to decompress a ureterocele. In cases where the ureterocele alone was present without reflux, no patient required additional surgery. If less than grade III reflux was present in only one ureter, 60% of their patients did not require further surgery. In contrast, a higher grade reflux than this into one or more renal moieties almost invariably led to further surgery (96%). It would appear this same logic would apply to primary endoscopic treatment. Thus, a very careful assessment of the VCUG performed at presentation becomes a critical factor in decision-making.

From this brief section, it can be readily deduced that there will not be one simple solution to all ureterocele problems. Minimizing the number of anesthetics and surgical procedures, as well as postoperative morbidity, becomes very challenging indeed.

Treatment of Intravesical Ureteroceles

Intravesical ureteroceles associated with a single ureter are more commonly seen in adults than children and may be an acquired lesion (Thompson and Kelalis, 1964). Although the severity of obstruction and hydroureteronephrosis is greater in children than in adults (Rabinowitz et al., 1978), single-system ureteroceles usually are associated with better function and less hydronephrosis than are duplex renal units and their more frequently associated ectopic ureteroceles. Thus, a separate discussion of the treatment of single-system ureteroceles appears appropriate. Although Snyder and Johnston (1978) felt that endoscopic incision of single-system ureteroceles was contraindicated because of the high incidence of a secondary ureteral reimplant being needed, it is important to remember that this was a review before the current era of better endoscopic techniques. Even if reflux were to follow, the decompressed ureter would be an easier one to later reimplant.

Endoscopic decompression of ureteroceles was suggested initially by Zielinski (1962) and Hutch and Chisholm (1966). Tank (1986) advocated unroofing of ureteroceles without regard for reflux and found that 50% showed improvement in function, and subsequent nephrectomy was not felt necessary. Lower tract reconstruction for recurrent infections was reported in only 10% of cases. The current modern approach to ureterocele incision with an effort to use a small incision to decompress the ureterocele with placement low on the ureterocele so that a flap valve to prevent vesicoureteral reflux is also achieved was suggested by Monfort and colleagues (1985, 1992), Rich and colleagues (1990), and Blyth and colleagues (1993). It is evident from the results experienced with intravesical ureteroceles that up to 90% of patients may be adequately treated by endoscopic incision alone. Thus, it would appear that for intravesical ureteroceles, whether associated with a single or duplex renal unit, a primary endoscopic approach today is preferred.

There are several *technical points* worth mentioning concerning *endoscopic treatment of ureteroceles*. As many ureteroceles are compressible with bladder filling, it may help to keep the bladder rather empty and massage the flank to distend the ureterocele to ensure

that one makes as low an incision as possible on the front wall of the ureterocele presenting just above the bladder neck (Fig. 46-16). A 3 F Bugbee using the cutting current at a high enough level so as to ensure a clean incision is utilized. If a clean cut is not achieved, one may end up pushing the inner layer of the ureterocele away from the outer layer, thus not achieving decompression. A perpendicular approach to the ureterocele is important to avoid a skiving incision that may likewise miss the lumen of the ureterocele. While a low incision is preferred in efforts to create a flap valve mechanism of the decompressed ureterocele, it must be borne in mind that if one incises too low, the incision will be potentially below the level of the ureterocele floor. A very small 2- to 3-mm incision is adequate in most cases, as the thermal effect of the incision will lead to an enlargement in the hole with healing. Only when the ureterocele appears to be very thick-walled would an incision any larger than this be appropriate. It may be a more prudent recommendation to make always as small an incision as possible with the acceptance of the fact that there will occasionally be a need for an endoscopic reincision. Confirmation of adequate decompression can usually be assured from seeing a jet of urine emerge from the incision site in the ureterocele. This can be augmented by massage of the ipsilateral flank.

In the open reconstruction of intravesical ureteroceles, if there is poor detrusor backing for the ureterocele, the bladder wall must also be repaired at the time of ureterocele excision. In single-system ureteroceles that are decompressed, it is hoped that the degree of ureteral dilation will go down to the point where a 5:1 ratio of submucosal tunnel length-to-diameter can be achieved to prevent vesicoureteral reflux. However, with massively dilated ureters associated with ureteroceles, even following decompression, a tailored reimplant may be required. Cohen's (1977) technique of cross-trigonal advancement is generally used because it permits the reimplant to be done away from the area of bladder wall reconstruction. On occasion, obstruction is very severe, and a nephrectomy may be justified to remove a destroyed renal unit (Fig. 46-22). As in the adult, occasionally a single-system ureterocele is small, with minimal obstruction, and requires no treatment.

When an intravesical ureterocele is associated with the upper pole of the duplex kidney, the upper pole often demonstrates poor function, and an upper pole partial nephrectomy and partial ureterectomy to below the level of the iliac vessels may be performed as described for ectopic ureteroceles in the following section. This approach is particularly attractive when there is no vesicoureteral reflux, as this "simplified approach" is likely to permit the avoidance of any bladder level surgery (Husmann et al., 1994). How-

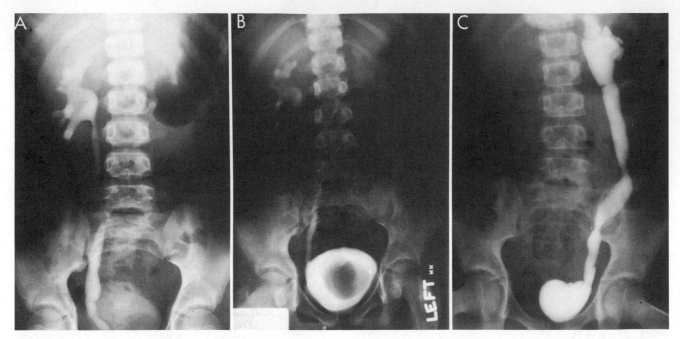

FIG. 46-22
Bilateral single-system ureteroceles. **A,** Early intravenous pyelogram (IVP) film shows left nonfunction and right minimal obstruction. In the bladder, cobra head deformity of ureterocele with good renal function is seen on *right.* **B,** Later IVP film demonstrates negative shadow of left ureterocele, but contrast obscures right ureterocele. **C,** Retrograde ureterogram of nonfunctioning left renal unit. Treatment was by left nephroureterectomy.

ever, it must be stressed that the incidence of vesicoureteral reflux after endoscopic incision of intravesical ureteroceles is sufficiently low (see above) to make the endoscopic approach perhaps even more attractive.

After partial nephrectomy, the ureter associated with the decompressed ureterocele is usually left open and drained. Attention must be paid to avoid damage to the lower pole ureter. Rarely, an intravesical ureterocele as part of a duplex unit may be associated with adequate function and a ureter small enough to permit ureterocele excision and a common sheath reimplant of the two ureters. More frequently, the associated ureter is too dilated to be reimplanted without tailoring. Here, if function justifies salvage, a renal level ureteroureterostomy or ureteropyelostomy may be used effectively (Fig. 46-23). The distal upper pole ureter in these salvageable cases is handled as previously discussed.

Treatment of Ectopic Ureteroceles

Ectopic ureteroceles are most commonly associated with the upper moiety of a duplex kidney and can be treated by a number of different surgical procedures (Fig. 46-24). In recent years the endoscopic approach to ureteroceles has been added to the various surgical approaches to these challenging cases, but not all issues have yet been settled, as will be evident from this presentation. *The endoscopic treatment of ectopic*

ureteroceles has not been as successful as intravesical ones (Blyth et al., 1993; Coplen and Duckett, 1994; Smith et al., 1994). The incidence of secondary surgery after endoscopic procedures is high, with Smith and colleagues (1994) reporting 80% and Blyth and co-authors (1993) reporting 50%. Nonetheless, the endoscopic approach would appear to be the preferred way of dealing with a neonate with this form of obstructive uropathy. In the antenatal ultrasound era, this is becoming increasingly the most common presentation for ureteroceles. Even if reflux were to follow, the likelihood of urosepsis is very likely (Etker et al., 1994), and reconstructive surgery can be electively carried out between 1 and 2 years of age, when complicated reconstructive procedures at the bladder neck are more safely accomplished and yet well before the age of toilet training, after which the bladder discomfort following a bladder neck procedure becomes more difficult for the child to tolerate.

There are *technical considerations* in the *endoscopic incision of an ectopic ureterocele* that are different from those for an intravesical ureterocele (Fig. 46-25). With the objective of achieving decompression of the ureterocele, a low puncture of the ureterocele to maintain a flap valve of the collapsed ureterocele continues to be a fairly uniform approach among different authors (Coplen and Duckett, 1994; Schlussel et al., 1994; Smith et al., 1994). Controversy exists about the treatment of the extension of an ectopic ureterocele

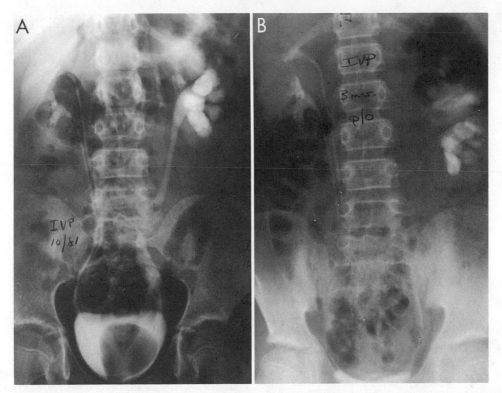

FIG. 46-23
Left ureteral duplication with ureterocele and function of upper pole treated by ureteroureterostomy. **A,** Preoperative intravenous pyelogram shows function of left upper pole and large ureterocele. **B,** After surgery, the left upper pole is well decompressed. The ureterocele collapsed and is no longer evident in the bladder.

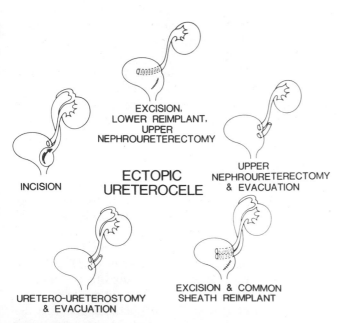

FIG. 46-24
Ectopic ureterocele: surgical options.

into the urethra. Concern has been expressed that following decompression, an obstructing distal portion might remain. However, Schlussel and colleagues (1994) and Smith and colleagues (1994) report no problems with the urethral extension of the ureterocele after puncture at the intravesical level only. Care was taken to make a low transverse small incision that was within the bladder with the bladder neck closed. When the technique is used as described by Blyth et al. (1993) of incising the intraurethral extension of the ureterocele upwards until the incision is clearly within the bladder (Fig. 46-25), one may be creating a situation where the opening of the bladder neck opens the orifice of the ureterocele, leading to a greater incidence of reflux. This may account for the increased incidence of postpuncture reflux seen in Blyth's versus Schussel's series. This concern about the distal extension of the ureterocele may be more germane to open ureterocele excision when the urethral extension could remain as a cusp, catching urine during voiding and thus obstructing the urethra (Ashcraft and Hendren, 1979).

The traditional method of treatment of an ectopic ureterocele associated with a duplex renal unit was total reconstruction with excision of the ureterocele, reconstruction of the detrusor, and reimplantation of

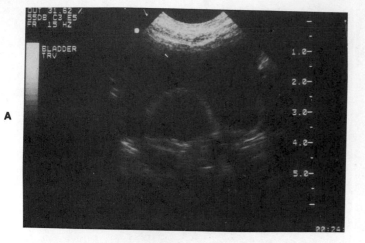

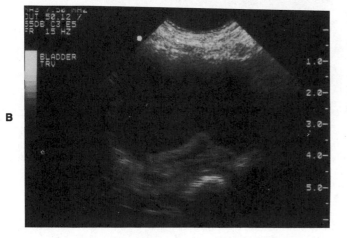

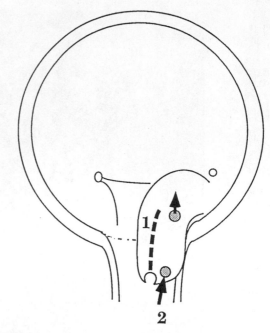

FIG. 46-25
Endoscopic incision of ectopic (extravesical) ureterocele. **A,** Ultrasound of bladder showing ureterocele with good detrusor support. **B,** Ultrasound of bladder showing collapsed ureterocele after endoscopic incision. **C,** Technique for endoscopic incision of ectopic ureterocele. 1. Vertical incision from orifice of ureterocele in urethra to above bladder neck probably promotes postincision reflux. 2. Second incision in urethral extension of ureterocele is not necessary. Small puncture low on ureterocele in bladder produces decompression without leaving cusp of residual ureterocele, which could act as valve and obstruct urethra.

the ipsilateral lower pole ureter and the contralateral ureter also, if required. Following this bladder operation, a separate flank incision was made and an upper pole partial nephrectomy completed (Hendren and Mitchell, 1971; Hendren and Monfort, 1979). If the upper pole had questionable function or the child was sufficiently ill to warrant a staged approach, the upper pole ureter could be exteriorized temporarily as a cutaneous ureterostomy. Monfort and colleagues (1992) used this technique in 18 patients with recovery of significant function in only three, indicating that this approach is rarely indicated. Since most ureteroceles present in the very young, often under 1 year of age, the total reconstruction approach requires a technically challenging excision of a ureterocele, often with a urethral extension. Complications are not rare (deJong, 1994). As mentioned, the urethral extension of an ectopic ureterocele may act as a urethral valve and produce bladder outlet obstruction. Also, if the ureterocele is excised but the bladder neck imperfectly reconstructed, incontinence may follow (Leadbetter, 1970). Incontinence can also rarely result from incomplete excision of a ureterocele that has an ori-

fice beyond the sphincter mechanism, leaving a channel that bypasses sphincteric control (Williams and Woodard, 1964).

Because of these considerable potential complications secondary to a total reconstruction early in life, alternate methods of treatment for ureteroceles were undertaken. In duplex renal units with an associated ectopic ureterocele, the upper pole unit usually has not demonstrated sufficient function to warrant salvage (Sen et al., 1992; Snyder et al., 1983). Because of this, a simplified "approach" based on a primary upper pole partial nephrectomy with ureterocele decompression and later a staged approach to bladder level surgery was an approach tried in several centers (Caldamone et al., 1984; Cendron and Bonhomme, 1968a; Cendron et al., 1981; King et al., 1983). The upper pole ureter was excised down to the level of the iliac vessels and left open to facilitate decompression of the ureterocele. The expectation was that decompression would simplify bladder surgery that would be carried out when the child was older or possibly could eliminate the need for an operation at the bladder level completely (Fig. 46-26). Ureterocele

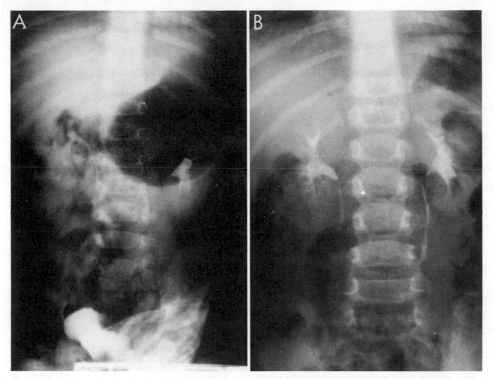

FIG. 46-26
Left ectopic ureterocele treated only by upper pole partial nephrectomy. **A,** Preoperative intravenous pyelogram (IVP) shows dropping lily sign, paucity of calyces, and absence of upper pole infundibulum. Ureterocele is just visible in the bladder. **B,** IVP 2 years following surgery shows excellent left kidney. Voiding cystourethrogram shows no reflux.

decompression by this technique was found to have the additional benefit that frequently ipsilateral lower pole reflux or obstruction and contralateral reflux or obstruction would subside. In the series of Husmann and colleagues (1994) the grade of reflux appeared to be important. If less than grade III reflux was present into the ipsilateral lower pole ureter or the contralateral ureter, 60% of their cases required no further surgery with spontaneous resolution of the reflux. However, a higher grade of reflux resulted in a 96% subsequent surgery rate for reflux. Other series have found the overall need for eventual bladder surgery to range from 25% to 50% (Caldamone et al., 1984; Cendron et al., 1981; King et al., 1983). Thus, it must be acknowledged that while the "simplified" approach of an initial upper pole partial nephrectomy provides very effective decompression, an incidence of subsequent bladder level surgery is likely to be significant, especially if there has been initial high-grade reflux. It was of interest to note that in Caldamone's series, ipsilateral lower pole vesicoureteral reflux first observed after decompression of the ureterocele was most likely to be persistent, suggesting that the filled ureterocele in some cases provided support for the submucosal course of the lower pole ureter. The ureterocele generally collapses so completely that it is difficult to subsequently visualize by a VCUG (Belman

et al., 1974; Caldamone et al., 1984; Cendron et al., 1981; Feldman and Lome, 1981). Occasional cases with poor detrusor backing for the ureterocele have been observed to have an improvement in bladder support after decompression.

Husmann and colleagues (1994) point out a rare complication of the "simplified" approach. They saw 6% of their patients treated with upper pole partial nephrectomy alone develop a stress pattern of urinary incontinence after toilet training. In these cases it would appear that the mass of the distended ureterocele distorted the bladder neck sufficiently to cause incompetence after decompression.

Experience with the "simplified" approach now has grown adequate to indicate that many pediatric urologists believe this staged approach to the treatment of ectopic ureteroceles with duplex systems will permit the majority of the children so treated to avoid a secondary bladder procedure, but that the need for lower tract reconstruction will continue to be significant.

In cases of ectopic ureteroceles where there is sufficient function of the associated upper pole to warrant a parenchyma-preserving approach, an endoscopic incision with an effort to avoid reflux (see above) may be undertaken. However, especially if there is no initial vesicoureteral reflux present, a ureteropyelostomy or high ureteroureterostomy may be a preferable alternative (see Fig. 46-23). This approach is less suitable if the lower pole pelvis is intrarenal or the lower pole ureter nondilated. Here the small amount of function represented in the upper pole would be better removed than to jeopardize the majority of renal function coming from the lower pole. Efforts at parenchymal salvage can be especially rewarding in the small infant, as recovery of function can occasionally be remarkable (Mayor et al., 1975).

Salvage of the upper pole renal unit by a primary bladder-level operation involving excision of the ureterocele and a common sheath reimplant has the disadvantage of requiring the reimplant of an often very dilated ureter into the small bladder of an infant. Amar and colleagues (1981) have also suggested ureterocele excision, lower pole ureteral reimplantation, and a low ureteroureterostomy of the upper pole ureter into the lower pole ureter. We have not been inclined to use this approach, because this procedure would appear to encourage the yo-yo phenomenon. In determining which upper pole units merit salvage, I have been inclined to agree with King and co-authors (1983) that usually examination of the delayed films from an IVP will demonstrate function in the cases worthy of salvage.

On occasion, a surgeon will begin a ureteral reimplantation for what appears to be simple primary vesicoureteral reflux into a single system, and as the ureter is mobilized, a second small ureter is found running to a small nonobstructed ureterocele. It is the small size of the ureter and associated lack of function in the diminutive upper pole unit that may lead to this intraoperative discovery (Bauer and Retik, 1978). Even though there is no function in the upper pole unit, treatment is usually satisfactory by a common sheath reimplant. It is uncommon to need to later remove the upper pole renal unit.

On occasion, an ectopic ureterocele from the upper pole of a duplex kidney will cause such a degree of lower pole obstruction or reflux that the lower pole is functionally destroyed. It has not been our experience that decompression of the ureterocele results in much return of function in the lower pole. In this situation a primary total nephroureterectomy may be justified.

In the performance of an upper pole partial nephrectomy to decompress a ureterocele in a duplex renal unit, several technical points bear mentioning. A relatively short transverse flank incision just below the tip of the twelfth rib permits complete mobilization of the kidney to facilitate surgery on the upper pole without difficulty in the majority of children. Because the upper pole renal vasculature is often anomalous and variable (Boijsen, 1959) when the kidney is mobilized, care should be taken to identify the frequently small vessels that course directly into the upper pole. If dissection is kept close to the upper pole to be removed, vessels running to this unit can be clearly identified before their division. In our experience this is the best way to avoid damaging the blood supply to the lower pole. I usually make no effort to dissect the renal vessels within the pedicle. Usually the ureter to the upper pole runs posterior to the renal vessels, but occasionally an aberrant vessel will be located behind the ureter. After the ureter to the upper pole has been clearly identified, it may be divided and the upper end of the ureter put on gentle traction to guide dissection of the upper pole parenchyma to be removed. The capsule may be stripped back to use later in closure if not too adherent from previous inflammation. Removal of the complete upper pole collecting system is the most important aspect of an upper pole partial nephrectomy. We make the parenchymal incision just on the upper pole side of the line of demarcation from the lower renal unit. Usually it is quite clearly evident following the division of the upper pole vessels. The hypoplastic or dysplastic upper pole can then be excised without a significant blood loss. Manual compression of the kidney provides adequate vascular control. I have not generally believed it was necessary to place a vascular loop or clamp on the pedicle.

Next, the distal end of the upper pole ureter should be dissected down to below the level of the iliac vessels, where it begins to assume a common adventitial sheath with the lower pole ureter. The upper pole ureter is usually dilated and tortuous; therefore, it may appear to wrap itself around and the more normal lower pole ureter. Dissection should be kept immediately on the wall of the upper pole ureter to prevent injury to the lower pole ureter. Patience with this often slightly tedious aspect of the dissection will gradually straighten the upper pole ureter, and the lower pole ureter will be well preserved. After dissection reaches the level of the iliac vessels, which is not difficult through the usual flank incision, the upper pole ureter is opened and the interior of the ureterocele gently irrigated with a feeding tube. If there is no reflux into the ureterocele, the stump of the excised upper pole ureter is left open. Occasionally, when the ureterocele is a large one, a small feeding tube may be left in the lumen of the upper pole ureter extending down into the ureterocele for a couple of days to act as a wick to help ensure that the ureterocele does indeed collapse. If reflux into the ureterocele has been noted to be present, the upper pole ureter should be ligated. Here there is an increased likelihood that a subsequent bladder operation to remove the ureterocele and upper pole ureteral stump may be required when the child is older. Last, the wound is irrigated and a small Penrose drain left to the area of the ureteral stump as well as to the area of the removed upper

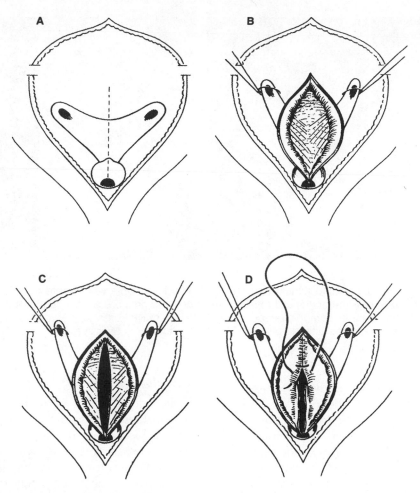

FIG. 46-27
Keeling repair of bladder neck after excision of ectopic (extravesical) ureterocele. Stephens' technique **(C, D)** involves a series of sutures placed to evert the detrusor at the bladder neck until the functional diameter of the bladder neck is restored to normal. The mucosal edge of the ureterocele provides a useful guide to the extent of eversion.

pole renal parenchyma. The child is usually ready for discharge from the hospital in 3 to 4 days.

In the minority of cases that come to the procedure of ureterocele excision and lower pole ureteral reimplantation, it is usually delayed electively until the child is about 2 years old and is most commonly needed for persistent ipsilateral lower pole reflux (Fig. 46-28). As excision of the ureterocele and bladder neck reconstruction are considerably more symptomatic than a simple ureteral reimplant alone, it is preferable to perform the surgery before the age of toilet training. Several technical points in this procedure are also worth bearing in mind. There are two basic methods for the intravesical excision for a ureterocele. If the detrusor backing for the ureterocele is solid, the back wall of the ureterocele can be left in place and the lower pole ureter tunneled beneath the mucosa. However, usually a bladder wall reconstructive procedure is warranted by detrusor weakness behind the ure-

terocele. It is usually possible to save a portion of the side walls of the ureterocele by separating the inner lining of the ureterocele to permit later mucosal coverage of the area of bladder wall reconstruction. If the ureterocele has a urethral extension, it is important not to leave a distal lip of mucosa that can be an obstructing flap valve. Either the entire urethral tongue of ureterocele can be excised and the bladder neck area carefully reconstructed before closing the mucosa, or if the bladder neck and urethra have not been dilated by the ureterocele, merely removing the ureterocele roof as it extends down the urethra will suffice. It is technically a simpler procedure, but one must be certain that a functionally intact urethra and bladder neck are left behind, because the primary reconstruction of these structures is easier than a secondary approach. As a ureterocele, especially ectopic ones, often widen the bladder neck, it is important to reconstruct this defect after ureterocele excision. The

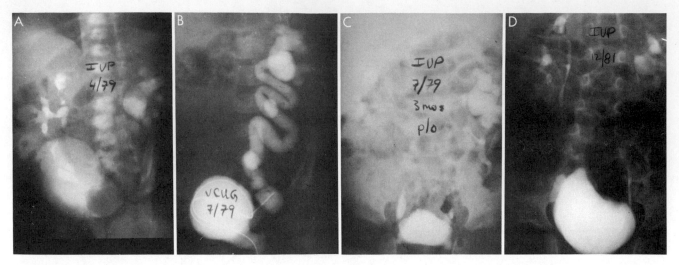

FIG. 46-28
Left ectopic ureterocele with upper pole nonfunction and ipsilateral lower pole vesicoureteral reflux treated by upper pole partial nephrectomy, excision of ureterocele, and reimplantation of lower pole ureter. **A,** Preoperative intravenous pyelogram (IVP) shows ureterocele and nonfunction of left upper pole. **B,** Preoperative voiding cystourethrogram shows left lower pole vesicoureteral reflux. **C,** IVP 3 months after surgery. **D,** Two and a half years after surgery.

technique of "keeling" as described by Stephens (1983) is particularly attractive (Fig. 46-27). A series of sutures is used to evert the detrussor ("keeling") until the bladder neck is reconstructed to a normal diameter. The mucosal edge of the ureterocele provides a good guide as to the amount of eversion needed. When the mucosa is reapproximated at the bladder neck, good bladder neck reconstruction can be ensured. Using this approach, I have yet to see a child with incontinence after ureterocele excision. To ensure that a small distal urethral mucosal cusp is not left to potentially obstruct the urethra (Ashcraft and Hendren, 1979), it is a simple matter at the end of the operation to use a small probe bent into a little hook from the perineal end of the urethra to catch a distal lip of ureterocele, draw it externally, and nip it with a fine pair of scissors.

As the ureterocele is mobilized, the upper pole ureteral stump will be mobilized with the lower pole ureter. This dissection in most cases can be accomplished totally intravesically. After the lower pole ureter has been sufficiently mobilized for an adequate reimplant, the upper pole ureter stump is opened on its wall opposite the common one shared with the lower pole ureter. No effort is made to excise the portion of the wall of the upper pole ureter that is contiguous with the lower pole ureter. In this way there should be minimal risk of injury to the lower pole ureter. A Cohen cross-trigonal reimplant is usually feasible and keeps the course of the ureter away from the area of recent bladder wall reconstruction. A ureteral stent is usually used only if the lower pole ureter is significantly abnormal.

Ectopic Ureter

An ectopic ureter is defined as one that opens at the bladder neck or more caudally rather than at its normal location on the corner of the trigone. As will be recalled from the previous embryologic presentation, an ectopic ureter forms when the ureteral bud has an abnormally high origin from the mesonephric duct with delayed or no separation from the duct. There are multiple sites for an ectopic ureter in both male and female humans (Fig. 46-29). However, in the male the ectopic ureter is always above the external sphincter, which accounts for the prime clinical difference in presentation between the sexes (see later discussion).

Incidence of Single and Duplex Systems

Our estimation of the incidence of ectopic ureters may be low, because not all cause symptoms. Campbell (1970) reported on 19,076 autopsies in children with a finding of 10 ectopic ureters, giving an incidence of one in 1900 children. Occasionally ectopy occurs in more than one family member (DeWeerd and Feeney, 1967; Musselman and Barry, 1973). In 80% of cases the ectopic ureter is attached to the upper pole of a duplicated renal system. The percent of ectopic ureters associated with duplication in females is even higher than 80%; as in males it is more common to see an ectopic ureter draining a single system (Johnston and Davenport, 1969; Schulman, 1976). Indeed, ectopic ureter is much more of a female clinical problem in general, with only approximately 15% of ectopic ureters having been reported in males (Schulman, 1972). Approximately 10% of ectopic ureters are bi-

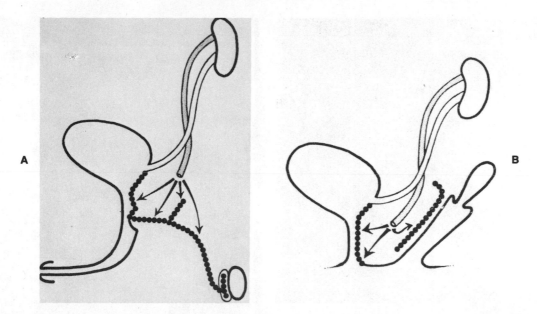

FIG. 46-29
A, Ureteral ectopia in male. Possible sites of ectopic ureter are above the external sphincter. **B,** Ureteral ectopia in female. Ectopic ureter may be located beyond continence mechanism and produce incontinence. (From Johnston JH: Problems in the diagnosis and management of ectopic ureters and ureteroceles. In Johnston JH, Scholtmejer RJ (eds): *Problems in Pediatric Urology.* Amsterdam, Excerpta Medica, 1972, p 57. Used by permission.)

lateral (Ellerker, 1958). When the ectopic ureter is part of a duplex system, the contralateral system is duplicated in approximately 80% of cases, and 21% will have duplication contralaterally with contralateral ectopy as well (Malek et al., 1972b).

The most frequently encountered anomaly associated with an ectopic ureter is hypoplasia or dysplasia of the renal moiety. There is a fairly good correlation between the degree of ectopia and the degree of renal abnormality, although it appears to hold better for duplex systems with ectopy than for single systems with ectopy (Schlecker et al., 1986). It may reflect the fact that a single ectopically placed ureteral bud has more potential for deviation in its course of growth toward the metanephric blastema than does an ectopic bud that is part of a pair of ureteral buds. According to this explanation, normal renal tissue might on occasion come to be associated with a quite ectopic system. Actually, severe ectopia with an orifice in the genital system is almost always associated with nonfunctioning renal tissue (Rognon et al., 1973; Schulman, 1972). A single ectopic ureter with a normal contralateral system usually does not result in any deficiency of the bladder neck. However, when two single ureters are ectopic, the bladder neck fails to form normally, and incontinence is a problem (see later discussion). Interestingly, when one single ectopic system is at the bladder neck and one is more distal, an intermediate level of bladder neck abnormality is present. In the series from the Philadelphia

Children's Hospital (Schlecker et al., 1985), most of the children in this intermediate group were continent.

Some series (Gill, 1980) have shown a higher incidence of other associated anomalies, especially imperforate anus, in single-system ectopy than in duplex ectopy.

Ectopic Ureter in the Female

The fundamental difference between ureteral ectopia in the female and male is accounted for by the fact that in females, ectopic ureters can come to terminate at a level distal to the continence mechanisms of the bladder neck and external sphincter and thus may be associated with incontinence (Fig. 46-29) (Johnston, 1972; Mogg, 1974). Approximately one third of ectopic ureters open at the level of the bladder neck (Fig. 46-30) or slightly more distally in the upper urethra (Kjellberg et al., 1968). The higher the orifice is, the less it will be associated urinary incontinence; however, obstruction is more common in higher ureters because they traverse a greater portion of the musculature of the bladder neck.

These more proximal ectopic ureters drain only during voiding when the continence mechanism is open. Vesicoureteral reflex occurs in 75% or more of these higher ectopic ureteral orifices, producing the paradox of both reflux and obstruction. By having the bladder neck repeatedly open, the cyclic VCUG of Lebowitz and Wyly (1984) provides an opportunity for the ob-

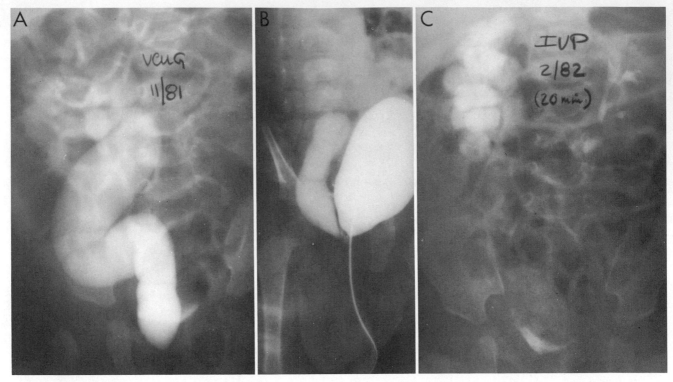

FIG. 46-30
Ectopic ureter at bladder neck in female who presented at 4 months of age with sepsis. **A,** Voiding cystourethrogram showing vesicoureteral reflux into very dilated right ureter. **B,** Oblique view from cystogram showing ectopic ureter entering at bladder neck. **C,** Intravenous pyelogram 3 months following tapered reimplant of right ureter.

structed ectopic ureter to drain before contrast is voided and thus increases the likelihood that the contrast will reflux into the ectopic system. When the ectopic ureter enters at the level of the external sphincter or more distally, reflux is less commonly seen.

Another frequent location for ureteral ectopy in the female is the area of the vaginal vestibule immediately around the urethral orifice (Fig. 46-31). Approximately one third of ectopic female ureters are found here. This area marks the terminal end of Gartner's duct—the mesonephric duct remnant in the female. Occasionally infant girls will present with an ectopic ureter entering what appears to be a urethral diverticulum, but that is actually a Gartner's duct cyst (Vanhoutte, 1970). In approximately 25% of ectopic ureters in females, the orifice opens into the vagina. More rarely, an ectopic ureter can end at a higher site on Gartner's duct with an opening at the level of the cervix or even uterus (less than 5%). These uterine, cervical, and vaginal cases presumably are the result of rupture of Gartner's duct into the urovaginal canal along their common wall. Ureteral ectopy into the rectum is very rare and usually is noted incidentally at autopsy (Uson and Schulman, 1972). Presumably it must result from an abnormal division of the cloaca by the descent of the urorectal septum or from an

abnormally placed mesonephric (wolffian) duct that empties into the posterior half of the cloaca.

Approximately one half of females with ectopic ureters present with a classic history of continuous dribbling incontinence despite what appears to be a normal voiding pattern (Malek et al., 1972b; Schlecker et al., 1986; Schulman, 1972). Not uncommonly, the problem in the female goes unrecognized until adulthood (Green, 1959). If the associated ureter is very dilated, the child may be continent when supine, and the pattern may be one of daytime wetting only. This reservoir effect may lead to an erroneous diagnosis of stress incontinence. Occasionally it is a persistent foul-smelling vaginal discharge that suggests an ectopic ureter. If the ectopic ureter ends in a Gartner's duct cyst, the child may present with a mass on the anterior vaginal wall. When the ectopic orifice is quite high and there is significant obstruction, reflux, or both, urinary infection is frequent and is the most common form of presentation for an ectopic ureter in the small child. An infant may present with an abdominal mass resulting from a severely obstructed ectopic ureter (Uson et al., 1972) (Fig. 46-32). There are well-documented cases of females with ectopic ureters entering the vestibule or distal urethra without incontinence, presumably due to obstruction of the ureter as it traverses the continence mechanism with emp-

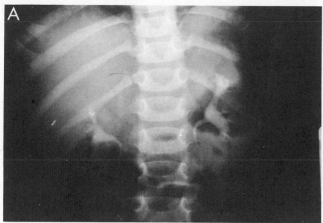

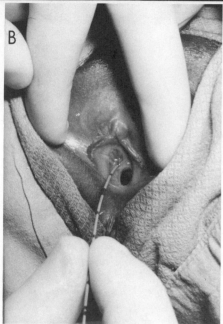

FIG. 46-31
Ectopic ureter in vaginal vestibule in female who presented with constant dribbling incontinence as well as normal voiding. **A,** Intravenous pyelogram shows right duplication with minimal upper pole function and down and outward displacement of lower pole (drooping lily sign). **B,** Ureteral catheter in ectopic ureter.

tying only during voiding (Ogawa et al., 1976). Flank pain may be the only symptom (DeWeerd and Litin, 1958). In this type of case, incontinence has been reported to develop after puberty or childbirth (Childlow and Utz, 1970; Davis, 1930).

The diagnosis of an ectopic ureter in the female may be obvious or may be very difficult. Particularly when there is ectopy into the external genitalia, there is likely to be nonvisualization of the associated renal unit (Grossman et al., 1967). When there is a duplicated drainage system, the presence of a nonvisualizing upper pole may be inferred from the effect of the dilated nonfunctioning system on the lower pole

of the kidney, the lower pole ureter, or both, as is seen with duplex systems and a ureterocele (see previous discussion). Ultrasound may be especially useful, detecting the dilated ectopic ureter behind the bladder. If there is little hydroureteronephrosis of the ectopic upper pole system, diagnosis may depend on recognizing the absence of an upper pole calyx or an apparent excessive thickness of the renal tissue on the medial aspect of the upper pole. Tomography during urography or a computed tomographic image of the kidney may be the most precise manner in which to make this diagnosis (Lebowitz, 1985). Bilateral ectopic ureters occur in approximately 10% of cases, and the radiographic findings may be very subtle, permitting one side to be easily missed (Fig. 46-33).

If the ureter is single and beyond the continence mechanism, the associated renal tissue frequently is nonfunctional, and the diagnosis may be made even more difficult by the fact that the associated kidney itself may be ectopic or even crossed and fused (Weiss et al., 1984). Renal function may be inadequate to permit visualization by either intravenous urography or renal scan (Scott, 1981). The finding of a hemitrigone at cystoscopy may lead to the erroneous diagnosis of renal agenesis. Associated genital and anal anomalies are seen in approximately one third of cases (Kesavan et al., 1977) and may also mask the presentation of single ectopia. Ultrasound looking for a dilated ureter behind the bladder may be particularly useful in this situation (Mascatello et al., 1977). Flush vaginograms carried out by occluding the introitus with a Foley balloon may demonstrate reflux into a vaginal ectopic ureter. The ectopic ureter alternatively may be able to be identified at vaginoscopy. However, there are cases where exploratory surgery is required, looking just above the bladder for the ureter. Once found, it can be traced upward to its associated renal unit.

When one is dealing with suspected ectopic ureters, dyes used to stain urine, such as indigo carmine and methylene blue, have a role. As function of renal tissue associated with ectopic ureters is usually poor, intravenous administration of dye often is not successful in demonstrating an ectopic ureteral orifice. However, in the investigation of an incontinent child, the presence of an ectopic ureter may be strongly suggested if the bladder is filled with indigo carmine- or methylene blue-stained saline via a Foley catheter, and observation of the perineum reveals a continued slow drip of clear urine. Phenazopyridine hydrochloride (Pyridium) appears to be a better color marker excreted by poorly functioning renal tissue than methylene blue or indigo carmine (Weiss et al., 1984), and thus, if a cotton swab is left high in the vagina overnight and it is stained orange, it may suggest the diagnosis of a vaginally ectopic ureter.

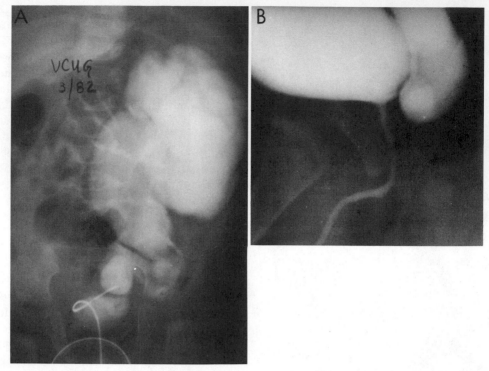

FIG. 46-32
Ectopic ureter to bladder neck in male infant who presented with an abdominal mass. **A,** Voiding cystourethrogram shows vesicoureteral reflux into massively dilated left renal unit. **B,** Oblique view shows ectopic ureter to bladder neck. Renal scan revealed the left kidney to constitute only 5% of total renal function. Treatment was by nephroureterectomy.

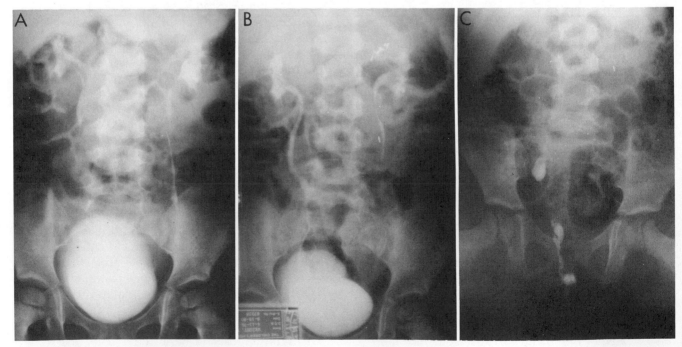

FIG. 46-33
Bilateral ectopic ureters in female who presented with constant incontinence as well as normal voiding. **A,** Initial intravenous pyelogram (IVP) shows down-and-outward displacement of left kidney and lateral displacement of ureter, suggesting duplication with ectopic ureter. Right kidney was not felt to be duplicated. Left upper pole partial nephrectomy did not correct incontinence. **B,** Follow-up IVP shows vertical axis to right kidney and mild tortuosity of right ureter, suggesting duplication with second ectopic ureter. **C,** Retrograde ureterogram of vestibular ectopic right ureteral orifice confirms suspicion of bilateral duplication with ectopia by showing upper pole ureter. Child was cured of incontinence by right upper pole partial nephrectomy.

Physical examination is also very important. Meticulous observation of the area around the urethral meatus and distal vagina will many times reveal a recurring drop of liquid over a very small opening that can be probed and then retrogradely injected to confirm the presence of an ectopic ureter (see Fig 46-33, *C*). Vaginoscopy with attention to the superior lateral aspect of the vagina may reveal vaginal ectopia. Sometimes the orifice is large and obvious. At other times it is hidden in a vaginal fold. Pressure on the anterior vaginal wall may produce a jet of cloudy fluid or pus from the ectopic orifice, revealing its presence.

The surgical treatment of an ectopic ureter in a female is dependent on the associated renal parenchyma. Single-system ureteral ectopia to the genital system usually has such poor parenchyma that a nephroureterectomy is appropriate, but when single-system ectopia is to the bladder neck or urethra, there is often adequate function to justify a reimplantation of the ureter into the bladder (Schlecker et al., 1986). When the ectopic ureter is associated with the upper pole of a duplex renal unit, function of the upper pole is usually inadequate to justify salvage, and a partial nephroureterectomy is most often performed. In the rare case where enough function is present to merit salvage of the upper pole, a ureteropyelostomy or ureteroureterostomy to drain the ectopic system into the lower pole system at the renal level is appropriate. If the lower pole pelvis is intrarenal and the lower pole ureter nondilated, this approach is less feasible. The ectopic ureter can be reimplanted into the bladder, although it may be sufficiently dilated to warrant tailoring.

With either duplex or single ectopic ureters, the entire distal ureter associated with ectopia into the introitus or vagina usually need not be removed. The distal ureteral segment is a rare source of later problems (Culp, 1960; Schlecker et al., 1986). If the distal segment becomes a source of stasis and infection, marsupialization of the ureter, usually a Gartner's duct cyst, into the vagina will correct the problem.

If instead of ending genitally in the vagina or introitus there is a urinary ectopic ureter ending in the bladder neck or urethra, then reflux of voided urine into the residual ureteral stump is likely to occur, and this may lead to a small amount of dribbling incontinence after micturition or, more commonly, to recurrent urinary infection. Thus, removal of the ureteral stump is more likely to be needed for urinary ectopic ureters. Although the dissection behind the bladder can be tedious, if dissection is kept immediately on the wall of the ureter, there is no reason for the bladder neck or external sphincter to be damaged. The transtrigonal approach can be very useful. In a postpubertal girl, excision may be accomplished transvaginally. If the ectopic ureteral stump is not too large, its lining can be destroyed endoscopically using a Bug-bee electrode, leading to obliteration of the ureteral lumen.

Ectopic Ureter in the Male

The ectopic pathway in the male extends from the bladder neck down the posterior urethra to the verumontanum and can lead to ureters ending in the mesonephric duct derivatives in the male: epididymis, seminal vesicle, and vas deferens (see Fig. 46-29). The most common location of an ectopic ureteral orifice in the male is the posterior urethra, where approximately one half of ectopic ureters will be found (Fig. 46-34) (Ellerker, 1958). In approximately one third of male patients, the ectopic ureter joins the seminal vesicle (Gordon and Kessler, 1972; Seitzman and Patton, 1960). Other ectopic sites are seen more rarely. Jona and colleagues (1979) have described a case of single ureteral ectopia to the epididymis. The connection of ectopic ureters to the male genital tract accounts for a presentation with epididymitis for males with ectopic ureters. Accordingly, any prepubertal male with epididymitis requires evaluation for an ectopic ureter (Siegel et al., 1987). In some males, symptoms caused by a genitally ectopic ureter do not present until the onset of sexual activity. At that time the male may present with epididymitis, prostatitis, seminal vesiculitis, or occasionally an infected seminal vesicle cyst that may lead to pain with a bowel movement or be tender on rectal examination (Bengmark et al., 1962). Because ectopic ureters in the male enter above the external sphincter, they generally do not produce incontinence as in the female. Symptoms of flank pain and urinary infection are more common. Occasionally there may be urgency or frequency due to the constant drip of urine into the posterior urethra. An occasional case of male incontinence may be due to reflux of urine into a dilated ectopic ureter with drainage after voiding into the posterior urethra and subsequent leakage out through a relaxed external sphincter (Williams and Royle, 1969).

A high index of suspicion may be required to diagnose an ectopic ureter in the male. An ectopic ureter entering the genital tract is often single and drains a nonfunctioning renal unit (Cendron and Bonhomme, 1968b; Rognon et al., 1973; Weiss et al., 1984). Since most ectopic ureters are at least a bit dilated, ultrasound may be very useful in locating the dilated ureter and its associated renal element. In the case of an ectopic ureter associated with a duplex renal unit, the indirect signs of hydroureteronephrosis of the upper pole unit described previously with respect to ureteroceles again apply. The greatest diagnostic difficulties arise in duplex renal units when there is a tiny upper pole unit draining into a minimally obstructed ectopic ureter with little dilatation (Babcock et al., 1977). Such renal units may be difficult to detect by ultrasound.

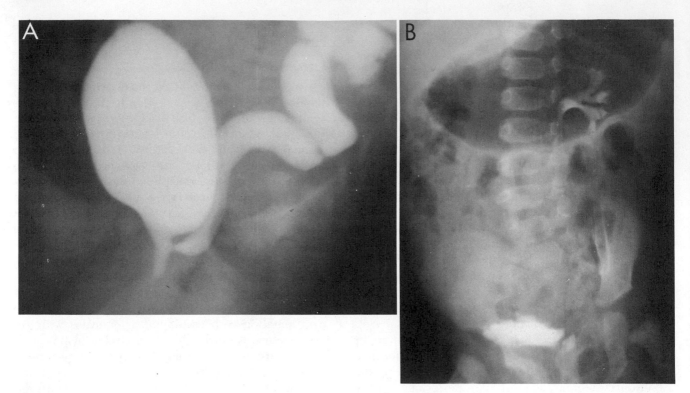

FIG. 46-34
Ectopic ureter to posterior urethra in a male who presented as an infant with sepsis. **A,** Voiding cystourethrogram shows vesicoureteral reflux into single ectopic ureter entering posterior urethra from solitary left kidney. **B,** Intravenous pyelogram after reimplant of ectopic ureter into the bladder.

The suspicion of a duplication with an ectopic ureter may be raised by finding a contralateral duplication, which is seen in approximately 40% of cases. Most ureters ectopic to the urethra or bladder neck will reflux (Lebowitz and Wyly, 1984; Schlecker et al., 1986), and thus careful examination of the oblique views from a VCUG and use of the cyclic voiding technique may enable the diagnosis to be made. In the male, as in the female, ectopic ureters at the level of the sphincters may demonstrate the paradoxic finding of both obstruction and reflux (Fig. 46-34). Occasionally, when the ectopic ureter is outside the urethra, the ejaculatory duct will be so dilated as to permit reflux (Williams and Royle, 1969).

Cystoscopy and examination with the patient under anesthesia are useful in establishing the diagnosis. A mass may be felt in the area of the seminal vesicle, or elevation of the floor of the bladder over a cyst (pseudo-ureterocele) may be noted as cystoscopy. The ectopic ureteral orifice may be seen at the bladder neck or urethra, or there may be an enlarged ejaculatory duct, permitting a retrograde study that will establish the diagnosis. When there is single ureteral ectopia, a hemitrigone is present. Occasionally a vasogram is useful in defining the anatomy (Schulman, 1976).

Treatment of ectopic ureters associated with duplex units in the male usually involves removal of the as-

sociated poorly functioning renal unit. Only rarely is function adequate to justify a ureteropyelostomy or ureteroureterostomy at the renal level. Because the ectopic ureter is usually dilated, a reimplantation of the duplex ectopic ureter into the bladder is a less attractive alternative. These issues come up only rarely in the male, since most duplex ectopic ureters occur in females.

In the treatment of single ureteral ectopy in the male, a functioning renal unit worthy of salvage is more likely to be present if the ectopia is to the urinary tract, namely, the bladder neck or urethra (Schlecker et al., 1986). When the single ectopic ureter is to a mesonephric remnant, the renal unit usually is not salvageable, and nephroureterectomy is appropriate. When an ectopic ureter enters the male genital duct, it may be unfit for the passage of sperm, and ligation of the vas may be required to avoid recurrent epididymitis.

Bilateral Single Ectopic Ureters

Bilateral single ectopic ureters are rare, and only slightly more than 50 have been reported in the medical literature in English (Cox and Hutch, 1966; Noseworthy and Persky, 1982; Schlecker et al., 1985; Williams and Lightwood, 1972). When bilateral single ectopic ureters are present at the level of the urethra or more distally, there is usually a poorly developed

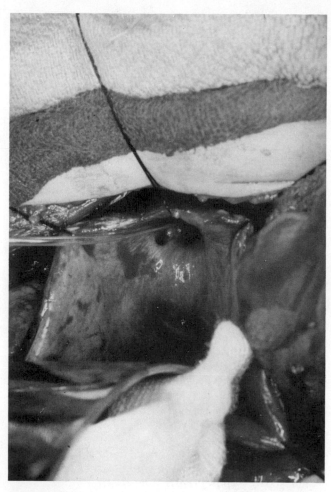

FIG. 46-35
Bilateral single ectopic ureters in incontinent male. View of opened bladder shows no trigone and poorly formed bladder neck. One ectopic ureteral orifice can be seen in the bladder neck.

bladder with an absent trigone and poorly developed bladder neck (Fig. 46-35). The embryologic explanation lies in the fact that the bladder neck and trigonal musculature appear to be derived from the tissue of the common stem of the mesonephric duct just below the point of origin of the ureteral bud. Thus if the bud takes its origin in a very cranial position, this critical area of the mesonephric duct never comes to be incorporated into the portion of the urogenital sinus that will form the bladder, and accordingly, no normal bladder neck and trigonal tissue are formed. Very rarely there is associated bladder agenesis (Glenn, 1959). Associated genital and anal anomalies are very common with bilateral single ectopic ureters (Kesavan et al., 1977).

Females most commonly are found to have bilateral single ectopic ureters located in the distal urethra. Infant girls usually present with urinary infection and are noted, incidentally, to have constantly wet diapers. Older girls most commonly present with incontinence. Females in general have poorer bladders and more severe renal anomalies than those seen in males with bilateral single ectopic ureters (Cox and Hutch, 1966; Williams and Lightwood, 1972). Although enough urine may enter the bladder in the male to permit some voiding to take place, males may also present with incontinence. Because some urine enters the bladder in the male, it is often slightly larger than the bladder seen in females.

This description represents the cases at the worst end of the spectrum of bilateral single ectopic ureters when both ureters are very distal from their normal point of entry into the bladder. When bilateral single ectopic ureters are present at the bladder neck level, the children may present with infection and upper urinary tract dilatation from obstruction, reflux, or both, but the bladder neck is generally better formed and continence more likely. When one ureter is ectopic to the urethra and one is ectopic at the bladder neck, there is an intermediate condition, but here incontinence is usually present (Schlecker et al., 1985).

Diagnosis is usually established by a carefully executed IVP and VCUG (Lebowitz and Wyly, 1984; Prewitt and Lebowitz, 1976). The reassociated renal units may show very poor function. The VCUG shows a small bladder with an open bladder neck. If the ectopic ureters are in the urethra, reflux is commonly present, and the VCUG usually makes the diagnosis. If the ureters are further down the ectopic pathway than the urethra, they usually are not demonstrated by VCUG. Again, an ultrasound examination may be useful. Saline into the vagina may enable reflux into a vaginally ectopic ureter to be recognized by the presence of refluxed air bubbles into the ureter, which can be picked up by ultrasound. A retrograde flush vaginogram with a Foley balloon occluding the introitus may similarly detect refluxing, vaginally ectopic ureters. At cystoscopy a child with bilateral single ectopic ureters usually is noted to have a poorly defined, funnel-shaped bladder neck and a small bladder capacity. In the male the ureteral orifices are usually located in the distal bladder neck or urethra, but in the female they may be more ectopic and thus more difficult to locate.

A child who is incontinent with bilateral single ectopic ureters presents a major challenge to reconstructive surgery. In the case where bladder capacity appears to be adequate, reimplantation of the ureters into the bladder and a Young-Dees-Leadbetter type of reconstruction of the bladder outlet may be appropriate (Leadbetter, 1964). If bladder capacity is inadequate, it may be feasible to turn the entire bladder into a long detrusor tube to provide continence and to create an adequate reservoir by a sigmoid cysto-plasty with antirefluxing anastomoses of the ureters to the colon segment (Arap et al., 1980). If the ureters are dilated, implantation into the bowel in an anti-refluxing fashion is less likely to succeed, and thus the use of an ileocecal augmentation anastomosing the di-lated ureters to the ileum and creating a nonrefluxing ileocecal valve (Hendren, 1980) may succeed in pro-ducing a nonrefluxing reservoir. More innovative ap-proaches to continent reconstruction of the lower uri-nary tract may be required (Duckett and Snyder, 1985; Mitrofanoff, 1980; see also Chapter 50). Although these reconstructions may require clean intermittent catheterization to empty, this would appear to be a reasonable price to pay to achieve continence in this vexing congenital anomaly.

REFERENCES

Albers DD, Geyer JR, Barnes SD: Clinical significance of blind-ending branch of bifid ureter: report of 3 addi-tional cases. *J Urol* 1971; 105:634.

Amar AD: Ureteropyelostomy for relief of single ureteral obstruction in cases of ureteral duplication. *Arch Surg* 1970; 101:379.

Amar AD: Simple ureterocele at the distal end of a blind-ending ureter. *J Urol* 1971; 106:423.

Amar AD: Treatment of reflux in bifid ureters by conver-sion to complete duplication. *J Urol* 1972; 108:77.

Amar AD, Egan RM, Das S: Ipsilateral ureteroureteros-tomy combined with ureteral reimplantation for treat-ment of disease in both ureters in a child with com-plete ureteral duplication. *J Urol* 1981; 125:581.

Ambose SS, Nicholson WP III: The causes of vesicoure-teral reflux in children. *J Urol* 1962; 87:688.

Ambose SS, Nicolson WP: Ureteral reflux in duplicated ureters. *J Urol* 1964; 92:439.

Arap S, Giron AM, Goes GM: Initial results of the com-plete reconstruction of bladder exstrophy. *Urol Clin North Am* 1980; 7:477.

Ashcraft K, Hendren W: Bladder outlet obstruction after operation for ureterocele. *J Ped Surg* 1979; 14:819.

Athey PA, Carpenter RJ, Hadlock FP, et al: Ultrasonic demonstration of ectopic ureterocele. *Pediatrics* 1983; 71:568.

Atwell JD, Cook PL, Howell CT, et al: Familial inci-dence of bifid and double ureters. *Arch Dis Child* 1974; 49:390.

Babcock JR Jr, Belman AB, Shkolnik A, et al: Familial ureteral duplication and ureterocele. *Urology* 1977; 9:345.

Barrett DM, Malek RS, Kelalis PP: Problems and solu-tions in surgical treatment of 100 consecutive ureteral duplications in children. *J Urol* 1975; 114:126.

Bauer SB, Retik AB: The non-obstructive ectopic uretero-cele. *J Urol* 1978; 119:804.

Belman AB, Filmer RB, King LR: Surgical management of duplication of the collecting system. *J Urol* 1974; 112:316.

Bengmark S, Nilsson S, Romanus R: Ectopic ureter draining into a seminal megavesicle causing defecation troubles: report of a case and review of the literature. *Acta Chir Scand* 1962; 123:471.

Berdon WE, Levitt SB, Baker DH, et al: Ectopic ureter-ocele. *Radiol Clin North Am* 1968; 6:205.

Blyth B, Passerini-Glazel G, Camuffo C, et al: Endo-scopic incision of ureteroceles: intravesical versus ec-topic. *J Urol* 1993; 149:556.

Boijsen E: Angiographic studies of the anatomy of single and multiple renal arteries. *Acta Radiol [Suppl] (Stockh)* 1959; 183:1.

Bordon TA, Martinez A: Vesicoureteral reflux associated with intact orthotopic ureterocele. *Urology* 1977; 9:182.

Britt DB, Borden TA, Woodhead DM: Inverted Y ure-teral duplication with a blind-ending branch. *J Urol* 1972; 108:387.

Brock WA, Kaplan WG: Ectopic ureteroceles in children. *J Urol* 1978; 119:800.

Caldamone AA, Snyder HM, Duckett JW: Ureteroceles in children: follow-up of management with upper tract approach. *J Urol* 1984; 131:1130.

Campbell JE: Ureteral peristalsis in duplex renal collect-ing systems. *AJR* 1967; 99:577.

Campbell MF: Ureterocele: a study of 94 instances in 80 infants and children. *Surg Gynecol Obstet* 1951; 93:705.

Campbell MF: Anomalies of the ureter. In Campbell MF, Harrison JH (eds): *Urology*, ed 3. Philadelphia, WB Saunders Co, 1970, pp 1487-1670.

Cendron J, Bonhomme C: 31 cas d'uretèrà abouchement ectopique sous sphincterien chez l'enfant du sexe fémi-nin. *J Urol Nephrol (Paris)* 1968a; 74:1.

Cendron J, Bonhomme C: Uretère à terminaison ecto-pique extra-vesicale chez des sujets de sexe masculin (à propos de 10 cas). *J Urol Nephrol* (Paris) 1968b; 74:31.

Cendron J, Melin Y, Valayer J: Simplified treatment of ectopic ureteroceles in 35 children. *Eur Urol* 1981; 7:321.

Childlow JH, Utz DC: Ureteral ectopia in vestibule of va-gina with urinary continence. *South Med J* 1970; 63:423.

Chwalla R: The process of formation of cystic dilatations of the vesical end of the ureter and of diverticula at the ureteral ostium. *Urol Cutan Rev* 1927; 31:499.

Cohen N, Berant M: Duplications of the renal collecting system in the hereditary osteo onychodysplasia syn-drome. *J Pediatr* 1976; 89:261.

Cohen SJ: The Cohen reimplantation technique. In Bergsma D, Duckett JW (eds): *Urinary System and Malformations in Children*. New York, Alan R Liss, Inc, 1977, pp 391-5.

Coplen D, Duckett J: The modern approach to uretero-celes. *J Urol* 1995; 153:166.

Cox CE, Hutch JA: Bilateral single ectopic ureter: a re-port of 2 cases and review of the literature. *J Urol* 1966; 95:493.

Cremin BJ, Funston MR, Aaronson IA: The intraureteric diverticulum: a manifestation of ureterocele intussus-ception. *Pediatr Radiol* 1974; 6:92.

Culp OS: Ureteral diverticulum, classification of the literature and report of an authentic case. *J Urol* 1947; 58:309.

Culp OS: Heminephroureterectomy: comparison of one-stage and two-stage operations. *J Urol* 1960; 83:369.

Davis DM: Urethral ectopic ureter in the female without incontinence. *J Urol* 1930; 23:4631.

deJong T, van Gool J, Valkenburg T, et al: Primary reconstruction of the urinary tract in large ectopic ureteroceles. Abstract 120, Section on Urology, American Academy of Pediatrics Meeting, Dallas, Texas, 1994.

DeWeerd JH, Feeney DP: Bilateral ureteral ectopia with urinary incontinence in a mother and daughter. *J Urol* 1967; 98:335.

DeWeerd JH, Litin RB: Ectopia of ureteral orifice (vestibular) without incontinence: report of case. *Mayo Clin Proc* 1958; 33:81.

Diard F, Eklof O, Lebowitz R, et al: Urethral obstruction in boys caused by prolapse of simple ureterocele. *Pediatr Radiol* 1981; 11:139.

Duckett JW, Snyder H McC: Use of the Mitrofanoff principle in urinary reconstruction. *World J Urol* 1985; 3:191.

Eklof O, Lohr G, Ringertz H, et al: Ectopic ureterocele in the male infant. *Acta Radiol [Diagn] (Stockh)* 1978; 19:145.

Ellerker AG: The extravesical ectopic ureter. *Br J Surg* 1958; 45:344.

Ericsson NO: Ectopic ureterocele in infants and children. *Acta Chir Scand (Suppl)* 1954; 197:8.

Etker A, Dhillon H, Duffy P, Ransley P: Prophylactic endoscopic puncture of ureteroceles in prenatally diagnosed duplex kidneys. Abstract 117, Section on Urology, American Academy of Pediatrics, Dallas, Texas 1994.

Fehrenbaker LG, Kelalis PP, Stickler GB: Vesicoureteral reflux and ureteral duplication in children. *J Urol* 1972; 107:862.

Feldman S, Lome LG: Surgical management of ectopic ureterocele. *Urology* 1981; 17:252.

Fenelon MJ, Alton DJ: Prolapsing ectopic ureteroceles in boys. *Radiology* 1981; 140:373.

Finkel LI, Watts FB Jr, Cobrett DP: Ureteral triplication with a ureterocele. *Pediatr Radiol* 1983; 13:343.

Gill B: Ureteric ectopy in children. *Br J Urol* 1980; 52:257.

Glassberg KI, Braren V, Duckett JW, et al: Suggested terminology for duplex systems, ectopic ureters and ureteroceles. Report of the Committee on Terminology, Nomenclature and Classification, American Academy of Pediatrics. *J Urol* 1984; 132:1153.

Glenn JF: Agenesis of the bladder. *JAMA* 1959; 169:2016.

Gordon HL, Kessler R: Ectopic ureter entering the seminal vesicle associated with renal dysplasia. *J Urol* 1972; 108:389.

Green LF: Ureteral ectopy in females. *Surg Clin North Am* 1959; 39:989.

Grossman H, Winchester PH, Muecke EC: Solitary ectopic ureter. *Radiology* 1967; 89:1069.

Hartman GW, Hodson CJ: The duplex kidney and related abnormalities. *Clin Radiol* 1969; 20:387.

Hendren HW: Reoperative ureteral reimplantation: management of the difficult case. *J Pediatr Surg* 1980; 15:770.

Hendren WH, Mitchell ME: Surgical correction of ureteroceles. *J Urol* 1979; 121:590.

Hendren WH, Monfort GJ: Surgical correction of ureteroceles in childhood. *J Pediatr Surg* 1971; 6:235.

Husmann DA, Ewalt DH, Glenski WJ, et al: Ureterocele associated with ureteral duplication and nonfunctioning upper pole segment: management by partial nephroureterectomy alone. *J Urol* 1995; 154:723.

Hutch JA, Chisholm ER: Surgical repair of ureterocele. *J Urol* 1966; 96:445.

Jona JZ, Glicklich M, Cohen RD: Ectopic single ureter and severe renal dysplasia: an unusual presentation. *Urology* 1979; 21:369.

Johnson DK, Perlmutter AD: Single system ectopic ureteroceles with anomalies of the heart, testis and vas deferens. *J Urol* 1980; 123:81.

Johnston JH: Problems in the diagnosis and management of ectopic ureters and ureteroceles. In Johnston JH, Scholtmeijer RJ (eds): *Problems in Paediatric Urology*. Amsterdam, Excerpta Medica, 1972, pp 57-78.

Johnston JH, Davenport TJ: The single ectopic ureter. *Br J Urol* 1969; 41:428.

Johnston JH, Heal MR: Reflux in complete duplicated ureters in children: management and techniques. *J Urol* 1971; 105:881.

Johnston JH, Johnson LM: Experience with ectopic ureteroceles. *Br J Urol* 1969; 41:61.

Kaplan N, Elkin M: Bifid renal pelves and ureters: radiographic and cinefluorographic observations. *Br J Urol* 1968; 40:235.

Kelalis PP: Ureterocele. In Kelalis PP, King LR, Belman AB (eds): *Clinical Pediatric Urology*. Philadelphia, WB Saunders Co, 1976, pp 503-35.

Kesaven P, Ramakrishnan MS, Fowler R: Ectopia in unduplicated ureters in children. *Br J Urol* 1977; 49:481.

King LR, Kozlowski JM, Schacht MJ: Ureteroceles in children: a simplified and successful approach to management. *JAMA* 1983; 249:1461.

Kjellberg SR, Ericsson NO, Rudhe U: *The Lower Urinary Tract in Childhood: Some Correlated Clinical and Roentgenologic Observations*. Chicago, Year Book Medical Publishers, Inc, 1968.

Klauber GT, Crawford DB: Prolapse of ectopic ureterocele and bladder trigone. *Urology* 1980; 15:164.

Klauber GT, Reid EC: Inverted Y reduplication of the ureter. *J Urol* 1972; 107:362.

Kohri K, Nagai N, Kaneko S, et al: Bilateral trifid ureters associated with fused kidney, ureterovesical stenosis, left cryptorchidism and angioma of the bladder. *J Urol* 1978; 120:249.

Kontturi M, Kaski P: Blind-ending bifid ureter with ureteroureteral reflux. *Scand J Urol Nephrol* 1972; 6:91.

Koyanagi T, Hisajima S, Goto T, et al: Everting ureteroceles: radiographic and endoscopic observation and surgical management. *J Urol* 1980; 123:538.

Kretschmer HL: Hydronephrosis in infancy and childhood: clinical data and a report of 101 cases. *Surg Gynecol Obstet* 1937; 64:634.

Leadbetter GW: Surgical correction of total urinary incontinence. *J Urol* 1964; 91:261.

Leadbetter GW Jr: Ectopic ureterocele as a cause of urinary incontinence. *J Urol* 1970; 103:222.

Lebowitz RL: Pediatric uroradiology. *Pediatr Clin North Am* 1985; 32:1353.

Lebowitz RL, Wyly JB: Refluxing urethral ectopic ureters: diagnosis by the cyclic voiding cystourethrogram. *AJR* 1984; 142:1263.

Lenaghan D: Bifid ureters in children: an anatomical, physiological, and clinical study. *J Urol* 1962; 87:808.

Leong J, Mikhael B, Schillinger JF: Refluxing ureteroceles. *J Urol* 1980; 125:136.

Livaditis A, Maureseth K, Skog PA: Unilateral triplication of the ureter and renal pelvis: report of a case. *Acta Chir Scand* 1964; 127:181.

Lund AJ: Uncrossed double ureter with rare intravesical orifice relationship: case report with review of literature. *J Urol* 1949; 62:22.

Mackie GG, Awang H, Stephens FD: The ureteric orifice: the embryologic key to radiologic status of duplex kidneys. *J Pediatr Surg* 1975; 10:473.

Mackie GG, Stephens FD: Duplex kidneys: a correlation of renal dysplasia with position of the ureteral orifice. *J Urol* 1975; 114:274.

Malek RS, Kelalis PP, Burke EC: Simple and ectopic ureterocele in infancy and childhood. *Surg Gynecol Obstet* 1972a; 134:611.

Malek RS, Kelalis PP, Stickler GB, et al: Observations on ureteral ectopy in children. *J Urol* 1972b; 107:308.

Mandell J, Colodny AH, Lebowitz R, et al: Ureteroceles in infants and children. *J Urol* 1980; 123:921.

Marshall FF, McLoughlin MG: Long-blind-ending ureteral duplications. *J Urol* 1978; 120:626.

Mascatello VJ, Smith EH, Carrera GF, et al: Ultrasonic evaluation of the obstructed duplex kidney. *AJR* 1977; 129:113.

Mayor G, Genton N, Torrado A, et al: Renal function in obstructive nephropathy: long-term effect of reconstructive surgery. *Pediatrics* 1975; 56:740.

Meyer R: Zur Anatomie and Entwicklungsgeschichte der Ureterverdoppelung. *Virchows Arch (Pathol Ant)* 1907; 187:408.

Mitrofanoff P: Cystostomie continente trans-appendiculaire dans le traitement des vessies neurologiues. *Chir Pediatr* 1980; 21:297.

Mogg RA: The single ectopic ureter. *Br J Urol* 1974; 46:3.

Monfort G, Guys J, Coquet M, et al: Surgical management of duplex ureteroceles. *J Ped Surg* 1992; 27:634.

Monfort G, Morrison-Lacombe G, Coquet M: Endoscopic treatment of ureteroceles revisited. *J Urol* 1985; 133:1031.

Musselman, BC, Barry JJ: Varying degrees of ureteral ectopia and duplication in 5 siblings. *J Urol* 1973; 110:476.

Nation EF: Duplication of the kidney and ureter: a statistical study of 230 new cases. *J Urol* 1944; 51:456.

Noe HN: Prolapsing single orthotopic ureteroceles in a boy: case report. *J Urol* 1978; 120:367.

Noseworthy J, Persky L: Spectrum of bilateral ureteral ectopia. *Urology* 1982; 19:489.

Nussbaum A, Dorst J, Jeffs R, et al: Ectopic ureter and ureterocele: their varied sonographic manifestations. *Radiology* 1986; 159:227.

Ogawa A, Kakizawa Y, Akaza H: Ectopic ureter passing through the external urethral sphincter: report of a case. *J Urol* 1976; 116:109.

Ossandon F, Androulakakis P, Ransley PG: Surgical problems in pelvioureteral junction obstruction of the lower moiety in incomplete duplex systems. *J Urol* 1981; 125:871.

Perkins PJ, Kroovand RL, Evans AT: Ureteral triplication. *Radiology* 1973; 108:533.

Perrin EV, Persky L, Tucker A, et al: Renal duplication and dysplasia. *Urology* 1974; 4:660.

Peterson LJ, Grimes JH, Weinerth JL, et al: Blind-ending branches of bifid ureters. *Urology* 1975; 5:191.

Prewitt LH Jr, Lebowitz RL: The single ectopic ureter. *AJR* 1976; 127:941.

Privett JTJ, Jeans WD, Roylance J: The incidence and importance of renal duplication. *Clin Radiol* 1976; 27:521.

Rabinowitz R, Barkin M, Schillinger JF, et al: Bilateral orthotopic ureteroceles causing massive ureteral dilatation in children. *J Urol* 1978; 119:839.

Rank WB, Mellinger GT, Spiro E: Ureteral diverticula: etiologic considerations. *J Urol* 1960; 83:566.

Rich MA, Keating MA, Snyder HM, et al: Low transurethral low incision of single system ureteroceles in children. *J Urol* 1990; 144:120.

Rognon L, Brueziere J, Soret JY, et al: Abouchement ectopique de l'uretère dans le tractus séminal: À propos de 10 cas. *Chirurgie* 1973; 99:741.

Royle MG, Goodwin WE: The management of ureteroceles. *J Urol* 1971; 106:42.

Schlecker BA, Snyder HM, Duckett JW: Bilateral single ectopic ureters (abstract 108). Presented at Mid-Atlantic Section of the AUA Atlanta, May 1985.

Schlecker BA, Snyder HM, Duckett JW: Ectopic ureters in children (abstract 153). Presented at AUA 81st Annual Meeting, New York, May 1986.

Schulman CC: Les implantations ectopiques de l'uretère. *Acta Urol Belg* 1972; 40:201.

Schulman CC: The single ectopic ureter. *Eur Urol* 1976; 2:64.

Schlussel R, Peters C, McClintock J, et al: Efficacy of transurethral incision of ureteroceles. Abstract 118 Meeting Section on Urology, American Academy of Pediatrics Meeting, Dallas, Texas, 1994.

Schultze R: Der blind endende Doppelureter. *Z Urol Nephrol* 1967; 60:271.

Scott JES: The single ectopic ureter and the dysplastic kidney. *Br J Urol* 1981; 53:300.

Seitzman DM, Patton JF: Ureteral ectopia: combined ureteral and vas deferens anomaly. *J Urol* 1960; 84:604.

Sen S, Beasley SW, Amed S, et al: Renal function and vesicoureteric reflux in children with ureteroceles. *Pediatr Surg Int* 1992; 7:192.

Sherwood T, Stevenson JJ: Ureteroceles in disguise. *Br J Radiol* 1969; 42:899.

Siegel A, Snyder HM, Duckett JW: Epididymitis in infants and boys: underlying urogenital anomalies and efficacy of imaging modalities. *J Urol* 1987; 138:1100-3.

Smith C, Gosalbez R, Parrott T, et al: Transurethral puncture of ectopic ureteroceles in neonates and infants. *J Urol* 1994; 152:2110.

Snyder HM, Johnston JH: Orthotopic ureteroceles in children. *J Urol* 1978; 119:543.

Snyder HM, Uri AK, Caldamone AA, et al: Ureteral duplication with ureterocele pathology of the upper pole (abstract 1). Presented at AUA Annual Meeting, Las Vegas, 1983.

Soderdahl DW, Shiraki IW, Schamber DT: Bilateral ureteral quadruplication. *J Urol* 1976; 116:255.

Stephens FD: *Congenital Malformations of the Rectum, Anus and Genitourinary Tracts,* London, E & S Livingstone, 1963.

Stephens FD: Caecoureterocele and concepts on the embryology and aetiology of ureteroceles. *Aust NZ J Surg* 1971; 40:239.

Stephens FD, Lenaghan D: The anatomical basis and dynamics of vesicoureteral reflux. *J Urol* 1962; 87:669.

Subbiah N, Stephens D: Stenotic ureterocele. *Aust NZ J Surg* 1972; 41:257.

Summer TE, Crowe JE, Resnick MI: Diagnosis of ectopic ureterocele using ultrasound. *Urology* 1980; 15:82.

Tacciuoli M, Laurenti C, Racheli T: Trigonal cyst in childhood. *Br J Urol* 1976; 48:323.

Tanagho EA: Embryologic basis for lower ureteral anomalies: a hypothesis. *Urology* 1976; 7:451.

Tanagho EA: Ureteroceles: embryogenesis, pathogenesis and management. *J Contin Educ Urol* 1979; 18:13.

Tanagho EA, Hutch JA: Primary reflux. *J Urol* 1965; 93:158.

Tank ES: Experience with endoscopic incision and open unroofing of ureteroceles. *J Urol* 1986; 136:241.

Thompson GJ, Kelalis PP: Ureterocele: clinical appraisal of 176 cases. *J Urol* 1964; 91:488.

Timothy RP, Decter A, Perlmutter AD: Ureteral duplication: clinical findings and therapy in 46 children. *J Urol* 1971; 105:445.

Tokunaka S, Gotoh T, Koyanagi T, et al: Morphological study of the ureterocele: a possible clue to its embryogenesis as evidenced by a locally arrested myogenesis. *J Urol* 1981; 126:726.

Tresidder GC, Blandy JP, Murray RS: Pyelopelvic and uretero-ureteric reflux. *Br J Urol* 1970; 42:728.

Uson AC, Lattimer JK, Melicow MM: Ureteroceles in infants and children: a report based on 44 cases. *Pediatrics* 1961; 27:971.

Uson AC, Schulman CC: Ectopic ureter emptying into the rectum: report of a case. *J Urol* 1972; 108:156.

Uson AC, Womack CE, Berdon WE: Giant ectopic ureter presenting as an abdominal mass in a newborn infant. *J Pediatr* 1972; 80:473.

Vanhoutte JJ: Ureteral ectopia into a Wolffian duct remnant (Gartner's ducts or cysts) presenting as a urethral diverticulum in two girls. *AJR* 1970; 110:540.

Weigert C: Ueber einige Bildungsfehler der Ureteren. *Virchows Arch (Pathol Anat)* 1877; 70:490.

Weiss JP, Duckett JW, Snyder HM: Single unilateral vaginal ectopic ureter: Is it really a rarity? *J Urol* 1984; 132:1177.

Weiss RM, Spackman TJ: Everting ectopic ureteroceles. *J Urol* 1974; 111:538.

Whitaker J, Danks DM: A study of the inheritance of duplication of the kidneys and ureters. *J Urol* 1966; 95:176.

Williams DI, Fay R, Lillie JG: The functional radiology of ectopic ureterocele. *Br J Urol* 1972; 44:417.

Williams DI, Lightwood RG: Bilateral single ectopic ureters. *J Urol* 1972; 44:267.

Williams DI, Royle M: Ectopic ureter in the male child. *Br J Urol* 1969; 41:421.

Williams DI, Woodard JR: Problems in the management of ectopic ureteroceles. *J Urol* 1964; 92:635.

Youngson GG: Ureteral triplication, contralateral duplication and bilateral extravesical ectopic ureter. *J Urol* 1985; 134:533.

Zielinski J: Avoidance of vesicoureteral reflux after transurethral ureteral meatotomy for ureterocele. *J Urol* 1962; 88:386.

Zoantz MR, Maizels M: Type I ureteral triplication: an extension of the Weigert-Meyer Law. *J Urol* 1985; 134:949.

CHAPTER 47

The Wide Ureter

H. Norman Noe

The therapeutic approach to the widely dilated ureter varies as to etiology and the pathologic significance associated with such dilatation. The wide ureter lacks effective peristalsis because of the inability of the ureteral walls to coapt; thus, it fails to properly propel a bolus of urine. This leads to urinary stasis, potential infection, predisposes to urinary calculi, and, in the extreme, results in renal parenchymal destruction. However, not all wide ureters carry this poor prognosis, and in some cases renal growth and development can proceed normally even in the presence of ureteral dilatation. Since successful surgical therapy of the wide ureter is currently possible, it becomes important to identify those patients with a dilated ureter who would benefit from such therapy. It is also equally important to identify those renal and ureteral units that will not benefit from surgery and can be observed safely. In this latter instance, surgical therapy can only serve as a source for potential complications and possible detriment without offering a significant change for benefit.

Much confusion has arisen as the debate regarding nomenclature for the wide ureter has continued. Caulk (1923) first used the term *megaloureter*. His original term has been shortened to simply *megaureter,* but the term itself has come •o mean different things to different observers. At its simplest it means only "big ureter." To achieve a more informed approach to management of the widely dilated ureter, it is essential to clarify the terms used to describe that ureter. Such precise classification allows treatment based on etiology and, thus, effective communication of the outcome of that treatment with our colleagues. The term "megaureter" should not bring to mind a specific disease process nor imply an etiology, but rather it should be used as a general term for the wide ureter. Descriptive and modifying terms can then be applied as a classification scheme is adopted.

The precise definition of what constitutes an abnormally wide ureter can be elusive. The diagnosis of megaureter inevitably is established based on some form of radiographic demonstration. Technically, any ureter whose width exceeds that of the upper limits of normal for any particular age group can be designated a megaureter. Cussen (1967) has established normal ureteral measurements in children from 30 weeks gestational age to 12 years of age. Using this scheme, any ureter greater than 7 mm in diameter technically becomes a megaureter. Practically speaking, however, there is little need to try to define megaureter in absolute diameter measurements. The radiographic appearance is usually striking, demonstrating more than just minimal ureterectasis. Marked ureteral dilatation is the usual case. Ureteral tortuosity also may be present. Pelvicalyceal dilatation is variable depending on the severity of the underlying disease process. Renal parenchymal scarring or loss may be present because of back-pressure atrophy or secondary to infection or calculi.

CLASSIFICATION

Several schemes for classifying the megaureter have been proposed (Belman, 1974; Glassberg, 1977; Whitaker and Johnston, 1976). The most pressing practical matter was to define the obstructive from the nonobstructive forms of megaureter, given that obstruction needs surgical correction as early as possible. Most observers easily accepted the difference between the obstructed and the refluxing megaureter, but it became less clear how to classify or categorize the so-called nonobstructive, nonrefluxing megaureter. Inherent in any discussion of the classification of megaureter is that one must accept that a wide ureter can exist without significant reflux or obstruction being present. Considerable confusion developed as this problem of classifying the megaureter was examined, and there was initial failure to accept a uniform terminology. As our understanding and experience with megaureters grew, it became possible for a more uniform terminology to be proposed and accepted.

In 1976, an international pediatric urologic seminar was held in Philadelphia. This was a combined meeting of the members of the Urological Section of the American Academy of Pediatrics, the Society for Paediatric Urological Surgeons, and the Society for Pediatric Urology. A committee was formed to develop a standard nomenclature and classification of wide ureters. This was accomplished and has been the classification scheme most widely adopted and used to the present (Stephens, 1977). Although many observers disagree regarding specific clinical instances for inclusion in this scheme, it offers the opportunity for all patients with wide ureters to be classified within the system. Many less complex systems are appealing but lack the ability to classify all patients clearly. It appears that some degree of complexity will have to be accepted to ensure completeness with any classification system.

The three major categories of classification in the aforementioned scheme are the refluxing megaureter, the obstructed megaureter, and, as noted earlier, the nonrefluxing, nonobstructed megaureter (Table 47-1). Each major category can be divided further into primary and secondary subcategories. A few pitfalls have already been pointed out. It is possible to have a wide ureter that shows both reflux and obstruction (King, 1980). This represents a special situation and should be kept in mind and specifically sought when evaluating the refluxing megaureter. Iatrogenic megaureter, the residual ureterectasis following urethral valve ablation, the prune-belly ureter, and other instances have been offered as examples for which classification is difficult or incomplete. It seems that with appropriate testing, most dilated ureters usually could be properly classified. One would also have to accept that it would be possible for the classification of the ureters to change depending on the results of therapeutic intervention. An example would be the secondary obstructive megaureter caused by urethral valves that improves following valve ablation and remains as a nonobstructive, nonrefluxing megaureter. Another instance could be the residual nonobstructive ureterectasis seen following successful ureteral reimplantation. Many patients may be properly classified only following serial evaluation or long-term observation. One should also remember that the testing procedures used to evaluate the wide ureter are prone to certain inaccuracies and may have to be repeated before proper classification can be achieved. Although imperfect, the international classification scheme seems to be the most comprehensive and widely accepted at present. This scheme is used in the discussion of the wide ureter in this chapter.

DIAGNOSTIC METHODS
General

All urologists are familiar with the fact that a ureter can appear normal on one testing circumstance and not on another. These differences can be accentuated further by different testing conditions; that is, the state of hydration, fluid load, or presence of urinary infection. The working party to establish the international classification agreed that any method that would demonstrate an abnormally wide ureter was sufficient to define the condition of megaureter. As mentioned previously, no definite measurement is used as an absolute point of definition for the diagnosis of megaureter because from a practical standpoint the diagnosis is usually quite clear radiographically.

The basic investigative procedure used by most urologists at present is the standard excretory urogram and voiding cystourethrogram. These tests will, first of all, define refluxing vs. nonrefluxing megaureter. In most instances, they also will be sufficient to identify many of the obstructive causes, both primary and secondary. These include such entities as the primary obstructive megaureter caused by a distal adynamic segment and the secondary obstructed megaureter attributable to valves, ureterocele, and other conditions. Fluoroscopy of the ureter during the initial excretory urogram also can be helpful if the radiologist is alerted to the need for doing such evaluation in children with large ureters. It also should be noted that certain variations in testing or screening for genitourinary pathology in children are evolving. In many instances, we are now substituting renal ultrasound for the excretory urogram in routine urinary tract infection evaluations. Likewise, the nuclear scan in the neonate is superior to the use of the excretory urogram. Appropriate information will still be obtained even in these instances, and usually an excretory urogram or an antegrade pyelogram will be obtained sometime during the diagnostic evaluation. In general, the next steps to be taken following the basic uroradiographic workup will depend on the information obtained from these initial information gathering procedures.

Endoscopic techniques generally are used only as

TABLE 47-1

Classification of Megaureter*

Refluxing megaureter
  Primary (congenital reflux)
  Secondary (urethral valves, neurogenic bladder, etc.)
Obstructed megaureter
  Primary (adynamic segment, urethral valves, etc.)
  Secondary (tumor, urethral valves, neurogenic bladder, etc.)
Nonrefluxing, nonobstructed megaureter
  Primary (idiopathic)
  Secondary (diabetes insipidus, infection, residual dilatation from
    surgery)

*Major categories within the international classification scheme for megaureter. Select examples are in parentheses. Note some conditions may appear in more than one category.

secondary procedures; more informative studies, which will be discussed further in the text, are relied on initially. Cystoscopy can be appropriate in the initial management of the entities such as posterior urethral valves, urethral stricture, or the evaluation of primary reflux, or it may be best deferred until the time of any planned definitive surgical procedure. In the past, retrograde ureteral catheterization noting any "hydronephrotic drip" has been used to help confirm a diagnosis or to add information in equivocal cases. This is now primarily of historical interest only. Retrograde pyelography with drainage films also can be beneficial, particularly if drainage is delayed for a substantial time. Drainage films following administration of a diuretic also can add useful information.

Once reflux has been excluded, the diagnostic dilemmas arise when it is unclear whether the wide ureter is truly obstructed or represents a nonrefluxing, nonobstructive megaureter. Two procedures are now widely used to help establish further information regarding the presence or absence of obstruction. These are the diuretic renogram and the pressure perfusion study as advocated by Whitaker (Ash et al., 1979; Koff et al., 1980; O'Reilly et al., 1978, 1979; Whitaker, 1973). Each test has advantages, disadvantages, and sources of error. In most settings, they can be considered complementary rather than competitive.

Diuretic Renogram

The diuretic renogram of furosemide-assisted nuclear scan attempts to quantitate or measure the ability of a system to empty following a diuretic challenge. It should be performed in a standard fashion with the patient being well hydrated. The most widely used radiopharmaceutical is technetium 99m diethylenetriamine pentaacetic acid (^{99m}Tc DTPA). Early images are recorded and interpreted as the angiographic phase of the study, with renal blood flow being estimated. During the first 3 to 4 minutes following injection, images are taken that reflect renal perfusion and can be used to calculate relative renal function. Over the next several minutes, images are made and data is gathered to generate a renogram curve. When the collecting system is well filled with isotope, images are then taken after intravenous (IV) administration of 1 mg/kg of furosemide (Lasix). When evaluating the megaureter, it must be remembered that areas of interest should include both the kidney and the lower ureter (Koff et al., 1984). In general, half-time clearance after furosemide should be accomplished in less than 15 minutes. If clearance is greater than 20 minutes, obstruction is likely. Clearance between 15 and 20 minutes is thought by many to represent equivocal test results.

Four types of renogram curves generally are recognized (Fig. 47-1). The normal pattern shows spon-

taneous washout of the tracer without the need for furosemide. The dilated, nonobstructive pattern shows progressive accumulation of the radionuclide prior to furosemide administration but prompt washout after its administration. The obstructed pattern shows no washout or progressive accumulation within the ureter and upper collecting system following administration of furosemide. In the equivocal pattern, there is some degree of washout following furosemide, but the rate of clearance is much slower than that in the nonobstructive system. Simultaneous imaging of the bladder and the ureter can be particularly helpful to define the point of obstruction if an abnormality at the ureterovesical junction is suspected (Fig. 47-2).

Several factors affect the accuracy of this test. The doses of both tracer and furosemide should be standard so that adequate comparison of test results can be made. Adequate hydration is essential to ensure clearance of the tracer, and if the child is not well hydrated this can serve as a source of error for interpretation of the test. IV fluid administration can be helpful and is advocated by many as a routine part of the test to ensure adequate hydration. IV fluids are essential when evaluating equivocal cases of obstructed megaureter. The degree of bladder filling influences the test, and during the procedure voiding should be initiated or catheterization performed to

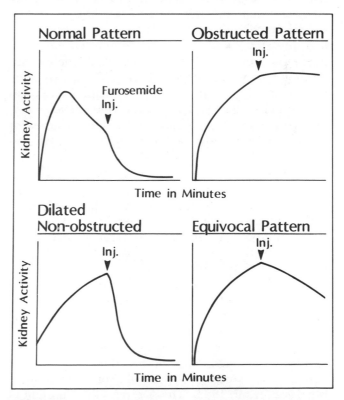

FIG. 47-1
Four major types of renogram curves generated during diuretic renography. Obstruction may be evidenced as a flat or even increased curve following furosemide injection.

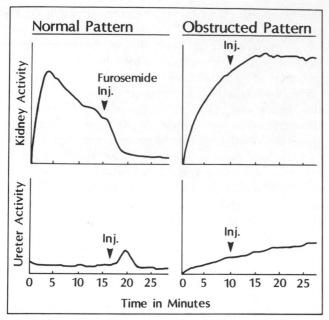

FIG. 47-2
Localization of the area of obstruction during diuretic renography by simultaneous renal and ureteral scanning. Note increased radioactivity in the ureteral region following furosemide injection when obstructed ureter is present.

ensure evaluation with both an empty and a full bladder. This is especially important when evaluating specific conditions involving obstruction at the ureterovesical junction or determining whether a hypotonic, high-pressure bladder may be responsible for some degree of ureteral dilatation. Poor renal function also can be an important source of error. The poorly functioning kidney may not generate enough of a diuresis to stimulate washout. By the same token, even a kidney with good function may not be able to diurese or empty an extremely capacious system if hydronephrosis is extreme (reservoir effect). In this situation, washout may be slow even if true anatomic obstruction is absent.

As we are seeing increasing numbers of children with diagnosed prenatal hydronephrosis, it is especially important to remember that renal function immaturity in the newborn can quite significantly alter the results of the diuretic renogram. Low levels of glomerular function lead to slow diuretic responsiveness, and when the degree extends to the ureterovesical junction it can make the timing of the diuretic and interpretation of the test quite difficult. When possible, it is best to obtain a diuretic renogram at 3 to 4 months of age, allowing time for renal maturity to occur and avoiding the possibility of a false-positive renal scan (Koff, 1988). This is especially important in the infant with either mild to moderate obstruction or an equivocal initial result as a newborn. The extraction factor component of the DTPA renal scan has been

advocated as a means of measuring clinically significant obstruction (Heyman and Duckett, 1988). Although this appears to be a reliable test, a broader experience will be required to determine its usefulness in this setting.

The advantages of the diuretic renogram are several. It provides information for renal function measurement, is minimally invasive, can be performed with standard equipment, does not require anesthesia, and, perhaps of greatest significance, can be easily used serially. The last can be particularly useful in evaluation of the equivocally dilated-obstructed system or in the postoperative patient.

Pressure Perfusion Studies

The pressure perfusion study is an attempt to define obstruction in terms of pressures generated when subjecting the system to a set flow rate. By definition, in an unobstructed setting a low pressure is maintained even when upper limits of normal flow are encountered. Thus, a volume of fluid can move "through" the system without difficulty and without the requirements of high pressure. With obstruction, however, a high pressure is generated with the same flow rate when an attempt is made to move the same volume of fluid through the system. It is the high pressure required to move a volume of fluid through the system that is thought to produce renal damage. This test was made popular by Whitaker (1973) and is accepted as an accurate method of determining upper urinary tract obstruction. Instances in which the results of the pressure perfusion study are difficult to interpret with certainty still remain.

The technique usually requires anesthesia in younger children, but it is possible with sedation and local anesthesia in the older, more cooperative child. It should be performed in the radiology suite where the test can be monitored radiographically. The system is represented diagrammatically in Figure 47-3. Access to the upper urinary tract is established by a percutaneous nephrostomy. An appropriate-sized urethral catheter is placed in the bladder. The system is then connected through a length of manometer tubing and incorporates a pressure transducer and recording apparatus. A series of stopcocks allows measurement of renal pelvic and intermittent bladder pressure at different phases of filling of the urinary system. A dilute contrast agent is added to the fluid used to fill the system. This allows images to be taken during perfusion to ensure a completely filled system. A perfusion pump is used to establish a standard fast flow of 10 ml/min, which is considered the upper limit of the physiologic range.

Prior to perfusion of the system, a baseline pressure is established as that measured at the kidney level. The bladder pressure is then checked against a base-

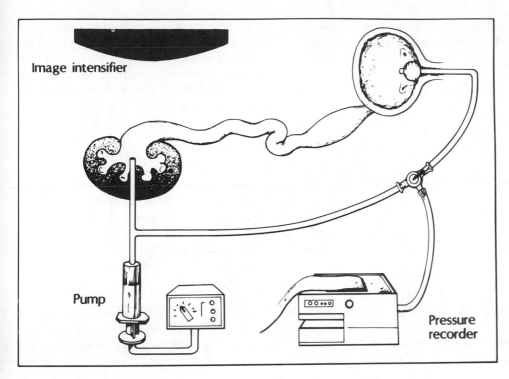

FIG. 47-3
Diagrammatic representation of
pressure perfusion study.

line and is usually somewhere between 3 to 5 cm H_2O pressure. Once perfusion of the urinary tract begins, spot radiographs are taken to afford anatomic information at various filling pressures; alternate renal and bladder pressures are recorded. When adequate measurements and radiographs have been obtained, the nephrostomy cannula can be removed or left, depending on the patient's therapeutic needs. The pressure generated when perfusing the cannula alone outside the body is measured so that this pressure can be subtracted from other readings to provide accurate calculation of the test results. In essence, one obtains renal pelvic pressure as a relative value. This relative renal pelvic pressure is the pressure recorded minus the cannula resistance and minus the bladder pressure.

A relative renal pelvic pressure less than 12 cm H_2O at a flow of 10 ml/min is thought to be normal when assessing a point of potential obstruction, such as the ureterovesical junction. A pressure differential of 13 to 20 cm H_2O is thought to be equivocal and to greater than 20 cm H_2O pressure difference to represent true obstruction. The test usually is considered most helpful in instances where impaired renal function and a large volume collecting system are present and the diuretic renogram is equivocal. When normal, the test is considered reliable. When equivocal or marginally elevated measurements are obtained, the results have to be interpreted with care.

Patients difficult to evaluate by this method are the same ones who are problematic by other methods. These include patients with noncompliant bladders, such as those with posterior urethral valves or refluxing ureters with residual ureterectasis following surgical correction. Such children may have normal relative renal pelvic pressures with the bladder empty but exhibit marked rises in pressure as the bladder fills. In these cases, the ureterovesical junction, by strict definition, is unobstructed, but a hypertonic detrusor generally acts as a form of obstruction once filling occurs. The result is the same as localized obstruction, but the treatment would be different and aimed at decreasing bladder pressures and increasing compliance as with augmentation cystoplasty. Large capacity systems also may have relatively low pressures even if obstruction exists. One must be certain that the urinary system to be tested is completely filled during the pressure perfusion studies to ensure accurate measurements. In addition, spot radiographs can ensure that no extravasation or leakage of fluid from the system has occurred, which could alter the accuracy of the results.

The main disadvantages of the pressure perfusion study are its invasive nature, the requirement for anesthesia in younger children, and that it is not easily applied in a serial fashion. It also gives no renal function information. As also noted above, the results at times are difficult to interpret. It has been noted experimentally that renal pelvic pressures do not always accurately reflect obstruction (Koff and Thrall, 1981). The determinants of the progression of hydronephrosis and possible renal damage include the rate of urine formation and the degree of duration of obstruction but, also importantly, must take into account the compliance of the pelvicalyceal and ureteral system. A large capacity collecting system can indeed tolerate larger volumes at lower pressures and thus give a certain measure of protection to an obstructed ureteral and renal unit once equilibration of urine formation and renal pelvic pressure has been reached. Thus, low pressures can be measured within a compensated system even though obstruction does exist. In these instances, pressure perfusion measurements may not be able to predict whether hydronephrotic progression can or will occur.

Despite the drawbacks and inaccuracies mentioned, the pressure perfusion study is still considered to be a very sophisticated method of demonstrating obstruction and should be viewed as complementary to other methods, specifically the diuretic renogram. The test can be applied intraoperatively, although this would seem to be applicable only in very selected instances to confirm a diagnosis or to check the immediate surgical result.

Comparisons of the diuretic renogram and the Whitaker test have been made. Kass and associates (1985) evaluated and compared the results of these two studies and have found an excellent correlation. In that series of 42 kidneys, the majority could clearly be defined as obstructed or unobstructed by either study. There were instances in which false-positives and false-negatives were encountered in both studies, although in less than 10% of the cases. Equivocal or indeterminate results also were obtained using both testing procedures, but again in less than 10%. It was through the complementary use of these tests and correlation with clinical, radiographic, and surgical findings that the final result could be established in these equivocal cases. Others have attempted to correlate the diuretic renogram and the pressure perfusion studies, with all investigators eventually concluding that there are certain limitations and technical considerations for each method (Gonzalez and Chiou, 1985). Both methods seem to have their advantages and disadvantages and sources of error. These must be kept in mind as test results are interpreted and surgical decisions are made.

Most agree, following the standard excretory urogram or ultrasound, to proceed with the diuretic renogram in evaluating possible obstruction. Its noninvasive nature and ready availability make it attractive. If the diuretic renogram shows prompt washout, obstruction can be excluded. If the scan shows obstruction, particularly with good renal function and a simple radiographic appearance being present, no further tests would be necessary, and surgery should be undertaken. If the results of the study are equivocal, if there is poor renal function or if there is a suspected error because of a capacious collecting system, then pressure perfusion studies would be next in order. If

the diagnosis is still unclear, repeat studies might have a role in the clinically stable patient. One should realize, however, that there will still be the unusual case where test results may remain unclear, and the decision will have to be based on clinical judgment and the final diagnosis sometimes made only at the time of surgery.

REFLUXING MEGAURETER
Primary

As shown in the earlier classification scheme, the refluxing megaureter may be divided into two basic categories, the primary and the secondary groups. Primary reflux refers to the circumstance in which only a ureterovesical junction malformation exists. There is inadequate ureteral tunnel length and free reflux is demonstrated on a voiding cystourethrogram (Fig. 47-4). Primary refluxing megaureters are more likely to be bilateral as opposed to the unilateral occurrence in the primary obstructed megaureter. Patients with refluxing megaureters most often present with signs and symptoms associated with urinary tract infection. Some will present with renal failure and azotemia, and a significant number of patients will be neonates and infants. Refluxing megaureters seem to be encountered more often in boys than girls. In addition to the classic symptoms of infection, in older children presentation also can involve findings associated with hypertension. Whereas most patients present in the classic symptomatic manner, some have been found to

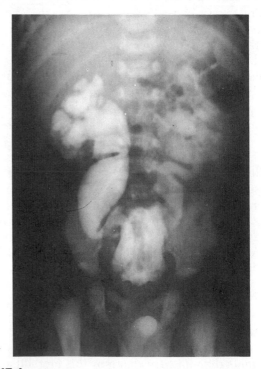

FIG. 47-4
Primary refluxing megaureter in a neonate presenting with urosepsis.

have refluxing megaureters without obvious clinical signs or symptoms. This usually has occurred as an incidental finding during other medical investigations, in prenatal screening or in conjunction with screening for familial reflux (Noe, 1992; Noe et al., 1992).

In many cases, the amount of renal parenchyma associated with the refluxing megaureter is reduced or renal scarring is already present at the time of discovery. The kidney may show changes of classic pressure atrophy similar to those with obstruction, or it may demonstrate a degree of dysplasia, if studied histologically. Secondary ureteropelvic junction obstruction can occur with severe reflux and a tortuous ureter (Fig. 47-5). This secondary obstruction in most cases resolves with correction of the reflux alone, and there is no need for secondary pyeloplasty.

Management of the primary refluxing megaureter depends on several factors. In my experience, most often the management has been surgical because the ureterovesical junction deformity has been severe, that is, the golf-hole orifice or ureteral insertion into the paraureteral diverticulum. Some children may be safely observed while on antimicrobial prophylaxis in hopes of spontaneous cessation. Realistically, however, experience has shown that with the more severe grades of reflux, spontaneous cessation is unlikely.

Surgical management of the refluxing megaureter usually involves primary reconstruction. In the past, ureteral reimplantation in these cases was prone to a high level of complication and failure and, for this

reason, ureterostomy or even permanent diversion was advocated. The latter is now thought to be inappropriate in most cases. Temporary diversion by cutaneous vesicostomy has proved useful in selected situations because of its ready reversibility and ease of performance (Allen, 1980; Duckett, 1974). This may be especially true in a sick neonate or in an infant with multiple congenital anomalies in whom definitive surgical correction is best delayed. When reflux is present with reasonable renal function and the clinical condition permits, definitive ureteral reimplantation and reconstruction is indicated, even in neonates and infants. It is in the infant and younger child that renal recovery and growth after successful surgery can be the most striking and gratifying.

Older children with refluxing megaureters often present with severe renal compromise with or without hypertension. Ureteral reimplantation in these instances seems to offer little in relationship to renal functional improvement. Surgery can be helpful; however, when frequent, difficult-to-control urinary tract infections are encountered because reimplantation in these patients can be performed successfully. Some have advocated this as a desirable alternative to later performance of pretransplant nephroureterectomy.

The unilateral refluxing megaureter can be associated with a degree of dysplasia or varying degrees of alteration of renal function, even to the point of nonfunction. In the case of the refluxing megaureter, a renal scan performed with an indwelling urethral catheter for maintenance of continuous bladder decompression can help determine the level of function in such a unilaterally affected unit. If renal function is poor to absent in the affected kidney and the contralateral kidney function is satisfactory, nephroureterectomy may be the therapy of choice.

Secondary

Secondary refluxing megaureters occur as a result of some primary abnormality involving the bladder or urethra. Common examples include the neurogenic bladder and outlet obstruction such as encountered with urethral valves (Figs. 47-6 and 47-7). Other less common conditions resulting in secondary reflux include ureteroceles, urethral strictures, cyclophosphamide and radiation cystitis, and the "nonneurogenic neurogenic bladder." The approach to the secondary refluxing megaureter is difficult in that the primary etiologic factors must be corrected before definitively dealing with the reflux.

With urethral valves only about 50% of patients will reflux at initial diagnosis and about one third of these will spontaneously resolve refluxing following successful valve ablation. Persistent reflux of lower grades can be observed with the patient on antibacterial prophylaxis. The more severe grades are usually due to

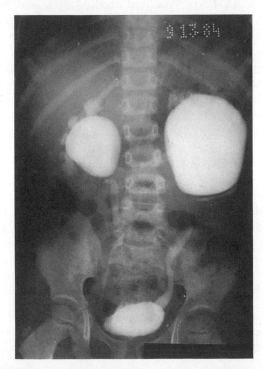

FIG. 47-5
Secondary ureteropelvic junction obstruction associated with reflux.

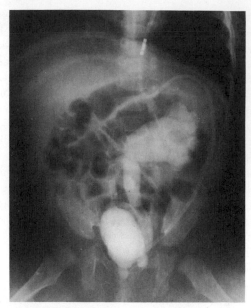

FIG. 47-6
Reflux associated with a neurogenic bladder.

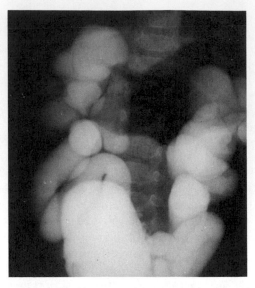

FIG. 47-7
Secondary refluxing megaureter attributable to posterior valves.

fixed anatomic deformities, such as paraureteral diverticula, and will usually require definitive reconstructive surgery. Persistent unilateral reflux following valve ablation is in many cases associated with a nonfunctioning kidney. As mentioned earlier, a renal scan with the bladder decompressed and catheterized will determine the level of renal function and give an idea as to whether reconstruction or nephroureterectomy is the appropriate course of action. In some instances of unilateral nonfunction where surgical treatment is required on the contralateral ureter, it can be helpful to delay nephroureterectomy until the success of the contralateral surgery has been determined. Many times the ureter to a nonfunctioning renal unit can be used to salvage an unsuccessful or complicated surgical result on what would be a solitary functioning kidney (Noe et al., 1984).

Management of reflux associated with the neurogenic bladder usually requires that a plan of definitive bladder management be established first. In the older child, this can involve clean intermittent catheterization with the appropriate pharmacologic manipulation and antimicrobial prophylaxis. In many cases, successful management of the bladder dysfunction will allow stabilization of the patient's condition and even lead to cessation of the reflux. In the neonate or infant, definitive bladder management may not be possible; in such cases, cutaneous vesicostomy has provided a temporary solution (Allen, 1980; Duckett, 1974). Closure of the vesicostomy with management of the bladder by clean intermittent catheterization and pharmacologic means can then be attempted before a final decision is required regarding the reflux. Even the higher grades of reflux have been observed to cease

in the neuropathic bladder after a period of vesicostomy drainage and with appropriate postvesicostomy bladder management (Noe and Jerkins, 1985). When required, ureteral reimplantation can be performed successfully in the presence of a neurogenic bladder. The success rate of ureteral reimplantation has reached a level where it now plays an important role in the management of this situation (Bauer et al., 1982; Jeffs et al., 1976; Woodard et al., 1981). A cross-trigonal procedure is preferred because the trigone is usually less trabeculated and the chance of postoperative obstruction is minimized in these thickened, abnormal bladders (Kaplan and Firlit, 1983). The improvement in the surgical management of even the refluxing megaureter in the neurogenic bladder makes it desirable, certainly in lieu of urinary diversion.

In the nonneurogenic neurogenic bladder or dysfunctional voider with severe reflux, appropriate bladder or sphincter management should precede any attempts at surgical correction to allow an optimum chance of surgical success. In the limited number of situations where severe reflux and cyclophosphamide or radiation cystitis coexist, attempts at ureteral reimplantation have not been successful. In this situation, augmentation cystoplasty has been used successfully and would seem to be a reasonable and attractive alternative to surface diversion (Noe and McSwain, 1983).

Primary and Secondary Reflux with Accompanying Obstruction

One criticism of the international classification is that it provides no separate category for those patients in whom reflux and obstruction exist in the same ure-

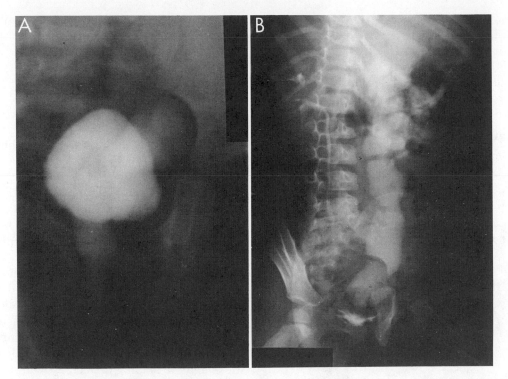

FIG. 47-8
A, Reflux into only the lower portion of a megaureter. **B,** Delayed intravenous pyelography film showing an obstructive element in addition to reflux.

ter. Although this is a small percentage of the total number of patients who will exhibit reflux, it is more likely to occur with the refluxing megaureter. This finding is of practical clinical importance in that ureters with both reflux and obstruction have been shown to be resistant to any form of treatment other than surgical correction (Weiss and Lytton, 1974). The obstructive component is thought to be more destructive; thus, surgery seems to be indicated in these situations.

Ureters with reflux and obstruction seem best classified as either primary or secondary refluxing megaureters since that is what most logically occurs initially. Subsequent obstruction results from ureteral wall fibrosis with muscle bundle disruption or fibrosis with fixed ureteral kinking as tortuosity develops. I have noted a particular association of this reflux-obstruction complex associated with paraureteral diverticula. This has been observed in both primary refluxing megaureters and in secondary refluxing megaureters associated with urethral valves. In fact, reflux may be low grade or may have ceased altogether in the older patient, resulting in a finding of a paraureteral diverticulum and altered ureteral orifice associated with ureteral fibrosis and fixation at the time of exploration and surgical correction of what was thought to be primary obstruction. In these cases, one can only infer that reflux began the disease process and, as the patient aged, the reflux ceased, leaving

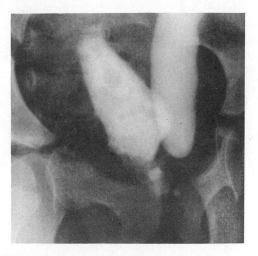

FIG. 47-9
Refluxing megaureter associated with secondary obstruction. (Note rounded appearance of the lower ureter characteristic of this finding on postvoiding film.)

the devastating effects of obstruction behind.

The possibility of this entity of reflux and obstruction must be kept in mind by both the urologist and the radiologist during the evaluation of the wide ureter. At the time of the voiding cystogram, reflux may not be demonstrated until the patient voids or it may extend only into a dilated, tortuous lower ureter (Fig. 47-8). Postvoiding films are important to obtain because they may show the rounded appearance of the distal obstructed ureter with a space between this point and the bladder. This space usually represents the fibrosed or stenotic segment of the distal ureter (Fig. 47-9). Other films may show a paraureteral diverticulum with reflux and poor drainage on delayed films. Diuretic renography or the Whitaker test may be necessary to define obstruction in selected patients.

OBSTRUCTIVE MEGAURETER
Primary

Primary obstructive megaureter refers to an intrinsic form of obstruction at or above the ureterovesical

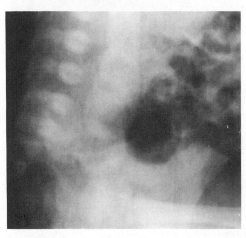

FIG. 47-10
Midureteral stricture in a solitary kidney discovered in a prenatal ultrasound. Lateral, delayed film during intravenous pyelography.

junction. Causes include ureteral stenosis or stricture, valves, atresia, ectopic ureteral orifice, and, perhaps best known, the distal adynamic segment.

Congenital Ureteral Strictures

Congenital ureteral strictures or stenosis can occur throughout the length of the ureter. They occur primarily at the distal ureterovesical junction but are seen occasionally in the midureter in the region of the pelvic brim (Figs. 47-10 and 47-11). Ureteral stricture at the ureteropelvic junction is discussed elsewhere in the text. A ureteral stricture or stenotic area should, by definition, be an anatomic narrowing that is defined by calibration. Such areas have been shown histologically to contain normal transitional epithelium with sparse muscle and a relative increase in collagenous tissue. These strictures primarily are thought to occur as a result of faulty muscularization during the development of the ureter at approximately the eleventh or twelfth week of embryogenesis. Vascular compression during a critical phase of development is thought to be responsible for this disturbed development of mesenchyme leading to decreased ureteral muscularization (Allen, 1970).

Ureteral Valves

Ureteal valves, like ureteral strictures, are rare. A true ureteral valve consists of a transverse fold of ureteral mucosa containing smooth muscle fibers above which are obstructive changes (Fig. 47-12). These are

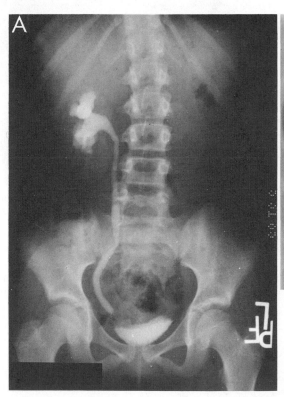

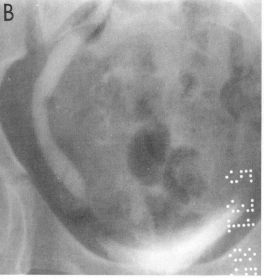

FIG. 47-11
A and **B,** Congenital distal ureteral stricture in child with solitary kidney. Child presented with flank pain and hematuria.

annular valves that may occur in either the upper or the lower ureter.

In the upper ureter, multiple transverse folds occur during normal fetal development (Ostling, 1942). These folds normally disappear with growth, but many believe that it is their persistence that is the source of valvular obstruction in the upper ureter (Albertson and Talner, 1972). Valvular obstruction in the lower ureter has been suggested to be secondary to persistance of Chwalla's membrane, but that theory will not account for the valves seen in the upper ureter.

Treatment of distinct ureteral valves will vary with the location. In the upper ureter, ureteropyelostomy or ureteroureterostomy can be used with excision of the valve and reimplantation being employed in the lower-most portion of the ureter.

In addition to the annular valves described above, eccentric cusplike valves also have been described as possibly obstructive, particularly in the lower ureter (Cussen, 1971). These cusplike folds are located at the junction of the proximal dilated ureter and the normal caliber distal ureter. Whether they are the primary source of obstruction or simply the result of a more distal obstruction is still unclear. A similar form of obstruction attributed to a tilt valve mechanism also has been described (Fowler and Kesavan, 1977). This tilt valve occurs where the proximal dilated ureter joins a normal caliber juxtavesical ureteral segment. The distal ureteral lumen meets the proximal dilated ureter in an eccentric fashion. That portion of the wall of the proximal ureteral segment that overlaps the distal ureteral segment, including the lip of the eccentric distal lumen, acts as a flap and causes obstruction according to this concept. Once again, whether this is a primary process or is a change secondary to more distal obstruction is, as yet, unclear. If indeed such a tilt valve mechanism exists, simple correction of the valvular obstruction could be performed and more extensive ureteral resection and reimplantation could be avoided. This would be especially attractive in such high-risk patients as children with posterior urethral valves and residual ureteral obstruction.

Ectopic Ureter

Ectopic ureters may prove to be destructive. This is especially seen in the case of the ectopic ureter at the bladder neck in which compression of the ureteral orifice by the bladder neck musculature acts to be obstructive (Fig. 47-13). Intrinsic abnormalities of the distal ectopic ureter also may contribute to the obstruction.

Distal Adynamic Segment

The distal adynamic segment is perhaps the best known of the causes of primary obstructed megaureter. This segment consists of the terminal 3 to 4 cm of ureter that does not conduct a peristaltic wave and thus fails to allow passage of a bolus of urine through this portion of the ureter (Fig. 47-14). This terminal ureteral segment is of adequate caliber anatomically

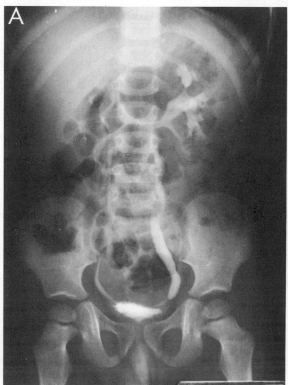
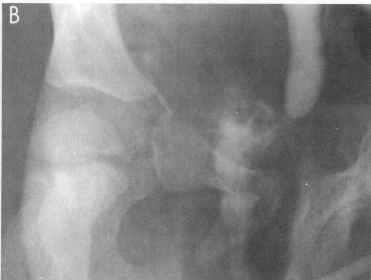

FIG. 47-12

A and **B,** Annular valve of distal ureter. (From Noe HN, Scaljon W: Case profile: ureteral valves. *Urology* 1979; 14:411. Used by permission.)

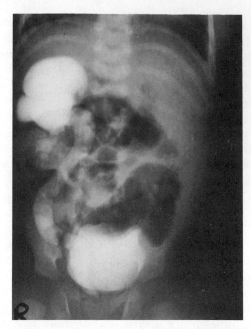

FIG. 47-13
Obstructive megaureter attributable to ectopic bladder neck insertion of upper pole ureter.

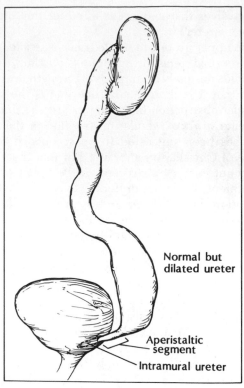

Normal but dilated ureter

Aperistaltic segment

Intramural ureter

FIG. 47-14
Distal adynamic segment as found in primary obstructive megaureter.

and can be readily catheterized using the appropriate sized ureteral catheter. Thus, the obstruction is functional rather than anatomic. Dilation appears proximal to this distal obstructive segment.

Caulk's (1923) original description likened this form of primary obstructed megaureter to Hirschsprung's disease. Although others attempted to further this concept, no neurologic deficit or absence of parasympathetic ganglia analogous to Hirschsprung's has ever been demonstrated. Several histologic studies, however, have been successful in demonstrating abnormalities in this distal adynamic segment. Increased collagenous tissue in the distal segment has been described (Gregoir and Debled, 1969). Others have described an area in this distal segment that is devoid of musculature (MacKinnon et al., 1969). Others have described predominantly circular muscle in this area (Murnaghan, 1957; Tanagho et al., 1970). Since the ureter is basically a smooth muscle meshwork of opposing helices, many have thought that the predominant circular pattern represents an exceptional tight helix formation at the distal end of the ureter, which has the same effect as a circular muscle. McLaughlin and colleagues (1973) reported histologic studies on light microscopy of 32 such ureters. In their study, 5 ureters were normal, 2 showed primarily circular muscle, and 3 showed mural fibrosis with essentially absent muscle. The largest single category in this study included 22 ureters that showed muscular hypoplasia or atrophy of widely separated muscle bundles interspersed with fibrosis (Fig. 47-15).

Electron microscopic studies of these ureters also have been performed (Hanna et al., 1976; Notley, 1972; Pagano and Passerini, 1977; Tokunaka et al., 1982). These early studies predominantly showed that collagenous tissue was observed in increased amounts between the muscle cells. It was thought that this would possibly alter the normal cell-to-cell contacts (intermediate junctions) thus disrupting electrical impulse propagation and peristalsis. More recently, quantitative histologic analysis of these dilated ureters has been performed (Lee et al., 1992). A color image analysis system was used to examine and compare collagen and smooth muscle components of the muscularis layers to more normal control ureters, primary obstructed megaureters, and primary refluxing megaureters. In patients with primary refluxing megaureters, there was a twofold increase in the tissue matrix ratio of collagen to smooth muscle when compared to patients with primary obstructed megaureter. In those with primary obstructed megaureters, the amount of collagen was increased but did not appear to be statistically different from the control ureters. These differences in the structural components (collagen and smooth muscle) may account for the difference in surgical outcomes as will be discussed later. Also, these histologic differences have been suggested to be a function of time. In an experimental study

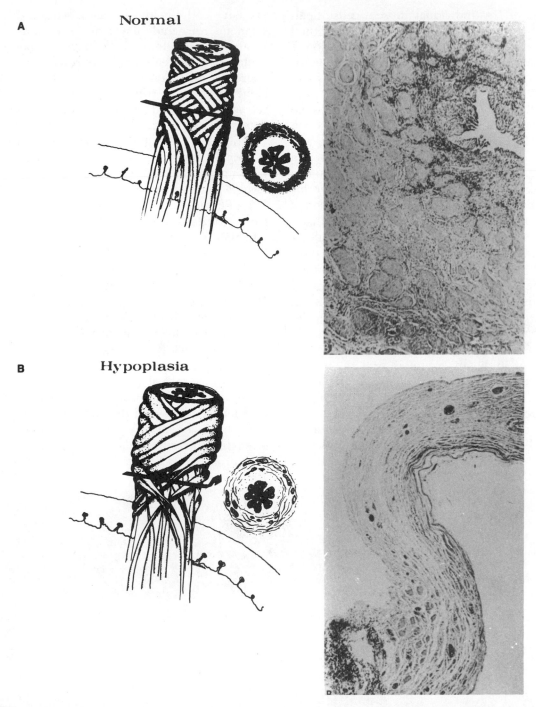

A Normal

B Hypoplasia

FIG. 47-15
Histopathologic findings in primary obstructed megaureter. **A,** Normal ureteral muscular orientation found in five ureters in McLaughlin's series. **B,** The most common abnormal finding of hypoplasia and atrophy of ureteral muscle seen in 22 patients in the McLaughlin series. (From McLaughlin AP III, Pfister RC, Leadbetter WF, et al: The pathophysiology of primary megaloureter *J Urol* 1973; 109:805. Used by permission.)

performed by Harada and associates (1992), 35 mongrel dogs in whom ureteral compliance and its relationship to histologic changes were studied over a period of 26 weeks following the establishment of partial ureteral obstruction demonstrated the initial response to be muscle hypertrophy with increased compliance up to 8 weeks following obstruction. Thereafter, the compliance significantly diminished and was proportional to the amount of connective tissue proliferation. Although most of these aforementioned studies have mentioned alteration in the collagen/smooth muscle ratio, to date no specific or consistent intracellular abnormalities of the individual muscle cells themselves have been shown in any of the ultrastructural studies. The distal thickened ureteral sheath also has been suggested as being partially obstructive and usually associated with bladder distention (Tokunaka and Koyanagi, 1982).

All of the above studies seem to point clearly to the fact that the predominant mechanism of obstruction of the ureter is disruption of muscular continuity and the prevention of proper muscular propulsion of a bolus of urine. Whether this can be blamed on a single anatomic finding or group of findings and whether this is at a gross or cellular level remain to be clarified.

Embryologically, the explanation of the distal adynamic segment is thought to rest with abnormal development involving the distal ureteral musculature. Tanagho (1973) noted that the distal ureteral musculature was the last to develop and, in particular, noted that the earliest development occurred primarily in muscle with circular orientation. Arrest later in development, such as by vascular pressure in the female or by the vas deferens in the male, could lead to diminished longitudinally oriented ureteral muscle and could result in the histologic changes noted (Tanagho, 1976).

The degree of ureteral dilatation proximal to the obstructing segment is variable. In many instances, only terminal ureterectasis is seen. In other instances, dilatation of both the renal pelvis and calyces also is present. As the bolus of urine reaches the obstructed segment, retrograde flow from that point leads to increased urine volume in the terminal portion of the ureter. This increased volume results in the variable degree of dilatation seen in the affected ureter. The ability of the upper ureter and pelvis to dampen this retrograde flow and maintain antegrade emptying will determine the effect, if any, on the renal parenchyma.

Clinically, presentation of patients with this entity is variable but is usually due to the symptoms accompanying urinary tract infection (Flatmark et al., 1970; Pagano and Passerini, 1977; Pfister and Hendren, 1978; Pfister et al., 1971; Rabinowitz et al., 1979; Williams and Hulme-Moir, 1970). In some instances, the infection is clearly related to the affected renal unit, but in others cystitis symptoms also may be present. With the latter, no relation to the ureteral anomaly is obvious and megaureter may be an incidental finding. Hematuria, abdominal pain, or abdominal mass also may be methods of presentation. Discovery also may be incidental during investigation for urinary incontinence or medical investigation for a nonurologic disorder. The signs and symptoms of renal failure are, fortunately, unusual modes of presentation in this disorder. The lesion appears to affect males more often than females except in the first year of life when they are roughly equal. The left ureter is affected more often than the right, and there is bilateral involvement in approximately 25% of the cases. Younger children

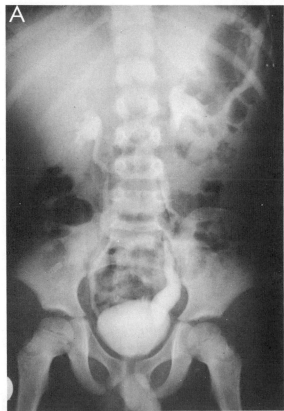
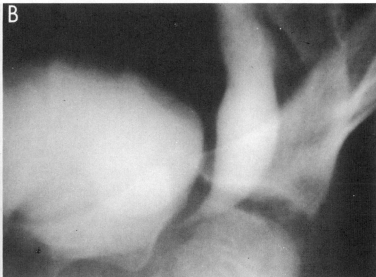

FIG. 47-16
Primary obstructed megaureter attributable to distal adynamic segment. **A,** Intravenous pyelogram showing terminal ureterectasis only, with otherwise normal renal unit. **B,** Oblique view of lower ureter showing area of distal adynamic segment.

(under 1 year of age) are more likely to have bilateral megaureters than are older patients. Contralateral renal agenesis occurs in approximately 10% of the cases. No hereditary basis is currently recognized for this entity.

Excretory urography or renal ultrasound is the means by which the diagnosis of primary obstructive megaureter secondary to the distal adynamic segment is made. Since the narrow distal obstructive segment is close to the bladder, oblique and postvoiding films may be helpful in visualizing this area (Figs. 47-16 and 47-17). Videofluoroscopic studies usually demonstrate active ureteral peristalsis down to the distal adynamic segment where the urine bolus then floods back up the ureter for a variable distance (Fig. 47-18). Upper ureteral or renal pelvic dilatation may or may not be present. The diuretic renogram or pressure perfusion studies can be useful in selected cases where the decision for treatment is unclear. Endoscopy performed at the time of surgery usually demonstrates a normal ureteral orifice and trigone. Retrograde ureteral catheterization is performed with ease, and a "hydronephrotic drip" can be noted in cases where significant obstruction is present. A retrograde ureterogram can confirm the diagnosis demonstrating poor emptying of the ureter, but this procedure usually is not required. If instrumentation is performed, it should be performed at the time of anticipated surgical correction to avoid introducing infection into a static system.

Treatment of these patients is dependent on the severity of the obstruction and the presence of symptoms. Those with only terminal ureterectasis and otherwise normal upper urinary tracts can be safely observed and usually do not progress. Surgical correction should be reserved for those with progressive or generalized hydronephrosis, parenchymal loss, cal-

culus disease, or persistent flank pain in patients with proven significant obstruction. Persistent or recurrent infections, particularly those that can be related to or lateralized to the affected renal unit, also form an indication for surgical treatment.

Secondary Obstructive Megaureter

Secondary obstructive megaureter occurs as a result of urethral obstruction, neurogenic vesical dysfunction, ureterocele, extrinsic compression, or fibrosis.

Urethral Valves

Urethral valves are the most commonly seen form of urethral obstruction leading to secondary obstructive megaureter. They can be due to a hypertonic detrusor muscle, ureteral fibrosis, or fibrosis and kinking associated with a paraureteral diverticulum. It should be remembered that ureteral dilatation can remain following valve ablation but not be associated with true obstruction. Marked improvement can occur in ureteral dilatation and tortuosity in a relatively short time following valve ablation (Fig. 47-19). In others, the diagnosis is less clear. In these latter instances, residual dilatation must be evaluated further to determine if true obstruction exists. The diuretic renogram is usually the first study obtained, and if it demonstrates a dilated but nonobstructed pattern, the patient may be observed. Serial studies, including renal function evaluation, are often helpful to confirm efficacy of a nonoperative approach. It should be remembered, as discussed earlier, that the state of hy-

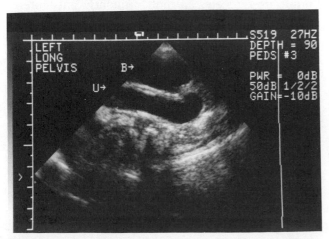

FIG. 47-17
Longitudinal ultrasound of an obstructed megaureter. Real-time image showed ureter clearly obstructed just at the ureterovesical junction. *B*-bladder; *U*-ureter.

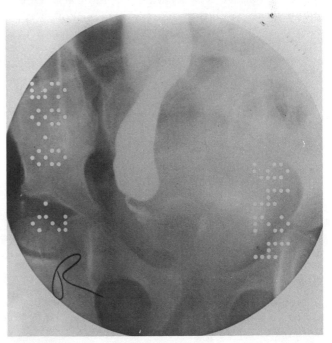

FIG. 47-18
Distal ureteral obstruction demonstrated on antegrade ureterogram at the time of percutaneous nephrostomy.

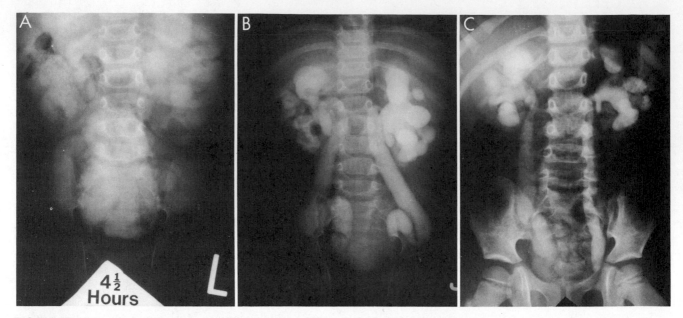

FIG. 47-19
A, Resolution of ureterectasis and hydronephrosis following valve ablation. Ureterectasis was present at diagnosis. **B,** Resolution of ureterectasis and hydronephrosis following valve ablation. Improvement was noted 12 months after valve ablation. **C,** Resolution of ureterectasis and hydronephrosis following valve ablation. There was further improvement 2½ years later.

dration, the level of renal function, the volume of the collecting system and, particularly, the degree of bladder fullness can influence the test results of the diuretic renogram. If the diuretic renogram is equivocal, the Whitaker test may be used. High relative renal pressures with the bladder empty indicate a significant amount of ureteral obstruction at the ureterovesical junction, and surgical treatment is indicated. One of the major difficulties in interpreting the Whitaker test in patients with urethral valves has been the effect of the degree of bladder filling on relative renal pressures (Glassberg et al., 1982). If pressures are low with the bladder empty but become rapidly abnormally elevated with bladder filling, the patient is potentially at risk for progressive renal damage. This pressure elevation is on the basis of the noncompliant bladder rather than on strictly what could be interpreted as an obstruction at the ureterovesical junction. In these cases, augmentation of the noncompliant bladder seems to be more appropriate than simply performing ureteral reimplantation into an abnormal lower urinary system. Diuretic renography or pressure perfusion studies usually are required to make this evaluation with accuracy.

Neurogenic Bladder

Neurogenic vesical dysfunction can result in obstructive megaureter. Management of the bladder by vesicostomy, clean intermittent catheterization, or pharmacologic manipulation usually results in resolution of the hydronephrosis without the need for di-

version. Once again, augmentation is sometimes required for the noncompliant bladder.

Successful ureteral reimplantation can be undertaken in the neurogenic bladder, as mentioned earlier. It is important to have the bladder stabilized in terms of function and emptying capabilities before attempting reimplantation.

Ureterocele

Obstructed megaureter can be secondary to ureterocele. Ureteroceles can involve the ipsilateral ureter or, in some cases, also be secondary to a contralateral ureter causing an element of obstruction. Simple ureteroceles are not frequently encountered in children but have been noted to occur. Ectopic ureteroceles tend to be more spectacular in their clinical appearance. Four major types of ectopic ureteroceles have been described (Stephens, 1971) and are discussed in greater detail elsewhere in the text. Although ureteroceles are included here as a secondary form of obstructive megaureter, it is obvious that ureteroceles potentially fall under several other categories in the classification scheme.

Mass: Vascular Compression

Extensive compression occurs with retroperitoneal masses or tumors (Fig. 47-20). Treatment usually consists of management of the primary condition with observation for resolution of the ureterectasis. Persistent ureterectasis following successful tumor treatment may require that additional studies be per-

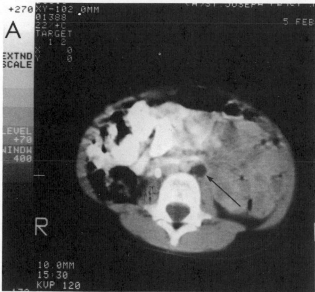

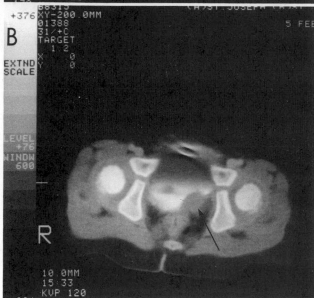

FIG. 47-20

A, Secondary obstructed megaureter due to tumor. CT scan shows hydronephrosis and enlargement of left ureter *(arrow).* **B,** Tumor recurrent at bladder wall at ureterovesical junction *(arrow).*

formed to determine if true obstruction remains. Vascular compression can occur as a result of aberrant or accessory vessels. In these instances, treatment is influenced by the vessel involved and the degree and location of the obstruction.

Fibrosis: Iatrogenic Causes

Fibrosis can result in ureteral obstruction and can be due to trauma associated with diverticula but is most often the result of prior surgery, that is, ureteral reimplantation. The assessment of postoperative residual ureteral dilatation following reimplantation can

be as challenging as in the similar situation involving posterior urethral valve patients. Once again, the diuretic renogram or pressure perfusion study is utilized when the diagnosis is unclear. As with valves, bladder compliance must be evaluated to ensure that accurate conclusions serve as a basis for treatment.

Occasionally, an unusual form of transient ureteral obstruction occurs following ureteral reimplantation. This is usually observed following surgery on the megaureter but also can be observed on ureters with less severe dilatation. Although anatomically the distal ureter is open and can be catheterized, a very high grade, if not almost complete, obstruction is observed postoperatively. This obstruction seems to be related more to ureteral dysfunction and altered peristalsis. A period of temporary drainage by either ureterostomy or short-term nephrostomy usually allows a return of ureteral function and resolution of the abnormality. Once ureteral function has been demonstrated to recover, simple undiversion or tube removal is all that is required to allow proper return of function of the urinary system.

NONREFLUXING, NONOBSTRUCTED MEGAURETER
Primary

The cause of isolated primary nonrefluxing and nonobstructed megaureter is not known. It could represent an intrinsic abnormality of ureteral development or perhaps a resolved obstruction leaving residual ureterectasis. The entire ureter is usually dilated from the bladder proximally. The degree of dilatation and the presence of caliectasis is variable. The distal ureter is not stenotic, nor is the remaining ureter especially tortuous. The diagnosis of a ureter in this category is, by definition, one of exclusion. In the absence of infection and with stable renal function, it seems safe to observe these patients. A case representative of this entity is shown in Figure 47-21.

In some cases, the prune belly syndrome can be considered in this category. Ureteral dilatation in the prune belly syndrome is secondary to abnormal ureteral muscular development, and the radiographic picture represents a degree of dysmorphism. It should be kept in mind that ureteral dilatation in the prune belly syndrome also may be demonstrated to be secondary to either obstruction or reflux. This entity is discussed in Chapter 49.

The concept of a dilated but nonobstructed urinary system has been brought keenly to the forefront with the advent and widespread use of fetal and maternal ultrasound. It has been shown, in many cases, that spontaneous resolution of mild intrauterine and postnatal urinary tract dilatation does occur (Grignon et al., 1986; Homsy et al., 1985; Johnson et al., 1987).

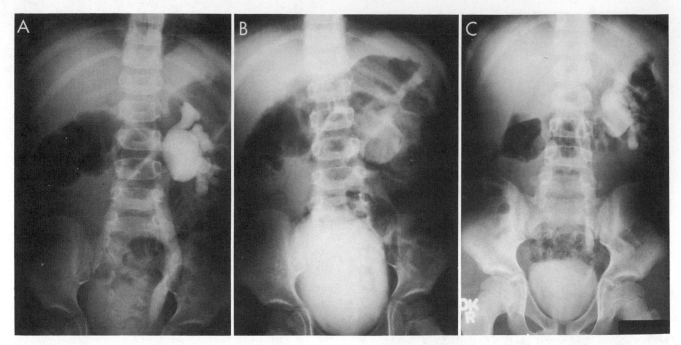

FIG. 47-21
A, Nonobstructive, nonrefluxing megaureter. Intravenous pyelogram (IVP) of solitary kidney with ureteral dilatation discovered on evaluation for hypospadias. **B,** Prompt washout shown 10 minutes after administration of furosemide. **C,** IVP 5 years later showing adequate renal growth without progression of hydronephrosis. Follow-up diuretic renograms have shown the system to be nonobstructed, and the creatinine clearance has remained stable.

The concept of a spontaneous resolution or improvement has been extended to a group of neonates discovered prenatally with megaureter that have been followed and evaluated (Vidal et al., 1988). Keating and co-authors (1989) have recently reported a large number of patients with megaureter discovered prenatally or serendipitously and who were followed without surgery. In that experience, 17 infants with 23 renal units were evaluated and followed without surgical intervention. Sixteen of these renal units were graded as moderate to severe, and the decision to manage them conservatively was made on the basis of renal function and the measurement of the extraction factor (Heyman and Duckett, 1988). Of the children followed, an improvement in the dilatation or sequential urograms in 15 of the megaureters occurred and none showed deterioration of function on renal scan. While at first this might seem to go against the advice of those advocating early surgical correction of obstruction (King et al., 1984; Mayor et al., 1975), it would seem on reflection that the real dilemma is in truly defining obstruction in the neonate or infant. There are numerous problems with precisely defining obstruction in this patient group, including the concept of renal functional maturity, which proceeds within the first few months of life (Koff, 1988). Thus, it would seem that when an asymptomatic mildly to modestly dilated system is discovered either serendipitously or through prenatal ultrasound that early

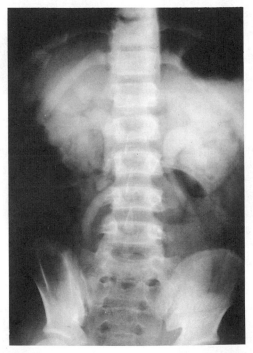

FIG. 47-22
Ureteral dilatation secondary to high urinary output in patient with diabetes insipidus.

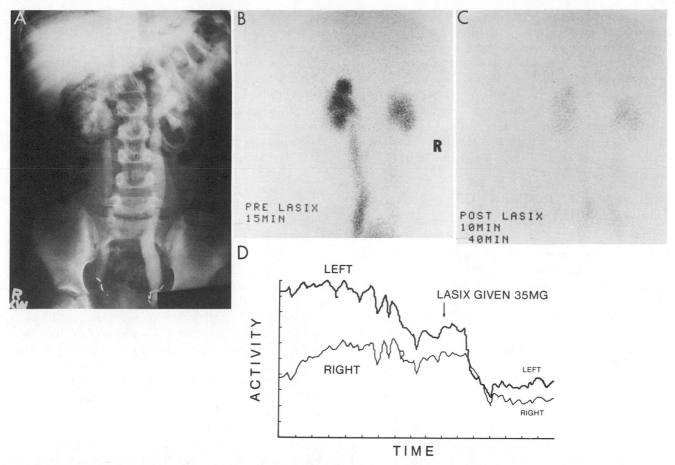

FIG. 47-23
A, Residual dilatation following ureteral reimplantation. Intravenous pyelogram shows ureteral dilatation postoperatively. **B,** Renal scan images before furosemide (Lasix) administration. **C,** Renal scan images showing prompt washout 10 minutes after furosemide administration. **D,** Renogram curves corresponding to images of the scan.

diagnostic studies attempting to define the degree of obstruction should be obtained. There appears to be no ill effect to at least a modest delay in reconstructive surgery in these children while waiting for renal function to mature (Dejter et al., 1988). If renal function is maintained and only mild to modest or improving obstruction is found, then careful but frequent followup can be offered as an alternative to surgical correction. It should be noted, however, that when significant obstruction, particularly with renal functional compromise, is present, it is still felt that early surgical correction to preserve renal function and prevent new insults is indicated. Whether the antenatally discovered megaureter that is asymptomatic turns out to be a different entity than those discovered in the past because of symptomatic infections, stones, abdominal pain, mass, etc., remains to be seen. It has been hypothesized that the fetal and neonatal ureter is more compliant with increased urinary output and that perhaps many of these children were simply unnoticed in the past because of their lack of symptoms. Only careful follow-up of such a series of patients

such as those reported can shed new light on this problem.

Secondary

Ureteral dilatation also can occur secondary to high urine flow and volume as in diabetes insipidus or in the compulsive water drinker (Fig. 47-22). Bacterial toxins also can affect ureteral muscular action leading to dilatation and diminished peristalsis.

Other conditions included in this classification are the residual dilatation following relief of the distal obstruction as in the patient with posterior urethral valves. Residual dilatation following ureteral reimplantation also may be categorized in this designation (Fig. 47-23). As mentioned earlier, the classification of the megaureter can be a dynamic process in that successful treatment of a primary condition can lead to residual changes that are no longer of clinical or surgical importance. Such seems to be the case in the remaining wide ureter after relief of distal obstruction or following certain instances of ureteral reimplantation. A word of caution for patients in this category is in order in that these patients should definitely be followed over a long term to ensure that no late renal deterioration or increase in hydronephrosis occurs.

Urinary tract infection as a result of urinary stasis is occasionally seen in patients in this category. If this is true, this can serve as an indication for surgical treatment. If ureteral muscular failure is suspected or peristalsis is absent, surgical remodeling of the ureter may be of no benefit. In these selected instances, replacement of the ureter with ileum or use of the ileal sleeve may be warranted.

SURGICAL MANAGEMENT OF THE MEGAURETER

Surgery to correct megaureter is directed at either the correction of reflux or the removal of obstruction. Indications for surgical treatment have been discussed previously in the individual categories, but, in general, with the obstructed megaureter, the indications are progressive hydronephrosis, parenchymal loss, or proven obstruction in those with lesser degrees of dilatation. Certainly, recurrent infections in the case of proven obstruction serve as an indication for surgery, but in the nonobstructed, nonrefluxing megaureter in which urinary stasis is leading to infection, surgery also might be appropriate. For those megaureters associated with reflux, surgery usually is indicated because of a fixed orifice abnormality or inability to control infections with or without renal parenchymal damage. Surgical treatment has become more and more sophisticated with current state-of-the-art ureteral reimplantation for megaureter becoming successful. This was not always the case, however, and the treatment of megaureter evolved from less successful approaches.

Caulk's (1923) treatment of his original case consisted of endoscopic ureteral meatotomy. It is not certain whether this was an obstructed or nonobstructed megaureter, but his results appeared to be good. Others tried similar surgical approaches with very poor results. Finally, in 1954, Nesbit and Withycombe concluded that megaureters should not be treated surgically.

Attempts in the treatment of megaureter then turned to methods to replace the ureter with small bowel. Several authors advanced techniques in this regard and good results were achieved, especially when using a nipple valve or intussusception technique to prevent reflux (Lewis and Cletsoway, 1956; Goodwin et al., 1959; Swenson et al., 1956). Others reported wrapping the entire dilated ureter either in denuded ileum or in the ileal wall in an effort to improve emptying (Grana and Swenson, 1965; Hirschhorn, 1964). Even though good long-term results were obtained, attention was still directed at surgery of the ureter itself.

In 1967, Creevy reported extensive ureteral tailoring with ureteral reimplantation. Also in 1967, Johnston reported surgical correction of megaureter and concluded that surgical treatment was, at that time, both practical and the indicated form of therapy. Hendren reported his positive results in 1969. In 1972, Bischoff first advocated tapering only the lowermost portions of the ureter at the time of ureteral reimplantation, and the results appeared satisfactory. Thus, the standard form of surgical therapy, that is, tailoring and reimplanting the lowermost portion of the megaureter, has evolved to its current state. This is now generally agreed to be the optimum initial approach. Usually the upper ureter improves and straightens with time and growth, and no further surgery is required. Upper ureteral tailoring and remodeling is done only when progressive obstruction remains and continued deterioration of the upper tract is observed following successful lower ureteral repair.

Although ureteral tailoring and reimplantation is now an accepted treatment when surgery is indicated for the megaureter, it has been noted previously that the surgical results can differ depending upon whether the etiology is obstructive or refluxing (Lee et al., 1992). Histologic differences shown in that study and others have consistently demonstrated an increased amount of collagen in the matrix of these ureters and an altered collagen/smooth muscle ratio, which probably affects function and effective peristalsis postoperatively. Although it may be anticipated that surgical results in severely refluxing megaureters are not as good as those obtained with obstructive megaureters, further study will be required to see if any different approach will improve the ultimate outcome.

The rationale for tailoring of the ureter relates to the basic pathophysiology of the inability of the ureteral walls to coapt and propel a bolus of urine. The dimensional changes on urine transport are best understood from the Laplace equation which describes the interrelationship of the variables that affect intraluminal pressure. The equation is as follows: pressure = tension × wall thickness/radius. By lowering the radius of the ureter with tailoring, the results would be an increase in intraluminal pressure and more efficient propulsion of urine through the system. To achieve this effect, two major technical procedures are used.

Surgical Techniques

As stated above, the lower ureter is the segment operated on first, planning to observe what, if anything, will be necessary for the upper ureter. Excisional tailoring has been considered the standard form of therapy for the past 10 to 15 years. The technique is represented in Figure 47-24. A transverse suprapubic incision is made, the bladder opened, and the

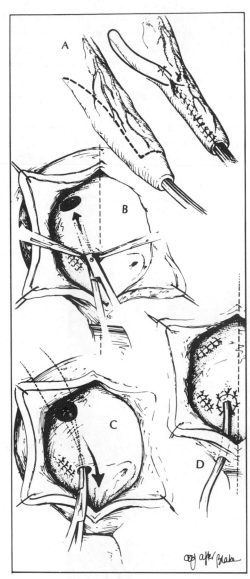

FIG. 47-24
Excisional tailoring and reimplantation of megaureter.

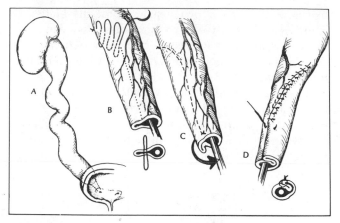

FIG. 47-25
Ureteral tailoring by the folding technique as proposed by Kalicinski.

ureter initially dissected intravesically. In reoperative cases, wider exposure may be required and a transperitoneal incision utilized. Once the ureter has been dissected free and drawn several centimeters into the bladder, it is then passed outside the bladder where dissection continues. The ureter is straightened as far as the blood supply allows. It is helpful to divide the obliterated hypogastric artery and sweep the peritoneum medially off the ureter. Gentle handling of the ureter with preservation of the ureteral blood supply on its medial aspect is essential to success. Any obstructive segment is ressected and the ureter shortened but not so as to produce tension on the reimplantation site. In the excisional technique, a portion of the lateral ureteral wall in the remaining distal 5 cm is then excised. This excision is opposite the vessels that course medially and longitudinally along the ureteral surface. Enough ureter is excised comfortably to narrow and tailor the ureter to approximately 12 F caliber. In addition to improving the efficiency of urine transport, narrowing the ureter allows one to more easily attain the desired ureteral tunnel length ratio in regard to ureteral width. If, for some reason, it is necessary to tailor a longer length of ureter, windows can be made in the ureteral adventitia and excision carried from window to window, thus better preserving the blood supply (Hanna, 1982). The ureteral closure is then performed in a watertight fashion in two layers using running 5-0 and 6-0 absorbable suture. Distal ureteral closure is by interrupted sutures to allow shortening of the ureter at the time of reimplantation should that be required. An adequate neohiatus is developed superiorly and medially to prevent angulation and narrowing and obstruction. If the tunnel is not placed in a superior and medial position, it can be brought through the original hiatus in a cross-trigone fashion (Ahmed, 1980). The latter has the theoretical advantage, at least, of being less likely to obstruct, particularly with bladder distention. A 4-cm tunnel is then constructed and the ureter reimplanted with the suture line rotated to face the detrusor muscle. Stenting catheters are left for 7 to 10 days and then removed one at a time, if bilateral ureteral surgery is performed. An excretory urogram or renal ultrasound is obtained at 4 weeks and repeated as needed if dilatation persists. A voiding cystogram is obtained in 6 months. A renal scan can be done in long-term follow-up, if renal changes or functional abnormalities are suspected.

Complications following this form of reimplantation are primarily either persistence of reflux or postoperative obstruction. Persistence of reflux can be caused by technical problems resulting in a shortened tunnel or a ureterovesical fistula. Obstruction can be due to ureteral angulation, ischemic atrophy, and fibrosis of the ureter or constriction at the hiatus. In some cases, extensive perivesical dissection can result in neurogenic vesicle dysfunction. As mentioned earlier, obstruction as a result of temporary ureteral dysfunction with altered peristalsis occurs in a few cases. Such temporary ureteral dysfunction or dysmotility is best managed by temporary diversion allowing resolution of the acute problem. With return of peristalsis, follow-up studies usually demonstrate no anatomic obstruction and simple undiversion is all that is required.

An alternative to excisional tailoring has been developed. Kalicinski and associates (1977) introduced a method of reducing the ureteral lumen by tailoring and folding the ureter, which still permits proper ureteral caliber reduction and reimplantation. Starr (1979) also reported a similar plication technique. The procedure as advocated by Kalicinski consists of excluding the excess ureteral lumen laterally with a running horizontal mattress suture of 4-0 or 5-0 absorbable suture. This lateral portion is then folded over

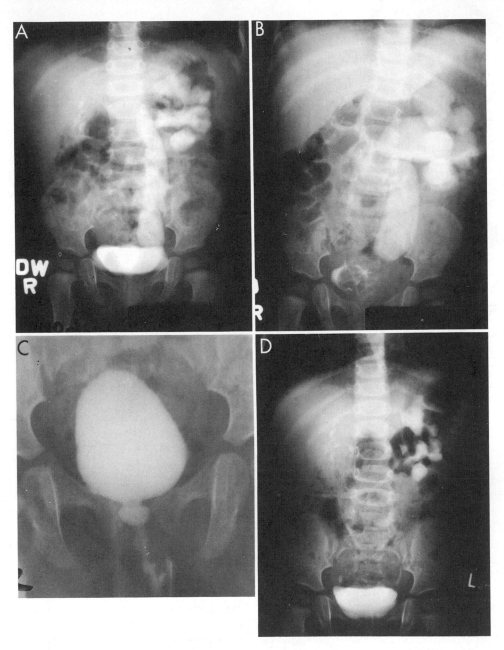

FIG. 47-26
A, Results of the ureteral folding technique in an infant. Intravenous pyelogram (IVP) shows ureteral dilatation, which proved to be an obstructive megaureter. **B,** Postoperative IVP at 1 week. Note large amount of edema and displacement of Foley catheter bulb to the right. Kidney functioned promptly and patient did well clinically. **C,** Postoperative voiding cystogram showing absence of reflux. **D,** Follow-up IVP 6 months after surgery. Marked reduction of ureteral caliber and improvement of left collecting system are seen. Ureteral bulk resolved without any long-term consequences.

the narrower medial portion of the ureter and secured with interrupted absorbable sutures (Fig. 47-25). The major advantages are better preservation of the ureteral blood supply, an ensured watertight ureteral closure, and the ability to remove the stenting catheters much earlier than with excisional tailoring. The last has benefits both from a patient comfort standpoint and the economic benefits of shorter hospitalization. "Modest" ureteral bulk, although initially a concern, has not proved to be a significant problem with ureteral folding (Fig. 47-26). Excess ureteral bulk can be a problem, however, especially in ureters with very poor peristaltic activity, and this must be kept in mind as experience with these new techniques grows. The ureteral folding or plication technique would seem to offer an attractive alternative to excisional tailoring also in that it might reduce the complications of ureterovesical fistula with ischemic changes or fibrosis or shortening of the tunnel (Bakker et al., 1988). Excisional tailoring also may be best applied in duplex systems with megaureter (Weinstein et al., 1988).

Although the infolding technique mentioned above has gained wide acceptance, it appears to have certain limits with extremely large and bulky ureters. A study by Parrott and colleagues (1990) compared excisional tailoring with that of the infolding technique. Although excellent results were obtained in both groups, it was suggesting that ureters larger than 1.75 cm in diameter met with a higher failure rate when attempts were made to infold these structures. Thus, it would seem that the extremely large, bulky ureter would be best served by wedge resection and perhaps would be the procedure of choice with the more dilated refluxing megaureters in an attempt to increase the success rate to that of surgery for the obstructed megaureter.

The results of ureteral tailoring have continued to improve as technical advances and experience have accumulated. Traditional excisional tailoring approaches a 90% success rate based on widespread reported experience. A large number of patients undergoing ureteral tailoring by the infolding technique have been reported, and that experience also has been favorable. Whereas both techniques have vastly improved our ability to help children with dilated ureters, excisional tailoring would still seem to be the procedure of choice for large, bulky ureters or large refluxing megaureters. It would thus seem that the ability to diagnose and properly classify the wide ureter has allowed us to select patients for surgery and also to select the proper technique for their correction. The continued thoughtful approach to the wide ureter will allow further advances to the management of this condition and enhance the lives of the children for whom we care.

REFERENCES

Ahmed S: Transverse advancement ureteral reimplantation: pull-through alternative in megaloureter. *J Urol* 1980; 123:218.

Albertson KW, Talner LB: Valves of the ureter. *Radiology* 1972; 103:91.

Allen TD: Congenital ureteral structures. *J Urol* 1970; 104:196.

Allen TD: Vesicostomy for the temporary diversion of the urine in small children. *J Urol* 1980; 123:929.

Ash JM, Kass EG, Gilday DL: Diuretic renal scans in pediatric hydronephrosis. *J Nucl Med* 1979; 20:263.

Bakker HHR, Scholtmeijer RJ, Klopper PJ: Comparison of two different tapering techniques in megaureters. *J Urol* 1988; 140:1237.

Bauer SB, Colodny AH, Retik AB: The management of vesicoureteral reflux in children with myelodysplasia. *J Urol* 1982; 128:102.

Belman AB: Megaureter: classification, etiology, and management. *Urol Clin North Am* 1974; 1:497.

Bischoff PF: Problems in treatment of vesicoureteral reflux. *J Urol* 1972; 107:133.

Caulk JR: Megalaureter: the importance of the ureterovesical valve. *J Urol* 1923: 9:315.

Creevy CD: The atonic distal ureteral segment (ureteral achalasia). *J Urol* 1967; 97:457.

Cussen LJ: Dimensions of the normal ureter in infancy and childhood. *J Invest Urol* 1967; 5:167.

Cussen LJ: The morphology of congenital dilatation of the ureter: intrinsic ureteral lesions. *Aust NZ J Surg* 1971; 41:185.

Dejter SW Jr, Gillis DF, Gibbons MD: Delayed management of neonatal hydronephrosis. *J Urol* 1988; 140:1305.

Duckett JW Jr: Cutaneous vesicostomy in childhood: the Blocksom technique. *Urol Clin North Am* 1974; 1:485.

Erhlich RM: Ureteral folding technique for megaureter surgery. *Soc Pediatr Urol Newslett* May 5, 1982.

Flatmark AL, Maurseth K, Knutrud O: Lower ureteric obstruction in children. *Br J Urol* 1970; 42:431.

Fowler R, Kesavan P: Extravesical reconstruction for ureterovesical obstruction in childhood. *J Urol* 1977; 118:1050.

Glassberg KI: Dilated ureter: classification and approach. *Urology* 1977; 9:1.

Glassberg KI, Schneider M, Haller JD, et al: Observations of persistently dilated ureter after posterior urethral valve ablation. *Urology* 1982; 20:20.

Gonzalez R, Chiou RK: The diagnosis of upper urinary tract obstruction in children: comparison of diuresis renography and pressure flow studies. *J Urol* 1985; 133:646.

Goodwin WE, Winter CC, Turner RD: Replacement of the ureter by small intestine: clinical application and results of the "ileal ureter." *J Urol* 1959; 81:406.

Grana L, Swenson O: A new surgical procedure for the treatment of aperistaltic megaloureter. *Am J Surg* 1965; 109:532.

Gregoir W, Debled B: L'etiologie du reflux congenital et du mega uretere primaire. *Urol Int* 1969; 24:119.

Grignon A, Filion R, Filiatrault D, et al: Urinary tract dilatation in utero: classification and clinical applications. *Radiology* 1986; 160:645.

Hanna MK: Recent advances and further experience with surgical techniques for one stage total remodelling of massively dilated ureter. *Urology* 1982; 19:495.

Hanna MK, Jeffs RD, Sturgess JM, et al: Ureteral structure and ultrastructure: Part II. Congenital ureteropelvic junction obstruction and primary obstructive megaureter. *J Urol* 1976; 116:725.

Harada T, Issa MM, Kigine T, et al: Ureteral compliance and histology in partial obstruction in a canine model. *J Urol* 1992; 148:1274.

Hendren WH: Operative repair of megaureter in children. *J Urol* 1969; 101:491.

Heyman S, Duckett JW: The extraction factor: an estimate of single kidney function in children during routine radionuclide renography with 99m technetium diethylene-triaminepentaacetic acid. *J Urol* 1988; 140:780.

Hirschhorn RC: The ileal sleeve: II. Surgical technique in clinical application. *J Urol* 1964; 92:120.

Homsy YL, Williot P, Danais S: Transitional neonatal hydronephrosis: fact or fantasy? *J Urol* 1985; 136:339.

Jeffs RD, Jonas P, Schillinger JF: Surgical correction of vesicoureteral reflux in children with neurogenic bladder. *J Urol* 1976; 115:449.

Johnson MJ, Gleave M, Coleman GU, et al: Neonatal renomegaly. *J Urol* 1987; 138:1023.

Johnston JH: Reconstructive surgery of mega-ureter in childhood. *Br J Urol* 1967; 39:17.

Kalicinski ZH, Kansy J, Kotarbinska B, et al: Surgery of megaureters — modification of Hendren's operation. *J Pediatr Surg* 1977; 12:183.

Kaplan WE, Firlit CF: Management of reflux in the myelodysplastic child. *J Urol* 1983; 129:1195.

Kass EJ, Majd M, Belman AB: Comparison of the diuretic renogram and pressure-perfusion study in children. *J Urol* 1985; 134:92.

Keating MA, Escala J, Snyder HM, et al: Changing concepts in the management of primary obstructive megaureter. *J Urol* 1989; 142:636.

King LR: Megalaureter: definition, diagnosis and management (editorial). *J Urol* 1980; 123:222.

King LR, Coughlin PW, Bloch EC, et al: The case for immediate pyeloplasty in the neonate with ureteropelvic junction obstruction. *J Urol* 1984; 132:725.

Koff SA: UPJ obstruction in neonates: renal scanning's role. *Dialogues Pediatr Urol* 1988; 11:10.

Koff SA, Shore RM, Hayden LJ, et al: Diuretic radionuclide localization of upper urinary tract obstruction. *J Urol* 1984; 132:513.

Koff SA, Thrall JJ: Diagnosis of obstruction in experimental hydronephrosis. *Urology* 1981; 17:570.

Koff SA, Thrall JH, Keys JW Jr: Assessment of hydroureteronephrosis in children using diuretic radionuclide urography. *J Urol* 1980; 132:531.

Lee BR, Partin AW, Epstein JI, et al: A quantitative histologic analysis of the dilated ureter of childhood. *J Urol* 1992; 148:1482.

Lewis EL, Cletsoway RW: Megaloureter. *J Urol* 1956; 75:643.

MacKinnon KJ, Foote JW, Wigglesworth FW, et al: The pathology of the adynamic distal ureteral segment. *Trans Am Assoc Genitourin Surg* 1969; 61:63.

Mayor G, Genton N, Torrado A, et al: Renal function in obstructive nephropathy: long-term effect of reconstructive surgery. *Pediatrics* 1975; 56:740.

McLaughlin AP III, Pfister RC, Leadbetter WF, et al: The pathophysiology of primary megaloureter. *J Urol* 1973; 109:805.

Murnaghan GF: Experimental investigation of the dynamics of the normal and dilated ureter. *Br J Urol* 1957; 29:403.

Nesbit RM, Withycombe JF: The problem of primary megaloureter. *J Urol* 1954; 72:162.

Noe HN: The long term results of prospective sibling reflux screening. *J Urol* 1992; 148:1739.

Noe HN, Jerkins GR: Cutaneous vesicostomy experience in infants and children. *J Urol* 1985; 134:301.

Noe HN, Jerkins GR, Spivey OS: Use of the ureter of a non-functional renal unit in pediatric urinary reconstruction. *Urology* 1984; 23:144.

Noe HN, McSwain HM: Management of severe reflux in the patient with cyclophosphamide cystitis. *J Urol* 1983; 130:769.

Noe HN, Scaljon W: Case profile: ureteral valves. *Urology* 1979; 14:411.

Noe HN, Wyatt RJ, Peeden JN et al: The transmission of vesicoureteral reflux from parent to child. *J Urol* 1992; 148:1869.

Notley RG: Electron microscopy of the primary obstructive megaureter. *J Urol* 1972; 44:229.

O'Reilly PH, Lawson RS, Shields RA, et al: Idiopathic hydronephrosis—the diuresis renogram: a new non-invasive method of assessing equivocal pelvoureteral junction obstruction. *J Urol* 1979; 121:153.

O'Reilly PH, Testa HJ, Lawson RS, et al: Diuresis renography in equivocal urinary tract obstruction. *Br J Urol* 1978; 550:76.

Ostling K: Genesis of hydronephrosis. *Acta Chir Scand (Suppl)* 1942; 72:5.

Pagano P, Passerini G: Primary obstructed megaureter. *Br J Urol* 1977; 49:469.

Parrott TS, Woodard JR, Wolpert JJ: Ureteral tailoring: a comparison of wedge resection with infolding. *J Urol* 1990; 144:328.

Pfister RC, Hendren WH: Primary megaureter in children and adults: clinical and pathophysiologic features of 150 ureters. *Urology* 1978; 12:160.

Pfister RC, McLaughlin AP III. Leadbetter WF: Radiological evaluation of primary megaloureter: the aperistaltic distal ureteral segment. *Radiology* 1971; 99:503.

Rabinowitz R, Barkin M, Schillinger JF, et al: Surgical treatment of the massively dilated primary megaureter in children. *Br J Urol* 1979; 51:19.

Starr A: Ureteral plication: a new concept in ureteral tailoring for megaureter. *Invest Urol* 1979; 17:153.

Stephens D: Caecoureterocele and concepts on the embryology and aetiology of ureteroceles. *Aust NZ J Surg* 1971; 40:239.

Stephens FD: The ABC of megaureters. In Bergsma D, Duckett JW Jr (eds): *Birth Defects, Original Article Series* vol 13. New York, Alan R Liss, 1977, pp 1-8.

Swenson O, Fisher JH, Cendron J: Megaloureter: investigation as to the cause and report on the results of newer forms of treatment. *Surgery* 1956; 40:223.

Tanagho EA: Intrauterine fetal ureteral obstruction. *J Urol* 1973; 109:196.

Tanagho EA: Embryologic basis for lower ureteral anomalies: a hypothesis. *Urology* 1976; 7:451.

Tanagho EA, Smith DR, Guthrie TH: Pathophysiology of functional obstruction. *J Urol* 1970; 104:73.

Tokunaka S, Koyanagi T: Morphologic study of primary nonreflux megaureters with particular emphasis on the role of ureteral sheath and ureteral dysplasia. *J Urol* 1982; 128:399.

Tokunaka S, Koyanagi T, Tsuji I, et al: Histopathology of the nonrefluxing megaloureter: a clue to its pathogenesis. *J Urol* 1982; 17:238.

Vidal V, Fremond B, Chaupis M, et al: Primary obstructive megaureter in infants: Medical or surgical treatment? Appropos of 24 cases. *J Urol* (Paris) 1988; 94:279.

Weinstein AJ, Bauer SB, Retik AB, et al: The surgical management of megaureters in duplex systems: the efficacy of ureteral tapering and common sheath reimplantation. *J Urol* 1988; 139:328.

Weiss RM, Lytton B: Vesicoureteral reflux and distal ureteral obstruction. *J Urol* 1974; 111:245.

Whitaker RH: Methods of assessing obstruction in dilated ureter. *Br J Urol* 1973; 45:15.

Whitaker RH, Johnston JH: A simple classification of wide ureters. *Br J Urol* 1976; 45:781.

Williams DI, Hulme-Moir I: Primary megaureter. *Br J Urol* 1970; 42:140.

Woodard JR, Anderson AM III, Parrott TS: Ureteral reimplantation in myelodysplastic children. *J Urol* 1981; 125:63.

CHAPTER 48

Vesicoureteral Reflux and Urinary Tract Infection in Children

R. Dixon Walker

Inasmuch as the upper urinary tract is aseptic when in its normal condition, the three prime questions to be answered in regard to inflammations are:

1. What are the bacteria of urinary infection?
2. How do they obtain access to the urinary tract?
3. Why do these bacteria sometimes cause infection and sometimes not?

E. L. Keyes (1926)

These questions were posed well before the combination of reflux and infection was recognized as the progenitor of pyelonephritis. Despite their apparent simplicity, they capture the significant queries about pyelonephritis that still perplex us today. Indeed, reflux had been recognized as abnormal in medieval times by Galen (Polk, 1965), who observed the competency of the ureterovesical junction in the dissected dog bladder when it was filled to capacity through the urethra. Others, including Pozzi (1893), recognized reflux in experimental animals and in humans but were unable to draw conclusions as to whether it was abnormal or not. Sampson (1903) observed that the normal obliquity of the ureter through the bladder prevented reflux, and in one operated patient with an end-to-side ureterovesical anastomosis, reflux occurred. He further recognized that in those instances where reflux occurred, it could conceivably be a cause of renal infection. Sampson's work was reviewed by Young, who stated that he had come to a similar conclusion in 1898 regarding the normal ureter and that in patients who had a normal ureterovesical junction there was no reflux, even when the bladder was forcibly distended through a catheter. It is of interest that, whereas reflux occupies a significant portion of a textbook on pediatric urology today, both major texts on pediatric urology from the early 1950s from the United States and Great Britain contained only one or two pages on reflux (Campbell, 1951; Higgins et al., 1951).

The point at which reflux became recognized as important had its genesis in Hutch's classic studies in 1952 demonstrating the effect of reflux in paraplegic patients and its relationship to chronic pyelonephritis. Prior to that time, operations on the ureterovesical junction had been performed and the methodology of cystograms had been developed; however, the clinical implications of reflux were not recognized. This work of Hutch was followed by the observation of Hodson (1959) that reflux was more common in children with urinary tract infection and that there was a high correlation between reflux and chronic pyelonephritis as seen on intravenous urogram (IVU). These classic studies ushered in a modern area of development of surgical techniques to treat this disease, and extensive studies on the natural history of reflux. More important, in a major way, they laid the foundation for the development of the specialty of pediatric urology.

PEDIATRIC URINARY TRACT INFECTION
Etiology and Classification

Urinary tract infection (UTI) is a common presentation in children with abnormalities of the genitourinary tract. Indeed about 50% of children under 12 presenting with UTI are found to have such abnormalities (Smellie and Norman, 1982). These children can be classified as having a complicated UTI. Conversely, an uncomplicated UTI is not associated with any congenital anomaly. The most common of these congenital abnormalities includes vesicoureteral reflux, obstructive uropathies, and neurogenic bladder. The significance of such abnormalities is that children with a complicated UTI have a higher incidence of pyelonephritis, whereas children with an uncomplicated UTI are more likely to have cystitis. Renal scarring, with its sequelae, is thus more common in children with a complicated UTI. Although this classification system is simplistic in that it does not incorporate other risk factors, such as host-bacterial interaction, it is still practical in defining the natural history and pathogenesis of UTI.

A controversial area is the relationship of UTI in male neonates to the presence or absence of foreskin. In 1985 Wiswell and associates presented their initial report of a decreased incidence of UTI in circumcised as compared to uncircumcised male infants. A follow-up study reviewing a larger number of patients showed a tenfold increase in UTI in uncircumcised male infants: 1.12% vs. 0.11% (Wiswell and Roscelli, 1986). Of interest was that a large number of these infected infants required hospital admission for management of clinical pyelonephritis. This study was the impetus for these investigators to look further at the relationship of UTI and circumcision with the finding that decreased numbers of routine neonatal circumcisions were being done and that this correlated with a rising number of neonatal male UTIs (Wiswell et al., 1987). Winberg and co-workers (1989) suggested that perhaps the prepuce was a "mistake of nature"; but rather than suggesting circumcision as a cure, it was suggested that the prepuce be colonized with a nonpathogenic anaerobic gastrointestinal bacteria from the mother. Wiswell and Geschke (1989) also have looked retrospectively at the sequelae of UTI in the uncircumcised male infant. They found a much higher incidence of bacteremia, renal failure, and death. This retrospective study has a serious flaw in that the results do not state whether these patients had any other associated risk factors, such as obstructive uropathy or vesicoureteral reflux. The unanswered question pertaining to this data is whether the increased incidence of UTIs in uncircumcised male infants is sufficient justification to return to the practice of routine neonatal circumcision. Although compelling, the aforementioned data does not support this. Rather it would seem prudent to consider circumcision in a male infant with a complicated UTI particularly if there has been a presentation with a febrile UTI. The benefit of the data by Wiswell and other authors is that they have presented objective data so that circumcision can be judged on scientific criteria rather than by emotion and bias.

Pathogenesis

The pathogenesis and effects of UTI can be broken down into two components: the pathogenesis of infection and the pathogenesis of renal scarring. The pathogenesis of UTI in children is very much like that which occurs in the adult and was discussed in Chapter 5.

Bacteria that cause urinary tract infection are most often aerobic gram-negative rods that are normal inhabitants of fecal flora. These organisms reach the bladder and kidneys through ascent from the rectum to the perineum, vagina, and urethra. The anatomic differences between male and female account primarily for the difference in incidence of urinary tract infections. These differences include the longer urethral length and the absence of the moist perineal-vaginal area in the male.

Bladder infection is the result of the relationship between virulent bacteria and the mucosal surface of the bladder. Factors that make bacteria virulent include the presence of pili, which may allow adhesion with uromucoid surfaces, and the nature of bacterial cell wall antigens and their association with hemolysin and colicin, which gives it a competitive advantage against other bacteria. Mutations on the surface of pili also may allow bacteria to adapt to changing conditions in the bladder.

Bacterial adherence is theoretically a vital link in the development of pyelonephritis. The subject has been reviewed nicely in the monograph by Schaeffer (1984). It has been common knowledge among bacteriologists for some time that bacterial adherence is a property that allows colonization of surfaces. Recently the role of adherence as a pathogenic phenomenon has been explored. Colonization of the alimentary tract and mucosally lined orifices takes place within the first few weeks after birth. The colonization of the gut by pathogenic organisms is the first step in the process that eventually produces renal scarring. The adherence of pathogenic bacteria to the perineum, vagina, urethra, or bladder wall resists the natural action of those structures to wash the bacteria away. Adherence is due to the interaction between binding molecules on the bacteria (ligands) and receptors on the host cells. This bond between bacteria and host cells is so well developed that it is almost impossible to reverse.

Bacterial ligands are located on fimbriae that provide the initial contact between bacteria and host cells. Fimbriae may be of several types, but any one bacterium will have only one type. Type 1, or mannose-sensitive fimbriae, are very common on nonpathogenic serotypes of *E. coli*. These fimbriae are so called because they react with a mannose sugar on the host cell surface. Mannose-resistant fimbriated bacteria are more likely to be pathogenic and have been implicated in pyelonephritis in children. Some mannose-resistant *E. coli* have fimbriae that possess P blood group bacterial adhesions and thus are referred to as *P pili bacteria*. The importance of these P pili bacteria is that they are implicated in a large number of children with clinical acute pyelonephritis. Kallenius and associates (1981) found P pili *E. coli* in 91% of children with acute pyelonephritis. Acute pyelonephritis was defined as urinary tract infection with temperature greater than 38° C, elevated C-reactive protein level, and elevated erythrocyte sedimentation rate.

The problem in relating this finding to renal scarring

is that many of the children in both studies did not have reflux; conversely, the study by Lombard and associates (1983) indicated that very few children with severe reflux and renal scarring have demonstrated infections with P pili bacteria.

Although renal scarring can occur in the absence of reflux (Roberts et al., 1985), the rate at which it does so is anecdotal. Thus, we are left with the conflicting data that suggest that the P pili *E. coli* is a very virulent strain, easily causing renal damage in experimental stiuations, and yet uncommonly is related to the renal scarring in children that is the focus of this chapter. Of course, other types of adherence may occur in severely refluxing children and may account for the development of renal scars. It has been shown that both capsular K and cell wall O antigens can cause adherence, and these antigens are present in a large number of *E. coli* organisms.

The bladder defense mechanisms include the mucosal surface of the bladder and the emptying capacity of the bladder. The mucosal surface of the bladder, its glycosoaminoglycan layer, and its propensity for infection may be determined genetically. Surface cells produce secretory IgA that may help to prevent bacterial colonization (Akerlund et al., 1979). Bladders that do not empty effectively leave urine behind; this promotes greater contact with bladder mucosa, which fosters bacterial growth. There are many conditions that may allow poor emptying of the bladder, including neurogenic bladder, vesicoureteral reflux, and obstructive uropathy. In the normal individual other factors inhibit the growth of bacteria, including the osmolarity and acidity of the urine.

Bacteria that reach the kidney and cause pyelonephritis have a similar relationship to the surface of the renal pelvis and collecting ducts of the renal medulla as bacteria do to the bladder. These bacteria reach the kidney more commonly when there is reflux or obstruction, but they also can reach the renal pelvis in a perfectly normal system. Pyelonephritis occurs when there is an inflammatory response in the medulla; leukocytes are mobilized to combat the infection, and the resulting phagocytosis of bacteria, with the release of high oxygen radicals, is a factor in eventual renal scarring.

The renal scar may develop very quickly or take quite a long time. Ransley and Risdon (1981) have proposed that some scarring in infants with intrarenal reflux takes place immediately after a severe pyelonephritic episode and have called it the "big bang" effect. They acknowledge that in some instances the process takes longer, perhaps in a series of "little bangs." Friedland (1979) has indicated that the full growth of a renal scar may take place over a period as long as 2 years.

The actual process of scarring probably is due to the normal cellular response to the invading bacteria. The same processes that come into effect to kill the bacteria also damage the tubular cell wall. Roberts (1983) has theorized that once bacteria adhere to renal tubular cells, an immune response is elicited. During phagocytosis, superoxide is released in a respiratory burst from the cell wall and damages both bacteria and tubular cells. This damage causes an interstitial inflammatory response that leads to renal scarring. In the monkey, the scarring and inflammatory response can be blocked by administering superoxide dismutase (Roberts et al., 1983). Further, Roberts and co-workers (1984) have been able to block adherence to tubular cells by immunization with an antifimbrial antibody. Immunization with a less purified *E. coli* mixture that had a mild protective effect against renal scarring also has been performed in piglets (Torres et al., 1984). All of these findings would suggest that immunization might be practical, but the complexity of doing it is discussed by Stamey (Schaeffer, 1984), who states that in the long run, antimicrobial agents may provide less expensive and better protection. Ischemic damage to renal tubular cells also can occur as a result of exposure to *E. Coli*. Anaerobic metabolism of *E. Coli* causes anoxia and consumption of the purine pool leading to release of superoxide radicals. This process can be blocked by allopurinal (Roberts, 1991). The complex mechanism of the development of renal scarring as described by Roberts is depicted in Figure 48-1.

Diagnosis

The diagnosis of UTI can be made on a urine culture obtained from a clean catch or a catheterized specimen. Clean-catch specimens are more likely to be contaminated, but if the growth is a single pathogenic bacteria, it is likely significant. Urine can be obtained easily from infants with a suprapubic bladder puncture. Colony counts of 100,000 colonies in a clean-catch urine are usually required to be significant, but any positive culture must be correlated with the symptoms that the patient presents with. Any urine culture greater than 5000 colonies from urine obtained on a suprapubic puncture or catheterized specimen is significant.

Presentation

Infants and young children with UTI are more likely to present with nonspecific signs or symptoms, two of the most common being failure to thrive and fever. Both of these are closely associated with complicated UTIs. Other symptoms in young children include vomiting, diarrhea, anorexia, and lethargy. Children of any age with renal scarring may present with hypertension. Older children and adolescents frequently will have symptoms of bladder irritability, anorexia,

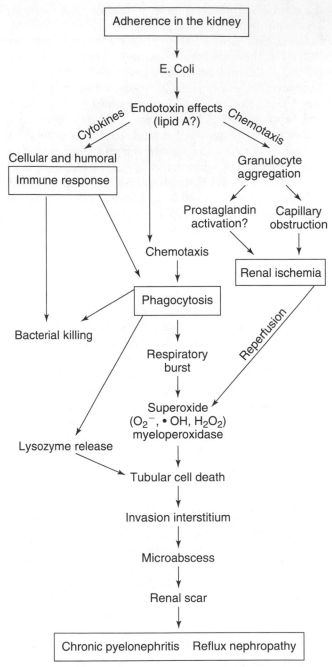

FIG. 48-1
Schematic representation of pathogenesis of pyelonephritis scar formation. (From Roberts JA: *J Urol* 1992; 148:1721. Used by permission.)

or abdominal pain (Smellie et al., 1964). Pain with sterile reflux may be colicky in nature. Older children may complain of flank pain with a full bladder. These symptoms are nonspecific as to localization of infection, but when associated with fever they are suggestive of upper urinary tract infection.

Fever is the key presenting symptom that helps to distinguish between children with pyelonephritis and those with cystitis, but it is not always a reliable de-

terminant. Since children with pyelonephritis are most likely to have reflux, this presenting symptom, if reliable, would be helpful in predicting which children would have a positive radiologic evaluation. Woodward and Holden (1976) evaluated 350 children with urinary tract infection and found that 90% of refluxing children had temperatures greater than 38.5° C, whereas only 40% of nonrefluxing children had similar temperatures. They noted that if only children with fevers had been evaluated, 10% of the refluxers would have been missed. Levitt and co-workers (1977) examined the IVUs of children with upper or lower tract symptomatology. Only 2 of 99 females with lower tract symptoms had abnormal IVUs, whereas 23 of 57 females with upper tract symptoms had abnormalities. The number of refluxing patients was not indicated in the study. Govan and Palmer (1969) found a high correlation between historical evidence of pyelonephritis (presumably fever) and reflux; there was a positive history in 79% of refluxing patients but only 39% of nonrefluxing patients. In the refluxing patients, only 7% still had symptoms of pyelonephritis after successful antireflux surgery. In addition, it was noted that the children with reflux tended to present with urinary tract infection an average of 2 years earlier than those without reflux. Smellie and colleagues (1982) presented data that are in conflict with some of these findings. In their large series of children with urinary tract infection, there was no age difference in those with or without reflux. Children with reflux were, however, more likely to present with fever, and it was particularly evident if there was also renal scarring.

It is difficult to localize infection on a clinical basis and although a number of laboratory tests have been suggested, most are not in standard usage. These tests have included urine concentrating ability, leukocyte excretion rate, antibody coated bacteria, LDH, and the measurement of β_2 microglobulin (Neal, 1989). The clinical diagnosis of pyelonephritis is best made with criteria of fever (>39° C), flank or costovertebral angle tenderness, and elevated white blood cell count. Jantausch and Rushton have advocated DMSA renal scanning as a means of making the diagnosis with a high degree of specificity (Anderson et al., 1994).

Radiologic Evaluation

The evaluation and management of children with UTI should allow initial treatment of the infection followed by evaluation after the urine is cleared. The exception is the child in which it is difficult to clear the infection or when obstructive uropathy is strongly suggested by history; in these instances an early ultrasound is appropriate. Standard radiologic evaluation of the child with urinary tract infection has traditionally been the VCUG and IVU. That protocol has been altered with the advent of ultrasound. The tremendous improvement in technique has modified urinary tract evaluation so that the current initial recommendation would be an ultrasound and a contrast VCUG. Ultrasound by itself is not sensitive enough to diagnose most cases of vesicoureteral reflux (Blane et al., 1993). Nuclear cystogram is a reasonable alternative in females. Children who have a normal ultrasound and no reflux need no further study. Children who have an abnormal ultrasound, particularly if anatomy is poorly defined, will require an IVU (Alon et al., 1989). These studies are indicated in any infant or child with a first infection. This dictum is being challenged for evaluation of older children and adolescents (Fair et al., 1979). The appropriate time to do these studies is after the urinary tract infection has cleared. Others, including Kaplan (1980), have advocated radiologic evaluation during or shortly after the urinary tract infection. Infection with coliform organisms may cause ureteral stasis so that an IVU or ultrasound performed while infection is present may demonstrate dilated ureters (Teague and Boyarsky, 1968). The length of time between treatment and radiologic study is empiric. Ideally, one should demonstrate absence of infection by urine culture 2 to 3 weeks prior to obtaining the VCUG. It is important that the VCUG be done in a physiologic manner so as not to produce artifact. The contrast material should be warmed if necessary and instilled by slow to moderate flow through a small urethral catheter. Only gravity flow should be used at no greater than 70 cm H_2O. Most often children are tested awake. Timmons and co-workers (1977) demonstrated that sleep cystograms could occasionally be useful, a view shared by Woodard and Keats (1973). The IVU is usually done after the VCUG to avoid contrast in the ureters. The IVU should have a good nephrogram phase so the renal outlines can be measured for parenchymal thickness and renal growth. Harrison and colleagues (1976) have stated that thinning of the medial edge of the superior pole of the kidney may be an indicator of reflux. Other indirect signs of reflux may be calyceal clubbing and ureteral dilation. Kuhns and co-workers (1977) felt that the presence of a ureteral jet on the bladder phase of the IVU precluded the finding of reflux. In situations in which the child continues a febrile course after treatment, renal ultrasound will demonstrate whether there is obstructive uropathy. Ultrasound also is useful as a screening tool in the older child with urinary tract infection and as a means of measuring renal growth and parenchymal volume.

Nuclear cystograms provide an alternative for the patient who may require multiple or longitudinal studies on an annual basis. The methodology is similar to contrast studies and has the advantage of a lowered radiation dosage. The advantages and disadvantages of nuclear cystography have been discussed in the section Classification of Reflux. Renal nuclear imaging (renal scan) is a better study than IVU in assessing patients with reflux. Objective functional information that can be used in following the patient or in comparing preoperative and postoperative function is obtained. Technetium 99m diethylenetriamine pentaacetic acid (^{99m}Tc DPTA) primarily is used to assess glomerular and tubular function; technetium 99m dimercaptosuccinic acid (^{99m}cDMSA) is best for visualizing cortical tissue and measuring renal function; and iodohippurate sodium ^{131}I is used to assess tubular function.

The Children's Hospital of Philadelphia outline of evaluation and management of UTI as depicted in Figure 48-2 is well thought out and would closely approximate evaluation and management by most pediatric urologists.

Cystoscopy

In the past cystoscopy has been considered part of the evaluation of the refluxing child, but this concept is changing. There are several reasons for the deemphasis on cystoscopy, primarily the added risk and cost of an anesthetic. The likelihood that low grades of reflux (grades I and II, International Classification) will disappear spontaneously is so great that cystoscopic information adds little to the diagnosis or management. For the higher grades of reflux with clear indications for surgical intervention, cystoscopy may be done at the time of reimplantation of ureters. The continued evidence against bladder neck or significant urethral obstruction in female patients obviates cystoscopy performed solely for the purpose of ruling out obstruction. Dilation of the urethra as a treatment for reflux is generally discouraged today.

What then are the indications for cystoscopy in the refluxing child, and what information can be gained by the procedure? There are no absolute indications for cystoscopy in the refluxing child. A relative indication is for the child with moderate reflux (grades III and IV, International Classification) when the information can be used to decide in favor of surgical management. Observation of the contralateral ureteral orifice in unilateral reflux is helpful to plan surgical therapy. The child with duplex ureters and reflux or an ipsilateral periureteral diverticulum may represent an indication for cystoscopy. Children with breakthrough urinary tract infections may require cystoscopy before a decision can be made about continuing medical therapy. Cystoscopy may be indicated in selected children who also are having urodynamic studies.

The information gained at cystoscopy includes information about the urethra, bladder wall, ureteral orifices and submucosal tunnels, and about the exter-

Childrens' Hospital of Philadelphia, Urology Algorithm for UTI

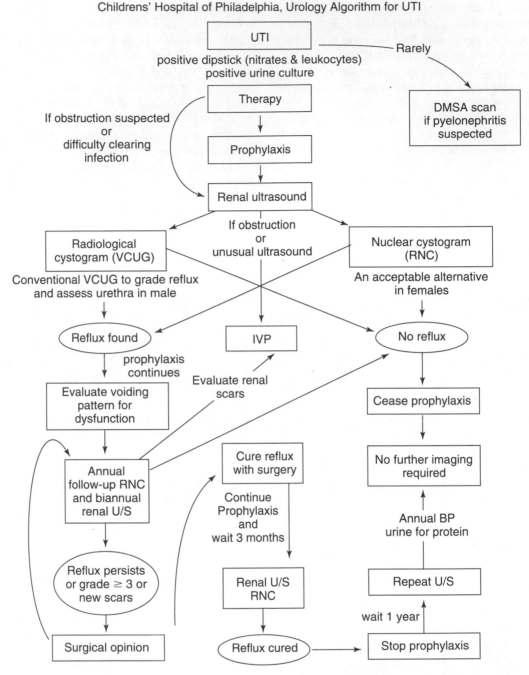

FIG. 48-2
Children's Hospital of Philadelphia algorithm for UTI. (Courtesy of John W. Duckett, M.D.)

nal genitalia and vagina. Even though urethral obstruction is rare, the urethra should be calibrated and compared with normal published standards (Immergut and Wahman, 1968). Urethras with calibration in the lower range of normal may be dilated to facilitate introduction of the cystoscope. Visualization of the bladder neck from the urethra may indicate the raised, small, cystic-appearing lesions that are consistent with cystitis cystica. Children with cystitis cystica may have

lower tract symptoms, such as urgency, frequency, and incontinence; however, associated reflux still has an excellent chance of spontaneous resolution (Brock et al., 1983). The description by Lyon and associates (1969) of orifice configuration is still widely used, although it does not correlate with spontaneous resolution as closely as once thought. Duckett (1983) found orifice configuration of only minimal value and indicated that even in the most abnormal orifices there was spontaneous resolution of reflux in 15% to 20% of patients. The tunnel length–ureteral diameter ratio can be measured nicely by using a 4 F whistle-tip ureteral catheter. The submucosal portion of the tunnel can be measured and an estimate of width obtained by comparing the width of the orifice to the width of the catheter (approximately 1 mm). A special fiberoptic transilluminating catheter that provides an objective measurement of both the submucosal and intramural portions of the ureter has been devised (Homsy et al., 1983). Data should be obtained with both a full and an empty bladder and should indicate whether the orifice is patulous, the degree of development of the trigonal muscle, the degree of trabeculation of the bladder wall, and whether the orifice moves laterally as the bladder fills. The position of bladder diverticula should be noted, particularly in relation to the ureteral orifice. Spontaneous resolution of reflux may occur with periureteral diverticula unless the ureter enters the diverticulum (Levitt and Weiss, 1985). Vaginoscopy and reinspection of the external genitalia also should be done at the end of the procedure; the pelvic organs can be palpated effectively with a rectal examination.

One of the major problems with cystoscopy in infants and children with reflux is the lack of consistency of observed findings among different examiners. Hjelmas and associates (in press), in evaluating the cystoscopic data from the International Reflux Study, found that there was a poor correction between cystoscopic finding and resolution of reflux.

Urodynamics

Urodynamics, including cystometrogram, perineal or periurethral electromyogram (EMG), and urinary flow studies, may be helpful in selected patients with vesicoureteral reflux. These studies, which have been done more often by our European colleagues, may be useful in patients with severe urgency and incontinence. Taylor and co-workers (1982) showed that 75% of refluxing girls had evidence of uninhibited bladder contractions. Allen (1979) has indicated that these uninhibited contractions yield higher intravesical pressures and that, when associated with reflux, may lead to greater renal damage. This assertion, however, is not supported by the data of Taylor and colleagues (1982). Koff and Murtagh (1983) have treated such patients with anticholinergic therapy and indicate that it may be helpful in resolution of reflux. Cystometric studies are more easily interpretable in the child with low grades of reflux. If uninhibited bladder contractions are detected, appropriate pharmacologic control will often arrest the reflux and associated infection. The cystometrogram is also difficult to do and is often uninterpretable in the very young child or infant.

DEMOGRAPHY

The demographic information that we have comes from three sources: (1) cystographic evaluation in normal children, (2) studies similar in children with urinary tract infection, and (3) the study of other animals. The first of these sources of information is largely closed to use now because of ethical constraints in obtaining studies in normal children. Studies in children with urinary tract infection allow us to look not only at the population but also at their siblings. Comparisons of experimental animals to humans let us look at those who are close phylogenetically and those that have a close anatomic resemblance.

Incidence

The incidence of vesicoureteral reflux (VUR) in normal infants and children is not known and probably varies depending on race and perhaps country of origin. Askari and Belman (1982) have reported on the infrequency of reflux in black children. In their studies of black children investigated for urinary tract infection, the incidence of reflux was only 25% of that seen in infected white children. Extrapolating these data with the lowered incidence of urinary tract infection in blacks, they concluded that the actual incidence of reflux in the normal black population was 10% of its occurence in a white population. Although the incidence of reflux was less in black children, its natural history, once discovered, is the same. Skoog and Belman (1991) described the distribution of grade of reflux and spontaneous resolution in black children and found it the same as in a larger group of white patients.

The incidence of reflux in other races or national groups is not known, although all of the large reported studies on refluxing patients seem to come from northern Europe, including the Scandinavian countries, Great Britain, and Ireland, as well as North America, Australia, and New Zealand. Manley (1981) suggested that reflux occurs more commonly in children with fair skin, blond hair, and blue eyes, although this was refuted by Urrutia and Lebowitz (1983), who believed that only red-haired children have a higher incidence of reflux.

A number of cystographic studies were done in normal children prior to the time at which constraints were rightly placed by human experimentation committees. Despite these constraints, the previously gained information is valuable. These studies must be examined critically since there was often no standardization of cystographic technique, and the patient populations were not well defined. We know now that it is particularly important because of the racial differences in incidence, and it is likely that in many of these studies the population chosen for study was unlike the population with urinary tract infection. In 1949, Gibson did 43 cystograms in children, using syringe injection of contrast, and found two causes of reflux. Iannaccone and Panzironi (1955) evaluated 50 infants without urologic disease and found only one instance of reflux. Although the patient population was not defined, they were all likely of Mediterranean origin. Jones and Headstream (1958) evaluated 100 children and found one who had reflux. Race was not defined, and 70% of the patients were males. Lich and co-workers (1964) did cystograms on 26 infants less than 48 hours old and found no reflux. Politano (1960) had similar findings in 50 normal children. Peters and associates (1967) defined race in 66 premature infants studied with cystography. They found no reflux in their group, 56 of whom were black. In contrast to these studies, all of which showed a very low incidence of reflux, is the study of Kollerman (1974), who found that reflux was more common. He examined 161 children with cystography. The technique was admittedly unphysiologic and involved filling the bladder with a syringe to capacities of 40 to 200 ml. No child had a history of urinary tract infection or of any urologic problem. Of the group, 18.5% had vesicoureteral reflux.

The incidence of reflux in children with urinary tract infection is suspected of being much higher than in the normal population, despite our difficulty in defining incidence in this latter group. Shopfner (1970) reviewed a large number of children defined as having a urinary tract infection by the culture of at least 100,000 colonies of bacteria/per milliliter of urine. Reflux was present in 14% of 1695 females and 29% of 523 males. Baker and colleagues (1966) had shown previously that reflux was most common in younger children with urinary tract infection, occurring in 70% of children less than 1 year of age, 25% of children at 4 years of age, 15% of children at 12 years of age, and 5.2% of adults. Compilation studies in children with asymptomatic bacteriuria yield similar results: 29% of preschool-age females and 23% of school-age females had reflux (Walker et al., 1977).

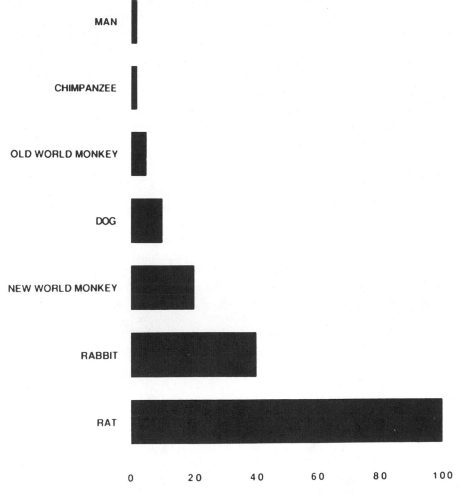

FIG. 48-3
Incidence of reflux in mammalian species (percentage). (From Roberts JA: *J Urol* 1992; 148:1721.

Reflux is a commonly occurring phenomenon in some animals as depicted in Figure 48-3. It occurs in almost all rats and many rabbit species. Christie (1971) found reflux in 80% of 3-month-old puppies, but it disappears spontaneously and is present in only 10% of adult dogs. It is not present in piglets or adult pigs. Roberts (1974) indicated that its presence in monkeys is variable and is both age- and species-related. In his studies on infant rhesus monkeys, reflux occurred almost all of the time in newborns but gradually disappeared, so that by 36 months of age it was uncommon. The disappearance curve was a gradual decline rather than a sharp change and was gone by the time the animal reached maturity. These studies are intriguing because the primates are close to us phylogenetically, and the disappearance curves closely parallel the disappearance of reflux in children with urinary tract infection. Figure 48-4 depicts a comparison between the disappearance of reflux in infant and maturing rhesus monkeys (Roberts, 1974) against the disappearance of reflux in a series of children with urinary tract infection (Baker et al., 1966).

Patterns of Inheritance

The observation that reflux occurs in siblings and parents of affected children has been known for the past two decades, but the actual mode of inheritance has not been determined.

Stephens and colleagues (1955) noted the occurrence of reflux in twins. Tobenkin (1964) reported on a family in which three different generations had evidence of reflux. He suggested that the mode of inheritance might be sex-linked, with incomplete penetrance. Mulcahy and coworkers (1970) reported three families in which two members had reflux and also noted that 18% of patients undergoing reimplantation had other family members with a history of urinary tract infection. Other investigators reported familial

reflux in series ranging from five to 20 families (Miller and Caspari, 1972; Schmidt et al., 1972; Zel and Retik, 1973).

Dwoskin (1976) reviewed 125 families of probands with reflux and found that 26.5% of siblings had reflux. In a similar study, Jerkins and Noe (1982) found 33% of siblings showing reflux. The conclusion from both of these studies was that the siblings of all children with reflux should be evaluated, particularly those less than 2 years of age. This conclusion has been confirmed now in studies that have gone on over a decade with the only change in recommendation being that aggressive screening should occur in all siblings less than 5 years of age (Noe, 1992).

Lewy and Belman (1975) believed that a pattern of autosomal dominance was suggested by the occurrence of reflux in a large number of siblings. The wide variability of reflux in siblings actually gives credence to a polygenic or multifactorial mode of inheritance, as has been suggested by Burger and Burger (1974). Polygenic modes of inheritance probably account for the variability of pathologic findings in many congenital urologic conditions of which reflux and hypospadias may be two of the best examples. The variable factor determined by this mode of inheritance appears to be submucosal ureteral tunnel length. Experimental data in puppies with reflux have indicated that in addition to ureteral tunnel length, a paucity of adrenergic nerve fibers may relate to reflux. The suggestion was that with maturation of the autonomic nervous system and the increase in the adrenergic nerve fibers, there was a concomitant decrease in the incidence of reflux (Kiruluta et al., 1986). The recent data from Noe and co-workers (1992) indicate that the transmission of reflux from parent to child is significant in that 66% of the offspring of affected parents have vesicoureteral reflux. These authors agree that the mode of transmission is almost certainly a multifactorial ge-

FIG. 48-4

Comparison of the disappearance of reflux in infant monkeys (Roberts and Riopelle, 1977) to that of children with urinary tract infection (Baker et al., 1966).

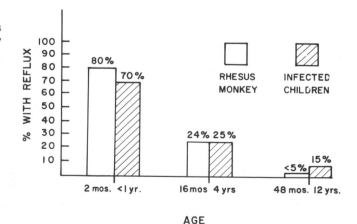

netic trait, but in some instances it may occur as an autosomal dominant pattern.

CLASSIFICATION AND TERMINOLOGY

Classification of Reflux

The earliest attempts at classification of reflux tended to broadly quantify the amount of reflux to the kidney or to classify by what was happening physiologically in the bladder. The former situation was represented by Rolleston and associates (1974), who classified reflux as being slight, moderate, or gross. These investigators noted that gross reflux was almost always associated with renal damage. Hinman and coworkers (1962) introduced the terms *high-pressure reflux* and *low-pressure reflux* to indicate reflux that occurred during bladder filling (low pressure) vs. that which occurred during voiding (high pressure). The implication from this distinction was that low-pressure reflux was congenital and would not resolve, whereas high-pressure reflux was more likely to resolve with time. The pressure effect on the kidney was not an issue at that time.

More precise measures of reflux were proposed in both the United States and Europe and have provided the nucleus for the International Classification System that is in current usage. Heikel and Parkkulainen (1966) proposed a five-category classification system that gained usage in northern Europe, whereas in this country the Dwoskin-Perlmutter (1973) classification system was commonly used. The International Classification System represented one of the first cooperative efforts of the International Reflux Study. It was the feeling of the original members of the study group that there were deficiencies in both the Heikel-Parkkulainen and the Dwoskin-Perlmutter systems that could be addressed only by a new system. Rather than discard the other two systems, the best characteristics of each were incorporated in the new system. Particular emphasis was placed on the fornices and calyces, and the anatomy of these structures provided the basis for classification. The International Classification System is shown in Figure 48-5. Despite the sophistication of this classification system, it was quickly recognized that clinical patterns of reflux were not neatly compartmentalized, and thus the subtle variation in each grade is illustrated in Figure 48-6.

Reflux also can be graded, although less precisely, by nuclear cystogram. There is no universally accepted grading system for nuclear cystography, with most radiologists simply using the terms mild, moderate, and severe. Majd and Belman (1979) have indicated that the clear advantage of nuclear cystography is the lower radiation dosage and because of this, it is an excellent tool for screening females and for follow-up studies in both sexes. The disadvantage is the dif-

GRADE OF REFLUX

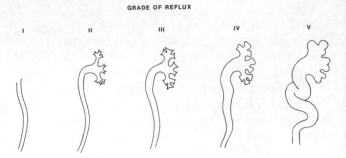

FIG. 48-5
International Reflux Classification.

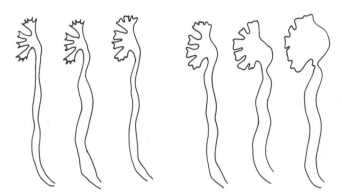

FIG. 48-6
Variations with grades III and IV of the International Reflux Classification.

ficulty in recognizing important associated bladder pathology, such as a bladder diverticula, or in viewing the male urethra.

Classification of Orifice Shape and Position

The shape and position of the ureteral orifice are important because of the probable relation of the ureteral orifice to the length of the intramural tunnel. Paquin (1959) has shown that the intramural tunnel is vital to the prevention of reflux. In normal nonrefluxing children, the tunnel length–ureteral diameter ratio was 5:1, whereas in refluxing children this same ratio was 1.4:1. It is likely that one needs at least a 3:1 ratio to prevent reflux, although this ratio is not satisfactory with ureters of a large diameter. Cussen (1967) has done an exacting study measuring normal submucosal and intravesical ureteral lengths in children of different ages. These data are partially presented and extrapolated in Table 48-1.

Lyon and associates (1969) described four basic orifice shapes: cone, stadium, horseshoe, and golf hole. These four shapes represent increasing levels of orifice incompetency. They believed that orifice shape rather than tunnel length determined valvular competency. One additional important observation is the position

TABLE 48-1

Mean Ureteral Tunnel Lengths and Diameters in Normal Children

Age (yr)	Intravesical Ureteral Length (mm)	Submucosal Ureteral Length (mm)	Ureteral Diameter at Ureterovesical Junction (mm)
1-3	7	3	1.4
3-6	7	3	1.7
6-9	9	4	2.0
9-12	12	6	1.9

Modified from Cussen LJ: *Invest Urol* 1967; 5:164.

of the orifice on the trigone and its relation to reflux. Those orifices that were laterally placed had a higher incidence of reflux and likely had shorter submucosal tunnels.

Mackie and Stephens (1975) developed a more complex classification of orifice position that was originally intended for duplex systems but not is generally used for single ureters as well. The system is a complicated one to remember because the authors have related orifice position to the original location of the ureteral bud on the wolffian duct. A diagram of the three zones of urethral orifice position is depicted in Figure 48-7.

Classification of Renal Scarring

Renal scarring can take a variety of forms (Smellie and Normand, 1979), as shown in Figure 48-8. Attempts to quantify the amount and character of renal scarring are important. Only if precise definitions of scarring and parenchymal thickness are made can one tell if there is progression of disease. This progression is important not only in investigational studies that compare treatments but, indeed, in the individual patient who is being followed with medical management. Equally important as the measurement of renal scarring is the measurement of renal growth. Some refluxing patients may exhibit only growth failure as an effect of their reflux. Claësson has developed an excellent method of measuring renal parenchymal volume and calculating renal growth (Winberg et al., 1979). This method uses the nephrogram phase of the IVU. By measuring the L1 to L3 intravertebral distance and the renal length, one can calibrate how close the kidney is to normal size. In addition, one can look at specific areas of the kidney and compare those to normal. The nomogram developed by Claësson is shown in Figure 48-9. The results of the International Reflux Study in Children (IRSC) showed that there was another type of injury related to reflux, which was parenchymal thinning (Olbing et al., 1992). Parenchymal thinning often preceded scar formation but, in some instances, was also reversible.

Recent evidence has indicated that DMSA scintigraphy is more sensitive than the IVU in detecting re-

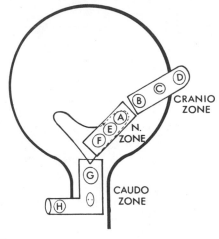

FIG. 48-7
Classification of the ureteral orifice position. (From Mackie GC, Stephens FD: *J Urol* 1975; 114:274. Used by permission.)

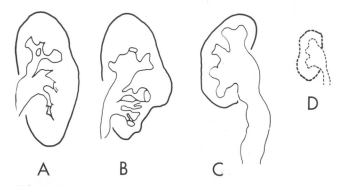

FIG. 48-8
Classification of renal scarring. (From Smellie J, Edwards D, Hunter N, et al: *Kidney Int* 1975; 8:S65. Used by permission.)

nal scarring. ^{99m}CDMSA is an excellent isotope for visualizing renal cortex. Elison and co-workers (1992) evaluated a large number of patients with both IVU and DMSA renal scanning and found a significantly larger number of scars detected by the latter method. In a related study Rushton and associates (1992) evaluated children with DMSA scanning after an episode of acute pyelonephritis and found that subsequent scarring occurred at the site of renal infection. Rushton and Majd (1992) reviewed an extensive array of studies and concluded that DMSA renal scanning is the most sensitive method of detecting renal scarring. It not only detects scars earlier than the IVU but also will detect smaller scars. Whether it will detect parenchymal thinning is as yet unclear, but studies in the piglet have suggested that it will (Giblin et al., 1993). The disadvantages of DMSA scintigraphy are cost and its current lack of availability worldwide and in many areas of the United States.

RENAL LENGTH AND PARENCHYMAL THICKNESS AND AREA IN NORMAL CHILDREN

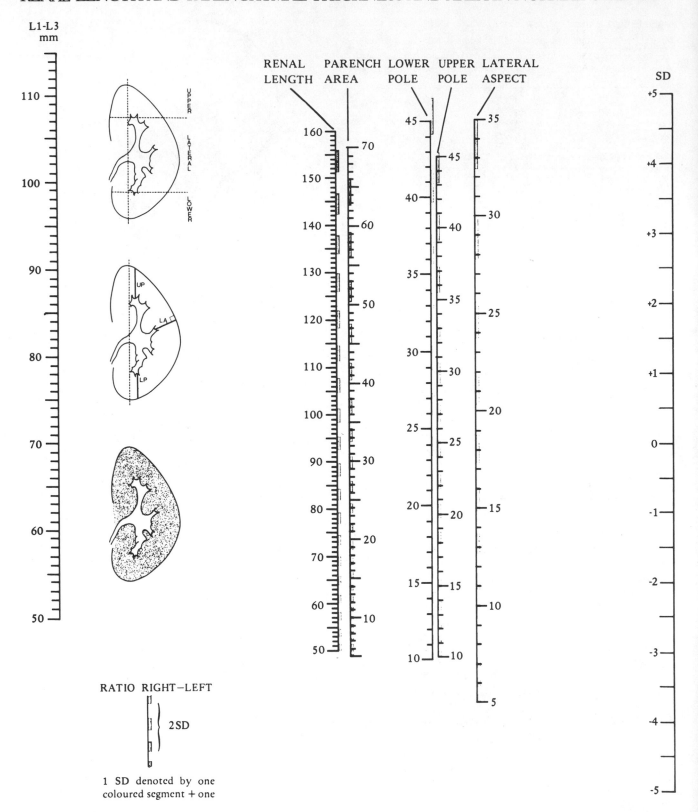

FIG. 48-9
Nomogram for measuring renal parenchymal thickness and area. (From Winberg J, Claësson J, Jacobsson B, et al: Renal growth after acute pyelonephritis in childhood: an epidemiological approach. In Hodson J, Kincaid-Smith P (eds): *Reflux Nephropathy.* New York, Masson Publishing USA, 1979, pp 309-322. Used by permission.)

NATURAL HISTORY
Etiology

Primary reflux is that which is due to an inadequate valvular mechanism at the ureterovesical junction unassociated with any obstruction or neurogenic bladder. *Secondary reflux* is that which occurs secondary to obstruction or neurogenic bladder.

The inadequate valve in primary reflux is the shortened submucosal tunnel. When the intramural and submucosal ureter have an adequate tunnel, the submucosal roof of the tunnel will compress as the bladder fills and will act as a flap valve. The mechanism is probably more passive than active. The role that the trigone plays is unclear. It was once thought that the distal ureter had to be fixed to the trigonal muscle to work, but the transverse bladder reimplant demonstrates that reflux can be corrected with no trigonal fixation. Nevertheless, it is probably important for the distal ureter to be attached to some muscle; if not, the tunnel appears to shorten with bladder filling, and reflux may occur.

The role that infection plays in reflux can be summarized by a review of both experimental and clinical data. Schoenberg and co-workers (1965) produced reflux in apparently normal puppies by infecting them with *Proteus*. Roberts and Riopelle (1978) observed that reflux resolved spontaneously in infected monkeys as often as in uninfected ones, but it took a longer time to do so. Their conclusion was that infection delayed maturation. Further, in adult monkeys, infection caused reflux only in damaged orifices, a finding that supported similar observations in the human. Shopfner (1970) and Blank and Girdany (1971) have stated that most nonobstructed reflux in man was secondary to infection, but most observers have disagreed with such a sweeping statement. Gross and Lebowitz (1981) could find no data in their large series of patients to suggest that infection causes reflux. Their conclusion was that both reflux and infection were independent variables that frequently coexisted and that the association was seen so often simply because the principal reason for doing a voiding cystourethrogram (VCUG) is urinary tract infection. Kaplan (1980) has indicated that some children will reflux only if the cystogram is done during an acute infection and that these children remain an unstudied population that may have a worsened prognosis. One can conclude from these data that infection does not cause reflux of the normal mature orifice and would be a factor only for those orifices that are immature or damaged.

As previously defined, secondary reflux occurs in association with obstruction or neurogenic bladder. Virtually all of the reflux that occurs secondary to obstruction occurs in males. Reflux in females associated with bladder neck obstruction is of historical interest only, and that which occurs with urethral obstruction is hard to define because of the controversial nature of the latter. Despite the best efforts of many to deemphasize the role of urethral stenosis in the female, it is nonetheless a diagnosis commonly made by the urologist. The data regarding reflux in obstructed males are likewise not clear. The incidence of reflux in infants with posterior urethral valves is 50%. Much of it is associated with abnormal ureteral orifices (Henneberry and Stephens, 1980). If obstruction caused reflux, a much higher percentage of valve patients should reflux. Several clinical investigators, including Hendren (1974) and Kurth and associates (1981), have tried to classify milder forms of urethral valves on the basis of degrees of reflux. The justification for it is questionable.

Secondary reflux is a common finding in both occult and true neurogenic bladders. Treatment is much more difficult and has a decreased success rate. Minimal voiding and urodynamic abnormalities are fairly common in primary reflux, and in some instances the spectrum is such that it may be difficult to differentiate between the patient with nonneurogenic/neurogenic bladder (Hinman-Allen syndrome) and the patient with urodynamic abnormalities secondary to reflux. The incidence of dysfunctional voiding is certainly more prevalent and more of a factor than has been appreciated previously. Unfortunately, the true incidence is not known and varies widely between investigators. Sillen and colleagues (1992) found elevated intravesical pressure in 17 of 18 infants with bilateral reflux of high grade as determined by urodynamic studies. On the other hand, the data from the International Reflux Study (IRSC) showed evidence of dysfunctional voiding in 18% of children with VUR whose parents responded to a questionnaire regarding voiding patterns (Van Gool, 1992). Koff (1992) indicated that these children with bladder instability had a different urodynamic pattern from those with nonneurogenic/neurogenic bladder, in that the former had a pattern of high end-filling pressure, whereas the latter had high voiding pressure. Thus reflux in this situation should not be considered either primary or secondary but is rather a combination of two factors, the high intravesical end-filling pressures and the immature ureteral orifice. The disappearance rate of this type of reflux is probably similar to that in children with normal bladder dynamics but may be delayed. Treatment with anticholinergics may be effective in decreasing uninhibited contractions and end-filling pressures while allowing the reflux to resolve spontaneously.

Bacteriuria and Renal Scarring

Hodson (1959) was the first to recognize the frequent occurrence of renal scars in children with recurrent urinary tract infections. Hodson observed that the scars were often polar and associated with calyceal clubbing. A number of questions were raised: Was it the reflux or the infection that caused the damage? Why did the scars occur in the polar areas? Why were children more susceptible to scarring than adults?

The relationship between renal scarring and reflux was strong, with 97% of children with renal scars showing evidence of reflux. This close relationship caused Bailey (1973) to use the term *reflux nephropathy* to describe the radiologic abnormality. Rolleston and co-workers (1970) made the observation that severe (gross) reflux in the infant was much more likely to be associated with renal damage. In 32 kidneys with severe reflux there was evidence of renal damage in 26. They theorized that the damage may have been related to the presence of intrarenal reflux. In a different series, Rolleston and colleagues (1974) demonstrated intrarenal reflux in 20 kidneys of 386 VCUGs. No intrarenal reflux occurred in any children more than 4 years of age. Of the 20 kidneys at risk, 13 showed renal scarring, always in the parenchyma overlying the segment with the intrarenal reflux. These data regarding intrarenal reflux are compelling; nonetheless, one must remember that it can be very hard to demonstrate on routine VCUG.

All of the aforementioned assertions assume that the renal scarring seen is acquired and indeed it is in most instances. There is historical evidence that the renal dysmorphism seen on IVU may represent both congenital and acquired lesions. In a small percentage of cases, renal scarring is present where there is no history of urinary tract infection. In fact, the development of renal scars in children with urinary tract infection and reflux occurs in only about 25% of those with severe reflux, in part because they are protected with antibiotics. Stecker and associates (1973) described the occurrence of renal dysplasia in a small series of patients with reflux. Sommer and Stephens (1981) evaluated children with severe reflux associated with hydronephrosis and found patterns of both dysplasia and obstruction. Habib (1979) states that three histologic patterns can occur in the scarred kidney: (1) renal dysplasia, (2) chronic pyelonephritis, and (3) segmental hypoplasia. Renal dysplasia is a common finding in refluxing patients with posterior urethral valves (King, 1985). It is also a common finding in patients with duplicated collecting systems and upper-pole pathology (Mackie and Stephens, 1975).

Countering this information is the majority of evidence that most renal scarring is acquired. The remarkable similarity between renal scarring in refluxing children and that which occurs in experimental animals lends credence to this hypothesis. Whether it is sterile reflux in pigs or infected reflux in pigs, monkeys, or dogs, the radiologic appearance is quite close to that of renal scarring in children. Hodson and Cotran (1982) have further stated that the histologic

appearance of renal scars does not satisfy the criteria for dysplasia. Bernstein and Arant (1992) examined 25 nephrectomy specimens from patients with reflux nephropathy and found linear scars extending from medulla to cortex. They believed these scars resulted from single papillary duct and medullary disruptions. A convincing observation by Winberg and associates (1975) is that renal scarring was acquired in the majority of children whom they observed. Only 4.5% of girls with a first-known infection had renal scarring, whereas scarring was present in 17% of girls with a second-known infection.

The most compelling evidence that sterile reflux causes renal scarring comes from studies of pigs. The pig is a good animal for comparative study because the anatomy of its kidneys so closely resembles human kidneys. Hodson and co-workers (1975) surgically produced reflux in Sinclair miniature pigs and in addition constricted the urethra with a silver wire ring. The latter maneuver produced higher intravesical pressures than normal and significant intrarenal reflux. The intrarenal reflux almost always occurred at the polar areas of the kidney. Renal scarring occurred in refluxing kidneys even when a sterile urine was maintained and consisted of interstitial fibrosis and aggregations of lymphocytes. The radiologic appearance of the scarring was remarkably similar to that seen in children with reflux. In those piglets infected with *Escherichia coli*, renal scarring that occurred also was very similar to that which occurred with sterile reflux, except that infected scars were more widespread and severe. Contrasting the findings of this study is the work of Ransley and Risdon (1981), who studied the relationship of intrarenal reflux to renal scarring and found that infection was necessary for the development of renal scarring and that the development of the scar could be altered by early microbial therapy. In monkeys, Roberts and colleagues (1982) examined the effect of sterile reflux and found no alteration in renal function as measured with iodohippurate sodium iodine 131 (Hippuran I 131).

The work of Hodson and co-workers (1975) in producing pyelonephritic scars in piglets led Ransley and Risdon (1975a) to examine the papillary anatomy of the piglet to seek an explanation for the polar location of most scars. Their findings were that the papillae in the polar areas were often confluent and that the flattened or concave area cribrosa had open papillary ducts that allowed intrarenal reflux. The middle areas of the renal medulla had papillae that were cone shaped, and papillary ducts were slits that closed with increased intrarenal pressure. They (Ransley and Risdon, 1975b) further discovered in examining kidneys of infants obtained at autopsy that these kidneys tended to have the same characteristics as the piglet kidneys (Fig. 48-10), although the fused papillae were

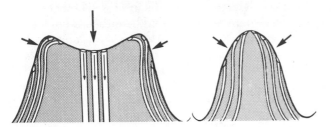

FIG. 48-10
Anatomy of confluent and simple papillae. (From Ransley PG: *Urol Res* 1977; 5:61. Used by permission.)

TABLE 48-2

Tubular and Glomerular Function Related to Grade of Reflux

Grade of Reflux*	Fasting Concentration, (mOsm/kg)	Creatinine Clearance, (ml/min)
Control	1,001 ± 104	130 ± 28
Grades I-II	864 ± 135	136 ± 43
Grade III	808 ± 119	127 ± 16
Grade IV	744 ± 129	108 ± 15
All grades with significant parenchymal scarring	543 ± 126	102 ± 41

Modified from Walker RD, Richard GA, Dobson D, et al: *Urology* 1973; 1:343. Used by permission.
*International Classification.

not as numerous. Roberts and associates (1981) indicated that in monkeys intrarenal reflux also occurred quite often even though most of the papillae are simple rather than compound or fused. They surmised that it was because even in simple papillae the tip can become flattened or concave, and when it occurs, the papillary ducts lose their normal valvular mechanism. Thus, it appears likely that bacteria gain access to the medulla through either normal compound polar papillae or flattened damaged simple papillae.

The controversy regarding sterile renal damage in experimental animals also occurs when one examines clinical data obtained from patients. The support for damage from sterile reflux comes from historical information, that is, that some patients with reflux and renal scarring have no past history of clinical urinary tract infection. These data are subjective and prone to error. Renal scarring often occurs early in life when the history is obscure, and the presenting symptoms of infection may be so generalized as to be mistaken for another illness. Additionally, the scarring may have been developmental rather than acquired. When new scars develop in followed reflux populations, they almost always occur in patients with recurrent infections. A study that counters this concept was conducted by Farnsworth and associates (1991) who evaluated a large number of infants with DMSA scintigraphy with a variety of presenting symptoms. They found two subgroups, one of 27 refluxing infants with scarring but no infection and another of 9 infants with scarring without either reflux or infection. Most studies, however, confirm the relationship between infection and scarring. Huland and Busch (1984) observed new renal scarring in 7 of 213 studied patients, all of whom had urinary tract infection. Smellie and coworkers (1975) studied 233 children with reflux, 10 of whom developed scarring in previously normal kidneys. All of these children had recurrent infections. Further studies were done by Smellie and Normand (1979) in which they reviewed the world literature to assess the development of renal scarring in previously normal kidneys. Of 1720 children studied, 83 developed renal scars. There was documentation of reflux in 80 of the children and infection in 79. The data

from the IRSC indicated that new renal scars developed in 12% of medically followed patients within 5 years; these scars were related to the number of episodes of pyelonephritis and the grade of reflux. The IRSC also designated a new classification of renal damage, parenchymal thinning; although reversible in some patients, it also resulted in renal scars in others (Olbing et al., 1992). Thus, the overwhelming clinical and experimental evidence is that renal scarring occurs primarily in association with severe reflux and infection and that the immature kidney is particularly susceptible. Thus, reflux, infection, and age are important risk factors for the pediatric population. The risk factors for an individual within this group further include bladder defense mechanisms and bacterial and host interrelationships.

EFFECTS OF REFLUX
Glomerular and Tubular Function

The effect of reflux on renal function is most analogous to that of partial ureteral obstruction in that tubular function is affected earlier than glomerular function. Reflux occurs in a retrograde fashion, and the increased pressure is felt first by the most distal nephron. The effect of reflux is difficult to distinguish from that of associated urinary tract infection. Defects in concentrating ability have been demonstrated in refluxing children with sterile urine, although almost all have had past histories of urinary tract infection (Walker et al., 1973). In experimental animals, the effect of infection on concentrating ability is felt no longer than 6 weeks after the infection is eradicated (Kaye and Rocha, 1970). The defects in concentrating ability in refluxing children are persistent even while the urine is sterile for long periods of time. Further, the concentrating defect is inversely proportional to the grade of reflux (Table 48-2). In many refluxing patients, there is improvement in concentrating ability after the reflux disappears. Impairment of concentration ability may be related to the anti–antidiuretic hormone (ADH) effect of increased medullary prostaglandin E (PGE) levels in patients with severe vesicoureteral reflux (Walker and Garin, 1990). Other parameters of tubular function, such as fractional excretion of sodium and magnesium, also may be affected (Kekomaki and Walker, 1988).

Glomerular function is usually not affected unless there has been parenchymal damage, and decreases in glomerular function are proportional to the amount of parenchymal loss. In the International Reflux Study there was no deterioration in glomerular function as measured by serum creatinine nor was there any decrease in glomerular filtration rate when measured by chromium-labeled ethylenediaminetetracetic acid (Smellie, 1992). Berg (1992) measured glomerular filtration rate and renal plasma flow in a large number of children with renal scarring and VUR. He found that decreases in renal function correlated with the degree of renal scarring, with decreased renal function being the most significant in those with bilateral, small, scarred kidneys.

Renal Growth

Small kidneys associated with reflux may have that morphology for a variety of reasons. Some kidneys may be small because of developmental arrest associated with, but not caused by, reflux. Expected renal growth is variable in this group of patients. Other small kidneys have acquired failure to grow related to reflux. Ambrose and colleagues (1980) reviewed the pathologic findings from kidney specimens of 63 patients with reflux and found a histologic pattern consistent with pyelonephritis in 51 (81%). Ibsen and co-workers (1977) found a relationship between the growth of the kidney and the persistence of reflux. In their study, patients with long-term reflux had kidneys that did not grow as well as normal. In contrast, Smellie and associates (1981) found that most refluxing kidneys grew at a normal rate if infection were controlled with prophylactic antibacterials. In 100 of 111 kidneys from 70 children who were followed for reflux, renal growth was normal. In the 11 kidneys in which growth was impaired, recurrent urinary tract infection was a problem in 10. McRae and co-workers (1974) found that kidneys with lesser degrees of reflux grew normally, but those with severe grades of reflux did not. Two studies have indicated that even small kidneys with significant renal scarring can grow after reflux resolves (Carson et al., 1982; Willscher et al., 1976). A recent study was, however, less encouraging with regard to the potential for renal growth (Shimada et al., 1988), showing that 75% of small kidneys remained small and that catch-up renal growth was the exception rather than the rule.

Physical Growth

Dwoskin and Perlmutter (1973) noticed in their series of patients that children with reflux tended to be in the lower-weight percentile groups. They reasoned that growth parameters should be measured in following children with reflux. Although no longstanding growth studies have been done in a large series of refluxing patients, Merrell and Mowad (1979) did find improvement in physical growth after reflux was surgically corrected in 35 patients. Sutton and Atwell (1989) compared physical growth while children with VUR were on medical therapy and also found that growth improved after subsequent reimplantation.

Hypertension

Refluxing patients with scarred kidneys are at greater risk for development of hypertension as young adults. Patients without renal scarring are probably not at any greater risk of becoming hypertensive than the normal population. Savage and co-workers (1978) found that elevated renins in patients with scarred kidneys may be an indicator for the eventual development of hypertension. Wallace and associates (1978) evaluated 166 patients who had successful reimplantation of the ureter for reflux and found 12.8% who were hypertensive 10 years after surgery. All of these hypertensive patients had renal scarring, and in a high percentage it was bilateral. Torres and colleagues (1983) evaluated 67 adults with bilateral reflux and found that 23 (34%) were hypertensive, most of whom had bilateral renal scarring or renal insufficiency. In the International Reflux Study only one patient developed hypertension in 5 years of follow-up (Smellie, 1992).

Renal Failure

Renal failure that develops with reflux and renal scarring occurs in a significant number of patients. It is difficult to determine the actual percentage of patients with scarred kidneys who will develop renal failure, but those with bilateral scarring and hypertension may be at particular risk. Bailey (1979) has indicated that as many as 30% of children may have end-stage renal failure because of reflux. That figure is higher than my personal experience. In the Children's Transplant Program at the University of Florida, between 7% and 10% of 110 children had scarred kidneys in which reflux may have been a factor. There were some, however, who had reflux unrelated to their renal failure, presenting with diseases such as nail-patella syndrome or asphyxiating thoracic dystrophy. The presence of a glomerulopathy associated with reflux and renal failure has been suggested by Kincaid-Smith (1979). Proteinuria was a common finding in the Mayo Clinic series in patients who had renal scarring and renal insufficiency (Torres et al., 1983). Although some have estimated that reflux may be a factor in as many as 20% to 30% of adults with end-stage renal failure, data were presented in 1977 from the

Transplant Registry and a large, single institution study that indicated an incidence of chronic pyelonephritis of 13% and 10%, respectively (Salvatierra and Tanagho, 1977). A recent review and update of infants with severe VUR followed for a long period indicates 80% have either unilateral or bilateral renal scarring, with 29% of these having either renal insufficiency, proteinuria, or hypertension (Bailey et al, 1992). Avant (1991) has stated that the mechanism for renal insufficiency or failure might be focal glomerular sclerosis brought on by renal hyperfiltration.

MANAGEMENT OF REFLUX

One of the most difficult decisions regarding the child with vesicoureteral reflux is deciding between medical and surgical management. Philosophy and bias with an admixture of fact combine in making the decision. Whether the child is managed medically or surgically is more often dependent on these intangible factors than on a rational review of what are reasonable certainties. If one believes that sterile reflux causes damage, that children are unlikely to outgrow reflux, and that long-term antibacterials have significant risks, the option is more likely to be surgical therapy. If, on the other hand, one believes that only infected reflux causes damage and that children are likely to outgrow reflux with little risk from prophylactic medication, medical treatment is the more likely option. Despite the fact that there are many unanswered questions about the natural history of reflux, there are some reasonable observations that, if considered, will allow us to make a rational decision.

1. *Reflux will disappear spontaneously in many children.* Spontaneous disappearance of reflux has been suggested by studies in both children and animals (Roberts and Riopelle, 1977; Shopfner, 1970). The disappearance is related to the age of the child and degree of reflux. Duckett (1983) reports that in his experience 63% of grade II, 53% of grade III, and 33% of grade IV reflux will resolve spontaneously if infection is controlled. This study did not differentiate between unilateral and bilateral reflux. Edwards and coworkers (1977) found that reflux resolved spontaneously in 85% of children with ureters of normal caliber on IVU. In children admitted to the Birmingham Reflux Study Group (1983) with severe reflux, 26% had either total or partial significant resolution within 2 years. Skoog and associates (1987) found that grades I, II, and III reflux had very similar disappearance curves when followed for a long period of time, and that by 5 years of age the reflux was gone in all but a small percentage of these patients. Arant (1992) found that in patients with grade I to III reflux, it had resolved in 5 years in 67%, decreased in 22%, and increased in 2%. All of these data give strong support to the concept that there is resolution of grades I to III

reflux in many growing children and indeed no evidence to refute it. The more pronounced grade III and grade IV reflux, especially when bilateral, has much less chance of resolution. The IRSC showed that patients with unilateral grade IV reflux had resolution 61% of the time, but in those with bilateral grade IV or grade IV-grade III combinations the resolution in 5 years was only 9% (Tamminen-Mobius et al., 1992). Grade V reflux is unlikely to resolve spontaneously. Reflux of this magnitude behaves quite differently from lower grades and is most often referred to as *refluxing megaureter*. The natural history of reflux after maturity is not known. Available evidence would indicate that primary reflux is unlikely to spontaneously resolve in older adolescents and adults.

2. *Sterile reflux is unlikely to cause renal damage. Persistent reflux of infected urine causes renal damage.* Despite the experiments in swine by Hodson and colleagues (1975), renal scarring rarely occurs in refluxing children if a sterile urine is maintained. The development of renal scarring in closely followed patients is almost always associated with breakthrough infections. Those incidents where sterile reflux is implicated in children are almost always anecdotal and retrospective. The only exception may be in grade V reflux, and in this situation, the refluxing megaureter is more analogous physiologically and pathologically to obstructive uropathy.

3. *Long-term antibacterial therapy is usually safe and well tolerated by children.* This fact does not imply that there is no risk, but simply that the risk is small. The physician who implements long-term therapy must monitor the patient to see if there are side effects. Nitrofurantoin frequently causes gastrointestinal distress in children and may be better tolerated in the macrocrystal form. Rare reactions include interstitial pneumonitis or pulmonary fibrosis, exfoliative dermatitis, hemolytic anemia, and peripheral neuropathies. Sulfa and trimethoprim-sulfa combinations have been associated with blood dyscrasias, Stevens-Johnson syndrome, gastrointestinal symptoms, and central nervous system abnormalities. Both drugs may cause allergic reactions. Monitoring requires alerting the patient and family to possible side effects and promptly ceasing therapy should severe side effects occur. Despite the rare side effect in isolated patients, most tolerate long-term antibacterial therapy for years with no problem. This minimal risk of medical therapy must be compared with the real and demonstrated risk of renal scarring and sepsis if antibacterials are not instituted. In the male with reflux, the risk of developing a urinary tract infection may be small enough to moderate the long-term therapy. In the older female with low-grade reflux, a similar course may be considered. In younger children followed with significant reflux, continuous antibac-

terial therapy will most likely provide protection against the development of renal scarring. Unfortunately, there is a high rate of noncompliance and being lost to follow-up in medically managed patients (Weiss et al., 1992).

4. *Most associated bladder abnormalities do not preclude the possibility that reflux may disappear spontaneously.* Such abnormalities include bladder diverticula, duplex ureter, cystitis cystica (cystitis follicularis), urethral obstruction, and uninhibited bladder. Although any of these abnormalities may lessen the chance for spontaneous disappearance, they do so in unpredictable fashion and are not contraindications to medical management (Aladjem et al., 1980; Peppas et al., 1991).

5. *Ureteral reimplantation surgery has a high success rate.* These success rates are discussed later in the chapter in the section dealing with surgical treatment; however, one should expect success rates of 95% to 98% in patients with normal-caliber ureters and normal bladders. Coleman and McGovern (1979) have indicated that success rates decline as the ureter and bladder become more abnormal. In their large series, the success rate in females was 98% when both bladder and ureter were normal, 54% when the ureter was markedly dilated, and only 40% when both the bladder and ureter were abnormal. The success rate for the American arm of the IRSC was 99% (Duckett et al., 1992).

6. *Reflux that persists in adolescence or adulthood is unlikely to disappear spontaneously.* Reflux in male adults may or may not be associated with significant morbidity. Reflux in adult females does carry a significant morbidity, particularly during pregnancy (Snyder and Duckett, 1981). This morbidity has been believed to occur only in pregnant females with reflux, but Austenfeld and Snow (1988) showed that in pregnant women with a past history of resolved vesicoureteral reflux, there was a higher rate of spontaneous abortion. This may or may not be related to associated urinary tract infection.

From the previous statements one can reach an assessment of the individual patient in deciding the course of management. Certainly for lower grades of reflux in infants and younger children every opportunity should be given for the reflux to disappear spontaneously. In those in whom it has not disappeared by late childhood or adolescence, consideration should be given to surgical therapy depending on the sex, likelihood of future infections, patient reliability for follow-up, and patient interest in a resolution to the problem. Patients with severe reflux that represent the more severe varieties of grade IV or V usually will require surgical management as the initial form of management. An exception to this is in the neonate where dramatic improvement can occasionally occur

in what appears to be severe reflux. This may be related to the increased compliance of the newborn collecting system. Patients with breakthrough urinary tract infections, particularly when associated with fever and regardless of the grade of reflux, probably should have ureteral reimplantation. Patients with high grade III and grade IV reflux who can be maintained with sterile urine can be followed for a time, but the failure of resolution in those with bilateral reflux is a strong factor in favor of earlier rather than later reimplantation.

Prospective Reflux Studies
International Reflux Study

An international collaborative study (Report of the International Reflux Study Committee, 1981) was initiated in 1979 that included centers in both Europe and the United States. The objective of the study was to answer the question as to whether surgical or medical therapy was the best for moderate to severe reflux. In the study, patients under 9 years of age with grade IV reflux were randomized to either medical or surgical therapy. Patients who had duplex ureters, a ureter entering a diverticulum, male urethral obstruction, neurogenic bladder, urinary tract calculus disease, and anorectal abnormalities were excluded. Children randomized to medical therapy were placed on prophylactic antibacterials, and the urine was monitored by culture at 3-month intervals. Radiologic studies, including IVU and contrast cystogram, were done at set intervals. The parameters followed include presence of hypertension, number of positive results for urinary tract infections, development of renal scarring, renal growth, and renal function. Children randomized to medical therapy who developed breakthrough urinary tract infections (two episodes of pyelonephritis) were allowed to switch to surgical therapy. For the safety and best interest of the patient, the entire study was reviewed frequently by an external monitoring committee. The principal conclusions of this study are as follows:

1. Bilateral grade IV reflux was unlikely to resolve within 5 years.
2. There was no difference in renal scarring between patients randomized to surgery or medical therapy at 5 years. There was a difference, however, in the pattern of scarring in that the scars in the surgical group occurred early, whereas those in the medical group were evenly distributed throughout the study. Also the incidence of clinical pyelonephritis was much higher in the medical group. Thus, since a number of medically followed patients still had reflux, it might be expected that scarring would be higher in two similarly constructed groups followed for another 5 years.

3. The surgical success rate, particularly when done by an experienced surgeon, was quite high.

Other Studies

Other independent investigators have performed studies that have attempted to answer these same questions, although not in a randomized manner. King (1977) began a clinical trial in 1963 that attempted to see if patients could be managed for long periods of time on medical therapy. After 10 years, he had 210 patients with 323 refluxing units followed for between 4 and 10 years on medical therapy. His conclusions were that reflux stopped in 51% and that 23% required surgery. The remainder were still being followed with their reflux without apparent harm to their kidneys. Those who required surgery did so because of either persistent breakthrough infection or because they had reached maturity. Edwards and colleagues (1977) followed 75 children with varying degrees of reflux and found a high likelihood of spontaneous disappearance except in patients with severe grades of reflux and intercurrent infections. Renal scarring only developed in children with infection. Dunn and co-workers (1978) attempted to follow medically 136 children with reflux, but they had failure in 96 children because of infection or worsening of the radiologic picture. Of these 96 children, 32 were believed to have worsened on IVP. It was the authors' conclusion that the more severe grades of reflux require surgical therapy.

The Birmingham Reflux Study (1983) has attempted to answer some of the same questions in a randomized study smaller in scope but with similarities to the International Reflux Study. Their report showed no clear advantage to either surgical or medical therapy in patients with reflux.

Medical Management
Choice of Antibacterial

The antibacterial chosen should be one that combines the following: is the least risk to the patient, has high urine concentrations, minimally alters vaginal-perineal flora, has a broad spectrum of action against most gram-negative bacteria, is available and well tolerated in liquid forms, and is available at minimal cost to the patient. No one antibacterial satisfies all of these criteria. Those in common usage are sulfas, sulfa-trimethoprim combinations, and nitrofurantoin. The antibacterial should be used in its lowest dose sufficient to keep the urine infection-free. Most often the initial prophylactic dose is one half to one third of the therapeutic dose. An example would be the use of 5 ml of sulfamethoxazole-trimethoprim suspension at bedtime rather than the normal twice-daily dosage. The lower prophylactic dose usually causes fewer side effects. The prophylactic medication should be given at bedtime if possible since it is that period when the child will retain the urine the longest and will more likely develop infection. All antibacterials should be continued as long as the patient is refluxing. Once the reflux has resolved, the antibacterials can be stopped. The patients will continue to require monitoring to make sure that infection does not recur. Recurrent infections are common after reflux resolves (Govan and Palmer, 1969), although most will now be associated with lower trct symptomatology rather than clinical pyelonephritis. Decter and co-workers (1988) have shown that males with reflux do equally well managed with observation alone as with antibacterial therapy. Thus, in this group no antibacterial therapy, but frequent monitoring of urine is an option.

Clinic Visits

Children with reflux should probably be seen at no more than 3-month intervals. Clinic visits should establish any history consistent with intercurrent infection or of reaction to the antibacterial. Physical examination should record parameters of physical growth and blood pressure. Laboratory studies should include urinalysis and culture at each visit, hemogram and white blood cell count at 6-month intervals, and serum creatinine clearance yearly. These tests represent only the minimum studies and must be altered depending on the condition of the child.

Home Culture Program

To ensure that the urine remains sterile, a number of methods have been developed to allow the parents to assess the urine at home. Our clinic has been most successful using the Bactercult method (Fennell et al., 1976). This method allows the parent to culture the urine at frequent intervals (1 to 3 months) at a fraction of the cost of coming to the clinic. Negative cultures are the most valuable. Positive cultures should be confirmed in the clinic and treatment altered accordingly. Additional advantages are that the child can be cultured when having an upper respiratory tract infection to make sure that the fever is not urinary tract in origin, and other siblings can be screened to see if they have positive urine cultures.

Frequency of Radiologic Studies

Intravenous urography or ultrasound should be performed initially in the infection-free patient and repeated at intervals of 18 to 24 months, but sooner, however, if repeated infections intervene.

Contrast VCUG is used as the initial study so as to grade the reflux and ascertain any associated bladder pathology. Subsequent studies should be done at about 12- to 18-month intervals. After the initial study is used for grading, subsequent studies may be done using radionuclide. Some have recommended two normal studies before the assumption that reflux is resolved; however, one study is usually adequate unless the patient continues to have febrile infections. DMSA scintigraphy is probably the most sensitive indicator of renal scarring and gives excellent assessment of differential renal function. It is indicated as both a baseline and for follow-up in patients with higher grades of reflux and when renal scarring is suspected on IVU or renal ultrasound. Its high cost and lack of universal availability have not allowed it to replace ultrasound or IVU.

Surgical Management

The evolution of surgical procedures designed to correct vesicoureteral reflux has been so successful that it has set a standard against which to measure medical therapy. Part of the reason is that the energies of the physicians treating the disease have been used more to seek a surgical resolution than to find out the natural history. Initially, there was a tremendous bias that reflux was deleterious, and indeed, it can be. Because it was discovered, however, that its effects, particularly if the urine was sterile, were unlikely to cause immediate damage, medical therapy became more appropriate. Nonetheless, the ingenuity shown by the pioneer surgeons in correcting reflux set a basis on which was built the framework of the specialty of pediatric urology.

Virtually all of the surgical procedures are based on one common denominator—the creation of a submucosal tunnel. Although some transplant urologists have had success with end-to-side ureterovesical anastomosis, this procedure is not used for primary reflux. Descriptions of surgical procedures currently in use must include a review of those procedures that were important in its evolution. Winter (1969) has nicely reviewed these historical aspects of reimplantation.

Extravesical Ureteroneocystostomy

Historical Aspects.—In 1896 Witzel was one of the first to develop an innovative procedure for tunneling the ureter (Payne, 1908). He accomplished this procedure by folding the bladder wall over the ureter after having first done an end-to-side anastomosis. Coffey's (1911) procedure was intended primarily for ureteral sigmoid anastomosis, but it also has been used by some for the bladder. In its original form, there was no anastomosis of the ureteral stump to the bladder mucosa; rather the distal ureter was pulled through a mucosal stab wound and anchored in the bladder with a large suture. It is unclear as to who

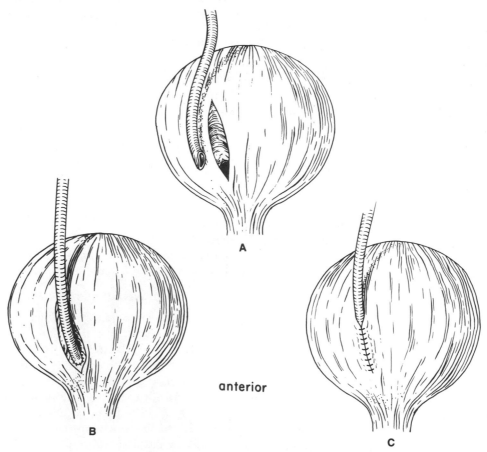

anterior

FIG. 48-11
Coffey's modification of anterior bladder reimplantation.

developed the refinement that allows the distal ureter–bladder mucosa anastomosis; however, it has been done by many surgeons in this manner and is described in transplant patients. The technique consists of first creating a 5-cm incision on the anterior lateral bladder wall through muscle. This incision is made with sharp dissection and is carried down until the mucosa bulges. At this point, a stab wound is made distally in the mucosa (Fig. 48-11, *A*), and the distal ureter is anastomosed to the mucosal edges with a fine absorbable suture (Fig. 48-11, *B*). The muscle is then closed over the ureter (Fig. 48-11, *C*). In 1910 Mann presented a technique discussed by Peterson (1918) that creates an extravesical submucosal tunnel by the development of a bridge of bladder muscle under which the ureter is passed.

Lich-Grégoir Repair.—The Lich-Grégoir repair (Grégoir and Van Regemorter, 1964; Lich et al., 1961) is an extravesical procedure for the repair of reflux developed almost simultaneously in both the United States by Lich and associates and in Europe by Grégoir. The procedure has enjoyed great popularity in Europe. Despite the initial concerns by Hendren (1974) and others that the procedure had a high recurrence of reflux, such has not been the experience of European surgeons or those who persisted with the procedure in this country. In this procedure, as described by Marberger and colleagues (1978), the patient is placed in the supine position with a Foley catheter in the bladder. The bladder is filled to moderate distention. A transverse incision is made above the pubis, and routine perivesical exposure is obtained. The obliterated hypogastric vessel is identified, ligated, and divided and the ureter identified where the obliterated vessel crosses it. The ureter is gently dissected free and isolated with a vessel loop. The ureter is dissected toward the bladder, carefully preserving the major vascular pedicles. With the straightest course of ureter marked against the posterior bladder wall, the bladder muscle is divided from the ureterovesical junction cephalad for a distance of

approximately 5 cm (Fig. 48-12, *A*). Bleeding points in the bladder muscle are electrocoagulated. Rents in the mucosa should be meticulously avoided but, if made, can be repaired with a fine running absorbable suture. The ureter is placed in the created furrow and the muscle closed over it with appropriate absorbable interrupted suture, such as 2-0 to 3-0 chromic catgut or 3-0 or 4-0 polyglycolic acid (Fig. 48-12, *B*). Any angulation of the ureter must be prevented. The Foley catheter may be removed early in these cases. No stents are required, and a drain is left in the perivesical space for a few days. Bilateral reimplants may be done at the same operation. Duplex ureters are left in their common sheath and treated as a single ureter. Daines and Hodgson (1971) have described a modification of the Lich-Grégoir procedure with ureteral advancement. In this modification, an absorbable suture is placed distally through the muscle of the bladder wall and the adventitia of the distal ureter to fix the ureter at or close to the trigonal muscle. Zaontz and co-workers (1987) described using the Lich-Grégoir repair with ureteral advancement technique in 120 refluxing ureters with a success rate of 93%.

The success rate of the Lich-Grégoir procedure has been comparable with that of other contemporary procedures. The initial poor success of 40% by Hendren (1974) influenced other American surgeons. The reports from Europe, however, do indicate the merit of the procedure. Grégoir and Schulman (1977) reported excellent results in 31 of 35 patients (89%). In a series of 429 ureters, Marberger and colleagues (1978) reported a success rate of 97.7%. In ten ureters that had postoperative reflux, it spontaneously disappeared in two, and eight required a further reimplantation. Two cases of ureteral obstruction required surgery. Houle and co-workers (1992) described their results with extravesical reimplant in 65 ureters. Success rate was 100% for grade I to III reflux, 93% for grade IV reflux and 67% for grade V reflux. Temporary difficulty in bladder emptying occurred in 16% of patients requiring clean intermittent catheterization. The problem was worse with bilateral extravesical reimplantation. Wacksman and colleagues (1992) described their experience in 211 ureters. Included in this were six megaureters that required tapering and nine duplex ureters. No obstruction was encountered, and only one patient had persistent reflux.

The disadvantages of the Lich-Grégoir procedure are related primarily to its lack of adaptability should one have an unexpected finding. Since the bladder interior is not visualized, preoperative cystoscopy may be important to evaluate the position of the orifices, place intraoperative stents, and ascertain that there is not associated pathology, such as a bladder diverticulum. Associated bladder diverticula may be difficult to repair as part of the procedure. The procedure

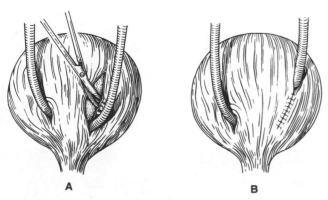

A   **B**

FIG. 48-12
Lich-Grégoir procedure; posterior aspect of bladder.

would be difficult in bladders of small capacity. Refluxing duplex ureters with associated pathology, such as ureterocele or ectopia, could not be managed with this technique.

Other Extravesical Reimplant Procedures.—The extravesical reimplant used by transplant surgeons is similar to that described by Coffey (1911). In a technique described by MacKinnon and associates (1968) and more recently by Wasnick and co-workers (1981), the distal ureter is simply brought through a mucosal stab wound with a fixing suture through the muscle wall. I prefer the more deliberate step of anastomosis of the distal ureter to the mucosal incision with a running 5-0 polyglycolic acid suture. Regardless, the success rate of this procedure in transplant patients is comparable with that of intravesical procedures.

Combined Intravesical and Extravesical Repair of Reflux

Historical Aspects.—The Manod-Vanverts repair, reported in 1908, was one of the first to use a combined intravesical and extravesical approach to reimplantation of the ureter (Councill, 1956). The operation was performed by extravesically dividing and ligating the ureter and passing the distal ureter through a stab wound in the bladder just above the previous orifice.

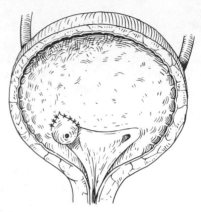

FIG. 48-13
Manod-Vanverts cuff procedure.

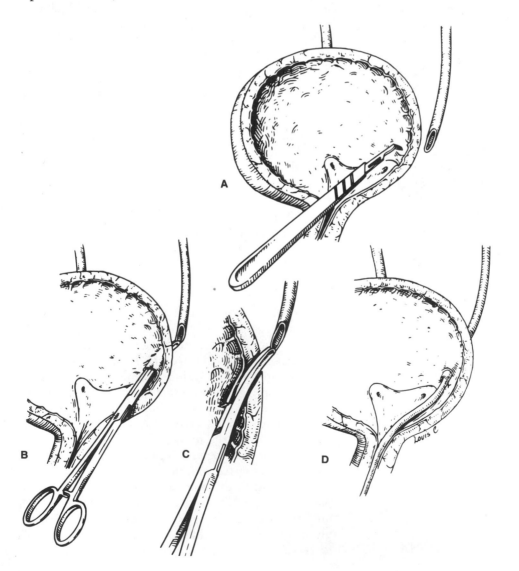

FIG. 48-14
Jewitt's procedure.

A cuff, which it was hoped would prevent reflux, was then developed (Fig. 48-13). This procedure led to a large number of cuff procedures by many prominent urologists, including Councill, Vest, Boyce, and Goodwin (Winter, 1969). Some of these procedures were done in experimental animals and some in patients, but in neither group were they very successful and they were soon abandoned.

Jewitt (1955) published a method of combined intravesical and extravesical repair of reflux that is similar to a procedure many urologists use today. This repair is used less commonly for primary reflux surgery, but is the procedure often used for a reimplant secondary to iatrogenic injury or trauma. The more modern version of the Jewitt repair has been called "ureteroneocystostomy simplex" by Poynter and associates (1967). Procedures very similar to the Jewitt, used in both refluxing and transplant patients, have been referred to as "Politano-Leadbetter repairs," which is inaccurate nomenclature since the latter is an entirely intravesical procedure. The Jewitt procedure is performed through a lower abdominal incision. The refluxing ureter is identified, divided, and the stump ligated. A submucosal tunnel is developed above the old orifice with scissors, knife, or grooved dissector (Fig. 48-14, A). A large clamp is then placed in the tunnel and bluntly pushed obliquely through the posterior bladder wall (Fig. 48-14, B), and the distal end of the ureter is grasped and brought back through the tunnel (Fig. 48-14, C). The distal end of the ureter is cut obliquely and sutured to the mucosa and superficial bladder muscle (Fig. 48-14, D).

The procedure described by Thompson and Patton (1971) is also a combined procedure that involves dividing the ureter extravesically at the ureterovesical junction without ligation of the distal stump. The distal ureter is brought through the old hiatus, laid in a raw, opened, muscular bed, and sutured to the mucosa and muscle of the trigone. The portion of the procedure that brings the ureter through the old hiatus is similar to the procedure described many years later by Ahmed (1983) to circumvent the problems with a thick-walled bladder.

Paquin Ureteroneocystostomy.—The Paquin (1959) procedure is a combined extravesical and intravesical approach to reimplantation of the ureter. The operation had as its basis Paquin's measurement of submucosal tunnel length. In his studies of the ureter in children, he found that most normal children had a ratio of 5:1 submucosal tunnel length–ureteral diameter. He tried to re-create this normal condition in the development of this operation. The procedure is still used today by former students of Paquin and his successors.

The procedure, as described by Woodard and Keats (1973), uses a transverse, suprapubic incision. The ureter is first identified extravesically after ligating the obliterated hypogastric vessels. The ureter is mobilized from the iliac artery to its junction with the bladder. It is divided and ligated at the bladder by first placing traction on the ureter prior to clamping so that no refluxing ureteral stump remains. The peritoneum is dissected from the posterior bladder wall. An anterior midline incision is made in the bladder so that adequate exposure is obtained. The anticipated tunnel site is selected posteriorly and the plane developed with Metzenbaum scissors through the muscle until the scissors can be identified submucosally. At this point, with continued dissection with the Metzenbaum scissors, a submucosal plane is developed down toward the trigone. A transverse incision is made in the mucosa at the area of the new meatus (Fig. 48-15, A). A clamp is placed through the submucosal tunnel, exiting the new meatus, and an 8 F red Robinson catheter is grasped and brought back through the tunnel and hiatus. The distal end of the ureter is sewn to the top of the red Robinson catheter and then brought back through the tunnel, being careful not to twist the ureter. The distal end of the ureter is excised, spatulated, splayed open, and sewn to the trigone with fine absorbable suture (Fig. 48-15, B). Extravesically, the ureter is fixed to the bladder with several fine absorbable sutures. Drainage of the extravesical space is with Penrose or Jackson-Pratt drains. Small Silastic or polyethylene stents may be used, if desired, and

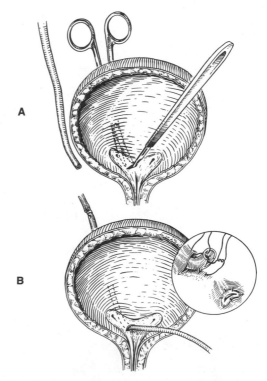

FIG. 48-15
Paquin's procedure.

the bladder is diverted with a urethral Foley or suprapubic catheter. The procedure lends itself well to be combined with a psoas hitch, and bilateral reimplants can be accomplished without difficulty.

The success rate of the procedure in the series of Woodward and Keats (1973) was 96%. Of 217 ureters, three had reflux and six had obstruction. Coleman and McGovern (1979) presented a large experience in which the success rate was much less when the ureter, bladder, or both were abnormal.

Intravesical Repair of Reflux

Suprahiatal Repair.—The Hess (1941) operation probably served as the basis for the Hutch I operation that was developed a decade later. The Hess operation was intended for distal ureteral stricture and yet embodied the same principles of creating a tunnel that are still used today.

Hutch (1952) presented the concept of the deleterious effects of reflux and at the same time an operation to correct the disease. The Hutch I operation was performed as an intravesical operation in which the mucosa and bladder muscle were divided above the level of the ureteral meatus for a distance of several centimeters in the line of the ureter (Fig. 48-16, *A*). The ureter is then retraced into the bladder and the

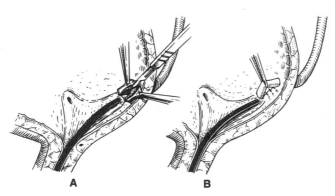

FIG. 48-16
The Hutch I procedure.

muscle and mucosa closed underneath the ureter (Fig. 48-16, *B*). The ureteral meatus is left undisturbed. The operation corrected the reflux in 83% of patients, but about 8% to 10% developed ureteral obstruction. Although for years the Hutch I was primarily of historical interest, it has been revived by Hackler (1977), who finds it a useful procedure in paraplegics. Evans and co-workers (1986) also have had commendable results in children with myelomeningocele.

The Mathisen (1964) procedure was developed as a combined intravesical and extravesical procedure but had its major component as an intravesical suprahiatal procedure and is important in the evolution of similar procedures done today. In this procedure a mucosal incision is made around the ureteral orifice and carried above the orifice for several centimeters. The muscular hiatus is divided in a cephalad direction so as to bring the ureter through a higher hiatus (Fig. 48-17, *A*). The muscular hiatus is tightened inferiorly with absorbable suture (Fig. 48-17, *B*). The ureter is then advanced and sewn distally to mucosa and muscle, following which the mucosal edges are closed over the ureter so as to form a tunnel (Fig. 48-17, *C*). Although the Mathisen procedure has received little notice, it is the original of almost all advancement procedures done today.

Politano-Leadbetter Repair.—The Politano-Leadbetter (1958) procedure is the most popular of the suprahiatal repairs and was probably the most common reimplant worldwide in the past.

The procedure is done through a short suprapubic incision. After adequate exposure, the bladder is opened through a vertical incision. The refluxing ureteral orifice is catheterized with an appropriate-size ureteral catheter or infant feeding tube. With a holding suture placed through the ureter, an incision is made around the orifice while traction is maintained on the holding suture by the surgeon and countertraction is maintained on the mucosa with fine, noncrushing forceps by the assistant (Fig. 48-18, *A*). The surgeon then develops a plane around the ureter and

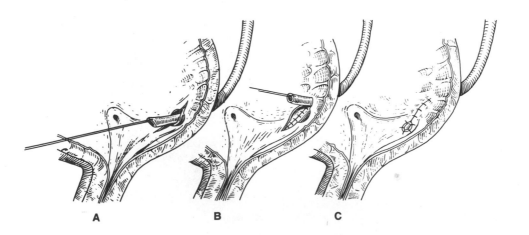

FIG. 48-17
Mathisen's procedure.

through the muscular wall of the bladder so that the ureter is freed from all of its muscular attachments. After the retrovesical space is entered, the ureter is dissected off of the peritoneum and the retroperitoneal fat with a cotton dissector. The retroperitoneal space can be directly visualized, if necessary, with a vein retractor (Fig. 48-18, *B*).

The submucosal tunnel is developed with tenotomy or Metzenbaum scissors (Fig. 48-18, *C*). If the bladder wall is badly scarred or adherent, the mucosa can be laid open to make this tunnel and later in the pro-

cedure reapproximated back over the ureter. The tunnel length should be five times the diameter of the ureter, and I prefer the ophthalmic calipers to make these measurements.

With adequate visualization in the retroperitoneal space and the line of the ureter, the new hiatus is created at the proximal end of the submucosal tunnel by incising onto the tip of a large right-angle clamp (Fig. 48-18, *D*). The traction suture is then grasped and the ureter brought through the new hiatus. The muscle of the old hiatus is closed with absorbable

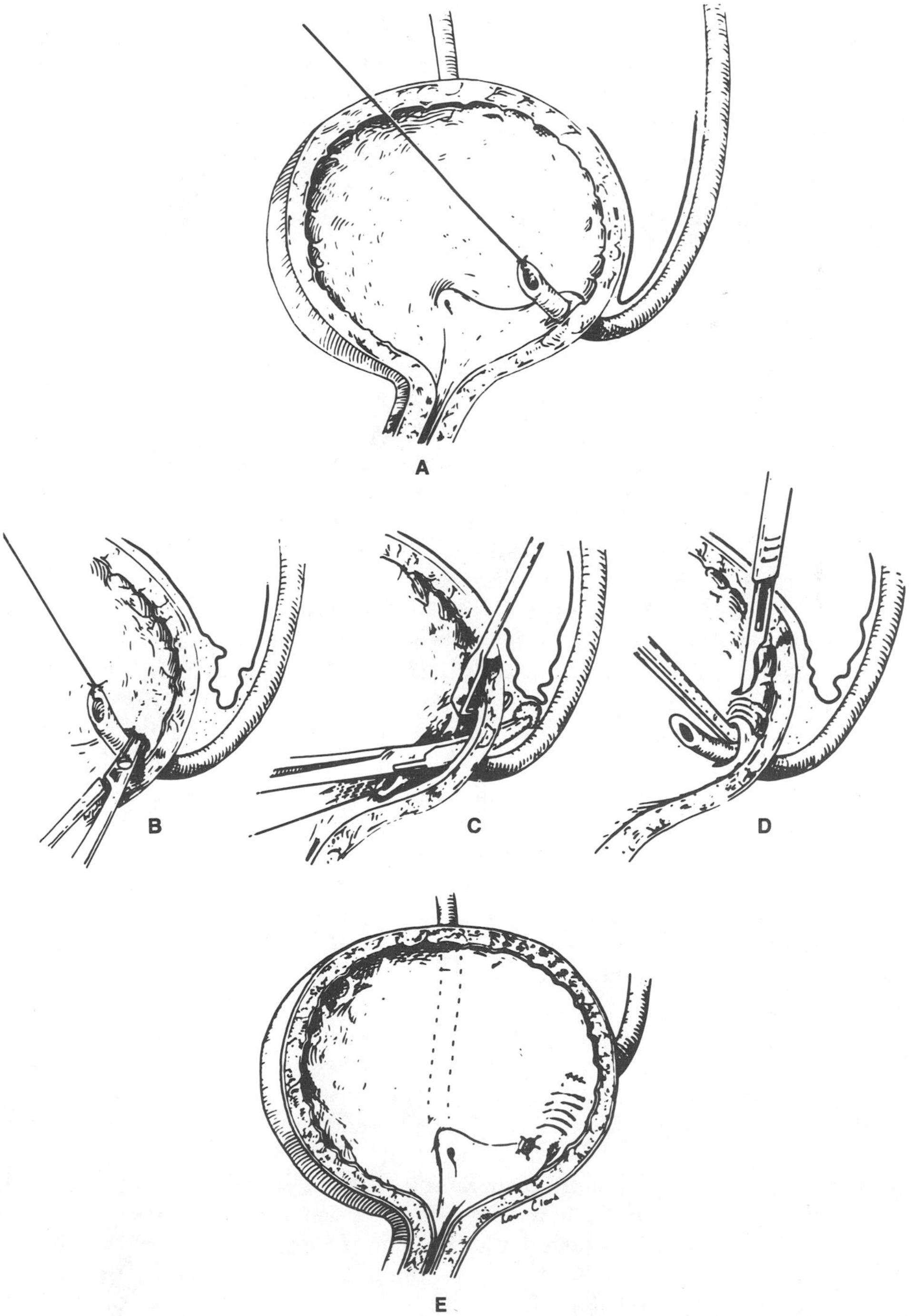

FIG. 48-18
Politano-Leadbetter procedure.

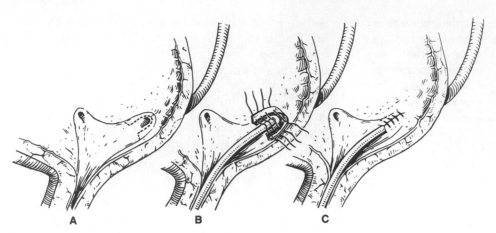

FIG. 48-19
Bischoff's procedure.

suture. The ureter is brought down through the new submucosal tunnel, the distal portion excised with Potts vascular scissors, and spatulated in its inferior margin. The distal ureteral orifice is then sewn to the mucosa at the site of the old orifice with interrupted fine absorbable suture, such as 5-0 polyglycolic acid suture (Fig. 48-18, *E*). The suture through the spatulated portion of the ureter should pick up muscle of the trigone so as to fix the distal ureter in this position. Both lateral sutures also may pick up small bites of bladder muscle. The mucosa at the proximal end of the tunnel is closed with fine absorbable suture, and the bladder is closed in layers. Urinary diversion is with the ureteral Foley or suprapubic catheter. The ureters may be stented with small catheters or feeding tubes depending on the preference of the surgeon.

The success of the Politano-Leadbetter procedure is comparable with other procedures, ranging between 97% and 99% (Brannon et al., 1973). The most severe complication has been ureteral obstruction because of kinking at the new muscular hiatus. If the new hiatus has too lateral a placement in the expandable portion of the bladder, hooking of the ureter may occur with a full bladder. Rarely, it has been reported that ureter has been brought through peritoneum or bowel wall (Tocci et al., 1976). These obstructions usually can be predicted by noting the ease with which a catheter will pass through the orifice to the kidney at the termination of the reimplantation. Any resistance to catheter passage should be interpreted as possible obstruction, and the site should be sought by extravesical exploration if necessary.

Infrahiatal Repair.—Almost all infrahiatal repairs have been advancement procedures; however, several have moved the ureteral meatus distal to the hiatus in other, unique ways. Bischoff (1957) described the creation of laterally based mucosal flaps (Fig. 48-19, *A*) that, when reapproximated over a ureteral stent, would move the meatus distally (Figs. 48-19, *B* and *C*). Witherington (1963) created mucosal flaps from above the hiatus (Fig. 48-20, *A*) which extended the meatus to a more caudad position (Fig. 48-20, *B*).

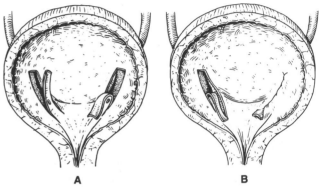

FIG. 48-20
Witherington's procedure.

Neither of these procedures has enjoyed wide use.

The Williams' operation was one of the first of the ureteral orifice advancement operations (Williams et al., 1961). The procedure did not involve significant mobilization of the ureter, which may have led to its abandonment. The procedure was performed by excising a distal wedge of mucosa (Fig. 48-21, *A*), mobilizing the orifice (Fig. 48-21, *B*), and sewing the orifice distally to the mucosa (Fig. 48-21, *C*). The Hutch (1963) II operation was another early advancement technique. In the first step of this operation, the ureteral orifice and a flap of distal mucosa were incised (Fig. 48-22, *A*). The ureter was then mobilized and distal mucosal flap excised (Fig. 48-22, *B*). Finally, the mucosal edges were reapproximated around the ureter and the orifice sewn in place distally (Fig. 48-22, *C*). Although the Hutch and Williams operations are not now used, they along with the Mathisen procedure, did spawn a number of other ureteral advancement techniques.

Glenn-Anderson Procedure.—The Glenn-Anderson (1967) procedure is most effective when the ureteral orifice is very laterally placed on the trigone. When the orifice is more medially placed on the trigone, the length of the submucosal tunnel may be limited by the distance between the orifice and bladder neck. In these instances the Allen (1973) proce-

FIG. 48-21
Williams' procedure.

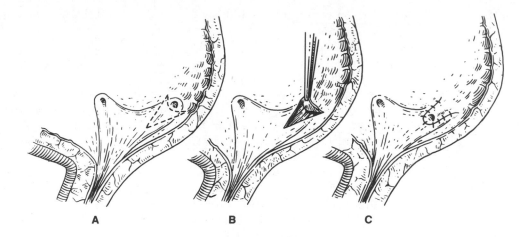

A   B   C

FIG. 48-22
The Hutch II procedure.

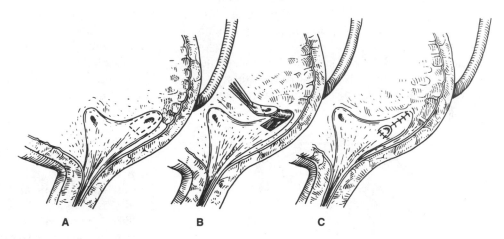

A   B   C

dure combines the hiatal enlargement of the Mathisen procedure with the advancement of the Glenn-Anderson extravesical procedure so that adequate tunnel length can be created.

The procedure is described as being done with the patient in the supine position and a sandbag or towel placed under the lower spine to thrust the bladder anteriorly, which also may help to flatten the posterior aspect of the bladder. Through a midline bladder incision, the ureter is identified and catheterized with a small feeding tube. An incision is made around the orifice and ureter mobilized by a combination of blunt and sharp dissection so that the distal 3 cm of ureter is freed (Fig. 48-23, *A*). A 15-mm submucosal tunnel is created from the hiatus toward the bladder neck. The muscular hiatus is tightened with appropriate absorbable sutures and the ureter passed through the tunnel, where the distal end is fashioned to appropriate length, spatulated, and sewn in place with absorbable sutures (Fig. 48-23, *B*). Stents may be used according to the preference of the surgeon and either ureteral or suprapubic drainage provided.

The advantage of this procedure is the low rate of obstruction resulting from it. The disadvantage is that reflux will still occur if patients are poorly selected and tunnel length is inadequate (Bellinger and Duck-

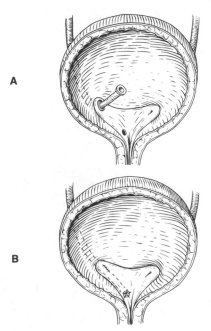

FIG. 48-23
Glenn-Anderson procedure.

ett, 1983). Proper selection of patients should result in success rates of 97% to 98%.

Cohen Procedure.—The Cohen (1975) procedure is a transverse advancement procedure that has achieved immense popularity since its introduction. The procedure has wide application but works particularly well in patients with small bladders.

The procedure involves placing the patient in the supine position with the buttocks and lower spine elevated by a towel. A transverse incision allows exposure to the bladder, which is opened through a midline incision. The refluxing ureter is catheterized with a small feeding tube and retracted with a suture ligature. A circumferential incision is made around the ureteral orifice, and the ureter is mobilized for 3 to 4 cm. A submucosal tunnel is developed across the trigone or bladder in such a fashion that the tunnel length is five times the diameter of the ureter (Fig. 48-24, A). The muscular hiatus is closed with absorbable sutures, and the ureter is brought through the new tunnel. The distal end of the ureter is excised and spa-

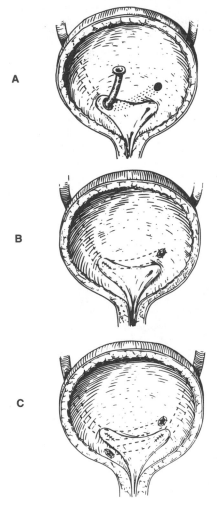

FIG. 48-24
Cohen's procedure.

tulated and the new meatus sutured with interrupted absorbable sutures (Fig. 48-24, B). Stenting and the method of diversion are left to the choice of the surgeon. Bilateral reimplantation also can be easily done (Fig. 48-24, C).

The advantage of this procedure is that an adequate tunnel length can be created to prevent reflux with very little chance of obstruction. Diverticula at the muscular hiatus have been reported (Ahmed and Tan, 1982), probably because of inadequate closing of the hiatus, although too tight a closure might result in obstruction. An additional complication is that these ureters can be difficult to catheterize by cystoscopy, although recent techniques have been described to accomplish it (Lamesch, 1981). The success rate of the Cohen reimplantation is 97% to 99%. Ahmed (1983) has proposed a technique that complements the Cohen reimplantation, which is of particular use in a thick-walled bladder. The procedure involves dividing the ureter at the hiatus (without dissecting the hiatus) and bringing the ureters through the hiatus before advancing them through a submucosal tunnel. The advantage of this technique is a decrease in incidence of obstruction.

Burbidge (1991) recently compared the results of reimplantation in 120 children, 50 of whom had a cross-trigonal repair and 70 of whom had a Politano-Leadbetter repair. The success rate was equal (97% to 98%) for both repairs, but a clear advantage to the Politano-Leadbetter repair was the ease of postoperative catheterization should that be required.

Other Recent Procedures.—Gil-Vernet (1984) presented a new technique of advancement of the ureteral orifice, with some similarities to the Williams' procedure, which does not mobilize the ureter but rather advances it toward the midline with a large absorbable suture. This procedure is not commonly done but De Gennaro (1991) reviewed their experience in 51 patients and found it successful in 91%.

Duplex Ureter Repair.—The procedure for repair of duplex ureters that I prefer is one that has the least likelihood of twisting or obstructing one of the ureters. The procedure is a combination of hiatal enlargement and advancement much in the fashion of Mathisen. The advancement can be either that described by Glenn and Anderson or by Cohen.

When this procedure is performed, the bladder is approached through a transverse abdominal incision. After the bladder is entered through a midline bladder incision, the relationship of the duplex orifices is noted. Most often the most cephalad and lateral orifice is to the lower pole and the smaller, most caudad and medial orifice is to the upper pole. The orifices are catheterized with feeding tubes. I prefer a 3.5 F feeding tube for the upper-pole ureter and a 5 F feeding tube for the lower-pole ureter (Fig. 48-25, A). The ureteral orifices are then tagged with a 4-0 monofilament figure-of-eight suture (Fig. 48-25, *B*). With traction on this holding suture, an incision is made around both orifices, and both ureters are mobilized. As the ureters are mobilized, the hiatus is enlarged (Fig. 48-25, *C*). The muscle of the hiatus is then closed with absorbable suture and distal tunnels made toward the bladder neck or across the trigone (Fig. 48-25, *D*). The two ureters may be separated in the most distal aspect or kept in continuity. Depending on which is done, either one or two separate submucosal tunnels are made, after which the ureters are brought through and sewn in place with interrupted fine absorbable suture (Fig. 48-25, *E*). The success of this procedure compares favorably with single ureters and is about 95%.

Associated Procedures.—Frequently other procedures must be done in conjunction with ureteral reimplantation to ensure a successful outcome. A commonly associated problem is a ureter that is dilated such that an adequate tunnel cannot be made. If the ureter is only minimally dilated (less than 8 to 10 mm), the area of the bladder base can be increased by doing a psoas hitch (Fig. 48-26). This procedure is also advantageous when the ureteral length has been compromised. Additionally, many urologists are arriving at the opinion that a psoas hitch, or some similar type of fixation of the bladder, should be used any time an extravesical repair is performed in order to fix the new hiatal area and prevent kinking of the ureter. Adequate exposure of the lower quadrant of the abdomen is important and can be achieved by making a slightly longer and more cephalad skin incision and mobilizing the peritoneal sac lateral to the rectus muscle much as one does in gaining exposure for a renal transplant. In a female, the obliterated hypogastric vessels and round ligament can be divided and the peritoneal sac mobilized so that the entire retroperitoneum in the lower quadrant is visualized. In the male, one should preserve the testicular vessels, which can be retracted with a vessel loop; however, if necessary, they also can be sacrificed with high ligation, allowing the testicle to survive off the vasa arterial supply. The bladder muscle is sutured to the psoas muscle with large absorbable suture that does not pass through the mucosa of the bladder. I prefer to do this procedure before making the submucosal tunnel. Some surgeons prefer to use nonabsorbable suture in attaching the bladder to the psoas muscle. If nonabsorbable suture is chosen, caution must be used in making sure the nonabsorbable suture does not enter the lumen of the bladder. In addition, one must be careful to avoid the genitofemoral nerve. Even if this nerve is avoided, patients will still frequently complain temporarily of pain in the thigh. The psoas hitch lends itself nicely to a Paquin type of reimplant (Middleton, 1980).

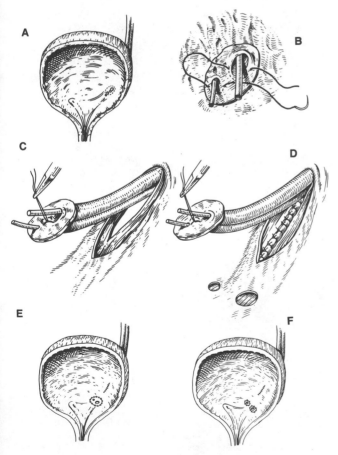

FIG. 48-25
Repair of duplex ureter.

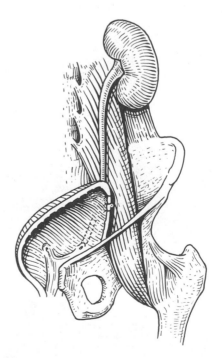

FIG. 48-26
Psoas hitch.

If the ureteral diameter is such that an adequate tunnel cannot be made, the ureter will need to be narrowed. In some instances the psoas hitch and ureteral remodeling are used in conjunction. Either the wedge resection (Hendren, 1969) or folding techniques (Kalicinski et al., 1977) can be used to narrow the ureter. Wedge resection is performed by excising a longitudinal strip of lower ureter maintaining the medial blood supply. The ureter is then reapproximated over a small stent with absorbable sutures prior to reimplantation. Folding techniques vary but have the common principle of decreasing both the luminal and exterior diameter of the ureter without any interruption of blood supply. Further details of these techniques are available in Chapter 47.

In instances where there is inadequate ureteral length, the Boari flap can be done as an alternative to the psoas hitch. A disadvantage of the Boari flap is that it is more difficult to achieve a nonrefluxing reimplantation. The transureteroureterostomy has had more success when a large gap has to be bridged and should probably be used when possible.

The occasional patient may require pyeloplasty for an associated ureteropelvic junction obstruction. Most often this obstruction is secondary to the reflux and will improve after reimplantation; therefore, that procedure should be done first. If obstruction is later identified by objective criteria (furosemide [Lasix] nuclear scan or percutaneous perfusion test), pyeloplasty may be indicated.

General Technical Considerations

A number of factors in technique that are essential to successful outcome of ureteral implantation are not included. Although the type of anesthesia is left to the anesthesiologist, it is important that adequate relaxation be maintained throughout the procedure. Unrelaxed patients tense the peritoneum behind the bladder, and exposure can be more difficult. An enema prior to surgery may be of help to void the patient with a large amount of stool in the rectum at the time of surgery. The bladder can be thrust forward and provide a more level base with a towel placed under the buttocks and lower sacrum.

The incision should be a transverse skin crease incision carried just beyond the lateral borders of the rectus muscle. The rectus fascia may be divided vertically in the midline to achieve adequate exposure. The classic Pfannenstiel approach with a transverse fascial incision will permit further lateral extension if needed. Minimal dissection extravesically is needed before the bladder is opened vertically in the midline down to 1 to 2 cm above the bladder neck. No manipulation of the interior of the bladder should be done with sponges or suction to avoid edema or mucosal bleeding. The Denis-Browne retractor is preferred for antireflux surgery in children (Fig. 48-27). Once this retractor is placed, all attempts should be made to avoid repeated moving and replacement since they cause mucosal hemorrhage and edema.

The bladder mucosa should be handled as minimally as possible and with atraumatic instruments. Holding sutures of 4-0 monofilament suture on atraumatic needles are advantageous and are used in figure-of-eight fashion through the refluxing orifice after first catheterizing it with a 3.5 F or 5 F feeding tube. Mucosal incisions around the orifice or in any location should be done with a sharp blade placed on a long knife

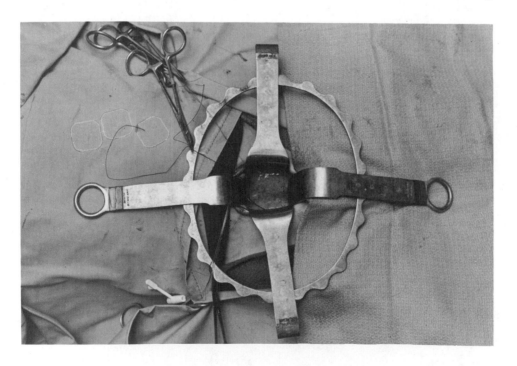

FIG. 48-27
Denis-Browne retractor.

handle. Dissection of the ureter should not skeletonize it. All muscle bundles must be cut and coagulated well away from the ureter. The ureter should be completely detached from its muscle attachments. The peritoneum must be pushed off the ureter with the dissector. Retraction through the hiatus with a vein retractor allows visualization of the peritoneum so that it can be pushed well away from the posterior bladder wall. Submucosal tunnels are made with fine scissors (Demartel or Metzenbaum). Division and spatulation of the ureter should be done with Demartel or Potts vascular scissors. The ureter should be handled either with a traction suture or a fine atraumatic vascular forceps, such as the Potts-Smith forceps. There should be no tension when the ureter is sutured to its new meatus, and any portion of ureter that appears to have a compromised blood supply should be excised back to normal tissue.

Stents should be soft and nonreactive and should not occlude the ureter. I prefer small Silastic stents or a 3.5 F or 5 F polyethylene feeding tube. Stents are most beneficial when the ureter has been tapered, when there has been extensive extravesical dissection, or when there is a great deal of edema. Their use remains at the discretion of the surgeon. Similarly, the diversion of the urine can be done with a urethral Foley or suprapubic tube. The former allows for early removal, and indeed some are reporting no diversion and a very short postoperative hospitalization (So et al., 1981). The suprapubic tube usually commits the patient to at least 1 week of diversion.

Follow-up and Management of Complications.— Postoperatively the patient is treated with a therapeutic dose of an antibacterial for several weeks and then maintained on antibacterial prophylaxis until it is demonstrated that there is no reflux. The common complications of reimplantation surgery are ureteral obstruction, persistent reflux, and bladder diverticulum. These complications usually are discovered on the postoperative radiologic studies. Ultrasound is now the best means to rule out postoperative obstruction and usually is done 6 to 12 weeks after surgery. The IVU and/or DMSA scintigraphy is used for specific indications in postoperative follow-up. If the initial ultrasound shows no obstruction, subsequent studies are done at 18- and 24-month intervals. Alternating IVU or DMSA scintigraphy and ultrasound can be used to follow the kidney structurally. If the patient has a 2-year film that shows no renal scarring, further measures of renal growth can be done with renal ultrasound. For patients with scarred kidneys, periodic assessment with IVU or DMSA scintigraphy will be useful in follow-up. The VCUG is done at 2 to 6 months postoperatively and will indicate whether the operation was successful in eradicating the reflux and also will show whether any diverticula are present.

Radionuclide cystography may be substituted for the contrast VCUG. If this study is normal, a repeat cystogram may be done in 1 year to be certain reflux has resolved. After that, no further cystograms are needed unless the patient develops recurrent infections.

Early mild obstruction on IVU or ultrasound is likely to improve and can be followed with serial ultrasound. If the obstruction is persistent, cystoscopic dilation of the intramural ureter with a ureteral catheter or balloon catheter may be of value. More severe obstruction, particularly when associated with J-hooking of a ureter through the peritoneum, will require exploration and repeat reimplantation.

Mild persistent reflux usually will disappear spontaneously and should be followed medically for at least 1 year unless the patient has breakthrough infections. The patient must be maintained on antibacterial prophylaxis. Severe persistent reflux will require reimplantation. In any patient who develops ureteral obstruction or reflux it is sage advice to reinvestigate the patient's original underlying symptoms to make sure the patient does not have a neurogenic bladder or dysfunctional voiding.

Bladder diverticula occur most often at the muscular hiatus. If small, they require no therapy. Larger diverticula may require surgical excision and necessitate reimplantation at the same time.

Periureteral Injection Techniques for Management of Reflux

The development of periureteral injection techniques to correct reflux has become an established procedure; however, its role in antireflux surgery is yet to be defined. Although the injection techniques have proved successful, there is still some question about the long-term results and the risk to the patient.

The injection of Teflon was developed in urology as a means to increase urethral resistance and to aid in the cure of incontinence. The basis for its use had been the relative safety of the procedure in otolaryngology. Success rates with periurethral injection for incontinence are quite reasonable (Walker, 1989), but serious objections were raised by Malizia and associates (1984), who showed both extensive granuloma formation locally, and migration of Teflon particles to vital organs. Despite the admonition regarding its use, procedures were developed for periureteral Teflon injection to cure reflux, and popularized by O'Donnell and Puri (1984). Subsequent presentations by Malizia and associates (1988), has shown similar problems with peri*ureteral* injection of Teflon as with peri*urethral* injection.

The concern about Teflon has led to the use of collagen as an injected substance to correct reflux. Although collagen does not appear to migrate and causes less foreign body reaction, there is a question about its long-term effectiveness since collagen may resorb over time. Other injection substances currently are undergoing both animal and human experimentation.

The success rate with injection techniques is 90%. There have been relatively few clinical complications reported. The indications for periureteral injection are ill-defined because of the possible long-term sequelae and the lack of an approved injectable substance by the Food and Drug Administration. However, if an acceptable substance is developed that can be injected with preservation of anatomic integrity and result in resolution of reflux in a majority of patients, it will almost surely change the course of reflux management. The likelihood would be that both parents and physicians would no longer accept long-term antimicrobial therapy if a safe outpatient surgical alternative were available.

Another experimental approach to surgical management of reflux is laparoscopic repair. Atala and coworkers (1993) described successful extravesical laparoscopic correction of experimentally induced reflux in pigs.

At this writing, one of the selected open operative procedures is the choice for patients with reflux who require surgical management, but the choice is likely to be altered in the future.

SUMMARY

Vesicoureteral reflux remains an enigmatic disease for which we have been more successful in defining a surgical cure than in understanding the natural history of the disease process. Longitudinal studies, such as the International Reflux Study, will continue to provide answers to some of our questions regarding the natural history of reflux. They also will raise new questions to be answered by future generations of investigators. Nonetheless, there is light at the end of the tunnel, and we are coming closer to providing answers to those queries posed by Keyes at the beginning of this chapter.

Acknowledgment

I would like to acknowledge Louis Clark, who did the artwork for this chapter.

REFERENCES

Ahmed S: Application of the pull-through technique of transverse advancement ureteral reimplantation. *J Urol* 1983; 129:787.

Ahmed S, Tan H: Complications of transverse advancement ureteral reimplantation. *J Urol* 1982; 127:970.

Akerlund A, Ahlstedt S, Hanson L, et al: Antibody responses in urine and serum against *Escherichia coli* O antigen in childhood urinary tract infection. *Acta Pathol Microbiol* 1979; 87:29.

Aladjem M, Boichis H, Hertz M, et al: The conservative management of vesicoureteral reflux: a review of 121 children. *Pediatrics* 1980; 65:78.

Allen TD: Modification of the ureteral advancement procedure for vesicoureteral reflux. *South Med J* 1973; 66:305.

Allen TD: Vesicoureteral reflux as a manifestation of dysfunctional voiding. In Hodson J, Kincaid-Smith P (eds): *Reflux Nephropathy*. New York, Masson Publishing USA, 1979, pp 171-180.

Alon U, Berant M, Pery M: Intravenous pyelography in children with urinary tract infection and vesicoureteral reflux. *Pediatrics* 1989; 83:332.

Ambrose SA, Parrott TS, Woodard JR, et al: Observations on the small kidney associated with vesicoureteral reflux. *J Urol* 1980; 123:349.

Anderson PA, Jantausch BA, Rushton HG, et al: Host-parasite interactions in urinary tract infections. *Dialogues Pediatr Urol* 1994; 17:Number 2.

Arant BS: Vesicoureteral reflux and renal injury. *Am J Kidney Dis* 1991; 17:491.

Arant BS: Medical management of mild and moderate vesicoureteral reflux: follow-up studies of infants and children. Preliminary report of Southwest Pediatric Nephrology Study Group. *J Urol* 1992; 146:1683.

Askari A, Belman AB: Vesicoureteral reflux in black girls. *J Urol* 1982; 127:747.

Atala A, Kavoussi LR, Goldstein DS, et al: Laparoscopic correction of vesicoureteral reflux. *J Urol* 1993; 150:748.

Austenfeld MS, Snow BW: Complications in pregnancy in women after reimplantation of vesicoureteral reflux. *J Urol* 1988; 140:1103.

Bailey RR: The relationship of vesicoureteral reflux to urinary tract infection and chronic pyelonephritis-reflux neuropathy. *Clin Nephrol* 1973; 1:132.

Bailey RR: Sterile reflux: is it harmless? In Hudson J, Kincaid-Smith P (eds): *Reflux Nephropathy*. New York, Masson Publishing USA, 1979, pp 334-339.

Bailey RR, Lynn KL, Smith AH: Long-term follow-up of infants with gross vesicoureteral reflux. *J Urol* 1992; 148:1709.

Baker R, Maxted W, Maylath J, et al: Relation of age, sex, and infection to reflux: data indicating high spontaneous cure rate in pediatric patients. *J Urol* 1966; 95:27.

Bellinger MF, Duckett JW: Vesicoureteral reflux: a comparison of non-surgical and surgical management. In Hodson J (ed): *Reflux Nephropathy Update*. Basel, S Karger, 1983, pp 81-93.

Berg UB: Long-term followup of renal morphology and function in children with recurrent pyelonephritis. *J Urol* 1992; 148:1715.

Bernstein J, Arant BS: Morphological characteristics of segmental renal scarring on vesicoureteral reflux. *J Urol* 1992; 148:1712.

Birmingham Reflux Study Group: Prospective trial of operative versus non-operative treatment of severe vesicoureteral reflux: two years observation in 96 children. *Br Med J* 1983; 2:171.

Bischoff PF: Megaureter. *Br J Urol* 1957; 29:46.

Blane CE, DiPietro MA, Zerin JM, et al: Renal sonography is not reliable screening examination for vesicoureteral reflux. *J Urol* 1993; 150:752.

Blank E, Girdany BR: Prognosis with vesicoureteral reflux. *Pediatrics* 1971; 48:782.

Brannon W, Oschner MG, Rosencrantz DR, et al: Experiences with vesicoureteral reflux. *J Urol* 1973; 109:46.

Brock WA, Smolko MJ, Evans KJ, et al: Cystitis follicularis in children with primary vesicoureteral reflux: a "conservative" analysis. *J Urol* 1983; 129:1020.

Burbidge KA: Ureteral reimplantation: a comparison of results with the cross trigonal and Politano-Leadbetter techniques in 120 patients. *J Urol* 1991; 146:1352.

Burger RH, Burger SE: Genetic determination of urologic disease. *Urol Clin North Am* 1974; 1:419.

Campbell MA: *Clinical Pediatric Urology*. Philadelphia, WB Saunders Co, 1951.

Carson CC, Kelalis PP, Hoffman AD: Renal growth in small kidneys after ureteroneocystostomy. *J Urol* 1982; 127:1146.

Christie BA: Incidence and etiology of vesicoureteral reflux in apparently normal dogs. *Invest Urol* 1971; 9:184.

Coffey RC: Physiologic implantation of the severed ureter or common bile-duct into the intestine. *JAMA* 1911; 56:397.

Cohen SJ: Ureterozystoneostomie, eine neue Antirefluxtechnik. *Aktvel Urol* 1975; 6:1.

Coleman JW, McGovern JH: A 20-year experience with pediatric ureteral implantation: surgical results in 701 children. In Hodson J, Kincaid-Smith P (eds): *Reflux Nephropathy*. New York, Masson Publishing USA, 1979, pp 299-305.

Councill WAH: Surgical treatment of vesicoureteral reflux. *South Med J* 1956; 49:1104.

Cussen LJ: Dimensions of the normal ureter in childhood. *Invest Urol* 1967; 5:164.

Daines SL, Hodgson NB: Management of reflux in total duplication anomalies. *J Urol* 1971; 105:720.

Decter RM, Roth DR, Gonzales ET: Vesicoureteral reflux in boys. *J Urol* 1988; 140:1989.

De Gennaro M, Appetito C, Lais A, et al: Effectiveness of trigonoplasty to treat primary vesicoureteral reflux. *J Urol* 1991; 146:636.

Duckett JW: Vesicoureteral reflux: a 'conservative' analysis. *Am J Kidney Dis* 1983; 3:139.

Duckett J, Walker R, Weiss R: Surgical results: International Reflux Study in Children—United States Branch. *J Urol* 1992; 148:1674.

Dunn M, Slade N, Gumpert JRW, et al: The management of vesicoureteric reflux in children. *Br J Urol* 1978; 50:474.

Dwoskin JY: Sibling uropathology. *J Urol* 1976; 115:726.

Dwoskin JY, Perlmutter AD: Vesicoureteral reflux in children: a computerized review. *J Urol* 1973; 109:888.

Edwards D, Normand ICS, Prescod N, et al: Disappearance of vesicoureteric reflux during long-term prophylaxis of urinary tract infection in children. *Br Med J* 1977; 2:285.

Elison BS, Taylor D, Van Der Wall H: Comparison of DMSA scintigraphy with intravenous urography for the detection of renal scarring and its correlation with vesicoureteral reflux. *Br J Urol* 1992; 69:294.

Evans R, Raezer D, Shrom S: Hutch-type reimplant in children with myelomeningocele. *Urology* 1986; 28:31.

Fair WR, McClennan BL, Jost RG: Are excretory urograms necessary in evaluating women with urinary tract infection? *J Urol* 1979; 121:313.

Fennell RS, Austin S, Walker D: Home culturing program for children with recurrent bacteriuria. *Am J Dis Child* 1976; 130:501.

Friedland GW: Post-reimplantation renal scarring. In Hodson J, Kincaid-Smith P (eds): *Reflux Nephropathy*. New York, Masson Publishing USA, 1979, pp 323-333.

Giblin JG, O'Conner KP, Fildes RD, et al: Diagnosis of acute pyelonephritis in piglet using single photon emission computerized tomography dimercaptosuccinic acid scintigraphy: pathological correlation. *J Urol* 1993; 150:759.

Gibson HM: Ureteral reflux in the normal child. *J Urol* 1949; 62:40.

Gil-Vernet JM: New technique for surgical correction of vesicoureteral reflux. *J Urol* 1984; 131:456.

Glenn JF, Anderson EE: Distal tunnel ureteral reimplantation. *J Urol* 1967; 97:623.

Govan DE, Palmer JM: Urinary tract infection in children. The influence of successful antireflux operations on morbidity from infection. *Pediatrics* 1969; 44:677.

Grégoir W, Schulman CC: Die extravesikale Antirefluxplastik. *Urologe [Ausg A]* 1977; 16:124.

Grégoir W, Van Regemorter GV: Le reflux vesicouretèral congénital. *Urol Int* 1964; 18:122.

Gross GW, Lebowitz RL: Infection does not cause reflux. *Am J Radiol* 1981; 137:929.

Habib R: Pathology of renal segmental corticopapillary scarring in children with hypertension: the concept of segmental hypoplasia. In Hodson J, Kincaid-Smith P (eds): *Reflux Nephropathy*. New York, Masson Publishing USA, 1979, pp 220-239.

Hackler RH: Modified Hutch I vesicoureteroplasty in paraplegia. *J Urol* 1977; 118:953.

Harrison RB, Howards SS, Thomas BR: Medical deviation of upper pole calix on intravenous urogram as indication of vesicoureteral reflux. *AJR* 1976; 126:1189.

Heikel PE, Parkkulainen KV: Vesicoureteral reflux in children. *Ann Radiol* 1966; 9:1.

Hendren WH: Operative repair of megaureter in children. *J Urol* 1969; 101:491.

Hendren WH: Reoperation for the failed ureteral reimplantation. *J Urol* 1974; 111:403.

Henneberry MO, Stephens FD: Renal hypoplasia and dysphagia in infants with posterior urethral valves. *J Urol* 1980; 123:912.

Hess E: Intracystic reimplantation of the ureter: a new operative technique. *J Urol* 1941; 46:866.

Higgins TT, Williams DI, Nash DFE: *The Urology of Childhood*. London, Butterworth, 1951.

Hinman F, Miller ER, Hutch JA, et al: Low pressure reflux: relation of vesicoureteral reflux to intravesical pressure. *J Urol* 1962; 88:758.

Hjelmas K, Duckett JW, Seppaenen J, et al: The value of cystoscopy in vesicoureteral reflux. (in press).

Hodson CJ: The radiologic diagnosis of pyelonephritis. *Proc R Soc Med* 1959; 52:669.

Hodson CJ, Cotran RS: Reflux nephropathy. *Hosp Pract* 1982; 17:133.

Hodson CJ, Maling TMJ, McManamon PJ, et al: The pathogenesis of reflux nephropathy. *Br J Radiol* 1975; 13(suppl):1-26.

Homsy YL, McSnyder H, Duckett JW, et al: Vesicoureteral reflux: the urodynamic dimension. *Dialogues Pediatr Urol* 1983; 6:1.

Houle AM, McLorie GA, Heritz DM, et al: Extravesical nondismembered ureteroplasty with detrusorraphy: a renewed technique to correct vesicoureteral reflux in children. *J Urol* 1992; 148:704.

Huland H, Busch R: Pyelonephritic scarring in patients with upper and lower urinary tract infections: long-term follow-up of 213 patients. *J Urol* 1984; 132:936.

Hutch JA: Vesicoureteral reflux in the paraplegic: cause and correction. *J Urol* 1952; 68:457.

Hutch JA: Ureteric advancement operation: anatomy, technique, and early results. *J Urol* 1963; 89:180.

Iannaccone G, Panzironi PE: Ureteral reflux in normal infants. *Acta Radiol* 1955; 44:451.

Ibsen KK, Uldall P, Frokjaer O: The growth of kidney in children with vesicoureteral reflux. *Acta Paediatr Scand* 1977; 66:741.

Immergut MA, Wahman GE: Urethral caliber of female children with recurrent urinary tract infections. *J Urol* 1968; 99:189.

Jerkins GR, Noe HN: Familial vesicoureteral reflux: a prospective study. *J Urol* 1982; 128:774.

Jewitt HJ: Upper urinary tract obstruction in infants and children: diagnosis and treatment. *Pediatr Clin North Am* 1955; 2:737.

Jones BW, Headstream JW: Vesicoureteral reflux in children. *J Urol* 1958; 80:114.

Kalicinski ZH, Kansy J, Kotarbinska B, et al: Surgery of megaureters—modification of Hendren's operation. *J Pediatr Surg* 1977; 12:183.

Kallenius G, Mollby R, Svenson SB, et al: Occurrence of P-fimbriated *Escherichia coli* in urinary tract infections. *Lancet* 1981; 2:1369.

Kaplan GW: Postinfection reflux. *Soc Pediatr Urol Newslett*, April 9, 1980.

Kaye E, Rocha H: Urinary concentrating ability in early experimental pyelonephritis. *J Clin Invest* 1970; 49:1427.

Kekomaki M, Walker RD: Fractional excretion of magnesium and renal concentrating capacity in refluxing renal units. *J Urol* 1988; 140:1095.

Keyes EL: *Urology*. New York, Appleton-Century-Crofts, 1926.

Kincaid-Smith P: Glomerular lesions in atrophic pyelonephritis (RN). In Hodson J, Kincaid-Smith P (eds): *Reflux Nephropathy*. New York, Masson Publishing USA, 1979, pp 268-272.

King LR: Current management of vesicoureteral reflux in infants and children. *J Contin Educ* 1977.

King LR: Posterior urethra. In Kelalis PP, King LR, Belman AB (eds): *Clinical Pediatric Urology*. Philadelphia, WB Saunders Co, 1985, pp 527-558.

Kiruluta HG, Fraser K, Owen L: The significance of the adrenergic nerves in the etiology of vesicoureteral reflux. *J Urol* 1986; 136:232.

Koff SA: Relationship between dysfunctional voiding and reflux. *J Urol* 1992; 148:1703.

Koff SA, Murtagh DS: The inhibited bladder in children: effect of treatment on recurrence of urinary infection and vesicoureteral reflux. *J Urol* 1983; 130:1138.

Kollerman VMW: Überbewertung der pathogenetischen Bedeutung des vesiko-ureteralen Refluxes im Kindesalter. *Z Urol* 1974; 67:573.

Kuhns LD, Hernandez R, Koff S, et al: Absence of vesicoureteral reflux in children with ureteral jets. *Radiology* 1977; 124:185.

Kurth KH, Alleman ERJ, Schroder FH: Major and minor complications of posterior urethral valves. *J Urol* 1981; 126:517.

Lamesch AJ: Retrograde catheterization of the ureter after antireflux plasty by the Cohen technique of transverse advancement. *J Urol* 1981; 125:73.

Levitt SB, Bekirov HM, Kogan SJ, et al: Proposed selective approach to radiographic evaluation of children with urinary tract infections. In Bergsma D, Duckett JW (eds): *Urinary System Malformations in Children*. New York, Alan R. Liss, Inc. 1977, pp 433-438.

Levitt SB, Weiss RA: Vesicoureteral reflux. In Kelalis PP, King LR, Belman AB (eds): *Clinical Pediatric Urology*. Philadelphia, WB Saunders Co, 1985, pp 355-380.

Lewy PR, Belman AB: Familial occurrence of nonobstructive, noninfectious vesicoureteral reflux with renal scarring. *J Pediatr* 1975; 86:851.

Lich R, Howerton LW, Davis LA: Recurrent urosepsis in children. *J Urol* 1961; 86:554.

Lich R, Howerton LW, Goode LS, et al: The ureterovesical junction of the newborn. *J Urol* 1964; 92:436.

Lombard H, Hanson AL, Jacobsson B, et al: Correlation of P blood group, vesicoureteral reflux and bacterial attachment in patients with recurrent pyelonephritis. *N Engl J Med* 1983; 308:1189.

Lyon RP, Marshall S, Tanagho EA: The ureteral orifice: its configuration and competency. *J Urol* 1969; 102:504.

Mackie GC, Stephens FD: Duplex kidneys: a correlation of renal dysplasia with position of the ureteral orifice. *J Urol* 1975; 114:274.

MacKinnon KJ, Oliver JA, Morehouse DD, et al: Cadaver renal transplantation: emphasis on urological aspects. *J Urol* 1968; 99:486.

Majd M, Belman A: Nuclear cystography in infants and children. *Urol Clin North Am* 1979; 6:395.

Malizia AA, Reiman HM, Myers RP, et al: Migration and granulomas reaction afer periurethral injection of polytef (Teflon). *JAMA* 1984; 251:3277.

Malizia AA, Woodard JR, Rushton HG, et al: Intravesical/suburetric infection of polytef: serial radiologic imaging. *J Urol* 1988; 139:185A.

Manley C: Reflux in blond haired girls. *Soc Pediatr Urol Newslett*, Oct 14, 1981.

Marberger M, Altwein JE, Straub E, et al: The Lich-Grégoir antireflux plasty: experiences with 371 children. *J Urol* 1978; 120:216.

Mathisen W: Vesicoureteral reflux and its surgical correction. *Surg Gynecol Obstet* 1964; 118:965.

McRae CU, Shannon FT, Utley WLF: Effect on renal growth of reimplantation of refluxing ureters. *Lancet* 1974; 1:1310.

Merrell RW, Mowad JJ: Increased physical growth after successful antireflux operation. *J Urol* 1979; 122:523.

Middleton RG: Routine use of the psoas hitch in ureteral reimplantation. *J Urol* 1980; 123:352.

Miller HC, Caspari E: Ureteral reflux as a genetic trait. *JAMA* 1972; 220:842.

Mulcahy JJ, Kelalis PP, Stickler GB, et al: Familial vesicoureteral reflux. *J Urol* 1970; 104:762.

Neal DE: Localization of urinary tract infections. *AUA Update Series* 1989; 8:Lesson 4.

Noe HN: The long-term results of prospective sibling reflux screening. *J Urol* 1992; 148:1739.

Noe HN, Wyatt RJ, Peeden JN, et al: The transmission of vesicoureteral reflux from parent to child. *J Urol* 1992; 148:1869.

O'Donnell B, Puri P: Treatment of vesicoureteral reflux by endoscopic infection of Teflon. *Br Med J* 1984; 289:7.

Olbing H, Claësson I, Ebel KD, et al: Renal scars and parenchymal thinning in children with vesicoureteral reflux: a 5-year report of the International Reflux Study in Children. *J Urol* 1992; 148:1653.

Paquin AJ: Ureterovesical anastomosis: the description and evaluation of a technique. *J Urol* 1959; 82:573.

Payne RL: Ureteral-vesical implantation. A new method of anastomosis. *JAMA* 1908; 51:1321.

Peppas DS, Skoog SJ, Canning DA, et al: Nonsurgical management of primary vesicoureteral reflux in complete ureteral duplication: is it justified? *J Urol* 1991; 146:1594.

Peters PC, Johnson DE, Jackson JH Jr: The incidence of vesicoureteral reflux in the premature child. *J Urol* 1967; 97:259.

Peterson A: The effect on the kidney of ureterovesical anastomosis. *JAMA* 1918; 71:1885.

Politano VA, Leadbetter WF: An operative technique for the correction of vesicoureteral reflux. *J Urol* 1958; 79:932.

Politano VA: Vesicoureteral reflux in children. *JAMA* 1960; 172:1252.

Polk HC Jr: Notes on Galenic urology. *Urol Surv* 1965; 15:2.

Poynter JH, Monger RH, Owens SB: Ureteroneocystostomy simplex: simple and effective approach to vesicoureteral reflux. *J Urol* 1967; 98:195.

Pozzi S: Ureteroverletzung bei Laparotomie. *Zentralbl Gynakol* 1893; 17:97.

Ransley PG: Intrarenal reflux: anatomical, dynamic and radiological studies. *Urol Res* 1977; 5:61.

Ransley PG, Risdon RA: Renal papillary morphology and intrarenal reflux in the young pig. *Urol Res* 1975a; 3:105.

Ransley PG, Risdon RA: Renal papillary morphology in infants and young children. *Urol Res* 1975b; 3:111.

Ransley PG, Risdon RA: Reflux nephropathy: effects of antimicrobial therapy in the evaluation of the early pyelonephritic scar. *Kidney Int* 1981; 20:733.

Report of the International Reflux Study Committee: Medical versus surgical treatment of primary vesicoureteral reflux. *Pediatrics* 1981; 67:392.

Roberts JA: Vesicoureteral reflux in the primate. *Invest Urol* 1974; 12:88.

Roberts JA: Pathogenesis of pyelonephritis. *J Urol* 1983; 129:1102.

Roberts JA: Etiology and pathophysiology of pyelonephritis. *Am J Kidney Dis* 1991; 17:1.

Roberts JA: Vesicoureteral reflux and pyelonephritis in the monkey: a review. *J Urol* 1992; 148:1721.

Roberts JA, Angel JR, Roth JK: The hydrodynamics of pyelorenal reflux: II. The effect of chronic obstructive changes on papillary shape. *Invest Urol* 1981; 18:296.

Roberts JA, Fischman NH, Thomas R: Vesicoureteral reflux in the primate: IV. Does reflux harm the kidney? *J Urol* 1982; 128:650.

Roberts JA, Hardaway K, Kaack B et al: Prevention of pyelonephritis by immunization with P-fimbriae. *J Urol* 1984; 131:602.

Roberts JA, Riopelle AJ: Vesicoureteral reflux in the primate: II. Maturation of the ureterovesical junction. *Pediatrics* 1977; 59:566.

Roberts JA, Riopelle AJ: Vesicoureteral reflux in the primate: III. Effect of urinary tract infection on maturation of the ureterovesical junction. *Pediatrics* 1978; 61:853.

Roberts JA, Roth JK, Domingue G, et al: Immunology of pyelonephritis in the primate model: V. Effect of superoxide dismutase. *J Urol* 1983; 128:1394.

Robert JA, Suarez GM, Kaack B, et al: Experimental pyelonephritis in the monkey: VII. Ascending pyelonephritis in the absence of vesicoureteral reflux. *J Urol* 1985; 133:1068.

Rolleston GL, Maling TMJ, Hodson CJ: Intrarenal reflux and the scarred kidney. *Arch Dis Child* 1974; 49:531.

Rolleston GL, Shannon FT, Utley WLF: Relationship of infantile vesicoureteric reflux to renal damage. *Br Med J* 1970; 1:460.

Rushton HG, Majd M: Dimercaptosuccinic acid renal scintigraphy for the evaluation of pyelonephritis and scarring: a review of experimental and clinical studies. *J Urol* 1992; 148:1726.

Rushton HG, Majd M, Jantauschm B, et al: Renal scarring following reflux and nonreflux pyelonephritis in children: evaluation with 99m technetium-dimercaptosuccinic acid scintigraphy. *J Urol* 1992; 147:1327.

Salvatierra O, Tanagho EA: Reflux as a cause of end-stage kidney disease: report of 32 cases. *J Urol* 1977; 117:441.

Sampson JA: Ascending renal infection: with special reference to the reflux of urine from the bladder into the ureters as an etiological factor in its causation and maintenance. *Johns Hopkins Hosp Bull* 1903; 14:334.

Savage JM, Dillon MJ, Shah V: Renin and blood pressure in children with renal scarring and vesicoureteral reflux. *Lancet* 1978; 2:441.

Schaeffer AJ: Bacterial adherence. In *Monographs in Urology*. Burroughs Wellcome Co, Research Triangle Park, NC. 1984, vol 5, no 5, pp 129-147.

Schmidt JD, Hawtrey CE, Flocks RH, et al: Vesicoureteral reflux: an inherited lesion. *JAMA* 1972; 220:821.

Schoenberg HW, Beisswanger P, Howard WJ, et al: Role of urinary tract infection in vesico-ureteral reflux. In Kass EH (ed): *Progress in Pyelonephritis*. Philadelphia, FA Davis Co, 1965, pp 632-640.

Shimada K, Matsui T, Ogino T, et al: Renal growth and progression of reflux nephropathy in children with reflux. *J Urol* 1988; 140:1097.

Shopfner CE: Vesicoureteral reflux. *Radiology* 1970; 95:637.

Sillen U, Hjalmas K, Aili M: Pronounced detrusor hypercontractility in infants with gross bilateral reflux. *J Urol* 1992; 148:598.

Skoog SJ, Belman AB: Primary vesicoureteral reflux in the black child. *Pediatrics* 1991; 87:538.

Skoog SJ, Belman AB, Majd M: A nonsurgical approach to the management of primary vesicoureteral reflux. *J Urol* 1987; 137:941.

Smellie JM: Commentary: management of children with severe vesicoureteral reflux. *J Urol* 1992; 148:1676.

Smellie J, Edwards D, Hunter N, et al: Vesicoureteric reflux and renal scarring. *Kidney Int* 1975; 8:S65.

Smellie JM, Edwards D, Normand ICS, et al: Effect of vesicoureteric reflux on renal growth in children with urinary tract infection. *Arch Dis Child* 1981; 56:593.

Smellie J, Hodson CJ, Edwards D, et al: Clinical and radiological features of urinary tract infection in childhood. *Br Med J* 1964; 2:1222.

Smellie J, Normand C: Reflux nephropathy in childhood. In Hodson J, Kincaid-Smith P (eds): *Reflux Nephropathy*. New York, Masson Publishing USA, 1979, pp 14-20.

Smellie J, Norman ICS: Urinary tract infection: clinical aspects. In Williams D, Johnston J (eds): *Paediatric Urology*. London, Butterworth Scientific, 1982, pp 95-112.

Smellie JM, Normand ICS, Katz G: Children with urinary tract infection: a comparison of those with and those without vesicoureteral reflux. *Kidney Int* 1981; 20:717.

Snyder HM, Duckett JW: Vesicoureteral reflux and pregnancy. *Soc Pediatr Urol Newslett*, Dec 21, 1981.

So EP, Brock WA, Kaplan GW: Ureteral reimplantation without catheters. *J Urol* 1981; 125:551.

Sommer JT, Stephens FD: Morphogenesis of nephropathy with partial ureteral obstruction and vesicoureteral reflux. *J Urol* 1981; 125:67.

Stecker JF, Rose JG, Gillenwater JY: Dysplastic kidneys associated with vesicoureteral reflux. *J Urol* 1973; 110:341.

Stephens FD, Joske RA, Simmons RT: Megaureter with vesico-ureteric reflux in twins. *Aust NZ J Surg* 1955; 24:192.

Sutton R, Atwell JD: Physical growth velocity during conservative treatment and following subsequent surgical treatment for vesicoureteric reflux. *Br J Urol* 1989; 63:245.

Tamminen-Mobius T, Brunier E, Ebel KD, et al: Cessation of vesicoureteral reflux for 5 years in infants and children allocated to medical treatment. *J Urol* 1992; 148:1662.

Taylor CM, Corkery JJ, White RHR: Micturition symptoms and unstable activity in girls with primary vesicoureteral reflux. *Br J Urol* 1982; 54:494.

Teague N, Boyarsky S: The effect of coliform bacilli upon ureteral peristalsis. *Invest Urol* 1968; 5:423.

Thompson IM, Patton JF: Pull-through ureteral reimplantation for reflux. *J Urol* 1971; 105:631.

Timmons JW, Watts FB Jr, Perlmutter AD: A comparison of awake and anesthesia cystography. In Bergsma D, Duckett JW (eds): *Urinary System Malformation in Children*. New York, Alan R Liss, Inc, 1977, pp 363-364.

Tobenkin MI: Hereditary vesicoureteral reflux. *South Med J* 1964; 57:139.

Tocci PE, Politano VA, Lynne CM, et al: Unusual complications of transvesical ureteral reimplantation. *J Urol* 1976; 115:731.

Torres VE, Kramer SA, Holley KE, et al: Effect of bacterial immunization on experimental reflux nephropathy. *J Urol* 1984; 131:772.

Torres VE, Malek RS, Svensson JP: Vesicoureteral reflux in the adult: II. Nephropathy, hypertension and stones. *J Urol* 1983; 130:41.

Urrutia EJ, Lebowitz TL: Re-reflux in blonde haired girls. *Soc Pediatr Urol Newslett*, Oct 14, 1983.

Van Gool JD, Hjalmas K, Tamminen-Mobius T, et al: Historical clues to the complex of dysfunctional voiding, urinary tract infection and vesicoureteral reflux. *J Urol* 1992; 148:1699.

Wacksman J, Gilbert A, Sheldon CA: Results of the renewed extravesical reimplant for surgical correction of vesicoureteral reflux. *J Urol* 1992; 148:359.

Walker RD: The injection of Teflon paste to correct urinary incontinence and vesicoureteral reflux. *AUA Update Series* 1989; 8:154.

Walker RD, Duckett J, Bartone FF, et al: Screening school children for urologic disease. *Pediatrics* 1977; 60:239.

Walker RD, Garin E: Urinary prostaglandin E_2 in patients with vesicoureteral reflux. *Child Nephrol Urol* 1990; 10:18.

Walker RD, Richard GA, Dobson D, et al: Maximum urinary concentration: early means of identifying patients with reflux who may require surgery. *Urology* 1973; 1:343.

Wallace DMA, Rothwell DL, Williams DI: The long-term follow-up of surgically treated vesicoureteral reflux. *Br J Urol* 1978; 50:479.

Wasnick RJ, Butt KMH, Laungani G, et al: Evaluation of anterior extravesical ureteroneocystostomy in kidney transplantation. *J Urol* 1981; 126:306.

Weiss R, Duckett J, Spitzer A: Results of randomized clinical trials of medical versus surgical management of infants and children with grades III and IV primary vesicoureteral reflux (United States). *J Urol* 1992; 148:1667.

Williams DI, Scott J, Turner-Warwick R: Reflux and recurrent infection. *Br J Urol* 1961; 33:435.

Willscher MK, Bauer SB, Zammuto PJ, et al: Renal growth and urinary infection following antireflux study in infants and children. *J Urol* 1976; 115:722.

Winberg J, Bergstrom T, Jacobsson B: Morbidity, age, and sex distribution, recurrences, and renal scarring in symptomatic urinary tract infection in childhood. *Kidney Int* 1975; 8:S101.

Winberg J, Bollgren I, Gothefors L, et al: The prepuce: a mistake of nature? *Lancet* 1989; 1:598.

Winberg J, Claesson I, Jacobsson B, et al: Renal growth after acute pyelonephritis in childhood: an epidemiological approach. In Hodson J, Kincaid-Smith P (eds): *Reflux Nephropathy*. New York, Masson Publishing USA, 1979, pp 309-322.

Winter CC: *Vesicoureteral Reflux and Its Treatment*. New York, Appleton-Century-Crofts, 1969.

Wiswell TE, Enzenauer RW, Cornish JD, et al: Declining frequency of circumcision: implications for changes in the absolute incidence and male to female sex ratio of urinary tract infections in early infancy. *Pediatrics* 1987; 79:338.

Wiswell TE, Geschke DW: Risks from circumcision during the first month of life compared with those for uncircumcised boys. *Pediatrics* 1989; 83:1011.

Wiswell TE, Roscelli JD: Corroborative evidence for the decreased incidence of urinary tract infections in circumcised male infants. *Pediatrics* 1986; 78:96.

Wiswell TE, Smith FR, Bass JW: Decreased incidence of urinary tract infections in circumcised male infants. *Pediatrics* 1985; 75:901.

Witherington R: Experimental studies on role of intravesical ureter in vesicoureteral regurgitation. *J Urol* 1963; 89:176.

Woodard JR, Holden S: The prognostic significance of fever in childhood urinary infections. *Clin Pediatr* 1976; 15:1051.

Woodard JR, Keats G: Ureteral reimplantation: Paquin's procedure after 12 years. *J Urol* 1973; 109:891.

Young HH: Editorial comment to ascending renal infection. *Johns Hopkins Hosp Bull* 1903; 14:334.

Zaontz MR, Maizels M, Sugar EC, et al: Detrusorrhaphy: extravesical ureteral advancement to correct vesicoureteral reflux in children. *J Urol* 1987; 138:947.

Zel G, Retik AB: Familial vesicoureteral reflux. *Urology* 1973; 2:249.

CHAPTER 49

Prune Belly Syndrome

Douglas E. Coplen
Brent W. Snow
John W. Duckett

Prune belly syndrome (PBS) consists of a constellation of three major findings associated with a number of other respiratory, gastrointestinal, musculoskeletal, and cardiovascular anomalies. A deficiency of abdominal musculature gives the child's abdomen a wrinkled, prune-like, appearance (Fig. 49-1). Bilateral nonpalpable undescended testes are present, and there is an abnormal urinary tract characterized by tortuous, dilated ureters, megalocystis, dilated prostatic urethra, and renal dysmorphism.

The syndrome was first described by Frolich (1839), and urologic interest began in 1895 with Parker's description. This syndrome has been called by many other names, including Eagle-Barrett syndrome (Eagle and Barrett, 1950), abdominal muscular deficiency syndrome (Welch, 1979), absence of abdominal musculature (Cremin, 1971; Culp and Flocks, 1954; Lattimer, 1958; McGovern and Marshall, 1959), triad syndrome (Nunn and Stephens, 1961), and mesenchymal dysplasia syndrome (Ives, 1974). Despite these many terms, the name PBS is the most widely accepted for this constellation of major and minor findings (Barnhouse, 1972; Carter et al., 1974; Duckett, 1976; Greskovich and Nyberg, 1988; Hammonds et al., 1974; King and Prescott, 1978; Rogers and Ostrow, 1973; Smith, 1976; Tuch and Smith, 1978; Waldbaum and Marshall, 1970; Woodhouse et al., 1982).

Stephens (1983) believes that the name prune belly syndrome has a negative effect on the patient and the family. Therefore, he has suggested that triad syndrome is a more appropriate name, especially in conversation with patients and their families.

SPECTRUM

The manifestations of PBS are varied widely. In some infants the disease is so severe that kidney development and urine production in utero are impaired. Subsequent oligohydramnios leads to pulmonary hypoplasia incompatible with life. These severely afflicted children may be stillborn or die shortly after birth. Before the 1970s, almost 50% of reported cases were postmortem reports (Barnhouse, 1972; Lattimer, 1958; McGovern, 1959). With aggressive management, including the judicious use of urinary diversion, peritoneal dialysis, and transplantation, some of these children may survive. On the other hand, there are children in whom renal function is normal even though the urinary tract has a markedly abnormal radiographic appearance. These children may grow up without much physical or physiologic impairment.

Attempts to correlate abdominal wall laxity with the degree of urinary tract abnormality or functional impairment have had little success. The appearance of either the abdomen or the urinary tract imaging should not lead one to draw conclusions about long-term prognosis or treatment options without careful evaluation of the functional status of the kidneys.

Some patients have the typical radiographic appearance of the urinary tract anomalies, but they may have one or both testes descended and a relatively firm abdominal wall. These cases are called "pseudoprunes" to distinguish their relationship from PBS (King, 1969; Williams and Parker, 1974; Williams and Taylor, 1969).

INCIDENCE

The incidence of PBS is estimated to be equal to that of exstrophy of the bladder (1 per 35,000 to 50,000 live births) (Baird and MacDonald, 1981; Garlinger and Ott, 1974). There is little data to support this estimation. However, in large centers, such as ours and Great Ormond Street, London (Williams, 1982), approximately equal numbers of PBS patients and exstrophy patients are seen. Clearly, the complete triad occurs only in males, but there is a subset of patients with two of three systems involved, and some of these are female.

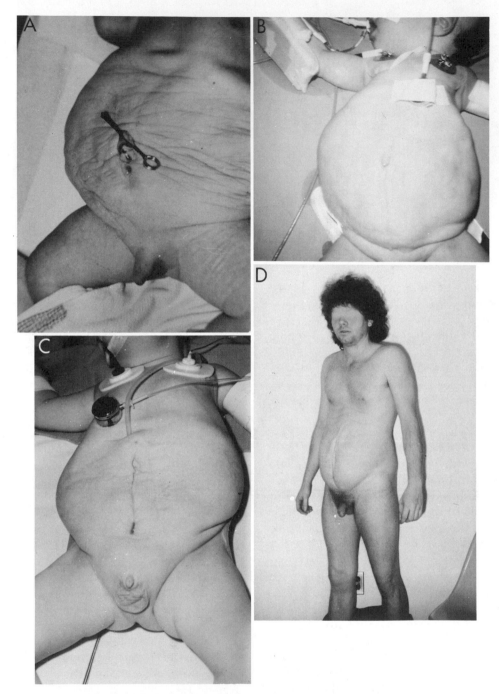

FIG. 49-1
A and **B,** Typical newborn abdominal appearance. Note wrinkling in **A** and laxity in **B. C,** A 1-year-old child with renal failure on chronic ambulatory peritoneal dialysis. **D,** A 24-year-old-man with typical potbelly. No surgery was done except for bilateral orchiopexies. Note pectus excavatum and prominent midline cutaneous infolding.

GENETICS

There is no evidence for a single gene or an autosomal recessive inheritance in PBS (Ives, 1974). Riccardi and Grum (1977) proposed a two-step autosomal dominant mutation with sex-limited expression and also proposed that different gene abnormalities might result in an identical phenotype. Harley and col-

leagues (1972) noted siblings with PBS and mosaicism, suggesting a genetic etiology. Subsequently, the occurrence of prune belly syndrome in siblings has been reported many times. Frydman (1993) reported a familial segregation of prune belly anomalies that appeared to follow an X-linked inheritance. Amacker and associates (1986) and Hoagland and co-workers (1988) described an association between prune belly syndrome and trisomy 21 and 18, respectively, whereas Watanabe and Yamanaka (1990) described two siblings with Beckwith-Wiedemann syndrome and prune belly syndrome. Despite the suggestion of chromosomal anomalies and associations with other syndromes, these still must be considered exceptions rather than the rule (Garlinger and Ott, 1974; Halbrecht et al., 1972). However, parents should be counseled with respect to potential occurrence in subsequent offspring, and the chromosomal analysis of PBS patients is recommended.

One of every 23 PBS patients is the product of a twin pregnancy (Ives, 1974). This is a much higher incidence than one would expect spontaneously (1 in 80). The majority of reported twins have been discordant for PBS and this again speaks against a genetic etiology for PBS (Ives, 1974). The cause in twins may be the result of an uneven division of the mesenchyma at a critical time of primitive streak development during the third week of embryogenesis.

EMBRYOLOGY

The embryologic explanation for the development of PBS is unknown. Four theories have been suggested.

1. It is possible that an intrinsic defect exists in the urinary tract that causes bladder and ureteral dilation. The consequent abnormal abdominal distention throughout embryogenesis would result in abdominal wall laxity and the characteristic appearance of a PBS patient. With this theory, the dilated bladder will mechanically block the testicle's descent into the scrotum. However, it does not explain the actual embryologic process of the urinary tract malformation, nor does the laxity of the abdominal wall necessarily correlate with the degree of urinary tract dilation.

2. We (Duckett, 1986a, 1986b) feel that most likely PBS results from an early prostatic membranous urethral obstruction that causes rapid bladder and ureteral distention at a critical time when the mesenchyme is moving into the developing musculature of the urinary tract and abdominal wall. Whether this is a functional (Hoagland, 1988; Moerman et al., 1984) or anatomic (Hoagland and Hutchins, 1987) obstruction is unclear. Either might cause the abdominal musculature laxity and prevent the testes from descending, as explained previously. This theory supposed that the delayed opening of the membranous obstruction recanalizes at a later time and the obstruction no longer persists. The overall incidence of urethral obstruction in reported autopsy cases is about 30% (Manivel et al., 1989; Wigger and Blanc, 1977). The outlet obstruction is clinically minimal in most patients at birth. This theory does not explain the more severe

changes in the distal urinary tract and the milder changes proximally.

3. Wigger and Blanc (1977) suggested that a primary myopathic or dysplastic process results in prune belly syndrome. The predominant involvement of medial and lower abdominal wall muscles and the dysplasia that is observed histologically indicate a problem with the development and differentiation of mesenchyme into striated muscle. The lateral thoracic somites have migrated to the midline (i.e., midline defects like exstrophy and omphalocele are not present) but the somites either fail to differentiate into myoblasts or the myoblasts did not migrate ventrally and caudally. The bladder arises from the same lateral somites, so the same defect could lead to the bladder findings in PBS. Similarly, the deficiency of smooth muscle and fibrosis in the ureters might interfere with normal peristaltic propagation and result in ureteral dilation. This theory, however, does not explain the discrepancy in upper and lower ureteral dilation or the presence of undescended testicles.

Gonzalez and colleagues (1990) studied second trimester urethral obstruction in the fetal lamb. In one animal this experimental manipulation resulted in musculoskeletal and genitourinary abnormalities and undescended testes as in PBS. It was hypothesized that the complete urethral obstruction in this model resulted in the findings that are distinctly different from the findings of the partial obstruction in posterior urethral valves.

Two histopathologic studies support an obstructive etiology for PBS. Serial sectioning of the intact bladder and urethra in infants with PBS (Hoagland and Hutchins, 1987) revealed a short segment of obstruction in the prostatic urethra just above the membranous urethra in some patients. In another patient (Hoagland, 1988), the hypoplastic prostatic urethra was dilated and the angulation at the level of the internal sphincter caused a functional obstruction.

4. Stephens (1983) suggested that the yolk sac perhaps could be at fault, since it holds a key relationship to the lateral folds of the discoid embryo as it enlarges and infolds into the chorionic cavity. If the yolk sac does not shrink and constrict, some may be retained inside the embryo, giving the abdominal wall redundance. This theory also would explain the bladder and urachal anomalies encountered since they arise from the allantois and yolk sac. This theory does not address the ureteral changes or the undescended testes.

However, Workman and Kogan's (1990) histologic evaluation of bladders from patients with PBS revealed two distinct groups. One group had marked muscle thickness consistent with obstruction, whereas the other group had thin bladders with increased connective tissue. This suggests either an obstructive or mesenchymal defect may be etiologic.

CLINICAL EVALUATION
Antenatal Diagnosis

Antenatal ultrasonography is now commonly obtained in most obstetrical practices. This leads to the in utero detection of anatomic urologic abnormalities, which may or may not require subsequent intervention. Bilateral dilation of the upper urinary tract in association with a large bladder that does not empty completely on real-time ultrasound is suggestive of PBS, but a similar presentation also would be seen with posterior urethral valves. Scarborough and colleagues (1986) suggested that the presence of fetal ascites early in gestation is suggestive of PBS and warrants more extensive evaluation. These anatomic abnormalities may be found as early as 15 weeks' gestation. Some have recommended in utero intervention for placement of a vesicoamniotic shunt to decompress the urinary tract and alleviate oligohydramnios (Estes and Harrison, 1993; Gadziala et al., 1982; Glazer et al., 1982; Nakayama et al., 1984). Others, on the basis of antenatal ultrasonographic evidence of PBS, have recommended pregnancy termination (Pescia et al., 1982).

It is our strong opinion that antenatal intervention or pregnancy termination for PBS is unwarranted on the basis of an antenatal ultrasound. Antenatal ultrasound is associated with both false-negative and false-positive findings that make in utero diagnosis sufficiently uncertain. There is no proof that relief of a functional obstruction in utero will affect renal function (Kramer, 1983). Renal dysplasia has been reported as early as 15 weeks' gestation making it difficult to justify in utero intervention (usually after 15 weeks) when there is no accurate way of determining the degree of dysplasia or assessing fetal renal function. In addition, the urinary tract dilation in PBS is not caused by obstruction but more often is the result of nonobstructive dilation in a functionally balanced system. There may be unusual circumstances in which abdominal distention or urinary tract dilation cause dystocia that may necessitate urinary tract decompression (Gadziala et al., 1982).

Diagnosis in the Newborn

Because of the typical features of a child with PBS, the diagnosis is usually obvious. Initially these patients should be monitored closely, with particular attention to their respiratory and renal function. We prefer to observe these patients for the first several days of life before radiographic evaluation, avoiding instrumentation that may lead to infection in the stagnant system. Bladder massage is helpful in getting the bladders to contract and empty.

ELEMENTS OF PRUNE BELLY SYNDROME
Abdominal Musculature

The abdominal musculature is unevenly involved. The lateral and inferior abdominal wall musculature is diffusely deficient, whereas the upper abdominal musculature and trunk musculature may be normal (Randolph et al., 1981). The musculature, however, may be totally absent in some cases (Manivel et al., 1989). The affected lower abdominal wall may consist of skin, subcutaneous fat, and condensation of fibrous tissue onto the peritoneum without evidence of organized muscle tissue (Afifi et al., 1972; Mininberg et al., 1973); however, the whole muscle may be simply thinned out within the fascia, replaced by thick bundles of collagen surrounded by fascia, or consist of fragments of muscle interspersed in collagen (Wigger and Blanc, 1977). The abdominal organs can be palpated easily through the abdominal wall in these infants.

Over the first year the wrinkled abdomen of the infant smooths. As the child begins to stand, a pear-shaped, or pot-bellied, appearance to the abdomen is manifested (see Fig. 49-1). The abdominal musculature weakness makes it difficult for these children to sit from a supine position. They typically roll over and use their arms to assist them. Developmental delays in other motor activities may be associated with their difficulty in axial balance when standing to walk.

Cryptorchidism

In PBS the undescended testicles are usually found at the level of the iliac vessels in the peritoneum on a long mesorchium. Kaplan and associates (1986) suggested a role for intraabdominal pressure in the process of testicular descent; however, Hutson and Beasley (1988) believe that the high intraabdominal pressure and bladder distension block descent. The underdevelopment of the inguinal canal also may contribute to the testicular nondescent (Hadziselimovic, 1983). The fact that "pseudoprune" patients can have normally descended testicles and firm abdominal walls sheds some doubt that mechanical forces are singly responsible for the cryptorchidism.

Histologic findings on testes biopsies vary. Case reports have described this testis as Sertoli cell-only (Uehling et al., 1984), hypospermatogonia with Leydig cell hyperplasia (Orvis et al., 1988), and normal for age-matched controls (Hadziselimovic, 1983). The most comprehensive review of testicular histology is the review from Children's Hospital of Philadelphia (Pak et al., 1993). This study compared PBS testes, other intraabdominal cryptorchid testes, and testes of age-matched controls. There was no significant difference in germ cell counts, Adult Dark (AD) stem cell, or Leydig cell counts found between the intraabdominal testes in PBS and other intraabdominal cryptorchid testes. The observation that germ cell counts approach normal in PBS patients less than one year of age suggests that the PBS testis, like other cryptorchid testes, is not a congenital malformation but the outcome of a disease state.

Occasionally the epididymis is detached from the testis, as noted in other circumstances of cryptorchidism. The ductus deferens may have a thickened wall of collagen with sparse musculature. The vas deferens may be tortuous and thin walled with atretic segments (Tayakkanonta, 1963).

The risk of testis tumor in PBS patients is poorly defined. Certainly the presence of germ cells in the young PBS patient testis places the patient at risk. Massad and colleagues (1991) showed histologic similarities with intratubular germ cell neoplasia in three infants with PBS. Two PBS patients have been noted to have testis tumors (teratoma and teratocarcinoma) of their intraabdominal testes at ages 24 and 30 years (Shockley, 1983; Woodhouse and Ransley, 1983). Parra and co-workers (1991) reported a seminoma in a 30-year-old who had undergone orchiopexy 6 years previously. Another PBS patient had a primary retroperitoneal embryonal cell tumor with normal testis biopsy results (Sayre et al., 1986).

ORTHOPEDIC ANOMALIES

The incidence of orthopedic abnormalities ranges between 30% and 45%, and it is the most commonly affected system outside the genitourinary tract (Green et al., 1993; Loder et al., 1992). The oligohydramnios in PBS is believed to produce limited intrauterine space, which in turn leads to fetal compression and resultant musculoskeletal deformities. Some of these compression effects are mild, such as elbow and knee dimples (Fig. 49-2), but other orthopedic anomalies have been noted. The involvement may be congenital (equinovarus (clubfoot), limb deficiencies, hip dysplasia, and vertebral anomalies) or developmental (renal osteodystrophy, scoliosis, and pectus deformities.) Loder (1992) believes that the embryologic characteristics of the congenital musculoskeletal problems correlate with an aberration of mesenchymal development around 6 weeks of gestation, but Green (1993) contends that the anomalies are a direct result of the oligohydramnios, based upon the unilaterality of many of the deformities.

GASTROINTESTINAL ANOMALIES

Gastrointestinal (GI) anomalies are seen in 20% to 30% of PBS patients. The majority of anomalies (malrotation, volvulus, atresia, and stenosis) result from persistence of the wide embryonic mesentery with absent fixation to the posterior abdominal wall (Silverman and Huang, 1950; Wright et al., 1986). The spleen has the same abnormal mesenteric attachment, and acute torsion has been reported in five patients (Heydenrych and DuToit, 1978; Teranoto et al., 1981).

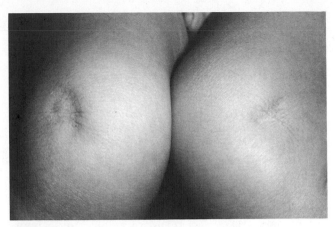

FIG. 49-2
Knee dimples seen in PBS. Dimples also may be seen on the elbows and are probably related to in utero compression.

Gastroschisis (Short et al., 1985; Wilbert et al., 1978), omphalocele (Peterson et al., 1972), Hirschsprung's disease (Cawthern et al., 1979) and imperforate anus (Morgan et al., 1978; Walker et al., 1987) have all been reported. PBS children may have problems with chronic constipation presumably secondary to the inability to generate intraabdominal pressure. This may require chronic intervention (Geary et al., 1986).

RESPIRATORY ANOMALIES

Significant respiratory problems have been observed in PBS. These may result from a combination of pulmonary hypoplasia secondary to in utero oligohydramnios and disordered thoracic mechanics resulting from scoliosis, rib cage abnormalities, and abdominal weakness (Crompton et al., 1993). Although the severe form of PBS pulmonary hypoplasia may be incompatible with life, the vast majority of patients have no baseline history of respiratory disease. Crompton and associates (1993) showed that the majority of patients with PBS had abnormal lung function when studied in a pulmonary function laboratory. Patients showed gas trapping secondary to poor expiratory effort, and half the patients showed significant restrictive lung disease that appeared to be secondary to musculoskeletal abnormalities rather than an interstitial lung problem. These pulmonary abnormalities must be considered before the elective treatment of PBS anomalies (i.e. musculoskeletal).

CARDIOVASCULAR ANOMALIES

Cardiovascular anomalies occur in about 10% of PBS patients (Adebonojo, 1973). Atrial and ventricular septal defects, as well as tetralogy of Fallot, are the most common anomalies seen.

The cardiovascular, pulmonary, or gastrointestinal anomalies may have far greater significance in the newborn period than the urologic manifestations of PBS. Urologists must individualize the approach for each patient's specific needs, realizing that the urologic anomalies are seldom a pressing problem in the newborn.

RADIOGRAPHIC EVALUATION

The introduction of infection during radiographic procedures is a real possibility, since the PBS urinary tract is dilated and urine may be stagnant. Caution should be used in all invasive diagnostic studies. Antibiotic coverage is recommended for radiographic instrumentation of the urinary tract.

Imaging of the urinary tract may be done with a voiding cystourethrogram, which usually fills the upper urinary tracts as a result of reflux. Some information about bladder functioning and emptying also can be gained from this study. The dilated tapered posterior urethra so characteristic of PBS also may be demonstrated.

Ultrasonography can be helpful in evaluating the size of ureters and the degree of the upper urinary tract hydronephrosis. It also may aid in distinguishing the amount of normal parenchyma from dysplastic parenchyma.

Upper urinary tract imaging is beneficial, but in the newborn it should be delayed for 2 to 4 weeks to allow for better visualization of the kidneys. A renal scan obtained with technetium 99m diethylenetriamine pentaacetic acid (^{99m}Tc DTPA) measures only gross function. Because of the dilation and tortuosity, furosemide (Lasix) administration and measures of half-time excretion are not valid in the PBS to demonstrate obstruction (Gordon, 1985).

KIDNEYS

Renal dysmorphism is a common finding. Cystic calyces are characteristic of PBS without narrowing of the infundibula. Incomplete renal rotation and an irregular renal outline may be present. Most kidneys display some degree of hypodysplasia. Four potential mechanisms for the development of hypoplasia and dysplasia have been proposed (Stephens, 1983).

1. The intermediate cell mass and metanephros may be devoid of its full complement of mesoderm from the primitive streak.
2. The ureteric bud may arise ectopically from the wolffian duct and lack induction capability (Mackie and Stephens, 1975).
3. A failure of the stepwise acquisition of mesonephric vessels by ascending kidney and ureter may lead to ischemia, resulting in ureteric atresia or stenosis and renal hypoplasia.
4. Early fetal obstruction to urine flow may cause these developmental changes.

In postmortem specimens, Stephens (1983) found hypoplasia and renal dysplasia (defined as any disorganization of the renal parenchyma consisting of embryonic tubules, cartilage, cysts, and mesenchymal connective tissue) in the majority of PBS patients. Renal cystic dysplasia is most commonly associated with some degree of distal obstruction (Wigger and Blanc, 1977), and those patients with urethral atresia usually have solid dysplastic kidneys, as described by Potter (1972). The involvement of the kidneys is variable and may be segmental; thus renal biopsy may not be accurately predictive of outcome. The autopsy patients evaluated by Stephens and Wigger were severely affected by the syndrome, and the prevalence of dysplasia in prune belly patients with "normal" renal function is unknown.

URETER

A radiographic hallmark of PBS is the characteristic ureteral redundancy, tortuousity, and dilation, with the distal portion being more involved than the proximal ureter (Berdon et al., 1977; Grossman et al., 1970) (Fig. 49-3). Segmental dilations of the midureter are found occasionally. Rarely, an obstructed ureteral segment is discovered. Fluoroscopic examination shows an ineffective churning peristalsis. With careful observation over time the ureters may straighten somewhat and the peristaltic activity may improve. Most of these ureters have free vesicoureteral reflux. It is difficult to incriminate an obstructive cause when the distal ureter is so much more involved with these changes than is the proximal ureter. Maizels and Stephens (1980) noted "pleat valves" in the caudal portion of these ureters, which may be obstructing at times (Cussen, 1971).

Histologic studies of the ureteral wall by Stephens (1983) show fibrocytes, collagen, and smooth muscle in varying proportion. Other histologic studies show that the ureteral wall is composed primarily of a thick hyaline ground substance that is acellular (Ehrlich and Brown, 1977; Hanna et al., 1977; Palmer and Tesluk, 1974). The degree of ureteral dilation did not correlate with the histologic findings.

BLADDER

The prune belly bladder is enlarged and thick walled but not trabeculated. The dome of the bladder may have a pseudodiverticulum where the urachus is attached (Fig. 49-4). Occasionally the urachus is patent, especially when there is complete urethral atresia. The bladder is irregular, and diverticula may be present. The trigone is splayed, the ureteral orifices are laterally placed (Stephens, 1983), and vesicoureteral reflux is present in 75% of the cases (Duckett, 1976).

The bladder wall has a variable histologic picture. Smooth muscle cells are intermixed with fibrocytes and collagen. Some portions of the bladder wall may

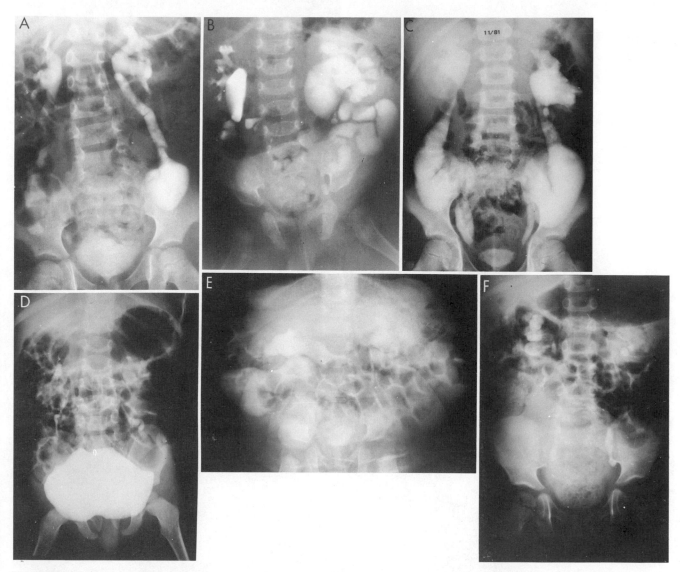

FIG. 49-3
A to **E,** Typical PBS urinary tract, representing a variety of cases with different degrees of dilation and tortuosity. All of these patients are being managed successfully without extensive reconstructive surgery. The patient in **B** is the same patient as in Figure 49-4. *B after* excision of the urachal diverticulum and partial cystectomy. Note the typical distal tortuousity and more prominent dilation. **F,** Patient shows cystic changes in the calyces and a large bladder.

be devoid of muscle cells completely. In some studies, actual muscle cell measurements show no evidence of hypertrophy (Cussen, 1971; Stephens, 1974); however, Workman (1990) showed that some bladders display smooth muscle hypertrophy consistent with an obstructive etiology.

During voiding, the intravesical pressures usually remain normal (Nunn and Stephens, 1961; Snyder et al., 1976; Williams and Burkholder, 1967). Some patients are able to empty their bladders completely; however, many have significant postvoid residuals. The latter may indicate abnormal bladder dynamics or a relative outflow obstruction (Snyder et al., 1976). In an analysis of 34 patients with PBS (Kinahan et al., 1992), three distinct uroflow patterns were identified.

Normal initiation and peak flow, prolonged steady low flow, and an intermittent pattern. The voiding pattern was not predictive of the ability to empty. Lee (1977) found that some bladders improve their tone and emptying with age.

PROSTATIC URETHRA

During voiding, the prostatic urethra markedly dilates, tapering down to the membranous urethra. These findings are characteristic of PBS (Fig. 49-5). To the inexperienced observer the PBS prostatic urethra may resemble posterior urethral valves (Fig. 49-6). Valvular obstruction in conjunction with PBS is rare. Most of the prostatic urethral dilation is posterior, and there is occasionally evidence of a small utri-

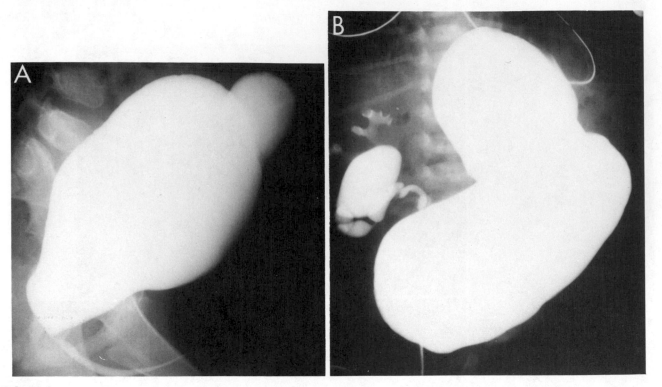

FIG. 49-4
A and **B,** PBS bladders with urachal diverticula. Note the wide open bladder neck in **A** with narrowed area at membranous urethra.

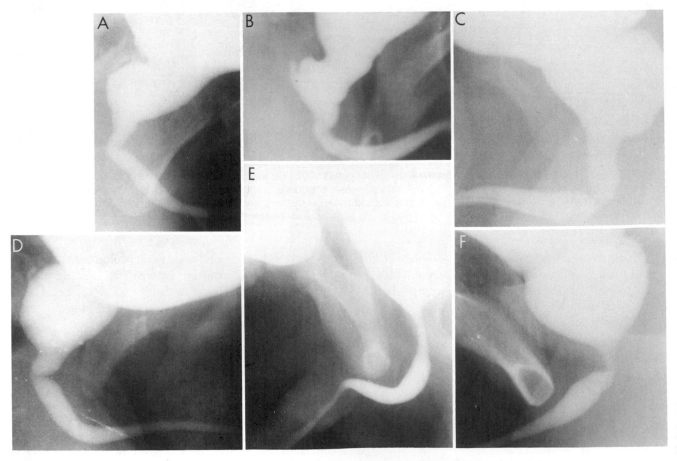

FIG. 49-5
Typical urethra of PBS. **A** to **F,** Six examples of the bladder neck, prostatic urethra, and anterior urethra.

cle. The verumontanum seldom can be seen on the voiding studies. The membranous urethra is usually of normal caliber, and the distinct diminution of caliber from the prostatic urethra to the membranous urethra has led many to assume that there is obstruction at this point.

Occasionally obstructive lesions have been found in the prostatic urethra. An autopsy series search by Wigger and Blanc (1977) revealed stenosis in 4 of 14 patients, atresia in 3 of 14 patients, and urethral valves in 4 of 14. Manivel (1989) found stenosis in 5 of 25 patients, atresia in 5 of 25, and urethral valves in 4 of

25. These findings are distinctly uncommon among living patients. Stephens (1983) carefully studied the prostatic urethra and noted anterior folding of the mucosa, which in some cases overlapped the urethral outlet, having a valvelike effect. He called this anterior folding a type IV posterior urethral valve and recommended a 12 o'clock incision of the redundant mucosa.

PROSTATE

Prostatic maldevelopment in PBS is the rule. Few normal epithelial elements are found on histologic evaluation (DeKlerk and Scott, 1978; Moerman et al., 1984; Popek et al., 1991). It is believed that the prostatic abnormalities are a result of disturbed mesenchymal-epithelial interaction. Since the prostates of posterior urethral valve patients also exhibit a disordered, yet distinct, mesenchymal-epithelial interaction, it is unclear whether the findings in PBS are the result of a primary mesenchymal problem or the result of obstruction (Popek et al., 1991). In PBS patients the contribution of the prostate to seminal fluid is unknown. However, the hypoplastic gland is likely the cause of the scant semen in these patients.

ANTERIOR URETHRA

The anterior urethra in PBS patients is usually normal. Occasionally a membranous urethral stenosis or atresia is present in the more severe cases. Without urethral or urachal patency these patients usually are stillborn or die in the newborn period. We have had two patients with severe stenosis and a patent urachus who survived with chronic renal failure.

The occurrence of megalourethra is seen more frequently in PBS than any other condition (Appel et al.,

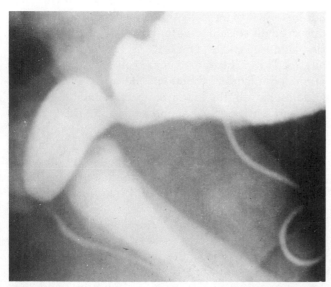

FIG. 49-6
Posterior urethral valve. This patient does not have PBS. This voiding study is shown to demonstrate the difference between posterior urethral valves and the typical PBS urethra.

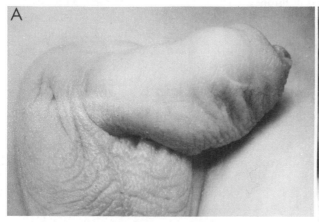
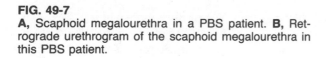
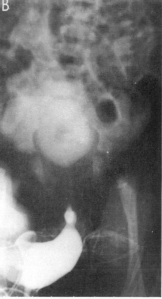

FIG. 49-7
A, Scaphoid megalourethra in a PBS patient. **B,** Retrograde urethrogram of the scaphoid megalourethra in this PBS patient.

1986; Mortensen et al., 1985; Shrom et al., 1981). Megalourethra occurs in two distinct types, fusiform and scaphoid (Sellers et al., 1976; Stephens and Fortune, 1993; Stephens, 1963). An absence of all three corporal bodies characterizes the fusiform type of megalourethra, which is the more severe defect. This results from a failure of the mesoderm in the urethral folds to develop, leading to an epithelium-lined urethra adjacent to a fibrous tunica albuginea (Dorairajan, 1963). The fusiform type of megalourethra has been strongly associated with PBS and stillbirths (Duckett, 1976; Shrom et al., 1981). The scaphoid type of megalourethra is less severe (Fig. 49-7) and results from failure of mesenchymal elements to invest the urethra, explaining the absence of spongiosal tissue in these patients. In a review of the literature (Shrom et al., 1981), nearly 50% of patients with scaphoid megalourethra had PBS.

Kroovand and associates (1982) described milder urethral abnormalities, including a fusiform dilation of the bulbous urethra and similar dilation of the pendulous urethra. These abnormalities are usually not significant. In general, the penises of PBS patients are long and slender with some curvature dorsally. Hypospadias has been reported.

MANAGEMENT

Therapeutic Considerations

Varied approaches to the management of the prune belly syndrome patient have been advocated.

1. Watchful waiting with selective surgical intervention (Duckett, 1976; Williams and Parker, 1974)
2. Early permanent urinary diversion (ileal conduit)
3. High loop ureterostomy or pyelostomy with subsequent urinary tract reconstruction (Randolph, 1977)
4. Nephrostomy with later reconstruction (Waldbaum and Marshall, 1970)
5. Immediate newborn reconstruction without prior diversion (Hendren, 1972; Jeffs et al., 1977; Parrott and Woodard, 1976; Welch and Kearney, 1974; (Adams and Hendren, 1992; Woodard and Parrot, 1978b)

In the 1950s, immediate surgical drainage followed by later reconstruction was the recommended management for PBS. McGovern (1959) believed that the "fact that a few patients have survived months or years without fundamental therapy is more a tribute to their good fortune in starting with fairly good kidneys. . . .than an argument for masterly inactivity." This approach supposes that the urinary tract dilation is secondary to obstruction and that massive reflux and residual urine leads to further renal damage, or both.

It is our opinion that the dilation in PBS is low pressure and nonobstructive and that reflux per se does not lead to renal damage without infection (Duckett, 1976, 1983, 1986; Snow and Duckett, 1984). Early intervention to create nephrostomy drainage, ureterostomies, or tube cystostomies may change a balanced though dilated urinary tract into one that will require reconstruction. It is our preference to give these patients prophylactic antibiotics and to watch them carefully, selectively intervening surgically, if necessary.

Our approach in the newborn includes careful monitoring of the child during the first several days of life. The creatinine level and electrolyte values should be followed and should stabilize at acceptable levels (creatinine <1.0 mg/dl). Spontaneous voiding should be observed for stream force and bladder emptying. Gentle bladder massage (Duckett and Harmon, 1994) usually leads to a bladder contraction and allows evaluation of bladder function. Because of the soft abdominal wall, the kidneys, ureters, and other structures are easily palpable and segmental dilations defined. With the urinary tract full of urine and easily palpable through a lax abdominal wall, it is difficult to avoid the temptation to achieve better drainage surgically. Catheter drainage should be discouraged since infection is likely to result. Prophylactic antibiotic coverage is mandatory.

There are patients during the newborn period with rising creatinine values, as well as acidosis, in whom intervention may be indicated. Although high diversion is rarely indicated, a cutaneous pyelostomy may be performed if the systems are redundant and stagnant (Randolph, 1977; Schmidt et al., 1973). Cutaneous ureterostomies should be discouraged in these patients, since the upper ureter is more normal and should be used in subsequent reconstruction (Woodard and Trulock, 1986).

Some authors encourage an extensive surgical reconstruction in the neonatal period in those infants they classify as mildly to moderately affected. This reconstruction includes excision of the distal half of the ureters with tapering reimplantation of the healthier upper portion of the ureters into the bladder. In addition, the size of the bladder is reduced, and the testes are brought into the scrotum without division of the spermatic vessels. The results of some of these reports are satisfactory in improving the radiographic appearance of the system, but the degree of renal dysplasia, not the degree of urinary tract dilation, is the limiting factor in these patients. Thus, the necessity for reconstruction from a functional and physiologic standpoint is debatable (Adams and Hendren, 1992).

We prefer a policy of watchful waiting in most cases (Fig. 49-8) based on the observation that the dilation of the urinary tract is not caused by obstruction, as in

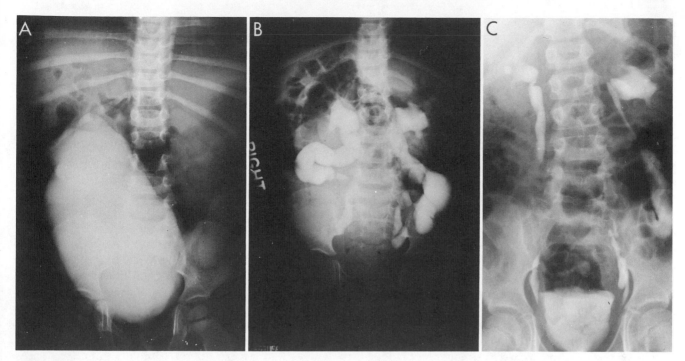

FIG. 49-8
A, Patient with PBS cystogram with large bladder but no reflux. **B,** Intravenous pyelogram with full bladder. **C,** Several years later when voiding dynamics balanced. No reconstruction was done.

the case of urethral valves. This is a congenital deficiency of smooth muscles of the pelvis, ureters, and bladder that allows the collecting system to distend to alarming proportions but without the significant pressure increase that would be associated with obstruction. Certainly there are bona fide indications for surgical intervention. Before embarking on such a course, however, remember that there are quite a few reported and unreported technical failures leading to permanent diversion or rapid renal failure (Dreikorn et al., 1977). Our initial experience with cases referred from elsewhere with this surgical approach have dictated our focus on bladder emptying as the key to reconstruction.

INFECTION

Infection can be devastating in the stagnant but balanced urinary tract of a PBS patient. Antibiotics in the neonatal period and long-term prophylactic antibacterial therapy with a sulfonamide or nitrofurantoin should prevent this complication. When urosepsis is present, the already poor ureteral peristalsis and bladder contractility are suppressed, and surgical drainage may become necessary.

ANESTHETIC CONSIDERATIONS

These anomalies present particular problems with anesthetic management and sedatives (Hannington-Kiff, 1970; Karamanian et al., 1974). It is recommended that newborns have apnea monitors. A 25-year review of the Great Ormond Street experience (Henderson et al., 1987) revealed a 6% incidence of postoperative upper respiratory infection. There were three postoperative deaths in 133 anesthetics. Only one of these was directly related to PBS. Normal doses of muscle relaxants may be used in these patients, but active physiotherapy is required postoperatively along with judicious use of analgesics.

BLADDER EMPTYING

The key to successful clinical management of PBS is assurance of bladder emptying. In the newborn and neonate, bladder massage by the nurses or mother is very effective in "assisted" voiding. Because of the bladder size, this is needed every 4 to 6 hours but is effective even more frequently. If infection or persistent upper-tract distention is unavoidable, then vesicostomy is indicated. After closure of vesicostomy, balanced voiding must be assured. Clean, intermittent catheterization (CIC) may be effective (Toronto) (Reinberg et al., 1989), but we believe it introduces the risk of infection and compliance problems. Finally, in older patients (7 to 15 years), sphincterotomy seems to be the most successful definitive treatment for balanced voiding and eliminates CIC.

CUTANEOUS VESICOSTOMY

When diversion of the dilated urinary tract is indicated, cutaneous vesicostomy is our preference (Duckett, 1974). Generally, this procedure vents the entire urinary tract with a pop-off system for decompression. The vesicostomy technique is simple and utilizes a small transverse incision midway between the symphysis and umbilicus. A button of skin and rectus fascia are excised, and the dome of the bladder is delivered into the field and sutured to the rectus fascia and skin. In contrast to other patients with vesicostomies, in PBS patients a rather generous stoma is made (28 F), since stenosis is found more frequently. If a urachal pseudodiverticulum is noted, it is excised at the time of cutaneous vesicostomy. The urine is simply allowed to drain into a diaper, and prophylactic antibiotics are continued.

REDUCTION CYSTOPLASTY

In some PBS patients the bladder is enormous. Emptying is infrequent and incomplete. Some investigators have recommended a reduction in bladder capacity in hopes of improving bladder emptying (Perlmutter, 1976). This procedure has been done in many ways. Generally, the dome and pseudodiverticulum of the urachus are excised, and the bladder is reapproximated in the midline (Woodard and Trulock, 1986). Williams and Parker (1974) recommended bladder plication rather than excision, whereas Hanna and colleagues (1977) proposed excision of bladder mucosa with overlapping detrusor flaps to augment the bladder emptying. We have not been impressed by the results of reduction cystoplasty, except for excision of urachal segments of pseudodiverticula (see Fig. 49-4).

URETHROTOMY

Despite the fact that the anterior urethra and membranous urethra in PBS patients are usually normal, a significant number of patients (30% to 50%) have difficulty with bladder emptying. Cukier (1977) proposed urethrotomy of the membranous urethra (Fig. 49-9) to improve bladder emptying. It is thought that the urethrotomy reduces the normal urethral outlet resistance that overbalances the diminished PBS detrusor contractile strength. Woodhouse and colleagues (1979) reported proper bladder emptying in 4 of 5 patients after urethrotomy and Williams (1979) reported urodynamic improvement following urethrotomy in the majority of patients. We favor this therapeutic procedure and have used it in 40% of our patients.

ANTERIOR URETHRA

PBS may be associated with either urethral atresia or megalourethra. Passerini-Glazel and colleagues (1988) reported a progressive soft dilation of the urethra (PADUA) that results in a normal caliber urethra. Great care is required to successfully pass a tiny wire or 3 F ureteral catheter initially to avoid extravasation and stricture. Each progressive step should be delayed 2 weeks to assure adequate enlargement. In cases where this is not successful or in cases of megalourethra, repair should be based upon sound principles of hypospadias repair.

VESICOURETERAL REFLUX

Three fourths of PBS patients demonstrate vesicoureteral reflux (Duckett, 1976). However, the indications for antireflux surgery in the PBS patient should be different (Duckett, 1976, 1983; Welch et al., 1975). Because the PBS patient has dilated ureters, the pressure from the vesicoureteral reflux is dissipated and does not reflect directly onto the renal papilla. It is technically difficult to prevent reflux and not cause some degree of obstruction at the

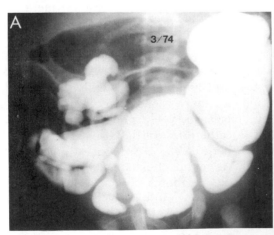
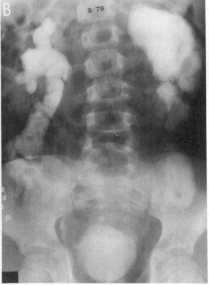

FIG. 49-9
A, Patient with PBS with cystogram at 1 month of age. **B,** Same patient 5 years later after a ureterocalycostomy of the left system and urethral sphincterotomy.

ureterovesical junction because of the poor peristaltic function of the ureters. Reflux without infection does not lead to renal deterioration. If infection becomes a problem in the young patient, cutaneous vesicostomy is the preferred temporary surgical procedure.

If an individual patient requires antireflux surgery as a result of recurrent urinary tract infections, it is best to use the more proximal portion of the ureter that comfortably reaches the bladder and to excise the redundant distal ureter. If ureteral tapering is necessary, we prefer imbrication rather than excision where appropriate. If the reflux is unilateral, a transureteroureterostomy may be considered and can effectively bypass the ipsilateral reflux. A psoas hitch also is recommended.

ABDOMINAL WALL PLICATION

The abdominal wall laxity usually improves as the child matures. However, Ehrlich and colleagues (1986) and Parrott and Woodard (1992) believe that the appearance may be "psychologically crippling" in many patients. Children may wear a corset, but abdominal wall plication has been utilized to correct this deformity. Stephenson (1953) reported that after vertical abdominal wall plication many of the patients returned to a more lax state. Ehrlich and colleagues (1986) described a midline abdominal incision with plication of the fascia rather than excision. A subsequent modification by Monfort and co-workers (1991) allows preservation of the umbilicus.

Initially, we tried vertical abdominal wall plications but were unsatisfied with the results (Duckett, 1976).

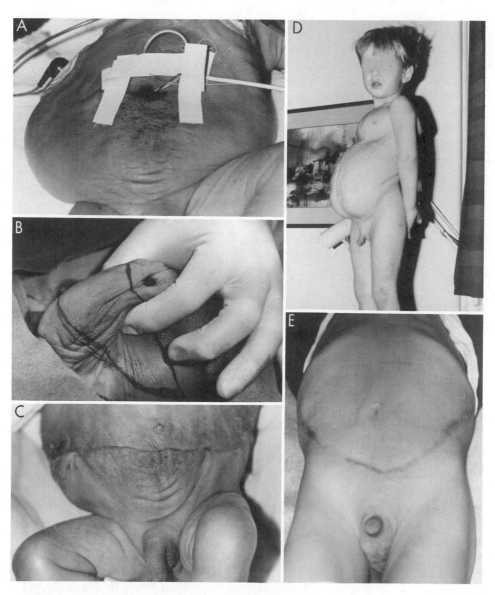

FIG. 49-10
Plastic repair of abdominal wall. **A,** Abdomen of neonate with PBS. **B,** Elliptic portion of the lower abdominal wall to be excised. **C,** Early postoperative result. **D** and **E,** Preoperative and postoperative appearance in an older child.

Randolph and associates (1981) studied the distribution of musculature and noted that the upper abdominal musculature was more normal. They used a transverse lower abdominal incision, removing the lower abdominal musculature, skin, and peritoneum. This technique nicely reconstitutes the patient's waistline, and in our own patients has a pleasing cosmetic result (Fig. 49-10). It can often be combined with orchiopexy or other reconstructive procedures when indicated.

Smith and associates (1993) reported that abdominoplasty resulted in improved urinary tract emptying; however, the procedure was performed in conjunction with major urinary tract reconstruction and tailoring and the relative contribution of the abdominoplasty must be questioned. It is possible that in the presence of repeated problematic pulmonary infections, plication may support a more effective cough.

ORCHIOPEXY

All male PBS patients have bilateral undescended testes. As previously mentioned, the fertility potential of these patients is in doubt (Uehling, 1982; Woodhouse and Snyder, 1985). However, orchiopexy is still recommended for these patients. The testicles are usually found in the abdomen on a broad mesorchium overlying the iliac vessels but may be found at any point along the pathway of normal testicular descent. In some patients the testis may be placed in the scrotum with conventional orchiopexy techniques. Woodard and Parrott (1978a) recommended a transabdominal neonatal orchiopexy in which the spermatic cord vessels can usually be mobilized to allow the testis to be positioned dependently in the scrotum without vascular compromise. It may be performed in conjunction with neonatal reconstructive surgery or at the time of abdominal wall plication. Fowler and Stephens (1959) described a technique wherein the spermatic vessels are divided and the testicle is placed in the scrotum on a vas and peritoneal pedicle blood supply. The success rate with this technique is approximately 75% (Boddy et al., 1991; Gibbons et al., 1979). This procedure allows the high intraabdominal testicles to be brought into the scrotum when the vessels are too short. The decision to do this procedure must be made before dissection around the testicle, which would disrupt the vasotesticular collateral blood supply. It has been recommended that the contralateral spermatic vessels be ligated at the time of the ipsilateral orchiopexy so that when the second orchiopexy is done at a later time, collateralization will have already developed. Microvascular autotransplantation, anastomosing the spermatic vessels to the inferior epigastric vessels, is feasible once the spermatic vessels are of sufficient size (5 years of age) with a success rate of approximately 80% (Boddy et al., 1991).

SEXUAL FUNCTION AND FERTILITY

Woodhouse and Snyder (1985) studied the sexual function of adult male PBS patients and found that erectile function was normal. Most patients had normal orgasm; however, seminal emission was absent in seven of eight patients. No male PBS patient has had documented fertility. This is most likely on the basis of poor prostatic function and seminal fluid, the abnormal configuration of the prostate and bladder neck, vasal anomalies, and abnormal spermatogenesis. Woodhouse and Snyder (1985) examined postejaculate urine for the presence of sperm, and none were found. However, in these patients, orchiopexy was performed in late childhood or early adolescence. The confirmation of germ cells in the PBS testis gives an indication for early efforts to place the testes in the scrotum (Pak et al., 1993). Even in the presence of retrograde ejaculation, if viable sperm were produced by the PBS testis, sperm harvesting and washing techniques might allow paternity.

RENAL FAILURE AND TRANSPLANTATION

Approximately 25% to 30% of PBS patients will develop renal failure. This is either a developmental (renal dysplasia) or acquired (urinary tract infection and pyelonephritis) problem. A histopathologic evaluation (Reinberg et al., 1991b) showed that the most severe renal changes in patients who developed renal failure after infancy were those of chronic inflammation and reflux nephropathy with less dysplasia when compared to kidneys of infants with renal failure. This stresses the importance of vigilant prevention of infection in these patients.

Reinberg and co-workers (1989) reviewed the Minnesota experience with renal transplantation. There was no significant difference in patient death, graft survival, or graft function between PBS patients and controls. Urinary tract undiversion was performed prior to transplantation, and intermittent catheterization was used routinely in the presence of chronic urinary retention. These results are in contrast to the results with renal transplantation from the same institution that show an adverse effect on allograft survival and function in posterior urethral valve patients.

CLINICAL EXPERIENCE

Over the last 20 years we have been involved in the care of 65 patients with PBS at the Children's Hospital of Philadelphia. Five patients died in the newborn period as a result of severe renal dysplasia, and three of these patients had urethral atresia. Two others subsequently died of renal failure. One patient with normal renal function died of pulmonary complications after 5 years with a tracheostomy.

Our clinical experience in primary cases is biased by our watchful waiting and selected surgical approach. One half of our patients, however, had aggressive management elsewhere before our involvement in their care. Therefore, we can subjectively compare a relatively conservative approach to the more aggressive approaches of other investigators.

Of the 32 patients managed entirely at Children's Hospital in Philadelphia that survived the neonatal period, 13 have had cutaneous vesicostomies as temporary diversion (40%). Ten of these patients have successfully been closed, and they have maintained stable renal function and a satisfactory clinical course. One patient was born with urethral atresia and urine spontaneously draining from his right flank and was treated initially with bilateral cutaneous ureterostomies. He presently has a vesicostomy and is awaiting reconstruction. Only four of these 32 patients required a pyeloplasty for ureteropelvic junction obstruction, one of which required a revision to a ureterocalycostomy to achieve success (see Fig. 49-9). Vesicoureteral reflux was noted in 24 of the 30 patients in whom voiding cystourethrograms were available for review. Five patients required nephroureterectomy for nonfunctioning kidneys, and histology showed dysplasia in all five. Ureteral reconstruction was deemed necessary in five of our 32 patients. Four patients had a relative ureterovesical junction obstruction, and the other patient had a large periureteral diverticulum of the bladder. Eight of the 32 patients (25%) initially

managed in Philadelphia have progressed to end-stage renal disease and had renal allografts placed. An additional eight patients have chronic renal insufficiency and three of these eventually will require renal transplantation.

Eleven patients had large residual urine volumes and difficulty voiding. Internal urethrotomies were performed; two patients required a second urethrotomy. Nine of these patients have benefited from this procedure, and no incontinence has developed.

Thirty-two patients had orchiopexies for a total of 60 undescended testes. Twenty-four testes were brought down by conventional techniques. A Fowler-Stephens technique (1959) was used to place 36 testicles in the scrotum (Gibbons et al., 1979). Five of these testes (14%) became atrophic. In one bilateral procedure, atrophy has necessitated hormonal replacement. Two patients with membranous urethral atresia underwent a foreskin island flap urethroplasty with excellent long-term results. The PADUA (Passerini-Glazel et al., 1988) procedure for urethral atresia has been used successfully in three patients since 1991. All three patients were successfully dilated up to 12 F over a 6-week time period. Twenty patients have had abdominal wall reconstructions. The initial six patients had vertical midline procedures with disappointing results. The last 14 patients have had a lower abdominal transverse incision and repair as suggested by Randolph and colleagues (1981) with good results.

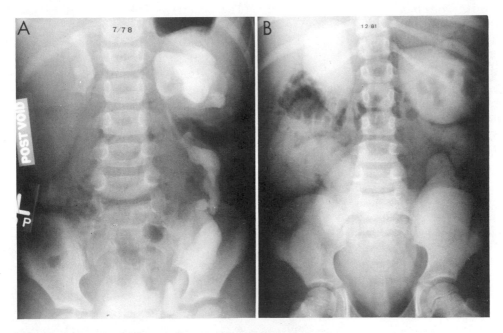

FIG. 49-11
A, This 8-year-old child was reconstructed from loop ureterostomies in the midureter with some reduction of the tortuousity of the ureters but no reimplantation of the ureter. **B,** The same patient 3 years later with relative outlet obstruction. The upper urinary tracts decompressed to their previous state after internal urethrotomy.

Of the 33 children initially managed elsewhere, 13 presented with urinary diversion, including end cutaneous ureterostomies (4), loop ureterostomies (5), pyeloileocutaneous diversion (1), and intubated diversions (3). Twelve of these 13 patients have since been undiverted (Fig. 49-11). Two of these patients have had primary ureteral reconstructions with tapering and reimplantations. One of these patients progressed to renal failure and died at 6 years of age, while two others have undergone successful renal transplantation (23%).

Woodhouse and associates (1982) reviewed 47 PBS patients cared for at the Great Ormond Street Children's Hospital in London over 35 years, beginning in 1947. Five newborns died within 1 month with severe renal compromise. Thirteen patients presented with infection or progressive renal compromise and underwent high diversion. In 10 patients renal function was stabilized. Of the group, only three achieved normal voiding and stable renal function. The implication was that reconstruction was not successful in this group. The remaining 29 patients (60%) were well at birth and stabilized without intervention. Twenty-one of these patients eventually had a urethral procedure, either resection endoscopy (six patients), a full-length urethrotomy (14 patients), or formal urethroplasty (one patient). Urethral obstruction sometimes recurred but could be reversed with another urethrotomy. Of the patients with renal complications, only three deteriorated as teenagers. Seventeen are into or past their pubertal growth spurt and with one exception are mature, well-motivated adults. Eleven (25%) of the group are considered unsatisfactory, with renal failure, hypertension, calculi, etc. One had a teratoma of the testis (Woodhouse and Ransley, 1983). They concluded that renal function could be improved by establishing proper bladder emptying. Upper urinary tract surgery was less rewarding, although deterioration could be halted.

A report of the 35-year experience from Babies Hospital, New York City (Burbige et al., 1987), reviewed 50 children. Fourteen patients died in the perinatal period of a combination of pulmonary and renal disease and two more patients died in the first 6 months of life of urosepsis. Overall mortality in the series was 32%. Thirty-four patients were available for long-term follow-up. Ten of the patients had upper tract diversion (all before 1975). Eight of 10 patients have stable renal function after reconstruction. After 1975, primary reconstruction was performed in 11 patients and all have stable renal function. Eleven patients did not undergo any diverting or reconstructive procedures and remain well. The authors concluded that the presence of dilated ureters on a standard IVP does not preclude a successful long-term result.

The clinical courses of 25 children with PBS from the Toronto Children's Hospital were reviewed (Geary et al., 1986). They demonstrated significant morbidity in 55% of patients ascribed to pulmonary, orthopedic, and gastrointestinal problems. There were three neonatal deaths. Growth retardation was seen in 30% and was not related to either plasma creatinine or extrarenal abnormalities. Five have severe renal insufficiency, and 17 have only mild renal insufficiency. No mention was made as to the method of urinary tract management with respect to diversion or reconstruction.

INCOMPLETE PRUNE BELLY SYNDROME

By definition, PBS must have the triad of an abnormal urinary tract, abdominal musculature laxity, and undescended testes. There is, however, an occasional patient who presents with two of the three elements required for the diagnosis. In our series, 15 patients had incomplete PBS. Twelve of these patients had the classic findings in the urinary tract and three of these (25%) developed end-stage renal disease. These patients frequently have a similar clinical course to PBS patients and need the careful follow-up demanded for patients with this syndrome.

Female patients with deficient abdominal musculature and the characteristic findings of the urinary tract have been seen (Rabinowitz and Schillinger, 1977; Reinberg et al., 1991a). The frequent occurrence of bladder outlet obstruction in the Reinberg series suggests a role in the pathogenesis of the syndrome. The occurrence of associated anorectal anomalies is high (40%) and the perinatal mortality was 40%. In addition, two of four surviving patients developed renal insufficiency. In the Philadelphia series, three patients (16%) were females, two of whom had moderately severely affected urinary tracts. One of these female patients has a moderate degree of renal insufficiency.

PROGNOSIS

In the past, PBS portended a poor prognosis, but PBS represents a wide spectrum of disease. The outcome depends to a great degree on the amount of renal hypodysplasia and the degree of respiratory embarrassment. The urinary tract is dilated and rarely obstructed and with better management of urinary tract infections, the outlook is brighter. Each patient must be dealt with on an individual basis. We prefer a watchful, waiting course, with selective surgical intervention as needed.

REFERENCES

Adams M, Hendren H: PBS reconstructions, abstract. *AAP* 1992.

Adebonojo FO: Dysplasia of the abdominal musculature with multiple congenital anomalies; prune belly or triad syndrome. *J Natl Med Assoc* 1973; 65:327.

Afifi AK, Rebeiz JM, Adonia SJ, et al: The myopathy of the prune belly syndrome. *J Neurol Sci* 1972; 15:153.

Amacker EA, Grass FS, Hickey DE, et al: An association of prune belly anomaly with trisomy 21. *Am J Med Genet* 1986; 23:919.

Appel RA, Kaplan GW, Brock WA, et al: Megalourethra. *J Urol* 1986; 135:747.

Baird PA, MacDonald EC: An epidemiologic study of congenital malformations of the anterior wall in more than half a million consecutive live births. *Am J Hum Genet* 1981; 33:470.

Barnhouse DH: Prune belly syndrome. *Br J Urol* 1972; 44:356.

Berdon WE, Baker DH, Wigger HJ, et al: The radiologic and pathologic spectrum of the prune belly syndrome. *Radiol Clin North Am* 1977; 15:8392.

Boddy SA, Gordon AC, Thomas DFM, et al: Experience with the Fowler Stephens and microvascular procedures in the management of intra-abdominal testes. *Br J Urol* 1991; 68:199.

Burbige K, Amodio J, Berdon WE, et al: Prune belly syndrome: 35 years of experience. *J Urol* 1987; 137:86.

Carter TC, Tomskey GC, Ozog LS: Prunebelly syndrome. *Urology* 1974; 3:279.

Cawthern TH, Bottene LA, Grant D: Prune belly syndrome associated with Hirschsprung's disease. *Am J Dis Child* 1979; 133:652.

Cremin BJ: The urinary tract anomalies associated with agenesis of the abdominal walls. *Br J Radiol* 1971; 44:767.

Crompton CH, MacLuskey IB, Geary DF: Respiratory function in the prune belly syndrome. *Arch Dis Child* 1993; 68:505-6.

Cukier J: Resection of the urethra in the prune belly syndrome. *Birth Defects* 1977; 13:95.

Culp DA, Flocks RH: Congenital absence of abdominal musculature. *J Iowa State Med Soc* 1954; 44:155.

Cussen LJ: The morphology of congenital dilation of the ureter: intrinsic ureteral lesions. *Aust NZ Surg* 1971; 41:185.

DeKlerk DP, Scott WW: Prostatic maldevelopment in the prune belly syndrome: a defect in prostatic stromal epithelial interaction. *J Urol* 1978; 120:341.

Dorairajan T: Defects of spongy tissue and congenital diverticula of the penile urethra. *Aust NZ J Surg* 1963; 32:209.

Dreikorn K, Palmtag H, Robal L: The prune belly syndrome: treatment of terminal renal failure by hemodialysis and renal transplantation. *Eur Urol* 1977; 3:245.

Duckett JW Jr: Cutaneous vesicostomy in childhood. *Urol Clin North Am* 1974; 1:485.

Duckett JW: The prune belly syndrome. In Kelalis PP, King LR, Belman AB (eds): *Clinical Pediatric Urology*. Philadelphia, WB Saunders Co, 1976, pp 615-635.

Duckett JW: Vesicoureteral reflux: a 'conservative' analysis. *Am J Kidney Dis* 1983; 3:139.

Duckett JW: Prune belly syndrome. In Holder TM, Ashcraft KW (eds): *Pediatric Surgery*. Philadelphia, WB Saunders Co, 1986a, pp 802-815.

Duckett JW: Prune belly syndrome. In Welch KJ, Randolph JG, Ravitch MM, et al (eds): *Pediatric Surgery*, ed 4. Chicago, Year Book Medical Publishers, 1986b, pp 1193-1203.

Duckett JW, Harmon T: Personal communication, 1994.

Eagle JF, Barrett GS: Congenital deficiency of abdominal musculature with associated genitourinary abnormalities: a syndrome: reports of 9 cases. *Pediatrics* 1950; 6:721.

Ehrlich RM, Brown WJ: Ultrastructural anatomic observations of the ureter in the prune belly syndrome. *Birth Defects* 1977; 13:101.

Ehrlich RM, Lesavoy M, Fine RM: A new abdominal wall reconstructive procedure for prune belly syndrome. *J Urol* 1986; 136:282.

Estes JM, Harrison MR: Fetal obstructive uropathy. Semin *Pediatr Surg* 1993; 2:129.

Fowler R, Stephens FD: The role of testicular vascular anatomy in the salvage of the high undescended testis. *Aust NZ J Surg* 1959; 29:92.

Frolich, F: Der Mangel der Muskeln, ins besondere der Seitenbauchmuskeln. Dissertation, Wurzberg, C.A. Zurn, 1839.

Frydman M, Cohen HA, Ashkenazi A, et al: Familial segregation of cervical ribs, Sprengel anomaly, preaxial polydactyly, anal atresia, and urethral obstruction: a new syndrome? *Am J Med Genet* 1993; 45:717.

Gadziala NA, Kavade CY, Doherty FJ, et al: Intrauterine decompression of megalocystis during the second trimester of pregnancy. *Am J Obstet Gynecol* 1982; 144:355.

Garlinger P, Ott J: Prune belly syndrome. Possible genetic implications. *Birth Defects* 1974; 10:173.

Geary DF, MacLusky IB, Churchill BM, et al: A broader spectrum of abnormalities in the prune belly syndrome. *J Urol* 1986; 135:324.

Gibbons MD, Cromie WJ, Duckett JW Jr: Management of the abdominal undescended testicle. *J Urol* 1979; 122:76.

Glazer GM, Filly RA, Callen PW: The varied sonographic appearance of the urinary tract in the fetus and newborn with urethral obstruction. *Radiology* 1982; 144:563.

Gonzalez R, Reinberg Y, Burke B, et al: Early bladder outlet obstruction in fetal lambs induces renal dysplasia and the prune belly syndrome. *J Ped Surg* 1990; 25:342-345.

Gordon I: The urological challenge to pediatric imaging, Meredith Campbell Lecture, AUA Annual Meeting, May 12, 1985, Atlanta.

Green NE, Lowery ER, Thomas R: Orthopaedic aspects of prune belly syndrome. *J Pediatric Orthopaedics* 1993; 13:496-501.

Greskovich FJ, Nyberg LM: The prune belly syndrome: a review of its etiology, defects, treatment and prognosis. *J Urol* 1988; 140:707-712.

Grossman H, Winchester PH, Waldbaum RS: Syndrome of congenital deficiency of abdominal wall musculature and associated genitourinary anomalies. *Prog Pediatr Radiol* 1970; 3:327.

Hadziselimovic F: *Cryptorchidism: Management and Implications*. New York, Springer-Verlag, 1983.

Halbrecht I, Komlos L, Shabtai F: Prune belly syndrome with chromosomal fragment. *Am J Dis Child* 1972; 123:518.

Hammonds JA, Van Den Ende EW, Boardman RG, et al: Prune belly syndrome. *S Afr Med J* 1974; 48:839.

Hanna MK, Jeffs RD, Sturgess JM, et al: Ureteral structure and ultrastructure: III. The congenitally dilated ureter (megaureter). *J Urol* 1977; 117:24.

Hannington-Kiff JB: Prune belly syndrome and general anesthesia. *Br J Anaesth* 1970; 42:649.

Harley LM, Chen Y, Rattner WH: Prune belly syndrome. *J Urol* 1972; 108:174.

Henderson AM, Vallis CJ, Sumner E: Anaesthesia in the prune-belly syndrome. A review of 36 cases. *Anaesthesia* 1987; 42:54.

Hendren WH: Restoration of function in the severely decompensated ureter. In Johnson JH, Scholtmeijer RJ (eds): *Problems in Paediatric Urology*. Amsterdam, Excerpta Medica, 1972, pp 1-56.

Heydenrych JJ, DuToit DE: Torsion of the spleen and associated prune belly syndrome—a case report and review of the literature. *S Afr Med J* 1978; 53:637.

Hoagland MH, Frank KA, Hutchins GM: Prune belly syndrome with prostatic hypoplasia, bladder wall rupture, and massive ascites in a fetus with trisomy 18. *Arch Pathol Lab Med* 1988; 112:1126.

Hoagland MH, Hutchins GM: Obstructive lesions of the lower urinary tract in the prune belly syndrome. *Arch Pathol Lab Med* 1987; 111:154.

Hutson JM, Beasley SW: Re: Association between abdominal wall defects and cryptorchidism (letter). *J Urol* 1988; 139:388.

Ives EJ: The abdominal muscle deficiency triad syndrome—experience with ten cases. *Birth Defects* 1974; 10:127.

Jeffs RD, Comisarow RH, Hanna MK: The early assessment for individualized treatment in the prune belly syndrome. *Birth Defects* 1977; 13:97.

Kaplan LM, Koyle MA, Kaplan GW, et al: Association between abdominal wall defects and cryptorchidism. *J Urol* 1986; 136:645-647.

Karamanian A, Kravath R, Nagashima H, et al: Anesthetic management of prune belly syndrome. Case report. *Br J Anaesth* 1974; 46:897.

Kinahan TJ, Churchill BM, McLorie GA, et al: The efficiency of bladder emptying in the prune belly syndrome. *J Urol* 1992; 148:600.

King LR: Idiopathic dilatation of the posterior urethra in boys without bladder outlet obstruction. *J Urol* 1969; 102:783.

King LR, Prescott G: Pathogenesis of the prune belly anomaly. *J Pediatr* 1978; 93:273.

Kramer SA: Current status of fetal intervention for hydronephrosis. *J Urol* 1983; 130:641.

Kroovand RL, Al-Ansari RM, Perlmutter AD: Urethral and genital malformations in prune belly syndrome. *J Urol* 1982; 127:94.

Lattimer JK: Congenital deficiency of the abdominal musculature and associated genitourinary anomalies: a report of 22 cases. *J Urol* 1958; 79:343.

Lee SM: Prune belly syndrome in a 54-year-old man. *JAMA* 1977; 237:2216.

Loder RT, Guiboux JP, Bloom DA, et al: Musculoskeletal aspects of prune belly syndrome: description and analysis. *AJDC* 1992; 146:1224-1229.

Mackie GG, Stephens FD: A correlation of renal dysplasia with position of the ureteral orifice. *J Urol* 1975; 114:274.

Maizels M, Stephens FD: Valves of the ureter as a cause of primary obstruction of the ureter: anatomic, embryologic and clinical aspects. *J Urol* 1980; 123:742.

Manivel JC, Pettinato G, Reinberg Y, et al: Prune belly syndrome: clinicopathologic study of 29 cases. *Pediatr Pathol* 1989; 9:691.

Massad CA, Cohen MB, Kogan BA, et al: Morphology and histochemistry of infant testes in the prune belly syndrome. *J Urol* 1991; 146:1598.

McGovern JH, Marshall VF: Congenital deficiency of the abdominal musculature and obstructive uropathy. *Surg Gynecol Obstet* 1959; 108:289.

Mininberg DT, Montoya F, Okada K, et al: Subcellular muscle studies in the prune belly syndrome: a functional urethral obstruction caused by prostatic hypoplasia. *Pediatrics* 1984; 73:470.

Moerman P, Fryns JP, Goddeeris P, et al: Pathogenesis of the prune belly syndrome: a functional urethral obstruction caused by prostatic hypoplasia. *Pediatrics* 1984; 73:470.

Monfort G, Guys JM, Bocciardi A, et al: A novel technique for reconstruction of the abdominal wall in the prune belly syndrome *J Urol* 1991; 146:639.

Morgan CL Jr, Grossman H, Novak R: Imperforate anus and colon calcification in association with the prune belly syndrome. *Pediatr Radiol* 1978; 7:19.

Mortensen PH, Johnson HW, Coleman GU, et al: Megalourethra. *J Urol* 1985; 134:358.

Nakayama DK, Harrison MR, Chinn DH, et al: The pathogenesis of prune belly syndrome. *Am J Dis Child* 1984; 138:834.

Nunn IN, Stephens FD: The triad syndrome: a composite anomaly of the abdominal wall, urinary system and testes. *J Urol* 1961; 86:782.

Orvis BR, Bottles K, Kogan BA: Testicular histology in fetuses with prune belly syndrome and posterior urethral valves. *J Urol* 1988; 139:335.

Pak LK, Ruchelli E, Ewalt D, et al: Testicular histology in prune belly syndrome: just another intra-abdominal testis? *J Urol* 1993; 149:226A.

Palmer JM, Tesluk H: Ureteral pathology in the prune belly syndrome. *J Urol* 1974; 111:701.

Parker RW: Absence of the abdominal muscles in an infant. *Lancet* 1895; 1:1252.

Parra RO, Cummings JM, Palmer DC: Testicular seminoma in a long-term survivor of the prune belly syndrome. *Eur Urol* 1991; 19:79.

Parrott TS, Woodward JR: Obstructive uropathy in the neonate. *J Urol* 1976; 116:508.

Parrott TS, Woodard JR: The Monfort operation for abdominal wall reconstruction in the prune belly syndrome. *J Urol* 1992; 148:668.

Passerini-Glazel G, Araguna F, Chiozza L, et al: The P.A.D.U.A. (progressive augmentation by dilating the urethra anterior) procedure for the treatment of severe urethral hypoplasia. *J Urol* 1988; 140:1247.

Perlmutter AD: Reduction cystoplasty in prune belly syndrome. *J Urol* 1976; 116:356.

Pescia G, Cruz JM, Werhs D: Prenatal diagnosis of prune belly syndrome by means of raised maternal AFP levels. *J Genet Hum* 1982; 30:271.

Peterson DS, Fish L, Cass AS: Twins with congenital deficiency of abdominal musculature. *J Urol* 1972; 107:670.

Popek EJ, Tyson RW, Miller GJ, et al: Prostate development in prune belly syndrome (PBS) and posterior urethral valves (PUV): etiology of PBS—lower urinary tract obstruction or primary mesenchymal defect? *Pediatr Pathol* 1991; 11:1.

Potter EL: Abnormal development of the kidney. In Potter EL (ed): *Normal and Abnormal Development of the Kidney*. Chicago, Year Book Medical Publishers, 1972, pp 154-220.

Rabinowitz R, Schillinger JF: Prune belly syndrome in the female subject. *J Urol* 1977; 118:454.

Randolph JG: Total surgical reconstruction for patients with abdominal muscular deficiency (prune belly) syndrome. *J Pediatr Surg* 1977; 12:1033.

Randolph JG, Cavett C, Geng G: Abdominal wall reconstruction in the prune belly syndrome. *J Pediatr Surg* 1981; 16:960.

Reinberg Y, Shapiro E, Manivel JC, et al: Prune belly syndrome in females: a triad of abdominal musculature deficiency and anomalies of the urinary and genital systems. *J Pediatr* 1991a; 118:395.

Reinberg Y, Manivel JC, Fryd D, et al: The outcome of renal transplantation in children with the prune belly syndrome. *J Urol* 1989; 142:1541.

Reinberg Y, Manivel JC, Pettinato G, et al: Development of renal failure in children with the prune belly syndrome. *J Urol* 1991b; 145:1017.

Riccardi VM, Grum CM: The prune belly anomaly: heterogeneity and superficial X-linkage mimicry. *J Genet* 1977; 14:266.

Rogers LW, Ostrow PT: The prune belly syndrome. *J Pediatr* 1973; 83:786.

Savre R, Stephens R, Chonko AM: Prune belly syndrome and retroperitoneal germ cell tumor. *Am J Med* 1986; 81:895.

Scarborough PR, Files B, Carroll AJ, et al: Interstitial deletion of chromasome 1 [del (1) (q25q32)] in an infant with prune belly sequence. *Prenat Diagn* 1988; 8:169.

Schmidt JD, Hawtrey CE, Culp DA, et al: Experience with cutaneous pyelostomy diversion. *J Urol* 1973; 109:990.

Sellers BB Jr, McNeal R, Smith RV, et al: Congenital megalourethra associated with prune belly syndrome. *J Urol* 1976; 16:814.

Shockley KF: Personal communication, 1983.

Short KL, Groff DB, Cook L: The concomitant presence of gastroschisis and prune belly syndrome in a twin. *J Pediatr Surg* 1985; 20:186.

Shrom SH, Cromie WJ, Duckett JW: Megalourethra. *Urology* 1981; 17:152.

Silverman FM, Huang N: Congenital absence of the abdominal muscle associated with malformation of the genitourinary and alimentary tracts: report of cases of review of literature. *Am J Dis Child* 1950; 80:9.

Smith CA, Smith EA, Gray M, et al: Voiding function in patients with prune belly syndrome after Monfort abdominoplasty. *J Urol* 1993; 149:260A.

Smith DW: Recognizable patterns of human malformation. In Smith DW (ed): *Major Problems in Clinical Pediatrics*. Philadelphia, WB Saunders Co, 1976, vol 70, p 5.

Snow BW, Duckett JW: The prune belly syndrome. In Retik AB, Curier J (eds): *Pediatric Urology*. Baltimore, Williams & Wilkins Co, 1984, pp 253-270.

Snyder HM, Harrison NW, Whitfield HM, et al: Urodynamics in the prune belly syndrome. *Br J Urol* 1976; 48:663.

Stephens FD: *Congenital Malformations of the Rectum, Anus and Genitourinary Tracts*. London, E & S Livingstone, 1963.

Stephens FD: Idiopathic dilatations of the urinary tract. *J Urol* 1974; 112:819.

Stephens FD: *Congenital Malformations of the Urinary Tract*. New York, Praeger Publishers, 1983.

Stephens FD, Fortune DW: Pathogenesis of megalourethra. *J Urol* 1993; 149:1512.

Stephenson KL: A new approach to the treatment of abdominal musculature agenesis and plastic reconstruction. *Surgery* 1953; 2:413.

Tayakkanonta K: The gubernaculum testis and its nerve supply. *Aust NZ J Surg* 1963; 33:61.

Teranoto R, Opas LM, Andrassy R: Splenic torsion with prune belly syndrome. *J Pediatr* 1981; 98:91.

Tuch BA, Smith RK: Prune belly syndrome: a report of 12 cases and review of the literature. *J Bone Joint Surg* 1978; 60:109.

Uehling DT: Testicular histology in triad syndrome. *Soc Pediatr Urol Newsletter*, Dec 30, 1982.

Uehling DT, Zadina SP, Gilbert E: Testicular histology in triad syndrome. *Urology* 1984; 23:364.

Waldbaum RS, Marshall VF: The prune belly syndrome: a diagnostic therapeutic plan. *J Urol* 1970; 103:668.

Walker J, Prokurat Al, Irving IM: Prune belly syndrome associated with exomphalos and anorectal agenesis. *J Pediatr Surg* 1987; 22:215.

Watanabe H, Yamanaka T: A possible relationship between Beckwith-Wiedemann syndrome, urinary tract anomaly and prune belly syndrome *Clin Genet* 1990; 38:410.

Welch KJ: Abdominal muscular deficiency syndrome (prune belly). In Ravitch MM, Welch KJ, Benson CD, et al (eds): *Pediatric Surgery*, ed 3. Chicago, Year Book Medical Publishers, 1979, pp 1220-1232.

Welch KJ, Kearney GP: Abdominal musculature deficiency syndrome: *prune belly*. *J Urol* 1974; 111:693.

Welch KJ, Stewart W, Lebowitz RL: Nonobstructive megacystis and refluxing megaureter in pre-teen enuretic boys with minimal symptoms. *J Urol* 1975; 114:449.

Wigger HJ, Blanc WA: The prune belly syndrome. *Pathol Annu* 1977; 12:17.

Wilbert C, Cohen H, Yu YT, et al: Association of prune belly syndrome and gastroschisis. *Am J Dis Child* 1978; 132:526.

Williams DI: Prune-belly syndrome. In Harrison JH, Gittes RF, Perlmutter AD, et al: (eds): *Campbell's Urology*, ed 4. Philadelphia, WB Saunders Co, 1979, pp 1743-1755.

Williams DI: The prune belly syndrome. In Williams DI, Johnston JH (eds): *Paediatric Urology*. London, Butterworth, 1982.

Williams DI, Burkholder GV: The prune belly syndrome. *J Urol* 1967; 98:1244.

Williams DI, Taylor JS: A rare congenital uropathy: vesicourethral dysfunction with upper tract anomalies. *Brit J Urol* 1969; 41:307.

Williams DI, Parker RM: The role of surgery in the prune belly syndrome. In Johnston JH, Goodwin WF (eds): *Reviews of Paediatric Urology*. Amsterdam, Excerpta Medica, 1974, pp 315-331.

Woodard JR, Parrott TS: Orchiopexy in the prune belly syndrome. *Br J Urol* 1978a; 50:348.

Woodard JR, Parrott TS: Reconstruction of the urinary tract in prune belly uropathy. *J Urol* 1978b; 119:824.

Woodard JR, Trulock TS: Prune belly syndrome. In Walsh PC, Gittes RF, Perlmutter AD, et al (eds): *Campbell's Urology*, ed 5. Philadelphia, WB Saunders Co, 1986, pp 2159-2167.

Woodhouse CR, Kellett MJ, Williams DI: Minimal surgical interference in prune belly syndrome. *Br J Urol* 1979; 51:475.

Woodhouse CR, Ransley PG: Teratoma of the testes in the prune belly syndrome. *Br J Urol* 1983; 55:580.

Woodhouse CR, Ransley PG, Williams DI: Prune belly syndrome—report of 47 cases. *Arch Dis Child* 1982; 52:856.

Woodhouse CR, Snyder HM: Testicular and sexual function in adults with prune belly syndrome. *J Urol* 1985; 133:607.

Workman SJ, Kogan BA: Fetal bladder histology in posterior urethral valves and the prune belly syndrome. *J Urol* 1990; 144:337.

Wright JR Jr, Barth RF, Neff JC, et al: Gastrointestinal malformations associated with prune belly syndrome: three cases and a review of the literature. *Pediatr Pathol* 1986; 5:421.

CHAPTER 50

PRINCIPLES OF URINARY TRACT RECONSTRUCTION

Curtis A. Sheldon
Howard M. Snyder III

"Please exercise the greatest gentleness with my miniature tissues and try to correct the deformity at the first operation. Give me blood and the proper amount of fluid and electrolytes; add plenty of oxygen to the anesthesia, and I will show you that I can tolerate a terrific amount of surgery. You will be surprised at the speed of my recovery, and I shall always be grateful to you."

—Willis J. Potts, 1959

Perhaps the child facing urinary reconstruction might further implore "Please provide definitive correction of my anomaly so that my kidney function might be preserved and so that I may live as normal a life as possible—dry, without tubes, without bags, and without dialysis that would distinguish me from my classmates. Please minimize the loss of intestinal or sexual function and maximize the potential for spontaneous voiding if you are able."

Major advances in surgical technique along with an ever-expanding understanding of the pathophysiology of pediatric urinary tract disease have resulted in tremendous strides in childhood urinary reconstruction over the past 2 decades. Surgical restoration of urinary tract function must be undertaken with specific goals in mind. The most obvious are preservation of the upper tracts and the attainment of the continence of urine. Consequently these concepts have received the greatest emphasis. It is critical, however, that the reconstructive surgeon also emphasize the potential for spontaneous voiding and minimize the disturbance of other organ system function.

Advances in the field of urinary reconstruction were slow in the 1950s and 1960s because of the popularity of Bricker's ileal conduit diversion (Bricker, 1950). Thought to be the ideal solution to bypass the abnormal bladder in children, ileal division failed long-term expectations. Not only was the negative body image a problem, but the silent deterioration of the kidneys was realized in the 15- to 20- year follow-up.

It was Hendren (1973, 1976) who popularized the concept of "undiversion" when he successfully rehabilitated dormant bladders. By solving many of the dilemmas of placing large ureters into bladders and preventing reflux, he demonstrated the feasibility of urinary reconstruction in children. This work, which provided the background for modern reconstructive efforts, has recently been reviewed (Hendren, 1990). For these contributions he was awarded the Pediatric Urology Medal by the American Academy of Pediatrics.

Childhood urinary reconstruction has since become an immensely complex endeavor as a result of a multitude of important patient variables and available technical options. It is therefore impossible to outline one reconstructive approach that is applicable to all or even a majority of patients. Instead the surgeon must be well founded in the physiologic principles of urinary reconstruction, competent in all of the technical options, and cognizant of the patient variables that so profoundly influence the potential for reconstructive success.

The modern approach to childhood urinary reconstruction is predicated on not only the preservation of renal function but on the preservation of quality of life. Objectives include total urinary continence, a 4-hour voiding or catheterization interval, riddance of external appliances, and complete self-sufficiency. These objectives are attainable by the creation of a balanced urinary system-unimpeded, nonrefluxing upper tract drainage into a low-pressure, large-volume reservoir with sufficient outlet resistance to allow continence and emptying by spontaneous voiding or clean intermittent catheterization.

PHYSIOLOGIC CONSIDERATIONS PERTINENT TO URINARY TRACT RECONSTRUCTION

The two most import physiologic considerations are the detrimental influence of high bladder pressure and the consequences of incorporation of gastrointestinal segments into the urinary tract.

Detrimental Influences of High Bladder Pressure

An obvious consequence of high bladder pressure is urinary incontinence. In this setting intravesical pressure exceeds bladder outlet resistance. Similarly, elevated intravesical pressure as a consequence of either detrusor instability or detrusor sphincter dyssynergia (volitional or in volitional) has been implicated as both a cause of both urinary tract infection and vesicoureteral reflux.

This is suggested by several observations. Koff in 1979 demonstrated the association of detrusor instability and detrusor sphincter dyssynergia with the diagnosis of urinary tract infection and vesicoureteral reflux. Additionally, treatment of detrusor instability with oxybutynin was demonstrated to allow resolution of both urinary tract infection and vesicoureteral reflux in a significant percentage of cases (Koff, 1983, Scholtmeijer, 1991). A similar, very important observation from the perspective of urinary reconstruction is the association of detrusor instability and detrusor sphincter dyssynergia with failure of antireflux surgery (Noe, 1985).

Intravesical pressure has also been demonstrated as an important prognostic variable for renal injury. Most data suggesting this relationship have come from a series of patients with neurovesical dysfunction secondary to myelodysplasia. McGuire in 1981 demonstrated a high risk of upper tract deterioration in children with myelodysplasia whose leak point pressure exceeded 40 cm H_2O. Patients with leak point pressures less than 40 cm H_2O appeared to have sparing of the upper tracts on follow-up. In a similar study (Churchill, 1987) a maximal urethral pressure on profilometry exceeding 35 cm of H_2O had a similar association. Thomsen (1984) showed that this pressure (40 cm H_2O) is also that which appears capable of altering renal papillary morphology and inducing intrarenal reflux of urine. Further, Jones and colleagues (1988) demonstrated that in chronic retention, bladder and renal pelvic pressures closely corresponded even in the absence of reflux.

There are less data available to quantitate an association between intravesical obstruction, elevated intravesical pressure, and renal injury. A relationship may be inferred by the known protective effects of several anatomic abnormalities occasionally encountered in patients with posterior urethral valves, which serve as "pop-off" mechanisms to diminish intravesical pressure (Rittenberg, 1988). Examples of such pop-off mechanisms include the VURD syndrome, urinary extravasation (e.g., urinary ascites), and large bladder diverticuli.

There are also supportive data from the transplant experience. A decreased survival and decrease in function of surviving allografts transplanted into posterior urethral valve bladders as compared with bladders of patients whose end-stage renal disease was due to vesicoureteral reflux has been demonstrated (Churchill, 1988, Reinberg, 1988). That this association is not simply due to the presence of an irregular distorted bladder with stasis is suggested by the observation that kidneys transplanted into Eagle Barrett (prune belly) syndrome bladders did not experience a similar reduction in allograft survival or function (Reinberg, 1989).

Successful surgical treatment of urinary incontinence and vesicoureteral reflux as well as the preservation of either native or transplanted kidneys is predicated upon medical or surgical control of intravesical pressure. It is important for the surgeon to recognize that intravesical pressure is a time-variable parameter that is strongly influenced by several factors. These include bladder wall compliance, urine output, frequency of voiding or catheterization, and residual urine. The surgeon must keep all these variables in mind to obtain low-pressure storage of urine.

An attempt is made to maintain intravesical storage pressure less than 35 to 40 cm H_2O during the accumulation of a volume of urine produced during a time period equal to a voiding or catheterization interval compatible with an acceptable lifestyle and compliance. This interval is generally 4 hours. Clearly, careful urodynamic assessment is critical in all patients for whom complex reconstruction is contemplated or for whom dysfunctional voiding is suspected. Medical control of intravesical pressure should be demonstrated prior to reconstruction, or consideration must be given to augmentation cystoplasty.

Consequences of Incorporating Gastrointestinal Segments Into the Urinary Tract

There are many consequences of the incorporation of gastrointestinal segments into the urinary tract. Examples include urinary tract infections, metabolic derangements, malignancy, urolithiasis, and alterations in gastrointestinal function.

Chronic infection and pyelonephritic renal destruction are well-recognized complications of enteric urinary diversion. Most notable was the early experience with *ureterosigmoidostomy* (Creevy and Reiser, 1952; Ferris and Odel, 1950; Spence et al., 1975; Zincke and Segura, 1975). Septic complications were particularly problematic prior to the development of an antirefluxing ureterocolonic anastomosis. Unfortunately, even with antirefluxing anastomotic techniques, chronic pyelonephritis and urolithiasis continued to be formidable problems for patients with a ureterosigmoidostomy.

This may be explained by two observations. The first is an extremely high bacterial count within the contents of the colon. The second is particularly high rectosigmoid pressures that may exceed 200 cm H_2O during defecation (Cher and Roehrborn, 1992). This high pressure may not only introduce fecal bacteria into the upper tracts but also may cause erosion of an initially successful antireflux mechanism over time. An additional problem contributing to upper tract injury was that of anastomotic obstruction in approximately 10% of cases.

Ureterosigmoidostomy was largely abandoned in favor of the ileal conduit (Bricker, 1950) as a result of these infectious complications and also because of a recognized risk of malignancy in patients with ureterosigmoidostomy. Theoretically the ileal conduit was felt to provide an ideal receptacle for urine. It was isolated from the fecal stream and had a direct cutaneous drainage that was thought to minimize receptacle pressure.

Unfortunately, long-term follow-up revealed that up to two thirds of children with this form of diversion would eventually have upper tract deterioration (Middleton and Hendren, 1976; Shapiro et al., 1975). This was felt to be due a high incidence of bacterial colonization of conduit urine and to the presence of freely refluxing anastomoses between the ureter and the ileal segment. As with the ureterosigmoidostomy, a high incidence of anastomic obstruction and urolithiasis was demonstrated. Of interest was the observation that conduit pressures could range up to 80 to 100 cm H_2O under conditions of conduit obstruction (Cher and Roehrborn, 1992). Such obstruction could be caused from stomal stenosis, mid-loop stenosis, occlusive clothing, or a full urostomy bag.

The realization of the importance of an antirefluxing urointestinal anastomosis led to the popularization of the colon conduit. The importance of preventing reflux was demonstrated experimentally in a canine model (Ritchie et al., 1974). These authors demonstrated an 83% incidence of histologically confirmed pyelonephritic renal injury in kidneys draining into refluxing ileal conduits as cpposed to a 7% incidence of those kidneys draining into a nonrefluxing colon conduit. Long-term follow-up of clinical series of colon conduits in children, however, continued to demonstrate a high incidence of urointestinal anatomic obstruction and stomal stenosis as seen with the ileal conduit (Elder et al., 1979).

The relatively high incidence of urointestinal anatomic failure seen in clinical series of colon conduits over time appears to be related to the duration of exposure of the colonic segment to urine. Obstruction as with the ileoconduit and ureterosigmoidostomy is perhaps explained by local inflammatory changes in the intestinal wall in the region of the urointestinal anatomoses. Reflux, perhaps, is due to erosion of the antireflux mechanisms resulting from the similarly high conduit pressures as seen with ileal conduits.

These data strongly suggest that renal preservation is best accomplished by maintaining a sterile, low-pressure upper urinary tract. This is best achieved by providing a reservoir that is highly compliant and stable over time, preventing reflux and minimizing bacterial colonization.

Metabolic Complications

The multiple and potentially devastating metabolic consequences of employing gastrointestinal segments in the urinary tract have been recently reviewed (Hall et al., 1991; McDougal, 1992). These metabolic derangements are due to solute flux, both active and passive, between the urine and blood across the gastrointestinal segment wall. The determinants of the character and severity of these metabolic derangements are a consequence of the nature of the segment employed, the absorptable surface area, the dwell time, and the metabolic reserve of the individual patient. Compensatory mechanisms for metabolic changes are provided by the kidneys, liver, and lungs. Significant compromise of function of any of these organ systems may accentuate the underlying metabolic defect. Syndromes include alterations in acid base status, disorders of serum electrolyte composition, hyperammonemia, and bone demineralization.

Systemic acidosis may be induced by the incorporation of jejunal, ileal, or colonic segments into the urinary tract. The mechanism for acidosis due to jejunal segments has been recently reviewed (Cher and Roehborn, 1992). In the jejunem, passive diffusion of solute occurs along concentration gradients. The passage of hypertonic urine into a jejunal segment will result in loss of both sodium chloride and water, resulting in hyponatremia, hypochloremia, and volume contraction with subsequent contraction acidosis. Additionally, diminished renal blood flow results in secondary hyperaldosteronism, resulting in a more hypertonic urine as well as hyperkalemia. The hyperkalemia is aggravated by the potassium shift of acidosis.

Clinically, jejunal conduits have been found to be associated with hypochloremia, hyponatremia, hyperkalemia, and acidosis in 20% to 40% of instances (Clark, 1974; Golimbu and Morales, 1973; Golimbu and Morales, 1975; Klein et al., 1986). Consequently jejunum is employed generally only as a last resort.

Figure 50-1 demonstrates the pertinent metabolic

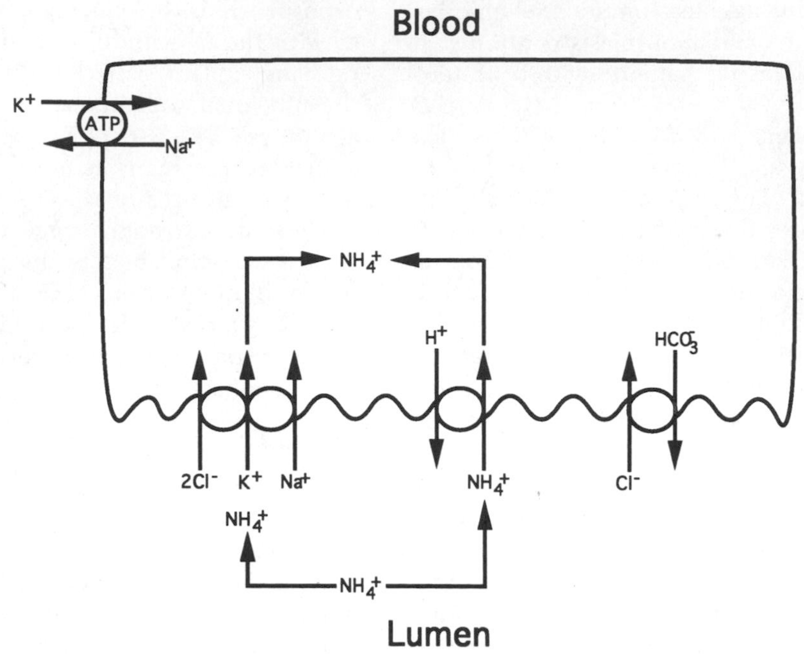

Blood

Lumen

FIG. 50-1
Proposed mechanism of hyperchloremic metabolic acidosis occurring in when urine is diverted through ileum or colon (see text). (Modified from McDougal WS: Metabolic complications of urinary intestinal diversion. *J Urol* 1992; 147:1201.

consequences of ileal and colonic segments interposed within the urinary tract. Active secretion of sodium (Na^+) and bicarbonate (HCO_3^-) as well as reabsorption of ammonium (NH_4^+), and chloride (Cl^-) is encountered. Absorption of ammonium appears to be quantitatively most important. Sodium is excreted in exchange for hydrogen, and bicarbonate is excreted in exchange for chloride. This results in absorption of ammonium chloride in exchange for carbonic acid (i.e. CO_2 and H_2O) (McDougal, in press). Probably some passive absorption of ammonia (NH_3) occurs as well.

Consideration of the effect of ammonium absorption explains many of the abnormalities encountered when ileum or colon has an interface with urine. Chloride is absorbed along with ammonia to maintain electrical neutrality, causing hyperchloremia. Ammonia is converted to urea by the liver. This generates hydrogen ions, which are buffered by serum bicarbonate, which produces water and CO_2. CO_2 is eliminated by the lungs resulting in a chronic compensatory respiratory alkalosis. The kidneys excrete the additional urea load and also contribute to hydrogen ion elimination. Additional buffering is provided by bone, resulting in variable demineralization and secondary hyperparathyroidism. This is manifest by hypercalciuria, hyperphosphaturia, hyperoxaluria, hypocitraturia, hypocalcemia, and hypomagnesemia. Osmotic diuresis and acidosis combine to result in total-body potassium depletion.

The ureterosigmoidostomy is prone to the devel-

opment of hyperchloremic metabolic acidosis. This is particularly problematic due to the massive surface area and the tendency for prolonged periods between evacuation. Hyperchloremic metabolic acidosis is reported in frequencies up to 80% (Ferris, 1950).

The incidence of clinically significant electrolyte abnormalities with ileal conduits is quite variable. Although most data published relate to adults, Malek and colleagues (1971) found clinically significant acidosis in 7% of children. However, more than two thirds of his patients demonstrated hyperchloremia. Similarly, Shapiro and co-authors (1975) found clinically significant acidosis in 13% of children with ileal conduits.

The published pediatric experience with respect to electrolyte abnormalities with colon conduits and intestinocystoplasty is less readily available. Elder and colleagues (1979) found clinically significant acidosis in 12% of pediatric patients with colon conduits, and Kass and Koff (1983) found an incidence of metabolic acidosis in 14% of children with intestinocystoplasty.

Of great concern is the recent observation that conventional measurement of serum electrolytes alone fails to detect many cases of absorptive acidosis (Nurse and Mundy, 1989). These authors reviewed 48 patients with various intestinal segments incorporated into the urinary tract. Thirty-three percent of patients had hyperchloremia; however, *all* had abnormal blood gases, predominantly metabolic acidosis with compensatory respiratory alkalosis.

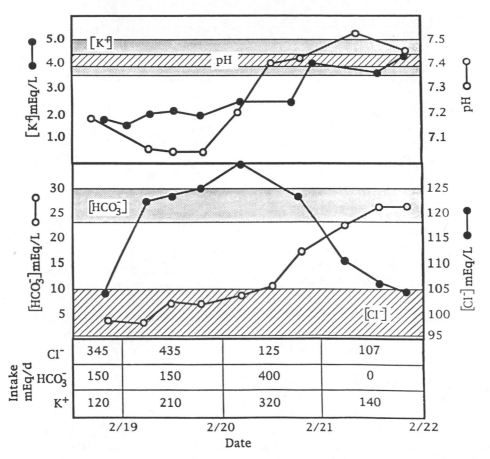

Cl⁻	345	435	125	107
HCO₃⁻	150	150	400	0
K⁺	120	210	320	140

Intake mEq/d

Date: 2/19 — 2/20 — 2/21 — 2/22

FIG. 50-2

Metabolic derangement secondary to absorptive acidosis associated with ureterosigmoidostomy. Response to therapy (see text). Note that initial resuscitation with sodium chloride resulted in increased hyperchloremia and acidosis.

Figure 50-2 demonstrates the approach to therapy of patients presenting with acute electrolyte derangement secondary to absorptive acidosis. Drainage of urine must be immediately ensured with the use of a rectal tube in the case of ureterosigmoidostomy, a conduit catheter if conduit stomal stenosis is present, or a urethral catheter in the presence of an intestinocystoplasty. Patients are typically dehydrated, and vigorous hydration will be necessary. Chloride must be avoided, and sodium lactate offers an excellent source for volume expansion. Potassium replacement is given by potassium acetate. Sodium bicarbonate may be administered cautiously to help correct acidosis. Chloride is subsequently introduced with caution.

Chronic acidosis may be treated by the administration of an oral alkali such as Shohl's solution or polycitra. Experimentally chlorpromazine (Kock et al., 1985a) and nicotinic acid (Koch et al., 1985) have been suggested as two clinically available agents which might have significant beneficial effect on clinical absorptive acidosis.

Metabolic alkalosis is a unique complication seen with gastrocystoplasty. Although uncommon, hypokalemic-hypochloremic metabolic alkalosis has been reported (Gosalbez et al., 1993; Kinahan et al., 1992). Of significance is the fact that these patients also appear to be quite vulnerable to dehydration during episodes of viral gastroenteritis. Although renal failure has been implicated as a risk factor for gastrocystoplasty-induced alkalosis (McDougal, 1992), series emphasizing the use of gastrocystoplasty for patients with end-stage renal disease have not demonstrated this syndrome (Sheldon et al., 1994a, 1994b). However, acid secretion has been documented to be sufficient to reverse the acidosis of azotemia (Fig. 50-3). Acute gastroenteritis appeared to precipitate alkalosis in two patients (Gosalbez et al., 1993). Both patients had normal renal function (GFR 91 and 111 ml/min/1.73 m²). Implicated etiologic factors included hypergastrinemia, dehydration, hypokalemia, and hypochloremia. Excessive bicarbonate absorption is postulated to occur secondary to the combination of mineralocorticoid excess and potassium/chloride depletion.

As reviewed by McDougal (1992) hypokalemia, hypocalcemia, and hypomagnesemia are significant potential sequelae of incorporating intestinal segments within the urinary tract. Severe depletion of total body potassium has been reported in some patients with

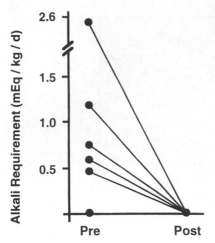

FIG. 50-3
Reduction of alkali requirement in children with end-stage renal failure following performance of gastrocystoplasty.

urinary intestinal diversion and may be potentiated in the face of renal dysfunction. Sufficiently severe hypokalemia to result in muscular paralysis has been reported.

Although hypocalcemia is rarely severe enough to be symptomatic, it may present with irritability, tremors, tetany, coma, and may even be fatal. Physical findings include positive Chevostek and Trousseau signs. Hypomagnesemia is also rarely severe enough to be symptomatic but may present with altered sensorium, personality changes, delirium, psychosis, weakness, tremors, tetany, seizures, and may also be fatal.

Hyperammonemia complicating urinary reconstruction with intestine has also been reviewed by McDougal (1992). Hyperammonemia may cause altered sensoria and coma. As previously noted, ammonium is actively absorbed from intestinal segments and may be present in large amounts in urine due to its generation by renal tubules and production from urea by urea-splitting organisms. The occurrence of significant hyperammonemia generally implies altered hepatic function (acute or chronic). It has, however, been seen in the absence of demonstrable hepatic disease, and in this instance bacteremia and sepsis should be suspected.

Perhaps the single most critical concern is the effect of the incorporation of intestinal segments on childhood growth and development. This concern is particularly worrisome in those patients with diminished renal function. Here, the metabolic insult is more likely and more severe because growth and development are often already significantly impaired.

Linear growth is difficult to assess due to large population variability and a dominant influence of genetic determinants on height and weight. Additionally, associated spinal and lower extremity pathology may confound the measurement of linear growth in many patients for whom urinary reconstruction is required. Consequently height and weight measurements, expressed as population means or compared only against extremes of population normal ranges, provide little meaningful data.

Several studies have, however, provided data strongly suggestive of defective linear growth. In 1971 Malek and colleagues published a series of 42 children followed with ileal conduits. They published the growth curves of these children, demonstrated that the majority remained within a range of normalcy defined as the third percentile to the ninety-seventh percentile, and concluded that growth was unimpaired. Analysis of their data, however, suggests that approximately 16% of these children actually experienced a considerable defect in linear growth. McDougal (1992) reported a series of 93 children followed with myelodysplasia in which those treated by urointestinal diversion were compared with those treated with intermittent catheterization of the native bladder. A decrease in linear growth in children with urointestinal diversion was demonstrated in all indexes reported. Of importance was a statistically significant decrease in the more objective measurements of biachromial span and elbow-hand length.

Mundy and Nurse (1992) reported an average of 20% reduction in growth potential in three of six children followed with colocystoplasty. Similarly, Wagstaff and co-authors (1992) reported a series of 60 children with intestinocystoplasty or continent diversion and noted delayed linear growth in 16 (27%) patients. Twelve patients experienced delayed growth in height in the absence of delayed growth in weight (20%). A mean loss of 25 percentile points was reported for these 12 patients.

Strong evidence exists for a primary effect of incorporating intestinal segments into the urinary tract on bone mineralization. That acidosis is the etiology of defects in bone mineralization, bone disease, and linear growth failure is suggested by several observations. Chronic metabolic acidosis in humans is known to cause increased urinary calcium excretion (Lemann et al., 1967). It is associated with hyperphosphaturia and secondary hyperparathyroidism. Also observed is a tendency toward decreased serum levels of calcium, phosphorous, and magnesium.

Decreased renal tubular calcium reabsorption is postulated to be a consequence of a direct effect of acidosis on the renal tubule. Additional, intestinal absorption of calcium and phosphorous is depressed by chronic acidosis (Cunningham et al., 1984; Gafter, 1980) as is vitamin D metabolism (Lee et al., 1987; Whiting and Draper, 1981). McDougal and Koch (1988) have demonstrated increased urinary sulfate

TABLE 50-1

Estimated Risk of Colon Cancer in Patients with Ureterocolic Anastomosis and in Patients Diverted for Benign Disease

Author	No. of Patients Followed Up	No. of Cases of Carcinoma	Incidence Per 100,000 Population	Risk
Urdaneta et al. (1)	23	3	13,000	550 × normal population
Parsons et al. (2)	29	2	6,900	280 × normal population
Eraklis and Folkman (3)	82	4	4,900	181 × whole population 7000 × population aged <25 yr
St Peter's cases (unpublished)	±200	7	3,500	80-100 × normal population

From Stewart M, Macral FA, and Williams CB: Neoplasia and ureterosigmoidostomy: a colonscopy survey. *Br J Surg* 69:414, 1982. The number of cases of colorectal cancer in the first three series gives a cumulative incidence of between 4.9% and 13%. When all are added together the cumulative, incidence is 9 out of 134 or 6.7%. The mean age at tumour diagnosis in the St Peter's cases is 46 years. The cumulative incidence of colon cancer in Birmingham is 0.11% in persons living up to 46 (4), of which approximately one-third occur in the rectosigmoid (5). Thus, the cumulative incidence of rectosigmoid cancer is 0.04%, giving an excess risk, in the St Peter's cases, of 80-100-fold.

excretion; this excretion is felt to cause impaired calcium reabsorption, which is magnified by acidosis.

Findings consistent with the diagnosis of rickets have been reported in children with ureterosigmoidostomy (Specht, 1967; Tobler et al., 1957). Osteomalacia has been reported in numerous instances with ureterosigmoidostomy (Harrison, 1958; Perry et al., 1977; Siklos et al., 1980). Additionally, biopsy-proven osteomalacia has been reported in two patients with ileal ureters (Salahudeen et al., 1984) and one patient with colocystoplasty (Hossain, 1970). These patients had in common hyperchloremic metabolic acidosis and mild to moderate renal insufficiency.

A very pertinent finding was the observation that myelodysplastic children with urinary intestinal interposition had an increased risk of bony fracture, number of fractures, need for surgery for spinal curvature, and complications from orthopedic procedures including delayed healing and nonunion (McDougal and Koch, 1991). Experimentally, urinary intestinal diversion in rats was found to be associated with a significant decrease in bone calcium content (McDougal and Koch, 1989).

The majority of patients reported with clinically evident bone disease have had either persistent or intermittent metabolic acidosis. Treatment with alkalinating agents has been partially capable of preventing or reversing demineralization disease in patients with urinary intestinal diversion (Hossain, 1970; Siklos et al., 1980). A similar effect has been demonstrated experimentally (McDougal and Koch, 1989).

The magnitude of the risk of bone disease in the reconstructed population is demonstrated by two important observations: (1) a 100% incidence of metabolic acidosis, of which approximately one third of cases are incompletely compensated (Nurse and Mundy, 1989), and (2) approximately 20% of patients undergoing reconstruction who have essentially normal electrolyte patterns will experience intermittent episodes of severe systemic acidosis (McDougal, 1992).

Malignancy

The risk of malignancy in patients undergoing urinary reconstruction with intestinal segments has recently been reviewed (Filmer and Spencer, 1990; Husmann and Spence, 1990; Rowland and Regan, 1992). A majority of our understanding of urointestinal malignancy following reconstruction comes from the ureterosigmoidostomy experience. This subject has been reviewed in detail (Husmann and Spence, 1990; Sheldon et al., 1983). Several clinical observations are of critical importance to the surgeon. The vast majority of tumors develop at or near the site of ureterocolonic anastomoses. Most have been adenocarcinoma; however, two patients diverted for bladder exstrophy have developed transitional cell carcinoma.

Although the risk of neoplasia is clearly much greater for these patients than the general population, the exact risk has been somewhat difficult to quantitate. Leadbetter and colleagues (1979) estimated a 5% lifetime risk. Zabbo and Kay (1986) estimated an 11% risk of malignancy and an 11% risk of noninvasive tumors. Colonoscopic surveillance has demonstrated a high incidence of premalignant findings such as adenomas and dysplasia (Starling et al., 1984; Stewart et al., 1982). Finally, the risk of malignancy has been estimated to be between 80 and 550 times that of the general population (Table 50-1). Eraklis and Folkman have estimated a 7000 times greater risk in those patients younger than 25 years of age.

There is a substantial interval between the performance of ureterosigmoidostomy and the presentation of malignancy (Fig. 50-4). The mean interval is 24 years with 69% of patients having malignancy detected between 15 and 30 years following reconstruction. This latency interval has several important implications. A carcinogenic effect is clearly implied. Moreover there is a potential for early surveillance diagnosis. Clearly, long-term follow-up is mandatory. These data raise an important concern as to the risk of malignancy in newer modalities of reconstruction for which follow-up is much shorter.

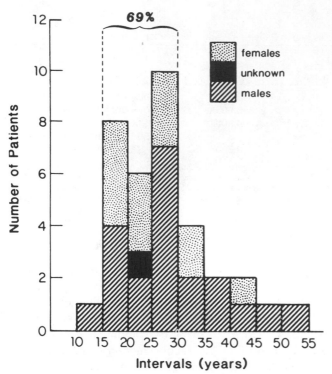

FIG. 50-4
Interval between ureterosigmoidostomy and diagnosis of malignancy. (From Sheldon CA, et al: Carcinoma at the site of ureterosigmoidostomy. *Diseases of Colon and Rectum* 1983; 26:58.

Of particular concern to the reconstructive surgeon is the observation of malignancy developing at the site of ureteral stumps years after ureterosigmoidostomy defunctionalization by either nephrectomy or alternate diversion (Husmann and Spence, 1990). Such cases account for approximately 17% of reported malignancies following ureterosigmoidostomy. The average interval from the original ureterosigmoidostomy was 21 years. Anastomoses were defunctionalized after a mean of 8 years but in two cases after only 6 or fewer months. Patients with previous ureterosigmoidostomy who undergo subsequent reconstruction should have the region of the ureterocolonic anastomoses resected (irrespective of their endoscopic appearance) at the time of surgery.

The incidence of malignancy developing in conduits and continent diversion has been comparably small (Filmer and Spencer, 1990; Rowland and Regan, 1992). One adenocarcinoma and one adenomatous polyp have been reported 20 and 22 years, respectively, after ileal diversion in children with exstrophy. Additionally, one adenocarcinoma has been reported arising 26 years after colon conduit diversion for bladder exstrophy. There have been several reports of malignancy when the primary disease requiring diversion was a pelvic malignancy. Most were of the same histologic type, suggesting recurrence. How-

ever, some were of completely different histologic type and with a long latency interval, suggesting a second malignancy.

Filmer and Spencer (1990) also reviewed 13 patients who had development of primary malignancies in bladders augmented for benign disease. There were seven adenocarcinomas, three transitional cell carcinomas, two undifferentiated carcinomas, and one oat cell carcinoma. Ten were reconstructed for bladder injury form tuberculosis, two from chronic cystitis, and one from neurovesical dysfunction. The interval ranged from 5 to 29 years with a mean of 18.5 years. Ten patients had undergone ileocystoplasties, and three had undergone colocystoplasties.

Because of the low incidence of spontaneous ileal malignancy, the occurrence of malignancy in the ileocystoplasty patient is particularly worrisome. It remains unknown, however, whether these data from patients with chronic inflammatory bladder injury can be extrapolated to children who undergo reconstruction for neurovesical dysfunction and exstrophy.

The pathogenesis of malignancy developing following urointestinal diversion has been reviewed by Husmann and Spence (1990). In 1980 Crissey and colleagues developed a rat model in which vesicosigmoidostomy was demonstrated to have a high incidence of tumor induction. Subsequent experimental data have demonstrated that Wistar-Furth and Sprague-Dawley rats are susceptible to such tumor induction, whereas Lewis rats are relatively resistant. Two differences in these species have led to theories of tumorogenesis. One difference relates to nitrate metabolism. As a consequence of this work, urinary nitrosamines, which are known to have a carcinogenic influence on colon, have been implicated. Nitrate is a normal urinary constituent. Several strains of bacteria found in feces and as a cause of urinary tract infection have been found to metabolize nitrate to nitrite and to nitrosamine. Although nitrosamines are not found in significant amount in either sterile urine or in normal feces, they are found in the feces of both rats and humans following ureterosigmoidostomy.

Although this potential etiology has gained rather wide acceptance, there are now data to refute nitrosamine as a dominant etiology for tumor induction in the ureterosigmoidostomy model. Agents known to block formation of nitrosamine such as vitamin C (Shands et al., 1989; Stribling et al., 1989), sodium-2-mercaptoethane sulfonate, and sodiumpentosanpolysulfate (Kalble et al., 1991) have not resulted in a significant protective effect from tumorogenesis.

A second implicated etiology relates to a difference in phagocytic activation among these strains of rats. Oxygen radicals from phagocytic activation have been implicated in carcinogenesis. Consequently an inflammatory response at the suture line itself could be a possible source of tumor induction and is consistent with the clinical observation of the vast majority of tumors occurring at the site of urointestinal anastomosis.

Of interest has been the observation that exclusion of urine or feces from the urointestinal anastomosis has a protective influence (Crissey et al., 1980). Additionally, the placement of an interposed segment of intestine between the urointestinal anastomosis and the fecal stream has been found to be protective (Gittes, 1986; Shands et al., 1989).

Clinically these observations underscore the need for surveillance with any intestinal interposition into the urinary tract. Probably an annual endoscopic evaluation after perhaps 10 years of exposure for any patient with ureterosigmoidostomy, continent diversion, or augmentation should be strongly considered. Patients with intestinocystoplasty might be at greater risk than those with simple conduits due to longer exposure of urine and larger urointestinal anastomosis.

Reconstructive alternatives to the use of intestinal interposition should be sought. When options are limited, augmentation cystoplasty and continent diversion would seem preferable to ureterosigmoidostomy. When ureterosigmoidostomy appears to be the best option, intestinal interposition as described by Hendren (1976), as well as Kim and coworkers (1988) would seem appropriate.

Hematuria-Dysuria Syndrome

An important complication of bladder reconstruction utilizing the stomach is the hematuria-dysuria syndrome. This is a syndrome of severe pain and urinary bleeding due to urothelial erosion from acid secreted in the urine following gastrocystoplasty (Nguyen et al., 1993). Additionally, peptic ulceration with perforation of the gastric patch segment of a gastrocystoplasty (Reinberg et al., 1992) and systemic alkalosis (Gosalbez et al., 1993; Kinahan et al., 1992) have been reported, presumably due to acid hypersecretion.

Three major factors appear to be operative in the genesis of this complication: acid hypersecretion, profound oliguria, and bladder neck incompetency. True acid hypersecretion would appear to be quite rare. Presumably the predominant mechanism for this would be hypergastrinemia, which has been reported in some incidences (Gold et al., 1992; Gosalbez et al., 1993; Kinahan et al., 1992). This could occur as a result of antral exclusion physiology if transposed antral tissue were exposed to a relatively alkaline environment. Other series, however, have failed to demonstrate more than minimal elevations in serum gastrin level (Adams et al., 1988; Sheldon et al., 1994). Efforts are directed at minimizing the incorporation of antrum in the gastrocystoplasty.

In some instances, however, it would appear that even basal levels of acid secretion may be problematic. Profound oliguria has clearly been demonstrated to be a precipitating cause of hematuria-dysuria syndrome within the end-stage renal disease population (Sheldon et al., 1994). Patients tolerating their gastrocystoplasty well have subsequently had development of hematuria-dysuria upon entering an oliguric phase only to have their symptoms completely resolve upon receipt of a renal allograft.

Endoscopic evaluation of children with the hematuria-dysuria syndrome suggests greater involvement of the urethra than the bladder itself. Consequently the presence of an incompetent bladder outlet may play an important role in the genesis of this complication. Additionally, some data would suggest that a particularly large gastric patch may be contributory (Dykes and Ransley, 1991).

Treatment focuses upon hydration to dilute the acid, insurance of bladder neck competence to avoid urethral exposure, and pharmacologic therapy directed at minimizing acid secretion. Bladder neck competence may be enhanced by administering anticholinergic agents, insurance of effective intermittent catheterization, and in some instances further bladder outlet reconstruction. Certainly one should pursue bladder reconstruction in any marginal bladder outlet in patients undergoing gastrocystoplasty. Anticholinergics may decrease urethral exposure by lowering intravesical pressure. In addition to affecting the smooth muscle of the bladder wall, oxybutynin chloride has been demonstrated to affect the smooth muscle of the gastric wall as well (Sheldon et al., 1994). Additionally, anticholinergic agents have the theoretic potential of lowering gastric acid secretion.

Specific pharmacologic therapy directed at lowering gastric acid secretion is important in some instances. Figure 50-5 outlines the current understanding of the mechanism of gastric acid secretion. Gastric acid is stimulated by activation of gastrin (G), histamine (H), and acetylcholine (Ach) receptors. These effects are mediated by second messengers such as inositol-tris-phosphate (IP_3), cyclic adenosine monophosphate (cAMP), and calcium (Ca^{++}). Acid secretion is then effected through the activity of the gastric proton pump (hydrogen-potassium-ATPase). Gastric acid secretion may be minimized by the use of histamine H_2-receptor antagonists or by the use of omeprazole, which inhibits the action of the gastric proton pump.

Patients who are anuric or have profoundly oliguria can experience dramatic alleviation of symptoms by periodic irrigation while awaiting subsequent transplantation. Removal of the gastric patch and augmentation with an alternate intestinal segment would be an additional theoretic therapeutic alternative but has not been considered in our experience.

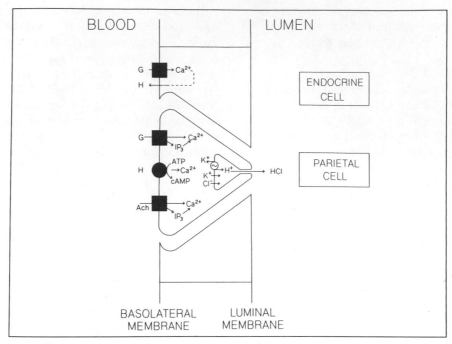

FIG. 50-5
Summary of the known parietal cell receptors, and their second messengers, which result in activation of acid secretion. (From Cuppoletti J and Malinowska DH: Gastric Secretion. In Sperelakis N. Banks RO (eds): *Physiology*. Boston, Little, Brown & Company, 1993, p 613.

Urolithiasis

A particularly significant problem in patients with both intestinal diversion and intestinocystoplasty is the development of urolithiasis. This occurs in the upper tracts at significant incidence, especially in those patients with urinary intestinal diversion. It is also being encountered in some patients following intestinocystoplasty.

The intestinocystoplasty bladder and the continent diversion pouch appear particularly prone to the development of reservoir calculi, particularly in those patients without dependent urine drainage, as with a Mitrofanoff continence mechanism to the abdominal wall. This complication has been seen in children (Blyth et al., 1992; Wagstaff et al., 1992). It has not been seen in any children who have undergone reconstruction with gastrocystoplasty (Sheldon et al., 1994), presumably due to altered solubility of stone constituents caused by aciduria.

Urolithiasis is a major contributor to renal injury by way of both obstruction and infection. Although the composition of calculi in such individuals is varied, struvite is particularly common. Also common are calcium oxalate and calcium phosphate. Uric acid has also been encountered, and stones containing mixtures of these elements are quite common.

Patients with intestinocystoplasty and with intestinal diversion experience metabolic changes that make precipitation of calculi more likely (Cher and Roehrborn, 1992; Steiner and Morton, 1991). These changes include hypercalciuria, hyperoxaluria, hypocitraturia, and decreased urinary magnesium. Increased urinary calcium and oxalate favor stone formation. Citrate and magnesium, which tend to have an inhibitory influence on calcium oxalate formation, are present in depressed levels, again facilitating stone precipitation.

Several other faciliatory conditions may contribute. The presence of urea-splitting organisms, which increase urinary pH, favor the precipitation of struvite calculi. This has been studied most carefully in patients with ileal conduits (Dretler, 1973). In this series 91% of patients had urea-splitting organisms in their urine, and 93% of the stones analyzed contained at least some struvite.

Another facilitatory condition is that of foreign bodies. These may include staples or nonabsorbable sutures used during reconstruction or hair introduced by intermittent catheterization. Mucous production may play a role as well.

Further, patients undergoing reconstruction appear to be particularly prone to dehydration. Often such patients have decreased renal concentrating ability, have greater vulnerability to the consequences of gastroenteritis, and may intentionally dehydrate themselves to achieve increased voiding or catheterization intervals or to enhance urinary continence. Urinary stagnation due to diverticuli, pouch irregularities, or nondependent reservoir drainage appears to be an important factor.

Altered Pharmacokinetics

The incorporation of intestinal segments also has the potential for altering the pharmacokinetics of several types of drugs. As reviewed by McDougal (1992), these would include any intestinally absorbed drug that is excreted unchanged by the kidney or any drug in which an active metabolite is excreted when these compounds may be reabsorbed through the intestinal segment. Such altered pharmokinetics have been observed for various antibiotics, phenytoin, and methotrexate. The surgeon must be cognizant of this potential complication.

Altered Gastrointestinal Function

Finally, the incorporation of intestinal segments into the urinary tract may result in significant alterations in gastrointestinal tract function. Alterations in gastric function have been reported following gastrocystoplasty (Gold et al., 1992). Functional alterations reported include weight loss, feeding intolerance, dumping physiology, delayed gastric emptying, and esophagitis. Some of these symptoms are consistent with simply a reduction in gastric capacity, which would be expected to resolve with time. Other symptoms suggest alterations in vagus innervation, loss of normal pyloric and antral motility function, and distortion of the gastroesophageal junction with resultant loss of competence and reflux esophagitis. These findings are a significant concern.

A recent review of gastrocystoplasty with emphasis on long-term follow-up (minimum follow-up of 1.5 years) failed to demonstrate any significant incidence of altered gastric function or altered acid base status in 23 consecutive patients (Sheldon et al., 1994). Technical emphasis must be placed on avoiding the vagus nerves, avoiding significant dissection in the region of the gastric pyloris, and avoiding traction-distortion of the angle of His (e.g., by gastrostomy tube), which may facilitate gastroesophageal junction incompetence.

Another theoretic concern is the potential for removal of sufficient parietal cell mass to interfere with vitamin B_{12} absorption secondary to decreased intrinsic factor production. Long-term follow-up will be necessary to make this determination.

Several potentially important sequelae of intestinal malabsorption may accompany intestinal resection. These include diarrhea, vitamin deficiency, and fecal incontinence. Diarrhea, or increased frequency of bowel movements, generally implies an alteration in intestinal transit time. This is most frequently due to alterations in bacterial colonization and impairment of

bile acid reabsorption (with or without accompanying steatorrhea). This subject has been reviewed in detail by Steiner and Morton (1991). The ileum is significantly less colonized with bacteria than is the colon. Loss of the ileocecal valve may alter ileal function both by decreasing transit time due to diminished regulatory control over ileal emptying into the colon and by allowing reflux of cecal bacteria, which may promote malabsorption. This effect appears to be exacerbated by concomitant ileal resection.

Malabsorption from ileal resection is directly related to the length of resection. Resection of less than 100 cm of ileum (adult equivalent) results in diminished bile acid reabsorption, which is generally compensated by increase hepatic synthesis. The bile salt pool is maintained and steatorrhea prevented. Bile salts, however, spill over into the colon, where they cause decreased colonic absorption of water and electrolytes, secretory diarrhea, mucosal injury with diminished effective absorptive surface area, and rectosigmoid irritation, which reduces rectosigmoid capacitance, promoting premature urge for fecal evacuation.

Resections of greater than 100 cm of ileum (adult equivalent) diminish bile acid reabsorption to a degree that cannot be compensated by increased hepatic synthesis. As a result the bile salt pool is diminished and steatorrhea develops. Another important sequelae of the diminished bile salt pool in this population is cholelithiasis, which like urolithiasis is clinically seen in a significantly increased incidence following ileal resection. Diarrhea induced by altered bile acid reabsorption with or without accompanying steatorrhea is further enhanced by the rapid emptying of ileal contents into the colon, causing a tendency for osmotic diarrhea.

The ileum is also the sole site of vitamin B_{12} absorption. Ileal resection has been demonstrated to be associated with vitamin B_{12} deficiency. This deficiency is manifested by macrocytic anemia and spinocerebellar degenerative disease but may take many years to become manifest due to body stores of vitamin B_{12}.

Significant pathophysiologic changes in gastrointestinal function have been demonstrated in patients following urinary reconstruction. A large body of data exist to demonstrate diarrhea following small-bowel resection. Large-bowel resection has been quite well tolerated. Associated bowel disease or treatment (e.g., radiation therapy) may exacerbate intestinal dysfunction.

Altered physiology can be demonstrated even after relatively small ileal resection in some instances. Jahnson and Pedersen (1993) reported a 22% incidence of vitamin B_{12} malabsorption following creation of an ileal conduit. These patients, however, received accompanying radiation therapy. Durrans and colleagues (1989) reviewed 16 patients with ileal conduits, only five of whom had malignancy and were potentially exposed to radiation therapy. Eighty-one percent of the patients demonstrated altered bile acid reabsorption, and a strikingly significant increase in bowel frequency was noted in these patients as well.

Although most of these data involve adult patients, King (1987) estimated that 10% of children undergoing resection of ileocecal valve segments will experience chronic diarrhea. Gonzalez and colleagues (1986) reported a patient with protracted diarrhea after creation of an ileocolonic neobladder. The diarrhea resolved after restoring intestinal continuity by returning the ileal cecal segment into normal position within the gastrointestinal tract.

Despite these data, use of intestinal and gastric segments appear to be extremely well tolerated in most children. It would, however, appear prudent to avoid removal of large segments of ileum or removal of the ileocecal valve for purposes of urinary reconstruction, particularly in otherwise compromised patients. Such patients would include those with preexisting malabsorption syndrome or short gut and patients with marginal fecal continence in whom fecal soilage may become incapacitating by loss of stool consistency. Such patients include those with myelomeningocele and imperforate anus who commonly required urinary reconstruction.

CONCEPTUAL APPROACH TO URINARY TRACT RECONSTRUCTION

Because of the high incidence of upper tract deterioration with time and the significant sequela of altered body image form cutaneous urinary diversion, incontinent diversion is no longer considered an acceptable alternative to childhood reconstruction. The exceptions to this would include temporary diversion for stabilization of renal function while awaiting ultimate reconstruction and extenuating circumstances where more formal continent reconstruction is not applicable.

There are four components to balanced urinary tract function that must be achieved to ensure long-term success with urinary reconstruction. The first component is that of adequate bladder (reservoir) capacity and compliance sufficient to provide low pressure storage. The maintenance of storage pressures less than 35 to 40 cm of water (Churchill et al., 1987; McGuire et al., 1981) will optimize upper tract preservation. Bladder capacity optimally should be sufficient to allow a 4-hour catheterization or voiding interval during the day and an 8-hour interval at night without achieving excess pressure and without precipitating incontinence.

The second component is that of adequate bladder outlet resistance sufficient to maintain urinary continence. Third, there must be a convenient, reliable mechanism for bladder (reservoir) emptying. Optimally this mechanism is spontaneous voiding. Otherwise intermittent catheterization is necessary. The native urethra may represent an acceptable conduit for this maneuver; however, if catheterization of the native urethra is either excessively difficult or uncomfortable to prevent optimal patient compliance, the provision of an alternate catheterizable conduit may be necessary. Finally, unobstructed and nonrefluxing sterile upper tract drainage of urine into the bladder (reservoir) is desirable to protect the upper tracts.

Urinary incontinence may be particularly difficult to assess and treat. The surgeon must be cognizant of the fact that multiple etiologies for incontinence exist and often coexist. Bladder outlet incompetence due to anatomic deformity or injury as well as deficiency in innervation may result in incontinence. Additionally, obstruction or detrusor failure and thus deficient bladder emptying may result in overflow urinary incontinence. A bladder with inadequate capacity due to uninhibited detrusor activity, a noncompliant detrusor wall, or inherent small volume may result in incontinence. Incontinence of urine may occur as a result of urine bypassing the urinary sphincteric mechanism as seen with urinary fistulas and with ectopic ureteral insertions. Pseudo incontinence (postvoid dribbling) may be seen with either urethral diverticuli or vaginal voiding. Finally, mixed pathology may occur with incontinence due to two or more of these mechanisms.

When contemplating urinary reconstruction, meticulous preoperative evaluation is critical. It is essential to tailor the reconstruction to the individual needs of the patient. Renal function is assessed by measurement of serum creatinine and by measurement of glomerular filtration rate to including measurement of differential function employing a radioisotope technique. Anatomy is assessed by intravenous urography or ultrasound, contrast voiding cystourethrography, and careful preoperative endoscopic evaluation. Bladder and sphincteric function evaluation assumes a dominant role. Here detailed urodynamic investigation as well as upright cystography to evaluate the competence of the bladder neck is performed. To interpret the results of urodynamic investigation it is important for the surgeon to know the patient's urine output, which is obtained by having the family keep a detailed diary of voided and/or catheterized volumes. Both average urine output per hour and maximal ranges of urine output are noted. This is of importance in designing an adequate-sized reservoir to allow a reasonable (4 to 5 times daily) emptying regimen. Finally, an assessment is made of the patient's potential for compliance with therapy. A careful history, physical examination, and counseling of the patient and family allows an assessment of the patient's intellect, dexterity, and potential for self-care.

Once this assessment has been undertaken, an exhaustive trial of nonoperative therapy is undertaken. This trial may include the use of one or a combination of two ore more pharmacologic agents (Table 50-2) in an attempt to achieve safe intravesical pressure from a perspective of upper tract preservation and continence (Bauer, 1987). This trial of therapy may also include intermittent catheterization. Intermittent catheterization, which was introduced by Lapidis and colleagues (1972), may result in sufficient stabilization of the urinary tract so as to avoid any reconstruction at all. Moreover this important therapeutic modality allows urinary reconstruction where spontaneous voiding would be unlikely. As a result of these two major influences of intermittent catheterization, cutaneous urinary diversion has been almost completely eliminated in the pediatric population. Intermittent catheterization has been proven to be a safe, reliable, and durable modality on long-term follow-up (Diokno and Sonda, 1981) and has also been proven to be successful when used in patients with intestinocystoplasty (Mitchell et al., 1987).

Several important caveats regarding prereconstruction urodynamic investigation merit emphasis. (1) An important goal is the achievement of a 4-hour dry interval between either spontaneous voiding or intermittent catheterization. The bladder (reservoir) must be sufficiently compliant to collect 4 hours of urine without exeeding storage pressures of 40 cm H_2O and without exceeding urethral resistance. Consequently measurement of urine output is an important component of urodynamic investigation. (2) Static urodynamic indexes such as leak point pressure and urethral pressure have not proven to be reliable predictors of continence. Stress indexes such as upright cystography, stress leak point pressure, and bladder cycling may yield superior results. (3) There are two sphincter mechanisms identifiable that may be independently abnormal and which may be independently investigated. Competence of one mechanism appears to be adequate in most patients to provide continence. An important secondary consideration is pertinent to that patient for whom gastrocystoplasty is anticipated. In this case bladder neck incompetence in the face of an adequate striated sphincter mechanism may still be unsatisfactory. This may allow sufficient exposure of the proximal urethra to acid urine as to allow precipitation of the hematuria-dysuria syndrome. (4) Significant problems may be encountered in the interpretation of standard urodynamic testing. Assessment of bladder compliance may be difficult in the presence of severe reflux and particularly in the presence of an incompetent bladder outlet. In the

TABLE 50-2

Types of Medicines that Modulate Lower Urinary Tract Function

Type	Minimum	Maximum
Cholinergic		
Bethanechol (Urecholine)	0.7 mg/kg t.i.d.	0.8 mg/kg q.i.d.
Anticholinergic		
Propantheline (Pro-Banthine)	0.5 mg/kg b.i.d.	0.5 mg/kg q.i.d.
Oxybutynin (Ditopan)	0.2 mg/kg b.i.d.	0.2 mg/kg q.i.d.
Glycopyrrolate (Robinul)	0.01mg/kg b.i.d.	0.03 mg/kg t.i.d.
Hyoscyamine (Levsin)	0.03 mg/kg b.i.d.	0.1 mg/kg q.i.d.
Sympathomimetic		
Phenylpropanolamine (alpha)	2.5 mg/kg b.i.d.	2.5 mg/kg t.i.d.
Ephedrine (alpha)	0.5 mg/kg b.i.d.	1.0 mg/kg t.i.d.
Pseudoephedrine (alpha)	0.4 mg/kg b.i.d.	0.9 mg/kg t.i.d.
Sympatholytic		
Prazosin (alpha) (Minipress)	0.05 mg/kg b.i.d.	0.1 mg/kg t.i.d.
Phenoxybenzamine (alpha)	0.3 mg/kg b.i.d.	0.3 mg/kg b.i.d.
Propranalol (beta)	0.25 mg/kg b.i.d.	0.5 mg/kg b.i.d.
Smooth muscle relaxant		
Flavoxate	3.0 mg/kg b.i.d.	3.0 mg/kg t.i.d.
Dicyclomine (Bentyl)	0.1 mg/kg t.i.d.	0.3 mg/kg t.i.d.
Other		
Imipramine (Tofranil)	0.7 mg/kg b.i.d.	1.2 mg/kg t.i.d.

From Bauer SB: Neuropathology of the lower urinary tract. In Kelalin PP, King LR, Belman AB (eds): *Clinical Pedatric Urology.* Philadelphia, WB Saunders, 1992, p 404.

latter instance, balloon occlusion of the bladder outlet may allow meaningful data. Evaluating the need of bladder outlet reconstruction in patients for whom bladder augmentation is anticipated may be difficult. Elevated bladder pressures from either small-capacity bladders or bladders with detrusor hyperactivity may falsely suggest sphincteric incompetence. Finally, it has been observed that bladder compliance may deteriorate with the development of excessive intravesical pressure following a bladder outlet procedure designed to achieve continence. This has been described with both artificial urinary sphincters and with urethral slings even in patients in whom preoperative studies documented normal compliance (Bauer, 1987; Kreder and Webster, 1992).

Wan and co-authors (1993) studied the leak point pressure and stress leak point pressure in 15 consecutive incontinent children. The mean leak point pressure was 19.9 cm H_2O, ranging from 5 to 50 cm H_2O. The mean stress leak point pressure (the intravesical pressure at which leakage occurred during valsalva maneuver) was 54.7 cm H_2O, ranging from 11 to 100 cm H_2O. These investigators studied stress leak point pressure before and after the injection of cross-linked collagen for treatment of urethral incompetence. The mean stress leak point pressure before and after injection was 39.4 cm H_2O and 96.4 cm H_2O, respectively. Those patients who became totally continent of urine experienced an average increase in stress leak point pressure of 59 cm H_2O, representing a 173% increase. A stress leak point pressure exceeding 100 cm H_2O was associated with an 83% continence rate. Leak point pressure itself did not provide adequate predictive data (Wan et al., 1993). Similarly, Kreder and Webster (1992) evaluated the problem of predicting the need for bladder outlet reconstruction in children for whom bladder augmentation was required. They evaluated urethral pressure profilometry and found this parameter to be unreliable.

Gonzales and Sidi (1985) reviewed 15 patients undergoing bladder augmentation from the perspective of predicting the need for bladder outlet procedures. They employed a combination of an erect lateral cystogram under fluoroscopic guidance to evaluate the bladder neck and direct electromyography to evaluate the striated sphincteric mechanism. In eight patients both mechanisms were incompetent. All of the patients underwent bladder outlet reconstruction, and those seven patients for whom follow-up was available were all continent of urine. Two patients had one mechanism demonstrated to be competent, and five had both mechanisms competent. These seven patients did not receive concomitant bladder outlet procedures, and six were ultimately continent of urine with one patient requiring subsequent bladder outlet reconstruction. Employing these criteria these investigators achieved a 93% continence rate.

Woodhouse (1992) employed a preoperative investigation consisting of bladder cycling through suprapubic catheters and video cystometrography and found their ability to predict sphincteric competence and the need for intermittent catheterization following augmentation to be 79% and 86%, respectively.

To achieve the previously outlined components of balanced urinary tract function, the surgeon must often compensate for inadequate bladder capacity or compliance, compensate for inadequate bladder outlet resistance, or provide a continent, catheterizable access to the bladder other than the native urethra. A unique aspect of achieving unobstructed and nonrefluxing urinary drainage into the bladder, which is particula common in the setting of complex urinary reconstruction, is compensating for inadequate ureteral length. Of additional importance is compensation for inadequate anorectal function and replacement of renal function in the setting of renal insufficiency. It is the achievement of these goals to which the remainder of this chapter is dedicated.

COMPENSATING FOR INADEQUATE BLADDER CAPACITY OR COMPLIANCE
Physiologic Considerations

The history of the incorporation of intestine to the genitourinary tract to produce urinary reservoirs goes back to an effort by von Mikulicz in 1898 (Thorne and Resnick, 1986). He utilized a segment of ileum as a patch to enlarge a small contracted bladder. During the first third of the twentieth century efforts centered more on the use of bowel in urinary tract reconstruction as a form of incontinent or cutaneous diversion. This work was summarized in the review by Hinman and Weyrauch (1937). By the 1940s experimental reports were emerging on the use of bowel as a substitute bladder (Bisgard, 1943; Rubin, 1948). In the 1950s and 1960s clinical results were reported (Couvelaire, 1951; Kuss et al., 1970; Winter and Goodwin, 1958). Interest in the use of bowel to create an adequate urinary reservoir was further stimulated by interest in undiversion in the early 1970s (Hendren, 1973, 1974, 1976; Lome and Williams, 1972). Clinical experience has provided insights into a better understanding of the physiology of intestinal use in the creation of a suitable urinary reservoir.

With the development of intestinal augmentation of the bladder it became evident early that this modality had a major effect on the dynamics of voiding. Gleason and colleagues (1972) carefully studied energy balance of voiding in six patients who had undergone a cecocystoplasty. They demonstrated that emptying took place primarily by means of increased intraabdominal pressure produced by straining. Two thirds of their patients had a significant postvoid residual urine volume. Such evidence made it clear the alternatives of spontaneous voiding were likely to be needed in most patients undergoing this type of urinary tract reconstruction.

Fortunately at approximately the time that the need for means of effective artificial emptying of the bladder arose, experience with intermittent catheterization was also being developed. In 1966 Guttman and Frankle reported the effectiveness of sterile intermittent catheterization in early management of traumatic paraplegia. This was followed in the early 1970s with the pioneering work of Lapides and associates (1972, 1976) on the use of clean, but not sterile, intermittent catheterization. This work demonstrated that it was the frequency of effective emptying of the reservoir rather than the sterile technique that was of critical importance in the avoidance of hydronephrosis and prevention of infection in patients unable to spontaneously empty their bladders.

The use of intermittent catheterization in children with a neurogenic bladder was a major advance (Charney et al., 1982; Duckett and Raezer, 1976; Kass et al., 1979; Tank, 1977). Ehrlich and Brem (1982)

TABLE 50-3

Classification of Augmentation, Neobladder and Continent Diversion Techniques

Augmentation
    Autoaugmentation
        Without seromuscular patch
        With seromuscular patch
    Intestinocystoplasty
        Ileocystoplasty
        Colocystoplasty
        Ileocecocystoplasty
    Gastrocystoplasty
    Ureterocystoplasty
Neobladder
    Ileal
    Colonic
    Ileocecal
    Gastric
Continent diversion
    External
        Ileal
        Colonic
        Ileocolonic
        Composite
    Internal
        Ureterosigmoidostomy
        Rectal bladder

showed that urinary infection was less common in children using clean intermittent catheterization than it was in children who had an ileal conduit urinary diversion. The technique of clean intermittent catheterization has even been effectively applied to both male and female infants younger than 1 year with a neurogenic bladder (Perez-Marrero et al., 1982). As clean intermittent catheterization gained recognition and acceptance as an effective means for producing low-pressure emptying of the bladder, it was a logical step to use the same technique to empty an intestinal reservoir with a catheterizable continent channel that exited on the perineum or on the abdominal wall. This then provided the key to the development of continent catheterizable urinary reservoirs.

Table 50-3 provides a classification scheme for various procedures directed toward compensation for inadequate bladder capacity or compliance that also allow urinary continence. Bladder augmentation can be performed with various donor tissues such as ileum, colon, ileocecal region, stomach, and ureter. As will be discussed later the concept of detubularization has had a major impact on intestinocystoplasty. A more recent concept is that of autoaugmentation either with or without an associated seromuscular patch overlying the denuded bladder uroepithelium.

For purposes of this discussion, the neobladder is defined as a bladder in orthotopic position that is entirely constructed of a segment of the gastrointestinal tract and which is drained either through the intact native urethra or through an orthotopically recon-

structed neourethra. Such neobladders may be constructed of ileum, colon, the ileocecal region, and stomach.

There are a large variety of continent urinary diversions that have greatly extended the percentage of patients who are candidates for continent reconstruction. Such diversion may be either external, involving a variety of segments of the gastrointestinal tract, or internal, such as the ureterosigmoidostomy, its multiple variations, and the rectal bladder.

There are several important reconstructive concepts pertinent to bladder augmentation. The first regards the management of the recipient bladder. If bowel augmentation is performed, leaving the detrusor essentially intact to generate high pressures, then the bowel segment will act urodynamically as a capacious diverticulum (Turner-Warwick and Ashken, 1967). Observation of this type of problem has led some authors (Tanagho, 1975) to advocate avoidance of the use of bowel segments in the closed urinary tract. This type of diverticular decompression instead of augmentation can occur with bowel added to either a neurologically intact or impaired bladder.

The problem can be avoided by an extended sagittal opening of the bladder ("clam cystoplasty"), in essence reconfiguring the bladder from a sphere into a flat plate, so that the detrusor is no longer capable of generating a contraction that produces a significant pressure elevation (Bramble, 1982) (Fig. 50-6). The alternative way of avoiding elevated detrusor pressure would be to perform a supertrigonal excision, as has been advocated by Gil-Vernet (1965) and Zinman and Libertino (1980b). If a wide bladder opening is used with augmentation, it would not appear important that the detrusor be excised, unless it is the source of unpleasant symptoms (Smith et al., 1977).

There are considerations that might lead to advantages in retaining a widely opened bladder remnant. Technically this facilitates the anastomosis of a bowel augmentation segment to the bladder. In neurologically intact patients the residual bladder may provide enhanced sensation. Additionally, it is possible that the detrusor may contribute to bladder neck opening and molding of the proximal urethra, improving voiding efficiency (Gleason et al., 1972). Appendicovesicostomy (Mitrofanoff principle) is more easily performed into detrusor than a bowel segment (Duckett and Snyder, 1986), as is ureteral implantation.

Just as pressure generated by the bladder detrusor is an important contributor to the pressure generated in an augmented urinary reservoir, so also is the pressure generated by the bowel segment itself. Bowel segments that are used in continuity to form a urinary reservoir continue to demonstrate peristaltic contractions. The pressure developed depends primarily on the degree of filling of the intestinal segment. Light

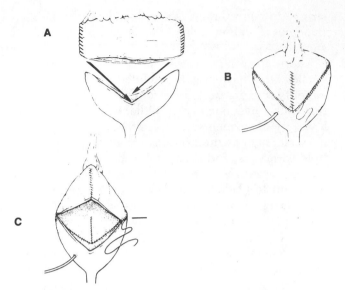

FIG. 50-6
"Clam cystoplasty" with "cup patch" of bowel. Sigmoid segment (20 cm) is opened on its antimesenteric side. The bladder is opened in a sagittal plane almost from anterior bladder neck to trigone (**A**). The bowel patch is reshaped to match size of opened bladder (**B**). Note bowel is closed beginning at open ends, effectively disrupting peristalsis (**C**). (From Mitchell ME: Use of bowel in undiversion. *Urol Clin North Am* 1986; 13:362.)

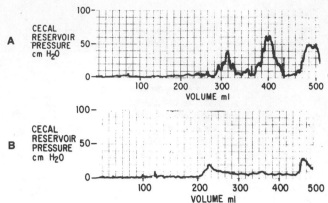

FIG. 50-7
Urodynamics of cecal reservoir. **A**, Tubular bowel produces high-pressure peristaltic waves. **B**, Cup patch bowel with peristalsis disrupted stores large volume without pressure rise. (From Goldwasser HR, Webster GD: Augmentation and substitution enterocystoplasty. J Urol 1986; 135:215. Used by permission.)

and Engelman (1985) studied pressures generated in intact (nondetubularized) ileocecal, cecal, and sigmoid augmentation of the bladder. With peristaltic waves, the pressure ranged from 60 to 100 cm H_2O. Kock (1969), in developing his continent intestinal reservoir, had previously observed that closed intact bowel segments were able to generate pressures of more than 100 cm H_2O regardless of whether the large or small bowel was studied. This observation led Kock to develop his concept of turning the intact bowel into a reservoir incapable of effective peristalsis by creating a "pouch" (Kock et al., 1985a). Opening the small bowel along its antimesenteric border and closing it with disruption of the circular muscle (detubularization) renders peristalsis ineffectual. Without the ability to undergo peristalsis, the bladder reservoir dilates and maintains a low pressure (Fig. 50-7).

The physiologic consequences of detubularization have been reviewed (Hinman, 1988; Koff, 1988; Schmidbauer et al., 1987). Detubularization with an incision along the antimesenteric border of the isolated bowel segment results in interruption of circular muscle fibers. The basic electrical rhythm of the bowel courses along the longitudinal muscle layer. As this electrical rhythm courses longitudinally, its activity is immediately spread to the adjacent circular muscle layer, which induces a contractile ring that increases intraluminal pressure and allows peristalsis. Detubularization interrupts this process and limits any con-

traction to a fraction of a surface area of the reconfigured bowel segment (Fig. 50-8).

Additionally, there is a very significant increase in the geometric capacity of the intestinal segment (Fig. 50-9) as reviewed by Hinman (1988). Because the volume of a cylinder is $\pi r^2 h$, a segment of bowel opened, folded, and retubularized will have a marked increase in its capacity. A similar increase will occur with each sequential reconfiguration.

This conceptual analysis is somewhat of an oversimplification due to the loss of volume with closure of the ends of such cylinders, but it is nonetheless useful for illustration. Schmidbauer (1987) and Koff (1988) took such closure into consideration and considered the effect of reconfiguration of a closed cylinder into a sphere whose volume is determined by $4/3\pi r^3$ (Fig. 50-10). These concepts demonstrate two important detubularization principles: (1) there is progressive widening of the increment in geometric capacity as the length of the donor bowel segment increases; and (2) the rate of incremental increase in geometric capacity is potentiated by an increased radius of the native donor bowel.

A third important concept is that of accommodation (Fig. 50-11). It is well known that over time, the reconstructed bladder will gradually enlarge. Such accommodation is a result of two physical principles: Pascal's Law, which states that within any intact chamber (simple or complex) there will be equilibration of pressure, and LaPlace's Law (T = Pr), which states that the greater the radius, the greater the wall tension for a given pressure. Thus at a constant pressure, a structure with a larger radius will accommodate a greater volume over time—again, an advantage for detubularized bowel segments.

Such physiologic concepts have been confirmed by

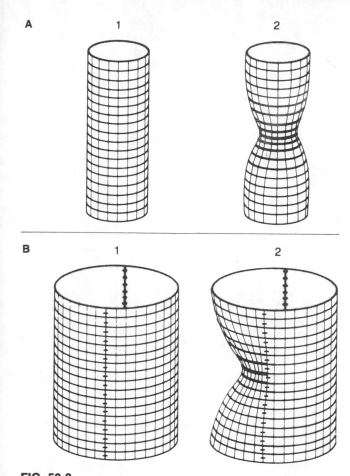

FIG. 50-8
A, Diagram of intact segment with effective contraction ring. **B,** Detubularized (folded) segment shows ineffective asynchronous contraction. (From Hinman F Jr: Selection of intestinal segments for bladder substitution: physical and physiological characteristics. *J Urol* 1988; 139:522.

overestimate resulting capacity if reconfiguration is not truly spheric, there also will be an effect of accommodation of volume over time. Traditionally, pediatric reconstructive surgeons have aimed at the achievement of normal capacity for age, which may be estimated by a variety of formulas such as bladder capacity (ounces) = age (years) + two. This formula, however, may not be adequate. The surgeon must keep in mind that the goal is to achieve a 4-hour daytime voiding or catheterization interval during which continence is maintained and pressures exceeding 40 cm H_2O are not generated. An additional goal is the ability to allow overnight urine collection with continence and without excessive pressure. Consequently such formulas may need to be modified according to the patients urine output and according to other therapeutic interventions such as nighttime tube feedings.

Several considerations must be entertained when choosing an *augmentation donor site*. There are anatomic considerations such as mobility of blood supply that favor the use of ileum, sigmoid, the ileocecal region, and the greater curvature of the stomach. The ability to implant a ureter or a Mitrofanoff neourethra may also be a consideration. Although good success with the LeDuc-Camey implantation of ureter into small bowel is reported by LeDuc and co-authors (1987), conventional implantations usually require the use of colon or stomach. Additionally, it may be important to avoid the peritoneal cavity so as to preserve peritoneal dialysis or a ventricular peritoneal shunt. Such considerations favor the use of ureteral augmentation or autoaugmentation.

The choice of augmentation donor site may be limited by the patient's primary disease. Patients with short gut may not tolerate loss of the ileocecal region or of a significant length of ileum. Patients with borderline fecal continence such as those with imperforate anus or myelodysplasia may not tolerate loss of ileocecal valve or the water reabsorptive capacity of the right colon. Metabolic consequences may assume an overriding influence. The risk of absorptive acidosis and growth retardation, which may be exacerbated by chronic renal insufficiency, may favor the use of autoaugmentation, ureteral augmentation, or gastrocystoplasty techniques.

There does not appear to be a significant difference between the various donor sites and the ability to achieve desired capacitance and compliance. Mitchell and Piser (1987) reviewed a large pediatriac series of bladder reconstructions employing both large and small bowel and found these procedures to result in similar urodynamic properties. Success was felt to be primarily dependent on the size and configuration of the resultant reservoir rather than on the origin of the bowel employed.

careful urodynamic investigation of tubularized and detubularized urinary reconstructive techniques. Goldwasser and colleagues (1987) compared cystoplasty compliance, capacity, and contraction with tubular and detubularized segments of both large and small bowel (Table 50-4). Cher and Roehrborn (1992) compared capacity, compliance, and contraction characteristics of continent reservoirs employing either tubularized or detubularized techniques (Table 50-5). These data demonstrate a significant increase in volume with all detubularization techniques. In addition, there is increased compliance manifested by an increased volume at first contraction, an increased volume at maximal contraction, a decrease in the maximal contraction pressure generated, and an increased voiding or catheterization interval.

The calculations of Koff (1988) offer a rough approximation of the length of ileum (R = 1 cm) or colon (R = 2 cm) required to achieve a desired capacity as a function of initial bladder volume in the pediatric setting (Table 50-6). Although these estimates will

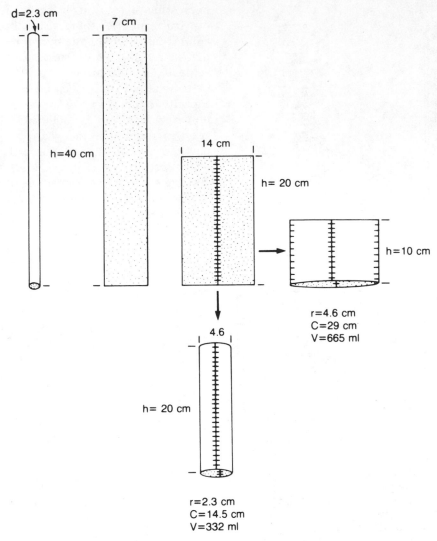

FIG. 50-9
Calculated capacity of 40 cm. segment opened and folded twice is 665 ml. (From Hinman F Jr: Selection of intestinal segments for bladder substitution: physical and physiological characteristics. *J Urol* 1988; 139:521.

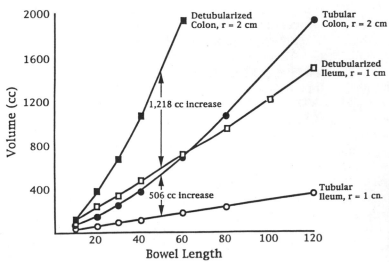

FIG. 50-10
Estimated influence of bowel length and radius on achievement of augmented bladder volume. (Data from Koff SA: Guidelines to determine the size and shape of intestinal segments used for reconstruction. *J Urol* 1988; 140:1151.

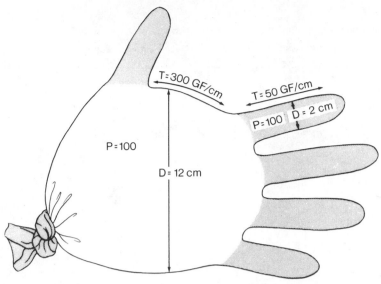

FIG. 50-11

Inflated surgeon's glove illustrates LaPlace's relationship. Although pressure *(P)* is equal throughout, tension *(T)* is greater in portion with greater diameter *(D)*. (From Hinman F: Selection of intestinal segments for bladder substitution: physical and physiological characteristics. *J Urol* 1988; 139:522.

TABLE 50-4

Effect of Detubularization of Colon and Ileum on Cystoplasty Compliance and Contraction

Cystoplasty	Mean Age (Years)	Mean F/U (Months)	Mean Cap (ml)	Mean Value At 300 ml cm H$_2$O	First Contr. Mean Vol (ml)	First Contr. Mean P cm H$_2$O	Max. Contr Mean Vol (ml)	Max. Contr Mean p cm H$_2$O
Tubular right colon	17.5	9.7	630	18.6	139	3:	467	63
Detubularized right colon	28.5	5.1	641	9.4	329	24	596	42
Tubular ileum	66.8	7.0	311	36	110	60	218	81
Detubularized ileum	20.0	5.7	403	14.4	197	22	265	28

Data from Goldwasser B et al: Cystometric properties of ileum and right colon after bladder augmentation, substitution or replacement. *J Urol*, part 2, 138:1007, 1987.

TABLE 50-5

Results of Urodynamic Studies After Various Forms of Urinary Diversion (Mean of Studied Patients in Each Group)

	Units	CIB n = 15	ICR n = 5	KP n = 4	PICR n = 7
Capacity	ml	362	278	666	687
Intraluminal pressure	cm H$_2$O				
At 200 ml	cm H$_2$O	26	14	7	13
At capacity	cm H$_2$O	37	45	28	25
Volume at first contraction	ml	150	50	53	41
Amplitude of contraction	cm H$_2$O	46	55	53	41
Voiding catheterization interval	hours	2.2	3.5	5.0	5.4

From Sher ML, Roehrborn CG: Incorporation of intestinal segments into the urinary tract. In Hohenfellner A and Wammack R (eds): *Continent urinary diversion*, Edinburg, Churchill Livingstone, 1992.
CIB, Camey ileal bladder; *ICR,* ileocecal reservoir; *KP,* Kock pouch; *PICR,* patched ileocaecal reservoir.

Because the reconstruction must be tailored to the individual needs of the patient, the surgeon must be familiar with a wide variety of reconstructive alternatives and have the patient prepared for all eventualities. This includes bowel preparation even when gastrocystoplasty, autoaugmentation, or ureteral augmentation are anticipated.

Small-Bowel Procedures

Camey Procedures

Couvelaire's (1951) early efforts at enterocystoplasty with small bowel after cystectomy were not successful. Camey's first small-bowel replacement of the bladder was performed in 1958. He gradually evolved his technique of using an incontinuity 35 to 40 cm segment

TABLE 50-6

Ultimate Augmentation Volume of Small Bladders Enlarged With Bowel Segments of Different Dimensions

Bladder Vol. (cc)	+	Bowel Length (cm)	Bowel Radius (cm)	=	Augmentation Vol. (cc)
50		20	1		250
50		30	1		382
50		40	1		532
50		50	1		697
50		60	1		877
50		10	2		250
50		20	2		532
50		30	2		877
100		10	1		203
100		20	1		327
100		30	1		470
100		40	1		630
100		50	1		804
100		10	2		327
100		20	2		630
100		30	2		992
150		10	1		380
150		20	1		530
150		30	1		695
150		40	1		875
150		10	2		530
150		20	2		875

From Koff SA: Guidelines to determine the size and shape of intestinal segments used for reconstruction. *J Urol* 1988; 140:1150.

of terminal ileum to replace the bladder after cystectomy for cancer (Fig. 50-12). A 25-year experience with this procedure was reviewed by Lilien and Camey (1984). After a cystoprostatectomy is done in the male patient, a U-shaped ileocystoplasty is performed with the midpoint of a 40 cm long ileal segment attached to the urethral stump. In only approximately 15% of cases has the mesentery of the ileum been inadequate to reach the urethral stump. Each ureter is anastomosed to one limb of the ileal segment. The ureteroileal anastomosis (LeDuc et al., 1987) is begun by incising each end of the loop along its antimesenteric border for 4 cm. The mucosa on the posterior wall is opened to create a mucosal trough 3 to 4 cm long. At the upper end of the trough the bowel wall is opened and the ureter drawn into the trough. The tip of the ureter is fixed with three stitches at the distal end of the trough, and the mucosa is sutured to the lateral ureteral wall with several sutures on each side. Secondary epithelialization of the ureter by bowel mucosa takes place. The 3 cm flap valve is effective in preventing urinary reflux in approximately 85% of cases (LeDuc et al., 1986).

In the most recent 3-year experience that Camey and colleagues (1987) reviewed, there have been complications in approximately one third of patients. Because the operation is being done after radiation therapy and total cystectomy, this would not appear to be unusual. Although ureteroileal fistulas were occasionally seen in the past, none has occurred since the addition of an antirefluxing technique of anastomosing the ureter to the ileal reservoir in 1977. Infectious complications have not been rare, but pelvic abscesses have not occurred since 1978, when closure of the pelvic peritoneum was eliminated from the procedure.

Results with the operation have shown a high level of patient acceptance. Voiding takes place by relaxation of the external sphincter and use of the Valsalva maneuver. It often requires two to three voiding attempts to produce effective bladder emptying. As long as voidings are performed every 2 to 3 hours, 90% of the patients are continent during the day. At night the patients are usually enuretic, unless they get up to void every 2 to 3 hours. An external condom device may permit the patients to be dry.

The reason for enuresis can be demonstrated by cystometrography. During filling, although the baseline reservoir pressure remains low, peristaltic waves occur that elevate the pressure to between 75 and 100 cm H_2O with an average leak pressure of 87 cm H_2O. As the reservoir fills, these peristaltic waves force urine into the urethra, resulting in enuresis. The usual reservoir capacity after a Camey procedure is 300 to 400 ml.

Recognizing the importance of detubularization and reconfiguration, the Camey procedure in recent years (Camey II) has undergone a detubularization modification with lessening of daytime frequency and improvement in nocturnal enuresis (Camey et al., 1987).

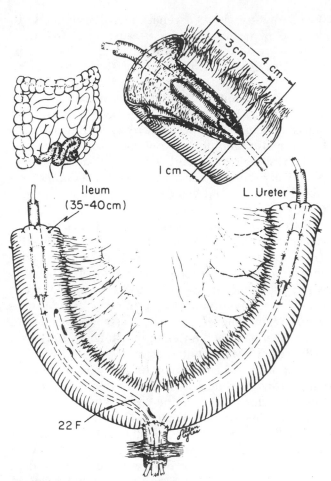

FIG. 50-12
Camey enterocystoplasty: 35 to 40 cm of intact ileum is anastomosed ot the urethral stump to create a continent intestinal reservoir. Note ureters are sutured into a 3 to 4 cm trough in the bowel mucosa in each limb of the reservoir to create effective antireflux flap valves. (From Lilien OM, Camey M: Twenty-five year experience with replacement of the human bladder (Camey procedure). *J Urol* 1984; 132:886. Used by permission.)

Kock Pouch

The other major surgical procedure to replace the bladder with small bowel is the Kock pouch (see Fig. 50-13). This procedure originally evolved from a detubularization technique for creating a continent and catheterizable intraabdominal fecal reservoir for patients with a permanent ileostomy (Kock, 1969). The success achieved in the gastrointestinal applications of this technique and patient acceptance led the technique to be applied to the urinary tract to create a continent catheterizable urinary reservoir. Introduced into the United States early in the 1980s, experience with this technique was rapidly gained (Kock et al., 1985a, 1985b; Montie et al., 1986; Skinner, 1987; Skinner et al., 1984a, 1984b).

A small-bowel reservoir is created from a 70-cm segment of ileum. The resection begins approximately

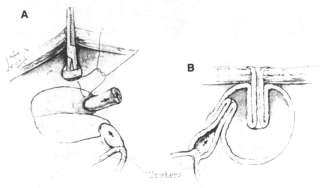

FIG. 50-13
Kock pouch: 70 cm segment of ileum is reformed into a peristaltic pouch with two nipple valves. Most recent modification involves fixation of nipple valve to reservoir wall changing it to a fixed flap valve. (From Kock NG, Norlen L, Phillipson BM, et al: The continent ileal reservoir (Kock pouch) for urinary diversion. *World J Urol* 1985; 3:146.)

50 cm above the ileocecal valve. The central 40-cm portion of the isolated ileal segment is opened and folded twice to create a reservoir pouch. This reservoir dilates postoperatively to create a large low-pressure reservoir with volumes measured up to 1500 ml. The 15 cm of ileum at each end is intussuscepted into this reservoir to form an afferent and efferent nipple valve to prevent reflux. The ureters are anastomosed in a standard Bricker fashion to the afferent limb, and with a low pressure in the reservoir, the nipple generally has been effective in avoiding reservoir-to-ileal (thus ureteral) reflux.

A reoperation rate exceeding 20% has complicated this procedure. The greatest problem has been the maintenance of an effective nonleaking nipple at the efferent end of the reservoir. With filling of the reservoir lateral pressure on the base of the nipple tends to efface it (Fig. 50-14), causing eversion of the nipple and loss of the continence mechanism. Various techniques have been evolved to stabilize the nipple, including the use of sutures, staples, and prosthetic cuffs. Fixation of the nipple to the inner wall of the reservoir by incising the mucosa on the nipple and reservoir wall and suturing the nipple down has improved the continence mechanism (Kock et al., 1985a; Olsson, 1985a, 1985b). In effect, this creates a flap-valve mechanism. Because the catheterization channel is the diameter of the normal ileum, the catheter occasionally catches on a fascial or muscle edge at the abdominal wall level, which leads to curling of the catheter before it reaches the reservoir.

Although asymptomatic bacteriuria is common, significant urinary tract infections have not been a major problem. Metabolic complications also are rare as long as the reservoir is emptied regularly. Emptying is performed three to six times a day with a 16 F to 20 F

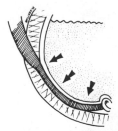 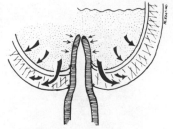

flap - valves   nipple - valves

FIG. 50-14
Flap valves, nipple valves. Nipple valves **(A)** are continent
because the nipple is circumferentially compressed by pressure within the reservoir. Unfortunately the intrareservoir
pressure also has a laterally disruptive force on the base of
the nipple, causing a shortening or total effacement of the
valve with loss of the continence mechanism. Flap valves **(B)**
are continent because the submucosal segment is compressed by filling of the reservoir (as for a reimplanted ureter
for vesicoureteral reflux). Unlike nipple valves, flap valves are
stable because they are fixed to the wall of the reservoir.
Thus reservoir filling does not tend to cause loss of the continence mechanism.

soft rubber catheter by means of the efferent limb into
the reservoir. Patient satisfaction with this continent
internal reservoir has been good (Boyd et al., 1987),
as had been seen previously with the Kock reservoir
for an ileostomy (McLeod and Fazio, 1984). The Kock
pouch is a technically complex procedure with a significant learning curve.

The Kock pouch, when used in a pediatric setting
for continent reconstruction, has proven to be a reliable alternative (Cumming and Woodhouse, 1989;
Hanna and Bloiso, 1987). There is, however, again a
high incidence of complications requiring reoperation
to control before an optimal final outcome was
achieved (Cumming and Woodhouse, 1989). Additionally, many pediatric urologists are concerned
about the long-term metabolic and nutritional consequences of the use of such a long segment of ileum.

Henriet and colleagues (1991) reported an attractive
alternative to the Kock pouch technique (Fig. 50-15).
Here an antirefluxing LeDuc-Camey ureteral implantation is employed instead of an afferent nipple valve.
A simplified stapling technique for the efferent nipple
resulted in a 96.2% continence rate. Further follow-
up will be necessary to determine the durability of
this modification.

Ileal Neobladder

A variety of ileal neobladder reconstructive alternatives have been described with encouraging results.
The urethral Kock procedure (Kock et al., 1989)
achieved a continence rate of 88% defined as spontaneous voiding, dry day and night, a daytime frequency no greater than 3 to 5 times daily, and nocturia

0 to 2 nightly. Eleven renal units deteriorated, 10
because of reflux and one because of obstruction.
There were 18 instances of reflux in the afferent nipple, 16 cases of which were associated with incontinence. The correction of reflux in these patients resulted in resumption of continence in each instance.
This important observation underscores the importance of accommodation. Early reflux in these patients
before maturation of the reservoir resulted in failure
of the reservoir to expand and prevent incontinence.
A similar result can occur in the face of a defunctionalized reconstructed bladder or with an incompetent
bladder outlet.

Pagano and colleagues (1992) reported their experience with the Padovana ileal bladder (Fig. 50-16).
This procedure results in a dependent funnel and a
spiraled detubularization. Thirty-seven of 41 patients
who underwent follow-up for at least 4 months were
proven to be continent during the day, and 33 were
dry at night. There were three instances of ureteral
stenosis employing the LeDuc implantation and seven
instances of bladder outlet stenosis.

Hautmann and colleagues (1993) reported 211 men
who received an ileal neobladder after radical cysta-
toprostatectomy. They employed a LeDuc-Camey antirefluxing ureteral implantation and a W loop of ileum.
Eighty-fiver percent were totally continent day and
night and voided spontaneously. Five percent were
wet at night only, and 6% were wet during the day.
Four percent required intermittent catheterization.
There was a significant complication rate with 32% of
patients experiencing complications sufficiently severe to require either hospitalization or reoperation.

Ileocystoplasty

As a technique for augmentation of the bladder,
Robertson and King (1986) used a "hemi-Kock pouch"
(Fig. 50-17). Here the detubularized ileal pouch is
sutured onto the bladder remnant with one nipple
only intussuscepted to permit the attachment of the
ureters to the reservoir as an effective antirefluxing
device. This procedure is particularly applicable when
the ureters are too short for reanastomosis to the bladder remnant or the bladder remnant is not suitable
for a ureteral reimplant. This technique also can be
used to create a continent catheterizable stoma to the
abdominal wall.

The greatest experience with ileum to augment the
bladder has been with the technique originally described by Goodwin and Winter (1959). Smith and
associates (1977) reviewed 45 ileocystoplasties with the
"cup-patch" technique. Although patients with a creatinine clearance less than 40 ml/min were excluded
from intestinal augmentation of the bladder, the authors found no electrolyte aberrations in their patients. The most common problem experienced was

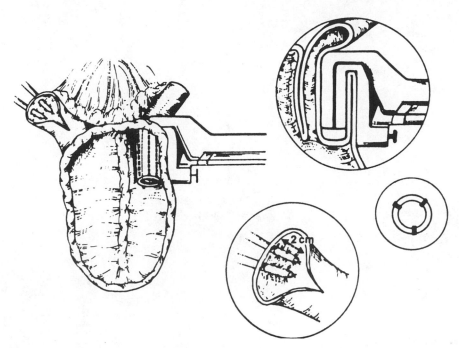

FIG. 50-15
Alternate technique for development of Kock pouch. (From Henriet MP, Neyra P, Elman B: Kock pouch procedures: Continuing experience in evolution in 135 cases. *J Urol* 1991; 145:17.

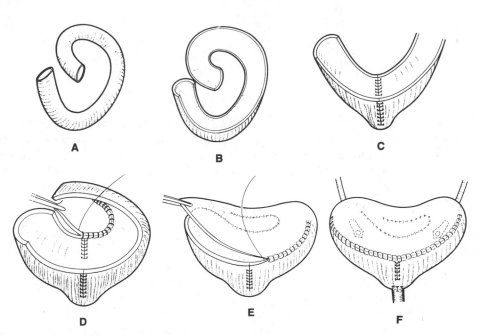

FIG. 50-16
The original configuration of vesica ileale padovana (VIP). **A,** 40 cm of terminal ileum. **B,** Detubularization. **C,** Construction of the lower funnel. **D-F,** Progressive shaping to the final geometry and bilateral uretero-ileal anastomosis according to LeDucCamey technique. (From Paganof et al: The vesica ileale padovana. In Holenfellner R, Wammack R (eds.): *Continent urinary diversion.* Edinburgh, Churchill Livingstone, 1992, p 122.)

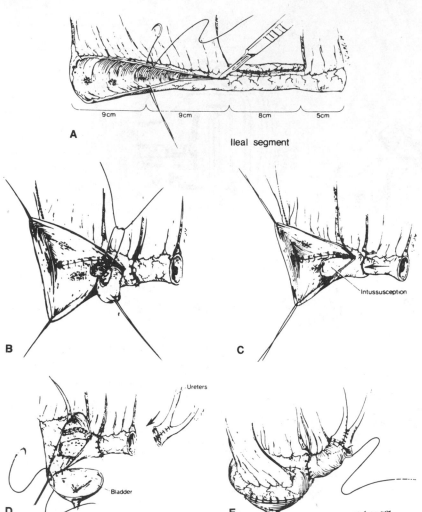

A

9cm   9cm   8cm   5cm

Ileal segment

B

C

Intussusception

D

Ureters

Bladder

E

FIG. 50-17
Hemi-Kock pouch: ileal pouch with one nipple fixed to wall of reservoir may be used to augment small bladder. Ureters are anastomosed to end of intact ileum. (From Robertson GN, King L: Bladder substitution in children. *Urol Clin North Am* 1986; 13:337.)

difficulty in bladder emptying. Intermittent catheterization has dealt effectively with this recently. Homsy and Reid (1974) also had a favorable experience with ileocystoplasty using the cup patch technique.

Ileocecal Segment Procedures
Ileocecocystoplasty

The ileocecal bowel segment has been attractive to urologists for reconstruction of the bladder because of the natural configuration of the cecum, which gave it the appearance of an ideal substitute for the bladder (Gilchrist et al., 1950; Gil-Vernet, 1965). Experience with the native ileocecal valve as an adequate antireflux mechanism has not been encouraging. At 25 cm of water pressure there is a 25% incidence of incompetence, with a 75% incompetence rate noted when the pressure reaches 50 cm of water (Rendelman et al., 1958). This high incidence was documented by Gil-Vernet (1965). Subsequently various surgical modifications of the ileocecal valve have been introduced in an effort to try to lessen the incidence of reflux.

Zinman and Libertino (1975, 1980a, 1986) wrapped the terminal ileum with a portion of the cecum (Fig. 50-18). Gittes sutured the terminal ileum around the base of the cecum, producing a form of a flap valve (Gittes, 1977; Whitmore and Gittes, 1983). Despite these modifications, a high incidence of reflux persisted.

Hendren (1980b) suggested cleaning the mesentery from approximately 8 cm of the terminal ileum and then intussuscepting this segment into the cecum to produce a long, antirefluxing nipple. Despite such efforts, about half of these nipple valves continued to reflux, pointing out the basic unsatisfactory nature of a nipple valve when compared with a flap valve (Hensle and Burbige, 1985; Wespres et al., 1986) (see Fig. 50-14). Hendren (1986) and Robertson and King (1986) modified the ileocecal nipple valve into a flap valve by taking the long intussuscepted segment and opening the mucosa on one side of the intussusception and on the inner wall of the cecum to tack the nipple down to one wall (Fig. 50-19). Robertson and King (1986)

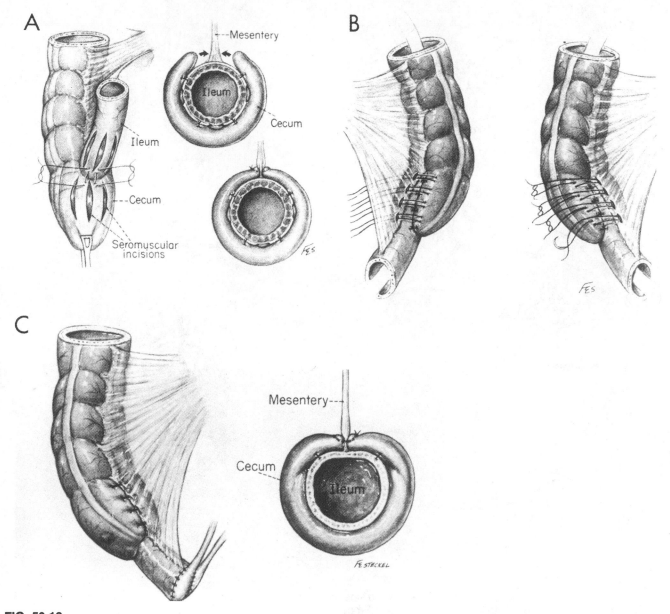

FIG. 50-18
Ileocecal intussusception: **A,** Scarification of cecum and ileum to help fix ileocecal 360-degree wrap. **B,** Sutures creating wraps are passed through windows in ileal mesentery. **C,** Completed ileocecal wrap. (From Zinman L, Libertino JA: Right colocystoplasty for bladder replacement. *Urol Clin North Am* 1986; 13:321-331.

prevented reflux in seven of eight cases. There was no obstruction to antegrade flow. This contrasts with 50% (two of four) reflux with the Gittes technique and 33% (three of nine) with ileocecal plication. In the latter group 33% were also obstructed to antegrade flow. At the present time the long intussuscepted ileal technique with fixation to the cecal wall to create a stable flap valve appears to have the best chance of producing a competent ileocecal valve.

When the cecal or ileocecal segment has been used intact for bladder augmentation, continence at night has been a significant problem in most series. Whitmore and Gittes (1983) reported enuresis in approx-

imately one third of their patients (17 of 55). Similar results were reported by Dounis and Gow (1979), although some of their patients' condition appeared to spontaneously improve with time. That this type of problem most likely reflects peristaltic waves in the intact bowel segment is reflected in the fact that when the cup patch technique is used, enuresis is rare (Light and Engelmann, 1986; Shirley and Mirelman, 1978; Thuroff et al., 1986). All of these authors have opened the ileocecal segment along the antimesenteric border and incorporated the ileum into the closure of the cecum, creating a large pouch with ineffectual peristalsis. Urodynamics in the series of Thuroff and col-

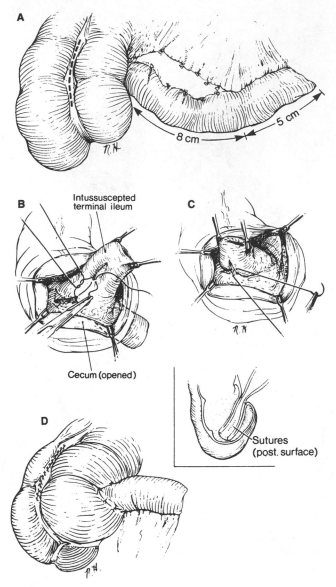

FIG. 5-19
Ileocecal intussusception with fixation of nipple down to side wall of cecum converting it into a stable flap valve. (From King LR, Robertson CN, Bertram RA: A new technique for the prevention of reflux in those undergoing bladder substitution or undiversion using bowel segments. *World J Urol* 1985; 3:194-196.)

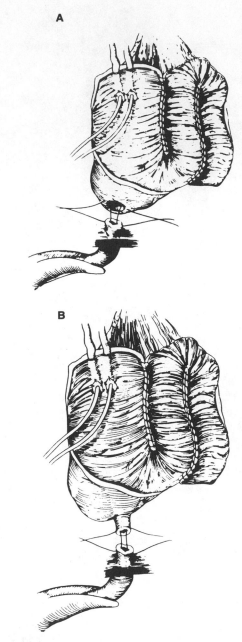

FIG. 5-20
Technique for bladder replacement employing Mainz pouch procedure. (From Wammack R, et al: The Mainz pouch. In Holenfellner R, Wammack R (eds.): *Continent urinary diversion.* Edinburgh, Churchill Livingstone, 1992, p 129.)

leagues and Light and Engelmann confirmed a low pressure in the reservoir.

Voiding in ileocecal augmented bladders occurs primarily through a pressure rise generated through abdominal straining (Gleason et al., 1972), and incomplete emptying is common. Intermittent self-catheterization may be required for effective emptying.

Ileocecal Neobladder and Ileocecal Continent Diversion

Wammack and colleagues (1992) reviewed their experience with the Mainz pouch neobladder (Fig. 50-20). Of 27 patients who underwent reconstruction, all were continent during the day, and all but three were continent at night. These authors also reported their experience with the Mainz pouch (Fig. 50-21) in 231 patients. They report a progressively improving experience in continence and excellent urodynamic characteristics of this continent diversion. The incidence of incontinence requiring revision has fallen from 84.5% with a sutured ileal invagination technique to 22.2% with a stapled ileal invagination technique

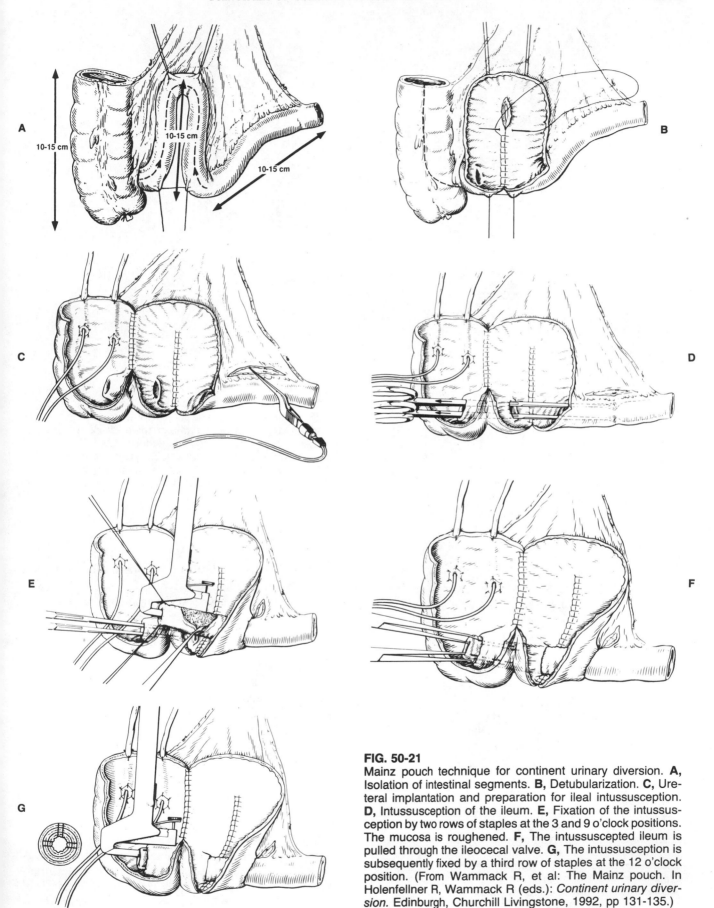

FIG. 50-21
Mainz pouch technique for continent urinary diversion. **A,** Isolation of intestinal segments. **B,** Detubularization. **C,** Ureteral implantation and preparation for ileal intussusception. **D,** Intussusception of the ileum. **E,** Fixation of the intussusception by two rows of staples at the 3 and 9 o'clock positions. The mucosa is roughened. **F,** The intussuscepted ileum is pulled through the ileocecal valve. **G,** The intussusception is subsequently fixed by a third row of staples at the 12 o'clock position. (From Wammack R, et al: The Mainz pouch. In Holenfellner R, Wammack R (eds.): *Continent urinary diversion.* Edinburgh, Churchill Livingstone, 1992, pp 131-135.)

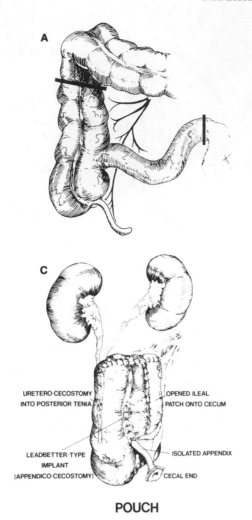
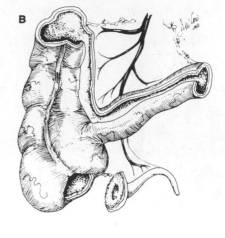

POUCH

FIG. 50-22
Penn pouch-continent appendicocecostomy. **A,** Ileocecal segment and appendix isolated, preserving bowel blood supply. **B,** Appendix is separated with preserved blood supply to be used as continent catheterizable channel. Ileocecal segment opened and closed together to disrupt peristalsis and ensure a low pressure reservoir. **C,** Ureters and appendix implanted in submucosal courses, creating effective flap valves. (From Duckett JW, Snyder HM: *Semin Urol* 1987; 5:55.)

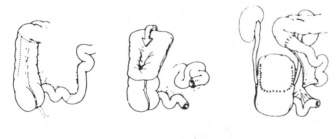
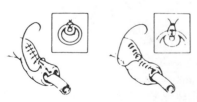

FIG. 50-23
Continent ileocecal reservoir dependent on hydraulic resistance form plicated ileal segment. Upper figures show right colon detubularized by vertical opening and transverse closure (Heineke-Mikulicz reconfiguration). Lower figures show double-layer imbrication of terminal ileum by nonabsorbable Lembert sutures. This narrowing may also be achieved with staples. (From Rowland RG, Mitchell ME, Bihrle R, et al: Indiana continent urinary reservoir. *J Urol* 1987; 137:1136. Used by permission.)

and to 13.8% with a stapled invagination plus a stapled fixation within the ileocecal valve.

Other continent diversions employing the ileocecal valve have included the Penn pouch (Duckett and Synder, 1985) depicted in Figure 50-22, the Indiana pouch (Ahlering et al., 1991; Rowland et al., 1987) demonstrated in Figure 50-23, and the Florida pouch (Lockhart et al., 1990).

Of these techniques, the Indiana pouch has been applied most frequently in pediatric practice and has been met with variable results. Leonard and colleagues (1990) reported a poor result from the perspective of incontinence requiring surgical revision, whereas Hensle and associates (1990) reported a very satisfactory outcome in their series.

Sigmoid Bowel Procedures
Colonic Neobladder

Use of a sigmoid colonic segment for bladder augmentation or replacement was reported experimentally by Rubin in 1948. He used an intact sigmoid segment in dogs with success and apparent continence. Gil-Vernet and colleagues (1962) presented a significant series of sigmoid segments used to replace the bladder. In 41 patients (one female, 40 male) an intact sigmoid segment was used to replace a bladder that had in most cases been removed for cancer. The midsection of the segment was sutured to the urethra, and the ureters were brought in with antirefluxing technique at either end of the U-shaped sigmoid segment. Although reflux was seen in all, clinical upper tract infection did not occur, and there were no electrolyte problems even in patients with preexisting renal failure. The patients were able to spontaneously empty their bladder well, as indicated by residual urine volumes no greater than 40 ml. Control, however, was more of a problem. Frequency of voiding was usual, with emptying required every 2 to 3 hours for daytime continence. Nocturnal enuresis was seen in virtually all cases, as with the Camey (1985) experience. Hradec (1965) reported on 60 sigmoid neobladders performed with a similar technique to that of Gil-Vernet with similar results.

Reddy and co-authors (1991) reported the construction of a colonic neobladder in 27 patients who underwent reconstruction following cystectomy. This reconstruction employed a detubularized segment of sigmoid colon. All patients voided spontaneously, and all were continent during the day. Sixty-seven percent were continent at night with two patients requiring insertion of an artificial urinary sphincter to achieve satisfactory nighttime continence. Three patients had vesicoureteral reflux, two of which resolved spontaneously.

Parra (1991) reported 27 colonic neobladders employing a right colon detubularized technique which, due to the fact that is was performed entirely with staples, was associated with a decrease in operative time. Twenty-six (96%) were reported as continent.

Colocystoplasty

Mathisen (1955) reported sigmoid augmentation of the bladder by the "open loop" technique, which is in essence the cup patch technique of Goodwin discussed earlier. This technique also was used by Dounis and Gow (1979) in their series in which the patch was an alternative to the intact sigmoid cystoplasty. Almost one third of patients had enuresis with the use of intact bowel, whereas with the sigmoid patch, the enuresis rate was zero. Eighty-seven percent of the patients in their series had a good result. Kvarstein and Mathisen (1981) used the same open-loop sigmoid patch technique for the treatment of persistent adult incontinence and were able to produce improvement in 90% of patients. In none of these reports did there appear to be any appreciable difference from other bowel segments with respect to ability to empty, infections, electrolyte abnormalities, or other significant variables. The striking improvement in continence caused by the use of a reconfigured and detubularized augmentation constitutes the most notable feature of the review of these different series.

Gastric Segment Procedures
Gastrocystoplasty

Interest in the use of gastric segments for purposes of bladder reconstruction is based upon the experimental work of Sinaiko (1956, 1960) employing a canine model. This concept was later applied to human bladder disease (Leong, 1978; Leong and Ong, 1972). Subsequent experimental work by Piser and colleagues (1987) and Kennedy and colleagues (1988) demonstrated that gastric bladder reconstruction was metabolically permissive, allowing its use in the face of acute acid loading or azotemia without the development of acidosis.

The work of Mitchell and co-investigators ushered in the modern era of the use of stomach in urinary reconstruction (Adams et al., 1988) (Fig. 50-24). They demonstrated the gastrocystoplasty technique to be highly successful, versatile, and well tolerated even in the face of azotemia.

As previously reviewed, reports of complications such as significant gastric symptoms, the hematuria-dysuria syndrome, and systemic alkalosis has raised questions as to the efficacy of this procedure. Long-term follow-up (minimum of 1.5 years) of 23 patients with gastrocystoplasty or gastric neobladder (Sheldon et al., 1994) revealed a continence rate of 91%, stable renal function in all patients, and upper tract deterioration in only one patient who became noncompliant with intermittent catheterization. There were no significant gastric symptoms and no incidence of electrolyte abnormality. Two patients with cases of hematuria-dysuria were encountered, one of which was mild and readily treated with hydration and histamine blockade and the other of which was transient, only occurring during a phase of severe oliguria while awaiting transplantation. Transplantation resulted in resolution of all symptoms. Gastrocystoplasty has proven to be an excellent alternative for patients with end-stage renal disease facing subsequent transplantation (Sheldon et al., 1994).

A recent modification of this procedure has been reported by Raz and colleagues (1993). This simplified version allows a segment of the greater curvature to be isolated, employing a stapled segment such that no resultant gastric defect is created requiring primary closure. This gastric patch is sutured to the bladder prepared by an inverted U-shaped bladder incision. Five patients were reported. Three were able to void spontaneously, and all were continent with stable upper tracts. One patient had histamine blockade resistant hematuria-dysuria syndrome. It is pertinent to

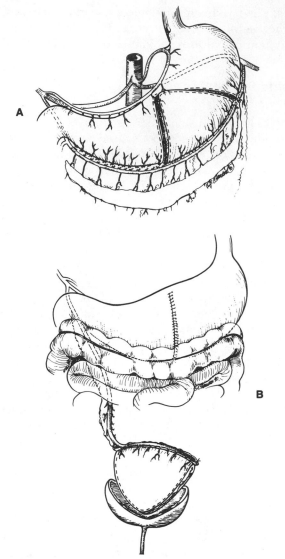

FIG. 50-24
Gastrocystoplasty. **A,** Development of right gastroepiploic pedicle and isolation of wedge of gastric fundus. **B,** Mobilization of right gastroepiploic pedicle through retroperitoneal plane into augmentation position. The stomach is closed. (From Mitchell ME: Gastrocystoplasty and bladder replacement with stomach. In Marshall FF (ed.): *Operative Urology.* Philadelphia, WB Saunders Co., 1991, pp 254-255.)

note that this procedure results in the inclusion of antrum within the gastric patch.

Gastric Neobladder and Continent Diversions

Gastric neobladder has been successfully employed for reconstruction with the native urethra (Mitchell, 1991), the orthotopic ureteral neourethra (Mitchell et al., 1988; Sheldon et al., 1994) and with the orthotopic appendocial neourethra (Sheldon et al., 1994).

Gastric composite continent reconstructions have been reported employing stomach and colon (Birhle et al., 1989) and stomach and ileum (Lockhart et al.,

1993). These procedures may be particularly appealing in the setting of complex diseases such as short-gut, chronic diarrhea, acidosis, azotemia, and severe pelvic radiation because of their versatility, potential for large capacity, and prospect for lessening of some side effects. Long-term experience will be necessary to document their utility.

Ureteral Augmentation

Sixteen patients undergoing ureteral augmentation (Fig. 50-25) have been recently reported by Churchill and co-authors (1993). Fifteen patients required intermittent catheterization, and one patient voided spontaneously. Excellent urodynamic characteristics were documented, and 10 patients were completely dry day and night. Five patients had significantly improved continence, and one patient was completely incontinent. There were five complications: transient extravasation (two cases), ureterovesical junction obstruction of the contralateral ureter (two cases), and Mitrofanoff stomal stenosis (one case). This procedure holds great promise, especially with respect to its ability to be performed as an entirely extraperitoneal procedure. It has demonstrated excellent compliance characteristics and has no known risk of absorptive electrolyte imbalance.

Autoaugmentation

Cartwright and Snow (1989) reported the use of an autoaugmentation technique employing excision of detrusor muscle over the bladder dome, leaving the underlying bladder uroepithelium intact (Fig. 50-26). Bilateral psoas hitches were performed to prevent approximation of the remaining muscular edges. The incision or excision of detrusor permits the mucosa to bulge like a large broad-based bladder diverticulum, increasing bladder volume and compliance. Seven patients were reported, of whom five demonstrated an excellent improvement in urodynamic characteristics. One experienced a modest improvement, and one, who had a failed result, required subsequent enterocystoplasty. Two patients experienced transient extravasation, and three patients had reflux in previously nonrefluxing units, two of which resolved. Most recently, these authors have considered this procedure most applicable for patients with poor compliance and with a preoperative bladder capacity ≥75% than expected for age. Further, if the intraoperative urodynamics fail to document at least a 30% to 50% increase in volume at pressures ranging from 20 to 40 cm H_2O, consideration is given to enterocystoplasty (Cartwright and Snow, 1994). Like the ureteral augmentation technique this procedure holds great promise due to its ability to prevent absorptive metabolic disorders and to be performed in an entirely extraperitoneal approach.

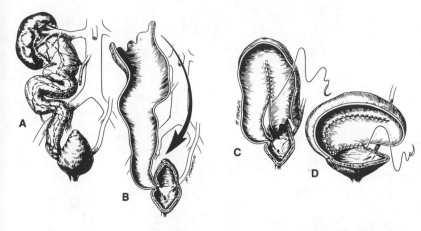

FIG. 50-25
Operative stages of ureteral bladder augmentation. **A,** Normal blood supply to ureter. **B,** Ureteral detubularization following mobilization. **C,** Reconfiguration of ureter into U-shaped path. **D,** Anastomosing ureteral patching to native bivalved bladder. (From Churchill BM, et al: Ureteral bladder augmentation. *J Urol* 1993; 150:717.

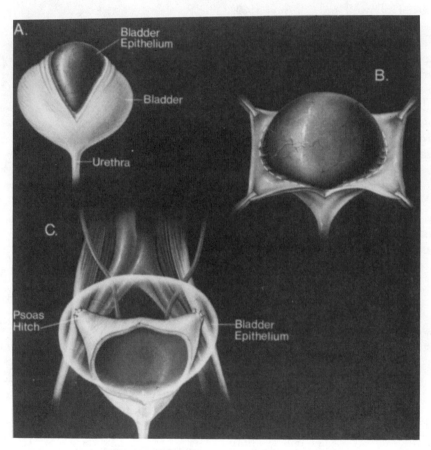

FIG. 50-26
Diagram of autoaugmentation. **A,** Detrusor incised. **B,** Detrusor stripped from intact bladder epithelium. **C,** Epithelium bulges with bladder filling. (From Cartwright PC, Snow BW: Bladder autoaugmentation: Early clinical experience. *J Urol* 1989; 142:505.

Internal Diversion—Procedures Providing Urinary Continence Via an Intact Ano-rectal Continence Mechanism

Ureterosigmoidostomy

Although abandoned by most institutions because of the risks of malignancy, acidosis, and upper tract deterioration, some centers continue to employ versions of ureterosigmoidostomy as a preferred modality for reconstruction in bladder exstrophy. Reports of series employing modern reconstructive techniques reveal quite acceptable results even with relatively long-term follow-up (Stockle et al., 1990). These authors report 46 children who underwent reconstruction with ureterosigmoidostomy and follow-up for a mean of 14.7 years. Daytime continence was achieved in 97.4% of patients, and nighttime continence was achieved in 92.3%. Endoscopic surveillance revealed one tubular adenoma, which was removed endoscopically. One patient had urolithiasis, and five patients had pyelonephritis. Five patients required treatment for metabolic acidosis. Upper tract deterioration sufficient to require conversion to colon conduit was encountered in three patients.

These authors use as an argument for employment of ureterosigmoidostomy in the exstrophy patient a high incidence of unsatisfactory outcome in patients reconstructed with conventional means included bladder neck reconstruction and augmentation (Hollowell and Ransley, 1991). This unsatisfactory outcome from the perspective of incontinence is attributed to a very high incidence of bladder instability in exstrophy (Hollowell et al., 1991; Hollowell and Ransley, 1991) and to a demonstrated poor response of the exstrophy bladder to anticholinergics. Also noted is a significant incidence of upper tract deterioration with primary exstrophy reconstruction on long-term follow-up (Mesrobian et al., 1988) and what appears to be a significant risk of adenocarcinoma developing in the bladder exstrophy plate itself (Mesrobian et al., 1988).

Proponents of ureterosigmoidostomy have attributed the high incidence of upper tract injury previously recorded to insufficient antireflux ureteral implantation techniques and to failure to achieve fixation to the sacrum, which allows ureteral kinking. To combat this, the sigmoid is fixed in position into the sacral promontory, and long, parallel, ureteral implantations are performed in the Goodwin fashion by means of an anterior sigmoid colotomy. (Goodwin et al., 1953).

Sigma-rectum

The incidence of nocturnal incontinence with ureterosigmoidostomy has been addressed by procedures designed to provide a detubularized segment of sigmoid colon at the level of the ureteral reimplantation. Examples include the Mainz sigma-rectum (Fig. 50-27) (Fisch et al., 1992). These authors have demonstrated improved pouch pressure characteristics and decreased nocturnal incontinence. A similar approach has been taken with the ileorectal Koch pouch where a Koch pouch is anastomosed to the side of the sigmoid colon (Koch et al., 1988).

It is of course imperative that anorectal competence be documented prior to such procedures. Sufficient anorectal competence to allow continence can be assumed if the patient can comfortably maintain continence, holding an enema of volume equal to approximately 8 to 10 hours worth of urine output during normal activities without leakage.

Rectal Neobladder

Some interest has been generated with respect to various modifications of the rectal bladder as reviewed by Ghoneim (1992). These procedures have in com-

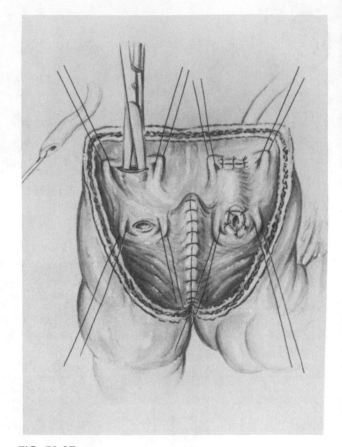

FIG. 50-27
The MAINZ pouch II (sigmoid-rectum. A longitudinal incision in the sigmoid colon is followed by a side-to-side anastomosis to create a detubularized segment. Sacral fixation is achieved and long ureteral reimplantation are performed in the Goodwin fashion. (From Wammack R, et al: The MAINZ pouch. In Hallenfellner R, Wammack R (eds.): *Continent urinary diversion.* Edinburg, Churchill Livingstone, 1992.)

mon a reliance upon the anorectal sphincter for continence. Additionally, the urinary reservoir is more compartmentalized. Figure 50-28 depicts the augmented and valved rectum (Ghoneim, 1992). This procedure was performed in 83 patients with a 100% daytime continence rate and a 99% nighttime continence rate.

Artificial Bladder

A permanently implanted, nonbiologic substitute for the bladder has been tried with such diverse materials as Vitallium, polyethylene, Teflon, polyvinyl, silicone rubber, Ivalon, Dacron, silver, Tantalum, and expanded polytetrafluoroethylene (Gor-Tex). This subject has been well reviewed by Kaleli and Ansell (1984). There have been basically two approaches. One was to have a nonbiologic material implanted to function as a mold around which urothelium could grow to reform a bladder. Early success with this technique in humans who had undergone a total cystectomy was reported by Tsulukidze and colleagues (1964), but no long-term results have been reported.

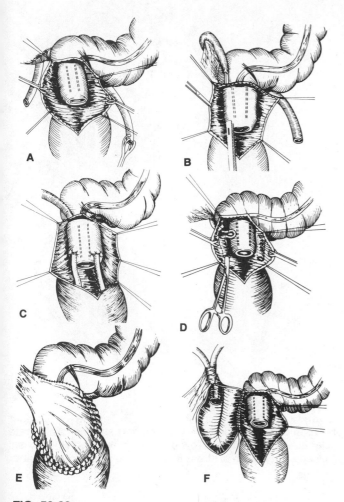

FIG. 50-28

The augmented and valve rectum. **A,** The anterior wall of the rectosigmoid is opened and a colorectal intussusception valve is created. **B,** The ureter is passed between the two layers of the intussusceptum. **C,** A stented mucosa to mucosa anastomosis is completed on both sides. **D,** An alternative (currently the method of choice) is to reimplant the ureters through a submucous tunnel following Goodwin's technique. **E,** The opened rectum is closed with an ileal patch. **F,** With dilated ureters a second intussusception valve from ileum is used for reflux prevention. (From Gonium MA: The modified rectal bladder (augmented and valved rectum). In Holenfellner R and Wammach R (eds.): *Continent urinary diversion.* Edinburg, Churchill Livingstone, 1992.)

The second approach has been to use an artificial bladder to which ureters and urethra could be attached. All efforts have failed because of the development of an inflammatory reaction with or without active bacterial infection.

COMPENSATING FOR INADEQUATE BLADDER OUTLET RESISTANCE

Urinary continence is maintained by a complex interrelationship between bladder outlet resistance and pressure. To maintain dryness, the bladder outlet resistance must exceed intravesical pressure not only at rest but during changes in posture, coughing, sneez- ing, and straining. There are several components to this mechanism. Certainly intrinsic urethral resistance due to inherit tension in the urethral wall as well as the length and diameter of the urethra play an important role (Lapides, 1958; Lapides et al., 1960). Other components include smooth and striated muscular activity and the fact that intraabdominal pressure may be reflected on the proximal urethra. This latter mechanism allows a balance to compensate for elevated intravesical pressure due to applied intraabdominal pressure by simultaneously applying similar pressure to the proximal urethra.

Based on these components of continence, it is not surprising that most surgical interventions designed for the achievement of incontinence include procedures to narrow the urethra, lengthen the urethra, suspend the bladder neck, and compress the urethra.

Urinary incontinence will commonly accompany denervation of a sphincteric mechanism. It may also accompay pelvic decent and the congenitally short, wide, or rigid urethra. Additionally urinary incontinence may be encountered secondary to increased intravesical pressure even in the absence of actual bladder outlet pathology.

Although anticholinergic agents can have a long-term effect to inhibit detrusor contraction and decrease intravesical pressure, α adrenergic agents suffer from tachyphylaxis and are of limited assistance in augmenting bladder outlet resistance. Most bladder outlet resistance augmentation is achieved with surgery, recognizing that clean intermittent catheterization may be needed to assist in bladder emptying.

Bladder Neck Keeling Procedure

Kelly (1913), a gynecologist, first suggested a vaginal approach to the plication of the bladder neck, which narrowed it and thus could be expected to increase bladder outlet resistance. Stephens (1970) described a keeling operation (Fig. 50-29), similar in principle, performed by a transvesical approach. A vertical incision is made posteriorly in the bladder mucosa from just above the interureteric line down into the urethra. The whole thickness of the trigonal muscle is then incised in the same line as the mucosal incision. Care is taken to avoid entry into the vagina. The cut edges of the trigonal muscle are everted posteriorly with a series of sutures beginning at the cranial end of the incision and running down into the urethra. Gentle upward traction of the sutures permits easier insertion of the more distal sutures. In this way the trigone, bladder neck, and urethra are narrowed. A second and third layer of sutures continue the process. Stephens believes this "bipenation" should be continued until the bladder outlet appears almost occluded. He recommends suprapubic drainage for 2 weeks to permit solid healing of the bladder in an undistended

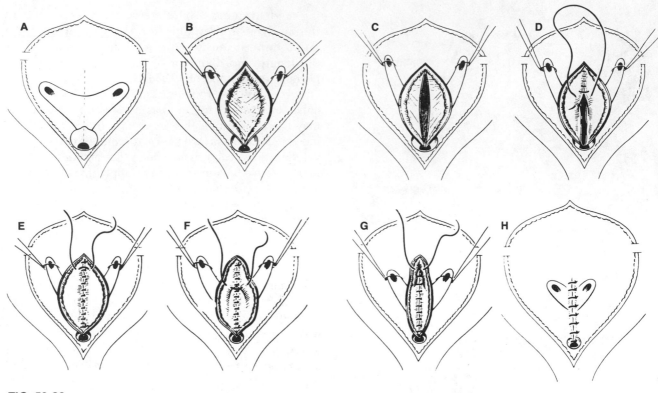

FIG. 50-29
Stephen's bladder neck keeling operation. Technique of bipenation and keeling. **A,** Incision in mucosa. **B,** Trigone and bladder neck muscle exposed. **C,** Incision, **D,** Keeling by Cushing suture. **E,** and **F,** Insertion of row of Lembert sutures to elongate the keel and to draw in the V of the bladder neck to make a smaller aperture. **G,** A third row of Lembert sutures. **H,** Mucosal sutures. Note narrowing of trigone and urethral meatus. (From Stephens FD: A form of stress incontinence in children: Another method of repair. *Aust NZ J Surg* 1970; 40:125.)

state. This approach to increasing bladder outlet resistance may be effective as an isolated procedure but would appear to have its greatest utility when performed at the time of the excision of an ectopic ureter or ureterocele to reconstruct a distorted bladder outlet. A particularly effective use of this procedure is in the reversal of incontinence due to previous Y-V plasty of the bladder neck.

Urethral Lengthening Procedures
Distal Vaginal Lengthening

Efforts to increase the distal urethral length by tubularization of the vaginal wall beyond the urethral meatus date back to Harris (1935). In this procedure a U-shaped incision was made around the urethral meatus and extended toward the clitoris. The vaginal wall was then rolled into a tube and the adjacent vaginal wall mobilized to be closed over it. The disadvantage of this procedure was the presence of overlapping suture lines that might increase the likelihood of a urethrovaginal fistula. Woodard and Marshall (1961) performed a similar urethral lengthening to treat posttraumatic female incontinence and described an eccentric vaginal flap intended to permit displace-

ment of the two suture lines and thus reduce the likelihood of fistula. Hendren (1980a) effectively used this approach in the treatment of incontinent girls. It has often been combined with a Young-Dees-Leadbetter type of bladder neck reconstruction. In his original series Hendren reported utilizing this approach for congenital or traumatic deficiency of the bladder neck and urethra. The causes included ureteral ectopia, severe female hypospadias, epispadias, infections, pressure necrosis from prolonged labor, nonsurgical trauma, and intentional resection for tumor. Hendren added to the previous operative procedure the use of a small buttock flap, which is rotated as a single pedicle flap to cover the neourethral vaginal tube. This permits good tissue coverage of the neourethra, especially high in the vagina where local tissue may be deficient. Several weeks after the flap has healed, it can be transected and the labia, which had to be divided to permit rotation of the flap, can be reconstructed. Hendren postulates that improved continence is produced not only by additional urethral length but also by the possible compression of the neourethra by bulbocavernosus and ischiocavernosus muscles, which are pulled around the neourethra as part of the repair. Although not every child was rendered perfectly continent by this procedure, the condition of all was significantly improved. This type of urethral lengthening has been applied to a normally situated urethra but has its greatest utility in assisting in the reconstruction of a urethra that is positioned high in the vagina, giving room for a significant distal tube to be constructed. This distal placement of the urethral meatus may facilitate intermittent catheterization. A labial or preputial (clitoromegaly of urogenital sinus) flap may be used instead of a buttock flap (Sheldon, 1994).

Proximal Urethral (Detrusor Tube) Lengthening

Young-Dees-Leadbetter Procedure.—Efforts to proximally lengthen the existing urethra through tubularization of the posterior detrusor grew out of the early work of Young (1919, 1922) and Dees (1949). In Young's procedure tissue in the posterior bladder neck was excised, and the bladder neck was then reconstructed with narrowing to the size of a silver probe. Dees' modification of this procedure involved excising more lateral mucosa and lengthening the proximal urethra toward the trigone, but it did not involve reimplantation of the ureters. Leadbetter (1964) extended the construction of a long posterior detrusor tube by reimplanting ureters higher in the bladder (Fig. 50-30). The mucosa was approximated to create a new urethra that would be 4 to 5 cm long. The detrusor muscle was overlapped to support the mucosal closure around an 8 F to 10 F catheter. In 1985 Leadbetter reported on a 10- to 22-year follow-up of this procedure in 27 children and seven adults. This series involved incontinence that stemmed from a combination of iatrogenic, traumatic, and congenital origins. Four (57%) of 7 adults were completely dry, and two (29%) required one to three perineal pads a day. Nineteen (70%) of 27 children were completely dry, and 1 (3%) had partial success, requiring several perineal pads a day. These results were somewhat better than those reported by Klauber and Williams (1974) in a group of 80 incontinent children with epispadias/exstrophy treated by the use of a simple Young-Dees procedure, supplemented in some cases by a Millan (1947) sling.

Other authors have had better success with the Young-Dees-Leadbetter type reconstruction using several modifications. Lepor and Jeffs (1983) attributed their success to a urethral suspension and use of urodynamic control at the time of surgery to ensure adequate urethral resistance. An 18 to 20 mm wide and 30 mm long posterior strip was tubularized and then suspended from the posterior surface of the rectus fascia in the fashion of a Marshall-Marchetti-Krantz procedure (1949) (Fig. 50-31). If intraoperative urethral pressure profilometry demonstrated a continence length of 3.5 cm and a urethral closure pressure

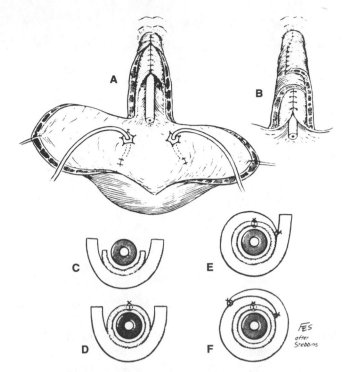

FIG. 50-30
Leadbetter technique of tubularization of posterior detrusor. Ureters are reimplanted higher in bladder to permit creation of a long detrusor tube. The detrusor is overlapped over the mucosal tube. (From Leadbetter GW: Urinary incontinence. In Libertino JA, Zinman L (eds.): *Reconstructive Urologic Surgery, Pediatric and Adult.* Baltimore, Williams & Wilkins, 1977, p 245. Used by permission.)

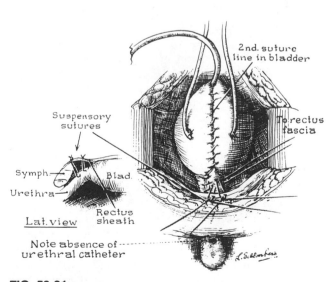

FIG. 50-31
Posterior detrusor tube suspended from posterior surface of pubic bone and rectus muscle. Suspension helps preserve both length and position of detrusor tube. (From Jeffs RD, Lepor H: Management of the exstrophy/epispadias complex, in Harrison JH, et al (eds.): *Campbell's Urology.* 5th ed. Philadelphia, WB Saunders Co, 1986, p 1902.)

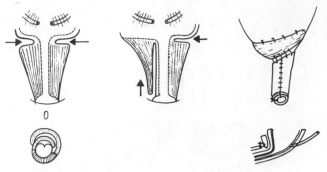

FIG. 50-32
Mollard's posterior detrusor tube. One wing of detrusor is wrapped around the bladder neck. **A,** Bladder incision for classic Young-Dees repair. *Shaded areas* represent removed mucosa. **B,** Bladder incision for Mollard repair. **C,** Completed repair of bladder neck with detrusor strip wrapped around top of repair. Bladder neck is not suspended. (From Mollard P: Precis D'Urologie de l'Enfant. Paris, Masson Publishing Co, 1984, p 237.)

between 60 and 90 cm H_2O with the bladder distended with 50 ml saline solution, the repair was believed to be satisfactory. Follow-up of 25 consecutive exstrophy cases who underwent posterior detrusor tube construction in this manner demonstrated that 86% of children had a daytime dry interval of more than 3 hours, and 80% reported less than one incontinent episode per day. Another review by Jeffs (1986) revealed a greater than 3-hour dry interval in 92% of cases.

Mollard (1980) modified the Young-Dees-Leadbetter procedure for exstrophy by creating an anterior muscular loop around the bladder neck. On one side of the detrusor tube a longitudinal muscle strip is made, while the other side is left adjacent to the lengthened urethra to roll over the mucosal closure (Fig. 50-32). Suspension of the neourethra was not performed. Mollard's results were good, with a dry interval of greater than 3 hours in 10 of 15 cases. These results, however, do not measure up to the reports from Jeffs.

Kramer and Kelalis (1982) reported their experience with reconstruction of children with episadias and performed repairs primarily by the Young-Dees-Leadbetter detrusor tube technique. Their results were good, with 10 (83%) of 12 female patients achieving complete continence and 37 (70%) of 55 male patients also dry. Two aspects of their report were particularly of interest. It was not until puberty that 19 of their 37 dry male patients achieved continence. It is clear that pubertal changes can assist in creation of outlet resistance after a detrusor tube repair. Additionally, the authors found that urinary retention immediately after a bladder neck operation was associated with improved continence subsequent to resolution of the retention. Temporary intermittent catheterization was used until the detrusor compensated adequately to produce effective emptying against the increased bladder outlet resistance that had been achieved.

Koff (1990) reported a modification of the Young-Dees-Leadbetter procedure, which he termed the "cinch" procedure (Fig. 50-33). Here a muscular flap encompasses the entire circumference of the neourethra and in addition is suspended to the anterior abdominal wall. He reported 10 patients, six of whom were dry during the day and night. Of these, three were are able to void and three are treated by intermittent catheterization. Two patients were dry during the day and wet at night, and two were wet both day and night. Essentially all of these patients had difficulties with the initiation of voiding postoperatively. Prolonged suprapubic drainage was required in several patients, and two had to be diverted by way of vesicostomy or ureterostomy.

Perlmutter and colleagues (1991) reported 22 patients undergoing bladder outlet reconstruction employing the standard Young-Dees-Leadbetter technique for exstrophy. Nine patients had a single bladder neck reconstruction, of whom eight (89%) were continent. Thirteen patients required additional surgeries. Of these, nine (69%) were continent. The additional surgeries included repeat bladder neck reconstruction (three cases) simultaneous augmentation (three cases), delayed augmentation (five cases), and insertion of an artificial urinary sphincter (two cases). The overall incidence of acceptable urinary continence was 77%.

Also in 1991, Hollowell and Ransley reported a large series of 86 patients who underwent bladder neck reconstruction for exstrophy. Of these, two patients were continent following their bladder closure only and did not require bladder neck reconstruction. Thirty-two underwent bladder neck reconstruction without augmentation, whereas 52 underwent bladder outlet reconstruction with augmentation, again with the Young-Dees-Leadbetter technique. Twelve patients who had reconstruction without augmentation achieved continence, whereas the remaining 20 required subsequent augmentation. The incidence of satisfactory continence in those patients treated by both bladder neck reconstruction and augmentation was 80%.

Hollowell and Ransley performed bladder augmentation in children whose estimated bladder capacity was less than 100 cc or for whom upper tract dilatation was identified. Other authors have augmented patients whose capacity was less than 60 cc (Gearhart et al., 1991; Perlmutter et al., 1991).

Hollowell and Ransley concluded that there were two significant advantages of combining bladder augmentation with bladder outlet reconstruction. The first was the achievement of almost immediate con-

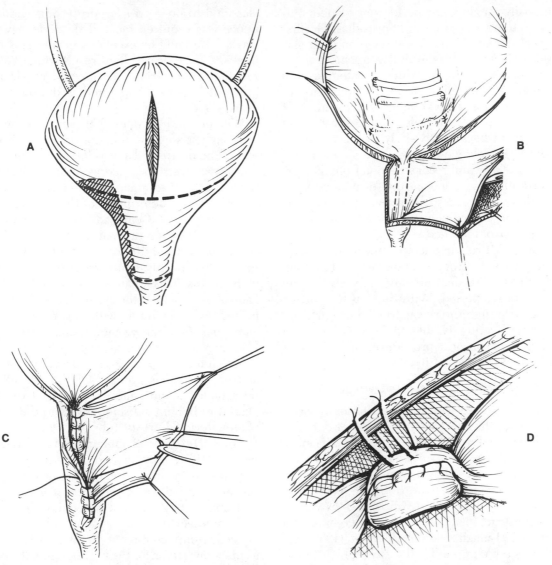

FIG. 50-33
The Cinch. **A,** Bladder incisions required to create bladder flap. **B,** Following transtrigonal ureteral reimplantation, mucosal strip is outlined to become neourethra. **C,** Mucosal layer of neourethra is closed followed by intramuscular closure. **D,** Outer muscular wrap has been sutured into position and the bladder neck suspended. (From Koff SA: A technique for bladder neck reconstruction and exstrophy: The Cinch. *J Urol* 1990; 144:547.)

tinence. The second was the achievement of a quality of ultimate continence that was superior to that of patients treated with bladder outlet reconstruction alone. The obvious disadvantages were the potential for spontaneous perforation of the bladder, the increased need for intermittent catheterization, and the development of urolithiasis.

Gearhart and co-authors (1991) evaluated the success of reoperations for patients with exstrophy who remained incontinent following a previous Young-Dees-Leadbetter bladder neck reconstruction. Eight patients underwent repeat bladder outlet reconstruction, of whom seven achieved a 3-hour dry interval with spontaneous voiding. One patient was continent

on intermittent catheterization. Nine patients were treated with augmentation. One of these underwent simultaneous Young-Dees-Leadbetter bladder neck reconstruction, four received a Mitrofanoff neourethra, and one received an artificial urinary sphincter. Eight of these patients have a continence interval exceeding 3 hours on intermittent catheterization, and six are dry both day and night. The one patient who is incontinent became so following erosion of an artificial urinary sphincter.

The placement of an adjuvant Mitrofanoff neourethra in patients undergoing Young-Dees-Leadbetter bladder neck reconstruction has several advantages (Sheldon, 1992). There are three important goals that are traditionally sought when performing bladder outlet reconstruction for exstrophy or epispadias. The first is urinary continence, which requires a long and narrow urethra. The second is the ability to achieve spontaneous voiding. This simply requires a patent urethra that is straight so that folds do not create occlusion. The third goal is the achievement of a urethra that can be catheterized should this be necessary (a not uncommon event particularly early in the postoperative period). To achieve this goal the surgeon may compromise the urethral reconstruction from the perspective of both length and narrow diameter. Additionally, catheterization of such a reconstructed neourethra may result in sufficient injury to cause either obstruction of incompetence.

The adjuvant Mitrofanoff neourethra allows a channel for intermittent catheterization, which has been useful for all such reconstructions especially in the early postoperative period. With time, as the patient learns to void through the reconstructed urethra, the Mitrofanoff neourethra is able to be removed in a simple outpatient surgical procedure, or because it does not leak, it can be left in situ.

Urethral Lengthening by Anterior Detrusor Tube

Tanagho Procedure.—Although posterior detrusor tubes have been the most common type of detrusor tube procedure performed to increase bladder outlet resistance, there has been a considerable experience with anterior detrusor tubes as well. The tubularization of an anterior strip of the detrusor to create a tube was begun by Flocks and Culp (1953) as a technique to reconstruct bladders in men undergoing total prostatectomy. Tanagho and colleagues (1969) extended this as a technique for the surgical treatment of urinary incontinence. Anatomic studies by Tangho and Smith (1966) showed that there was a condensation of the middle circular fibers of the bladder wall above the bladder neck for a 2 cm segment. They believed that a flap formed from this tissue and turned into a tube would have sufficient muscle tone to create an effective urethral closure pressure. The anterior detrusor tube is begun at the level of the bladder neck after transecting the urethra. It is made 1 inch wide and 1 inch long. After the tube is developed, the flap is tubularized, paying attention to be certain to include the middle circular muscle fibers. The tube is then reanastomosed to the distal urethra. The new detrusor tube is suspended anteriorly from the back of the pubic bone or abdominal wall. In 1981 Tanagho reported a 10-year experience with this procedure. Of the 56 patients undergoing an anterior detrusor tube procedure, 44 had postprostatectomy incontinence. However, five had epispadias or other congenital anomalies leading to incontinence. Five represented posttraumatic incontinence. Results were

classified to be good if no protection against incontinence was required most of the time. Overall there was a 70% good or excellent result. This contrasted to a 50% good or excellent result with a Young-Dees-Leadbetter posterior detrusor tube repair in a similar group of 25 patients operated on during the same 10-year period.

Williams and Snyder (1976) reported a modification of Tanagho's anterior detrusor tube in which the distal end of the detrusor flap was left in continuity with the dorsal urethra, thus making the muscular strip a bipedicle graft, presumably with a more reliable blood supply. In the description of their procedure an anterior strip 2 to 3 cm wide and adequately long to permit a detrusor tube of 3 to 4 cm in length was constructed around a 10 F catheter. They also suspended the detrusor tube from the posterior surface of the rectus. This repair is most suitable for congenital anomalies in which the posterior bladder wall is deficient (as in children with severe urogenital sinus anomalies) or when previous damage to the posterior bladder wall occurred during ureterocele surgery or after a fractured pelvis, as opposed to the exstrophy and/or epispadias groups. Of the 12 children with intractable incontinence reported, two thirds appeared to benefit substantially from the construction of an anterior detrusor tube.

Total Detrusor Tubularization.—Arap and colleagues (1976, 1980) extended the concept of a detrusor tube to include a total detrusor tube made from the entire bladder in the reconstruction of bladder exstrophy. They reported a staged procedure in which a 20 cm intact sigmoid segment with Leadbetter-type antireflux implantation of the ureters into a tenia and a cutaneous stoma for the bowel segment were created as a first stage. The reconstruction of the bladder into a long detrusor tube was performed at the same time. Tubularization of a mucosal strip with a wrap of the detrusor around it constituted the continence reconstruction. Subsequently the end of the detrusor tube was anastomosed to the intraabdominal end of the sigmoid conduit, and finally, the cutaneous sigmoid stoma was closed to allow voiding through the long detrusor tube. Voiding occurs through elevation of intraabdominal pressure (Valsalva's maneuver). Of 29 patients who have had follow-up between 1 and 11 years, 9 are younger than age 5 years and were believed to be too young to be evaluated conclusively for continence. Of the remaining 20 patients, 15 are continent, which means they stay dry between micturitions during the day. Thirteen of the 15 void at hourly intervals or longer. Two have only a 30-minute interval of dryness.

A similar conceptual approach employs tubularization of the exstrophy plate as a urethra and the creation of a neobladder employing a modification of the Maintz pouch (Fisch, 1992). Of eight patients reported only one is completely continent, and two are dry during the day but wet at night. Three patients were converted to other forms of urinary drainage due to either complete incontinence (two patients) or urinary retention (one patient).

Bladder Neck Suspension and Fixation
Open Bladder Neck Suspension

These procedures were designed primarily for the correction of stress urinary incontinence related to abnormally low positioning of the urethrovesical junction. Increased intraabdominal pressure thus could not be transmitted to the urethra, with a resultant low-pressure gradient between the bladder and the urethra leading to stress urinary leakage during periods of increased intraabdominal pressure. This is a specifically defined abnormality and, if anatomically corrected, should lead to correction of stress incontinence in the female without the production of problems with bladder emptying, provided that detrusor function is normal. The urethral suspension procedures may also produce urethral stretch and thus lengthening, urethral narrowing, and/or urethral compression, which may also increase bladder outlet resistance.

The urethral suspension and fixation procedure that has become the standard against which others have been compared is the Marshall-Marchetti-Krantz operation (1949). In this open operation the urethra is suspended from the posterior aspect of the pubic bone or rectus fascia with a series of absorbable sutures, which most surgeons today place into the periurethral tissues adjacent to the urethra. In elevating this tissue the endopelvic fascia is also tightened. This suspension brings the urethrovesical junction to a position where increases in intraabdominal pressure are directly transmitted to the urethra. A high-pressure gradient between the bladder and urethra is maintained during increases in abdominal pressure, thus correcting stress incontinence. A 96% success rate has been reported recently (Krantz, 1980) in patients who were properly selected.

The Burch procedure (1961) is a similar operation to elevate the urethrovesical angle; however, in this operation vaginal fascia near the urethra is sutured to Cooper's ligament (ileopectineal ligament). The initial phases of this and the Marshall-Marchetti-Krantz operation are identical. Adequate dissection in Retzius' space is performed to permit exposure of the ileopectineal ligament. An assistant's fingers are used transvaginally to elevate the anterior vaginal wall to a position at which it lies comfortably against the ileopectineal ligament without tension. At this point the vaginal wall is sutured to the ligament with all layers except the vaginal mucosa. Two or three per-

manent sutures are used on each side, taking care to palpate the Foley catheter in the urethra to avoid sutures being placed too close to the urethra. The possible advantages of this operation are that the ileopectineal ligament may provide a more reliable anchor for sutures than the periosteum of the pubic bone. Additionally osteitis pubis is avoided. A disadvantage is that if there is rigidity of the tissues to be used because of previous surgery, infection, or radiation therapy, the procedure may inadequately elevate the urethra. It is theoretically possible by drawing stitches from a periurethral location laterally to actually suture the bladder neck open, leading to worse incontinence. However, properly done, the procedure has an excellent success rate (Stanton and Cardozo, 1979). As a primary procedure, there was a 96% success rate. Previous operations reduced this to 75%. The overall cure rate at 2 years was 85%.

Endoscopic Bladder Neck Suspension

As it became clear that urethral suspension operations had much to offer in the treatment of stress urinary incontinence, the development of semiclosed needle suspensions became a logical progression in technique. The original Pereyra procedure (1959) used number 30 stainless steel wire, which was looped through the vagina without a vaginal incision by the blind passage of a specially designed needle through a small suprapubic incision. Subsequently the technique has been modified in a number of ways.

Endoscopic suspension was first described in 1973 by Stamey. His innovation was to emphasize the use of the cystoscope to control accurate placement of the suspending sutures exactly at the urethrovesical junction so as to ensure appropriate urethral suspension. The procedure is performed with the patient in the dorsal lithotomy position. A T-shaped vaginal incision is made and the periurethral tissues exposed, taking care to leave the tissue on either side of the bladder neck and urethra undisturbed to avoid injury to the endopelvic (pubocervical) fascia, which is essential to the suspension of the urethra. Through a short suprapubic incision the specially designed Stamey needle is introduced through the rectus fascia. The surgeon's index finger is then used to guide the tip of the needle into the vaginal incision, ensuring that the needle passes sufficiently close to the bladder neck to go through the endopelvic fascia, which is attached to the urethra. With the needle in place, cystoscopic inspection is performed with movement of the needle to ensure that the appropriate tissues have been penetrated, while the lumen of the bladder and urethra have been avoided. A number 2 monofilament nylon suture is threaded through the eye of this special Stamey needle and drawn back suprapubically. The procedure is then repeated, passing the needle 1 cm lateral to the first puncture. A 1-cm segment of knitted Dacron graft material is placed at the end of the looped suture to ensure that the nylon stitch does not pull through the periurethral tissues. This lies in the vaginal vault beneath the mucosa. Endoscopic suspension is then performed on the opposite side. The successful closure of the bladder neck is confirmed by filling the bladder to 300 to 500 ml and ensuring that urethral leakage ceases with appropriate elevation of the suspending sutures. They are then tied over the rectus fascia. At the end of the procedure a percutaneous suprapubic tube is placed. On the second or third day after surgery efforts at voiding are begun, and use of the suprapubic tube is discontinued when there appears to be effective bladder emptying. In half of the patients in Stamey's report (1980) it was possible to remove the suprapubic tube by the seventh day after surgery. In fewer than 10% of cases more than 1 month was required to establish satisfactory bladder emptying. This technique has produced a cure in 91% of 203 consecutive patients, suggesting it is a reliable alternative to open urethral suspension procedures.

Gittes and Loughlin (1988) modified the Stamey endoscopic suspension by making no vaginal incision at all. Instead they allow the monofilament nylon suture to bury itself by gradually cutting the vaginal epithelium. They have not had a problem with infection and report comparably good results.

In the Raz needle suspension procedure (Hadley et al., 1985), Stamey's technique has been modified in several ways. In the vaginal dissection through an inverted U-incision, the retropubic space is entered, and mobilization of the urethra and bladder neck is performed to be certain that the urethra can be moved intraabdominally enough to expose it to intraabdominal pressure. This is particularly important in patients who have had scarring of the periurethral tissues from previous surgery. To ensure adequate fixation of the suspension sutures to the periurethral tissues, a serial helical stitch encompassing the endopelvic fascia as well as the full thickness of the vaginal wall except for the epithelium is used to produce a broadly secured anchoring of the suture to the periurethral tissues.

Suprapubically the suspending sutures are elevated to be certain that closure of the bladder neck is occurring as confirmed by cystoscopic inspection. If considerable tension must be placed on the suspending sutures, this suggests that inadequate mobilization of the urethra and bladder neck area has been performed through the vaginal incision. The suspending sutures are tied over a small pledget of Silastic mesh and then tied to one another. As reported in 1983 (Leach et al.), experience with 250 patients has shown a 96% excellent result. Fifty-two (94%) of 55 patients who had undergone previous failed operative attempts to correct stress incontinence were cured with this ap-

proach. The greatest merit to this approach would seem to lie in its thorough mobilization of the urethra and then secure fixation of the periurethral sutures to ensure reliable suture suspension.

Fascial Sling Procedures

There is a significant difference between the suspension-type procedures and those that involve some form of sling suspension of the urethra. This type of approach dates to the Millan suspension (1947). In this operation a Pfannenstiel incision is made, exposing the rectus fascia. Two longitudinal strips of rectus fascia are defined just above the insertion of the rectus into the pubic bone. These are approximately 1 cm wide and as long as possible. The flaps are dissected, maintaining their continuity with the rectus fascia laterally on each side. The rectus muscles are then split in the midline and Retzius' space dissected to expose the urethra, which should have an indwelling Foley catheter.

The bladder neck region and urethra are separated from the vaginal wall, taking care not to enter either urethra or vagina. The two rectus strips are brought into Retzius' space lateral to the rectus muscle, passed beneath the urethra at the bladder neck, brought back suprapubically through the midline incision between the rectus muscles, and then sutured to the anterior rectus fascia with sufficient elevation of the bladder neck to ensure intraabdominal positioning of the urethra. Millan reported an 80% success rate with this procedure. Its biggest drawback has been a significant problem with long-term urinary retention. Beck (1978) reported using a simple free fascia strip as a sling. Up to one third of his cases have significant retention for as long as 2 years after surgery. Another disadvantage is that sling procedures, particularly if a foreign material is used, can occasionally result in erosion of the urethra or bladder neck. It would appear that sling procedures add a compressive element not present with simple periurethral suspension of the urethra. Direct compression of the urethra by the fascial strip would add to bladder outlet resistance and explain the different outcome from simple suspension.

Sling urethral suspension procedures have been modified by combining them with needle suspension. In the Raz technique of transvaginal needle suspension of the bladder neck with a fascial sling (Hadley et al., 1985), a rectus fascial patch is fashioned like a hammock to cover the length and width of the urethra. Four polypropylene (Prolene) sutures placed at each corner of the graft are drawn suprapubically with four passes of a Stamey-type needle as in an endoscopic suspension. Upward elevation of the suspending sutures lifts the entire urethra and/or bladder neck unit upward and compresses it through the action of the patch. Raz reserves this approach for female patients with an ineffective intrinsic urethral sphincter unit and expects the compression to improve urethral closing pressure. Of 22 patients with short-term follow-up, 21 are dry; however, 15 of the 21 require intermittent self-catheterization to effect bladder emptying. All but one of the patients in this series had undergone between two and eight previous suspension procedures to the urethra or bladder neck.

McGuire and colleagues (1986) modified this technique by using only two sutures with bolsters to pull upward a smaller rectus fascial strip with the same technique as a Stamey suspension (Fig. 50-34). This modification appears to effectively increase bladder outlet resistance despite the fact that a urethral pressure profile generally does not rise much above 30 cm of water. Endoscopically the bladder neck is closed. McGuire's original publication reported success with eight girls with neurogenic bladder secondary to myelodysplasia. All girls continue on intermittent catheterization. Subsequently he has expanded this series successfully to a total of 17 patients, 15 girls and two boys with spina bifida, with success in all cases (McGuire, 1986). Although a straightforward Stamey suspension has been reportd to be successful in increasing outlet resistance in girls with a neurogenic bladder (Woodside and Borden, 1986), it would appear that the compressive aspect of sling procedures contributes an element to a urethral suspension that improves the success of procedures in the myelomeningocele group.

An innovative but slightly different approach to the issue of urethral suspension has been contributed by Sexton (1978). He uses a silicone strip 4 mm wide as a loop from the rectus fascia through Cooper's ligament. In this suspension procedure the silicone strip is brought around a full-thickness segment of vaginal wall on either side of the urethra but crosses dorsal to rather than ventral to the urethra. With traction upwards on the silicone strip ends suprapubically, the urethra and bladder neck are elevated with the elevation of the vaginal wall, but the urethra is not directly suspended as in the previous fascial sling procedures. If anything, this suspension procedure compresses the urethra downward against the vaginal wall. In Sexton's hands, this procedure has been highly successful in a series now encompassing 1000 patients. It has the advantage of lowering the risk of urethral erosion. The silicone strip, which actually enters the vagina, becomes secondarily epithelialized with few complications.

Herschronn and Radomski (1992) reported 13 adult male patients who underwent reconstruction for incontinence in the face of neurovesical dysfunction who received simultaneous bladder neck tapering, placement of a urethral sling, and bladder augmentation (Fig. 50-35). In two patients the sling was composed

of marlex, and both eroded. In the 11 remaining patients, rector fascia was employed, and no erosions were encountered. A 1.5-cm wide strip of fascia was developed that retained its attachment at the level of the pyramidalis on one side. It was swung around beneath the bladder neck and sutured to the level of the pyramidalis on the contralateral side. Nine (69%) patients were totally dry on intermittent catheterization, while an additional two (15%) patients required less than two pads daily. One patient required an artificial urinary sphincter, and one patient continues to be incontinent. Additional complications encountered included bladder neck stricture (two cases) bladder calculi, and epididymitis (one case each).

Elder (1990) reported 14 children with myelomeningocele who were treated employing a free rectus fascia graft sling that was 1 to 1.5 cm × 4 to 6 cm. Of these 13 patients were augmented. Twelve patients (86%) were completely dry on intermittent catheterization, while one is dry during the day and wet at night. The remaining patient is completely inconti-

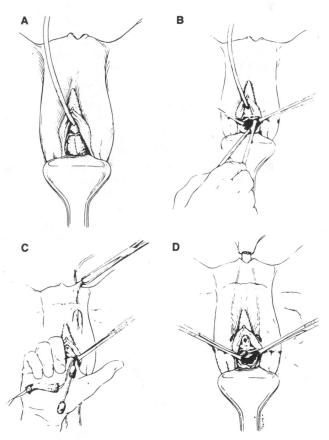

FIG. 50-34
McGuire's modified pubovaginal sling. A 1 × 3 cm rectus fascial strip is pulled up by techniques of a Stamey endoscopic suspension to add a compressive element. (From McGuire EJ, Wang C, Usitalo H, et al: Modified pubovaginal sling in girls with myelodysplasia. *J Urol* 1986; 135:94. Used by permission.)

nent. This series clearly demonstrates the utility of this technique in patients with neurogenic bladders.

Direct Urethral Compression by Foreign Body

There has been considerable interest and progress in the production of increased bladder outlet resistance through the use of external compression of the urethral lumen during the last 20 years as nonreactive polymers of varying types have been developed. Passive compression of the bulbar urethra was begun by Kaufman (1970, 1972). In the Kaufman I procedure (crural cross), the insertion of the corpora into the pubic bone was divided on each side, and the crura was then crossed over the bulbar urethra and reattached to the pubic bone on the opposite side. In the Kaufman II procedure (crural approximation), the crura were compressed against the bulbar urethra by a Marlex tape, which surrounded the crura and urethra. An additional modification was made with the addition of a Marlex pad between the crura and the urethra to increase urethral compression. In his report of this modification, Kaufman (1972) noted in 42 consecutive cases a success rate of approximately 60%. In an effort to improve on these results Kaufman abandoned crural approximation in 1972 and began implanting a prosthesis containing a silicone gel (Kaufman, 1973). This prosthesis contained a polyurethane velour capsule around all of the prosthesis, except for the portion in direct contact with the bulbar urethra, to encourage fixation by fibrous tissue ingrowth. Four Dacron straps were placed around the corporal bodies (two each) and stapled into bone at the base of the crura for fixation. An advantage of this prosthesis was the ability to postoperatively inject more fluid into the device with a fine needle to increase urethral compression. Because the only unsupported side of the prosthesis was the bare portion in contact with the bulbar urethra, further filling of the prosthesis resulted in selective bulbar urethral compression. Urethral pressure profilometry was used to monitor the increase in outlet resistance produced intraoperatively. Moderate tension was adjusted with the straps to try to achieve a pressure of 70 to 90 cm H_2O. If the closing pressure was less than 60 cm H_2O, the prosthesis was injected on the table to bring the pressure up to 70 to 90 cm H_2O. In their report of 184 cases, there were 125 primary cases and 59 cases with previous unsuccessful surgery for urinary incontinence (postprostatectomy, 168; neurogenic bladder, 16). Early postoperative continence was better than that seen on longer term follow-up. However, after one or more injections of the prosthesis, usually adding 5 to 10 ml of fluid each time, a 60% excellent or good result was achieved.

The most serious of the 20 major complications seen with the Kaufman prosthesis was urethral erosion, which occurred in 12 patients, two of whom had associated osteomyelitis requiring a prolonged hospitalization. Three of the patients with urethral erosion required a supravesical urinary diversion. Eight other patients had infection without erosion that required removal of the prosthesis. Other (Graham et al., 1982) have had roughly similar success (47%) with a high complication rate, particularly in patients incontinent following surgery to remove malignant disease.

Periurethral Injection

Direct passive urethral compression through the periurethral injection of Teflon (polytetrafluoroethy-

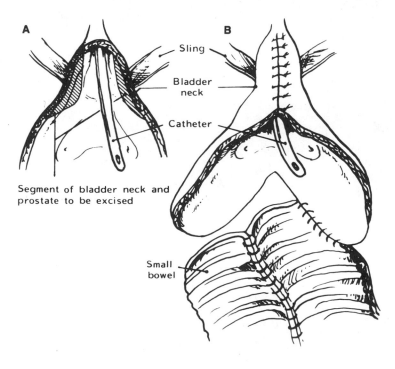

FIG. 50-35
Fascial sling and bladder neck tapering. **A,** Extension of midline vesical incision through bladder neck with mobilization of bladder neck. **B,** Approximation of outlet with two layers of interrupted absorbable suture after excision of wedges of bladder neck. Fascial sling is placed around the bladder neck and augmentation cystoplasty completed. (From Herschorns, Radomski SB: Fascial slings and bladder neck tapering in the treatment of male neurogenic incontinence. *J Urol* 1992; 147:1073-1075.)

lene) paste was suggested initially by Politano and colleagues in 1974. The raising of a submucosal wheel of Teflon paste coapts the urethral wall, increasing bladder outlet resistance and preventing the transmission of intraabdominal pressure to the urethra through a column of urine in an open bladder neck and/or posterior urethra.

In the female, a 17-gauge needle attached to a mechanical syringe is inserted at the urethral meatus and advanced periurethrally toward the bladder neck. Several cubic centimeters of Teflon paste are injected, and the injection is continued as the needle is withdrawn. The procedure is performed usually at the 3 o'clock, 6 o'clock, and 9 o'clock positions around the urethra. A total of 10 to 15 ml of paste is usually injected. During injections a cystoscopic inspection of the bladder and urethra ensures that perforation of the needle into the lumen has not occurred. In the male a cystoscope is left in the urethra to inspect the area of the bladder neck and prostatic urethra while the injection is performed by means of a needle tip placed in the area of the external sphincter. Approximately 15 ml of paste is injected in the male, with the goal being to create closure or significant narrowing of the lumen.

In a report of 165 patients treated for incontinence caused by various factors, Politano (1982) reported an overall good to excellent result in 75% of cases. In male patients the greatest number of treated patients had postprostatectomy incontinence. In female patients stress incontinence was the most common problem, although a wide range of other causes for incontinence was also noted. The main cause of failure was the injection of inadequate amounts of Teflon paste. Second injections corrected may initial poor results. This same technique has been used in female patients who have neurogenic bladder disease (Lewis et al., 1984). Five of the six patients treated have achieved total continence but do require intermittent catheterization. Ten injections were required in the six patients.

Complications from this technique have been reported by Politano's group to be minimal. Some patients without a neurogenic bladder have had transitory urinary retention. Approximately one fourth of the patients experience symptoms of dysuria and occasionally perineal discomfort, which generally subside after a few days. Possible worrisome complications have been reported by Malizia and colleagues (1984) and Claes and colleagues (1989). These authors studied migration and granulomatous reaction after the periurethral injection of Teflon paste in experimental animals. They found, on short-term follow-up, that there was evidence of migration of the Teflon particles to the pelvic lymph nodes and lungs. In animals studied for a longer period (10½ months) Teflon particles were found in the pelvic nodes, lungs, and brain of all, in the kidneys of four of the seven animals, and in the spleens of two. Generally the reaction to Teflon particles was minimal on short-term follow-up, but in the animals studied long-term, the particles were noted to be surrounded by a pronounced chronic inflammatory reaction. These findings have raised significant questions about the use of Teflon injections, particularly in children. The Food and Drug Administration has not yet cleared the use of Teflon paste in the urinary tract. The initial experience with the use of a collagen implant in a similar manner has been reported (McGuire et al., 1990). Early experience appears encouraging.

Artificial Urinary Sphincter

There have been several devices created for the active mechanical compression of the urethra to increase urethral resistance. The Rosen prosthesis (1978) consists of a three-pronged clamp, two arms of which are parallel on one side, with a third single arm carrying a balloon opposing them. The bulbar urethra is threaded between the limbs of the clamp, and the balloon is inflated by a scrotally placed reservoir balloon with a release valve incorporated into its neck. With inflation of the balloon the urethra is kinked and compressed. There is no mechanism to control the pressure achieved. The device has been placed around the bulbar urethra in males, usually for postprostatectomy incontinence or incontinence arising as a result of abdominoperineal resection or neurogenic bladder. In Rosen's report (1978), 18 (77%) of 23 patients were cured. There were three device failures that were corrected successfully. Rosen experienced only two urethral fistulas, which required removal of the device and the placement of a suprapubic tube. The fistulas then closed. One patient experienced skin necrosis in the scrotum. Other authors (Augspurger, 1981; Giesy et al., 1981; Light and Pietro, 1986) have not reported such a satisfactory experience. Only nine (53%) of Augspurger's 17 patients had a functioning prosthesis with a follow-up of just over 2 years. One quarter had to have the prosthesis removed. The major complication was aneurysmal formation in the balloon. There were two cases of infection; one resulted in urethral erosion. In the series by Giesy and colleagues of 19 patients, 26 secondary operations were required during a follow-up period ranging from 9 to 34 months. The main complications were balloon leakage, aneurysmal changes in the balloon, tubing leaks, reservoir malfunction, and urethral erosion (five patients). The actuarial survival of a first Rosen implant in this series was under 20% at 18 months' follow-up. Because of this experience, the use of this particular prosthesis has been abandoned in most centers.

A more complex form of artificial urinary sphincter

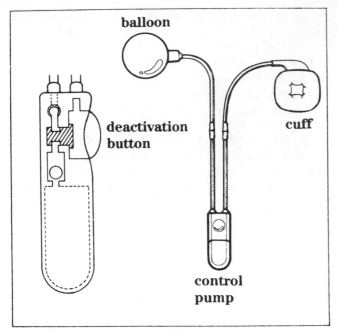

FIG. 50-36
American Medical Systems model 800 artificial urinary sphincter. Much simplified model with deflation pump, delay-fill resistor, and deactivation button in one control unit that can be implanted in the scrotum or labia. (From American Medical Systems, Minnetonka, Minn, Publication 30831.)

was introduced by Scott and colleagues (1974). This was a hydraulic device constructed of medical-grade silicone consisting of a cuff placed around the bladder neck or bulbar urethra, a reservoir that was placed intraabdominally, and an activating pressure bulb located in the scrotum or labia. A specially designed valve controlled the pressure in the cuff. Improved models were introduced by American Medical Systems (AS 721, 791, and 792) until the current AS 800 model (Fig. 50-36) was introduced in 1984 (Montague). Controlled pressure is maintained in the cuff until the pump is squeezed, transferring fluid from the cuff into the reservoir balloon and permitting bladder emptying to take place. A delay-fill resistor in the control mechanism provides 1 to 2 minutes of lowered intraurethral pressure before automatic refilling of the cuff takes place from the reservoir balloon. The model AS 800 sphincter also incorporates in the control device a deactivation button as well as the deflation pump. This device is placed in the scrotum or labia. The concept of primary deactivation permits healing and reestablishment of good blood flow to take place before external compression is applied to the urethra. Activation of the sphincter is carried out by a brisk squeeze of the deflation pump.

Multiple mechanical problems have occurred in patients with the artificial sphincter in place. The most common problems have been fluid leaks from the cuff

or tubing kinks requiring a surgical revision. The most serious complications are erosion of the sphincter into the urethra or the development of infection around the cuff. The latter problems generally require removal of the device. The latest modification in manufacture, which involves dip-coating the cuff with silicone and emphasis on placement of a low-pressure cuff with primary deactivation, may improve results.

In the selection of patients for the genitourinary sphincter, it has been emphasized that sterile urine, low-pressure storage, and an ability to spontaneously and fully empty the bladder are important (Light and Scott, 1984). Scott and co-workers have always advocated the creation of total incontinence by means of a transurethral sphincterotomy in boys or a bladder flap urethroplasty in girls before the implantation of the sphincter. Others using the device prefer to use intermittent self-catheterization with the artificial sphincter in place to ensure complete bladder emptying, avoiding ablative surgery on the outlet (Diokno and Sonda, 1981).

There are a number of technical points that merit emphasis in the placement of the Scott artificial sphincter. The bladder neck position is usually preferable. Sidi and colleagues (1984) reported a 55% incidence of stress incontinence as a major problem with bulbar urethral placement contrasted with a 21% incidence of mild stress incontinence when the sphincter was implanted around the bladder neck.

The large series reported by Montague (1992) in which 166 adult and pediatric patients were reported is noteworthy for the achievement of a very high continence rate employing the artificial urinary sphincter in the region of the bulbous urethra in men. This, in contrast to earlier reports, clearly demonstrates the utility of this technique.

The need to avoid bacterial contamination of the wound cannot be overemphasized. Preoperative antibiotic coverage is routinely administered, and an antibiotic irrigant for the surgical field is employed.

The most critical step in the discussion lies in the creation of an adequate space around the bladder neck to place the cuff. Conventional wisdom would dictate that if dissection posterior to the bladder neck opens either urethra, bladder, or vagina, it is wise to postpone placement of the sphincter. Recent evidence would suggest that this may not always be necessary (Salisz and Diokno, 1992).

The reservoir balloon is placed such that it is subjected to intraabdominal pressure. When coughing or straining occurs, increased balloon pressure is transmitted to the cuff, preventing leakage. Connections of the tubing are made above the level of the rectus fascia in the deep subcutaneous tissue to facilitate later revision, if necessary.

The intraoperative use of urethral pressure profile

measurement may be useful to demonstrate that the sphincter is active in compressing the urethral tissue. The use of as low as pressure cuff as is consistent with achieving continence is important. Mitchell and Rink (1983) recommended the routine use of a 60 to 70 cm H_2O pressure balloon initially in children. It has been a common experience that the higher the pressure in the balloon is, the greater the erosion rate is, (Barrett and Furlow, 1984; Sidi et al., 1984).

Primary deactivation to permit healing of the surgical area before subjecting the urethra to pressure appears to lower the incidence of sphincter erosion (Furlow, 1981). After waiting approximately 6 weeks the sphincter is activated. The AS 800 model design, which permits secondary activation without surgery, is a particularly encouraging advance.

It is critical that patients recognize that compliance with a program of regular bladder emptying is essential to avoid the transmission of high intravesical pressures to the upper tracts. It is paradoxic that our experience with compliance has been the worst in children who were rendered incompletely dry with a sphincter. Several have become discouraged and simply stopped opening the sphincter, resulting in a high-pressure bladder with secondary upper tract damage. Long-term surveillance is critical in patients with a genitourinary sphincter in place, as late changes in the dynamics of the bladder have been reported and silent damage to the upper tracts can follow (Bitsch et al., 1988; Light and Pietro, 1986). We recommend a semiannual ultrasound surveillance of the urinary tract indefinitely, even if the patient appears clinically well.

Reports of results with the use of the Scott artificial sphincter have accumulated as experience has been gained during the last 10 years. In a report from Scott's center (Light and Scott, 1984), an experience with 132 children is reviewed. Four underwent implantation of the AS 800 model, and the rest had the AS 792 model implanted. The most common cause of incontinence was a neurogenic bladder secondary to spina bifida. Ninety-two (70%) patients are completely continent. An additional 10% have mild stress incontinence and require no more than one incontinence pad per day. Only 9% were considered treatment failures.

Light and Scott (1983) also reported their experience with the use of the artificial sphincter in children with the epispadias and/or exstrophy complex. In 11 patients (eight male and three female) total continence was achieved in 10, whereas one was removed because of infection. Sidi and colleagues (1984) reported 72% satisfactory results in 36 male and seven female children using the AS 791 and AS 792 sphincters. Thirty-five percent had mechanical failure and 17% erosions. Mitchell and Rink (1983) reported on their experiences in 41 children, with 80% achieving complete

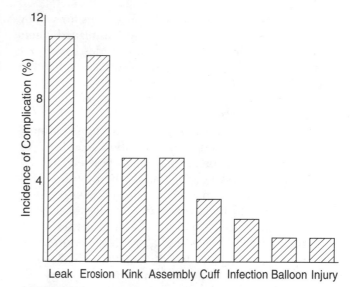

FIG. 50-37
Complications encountered in 279 patients reported in five recent large series. (See text.)

continence. Barrett and Furlow (1984) reported their experience with 22 children, with only two treatment failures, both occurring secondary to bladder neck erosion using sphincters with a balloon pressure of greater than 90 cm water.

Figure 50-37 outlines the complications encountered in five of the most recent large series. These series cover 279 patients, of whom 224 (80%) achieved continence (Belioli et al., 1992; Bosco et al., 1991; Churchill et al., 1989; Gonzalez et al., 1989; Montague et al., 1992). The most common complications were those of leakage of sphincteric fluid and erosion. Other important mechanical problems included those related to tube kinking and assembly malfunction.

The experience of Bosco and colleagues (1991) demonstrated that patients in whom a balloon pressure between 51 and 80 cm H_2O was employed achieved success much more often than those for whom a pressure between 81 and 100 cm H_2O was employed. These authors also reported a mean survival of the artificial urinary sphincter of 7.2 years and demonstrated that the AS 800 model had a significantly lower reoperation rate than the earlier models. A similar finding was reported by Gonzalez and colleagues (1989) where the incidence of reoperation fell from 19 per 1000 patient months (models AS 791, 792) to seven reoperations per 1000 patient months with the AS 800 model.

Alibadi and Gonzalez (1990) further demonstrated the utility of the artificial urinary sphincter in patients in whom the sphincter was placed following earlier failed reconstruction for incontinence. In 11 patients who had undergone previous Young-Dees-Leadbetter reconstructions or bladder neck suspension, eight (73%) had a long-term successful outcome. Noteworthy was a very poor success rate in patients for whom a second artificial urinary sphincter was placed when a previous one had eroded. Several series have documented the utility of the artificial urinary sphincter in patients who have bladder augmentation (Gonzalez et al., 1989; Kreder and Webster, 1992; Mitchell and Rink, 1983; Strawbridge et al., 1989).

An assessment of the ability to predict those patients who will require bladder augmentation in addition to artificial urinary sphincter placement was reported by deBadiola and colleagues (1992). These authors reported 33 pediatric patients with neurovesical dysfunction assessed by preoperative urodynamics (Fig. 50-38). Eight patients had a capacity exceeding 60% of that predicted by age, and all achieved continence without enterocystoplasty. Fifteen patients had a measured capacity less than 60% predicted by age. Of these, eight had a compliance at capacity exceeding 2 ml/cm H_2O. All were dry without the need for augmentation. In contrast, seven patients with capacities less than 60% of predicted had a compliance less than 2 ml/cm H_2O. These patients required bladder augmentation for persistent incontinence (six patients) and upper tract deteriorations (one patient).

The ability to predict those patients who will require bladder augmentation is confounded by the demonstration of the potential for such bladders to lose compliance over time (Bauer, 1986). Such patients are at risk for both urinary incontinence and upper tract de-

terioration. Possible physiologic explanations may include an overestimation of bladder compliance on preoperative urodynamic study secondary to urethral incompetence or vesicoureteral reflux, alterations in bladder compliance secondary to a changing neurologic status with growth and tethering of the spinal cord, and likely to actual change in the detrusor in response to bladder outlet occlusion.

A concern for some time has been the effect of placing an artificial urinary sphincter around the bladder neck in the male from the perspective of prostatic and sexual development. This question was addressed by Jumper and colleagues (1990). These authors evaluated 13 teenage male patients with myelomeningocele in whom an artificial urinary sphincter was positioned around the bladder neck for a period exceeding 3 years. These patients were compared with 12 age-matched patients in a control group also with myelomeningocele. No evidence for alteration in sexual development or function and no evidence for alterations in prostatic growth or morphology was detected in this study employing transrectal ultrasonography.

A finding of unknown significance is that of particles shedding and migration in patients with artificial urinary sphincters (Barrett et al., 1991). These authors reviewed 26 patients who at the time of revision of a genitourinary prosthesis underwent selective biopsy of the reactive fibrous capsule (25 patients) and draining lymph nodes (four patients). Eighteen of 25 patients demonstrated shed silicone particles within the periprosthetic tissue, and all biopsied lymph nodes demonstrated such particles. Fourteen of these 29 specimens revealed evidence for foreign body granulomas.

Although some groups have tried placement of the artificial sphincter around a bowel catheterizable channel to create continence, this has usually resulted in erosion, and only bladder neck placement in children is recommended (Bruskewitz et al., 1980). Some recent data suggests the potential use of the artificial urinary sphincter in such intestinal segments if the pressure is kept to less than 80 cm of water (Light, 1989; Mitrofanoff et al., 1992; Weston et al., 1991). Despite these observations, this application would continue to be one of last resort.

Creation of Urethral Flap Valve of Detrusor

In the aforementioned techniques, urethral resistance was incurred by either narrowing, lengthening, or compression. Another approach to produce a competent urethra is to turn the junction of the urethra with the bladder into an effective flap-valve as is seen at the normal ureterovesical junction. This technique has been described by Kropp and Angwafo (1986) (Fig. 50-39). A detrusor tube is formed anteriorly or pos-

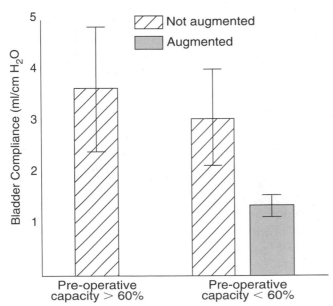

FIG. 50-38
Pre-operative capacity and bladder compliance is predictive in the need for augmentation. (See text.) (From Badiola FI, et al: Influence of pre-operative bladder capacity and compliance on the outcome of artificial sphincter implantation in patients with neurogenic sphincter incompetence. *J Urol* 1992; 148:1493-1495.)

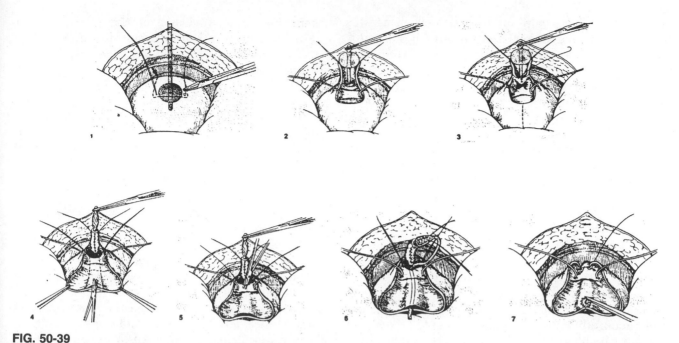

FIG. 50-39

Detrusor flap valve. A detrusor tube is created (anterior shown, posterior tube also possible) and tunneled submucosally in bladder to create a competent flap valve. (From Kropp KA, Angwafo FF: Urethral lengthening and reimplantation for neurogenic incontinence in children. *J Urol* 1986; 135:534. Used by permission.)

teriorly in continuity with the bladder neck and urethra. The blood supply to this mobilized tube is maintained through the bladder neck. The tube is reimplanted submucosally in the bladder. Compression of the detrusor tube as the bladder fills creates an effective flap-valve mechanism, producing continence. Increased intravesical pressure results in increased compression of the detrusor tube, thus preventing leakage. Spontaneous voiding is not possible in this situation, and intermittent catheterization is required for bladder emptying.

In the report by Kropp and Angwafo (1986) anterior detrusor tubes were created in 10 patients and posterior tubes in three patients. The length of the tubes ranged from 3 to 7 cm, with the majority between 4 to 5 cm length. With intermittent catheterization none of the children need diapers either day or night. Three have an occasional minor dribble, but only one requires a minipad. The main postoperative problem in this group was difficulty with catheterizations mostly in males, which could occur late. This generally was the result of hang-up of the catheter just proximal to the detrusor tube. Two boys required a perineal uretherostomy for easier catheterization, and in one a 5 mm transurethral resection of the roof of the proximal end of the tube satisfactorily restored easy catheterization. The excellent results achieved with a flap-valve mechanism suggest that in children who have a urethra sufficient for instrumentation, this technique of flap valve creation may be a useful technique in

constructing a continent, catheterizable access to the urinary bladder.

The utility of the Kropp urethral reconstruction was further evaluated by Belman and Kaplan (1989). Fourteen (78%) of 18 patients achieved a 4-hour continence interval. Eight patients had difficulty with intermittent catheterization, which is mandatory following this procedure. Four patients developed new vesicoureteral reflux in the postoperative period. These authors now recommend leaving the urethral catheter in for 5 weeks following reconstruction and consider prior bladder neck surgery to be a relative contraindication to this procedure.

PROVIDING FOR ALTERNATE CONTINENT URINE DRAINAGE

Physiologic Considerations

Procedures directed at urethral functional replacement have in common the creation of a tubular conduit with sufficient length and exposure to external compressive forces to provide outlet resistance that cannot be overcome by intravesical (intrareservoir) pressure. The success of these procedures in terms of continence depends on the achievement of controlled reservoir-neourethral balance. Neourethral resistance to reservoir outflow must be sufficient to not only exceed resting intravesical pressure but also to exceed the intermittent intravesical pressure elevation associated with gravity (upright posture) as well as episodic additive intraabdominal pressure spikes (coughing, sneezing, straining, and sudden postural changes). The functional characteristics of various types of continent conduits has been recently reviewed (Hinman, 1990).

The creation of neourethral resistance must be complemented by low intravesical (intrareservoir) pressure. This may entail bladder augmentation or replacement by bowel and should include reconfiguration by detubularization. A large capacity is imperative, as is intermittent catheter drainage before the low-compliance portion of the reservoir's pressure-volume curve is entered. As the reconstruction of outlet resistance to permit spontaneous balanced voiding is most difficult, the construction of a neourethra should not be used with the anticipation of spontaneous voiding. The patient should anticipate a possible permanent need for intermittent catheterization.

The mechanisms underlying the creation of a continent neourethra involve combinations of all the manipulable variables that influence tubular conduit hydraulic resistance. These include not only long length and small radius but most important the controlled application of external compressive pressure. Continuous hydraulic resistance may be applied by plication or tapering. Variable resistance is achieved by the exposure of the neourethra to intraabdominal pressure with or without exposure to intrareservoir pressure. These mechanisms all have in common a long, small diameter conduit that is pliable and thereby collapsible. In addition to these considerations, a small diameter facilitates catheterization without kinking or coiling of the catheter.

Although a transabdominal tube of bladder, bowel, appendix, or ureter with a sufficient length exposed to intraabdominal pressure may provide continence through hydraulic principles, greater success is achieved by supplementation with a valve mechanism, whereby a portion of the neouretheral length is exposed to intravesical hydrostatic pressure. Nipple and flap valve mechanisms are used most commonly.

A *nipple valve* is a lumen within a reservoir created by the inversion of a tubular conduit. This most commonly takes the form of ileocecal or ileal-ileal intussusception. The circumferential application of intrareservoir pressure causes luminal collapse and sufficient resistance to prevent egress of urine. Because normal anatomy readily lends itself to this mechanism, such procedures are technically easy, fast, and associated with minimum early complications. They are, however, subject to an inherent instability resulting from the fact that the same forces that achieve luminal collapse cause anatomic distraction at the base of the nipple, resulting in valve shortening and often eventual incompetence (see Fig. 50-14).

The *flap valve* is, again, a lumen within a reservoir,

but in this instance all or a portion of the smaller internal conduit is supported against the inner surface of the wall of the urinary reservoir. Here intrareservoir pressure collapses the internal lumen, and if the compressed channel is well anchored to the wall of the reservoir, additional intrareservoir forces simply further compress the channel and are not disruptive to the flap valve mechanism. This is the mechanism that underlies the normal competence of the ureterovesical junction.

Several embellishments have been added to the nipple valve in an attempt to enhance stability. Serosal scarification and sequential seromuscular suture fixation (Hendren, 1980a) have been used to enhance apposition of the adjacent serosal surfaces of a bowel intussusception but have not been proven sufficiently durable. Internal transmural longitudinal stapling of the intussusception's adjacent walls (Thuroff et al., 1986) has proven durable but has been complicated by intravesical foreign material and stones. Additionally, rings fashioned from fascial or prosthetic strips have been used at the intussusception entrance to strengthen suture fixation (Skinner et al., 1984a), but erosion has been a common problem.

The most appealing embellishment of the nipple valve is its conversion to a flap-valve mechanism. This has been performed by opening the mucosa and suturing the nipple down against one wall of the reservoir. This has been used for ileocecal segments (Hendren, 1978b; King, 1987) as well as for ileal-ileal segments (Olsson, 1985a, 1985b; Robertson and King, 1986). This change of an unstable nipple valve to a fixed flap valve appears to hold up better as an antireflux valve on follow-up.

Probably the most important adjunct to the efficiency and longevity of these valvular mechanisms is their exposure to low reservoir pressures. Thus the creation of a low-pressure reservoir, as reviewed previously, is an essential component in the construction of a competent neourethra. Once constructed, these neourethras have the potential for anastomosis to the residual native urethra, if present, or for the creation of a continent anterior abdominal or perineal stoma.

Bladder Tubes for Neourethra
Hydraulic Resistance

In 1958 Lapides first described an operation designed to create a detrusor tube from the bladder dome that exited on the anterior abdominal wall. A flap of the front wall of the bladder is incised, leaving it attached at the dome. This flap is then formed into a tube and brought through the rectus muscle to create a stoma positioned just below the umbilicus. The length of this detrusor tube and its diameter provide the resistance to outflow needed to produce continence.

Lapides (1978) reported the follow-up of seven patients for as long as 17 years. Most had sustained a loss of the posterior urethra secondary to trauma. Five of the seven patients were male. All of these patients maintained urinary continence for 2 to 4 hours during the day and were completely dry at night. There was no stress incontinence. Six of the seven patients were able to void spontaneously, and one required intermittent catheterization. Although bacteriuria was seen in all of the patients, none had any evidence of upper tract deterioration.

Koff (1985) reported on the use of this technique in children. In his technique the detrusor flap is made as long as possible (9 to 11 cm). At the apex the flap is 2 cm wide and its base at the dome of the bladder 1 to 2 cm wider to ensure a good blood supply. The detrusor tube is placed again through the rectus muscle and brought out as high near the umbilicus as possible. Koff believes that continence is contributed to not only by the hydraulic resistance of the tube but also by the pressure created by the rectus muscle as it contracts in response to increases in intraabdominal pressure. Additionally, because the stoma is always superior to the bladder, gravitational forces lesson the likelihood of leakage.

Nipple Valve

After experimental work done in dogs (Schneider et al., 1975a, 1975b) the same group created a continent vesicostomy in a series of 17 adult patients (Schneider et al., 1977). Fifteen of the 17 patients had a neurogenic bladder. Similar to the detrusor tube created by Lapides, a long muscular tube of bladder based on the dome was fashioned. It was 9 cm in length, with a width of 5 cm at the base and 3 cm at the tip. The detrusor flap was tubularized, with the base segment of 3 to 4 cm being fixed as an intussuscepted nipple in the bladder. Nonabsorbable sutures for fixation of the nipple were recommended because of experience with loss of the intussusception with absorbable sutures. The nipple was further reinforced by nonabsorbable sutures between the detrusor tube and the bladder. The bladder was also secured to the anterior abdominal wall where the detrusor tube passes through the rectus in an effort to maintain a stable reconstruction. With a maximum follow-up of 26 months, there was a continent vesicostomy created in 13 of the 17 patients. All patients practiced clean intermittent catheterizations with intervals ranging from 3 to 8 hours. Two of the patients had failure associated with necrotizing fasciitis, and two had failure because of reduction of the intussusception. Bladder calculi related top the nonabsorbable sutures to fix the nipple valve formed in two patients, but these were removable by endoscopy.

Intestinal Tubes for Neourethra
Hydraulic Resistance

Rowland and colleagues (1985, 1987) described an ileocecal form of continent diversion that depends on hydraulic resistance from a plicated or tailored ileal segment for continence (see Fig. 50-23). In their most recent modifications, the Indiana group used the entire right colon opened out and then folded down on itself to create a detubularized reservoir. Continence is provided by the hydraulic resistance in the terminal 15 to 20 cm of ileum above the ileocecal valve, which is tapered with staples. The catheterizable ileal stoma is brought out through the rectus in the right or left lower quadrant. The smaller diameter of the tapered ileum facilitates catheterization by helping to avoid kinking or coiling of the catheter. Because the hydraulic resistance in the ileal segment was not felt to vary with increasing pressure in the right colon reservoir, leakage might be expected with sufficient filling. However, Rowland and colleagues (1987) reported a dry interval of at least 3 hours in 90% of their patients, most of whom are adults who have undergone cystectomy for bladder cancer. The simplicity of this continent reconstruction adds to its attractiveness.

The mechanism of continence with the Indiana pouch has recently been investigated (Carroll et al., 1989; Juma, 1990). Continence is achieved by a combination of low pouch pressure and elevated resistance to urine flow through the tapered ileal conduit. This resistance is not only generated by the length of the conduit and its small diameter but is also contributed to by a natural resistance generated by the ileocecal valve. Of most interest was the finding of intermittent muscular contraction, which occurred more frequently in the conduit than in the reservoir and tended to occur either simultaneously with or immediately preceding reservoir contraction.

Nipple Valve

Success with the use of nipple valves to create a continent catheterizable channel is closely related to the development of a nipple valve to prevent reflux from the reservoir to the upper tracts. Work with this problem was part of the development of ileocecal augmentation of the bladder with the ureters attached to the ileum. Because the ileocecal valve was incompetent 75% of the time at pressures above 50 cm H_2O (Rendleman et al., 1958), it was evident that efforts to improve this valve mechanism were required for its effective use in the genitourinary tract. A wrap of the terminal ileum by the cecum around approximately 300 degress of the terminal ileum was proposed by Zinman and Libertino (1975). Gittes (1977) proposed fixing the terminal ileum around the convex surface of the cecum so that as cecal distention took place, the terminal ileum would be compressed, producing an antireflux mechanism. Unfortunately this modification still was associated with reflux in approximately 33% of cases. Hendren (1980a, 1980b) proposed trying to form a more stable nipple valve by denuding the mesentery from 8 cm of the terminal ileum to produce a 4 cm nipple into the cecum. Scarification of the serosa of the ileum was performed to try to promote fibrosis to fix the nipple. Despite these efforts, King and colleagues (1985) and Mitchell and Rink (1985) continued to find reflux rates approaching 50%. Hendren has most recently taken the intussuscepted ileocecal segment and opened the mucosa along one wall as well as along the wall of the cecum and fixed the intussusception to the wall of the cecal segment, thus effectively changing a nipple technique of antireflux into a flap-valve technique. This finally appears to be a reliable technique to prevent reflux. This experience also has been verified by King (1987), who reported that five of six ileocecal intussusceptions sutured to the inner wall of the cecum appeared to be successful in preventing reflux.

Procedures intended to create a continent, catheterizable intestinal tube attached to a urinary reservoir reflect many of the problems with incompetence of the ileocecal valve that have just been discussed (Ashken, 1982; Mansson et al., 1984, 1986; Sullivan et al., 1973; Zingg and Tscholl, 1977). The more successful variations of the nipple valve technique have involved modifications that actually create a flap-valve mechanism.

Benchekroun (1982) described still another variant on the use of the ileocecal segment for continence (Fig. 50-40). A 14-cm segment of ileum is turned in on itself so that the two mucosal surfaces lie opposed. The mucosa of the two ends is sutured together in two places, leaving an inner space open for the drainage of mucus. It is into this inner space that urine can also flow from the reservoir as it fills, producing compression of the serosa-lined catheterizable channel. The series of Benchekroun (1987) was extended to 62 patients. The greatest complication has been ileal devagination, which has occurred in 18 of 62 patients. In most patients this could be repaired at reoperation. Overall 56 of the 62 patients are continent on clean intermittent catheterization.

Benchekroun and colleagues (1989) have since reported a larger series of 136 patients. Of these 105 (75%) were immediately continent of urine, and 24 (17.6%) became continent with a revision of the valve mechanism. The valve mechaism was found to be easily catheterized in 88.3%, and the overall continence rate was 92%. In a recent study, Quinlan and colleagues (1991) employed the Benchekroun continence mechanism in nine patients with complicated urinary tract disease, all of whom became continent. Com-

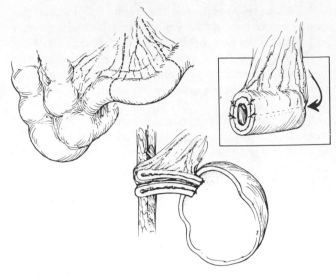

FIG. 50-40
Continent ileocecal reservoir—Benchekroun. Separate ileal segment is inverted so the mucosal surfaces lie opposite. Filling of the mucosa-lined space from the reservoir compresses the catheterizable channel, which is serosa-lined and produces continence. (From Duckett JW, Snyder HM: Use of the Mitrofanoff principle in urinary reconstruction. *World J Urol* 1985; 3:191.)

plications included valve fistula (one case), difficulty with catheterization due to false passage (one case), and stomal stenosis requiring dilatation (three cases).

Flap Valve

The possibility of using a flap-valve mechanism of tunneled ileum into a large bowel reservoir to prevent reflux has been examined experimentally by Vinograd and colleagues (1984). In dogs, untapered, terminal ileum was placed in a submucosal tunnel in the ascending colon in an effort to surgically recreate a competent ileocecal valve. Submucosal tunnel lengths were 2, 4, and 6 cm. In barium enemas done to evaluate reflux, only submucosal segments of 2 cm were shown to be incompetent. At 3 months reoperation and cross-clamping of the cecum to permit infusion of the right colon with saline solution for measurement of the pressure at which the ileocecal valve would reflux was performed. Not one of 19 dogs with a 4 cm or greater submucosal tunnel had any leakage at pressures less than 50 cm H_2O. Only three valve mechanisms refluxed at pressures less than 100 cm H_2O. This concept has had limited clinical experience but has failed to gain general acceptance (Ashken, 1982; Lobe, 1986).

In 1980 Mitrofanoff first reported the use of the appendix and the ureter as a catheterizable conduit attached with a flap-valve antirefluxing technique to the bladder with the proximal end brought out to the skin for clean intermittent catheterization. In his orig-

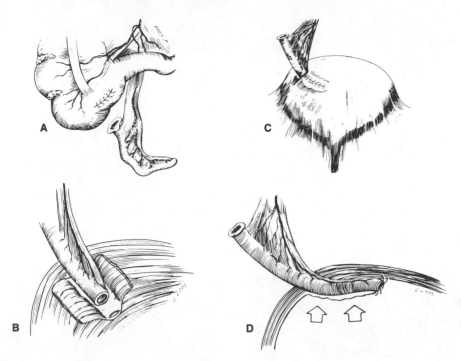

FIG. 50-41

Mitrofanoff procedure. **A,** Appendix has been mobilized on its mesentery, and cecal segment is closed. **B,** Extravesical dissection shows mucosal orifice in which distal end of appendix will be implanted. **C,** Finally, detrusor is closed over implanted appendix, and its proximal end is then brought to skin to serve as catheterizable stoma. **D,** This diagram depicts resulting continent flap-valve mechanism of Mitrofanoff procedure; similar to reimplanted ureter, rise in intravesical pressure compresses conduit against detrusor, occluding its lumen and achieving continence. (From Sheldon CA, Gilbert A: Use of the appendix for urethral reconstruction in children with congenital anomalies of the bladder. *Surgery* 1992; 112:805-812.)

inal experience the only failures followed hydrone-phrosis resulting from failure to create an adequate low-pressure urinary reservoir. The Mitrofanoff principle can be summarized as consisting of two components. (1) A narrow supple conduit (most frequently the appendix or ureter) is brought to the skin as a catheterizable stoma. (2) An antirefluxing connection of this conduit to the reservoir provides continence by a flap-valve mechanism (Fig. 50-41).

This principle, originating from Mitrofanoff's concept, and the extension of the above principles have permitted the continent reconstruction of the lower urinary tract in a wide variety of situations (Duckett and Snyder, 1985, 1986). The small caliber of the catheterizable conduit facilitates catheterization by helping to avoid problems with kinking and coiling catheters. The small diameter and supple nature of the catheterizable conduit permits the simple creation of an effective flap-valve mechanism by placing a portion of the conduit in a submucosal position within the reservoir. The operative technique is straightforward and has been successful in many different hands (Mollard et al., 1983; Monfort et al., 1984).

Table 50-7 (Borzi et al., 1992; Duckett and Lotfi, 1993; Dykes et al., 1991; Sheldon and Gilbert, 1992;

Sumfest et al., 1993; Woodhouse et al., 1989) outlines the recent experience with various modifications of the Mitrofanoff principle. This experience encompasses 159 patients, of whom 98 (62%) had their neourethra constructed from appendix. Ureter was used in 42 (26%) and tapered ileum in 10 (6%). Also employed were tubes constructed of bladder, hind gut, stomach, vas deferens, and fallopian tube. Ninety-six percent of patients were reported as achieving ultimate continence. The most common complication was that of stomal stenosis, requiring stomal revision. Rarely encountered were Mitrofanoff neourethras that could not be negotiated or which were lost due to ischemic necrosis. The appendix was found to be the most reliable conduit for achieving continent catheterization access (Sumfest, 1993).

The Mitrofanoff neourethra concept has been proven to be extremely versatile. The neourethra has been implanted into bladder, colon, and stomach with equal efficiency (Elder, 1992; Sheldon and Gilbert, 1992). The flexibility of this technique is also exemplified by the ability to externalize the Mitrofanoff neourethra at either the anterior abdominal wall (Fig. 50-42), the umbilicus (Fig. 50-43), and the perineum (Fig. 50-44) as reviewed by Sheldon and Gilbert

TABLE 50-7

Source of Mitrofanoff Neurothra and Outcome in 159 Patients from Six Recent Large Series

Series	Woodhouse, 1989	Dykes, 1991	Sheldon, 1992	Borzi, 1992	Sumfest, 1993	Duckett, 1993	Total
Number of Cases	16	28	17	10	47	41	159
Appendix	5	19	14	9	26	25	98 (62%)
Ureter	10	8	2	—	11	11	42 (26%)
Tap. ileum	—	—	1	—	4	5	10 (6%)
Bladder	—	—	—	—	4	—	4
Hindgut	—	—	—	—	2	—	2
Gastric	—	—	—	1	—	—	1
Vas deferans	—	1	—	—	—	—	1
Fallopian tube	1	—	—	—	—	—	1
Continence	14	27	17	8	44	41	152 (96%)
Stenosis	3	4	2		9	3	21 (13%)

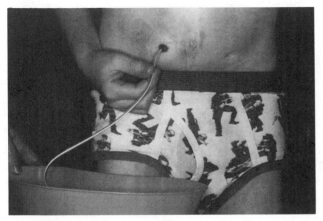

FIG. 50-42
Typical Mitrofanoff neourethra with catheter in position. (From Sheldon CA, Gilbert A: Use of the appendix for urethral reconstruction in children with congenital anomalies of the bladder. *Surgery* 1992; 112:805-812.)

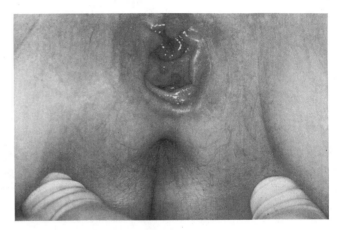

FIG. 50-44
Neourethra brought to perineum in orthotopic position. (From Sheldon CA, Gilbert A: Use of the appendix for urethral reconstruction in children with congenital anomalies of the bladder. *Surgery* 1992; 112:805-812.)

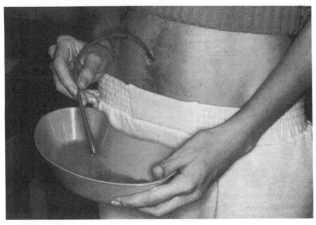

FIG. 50-43
Inconspicuous umbilical stoma is easily catheterized by patient. (From Sheldon CA, Gilbert A: Use of the appendix for urethral reconstruction in children with congenital anomalies of the bladder. *Surgery* 1992; 112:805-812.)

(1992). The versatility of this technique has been enhanced by the use of cecal tubularization to extend the length of the appendix (Cromie et al., 1991; Sheldon and Gilbert, 1992; Sumfest et al., 1993).

An important technical concept concerns the construction of an ureteral Mitrofanoff neourethra. When a segment of distal ureter associated with vesicoureteral reflux is employed to create a Mitrofanoff neourethra, antireflux (i.e., continence) of this catheterized ureter may be augmented when necessary by utilizing the technique of Hutch (1952) (Fig. 50-45) or Lich-Gregoir (Gregoir, 1964) (Fig. 50-46), all of which do not disturb the junction of the ureter with the trigone. This preserves ureteral vascularity while increasing the ureter's submucosed segment length (flap valve). Free segments of ureter, however, have been successfully used with the Mitrofanoff principle, maintaining a blood supply on a "ureteral mesentery" (Mitchell, 1988; Sheldon and Gilbert, 1992). Another important technical consideration is that of an inser-

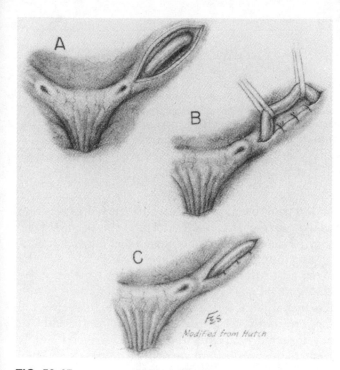

FIG. 50-45

Hutch ureteral reimplant. The distal ureter is left attached to the bladder muscle to preserve the ureteral blood supply. By transposing a segment of the ureter to the inner wall of the bladder, an effective flap valve is created. (From Politano VA: Management of vesicoureteral reflux. In Libertino JA, Zinman L (eds): *Reconstructive Urologic Surgery, Pediatric and Adult.* Baltimore, Williams & Wilkins, 1977, p 127. Used by permission.)

tion V or U skin flap when constructing the Mitrofanoff stoma. This can be used either to prevent or to treat stomal stenosis.

The important potential complication of reservoir rupture subsequent to noncompliance with catheterization of a watertight urinary reservoir has been experienced (Borzi et al., 1992). Patients and families must be strictly cautioned against this. This eventuality argues for the preservation of the native urethra as a "pop-off" mechanism rather than simply dividing the bladder outlet.

Technical modifications of the Mitrofanoff principle have included that of Keetch and co-authors (1993) in which the entire appendix is placed intravesically with only its tip exiting the bladder and then directly exiting the anterior abdominal wall. Borzi and Gough (1993) have reported the use of a pedicled gastric tube as a continent catheterizable neourethra. As previously discussed, Duckett and Snyder (1985) have extended this concept into the development of the "Penn pouch" (See Fig. 50-22). The Mainz pouch has recently been given a successful alternate continence mechanism that is similar to the Penn pouch except that the appendix is left attached to the cecum with its distal end brought out as the catheterizable stoma. The appendix is placed submucosally in the cecal wall as in a Lich-Gregoir ureteral implant to create an effective flap-valve continence mechanism.

A direct comparison of nipple valve and flap valve mechanism was made by Cumming and colleagues

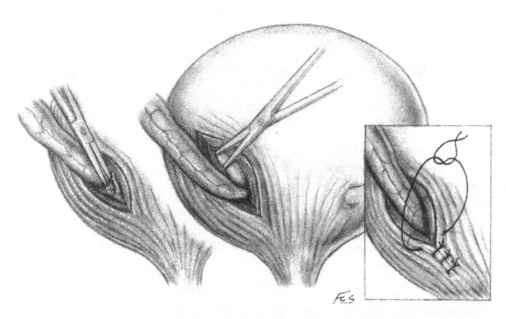

FIG. 50-46

Lich-Gregoir ureteral reimplant. Distal ureter left attached to bladder muscle as in Hutch reimplant. Extravesical dissection permits lengthening of submucosal course of ureter preventing reflux. Bladder muscle is closed behind ureter to support flap valve. (From Politano VA: Management of vesicoureteral reflux. In Libertino JA, Zinman L (eds): *Reconstructive Urologic Surgery, Pediatric and Adult.* Baltimore, Williams & Wilkins, 1977, p 130. Used by permission.)

TABLE 50-8

Lower Urinary Substitution (Bladder and Urethra)

Series	Number of Patients	Neourethra	Neobladder	Continence
Mundy, 1988	8	Labia (6)	Colon	5 (83%)
		Prepuce (2)	Colon	
Mitchell et al., 1988	4	Ureter (2)	Colon	7 (88%)
		Ureter (2)	Stomach	
Sheldon and Gilbert, 1992	2	Ureter (1)	Stomach	2 (100%)
		Appendix (1)	Stomach	

(1987). These authors compared six patients undergoing continent reconstruction employing the Koch technique with seven patients reconstructed employing the Mitrofanoff principle. Of the six patients undergoing nipple valve construction (Koch pouch), only two were completely continent, and 10 revisions were undertaken in four patients. Among seven patients with a flap valve (Mitrofanoff), six were completely continent of urine, and three revisions were required in two patients.

Total urethral replacement in the female and partial urethral replacement in the male is possible employing cutaneous tubularized pedicle grafts, ureter, and appendix extended with cecum (Mitchell et al., 1988; Mundy, 1989; Sheldon and Gilbert, 1992) employing a flap-valve principle. Replacement of the entire lower urinary tract with substitution of both bladder and urethra is now possible with success as outlined in Table 50-8 (Mitchell et al., 1988; Mundy, 1988; Sheldon and Gilbert, 1992).

COMPENSATING FOR INADEQUATE URETERAL LENGTH

In the reconstruction of the urinary tract, the method by which the upper urinary system is connected to the reservoir is of great importance. Because of the high number of patients who have had continent reconstruction requiring clean intermittent catheterization, the incidence of bactiuria is high. It seems wise, in children particularly, to protect the upper urinary tract by a nonrefluxing attachment of the ureter or ureteral substitute to the reservoir. When the ureter is short or abnormal, this can be challenging. It is the purpose of this section to review a number of the techniques that have been utilized to deal with this problem.

Nephropexy

Every effort must be taken to attach the upper urinary tract to the lower without tension. In the past, extensive mobilization of the kidney and ureter together to achieve a downward displacement was rarely undertaken because of fear that such mobilization would devascularize the ureter. Hendren (1978a) showed that by widely mobilizing the kidney and ureter as a unit, an additional several centimeters can be obtained in the infant or up to 2 to 3 inches in an older individual (Fig. 50-47). Essential to success with this technique is a meticulous dissection sweeping all the retroperitoneal tissues toward the ureter and kidney to avoid damaging the segmental blood supply going to the ureter. A plane of dissection is established immediately behind the mesentery of the colon. The dissection along the pelvic wall and iliac vessels is similar to that for a radical pelvic lymphadenectomy, skeletonizing those structures and maintaining all the retroperitoneal tissue with the ureter. The aorta and vena cava similarly are swept clean, displacing the tissue laterally with the ureter. This leaves the lateral gutter bare. The gonadal vessels may be divided distally and also kept with the ureter, helping to preserve a segmental blood supply. Next the kidney is mobilized laterally, superiorly, and posteriorly just as it would be for a radical nephrectomy. It maintains its attachments only through the renal hilus. Care is taken not to disturb the medial attachments at the hilus. With this extended mobilization, the kidney can then be displaced to some extent in virtually all cases. The lower pole of the kidney is sutured to the psoas muscle with nonabsorbable sutures as low as it may comfortably be placed without undue tension on the pedicle. As there is not a major amount of extra length achieved with this extensive surgery, it is appropriate to reserve this maneuver for those cases in which some of the techniques to be mentioned below have come up just short of being adequate, and a small amount of further ureteral length is all that is required to ensure a good result.

Transureteroureterostomy

One of the most useful techniques in urinary tract reconstruction is the transureteroureterostomy (TUU) (Fig. 50-48). Since the report by Hodges and colleagues (1963) was published, the technique has be-

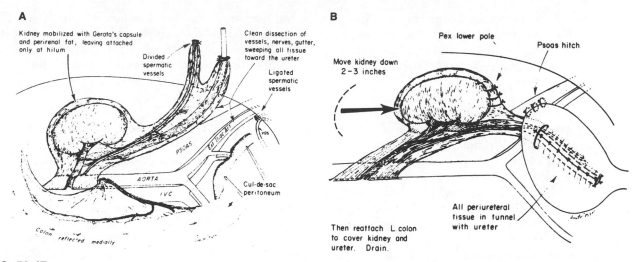

FIG. 50-47
Nephropexy—Hendren's technique. (From Hendren WH: Some alternatives to urinary diversion in children. *J Urol* 1978; 119:654. Used by permission.)

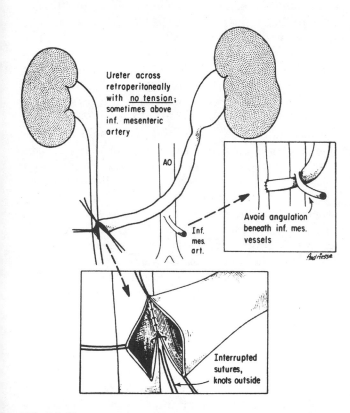

FIG. 50-48
Transureteroureterostomy. Meticulous attention to technical detail and avoidance of tension gives a high success rate. (From Hendren WH, Hensle TW: Transureteroureterostomy: Experience with 75 cases. *J Urol* 1980; 123:826. Used by permission.)

come increasingly popular. Although there have been some reports of complications with this technique (Ehrlich and Skinner, 1975; Sandoz et al., 1977), most reports have been overwhelmingly favorable (Halpern

et al., 1973; Hendren and Hensle, 1980; Hodges et al., 1980). In both adult and pediatric series, reported success rates have been more than 90%. In a review of these experiences several principles essential to the successful execution of a TUU have emerged. Wide exposure is essential and usually should be achieved transabdominally. Adequate mobilization of the donor ureter so that a tension-free anastomosis can be established is similarly important. Wide ureteral mobilization, including the gonadal vessels in some cases, permits the ureter to be brought to the opposite side without tension. If the ureter is too short to lie comfortably under the inferior mesenteric artery, then the ureter should be placed above this vessel. The anastomosis should be placed on the medial wall of the recipient ureter. Whenever possible, the recipient ureter should be left in situ without mobilization. This ensures a better blood supply to the area of the anastomosis. Spatulation of the donor ureter should ensure a generous anastomosis with the recipient ureter. Size discrepancy between the ureters is not a problem. If the donor ureter is larger than the recipient ureter, it simply is cut straight across. The length of incision in the recipient ureter can be varied as needed. Drainage is particularly critical to avoid extravasation of urine and subsequent fibrosis with wound contracture around the TUU. Urine has a remarkable ability to induce the formation of fibrous tissue (Peacock and Van Winkle, 1970). Accordingly, ureteral wounds from which urine has been diverted have considerably less fibrosis surrounding them. In a TUU either an internal stent to divert the urine from each kidney or a nephrostomy tube would appear advisable. Adequate local drainage is essential but is not as effective in avoiding fibrosis around the anastomosis as preventing urinary leakage in the first instance. Meticulous attention to technique clearly contributes to the achievement of this goal.

Hendren and Hensle (1980) also point out that a segment of intestine can be successfully used as a high form of pyelopyelostomy to effect drainage of a kidney with a totally lost ureter through its contralateral mate.

The usefulness of TUU lies primarily in letting one good ureter serve as effective drainage for two renal units. One good long reimplant with a TUU is better than two compromised reimplants. The vesicopsoas hitch, mentioned below, contributes to success in this endeavor. In general, the better ureter with the least dilation is the one that should be reimplanted into the bladder. Used in this way transureteroureterostomy can make a major contribution to successful nonrefluxing reconnection of the upper urinary tract to the bladder or to a urinary reservoir.

Psoas Hitch and Boari Flap

When the bladder is large and supple, it can contribute in a major way to successfully dealing with a short ureter. Even when a bladder is quite small and thick-walled, it can often be gently stretched and surgically reshaped to permit a ureteral reimplant to be performed. In general, it is more satisfactory to use up bladder in achieving a nonrefluxing uroepithelial-to-uroepithelial anastomosis than being concerned about the lack of bladder volume that could follow. Augmentation of the bladder effectively deals with the bladder problem without difficulty.

The immobilization of a portion of the bladder by suturing it upward against the psoas muscle above the iliac vessels was popularized in the late 1960s (Prout and Koontz, 1970; Turner-Warwick and Worth, 1969). This vesicopsoas hitch facilitates reimplantation of a shortened ureter and permits replacement of at least the distal third of the ureter without difficulty (Fig. 50-49). By permitting a longer submucosal tunnel, it may permit a successful ureteral reimplant with a dilated ureter, which would not be feasible in a bladder without this maneuver.

In performing a vesicopsoas hitch it is useful to open the bladder on the side away from the proposed hitch to permit more bladder to be stretched up toward the psoas muscle. To facilitate a permanent fixation of the bladder to the muscle, fat is cleared off the psoas and bladder wall to ensure good muscle-to-muscle apposition. Although absorbable sutures usually have been used, we prefer nonabsorbable sutures placed through a generous bite of the bladder wall but excluding the mucosa. After seeing where the bladder will lie comfortably against the psoas, it is generally easier to make the hiatus at this point and create the submucosal

tunnel before fixing the bladder into position. The surgeon can hold the stretched bladder up against the psoas, relieving tension, while the assistant ties down the three to five sutures usually used to hitch the bladder. With a little care there is no need to injure or entrap the genitofemoral nerve. The ureter is then drawn into its submucosal tunnel, taking care that there is no angulation or torsion at the hiatus. Although there is disagreement about the use of a ureteral stent to ensure renal drainage after this maneuver, it is our practice to usually employ a small feeding tube for this purpose.

The Boari flap is an extension of the concept of a vesicopsoas hitch. Although originally performed successfully by Casati and Boari (1894) in experimental dogs, the popularization of the use of a bladder flap for ureteral replacement is the result of the work of Ockerblad (1947). In this procedure a bladder flap is formed from the front wall of the bladder with its hinge at the lateral dome of the bladder, permitting the flap to be rotated upward toward the kidney. By combining this flap with a vesicopsoas hitch, a nearly complete replacement of the ureter can be performed. There is a report of an 18 cm distal ureteral replacement with this combination technique (Kelami et al., 1973). Essential to the success of this flap is the preservation of a good blood supply to the bladder muscle that constitutes it. The base of the flap should be wider than the apex, and following the principles of plastic surgery, it is best to maintain a length-to-diameter ratio of not greater than 2:3 to 2:1. Boxer and colleagues (1978) recommended a base with a width of at least 4 cm and an apex of at least 3 cm. It is wise to fix the length of this muscular flap posteriorly against the muscle of the gutter to maintain its position. After the attachment of the ureter it is tubularized as part of the bladder closure. An antirefluxing submucosal course for the ureter in the upper protion of the flap can be created as recommended by Gil-Vernet (1969).

Ureterocalycostomy

Although Neuwirk (1947) was probably the first to describe a ureterocalycostomy, pulling the ureter into the cortex, and suturing the ureter to the renal capsule, later experience showed that this approach lead to obstruction of the intrarenal ureteral segment because of fibrosis of the cortex. Jameson and colleagues (1957) recognized that amputation of enough of the lower pole cortex to permit the ureter to be safely joined to a tangential opening of the lower pole calyx was required for success (Fig. 50-50). Hawthorne and colleagues (1976) emphasized this along with spatulation of the ureter to create a maximum diameter patient anastomosis. A stent and nephrostomy tube are usually used.

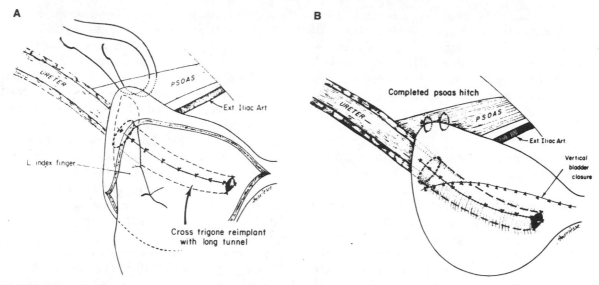

FIG. 50-49
Vesicopsoas hitch. Stretch of the bladder and fixation to psoas muscle permits a good reimplant of a short or dilated ureter. The Boari flap is an extension of this technique with a broad flap of detrusor hinged at the bladder dome. (From Hendren WH: Some alternatives to urinary diversion in children. *J Urol* 1978; 119:653. Used by permission.)

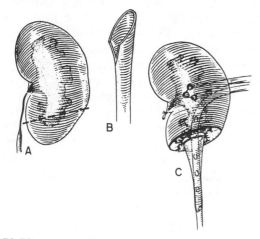

FIG. 50-50
Ureterocalycostomy. Essential to success with this useful technique is **(A)** amputation of lower pole cortex to widely expose lower pole calyx; **(B)** spatulated ureter for wide anastomosis; **(C)** good drainage, usually nephrostomy and stent. (From Hawthorne NJ, Zincke H, Kelalis PP: Ureterocalycostomy: An alternative to nephrectomy. *J Urol* 1976; 115:585. Used by permission.)

Although not as frequently used as some other techniques for dealing with a short ureter, a ureterocalycostomy can be particularly useful in the reoperative situation in which the pelvis and upper ureter have been destroyed secondary to previous surgery or trauma.

Renal Autotransplantation

The first successful renal autotransplants were performed for ureteral loss secondary to injury (Marshall et al., 1966); however, this is a relatively rare way of dealing with the short ureter. Stewart and colleagues (1977) reported an experience with eight ureters in six patients who underwent autotransplantation for benign ureteral disease. There was a 25% failure rate emphasizing the formidable nature of this surgery. Their experience also showed that when the renal hilus is badly scarred as part of advanced pyelonephritis, the dissection is likely to be difficult, with a lowered success rate. Diseased kidneys also appear to tolerate ischemia relatively poorly. Having raised these warnings, autotransplantation may be an ideal way to deal with certain isolated situations. Colodny (1980) performed an undiversion in a child with two short ureters by autotransplanting one kidney into the contralateral iliac fossa. This permitted the kidney in the renal fossa to have its ureter hooked to the upper end of the transplanted kidney's renal pelvis. The transplanted kidney's ureter was able to be attached in an antirefluxing fashion to the bladder.

A large, much more encouraging, series of autotransplantations was reported by Novick and colleagues (1990). These authors reported 108 patients who had undergone renal autotransplantation. This procedure was performed for renal artery disease (67 patients), ureteral defects (27 patients), and renal cell carcinoma involving bilateral or solitary kidneys (14 patients). Twenty-eight autotransplantations were performed in 27 patients for ureteral disease. Of these, 15 were reconstructed employing a ureteroneocystostomy. Eight received pyelovesicostomy, two ureteroureterostomy, two pyeloureterostomy, and one ureterosigmoidostomy. The success rate was 89%. Twenty-four patients are presently alive with a well-functioning autotransplant kidney, all of whom are normotensive and have stable renal function. One kidney never functioned following the procedure, and two were subsequently lost secondary to hemorrhage (one at 1 day and one at 12 days postoperatively).

Intubated Ureterotomy

The Davis intubated ureterotomy, first described in 1943, is now infrequently used. This procedure, which depends on secondary epithelialization from an incised ureter, however, can be effective and should be held in reserve for the rare situation in which it appears to be needed. Its greatest use might be for correcting strictures in the lumbar ureter when the defect is too great to bring the kidney down or the distal ureter up for a primary anastomosis and insufficient upper ureter is present for a direct transureteroureterostomy. As mentioned above, however, Hendren's small-bowel pyelopyelostomy or segmental intestinal interposition (discussed below) may be an attractive alternative to the more uncertain secondary healing that the intubated ureterotomy requires.

The technical aspects of an intubated ureterotomy remain little changed from the thorough description of Smart (1961). The strictured portion of the ureter should be adequately exposed while minimally disturbing it from its bed to preserve whatever local blood vessels are present. A ureterotomy from at least 1 cm above the stricture to 1 cm below must be performed meticulously. Proximal diversion must be established with a well-located nephrostomy tube. Failure of adequate proximal diversion is one of the common causes of failure with this procedure. Inadequate stenting is another source of failure. A stent that is of minimally reactive foreign material, such as Silastic, and of a size to fill the lumen of the normal ureter well above and below the intubated area is appropriate. It is critical that the stent not be so large as to induce ischemia in the normal ureter, or the cure will produce its own recurrent problem. Self-retaining catheters provide a good form of stent. The length of time for stenting is uncertain. Davis recommended 4 to 6 weeks. The internal Silastic stents may permit a longer period of stenting without previously seen complications. As indicated by the report of Ackermann and Frohmuller (1973), in which the authors achieved a 70% satisfactory result in 68 cases of ureteral intubation, this technique does have sufficient success to warrant holding it in the reconstructive urologist's armamentarium.

Free Grafts

Of all the free graft materials used in experimental ureteral replacement, only the bladder mucosal graft has shown much promise. Hovnanian and colleagues (1965) and Hovnanian and Kingsley (1966) were able to show in dogs that bladder mucosa formed around a stent and used to fill in a ureteral gap was capable of picking up blood supply from its bed and regenerating a uroepithelially lined tube, which surprisingly had evidence of muscular fibers supporting it as well. The biggest problem in their model was a lack of reliability. Their 29% failure rate from a variety of causes makes it difficult to advocate this for clinical use. Other researchers have had trials with parietal peritoneum (Esposti, 1956), stomach, small and large intestine (Tosatti, 1963), homologous and autologous freeze-dried ureteral segments (Harvard et al., 1961), and split-thickness skin grafts (Horton and Politano, 1955), all without significant success. Autogenous vein grafts (Rosenberg and Dahl, 1953) and homologous arteries (Sewell, 1955) have had no better success. For the present, free grafting appears to have little clinical applicability.

Pedicle Grafts

Experimental work with various pedicle grafts also has been frustrating, although perhaps with a glimmer of more hope than free grafts. Schein and colleagues (1956) used a pedicled appendix as a ureteral substitute and produced a viable graft. However, the experiment failed physiologically when the animal developed hydronephrosis. There have been isolated reports of success in the human with ureteral replacement with appendix, one with a 20-year follow-up (Martin, 1981; Wesolowski, 1981). Some authors have had limited success with full-thickness abdominal wall skin to form a tube for ureteral replacement (Keshin and Fitzpatrick, 1962). Greater success has been experienced correcting stenosis around the ureteropelvic junction by flaps constructed from the renal capsule (Thompson, 1977). Although this technique does not permit correction of ureteral defects much beyond the ureteropelvic junction, Kheradpir (1983) reported three cases in which a giant hydronephrosis associated with ureteropelvic junction obstruction was successfully reconstructed by forming a total ureteral replacement out of the redundant pelvic tissue. Thus there may be a use for an occasional autogenous pedicle graft repair in clinical practice.

Intestinal Ureter

Although earlier animal experimentation had been done, it was Shoemaker who was credited (Melnikoff, 1912) with replacement of the ureter in an 18-year-old woman who had a tubercular stricture in a two-stage procedure using the ileum. Although colon (Struthers and Scott, 1974) and jejunum (Golimbu and Morales, 1975) have been used for ureteral replacement, the principal intestinal segment used has been ileum. Swenson and colleagues (1956) reported early work in children. The Urology Service at The University of California in Los Angeles popularized the ileal ureter early (Goodwin et al., 1959; Moore et al., 1956) and continues to report a good experience (Boxer et al., 1979). Although the primary indication for ureteral replacement by intestine has been recurrent renal calculi, the second most common use of this technique has been in the treatment of damaged ureters, usually iatrogenic, that require replacement. In recent years there has been an increased use of small bowel as part of urinary reconstruction in children and young adults (Hendren, 1978b) (Fig. 50-51).

There have been a number of points that have emerged with experience with the ileal ureter that bear emphasis. Although it appears to make no difference whether the ileal ureter is placed intraperitoneally or extraperitoneally, it is critical that it be isoperistaltic. For replacement of the right ureter the mesentery of the ileum must be rotated 90 degrees. A widely spatulated anastomosis to the renal pelvis or lower pole infundibulum and a direct anastomosis to the back wall of the bladder near the trigone usually has been performed (Boxer et al., 1978). Approximately 25 cm of ileum is used, beginning at least 20 cm above the ileocecal valve. This length may be

shortened by using a vesicopsoas hitch. The bladder must be able to effectively empty. On review of the UCLA experience with children (Boxer et al., 1978), much of the low success with a refluxing ileal ureter in children (failure in six of 11) can be attributed to poor bladder emptying. The ability of the ileum to reabsorb urea and electrolytes may cause complications in the patient with significant renal failure, particularly if compounded by poor drainage of the system. In the UCLA experience hyperchloremic acidosis was generally not seen as long as the serum creatinine level before ileal ureter construction was less than 2 mg/dl. If intrahepatic disease limits urea metabolism, hyperammonemia can be a problem (McDermott, 1957). Middleton (1977) demonstrated that the absorption of urinary solutes is directly proportional to the surface area of the ileum exposed and the transit time. He has shown that tapering reduces the surface area significantly and thus theoretically should be advantageous in the creation of bowel ureters in patients in renal failure. Waters and colleagues (1981) and Vatandaslar and associates (1984a, 1984b) showed that tapering does not appear to significantly affect drainage. Tapering of the lower ureter appears to be important in achieving an antirefluxing anastomosis of the ileal ureter to the bladder (Hendren, 1978b).

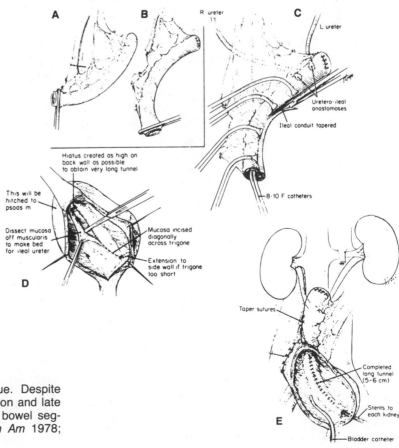

FIG. 50-51
Tapered intestinal ureter—Hendren's technique. Despite meticulous technique, persistent reflux is common and late strictures occur. (From Hendren WH: Tapered bowel segment for ureteral replacement. *Urol Clin North Am* 1978; 5:607.)

The issue of whether the bowel ureter should be attached to the bladder in an antirefluxing fashion has been much debated. In the adult reflux appears to be well tolerated. In the UCLA series (Boxer et al., 1978), of the 55 patients studied by cystogram, 40 experienced vesicoileal reflux, but 39 (97.5%) of the 40 had a good outcome. Experimental work in the dog (Vatandaslar et al., 1984a) would tend to support this experience. Ninety percent of the dogs had intermittent or persistently positive urine cultures but a good outcome. The issue of reflux with ileal ureters in children continues to be debated. Firlit and associates (1980) had a high incidence (six of seven) of reflux in children undergoing undiversion with ileal ureters. In their follow-up these patients did well, and Firlit questioned the need for an antirefluxing anastomosis. However, this group had little problem with urinary infection. Because positive urine cultures are so common in the reconstructed urinary tract requiring intermittent catheterization for effective emptying, a more aggressive attitude toward reflux prevention, as Hendren has always advocated, may be justified.

There are a number of technical points that have been emphasized (Hendren, 1978a) and that should be kept in mind during efforts to create an antirefluxing ileal ureter implantation into the bladder. A suitable bladder is critical. A contracted, fibrotic bladder is not suitable for implantation of an ileal ureter. In this circumstance, use of the ileocecal segment with dependence on the reinforced ileocecal valve for an antirefluxing mechanism is perhaps more likely to succeed. By tapering the ileal segment on its antimesenteric border by 30% to 40% and closing the taper in two layers with absorbable sutures, the diameter of the ileum can be reduced by approximately 50%. In the nondilated ileum this would give a diameter of approximately 1 cm. To achieve at least a 5:1 length-to-diameter ratio for an effective flap-valve mechanism, a bowel reimplant that is 5 to 8 cm long is appropriate. To achieve this Hendren recommends the routine use of the vesicopsoas hitch. The reimplanted ileal ureter can be stretched completely across the bladder and up the far side wall, if necessary. The use of the vesicopsoas hitch not only permits a longer submucosal tunnel but also fixes the new hiatus, helping to avoid angulation and kinking with bladder filling. Even if all these points are meticulously followed, success is not universal. In Hendren's experience there is a 25% reflux rate after ileal ureter tapering and implanting into the bladder (Hendren, 1978b). Others have had a similar experience, both in adults (Heaney et al., 1980) and children (Firlit et al., 1980).

Bajany and colleagues (1991) reviewed 29 patients who had undergone ileal segment reconstructions. Of these, nine patients received ileal sleeves and the remaining 20 either partial or total ileal replacement of the ureter. Of these, 15 (75%) have demonstrated stable renal function on long-term follow-up. Electrolyte abnormalities and acidosis were encountered only in patients with renal insufficiency. Of particular note was the incidence of reflux. These authors demonstrated a very successful antireflux reconstruction employing the Le Duc technique for which the incidence of reflux was only 17%. In contrast, 12 patients reconstructed with an intravesical nipple and four patients reconstructed with an ileocecal intussusception experienced a 50% incidence of reflux.

An additional complication that is emerging with the use of ileal ureters is the late development of a ureteral stricture. Hendren and McLorie (1983) reported five cases, one as long as 20 years after ileal ureter construction. Tapper and Folkman (1976) showed that bowel exposed to urine develops lymphocyte depletion, and it is postulated that this may lead to transmural bacterial invasion with episodes of bacteriuria, which in turn produces an inflammatory response leading to a late stricture. This is presumably the same mechanism that is seen in the late strictures that occur with ileal conduits. Perhaps the problem could be avoided if urine sterility could be maintained consistently, but this is difficult to achieve in the reconstructed urinary tract that is often subject to emptying by clean intermittent catheterization.

Greater success with bowel ureters may be achieved if they are not required to be anastomosed to the bladder. Casale and associates (1985), in performing undiversion, and Lytton and Schiff (1981), in dealing with ureteral injury, have had success with the interposition of a bowel segment to bridge a ureteral gap. The bowel segments were not tapered and did appear to drain well. Neither group has reported problems with mucous production, infection, calculi, or upper tract deterioration. Although follow-up in these series is limited, this may be a promising technique when there is a useful distal ureteral segment that cannot be joined to the upper urinary tract by the means covered earlier.

In situations in which the use of a bowel ureter would necessitate a tapered ileal ureter implantation into the bladder, the problems of persistent reflux and late strictures would make the bowel ureter a less attractive reconstructive option. Uroepithelial-to-uroepithelial anastomosis is generally preferable, even if this requires the use of most of the bladder to create a satisfactory antirefluxing anastomosis of the upper urinary tract to the bladder. Bladder capacity can be augmented by intestinocystoplasty.

OPTIMIZING ANORECTAL FUNCTION

The management of anorectal function imbalance is commonly underaddressed in the pediatric popula-

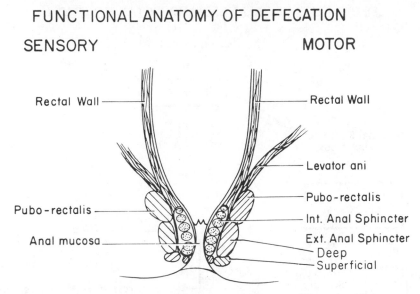

FUNCTIONAL ANATOMY OF DEFECATION

SENSORY **MOTOR**

FIG. 50-52
Main anatomical mechanism responsible for fecal continence. (From Leape LL: Other disorders of the rectum and anus. In Welsh KJ, Randolph JG, Ravitch MM, et al (eds.): *Pediatric Surgery.* 4th ed, Yearbook Medical Publishers, 1986, p 1039.)

tion. This area has tremendous significance for the reconstructive pediatric urologist and has been reviewed from a surgical perspective (Leape, 1986). Failure to address deficiencies in anorectal function may result in failure of urinary reconstruction both from the perspective of complications within the urinary tract but also because of the fact that the achievement of urinary continence is hardly a significant improvement in the patient's life if he or she continues to be incontinent of stool.

Coexistent anorectal and urinary tract disease is common and accounts for a large percentage of patients who require major urinary reconstruction. Examples include patients with myelomeningocele, sacral agenesis, other spinal abnormalities, Vater's complex (Sheldon et al., 1994a), and behavioral abnormalities such as encopresis and constipation, which is often associated with children with infrequent voiding as well as volitional or nonvolitional dyssynergia.

Alteration in function of either the gastrointestinal tract or the genitourinary tract may profoundly influence the function of the other. Fecal retention may interfere with bladder emptying, and fecal soilage may result in urinary tract infection. Additionally, patients with persistent fecal soilage may have little incentive to work on their urinary tract regimen to achieve continence of urine.

Further, treatment of one system may adversely affect function of the other system. For example, the use of Ditropan to diminish detrusor activity commonly causes constipation. Conversely, the use of Cisapride to treat hypomotility disorders of the intestinal tract may result in excessive detrusor activity and its

sequellae (Carone et al., 1993). As previously discussed, resection of the ileum or resection of the ileocecal valve for purposes of urinary reconstruction may result in significant dysfunction of the gastrointestinal tract.

There are several important components of balanced anorectal function. Figure 50-52 demonstrates the predominant anatomic mechanisms responsible for fecal continence. Demonstrated is the internal and sphincter, which is smooth muscle in composition, is normally in a state of near-maximum tonic contraction, relaxes reflexually in response to rectal distension, and is not under voluntary control. The striated sphincter complex consists of the puborectalis and the components of the external anal sphincter, all of which are under volitional control. These structures serve to achieve anorectal continence by concentric synergic contraction as well as anterior angulation. The puborectalis exists in a state of tonic contraction and undergoes reflex-increased contraction in the face of increasing intraabdominal pressure to prevent stress incontinence. The external sphincter contracts reflexly in response to stimulation of the anal mucosa as well as to increased abdominal pressure and rectal distention. Of critical importance is the anal mucosa, which is densely intervated and is extremely sensitive to tactile sensation.

Figure 50-53 outlines the normal physiologic events ensuring fecal continence. Colonic motility results in filling of the rectum and is sensed by the patient as a predefecation urge. Filling of the rectum reflexually results in relaxation of the internal sphincter. As a result of this relaxation, stool enters the anal canal,

COMPONENTS OF BALANCED ANORECTAL FUNCTION

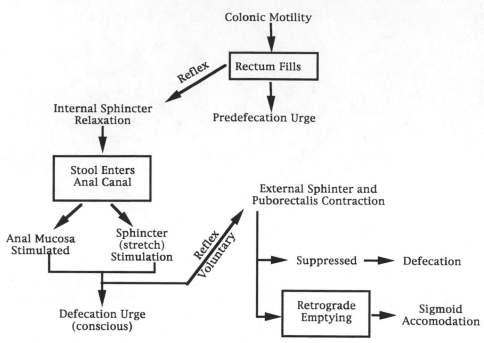

FIG. 50-53
Interaction of components of balanced anorectal function. (See text.)

TABLE 50-9

Functional Classification of Anorectal Disorders

	Fecal Retention	Fecal Soilage
Anatomic	Stricture Stenosis	Overflow incontinence Injured/congenitally deficient sphicter
Neuropathic	High pressure anal canal Hirschprung's disease	Overflow incontinence Low pressure anal canal
Behavioral	Constipation	Encopresis
Constitutional	Constipation	Diarrhea

resulting in stimulation of the anal mucosa and stretch of the striated sphincteric mechanism. These two events in combination provide the patient with an exquisite urge for defecation. In response to reflexive stimuli as well as voluntary control, the striated sphincteric mechanism undergoes increasing contraction. Should the patient suppress this contraction, defecation will follow. When defecation is not desired, striated sphincteric contraction results in retrograde emptying of the anal canal, which is facilitated by reflex accommodation of sigmoid capacity. Alteration in any of these mechanisms may result in anorectal dysfunction sufficient to complicate the management of children requiring genitourinary reconstruction.

Table 50-9 provides a functional classification of the most common types of anorectal dysfunction pertinent to the management of urinary tract pathology. Anorectal dysfunction resulting in both retention as well as fecal soilage may be due to anatomic, neuropathic, behavioral, and constitutional etiologies. Commonly a combination of etiologies coexist.

The evaluation of patients with anorectal dysfunction is primarily performed through a careful history of defecation and treatment of defecation disorders as well as a physical examination including rectal examination to estimate caliber and tone. In selected instances a barium enema or defecography as well as anal manometric analysis may be necessary. In the evaluation of the anal sphincter electromyogram, one must be cognizant of the fact that significant functional disassociation between the anorectal striated sphincter function and the urinary striated sphincter function has been demonstrated for a number of neurologic disorders including spina bifida (Nordling and Mayhoff, 1979).

Nonoperative management, if appropriately applied, is capable of controlling anorectal dysfunction in the majority of children. Management is directed at the control of constipation, diarrhea, colonic decompensation, and fecal soilage.

Constipation is generally readily controlled through a combination of dietary influences (Table 50-10) and the administration of selective laxatives or cathartics (Table 50-11). Diarrhea is rarely problematic in children requiring urinary reconstruction, unless it is antibiotic-induced, related to short-gut physiology, or bypass diarrhea secondary to impaction.

Decompensated bowel is a common problem encountered within this population. Chronic fecal retention results in progressive colonic decompensation presenting as constipation, bypass diarrhea, and encopresis. The goal is to achieve recovery of motor and sensory function and painfree defecation to encourage patient compliance. Treatment has three components: (1) evacuation of retained feces, (2) softening of the stool consistency, and (3) bowel training.

Evacuation may be achieved by manual extraction and by the administration of enemas. Generally large-volume retention enemas administered in the knee-chest position will be necessary to evacuate the colons in such children. In infants saline solution enemas are preferred and in older children soap suds enemas (1 to 2 quarts), milk and molasses enemas (4 oz of molasses in 1 qt of milk), and mineral oil enemas (60 to 90 ml) may be administered.

Once evacuation has been achieved, stool softening is obtained through dietary measures to loosen and bulk the stool. Bran, colace, and milk of magnesia are all effective in this regard. The goal is a soft stool. The dosage of these medications are not altered to attempt to achieve any specific stool frequency.

Bowel training, usually requiring several months of therapy, is then undertaken. This therapy involves primarily behavior modification; however, biofeedback techniques have been employed by a number of investigators. Data would suggest, however, that behavior modification has the dominant influence (Whitehead et al., 1986). A program of daily timed defecation planned to occur 20 to 30 minutes after a meal (usually the evening meal) is employed to take advantage of the gastrocolic reflex. The patient attempts for several minutes to defecate, and if unsuccessful, is assisted by digital stimulation, the administration of a glycerin suppository, or occasionally the

TABLE 50-10

Examples of Dietary Influences on Stool Consistency

Loosen Stool	Firm Stool	Bulk Stool
Juices (except apple)	Refined bread	Whole grain bread
	Crackers	Bran, popcorn
Sugar: Punch, lemonade, candy, popsicles	Skim milk, yogurt	Nuts, seeds
	Poached eggs	Prunes, figs, dates
	Apples, bananas	Fruit pulp
Water	White rice, cream of rice	Beans, lentils, peas

administration of a Ducolax suppository. It is important that such suppositories be accurately placed so that they are not buried within the bulk of the stool but rather are positioned between the stool and the rectal wall.

Occasionally the administration of enemas at this time will also be useful. An expansion enema with either water or saline solution may help stimulate the anorectal reflex and irritative enemas such as hypertonic saline solution or Ducolax enemas may be given to further stimulate defecation. In refractory cases (especially early on in the course of bowel training) oral cathartics may be beneficial. Such compounds as Senekot or Ducolax may be administered 6 to 12 hours prior to the anticipated time of defecation to aid in this process.

Fecal soilage is particularly devastating to the child with voiding dysfunction. Perineal inflammation and colonization greatly facilitate the genesis of urinary tract infection and dysfunctional voiding pathology. Soilage due to overflow incontinence such as encopresis is managed as outlined for decompensated bowel, and in selected cases mineral oil may dramatically reduce the tendency for retentive pathology.

A particularly difficult problem, however, involves the management of fecal soilage associated with a low-pressure anal canal either of anatomic or neuropathic etiology, as is often seen with myelomeningocele or imperforate anus. Bulking agents and hydroscopic agents should be used to provide a soft stool that is sufficiently formed to maximize retention. Time defecation and expansion enemas to intermittently evacuate the colon can result in dramatic improvement in fecal continence even in this difficult population. Because of the lack of sufficient predictability, oral cathartics should be avoided.

Expansion enemas may be difficult due to the tendency of the enema material to leak around the catheter secondary to the loose, patulous anus. However, very effective enema continence catheters have been developed and proven effective (Liptak and Revell, 1992; Shandling and Gilmour, 1987). Through these catheters approximately 20 ml/kg of lukewarm tap water containing 1 tsp of table salt per 500 ml is ad-

TABLE 50-11

Examples of Laxatives and Cathartics

Class	Examples	How Supplied	Dosage
Emollients	Dioctyl sodium sulfosuccinate (Colace)	Capsules: 50 mg; 100 mg Liquid: 10 mg/ml Syrup: 4 mg/ml	<3 y.o.: 10-40 mg/day 3-6 y.o.: 20-60 6-12 y.o.: 40-120 >12 y.o.: 50-200
	Mineral oil	—	<5 y.o.: not recommended 5-11 y.o.: 5-15 ml q.d. ≥ 12 y.o.: 15-45 ml q.d.
Bulk formers	Bran	—	1 tbs/day adv. as needed
	Psyllium hydrophilic mucilloid (Metamucil)	—	1 tsp/day adv. as needed
Osmotic cathartics	Dark Karo syrup	—	Infant: 1/4-1/2 tsp in bottle b.i.d. to t.i.d.
	Magnesium hydroxide (Milk of Magnesia)	—	Child: 1/2-2 tbs/day
Stimulant cathartics	Bisacodyl (Ducolax)	5 mg tablet	3-11 y.o.: 1-2 tablets simple dose ≥12 y.o.: 2-3 tablets simple dose
		10 mg suppositories	<2 y.o.: 1/2 supp. simple dose 2-11 y.o.: 1/2-1 supp. simple dose ≥12 y.o.: 1 supp. simple dose
	Senna (Senokot)	Syrup	1 mo-1 yr: 1/4-1/2 tsp hs 1-5 yr: 1/2-1 tsp hs 5-15 yr: 1-2 tsp hs >15 yr: 2-3 tsp hs

ministered. Because early prototypes of these catheters were made of latex, they are unsuitable because chronic use may have led to latex allergy. New non-latex-containing catheters are now available and should be preferentially employed.

Operative management of anorectal function is occasionally necessary. Most often this involves re-operative surgery for imperforate anus or cloaca where magnetic resonance imaging of a persistently incontinent patient demonstrates that previous surgery did not result in positioning of the rectum within the striated sphincteric complex. Such patients may be dramatically improved by posterior sagittal anorectal reconstruction. Patients with retentive disease secondary to scarring or stricture from previous surgery may benefit from anoplasty. Additional available procedures, whose effectiveness is less well demonstrated, include the gracillis sling (Braudesky and Holschneider, 1976; Pickrel et al., 1959; Raffensperger, 1979) and free muscle transplant (Hakelius et al., 1978) for fecal incontinence and sphincterotomy or myectomy (Martelli et al., 1978; Shandling, 1969) for fecal retention.

A very important surgical development in the treatment of such complex patients has been the nonrefluxing appendicocecostomy, which allows the administration of an antegrade continence enema (ACE) (Malone et al., 1990). In this procedure a nonrefluxing anastomosis between the appendix and cecum is performed with the opposite end of the appendix exteriorized to the abdominal wall. Patients are managed with the administration of saline solution enemas through the appendicocecostomy in a manner similar to that used for expansion enemas with enema continence catheters. No fecal stomal leakage was noted, and dramatic improvement in anorectal competence was noted in each case.

Squire and colleagues (1993) reported 25 patients receiving the Malone continent cecostomy. One appendicocecostomy was abandoned due to severe stenosis. Three patients developed stomal stenosis responding to dilatation, and three additional patients experienced occasional difficult catheterization. The remaining 19 patients experienced no problem, and all 24 had markedly improved fecal continence.

We have used this technique and have also experienced dramatic improvements in anorectal function and secondary improvements in urinary tract function. Obviously the surgeon must strongly weigh the importance of this procedure against the need for a Mitrofanoff neourethra in patients with complex, coexistent anorectal and bladder anomalies requiring surgical intervention. We have, however, used tapered ileal segments for either a Mitrofanoff neourethra or a continence cecostomy.

REPLACEMENT OF INADEQUATE RENAL FUNCTION

Rational For Early Transplantation in Children

As previously reviewed (Ettenger, 1992; Harmon and Jabs, 1992; Sheldon, 1987), children in contrast to adults have very poor tolerance to the sequelae of uremia. Linear growth retardation is almost a universal complication of chronic renal failure in children. Implicated factors include metabolic acidosis, sodium deficiency, secondary hyperparathyroidism, vitamin D deficiency, calorie and protein malnutrition, hormonal disturbances, anemia, and uremia itself. As repoted by Sharer and Gilli (1984), approximately 30% to 40% of children are below the third percentile for height before the onset of dialysis. Growth velocity below the third percentile is seen in almost 70% of children on hemodialysis. Further prepubertal children on dialysis for more than 1 year have mean height loss of approximately 0.4 standard deviations per year with one third losing more than 0.5 standard deviations per year. After 5 or more years on dialysis, prepubertal children lose an average of 2.4 standard deviations in height compared with 0.4 standard deviations following transplantation.

Dramatic improvements in this linear growth have been seen with emphasis directed at nutritional support and the correction of acidosis, anemia, and electrolyte abnormalities. Most important, the administration of growth hormone has proven very beneficial. Despite these advances, the most advantageous event in maximizing growth in children with chronic renal failure is transplantation. A recent review by NAPRTCS revealed that the most positive effect of transplantation occurs in children younger than 2 years of age. Significant catch-up growth was possible in children younger than 6 years of age and was much less common in older individuals (Tejani, 1993).

Chronic renal failure also has a major impact on neurologic development. This subject has been recently reviewed by Hobbs and Sexson (1993). Although studies assessing the impact of chronic renal failure on ultimate intellectual compacity are extremely difficult to interpret, several pertinent observations have been made. The brain is most vulnerable during the first 2 years of life. This is demonstrated by the profound effect of malnutrition in infancy, which is associated with both a diminished head circumference and diminished ultimate intellectual performance.

Rotundo and colleagues (1982) reviewed 23 patients with end-stage renal disease developing in the first year of life. Ninety-five percent of patients demonstrated developmental delay with hypotonia, seizure activity, and dyskinesia noted in 65%, 65%, and 55%, respectively. McGraw (1983) reviewed 12 children with end-stage renal disease presenting in infancy. Although the head circumference was normal at birth in these infants, this parameter was more than two standard deviations below mean in 75% of patients and more than three standard deviations below mean in 50% of patients by age 1 year.

Recent data suggest that renal transplantation in infancy has a potentially dramatic impact on ultimate neurologic development. So and co-authors (1984) reviewed 16 infants who underwent renal transplantation between 6 and 11 months of age. Patients were followed by 2 to 7.5 years, and a mean increase in head circumference of 2.2 standard deviations was noted. Also documented was excellent recovery of mental and motor development. These findings are consistent with those of Polinsky (1987), who reported developmental delay in 85% of children on long-term dialysis as opposed to 31% of those with a functioning allograft.

Outcome analysis unquestionably supports the positive impact of pediatric renal transplantation. Renal transplantation remains the preferred modality of therapy for childhood end-stage renal disease. Patient survival has proven to be excellent with a 2-year survival rate of 95% for living-related donor recipients and 92% for cadaveric recipients (McEnery, 1992). A 15-year patient survival rate of 81% has been reported by Kim (1991). This contrasts favorably with adult survival data ranging between 27% to 67% at 10 years (Mahony, 1986).

Graft survival, however, has generally been reported lower than that of adult counterparts (Cecka, 1991). More recent data suggest more comparable allograft survival with 88% of living-related donor grafts and 71% of cadaveric grafts functioning at 1 year (Alexander, 1990).

Rehabilitation of pediatric transplant recipients has been excellent (Offner, 1988; Potter, 1991). Ninety-six percent of children with a functioning renal allograft are capable of attending school. Adult recipients, undergoing transplant during childhood, are capable of full-time employment in 70% to 84%. Approximately one half of such individuals are married, and one fourth have children.

Perhaps the greatest impairment to the development of pediatric renal transplantation has been the reluctance to recognize that pediatric renal tansplantation is significantly different than transplantation in adults (Ettenger, 1992; Harmon and Jabs, 1992). Important and unique considerations in childhood renal transplantation include the urgency of transplantation with respect to maximizing growth and neurologic development. Additionally, the primary disease causing end-stage renal disease is considerably different and has a profound impact on patient management and prognosis. Choice of donor also has a critical impact. A review by the North American Pediatric Renal Transplant Cooperative Study (NAPRTCS) reveals that 43% of pediatric transplantations come from a living-related donor source (McEnery, 1992). This important allograft source has proven to be particularly valuable in the very young, in whom outcome with living-related donor grafts is clearly superior to that with cadaveric grafts (Briscoe, 1992; Ehrich, 1992; Ismail-Allouch, 1993; Najarian, 1991).

Another important consideration with respect to donor choice is the increased adverse effect of early ATN on ultimate graft survival in children as compared with adults (Ettenger, 1992). Another important component to the lower graft survival seen in some pediatric series appears to be related to a preferential distribution of kidneys from young donors to pediatric recipients. Recent data demonstrate that kidneys from donors less than 5 years of age and especially those from donors less than 2 years of age are associated with an inferior prognosis (Alexander, 1991; Harmon, 1992).

Additional important differences include cyclosporin metabolism and absorption, which make dosing more difficult, an increase propensity for graft thrombosis, and high immunologic responsivity increasing rejection risk. Of great concern is the risk of noncompliance, which has been particularly problematic in the adolescent population.

Of particular importance is the unique nature of primary disease in the pediatric end-stage renal disease population. The NAPRTCS report reviewing 1550 children receiving 1667 renal allografts found that 42% of patients had end-stage renal disease secondary to congenital malformations and 12% due to focal segmental glomerular sclerosis (McEnery, 1992). Focal segmental glomerulosclerosis has a strong propensity for graft recurrence. Allograft failure secondary to recurrent disease is reported in 7% of pediatric transplants (McEnery, 1992) as opposed to 2% in adult series (Mathew, 1988).

Congenital urologic disease is reported to occur in 20% to 30% of pediatric patients with end-stage renal disease (Burns, 1992; Churchill, 1988; Kabler, 1983; McEnery, 1992). The NAPRTCS review reported an incidence of obstructive uropathy of 16% with patients younger than 5 years of age having an incidence of obstructive uropathy exceeding 20% (McEnery, 1992). Churchill (1988), in a review of 300 cadaveric pediatric renal transplants, found the incidence of reflux nephropathy to be 20%. The presence of vesicoureteral reflux itself and most important, the often associated dysfunctional voiding pattern (with high bladder pressures or poor emptying), has significant implications with respect to transplantation in children. These problems must be corrected before successful transplantation can be anticipated (see the following text).

Consequences of Urologic Disease on Transplantation

That the presence of congenital urologic disease may have on adverse influence on the success of renal transplantation is demonstrated by the increased risk of urinary tract infection, allograft dysfunction, technical complications, and graft loss experienced in such patients.

Urinary tract infection can be particularly deleterious to both graft and recipient in the face of immunosuppression. The risk of urinary tract infection is potentiated in transplant recipients who have posterior urethral valves as the etiology of their renal failure. Mochon (1992) reported an infection risk of one in 30 patient months in valve recipients as contrasted to one in 216 patient months in controls. Similarly, Groenewegen (1993) reported an incidence of urinary tract infection of 55% in valve recipients as opposed to 24% in controls. An analagous problem is seen in patients whose primary disease is vesicoureteral reflux and who continue to have reflux into the native kidneys at the time of transplantation. The incidence of acute symptomatic urinary tract infection in this population is 43% as contrasted to 18% in controls (Bouchot, 1991).

A definite tendency for progressive allograft dysfunction over time is seen in posterior urethral valve patients when compared with controls, implying a deleterious effect of chronic elevated intravesical pressure similar to that described earlier in this chapter for native kidneys (Bryant, 1991; Cairns, 1991; Reinberg, 1988). Groenewegen (1993) reported a risk of urinary extravasation of 15% in posterior urethral valve patients as compared with 4% in controls, suggesting another adverse effect of elevated intravesical pressure. Also seen more commonly in valve patients was ureterovesical junction obstruction and urinary fistula, although these differences did not reach statistical significance.

These data demonstrate that patients with a history of significant urologic disease must be extensively evaluated prior to transplantation, vesicoureteral reflux resolved by either ureteral reimplantation or nephrectomy, and elevated intravesical pressure stabilized by either pharmacologic measures or, when necessary, augmentation cystoplasty. Complete low-pressure bladder emptying must be ensured prior to transplantation.

The surgical transplant evaluation of the child has previously been summarized (Sheldon et al., 1992). Prior to undertaking transplantation, the surgeon must document that the bladder is sufficiently compliant to prevent deterioration of the allograft, that there is adequate capacity to allow for social continence with acceptable urinary frequency, and that the bladder outlet is sufficiently competent to allow continence of urine. Adequate bladder emptying by either spontaneous voiding or intermittent catheterization must be documented, and compliance with bladder management should be demonstrated prior to transplantation. This is especially true if intermittent catheterization will be necessary.

All patients undergo a detailed surgical screening

beginning with a history and physical examination, assessment of blood pressure, urine culture, and measurement of 24-hour urine output and protein excretion. A renal ultrasound and contrast voiding cystourethrogram are obtained in each case. Selected patients will then undergo urodynamic investigation including uroflometry-electromyography, cystometrography, and urethral pressure profilometry. This is indicated in any patient who has a history of voiding symptoms or who has undergone prior treatment for known urologic disease.

A therapeutic trial should be provided for children who have dysfunctional bladders demonstrated preoperatively. Most patients can be stabilized with a combination of anticholinergics and/or intermittent catheterization. Those who fail to be stabilized and meet the previously outlined goals are considered for surgical reconstruction of their bladder.

Those patients who present with a defunctionalized bladder are the most difficult to evaluate. Those patients whose bladder is defunctionalized due to anuria or severe oliguria secondary to primary renal disease can be safely assumed to have an adequate bladder for purposes of transplantation. This is particularly true if the patient was free of any voiding symptoms prior to the loss of his or her urine production.

In the case where a bladder is defunctionalized due to previous urinary diversion, one must assume primary bladder dysfunction. If urodynamically the bladder is demonstrated to be sufficiently compliant and the bladder outlet to be sufficiently competent, one may proceed directly with transplantation. When this is not the case, we prefer to perform urinary undiversion before transplantation to refunctionalize the bladder. This has proven to be safe and well tolerated (Gonzalez et al., 1984). In this study 13 patients with chronic renal failure underwent urinary undiversion. In no instance was renal function significantly further impaired, and in no case did surgery itself precipitate the need for dialysis or transplantation earlier than anticipated by the natural history of the disease.

Such undiversion allows assessment of urinary continence and allows bladder function to be stabilized pharmacologically and, if necessary, by intermittent catheterization. Should this be unsuccessful, bladder reconstruction is then undertaken.

In instances where the kidneys have been removed, it is not feasible to perform undiversion. If the bladder does not demonstrate adequate compliance characteristics, it is possible to undertake bladder cycling to see if exposure to filling will alow accommodation. This is generally done employing an intermittent catheterization regimen or a suprapubic catheter.

One unique aspect of pediatric renal transplantation is the relatively common need for pretransplant sur-gical intervention. In addition to the need for dialysis access in many instances, nephrectomy, ureteral reimplantation, urinary undiversion, and bladder augmentation are occasionally necessary as well. Rarely a neobladder creation, continent urinary diversion, or creation of an intestinal conduit will be necessary. When undertaking such pretransplant surgery, it is important to plan the surgical incision to minimize interference with current or anticipated peritoneal dialysis as well as subsequent transplantation itself. The best means for avoiding loss of access to the peritoneal cavity for purposes of dialysis is an extraperitoneal approach to the urinary tract, which can readily be attained for nephrectomy and ureteral reimplantation.

To minimize interference with subsequent transplantation, peritoneal dialysis catheters are placed such that the exit site is opposite the side of anticipated subsequent transplantation. Transverse upper abdominal incisions, which may divide the superior epigastric vessels, are specifically avoided. With a subsequent Gibson incision (especially if bilateral) the inferior epigastric vessels and lateral collateral blood supply may be compromised, resulting in poor wound healing.

Whenever possible, nephrectomy is avoided to allow production of urine output that maintains a functionalized bladder and facilitates dialysis therapy either before transplantation or after transplantation if the graft fails. Any endogenous erythropoietin production will be maintained and helps to avoid presensitization by frequent transfusions. In addition, the ureters are preserved, which may be necessary for subsequent transplant reconstruction should ureteral complication occur.

Indications for nephrectomy include the presence of recurrent urinary tract infections, urinary tract infection-prone upper tract anatomy, refractory hypertension, severe proteinuria, and severe polyuria. In these instances preservation of kidneys may complicate posttransplant therapy and compromise allograft outcome.

When necessary, nephrectomy is performed through lateral flank incisions or through dorsal lumbotomy incisions through which the peritoneal cavity is rarely, if ever, entered. Such procedures can be performed without interruption of peritoneal dialysis. In those instances where bilateral nephrectomy is felt necessary and preemptive (avoiding dialysis) transplantation desired, one may remove the kidney with the worst function first, and if the second kidney provides adequate function, dialysis can be avoided. At the time of transplantation the remaining kidney can be removed through the transplant incision.

Ureteral reimplantation may be necessary to correct vesicoureteral reflux or vesicoureteral obstruction. As previously outlined, these problems may predispose to urinary tract infections following transplantation. These procedures are justified if nephrectomy is not indicated due to hypertension, infection, polyuria, etc.

As noted previously, urinary undiversion, bladder augmentation, creation of a neobladder or creation of a conduit may be required. Should a conduit be necessary, a colon conduit is preferred to allow a nonrefluxing ureteral implantation.

Of particular importance is the timing of surgery for urethral obstruction. Surgeries (including transurethral procedures) for such pathology as valves and stricture should not be performed in the face of a defunctionalized bladder, as a dry urethra is prone to stricture in this setting. Whenever possible, such surgery is performed as part of undiversion. Endoscopic procedures such as fulguration of urethral valves or internal urethrotomy for stricture can also be performed at the time of transplantation to avoid this complication. In the setting of a severe urethral stricture requiring urethroplasty, we have preferred a staged approach unless urine flow can be established by undiversion. In this instance, a first-stage procedure is performed to allow free drainage of the urethra. The transplant is performed, and after the child is stable and on maintenance immunosuppression, the second stage of the urethroplasty can be undertaken.

The surgical techniques for pediatric transplantation represent simple variations of those used in adults. The physiologic disturbance created by such transplantation, however, is substantially different and requires careful attention.

After the induction of anesthesia, venous access is obtained to allow rapid transfusion and to allow central venous pressure monitoring and blood sampling. A Foley catheter is placed, and the bladder is filled to capacity with an antibiotic-containing saline solution under gravity-dependent flow. Particularly in the child with a reconstructed bladder, it is important to have access to the catheter to allow filling and deflation of the bladder to facilitate surgery.

The incision for transplantation varies with the status of the recipient and the size of the allograft. This incision must occasionally be modified because of the existence of previous incisions. If, for example, the patient underwent pretransplant nephrectomy through an upper abdominal transverse incision, the transplant incision should be altered so as to preserve caudal and lateral blood flow. In some instances this will necessitate a midline incision. In others a more lateral Gibson incision may be sufficient. In the normal circumstance, however, the transplant incision is performed as a hockey stick incision, coursing just lateral to the rectus abdominous superiorly and coarsing medially toward the rectus inferiorly to terminate approximately 1 cm superior to the pubis. Generally the rectus fascia is divided while the rectus muscle is retracted medially without division.

The retroperitoneum is entered, the inferior epigastric vessels are doubly ligated and divided (unless preservation is deemed necessary), and the spermatic cord in males is isolated and retracted free from injury. The retroperitoneal space is then developed by blunt dissection, reflecting the peritoneum medially with care directed at avoiding entry of the peritoneal cavity. Many children will be on peritoneal dialysis, and this modality can be used in the perioperative period to control fluid and electrolyte imbalances if graft dysfunction is encountered, unless the peritoneum is violated.

In children weighing more than 20 kg, the retroperitoneal space will generally accept an adult kidney with the vascular anastomosis performed at the level of the common iliac artery and vein. In some children who weigh 10 to 20 kg, the retroperitoneal space will accept a small adult kidney or child cadaver kidney retroperitoneally, with the vascular anastomoses usually performed directly to the distal aorta and the common iliac vein. In most patients who weigh less than 20 kg or in patients receiving concomitant bilateral nephrectomies, a mid-line transperitoneal technique may be useful (Fig. 50-54). The ascending colon is mobilized to allow anastomosis to the aorta and vena cava. Upon completion of the transplantation, fixation of the cecum and ascending colon over the kidney allows retroperitonealization of the allograft. Attention is directed at intentionally leaving the lower pole of the allograft exposed for subsequent needle biopsy.

An additional consideration in the face of significant patient-allograft size discrepancy is that of surgical mass reduction (Takahashi et al., 1993). This may be considered in those incidences where a small child has compromised cardiac reserve and may not tolerate placement of an adult kidney. It may also be considered when it may be particularly important to avoid a transperitoneal approach. This, for example, may be necessary to preserve peritoneal dialysis access but may be especially important in the child who has a ventricular peritoneal shunt.

Once exposure has been achieved by any of the previously mentioned routes, the appropriate vessels are mobilized with strict attention directed at sequential ligation of the lymphatic vessels as they course over the arteries and veins. Proximal and distal vascular control is achieved with vessel loops or vascular clamps. The kidney, which has been submerged in ice saline solution, is flushed with cold preservation solution, and any necessary vascular reconstruction is undertaken while the kidney is on ice. The kidney is brought to the operative field to confirm adequate retroperitoneal volume for placement of the kidney and to determine at what point along the aorta, vena

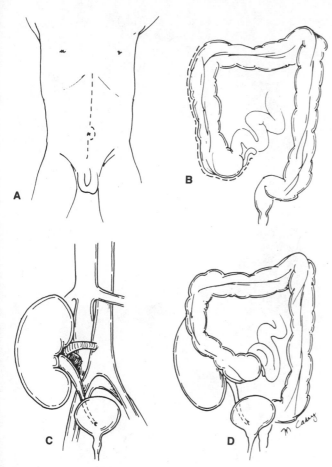

FIG. 50-54
Surgical approach to renal transplantation in the infant. (From Sheldon CA, Najarian JS, Mauer MS: Surg Clin North Am 1985; 65:1589-1621.)

cava, or iliac vessels the donor renal vessels can be anastomosed without kinking or tension. The vascular anastomosis is often more difficult in children secondary to the small size of the recipient vessels. One generally attempts to attain as high as of an anastomosis as possible (aorta, vena cava, proximal common iliac vessels) to technically facilitate the anastomosis but also to help maximize available blood flow to the allograft.

It is important to recognize that patients who require urologic surgery for a dysfunctional bladder may provide an additional challenge from the perspective of their vascular anastomoses. This is especially true in the instance of Vater's Syndrome, where anomalous retroperitoneal vessels may be encountered, and in the case of neurovesical dysfunction, where very small retroperitoneal vessels may be encountered (Forsyth et al., 1990).

The kidney is resubmerged in ice saline solution while any necessary adjustments in exposure are made. The vascular anastomoses are made in donor-

spatulated end-to-recipient side fashion with simple running 6-0 prolene sutures. The recipient vessels are thoroughly irrigated with heparinized saline solution and trimmed free of loose adventitia before anastomosis. Cadaveric kidneys harvested from young donors are implanted with the use of the aortic and caval cuffs to facilitate anastomosis and avoid luminal compromise. Optical magnification facilitates the accuracy of anastomosis. In those cases where the aorta is cross-clamped, systemic heparinization is undertaken prior to this event.

The unclamping of the recipient vessels and onset of renal allograft flow set the stage for the first major physiologic disturbance. For example, an adult kidney that may acutely sequester a blood volume of 250 to 300 ml, when placed in a small child (estimated blood volume 80 ml/kg) will drain a substantial portion of blood volume and cardiac output. The prevention of severe hypotension, ischemic injury to the kidney, and even vascular thrombosis of the allograft is a coordinated effort between the surgeon and anesthesiologist. As the anastomoses are completed, the patient is volume-loaded to a central venous pressure of 12 to 16 cm H_2O. In addition, if aortic and caval occlusion has been used, one mEq/kg of sodium bicarbonate is administered. During the performance of the anastomosis, lasix (0.5 mg/kg) and mannitol (0.5 g/kg) are administered. The vascular loops or clamps are released, and finger compression is temporarily maintained over the renal artery to prevent renal embolization as well as to prevent a sudden massive drain-off of cardiac output. In the very small recipient, renal arterial flow is progressively established by release of this compression as tolerated by the patient's vital signs. In children weighing less than 10 kg, the average and maximal fall in central venous pressure is approximately 4 and 7 cm H_2O, respectively (Miller et al., 1983). Resumption of adequate peripheral tissue perfusion is most conveniently documented by measuring central venous pressure as well as venous oxygen tension and saturation (blood drawn from the central venous line).

The ureteroneocystostomy is then performed similar to that performed in the adult. The difference here is that the length of the suburothelial tunnel required to ensure no reflux (between 4 to 5 times the ureteral diameter) may be difficult to achieve a small-capacity pediatric bladder. The ureter may be implanted into the bladder with a variety of techniques. Traditionally, a transvesical procedure has been used. In the setting of a relatively normal bladder (normal capacity, not massively trabeculated, no thickened or reactive mucosa), we prefer to use an extravesical ureteral implantation technique. This avoids the need for a midline cystostomy (the most common site of urinary extravasation) and minimizes postoperative hematuria and the risk of clot retention, which is a particularly important consideration in the very young recipient whose urethral catheter is of very small diameter. The extravesical implantation can be performed employing a longitudinal incision as demonstrated in Figure 50-55 (Wasnick et al., 1981) or a two-incision technique shown in Figure 50-56 (Mesrobian et al., 1992).

An additional consideration is that of ureteral stenting. We advocate stenting in the setting of prior bladder reconstruction. Routine stenting in pediatric transplantation, however, offers several potential advantages as well. Bergmeijer and associates (1990) reported a series of 36 children ranging in age from 2 to 18 years. Eighteen patients underwent a stented allograft implantation, and 18 underwent a nonstented implantation. Both groups were similar in age and sex ratios. The nonstented group experienced six severe urologic complications. These included extravasation (two cases), obstruction (three cases), and one case with both extravasation and obstruction. Two allografts were lost directly as a consequence of these complications. In contrast, only one patient in the stented group experienced a urologic complication, and this was a late ureterovesical junction stenosis that required surgical revision.

Although this complication rate in patients without stents seems unusually high, it does support our contention that more subtle changes at the ureterovesical junction in the absence of stenting may complicate the patient's course. Early graft dysfunction due to anastomotic edema may be confused with early rejection and result in an unnecessary renal biopsy or unnecessary alterations in immunosuppressive therapy. Additionally, we postulate that transient obstruction may contribute to the ischemic insult already experienced by the allograft due to acute tubular necrosis, which is usually present to some degree even with optimal cold preservation. The presence of any element of rejection or limitation in cardiovascular reserve, especially in the small child, may compound the resultant ischemia. Although these risks remain to be proven, we advocate the routine use of an indwelling double-J ureteral stent.

The ureteral anastomosis is performed with interrupted 5.0 or 6.0 absorbable suture material, and the wound is closed without drainage. We prefer a running prolene fascial closure reinforced with interrupted polyglycolate sutures to ensure a dry wound free from accumulating transudate (lymphatic fluid and peritoneal dialysis fluid), which may potentiate infection in the immunosuppressed patient.

Transplantation into Conduits

Patients who do not have a bladder available for transplantation may be transplanted into an intestinal conduit. This was first reported in 1966 by Kelley and

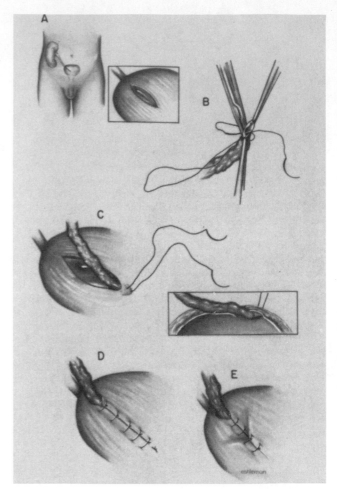

FIG. 50-55
Technique of anterior extravesical ureteroneocystostomy. (From Wasnick RJ, Butt KM, Laungani G, et al: Evaluation of anterior extravesical ureteroneocystomy in kidney transplantation. *J Urol* 1981; 126:307.)

colleagues. Glass and associates (1985) reviewed their cases and the literature and reported 68 cases of renal transplantation into intestinal conduits. Sixty-four were ileal conduits, whereas four were colon conduits. The majority of these patients were children. Thirty-four grafts were living-related donor, and 29 were cadaveric. The source of the allograft was unkown in five patients. The reported graft survival was 52% (35% for cadaveric and 70% for living related donor grafts). Thirty-two percent of patients experienced complications attributable to the urinary conduit. Eight patients experienced septic complications, none of which were fatal. Ureteral strictures or upper tract stones were encountered in five patients, and four patients developed pyelonephritis in their allograft. Six patients developed either stomal or intestinal complications. One patient developed florid metabolic acidosis.

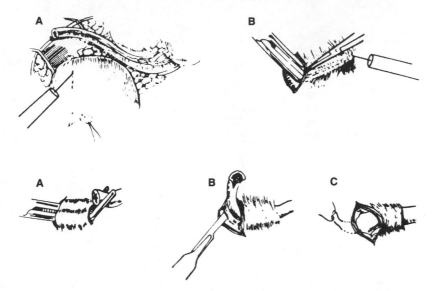

FIG. 50-56
Extravesical ureteral reimplantation. (From Mesrobian HG, et al: Modified extravesical ureteral reimplantation in pediatric renal transplantation: Five years of experience. *J Urol* 1992; 147:1340.)

Nguyen (1990) reported eight patients transplanted into conduits (seven ileal conduits and one colon conduit) along with two patients transplanted into enterocystoplasties. They compared the results of these transplantations with those of patients who had intestinal conduits but were transplanted into their native bladder. Although graft survival was not significantly different, the incidence of complications was dramatically different. No surgical complications occurred in the group transplanted into the native bladder. In contrast, those patients transplanted into conduits experienced extravasation (three cases) and ureteral stenosis, urolithiasis, sepsis, acidosis, and wound dehiscence (one case each).

Hatch (1991) summarized the data collected by the urologic society for transplantation and vascular surgery. He reported 55 renal transplants performed in 50 patients with intestinal conduits from 16 different centers. Sixteen patients were children, and 34 were adults. Patient survival was 92%, and the 2-year graft survival was 81% for cadaveric grafts and 79% for living-related donor grafts. Eleven (20%) transplanted procedures were associated with significant surgical complications. These included abscess (four cases), urinary extravasation (three cases), and stomal stenosis, wound dehiscence, small-bowel obstruction, and ureteropelvic junction obstruction (one case each).

Additionally, 23 (46%) patients experienced significant infectious complications, of which 10 (20%) involved pyelonephritis.

As a result of the available data it would appear that renal transplantation into intestinal conduits should be minimized. It is, however, acceptable in those instances where the bladder cannot be rehabilitated.

Transplantation into Reconstructed Bladders

Surgical reconstruction of a dysfunctional bladder has been demonstrated to allow transplantation with acceptable results. Such an approach allows optimal allograft preservation and appliance-free continence and is preferable to the alternative of transplantation into an intestinal conduit. Because many such patients will have difficulty with spontaneous voiding, the work of Barnett and colleagues (1985) demonstrating the safe and effective application of clean intermittent catheterization in transplant recipients was instrumental.

Table 50-12 summarizes 33 transplantations performed in 28 patients younger than the age of 21 years reported in the literature. Although these data are difficult to interpret due to variable lengths of follow-up, several observations seem particularly pertinent. The patient survival rate was 100%, and the overall allograft survival rate was 79%. Graft survival was identical for the 25 living-related donor grafts and the eight cadaveric grafts. Twenty-six (93%) of 28 of the patients had a functioning allograft at the time of report. Seven grafts were lost. No graft was lost to a technical complication or to an infectious complication. In each instance allograft loss was due to chronic rejection. Three (43%) of the seven grafts lost occurred in recipients younger than 10 years of age.

The incidence of graft loss due to chronic rejection may be somewhat higher than expected, especially in those patients undergoing more complex reconstructive surgery. It is interesting to speculate that the

TABLE 50-12

Renal Transplantation in Augmented Bladders

Series	Age (Years)	Diagnosis	Augment	Source	Follow-up (Mo)	Function	Cause of Graft Loss
Thomalla et al., 1989	14	EXSTR	ICC	LRD	—	Yes	—
	11	PUV	C	LRD	—	Yes	—
	14	PUV	C	LRD	—	Yes	—
	16	NVD	I	LRD	—	Yes	—
	16	PUV	IC	CAD	—	No	CHR REJ
Zaragoza et al., 1993	17	NVD	IC	LRD	92	Yes	—
	13	VUR	I	LRD	16	Yes	—
	13	NVD	IC	LRD/CAD	50	No/Yes	CHR REJ
	14	PUV	I	LRD	10	Yes	—
	10	PUV	I	LRD	8	Yes	—
	18	VUR	I	LRD/CAD	14	No/Yes	CHR REJ
	13	PUV	I	LRD	5	Yes	—
	12	PUV	I	CAD	25	Yes	—
Barnett et al., 1987	16	NVD	IC	LRD	46	Yes	—
	14	NVD	IC	LRD	34	Yes	—
	11	—	IC	LRD	19	Yes	—
Sheldon et al., 1994	2	PUV	G	CAD/CAD	30	No/Yes	CHR REJ
	8	UGS	G	LRD	22	Yes	—
	20	CL EXSTR	GN	LRD	24	Yes	—
	3	UGS	GN	LRD	19	Yes	—
	7	PUV	C	LRD/CAD	54	No/Yes	CHR REJ
	18	VATER	PU	LRD	35	No	—
	9	NVD	G	LRD	36	Yes	—
	10	PUV	G	CAD	24	Yes	—
	9	BSEU	G	LRD/LRD	27	No/Yes	CHR REJ
Sheldon, unpublished	12	CLOACA	G	LRD	5	Yes	—
	17	VATER	G	LRD	3	Yes	—
	9	PUV	G	LRD	3	Yes	—

Diagnoses: EXSTR, exstrophy; PUV, posterior urethral valves; NVD, neurovesicle dysfunction; VUR, vesicoureteral reflux; UGS, urogenital sinus; CLEXSTR, cloacal exstrophy; VATER, VATER's complex; BSEU, bilateral single extopic ureters; CLOACA, cloaca. *Sources:* LRD, living related donor; CAD, cadaveric. *Causes of graft loss:* CHRREJ, chronic rejection.

incorporation of a gastrointestinal segment into the urinary tract may alter the efficacy of immunosuppressive agents. Also possible would be a degree of presensitization (unrecognized by current immunosurveillance techniques) due to the administration of blood transfusion during previous reconstructive procedures.

That transplantation is applicable to even the most complicated children with end-stage renal failure is suggested by the data of Sheldon and colleagues (1994b). In this series seven (78%) patients were recipients younger than 10 years of age. Most required significant additional reconstructive surgery for continence or for bladder access. Six patients underwent creation of a Mitrofanoff neourethra, two underwent insertion of an artificial urinary sphincter, and four required intermittent catheterization. All patients were totally continent, and eight (89%) had a functioning allograft at the time of report.

Six of the 33 reported transplants into reconstructed bladders experienced a significant surgical complication. These included distal ureteral obstruction requiring revision (two cases), loss of bladder compacitance during defunctionalization, renal artery stenosis requiring transluminal angioplasty, small-bowel obstruction, and Mitrofanoff stenosis (one case each).

The principles of transplantation into a reconstructed bladder include the following. (1) Avoid a dry reconstruction. The capacity and compliance of a reconstructive bladder can be lost while awaiting transplantation if the interval is long. This can be avoided by undiversion of native kidneys, if present, by bladder cycling, or by using a living related donor allograft where timing can be optimized. (2) The risk of reabsorptive acidosis occurring either prior to transplantation with drainage of the native kidneys into the reconstructed bladder or following transplantation if the allograft fails over time can be minimized by avoiding the use of small intestine and colon; specifically, gastrocystoplasty, augmentation with ureter and pelvis, and autoaugmentation all have the potential for minimizing reabsorptive acidosis. (3) Two procedures designed to increase bladder capacity and compliance have the potential for being performed retroperitoneally, avoiding interference with present or future peritoneal dialysis or with ventricular peritoneal shunts. These are autoaugmentation and augmenta-

TABLE 50-13

Complications of Urinary Reconstruction

Previously Reviewed
  Metabolic
  Oncogenic
  Intestinal dysfunction
    Fecal incontinence
    Malabsorption
Reconstructive failure
  Upper tract deterioration
  Failure to empty
  Failure to store
  Inability to catheterize
Acute abdominal surgical illness
  Extravasation/rupture
  Bowel obstruction
  Pseudomembranous enterocolitis
  Toxic shock
Urolithiasis
Renal transplant complications
  Mortality
  Morbidity
  Graft Loss
    Vascular
    Nonvascular
Latex Allergy
Obliteration of peritoneal cavity
Wound complications
  Infection
  Dehiscence
  Blood supply
Pregnancy complications

tion employing ureter and pelvis. (4) Because antirefluxing ureteral implantation is important, choices for augmentation may be limited in some patients. Whenever possible, implantation into the native bladder is preferable. If this is not possible, only augmentation with colon, the ileocecal segment, and stomach allow the potential for reliable antirefluxing anastomosis. (5) During the performance of such transplantations, the blood supply of the augmented bladder and of any associated Mitrofanoff neourethra must be meticulously identified and preserved.

COMPLICATIONS

Table 50-13 outlines the most common and significant surgical complications associated with urinary tract reconstruction. Complications related to metabolic derangements, carcinogenesis, and intestinal dysfunction have been previously reviewed. Urolithiasis, particularly as it involves the upper urinary tract, has been reviewed. However, further discussion regarding urolithiasis in the reservoir is pertinent. Other complications include reconstructive failure (upper tract deteriorization, failure to store, or failure to empty), acute abdominal surgical illness (e.g., perforation), renal transplantation complications, latex allergy complications, obliteration of the peritoneal cavity, wound complications, as well as pregnancy complications.

Reconstructive Failure

Reconstructive failure may be expressed as upper tract deterioration, failure to store, and/or failure to empty. Upper tract deterioration may be associated with obstruction, reflux, infection, or inadequate reservoir function. Obstruction of the kidney may be due to acute angulation of the ureter, ischemic contracture, urolithiasis, or inflammatory changes. The need for resectional ureter tapering, extensive ureteral mobilization, division of the ureter at more than one level, and reconstruction resulting in other than a urothelial to urothelial anastomosis appears to enhance this risk.

Ureteral reflux is most commonly encountered due to failure to achieve sufficiently low intravesical (intrareservoir) pressures. Additional risk factors include the employment of nipple valve antireflux techniques as opposed to flap valve techniques. Again a urothelial to urothelial anastomosis appears superior for this purpose. Prevention of reflux appears important because patients who have a portion of the gastrointestinal tract incorporated into their genitourinary reconstruction and intermittent catheterization have a high incidence of bacteriuria.

Burbige and Hensle (1986) reported that 19 of their 56 reconstruction patients had either intermittent or chronically colonized urine. This was most common in those with bowel as part of their reconstruction. Nine of the 19 had a history of recurrent pyelonephritis before their reconstruction. Gil-Vernet and colleagues (1962) found that 90% of their patients with an intestinal cystoplasty had positive cultures, but there were no episodes of pyelonephritis with a follow-up of at least 3½ years in their patients. Kass and Koff (1983) found that all 14 of their patients with augmented neuropathic bladders had positive cultures, but only two developed symptoms of pyelonephritis. Findings are similar in patients who have continent reservoirs that are being catheterized. Benchekroun (1986) reported that half of his patients undergoing reconstructions had positive cultures after surgery, but only two out of 62 developed clinical pyelonephritis; both were patients who were emptying their reservoirs only twice a day. Mansson and colleagues (1986) made a careful study of the bacteriuria commonly seen in continent reservoirs. In their nine patients with continent cecal reservoirs, 20 of 34 catheterized urine samples were positive, usually for an aerobic or facultative anaerobic bacteria in pure culture. They found that the stomal and peristomal bacterial flora remained fairly stable. They postulate that, as with clean intermittent catheterization through the normal urethra, bacteria may be inoculated into the reservoir with instrumentation (Ehrlich and Brem, 1982). Mansson (1987) performed follow-up on 27 patients with continent reservoirs for a total of 1040 months, with only two having symptomatic urinary tract infection. Both of these patients had a stricture. They postulate that high levels of secretory IgA in the reservoir may help to prevent bacterial adherence. Also, mucin might act as a receptor analog to trap bacteria.

From this information it is clear that bacteriuria is a common finding in patients who undergo major urinary tract reconstruction. This may supply further evidence for those who believe that at least in children, an antirefluxing attachment of the upper urinary tract to the reservoir is appropriate. When a symptomatic infection occurs, a careful search for an anatomic obstruction, calculus, reflux, or inadequate reservoir compliance or emptying is appropriate.

Acute Abdominal Surgical Illness

Acute abdominal surgical illness is a grave concern in the patient who has undergone urinary reconstruction, particularly that associated with bladder augmentation or creation of an intestinal reservoir. The most common causes of an acute surgical abdomen in this setting are perforation of the augmented bladder or intestinal reservoir or small-bowel obstruction. Less common but important members of this differential diagnosis include pseudomembranous enterocolitis, toxic shock syndrome, and ventricular peritoneal shunt complications.

As large series of augmentations and intestinal reservoir construction are developed, it is becoming clear that perforation of the reservoir is a risk that must be emphasized to both patients and their families. Deaths have occurred in several series (Elder et al., 1988; Rushton et al., 1988). The presentation is usually that of an acute abdomen. The symptoms, however, may be quite nonspecific, and a high index of suspicion is essential. Diffuse abdominal pain, fever, abdominal distention, and diminished urine output are characteristic. It is important to be cognizant of the fact that the rupture may occur many years after reconstruction. Altered sensation in patients with dyraphic states or spinal cord injury and steroid administration in renal transplant patients may confound the diagnosis.

In establishing the diagnosis, various diagnostic studies may be useful. A cystogram is essential but may not demonstrate the leak, if the perforation is confined and under sufficient pressure to prevent contrast from freely entering the extravesical collection. Complete distention of the augmented bladder or reservoir is imporant, as are oblique views. Further films should be obtained after drainage of the reservoir, looking for residual extravesical collections. Unfortunately because augmented bladders often are irregular and they empty imperfectly with catheterization, it may be quite difficult to determine whether a small area of residual contrast represents extravasation. Cystography has a 50% false-negative rate (Table 50-14).

Abdominal ultrasound may be most useful in estab-

TABLE 50-14

Cystographic Diagnosis of Reservoir Perforation

Series	Number of Episodes	Cystogram Result	
		Positive	Negative
Elder, 1988	4	2	2
Rushton et al., 1988	3	0	3
Sheiner and Kaplan, 1988	2	0	2
Rosen and Light, 1991	6	6	0
Mevorach et al., 1992	1	0	1
Total	16	8	8

lishing the diagnosis, although gaseous distention of the small and/or large bowel may make imaging a reservoir difficult. The techniques of utilizing a "champagne cystogram" in which microscopic air bubbles are introduced into the augmented bladder by irrigating in saline solution rapidly through a catheter may be useful. The microspheres of air create an echogenic pattern that is easily visualized by ultrasound. If they are extravasated, it may be possible to recognize the bladder perforation. Also, the microspheres allow for the limits of the bladder or reservoir to be identified, and a contiguous fluid collection without microspheres may indicate a confined urinoma. A computed axial tomographic study of the abdomen with contrast in the bladder or reservoir may be the most accurate method of making the diagnosis. However, any patient with an augmented bladder on intermittent catheterization who has abdominal pain, fever, or vomiting should be presumed to have a bladder perforation, unless the symptoms can be conclusively demonstrated to be of some other cause. Exploratory laparotomy may be required to make the diagnosis.

If a perforated augmented bladder is found, a debridement of the edges of the perforation should be performed to ensure healthy tissue for closure. Closure with at least two layers in a watertight fashion is appropriate. Copious irrigation of the abdominal cavity on the presumption that the extravasated urine is infected is appropriate. Adequate drainage postoperatively helps to avoid the development of an intraabdominal abscess. An attempt is made to avoid entry of the fibrous capsule surrounding an artificial urinary sphincter, if present. Although healing of bladder perforation by draining the bladder alone may be successful, we believe that in general, operative treatment is more prudent.

The possible causes of these perforations remains conjectural. Bladder perforation secondary to clean intermittent catheterization without augmentation has been reported (Reisman and Preminger, 1989) and has been implicated in the augmented bladder as well. However, perforation of augmented bladders in the absence of intermittent catheterization has been reported (Rosen and Light, 1991). As Tapper and Folkman (1976) demonstrated, bowel in contact with urine may become lymphoid-depleted and thus may be more susceptible to invasive bacterial infection with the potential for inflammatory weakening of the bowel wall. This has been implicated both in perforation and failure of ureteral reimplantation into bowel segments. However, studies addressing this question by intraoperative fluid culture have demonstrated that many such perforations involve sterile urine (Rosen and Light, 1991). Other implicated etiologies include torn adhesions during bladder filling, "blow out" from failure to catheterize, and ischemic injury secondary to increased intravesical pressure.

Essig and colleagues (1991) demonstrated that increased intravesical pressure in an acute canine model of colocystoplasty resulted in perfusion indexes in the colon patch compatible with ischemic necrosis. That this etiology is plausible is suggested by the work of Wangensteen (1955), who, during his studies on small-bowel obstruction in a canine model, found that an intraluminal pressure of 20 cm H_2O applied for 28 hours or an intraluminal pressure of 40 cm H_2O applied for 17 hours resulted in bowel wall necrosis. Similarly, Boley and colleagues (1969) demonstrated in both large and small bowel that intraluminal pressures less than 40 cm H_2O did not interfere with intestinal blood flow. Beyond 40 cm H_2O an incremental compromise in blood flow was noted. Clinically intravesical pressures up to 100 cm H_2O with tubularized augmentation and up to 90 cm of H_2O with detubularized augmentation have been reported (Decter et al., 1987; Goldwasser et al., 1987).

Although the etiology remains conjectural, the majority of perforations have been associated with augmentation onto a neurogenic bladder remnant. More than two thirds of patients have been on intermittent catheterization, and total continence appears to be a common factor in such individuals. Perforations have been described over a wide age range, ranging from infancy into adulthood. Ileal, colonic, and gastric augmentations have been associated with perforation, and both tubularized and detubularized augmentation techniques have been employed in these individuals. Histologic evaluation of the resected site of perforation has generally revealed inflammation, fibrosis, and sclerosal adhesions, but has on occasion demonstrated evidence of ischemic necrosis (Sheiner and Kaplan, 1988).

Small-bowel obstruction following any transperitoneal procedure may be encountered secondary to adhesions. Particularly problematic in the setting of complex urinary reconstruction is the potential for internal hernias. Internal hernias behind segments of ureter and vascular pedicles to neourethras and augment patches are possible but avoidable, if retroperitonealization techniques are employed. Such problems may be very difficult to prevent in patients who have previously undergone chronic peritoneal dialysis or who have had a long-term indwelling ventricular peritoneal shunt where the peritoneal surface may be inflamed, firm, and difficult to mobilize.

The diagnosis of small-bowel obstruction is best made by clinical evaluation and is aided by flat, upright, and occasionally lateral decubitus or cross-table lateral films of the abdomen. The distinction of small-bowel obstruction from ileus and from delayed perforation may be difficult. Evidence for peritonitis requires laparotomy. Particularly problematic may be the high small-bowel obstruction where plain film studies may demonstrate very unimpressive degrees of dilatation. As closed loop obstructions in this setting may cause ischemic bowel compromise, an aggressive approach to diagnosis in this setting employing GI contrast is indicated.

Treatment of any patient suspected of having a small-bowel obstruction includes effective nasogastric suction and frequent serial abdominal examinations. Evidence for clinical deterioration (peritonitis, systemic illness) or failure of the obstructive pattern to resolve within 24 to 48 hours of presentation warrants laparotomy.

Pseudomembranous enterocolitis may occur as a result of antibiotic administration in the perioperative period. Although this is generally associated with copious diarrhea and is readily diagnosed by positive cultures for clostridium difficele and positive assays for *C. difficile* toxin, patients with relatively minimal diarrhea and with significant abdominal distention and pain may be encountered. Early in the course of illness, C. difficile culture and toxin assays may be falsely negative, allowing such illness to be confused with small-bowel obstruction and perforation.

An interesting complication that has only been recently reported is that of toxic shock syndrome related to bladder augmentation (McCahill et al., 1992). Because *Staphylococcus aureus* is a rare cause of urinary tract infection and because only approximately 10% of *S. aureus* strains are capable of toxic shock syndrome toxin-1 production, the overall risk should be small. The morbidity is, however, high. Patients present with fever, hypotension, a sunburn-like rash, myalgia, weakness, confusion, vomiting, diarrhea, and renal and hepatic dysfunction. Pealing from the palms and soles is common. Diagnosis is confirmed by toxic shock exotoxin assay, and treatment includes vigorous volume resuscitation, maintenance of blood pressure, and antistaphylococcal therapy.

Toxic shock syndrome toxin-1 is a 193-amino acid peptide. This peptide is presumably permeable to bowel (or at least inflamed bowel) due to the previous reports of toxic shock syndrome associated with *S. aureus* enterocolitis. This is presumably the etiology of this syndrome when associated with augmentation.

Patients with ventricular peritoneal shunts may present with complications associated with acute abdominal surgical illness, and a high index of suspicion is warranted. Even in the absence of urinary reconstruction, such shunts may be associated with acute abdominal syndromes due to infection, small bowel obstruction, and pseudocyst formation. These risks appear to be enhanced following transabdominal surgery. Shunt tubing is covered with a biofilm. Thus, minimizing handling of the shunt tubing will thus minimize the likelihood of infecting the tubing.

The conduction of a laparotomy following urinary reconstruction is of critical concern. Certainly the elective laparotomy should be preceded by formal bowel preparation in the face of augmentation or continent diversion. The surgeon should have access to a catheter in the bladder to allow insufflation and desufflation for identification purposes, and a catheter should be placed in any catheterization conduit such as Mitrofanoff neourethra. Efforts directed at identification and preservation of mesenteric blood supply to any gastric or intestinal segments employed in reconstruction should be made. Whenever possible, an experienced reconstructive urologist should be present.

Urolithiasis

In patients who have augmented bladders or continent intestinal reservoirs, the development of reservoir or bladder stones, often a number of years after the procedure, is fairly common. Hradec (1965), reporting on 114 patients, found a 10% incidence of bladder calculi. In his series most could be dealt with endoscopically. In the series of 74 patients reported from UCLA (Smith et al., 1977), there were three bladder calculi and two renal calculi that developed as late complications. In the series of 18 cecal reservoirs reported by Mansson and colleagues (1984), there were three cases of reservoir stones that developed during a mean follow-up period of 39 months. A high incidence of reservoir stones has been reported by Benchekroun (1987) from Morocco, where 15 of his 62 patients developed reservoir calculi.

Ginsberg and colleagues (1991) reported the occurrence of 64 stones in 383 patients undergoing a Koch pouch procedure (16.7%). Many of these were associated with eroded Marlex or with staples. Techniques eliminating the use of Marlex and decreasing the amount of staples resulted in a reduction risk of stone formation to 10%. A notable finding in this series, which encompassed a wide age range, was that the incidence of stones developing in patients undergoing Koch pouch creation for urothelial cancer was 13.1%. In contrast, the incidence in patients whose primary diagnosis was neurovesical dysfunction or bladder exstrophy was 38.2% and 28.6%, respectively, suggesting an increased risk in the pediatric population.

Blyth and co-authors (1992) reported urolithiasis in 26 (30%) of 87 patients undergoing enterocystoplasty. Twenty-three of these 26 stones occurred in the urinary reservoir. These stones typically were triple-phosphate in composition. The authors found that the most successful therapy for upper tract stones was extracorporeal shock wave lithotripsy, and the most successful therapy for reservoir stones was open surgical extraction. Attempts at extracorporeal shock wave lithotripsy or electrohydraulic lithotripsy for stones in the reservoir resulted in extensive fragmentation and residual fragments that resulted in recurrence of stone formation. The authors also note an increased risk of urolithiasis in patients undergoing Mitrofanoff reconstructions possibly associated with loss of dependent drainage of the bladder.

As these authors review, in urinary tract reconstruction with intestinal segments, urine tends to be undersaturated for both struvite and carbonate appetite. It may be intermittently supersaturated, however, with calcium phosphate. Struvite and carbonate appetite crystallization requires significantly elevated levels of hydroxyl ion, ammonium ion, and carbonate ion. In general, this only occurs in the setting of ureolysis, as seen often in the setting of proteus and providencia infections and occasionally with klebsiella infections.

Loss of dependent reservoir drainage results in accumulation of mucus and other particulate debris. A biofilm that facilitates the precipitation of struvite calculi is allowed to form. Consequently, vigorous hydration with irrigation of the reservoir with sterile saline solution or boiled water on a regular (daily) basis and perhaps the administration of acetohydroxamic acid (Lithostat) may be preventative (Griffith, 1979). Some stones have been dissolved with hemiacidrin irrigation (Jacobs and Gittes, 1976). In our series of 23 consecutive gastrocystoplasties followed for a minimum of 1.5 years, we have encountered no instance of reservoir calculus (Sheldon et al., 1995). Presumably this occurs due to acidification of urine from the gastric patch. Additionally, patients whose course had been complicated by both recurrent upper tract calculi and bladder calculi have remained stone-free following gastrocystoplasty.

Renal Transplant Complications

A detailed analysis of 39 deaths in 215 pediatric renal allograft recipients followed long-term revealed a significant increased risk in the very young (Sheldon et al., 1992a). In patients older than 6 years of age, the 2-year patient survival and graft survival exceeded 90% and 70%, respectively. In contrast, those within the population younger than 6 years of age a 75%

patient survival rate, and a 45% graft survival rate was noted. This series was primarily cadaveric in nature and spanned many years. Loss of allograft function preceded death in 67% of patients. Allograft loss was due to rejection (61%), renal vascular thrombosis (35%), or recurrent disease (4%). In 17 (44%) patients the death was attributed to the primary disease. Here patients died from dialysis complications, the effect of chronic uremia, and from fluid and electrolyte complications following loss of their allograft. In nine (23%) patients death occurred from a variety of causes with functioning allograft. Four patients died of sepsis, and one patient died of cancer.

Thirteen (33%) deaths were felt to be potentially preventable had modern standards of therapy been applied. The most common cause of death was inappropriate rejection therapy (where rejection had not been biopsy-documented) and failure to withdraw rejection therapy in the face of known infection. Such potentially preventable deaths accounted for 54% of deaths in children younger than 5 years of age and 26% of deaths in children older than 5 years of age.

The authors concluded that the leading causes of death were cardiovascular complications of chronic renal failure and overwhelming sepsis secondary to immunosuppression. Additionally, survival in the very young was very dependent upon graft survival, a finding which strongly supports the use of living-related donor allografts within this population. Further, rejection therapy without biopsy documentation, overaggressive therapy of the chronically failing graft, and failure to withdraw immunosuppression in the face of infection was especially poorly tolerated in the very young.

In a series of 303 pediatric renal transplantations, 39 complications of surgical significance were encountered (Sheldon et al., 1992b). Renovascular complications were encountered in 7.6% of patients, and nonrenovascular complications were encountered in 5.3%. Of these, 54% were felt to have a technical etiology, and 46% were surgically significant due to the fact that management required surgical intervention.

Figure 50-57 demonstrates the relationship between the incidence of renovascular complications and recipient age. Clearly the highest risk for renovascular complication occurs in the very young. Renal artery thrombosis was encountered in 10 patients, renal vein thrombosis in six patients, renal artery stenosis in four patients, and primary nonperfusion in three patients. A technical etiology could be implicated in only a small minority of patients whose graft was lost due to renovascular thrombosis. It was postulated that the increase in intrarenal vascular resistance from ATN combined with the limited cardiac reserve of the small child sets the stage for these thrombotic events.

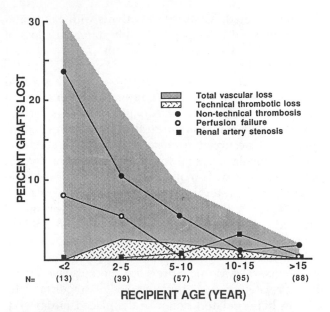

FIG. 50-57
Vascular graft loss as a function of recipient age in pediatric cadaveric renal transplantation. (From Sheldon CA, et al: Complications of surgical significance in pediatric renal transplantation. *J Ped Surg* 1992; 27:486.)

Nonrenovascular complications included symptomatic lymphoceles (three cases), ureteral necrosis (two cases), ureteral obstruction (one case), small-bowel obstruction or inadvertent enterotomy (two cases), and popliteal thromboembolism and urinary extravasation (one case each). Six cases of posttransplant hemorrhage were encountered (one due to an anastomotic defect, one due to hilar injury during harvesting, and one of unknown etiology). Three instances of hemorrhage were due to acute renal rupture secondary to acute rejection.

The problem of graft thrombosis in pediatric renal transplant recipients was studied by the North American Pediatric Renal Transplant Cooperative Study (Harmon et al., 1991). These authors found that within the living-related donor transplant population, there was a significantly increased risk in thrombosis in recipients younger than 6 years of age. In fact, if thrombosis was eliminated, graft survival in these patients was very similar to that of any age group. Also noted was a possible association between graft thrombosis and lack of prior dialysis before transplantation. An increased risk of thrombosis was noted within the cadaveric transplant population. Young age of donor and long cold storage time were strongly associated with thrombotic risk, and these risks were additive. Of significance was the finding that younger grafts are often associated with longer storage times. Patients whose original disease was either oxalosis or congenital nephrotic syndrome had a 14.8% risk of graft thrombosis compared with 3% in the remainder of the pediatric patients studied. This risk in patients with congenital nephrotic syndrome is presumably due to the loss of antithrombin 3 and perhaps protein C and protein S in the urine.

Nelson and colleagues (1989) reviewed surgical complications in their series of pediatric renal transplantaion. Breakdown of the ureteroneocystostomy was the most common surgical complication encountered and occurred exclusively in small recipients whose transplant was performed intraperitoneally and whose bladder was small or otherwise abnormal. The incidence of ureteral complication in this series was 10%. These authors concluded that there was an increased risk of surgical complications in small children receiving intraperitoneal grafts (35% vs 9%). The risk of graft loss in this population was higher as well. Good graft survival was encountered in both cadaveric and living-related donor grafts placed extraperitoneally and in living-related donor grafts placed intraperitoneally. Significantly poorer results were obtained with cadaveric grafts placed intraperitoneally into small recipients.

Kashi and colleagues (1992) reviewed a series of 507 transplantations in which 45 urologic complications were encountered. Of these, 39 (87%) complications were ureteral. Obstruction was encountered in 30 instances and necrosis in nine. These complications were manageable through percutaneous techniques in the majority of patients; however, a number required open surgical interventions. The 1-year graft survival rate was not influenced by the occurrence of ureteral complications. Of note, however, is the fact that renal function was significantly worse within the population suffering ureteral complications ($p = 0.01$).

Many ureteral complications are felt to be of a vascular etiology. As the blood supply of the transplant ureter originates from the main renal artery, the blood supply to the distal-most ureter is most vulnerable. These authors found that kidneys with delayed primary function had an increased risk of ureteral complications supporting a vascular etiology. Of particular note was the lack of association of HLA matching, cystotoxic antibody formation, and rejection episodes, indicating an immune etiology is unlikely.

Shokeir and colleagues (1993) reported 41 ureteric complications in 650 living-related donor transplants, an incidence of 6.3%. Fistula was encountered in 17 patients and obstruction in 24. This series is noteworthy for the fact that five complications were managed by ileal ureter substitution. No graft loss was encountered within this population, and there was no mortality. As previously discussed, the placement of a ureteral stent at the time of pediatric transplantation has been shown to decrease the risk of ureteral complication. Additionally, it helps limit the differential diagnosis of early graft dysfunction. As the renal allograft is particularly vulnerable to the effects of obstruction, the application of this technique may maximize graft function.

The occurrence of ureteral complication can be further minimized by careful harvesting techniques to preserve ureteral blood supply. Additionally, the shortest length of ureter allowing an antirefluxing anastomosis without tension should be utilized. The incidence of reported ureteral complications provides another argument for preserving native kidneys and ureters when possible. A ureteroureterostomy between the transplant ureter and the ipsilateral native or even contralateral native ureter is certainly preferable to the use of an ileal ureter. An ipsilateral anastomosis can be performed without entry of the peritoneal cavity, which allows for preservation of peritoneal dialysis access.

As previously discussed, there appears to be an increased risk of rejection in patients receiving transplantation following complex urinary reconstruction. While the etiology of this remains speculative, certainly blood product administration during such procedures should be minimized. In addition to employing cytomegalovirus-negative blood in CMV-naive potential recipients, it is preferable to optimize red cell mass with erythropoietin administration, using autologous blood if possible and otherwise employing a white cell filter and azathioprene with transfusion to minimize the risk of presensitization.

Latex Allergy Complications

Intraoperative collapse secondary to latex-induced anaphylaxis has been reported with an alarming incidence (Gold et al., 1991; Nguyen et al., 1991; Pasquariello et al., 1993; Slater, 1989). Both patients reported by Nguyen and colleagues (1991) subsequently underwent an uncomplicated anesthesia and surgery employing a latex-free environment and preoperative preparation employing steroids and antihistamines. Postoperative evaluation of 15 patients experiencing antiphylaxis by Gold and colleagues (1991) revealed, in retrospect, a positive history of skin reaction to rubber (47%) and a positive skin test for latex allergy in 100%.

The incidence of presensitization to latex products is a major concern. Slater and colleagues (1991) assayed for rubber-specific IGE by radioallergosorbent testing and found elevated levels in 34% of 32 preoperative children with myelomeningocele. In contrast, elevated levels were found in only 11% of 35 preoperative age-matched controls and 2% of 45 outpatient controls studied. Yassin and colleagues (1992) screened 76 patients with myelomeningocele by skin testing employing latex extracts. Forty-nine (64.5%) patients were found to be positive. Careful review for symptoms of latex allergy revealed the presence of symptoms in 49% of patients with a positive test and no patient with a negative test. There was no significant correlation among age, sex, or intermittent catheterization and positive skin testing. A significant association, however, was an increased incidence of surgical procedures ($p < 0.001$).

In a similar study by Ellsworth and colleagues (1993), no significant correlation between latex allergy and intermittent catheterization was identified. Again there was a significant correlation between the incidence of surgical procedures and latex allergy ($p = 0.03$). There was, however, no significant correlation when intraabdominal procedures were evaluated in isolation. These authors suggest that it is primarily a blood-tissue barrier breakdown that presensitizes these patients, and they suggest that all surgeries in patients with myelomeningocele be performed employing a latex-free environment.

Obliteration of the Peritoneal Cavity

Transperitoneal surgery may obviate the effectiveness of peritoneal dialysis and ventricular-peritoneal shunt drainage secondary to loculation from adhesions. Additionally, peritoneal inflammatory changes even in the absence of loculation may render these modalities ineffective secondary to loss of ultrafiltration capacity. Although we have been successful in a few instances in laparoscopically relieving intraperitoneal adhesions to allow peritoneal dialysis, this complication is best avoided by minimizing transperitoneal surgery, when possible, in the patient population at risk.

The small child with chronic renal failure may be particularly at risk. Here fistula or graft surgery for hemodialysis access is less reliable than in the older patient. Additionally, indwelling central venous catheters for hemodialysis may induce severe and progressive thrombosis, ultimately eliminating this access. Similarly, options for central spinal fluid drainage in patients with hydrocephalus may be limited in the very young. In this setting both ventricular-venous and ventricular-plural shunting may be significantly more problematic. Also potentially of concern is the use of ventricular-plural shunting in patients with chronic pulmonary disease.

These concerns argue for delayed transperitoneal reconstruction in patients requiring ventricular-peritoneal shunting or those with chronic renal failure until the patient reaches an age when dependence upon the peritoneal cavity is less critical. Such patients, for example, are often best treated by temporary vesicostomy.

There is a small but significant risk of ventricular-peritoneal shunt malfunction following transabdominal surgery (Pittman et al., 1992). Kreder and colleagues (1990) reported two patients with shunt infections encountered in 54 patients undergoing bladder augmentation in the face of ventricular-peritoneal shunting. These authors recommend closed-suction drainage and removal of the drainage catheters in the early postoperative period (2 to 3 days). In addition, they recommend the use of a broad spectrum of antibiotics for a 7- to 10-day period. As shunts are covered by a biofilm that tends to protect them, it is important to handle them as little as possible and avoid air exposure by exteriorization during surgery.

White and colleagues (1991) reported six symptomatic abdominal pseudocyst occurring in 27 (22%) of myelomeningocele children with ventricular-peritoneal shunts following transabdominal urologic surgery. Only one (1.3%) pseudocyst was encountered in 76 such patients who did not undergo transabdominal surgery. Merovach and co-authors (1991) reported the erosion of a ventricular peritoneal shunt into the augmented bladder presenting with the catheter exiting through the urethra.

The nature and significance of abdominal complications from ventricular-peritoneal shunts in general was reviewed by Bryant and co-authors (1988). These authors report a 10% to 30% incidence of intraabdominal complications of ventricular-peritoneal shunts. Complications include visceral perforation. Perforation of bowel, bladder, vagina, gallbladder, and scrotum have been reported. Additionally, peritonitis, ascites, and pseudocysts may occur. Acute visceral perforation may present with peritonitis, whereas chronic perforation generally presents as a shunt infection. Occasionally a shunt catheter will found to be presenting through the anus, vagina, or urethra.

Evaluation of such a patient presenting with an acute abdomen begins with the attainment of a plain film of the abdomen, a CBC, and a culture and analysis of the central spinal fluid (CSF). Evidence for shunt infection necessitates externalization of the shunt. The presence of free air, persistence of abdominal symptoms despite antibiotic therapy, and/or clinical deterioration may warrant laparotomy.

A mass encountered on plain film analysis is evaluated by ultrasonography, whereas evidence for bowel obstruction is evaluated by contrast CT scanning. If the plain film and CSF analysis are normal, a radionucleotide shunt scan is undertaken. Those patients whose presentation is primarily that of neurologic symptoms are evaluated employing cranial computed tomography and a radionucleotide shunt scan.

Wound Complications

As with any major transabdominal surgery, wound infections and wound dehiscence may occur but are rare when careful surgical technique is employed. Of particular concern, however, is the planning of surgical incisions so as not to interfere with the blood

TABLE 50-15

Principles of Pediatric Urinary Reconstruction—Operative Strategy

Problem	Principles	Sample Solutions

I. Urine is diverted	1. Careful assessment of prediversion status.
	2. Complete preoperative evaluation: Consider reflux, obstruction, high-pressure storage, and incontinence.
	3. Surgical strategy with options prepared before surgery.
	4. Uroepithelium to uroepithelium anastomosis preferred.
		1. Preoperative evaluation:
		  a. Renal function assessment (renal scan, GFR, differential function).
		  b. Complete anatomic delineation:
		    1. IVU and VCUG with upright film.
		    2. Retrograde conduit and ureterostomy studies.
		    3. Endoscopy (retrograde injection of ureteral stumps if necessary).
		  c. Functional assessment:
		    1. CMG, urine output measurement.
		    2. UPP, LLP, stress LPP.
		    3. Urethroscopy, cystoscopy.
		    4. Periurethral EMG.
		    5. Bladder cycling (CIC vs. SP tube).

II. Ureter is too short	1. Avoid interposed bowel segment if possible.
	2. Avoid tapered bowel segment implantation into bowel or bladder if possible.
	3. Uroepithelium to uroepithelium anastomosis is best, even if it requires use of most of the bladder.
		1. One ureter too short:
		  a. TUU.
		  b. Psoas hitch/Boari flap.
		  c. Downward mobilization of kidney.
		  d. Autotransplantation.
		  e. Ileal ureter.
		2. Both ureters too short:
		  a. Psoas hitch/Boari flap plus TUU.
		  b. Autotransplantation plus ureteropyelostomy.
		  c. Ileal ureter.

III. Ureter is too wide	1. Two wide ureters are often best managed by one long tunnel and TUU.
	2. Tailored ureteral implantation into bladder is preferable to any implantation into bowel.
	3. Use of ileocecocystoplasty may be preferable to implantation of tapered ureter into colon.
	4. Previously tapered ureter should not be retapered (nonresectional tailoring acceptable).
		1. Attempt direct ureteral implantation into bladder:
		  a. No tailoring necessary if ureter <1 cm.
		  b. Otherwise, tapered/tailored bladder implantation.
		2. If ureter is too short or has been previously tapered, consider ileocecocystoplasty with modified ileocecal intussusception to create flap-valve antireflux mechanism.

IV. Ureterovesical junction is incompetent	1. Ureteral reimplantation into a high pressure reservoir has a high risk of failure.
	2. Concomitant upper ureteral undiversion and lower ureteral reimplantation is acceptable with meticulous preservation of ureteral blood supply.
	3. Direct ureteral implantation into bladder if possible is always preferable to bowel implantation.
		1. Attempt ureteral implantation into bladder even if augmentation is necessary.
		2. With concomitant proximal diversion and distal reflux:
		  a. Staged approach considered if blood supply tenuous.
		  b. Avoid dry reimplant. Do upper ureteral undiversion first if staged.

V. Bladder too small or hyperreflexic	1. Persistent noncompliant hypertonic CMG curve or inadequate capacity below 40 cm H_2O pressure indicates need for augmentation.
	2. Intermittent catheterization is always anticipated with bladder augmentation.
	3. Liberal use of bladder augmentation increases chance of success with major reconstruction.
	4. Avoid tubular bowel segment for augmentation.
	5. Loss of accommodation may accompany:
	  a. Dry augmentation.
	  b. Severe reflux.
	  c. Bladder outlet incompetence.
	  d. Hour-glass bladder.
		1. A detubularized bowel segment is always used for augmentation (e.g., small or large bowel cup patch or ileal to cecal longitudinal inlay).
		2. Capacity <60% expected for age or compliance <2 ml/cm H_2O suggests need for augmentation.
		3. Clam-shell preparation of native bladder.
		4. Aggressively prevent incontinence and reflux.

VI. Bladder absent or unreconstructable	1. If urethra and continence mechanism is intact, attempt to reestablish urethral continuity. 2. Because of real incidence of failure with urethral drainage, alternative options (Mitrofanoff principle) must not be sacrificed. 3. Urothelial-intestinal anoatomosis with admixture of urine and feces enhances risk of malignancy. 4. If neurologically normal and rectal continence proven by 500 ml saline enema, consider internal diversion.	1. Neobladder. 2. Continent diversion. 3. Ureterosigmoidostomy or ureterosigmoidostomy variant.

TABLE 50-15 (cont.)

Problem	Principles	Sample Solutions

VII. Urethra incompetent	1. UPP or LPP <40-60 cm H_2O or stress LPP <100 cm H_2O, quiet EMG, and incompetent bladder neck on upright cystogram—likely requires bladder outlet reconstruction.
	2. Success of urethral reconstruction without concomitant bladder augmentation is low if low-volume and/or high pressure reservoir used.
	3. Benefits of AUS consistently outweigh risks only if spontaneous voiding is likely and if no previous bladder neck reconstruction has been performed.
	4. Anticipated need for CIC is not contraindication for AUS.
	5. Adjuvant Mitrofanoff neourethra may optimize success of bladder outlet reconstruction.
	6. Loss of native urethra avoided if possible:
	  a. Loss of "pop-off" mechanism may facilitate spontaneous bladder rupture.
	  b. Loss of dependent drainage may facilitate stone formation.
	7. Flap valve mechanism inherently more stable than nipple valve.
		1. Urethral lengthening (detrusor rube) with suspension is widely applicable.
		  a. Neourethra should be narrow and long (>4 cm) for adequate hydraulic resistance.
		  b. Consider appendix, ureter, gastric or detrusor tube as alternate catheterizable channel with flap valve for continence (Mitrofinoff).
		2. A motivated and functional patient, able to empty bladder spontaneously, with an unscarred bladder neck who does not require concomitant major reconstruction is an ideal candidate for AUS.
		3. Fascial sling.
		4. Consider urethral interruption and Mitrofanoff in selected cases.

VIII. Urethra inaccessible or unreconstructable	1. Success of reconstruction may be directly dependent on frequent CIC of continent catheterizable channel.
	2. Compliance directly dependent of patient convenience:
	  a. Accessible, easily catheterizable conduit.
	  b. Compatable with self-care.
	  c. Not painful.
		1. Mitrofanoff principle:
		  a. Appendix available—appendicovesicostomy.
		  b. Appendix not available:
		    1. Distal cutaneous ureterostomy (nonrefluxing system).
		    2. Tapered ileum.

IX. Patient has ventricular-peritoneal shunt	1. Incidence of shunt contamination is low but significant.
	2. Morbidity of shunt contamination is high:
	  a. Loss of mental capacity.
	  b. Increased risk of seizure.
	3. Extraperitoneal procedures should be sought.
	4. Delay procedure until age allows safe application of alternative CSF drainage
	  a. Ventricular-pleural shunt.
	  b. Ventricular-venous shunt.
		1. Avoid use of bowel when possible.
		2. If augmentation is necessary, in addition to routine bowel preparation, perform intraoperative intraluminal antiseptic irrigation before opening bowel.
		3. Closed drainage only is employed and used on a short-term basis.
		4. Effective temporary urinary diversion (stents, nephrostomy, or SP tube) important to avoid urinary leakage.
		5. Antibiotic coverage is begun preoperatively.
		6. If augmentation is necessary, consider autoaugmentation, ureteral augmentation and possibly gastric augmentation (if applicable).

X. Patient has PD catheter or PD catheter anticipated	1. Extraperitoneal procedures should be sought.
	2. If transplantation anticipated and transperitoneal reconstruction necessary:
	  a. LRD–Plan to allow short interval on hemodialysis.
	  b. CAD–Consider deferring until age at which hemodialysis reliably applied on long-term basis.
		1. If augmentation necessary, consider autoaugmentation or ureteral augmentation (if applicable).

XI. Patient has marginal fecal continence	1. All patients with myelodysplasia or imperforate anus are considered to have marginal fecal continence.
	2. Avoid removal of ileocecal region or large ileal resection.
	3. Consider preservation of appendix if appendicocecostomy may be required to facilitate fecal continence.
		1. Bladder augmentation required:
		  a. Sigmoid or lileal patch.
		  b. Gastrocystoplasty.
		2. Bladder replacement required:
		  a. Colonic neobladder.
		  b. Gastric neobladder.
		  c. Mitrofanoff principle.

(Continued.)

TABLE 50-15 (cont.)

Problem	Principles	Sample Solutions

XII. Patient has chronic renal failure	1. Incorporation of intestine into urinary tract may result in metabolic disturbance.
	2. Pretransplant augmentation may markedly benefit some patients:
	  a. Facilitation of ureteral implantation.
	  b. Reduction of post-transplant voiding disturbance.
	  c. Post-transplant augmentation runs risk of septic complications.
	3. Blood transfusion may presensitize patient for subsequent transplantation.
	4. Transverse abdominal incisions may compromise subsequent transplantation.
		1. If transplantation anticipated and augmentation necessary:
		  a. Frequent cateterization and overnight continuous drainage may minimize metabolic insult.
		  b. Stomach, ureter or autoaugmentation preferred options.
		2. If blood transfusion required:
		  a. CMV negative blood in CMV naive patient.
		  b. Consider erytropoetin-autologous transfusion.
		  c. Consider azothiprine coverage and WBC filter.

supply of the anterior abdominal wall. Particularly problematic are upper abdominal transverse incisions that interrupt the superior epigastric blood flow in patients at risk for chronic renal insufficiency. Patients requiring subsequent renal transplantation may require incisions that compromise inferior epigastric blood flow and lateral collateral blood flow, which may significantly compromise wound healing. Within this population renal procedures are best performed through lateral flank or dorsal lumbotomy incisions. Transabdominal surgery is best performed through a midline approach.

Pregnancy Complications

The risk of pregnancy complications in patients who have previously undergone bladder augmentation has been reviewed by Hill and Kramer (1990). As these authors review, complications are expected due to the experience with pregnancies in patients who have undergone urinary conduits and ureterosigmoidostomy. In this setting premature birth has been reported in an incidence ranging from 20% to 50%. Urinary tract infections are seen in approximately 15% of patients, with urinary obstruction and intestinal obstruction encountered in 13% and 10% of patients, respectively.

These authors reviewed 15 patients who became pregnant following bladder augmentation. Urinary tract infection was encountered in nine (60%), and premature birth was encountered in four (27%). Based on their experience, these authors conclude that, in the face of bladder augmentation alone, a vaginal delivery can be pursued without undo risk. In the setting of previous bladder outlet reconstruction or an artificial urinary sphincter, a cesarean section is recommended. The cesarean section is preferably performed in an elective setting and preferably in the presence of an experienced reconstructive urologist.

RECONSTRUCTIVE PRINCIPLES

On the basis of all the information reviewed in this chapter, certain themes have emerged that underlie our approach to reconstructive pediatric urologic surgery. They can be summarized as follows:

1. The presurgical evaluation in each case must be meticulous from both an anatomic and functional point of view. Today, most of the physiologic consequences of reconstructive efforts can be anticipated.

2. Compromise of renal function need not preclude reconstructive efforts. However, if intestine is incorporated into the genitourinary tract, the risk of at least transitory hyperchloremic acidosis is increased. This can generally be dealt with by sodium bicarbonate supplementation. Stomach may offer the useful alternative when the glomerular filtration rate is less than 40 to 50 mm/min/1.73 m². Also, considered in this setting should be autoaugmentation and ureteral augmentation procedures.

3. One-stage reconstruction is usually possible and preferable. Wide exposure is routine, and meticulous attention to technique is essential. A one-stage reconstruction avoids problems with a "dry" ureteral and urethral procedure. Sometimes the possibility of a secondary procedure to achieve a final measure of complete continence cannot be avoided.

4. Uroepithelium to uroepithelium attachment of the upper urinary tract to the bladder or reservoir usually produces the lowest complication rate and best result. A sacrifice of bladder volume to achieve a direct nonrefluxing connection of the upper urinary tract to the bladder is justified, as intestinal augmentation usually restores volume. The high incidence of bacteria in reconstructions using segments of the gastrointestinal tract emphasizes the need to avoid reflux of urine into the upper urinary tract.

5. In the surgical creation of a continence mechanism, the greatest long-term success rates appear to result from the use of a flap valve as opposed to a nipple valve or hydraulic resistance.

6. Inadequate low-pressure (less than 40 cm H₂O) storage reservoir is essential. In bladder augmentation it is essential to widely open to bladder to disrupt the

ability of the detrusor to achieve a high pressure. Bowel should be routinely detubularized.

7. Effective, intermittent, low-pressure emptying of the bladder or reservoir is essential. Spontaneous voiding after major continent reconstruction is frequently impossible. The use of short- or long-term, clean, intermittent catheterization should be anticipated.

8. In the setting of complex bladder outlet reconstruction, even when spontaneous voiding is anticipated, the use of an advantant Mitrofanoff neourethra may be indicated to allow temporary intermittent catheterization that would otherwise run risk to compromise or injury to the bladder outlet.

Table 50-15 outlines the principles of pediatric urinary reconstruction with sample solutions for operative strategy presented.

REFERENCES

Ackerman R, Frohmuller H: Experiences with intubated ureterotomy and its indications. *Urology* 1973; 12:112.

Adams MC, Mitchell ME, Rink RC: Gastrocystoplasty: An alternative solution to the problem of urologic reconstruction in the severely compromised patient. *J Urol* 1988; 140:1152-1156.

Alexander SA, Arbus GS, Butt KMH, et al: The 1989 report of the North American Pediatric Renal Transplant Cooperative Study. *Pediatr Nephrol* 1990; 4:542-553.

Aliabadi H, Gonzalez R: Success of the artificial urinary sphincter after failed surgery for incontinence. *J Urol* 1990; 143:987-990.

Arap S, Giron AM, DeGoes GM: Complete reconstruction of bladder exstrophy. *Urology* 1976; 7:413-416.

Arap S, Giron AM, deGoes GM: Initial results of the complete reconstruction of bladder exstrophy. *Urol Clin North Am* 1980; 7:477-491.

Ashken MH: Urinary caecal reservoir. In Ashken MH (ed): *Urinary Diversion*. New York, Springer-Verlag, 1982, p 112.

Augspruger RR: Pitfalls of the Rosen anti-incontinence prosthesis. *J Urol* 1981; 125:201-203.

Badiola FI, Gastro-Diaz D, Hart-Alustin C, et al: Influence of preoperative bladder capacity and compliance on the outcome of artificial sphincter implantation in patients with neurogenic sphincter incompetence. *J Urol* 1992; 148:1493-1495.

Bajany DE, Lockhart JL, Politano VA: Ileal segment for ureteral substitution or for improvement of ureteral function. *J Urol* 1991; 146:302-305.

Barnett M, Bruskewitz R, Glass N, et al: Long-term clean intermittent self-catheterization in renal transplant recipient. *J Urol* 1985; 134:654-657.

Barrett DM, Furlow WL: Incontinence, intermittent self-catheterization and the artificial genitourinary sphincter. *J Urol* 1984; 132:268.

Barrett DV, O'Sullivan DC, Malizia AA, et al: Particle shedding and migration from silicone genitourinary prosthetic devices. *J Urol* 1991; 146:319-322.

Bauer SB: Neurogenic bladder dysfunction. *Ped Clin NA* 1987; 34:1121-1132.

Bauer SB, Reda EF, Colodny AH, et al: Detrusor instability: a delayed complication in association with the artificial sphincter. *J Urol* 1986; 135:1212.

Beck EP: The sling operation. In Buchsbaum HJ, Schmidt JD (eds): *Gynecologic and Obstetric Urology*. Philadelphia, WB Saunders Co, 1978.

Belloli G, Campobasso P, Mercurella A: Neuropathic urinary incontinence in pediatric patients: Management with artificial sphincter. *J Pedr Surg* 1992; 27:1461-1464.

Belman AB, Kaplan GW: Experience with the Kropp anti-incontinence procedure. *J Urol* 1989; 141:1160-1162.

Benchekroun A: Continent caecal bladder. *Br J Urol* 1982; 54:505-506.

Benchekroun A: The ileococcal continent bladder. In King L, Stone AR, Webster GD (eds): *Bladder reconstruction and continent urinary diversion*. Chicago, Year–Book Medical Publishers, 1987; 224-237.

Benchekroun A, Essakalli N, Fail M, et al: Continent urostomy with hydraulic ileal valve in 136 patients: 13 years of experience. *J Urol* 1989; 142:46-51.

Bergmeijer J, Nijman R, Kalkman E, et al: Stenting of the ureterovesical anastomosis in pediatric renal transplantation. *Transpl Int* 1990; 3:146-148.

Bihrle R, Brito CG, Adams MC, et al: Construction of an antirefluxing urinary conduit using a plicated ileocecal segment. *J Urol* 1989; 142:1564-1569.

Bisgard JD: Substitution of the urinary bladder with a segment of sigmoid. *Ann Surg* 1943; 117:106-109.

Blyth B, Ewalt DH, Duckett JW, et al: Lithogenic properties of enterocystoplasty. *J Urol* 1992; 148:575-577.

Boley SJ, Agrawal GP, Warren AR, et al: Pathophysiologic effect of bowel distention on intestinal blood flow. *Am J Surg* 1969; 117:288.

Borci PA, Bruce J, Gough DC: Continent cutaneous diversions in children: experience with the Mitrofanoff procedure. *Br J Urol* 1992; 70:669-693.

Borzi P, Gough DCS: Pedicled gastric tube as a catheterising conduit. *Eur Urol* 1993; 24:103-105.

Bosco PJ, Bauer SB, Colodny AH, et al: The long-term results of artificial sphincters in children. *J Urol* 1991; 146:396-399.

Bouchot O, Guillonneau B, Cantarovich D, et al: Vesicoureteral reflux in the renal transplantation candidate. *Eur Urol* 1991; 20:26-28.

Boxer RJ, Fritzsche P, Skinner DG, et al: Replacement of the ureter by small intestine: Clinical application and results of the ileal ureter in 89 patients. *J Urol* 1979; 121:725.

Boxer RJ, Johnson SF, Ehrlich RM: Ureteral substitution. *Urology* 1978; 269-278.

Boyd SD, Feinberg SM, Skinner DG, et al: Quality of life of urinary diversion patients: Comparison of ileal conduits versus continent Koch ileal reservoirs. *J Urol* 1987; 138:1386.

Bramble FJ: The treatment of adult enuresis and urge incontinence by enterocystoplasty. *Br J Urol* 1982; 54:693-696.

Braudesky G, Holschneider AM: Operations for the improvement of fecal incontinence. *Prog Pediatr Surg* 1976; 9:105.

Bricker EM: Bladder substitution after pelvic evisceration. *Surg Clin North Am* 1950; 30:1511-1521.

Briscoe DM, Kim MS, Lillehei C, et al: Outcome of renal transplantation in children less than two years of age. *Kidney International* 1992; 42:657-662.

Bruskewitz R, Raz S, Smith RB, et al: AMS 742 Sphincter: UCLA experience. *J Urol* 1980; 124:812-814.

Bryant JE, Joseph DB, Kohaut EC, et al: Renal transplantation in children with posterior urethral valves. *J Urol* 1991; 146:1585-1587.

Bryant MS, Bremer AO, Tepas JJ, et al: Abdominal complications of ventriculoperitoneal shunts-case reports and review of literature. *The American Surgeon* 1988; 50-55.

Burbige KH, Hensle TW: The complications of urinary tract reconstruction. *J Urol* 1986; 136:292.

Burch JC: Urethrovaginal fixation to Cooper's ligament for correcton of stress incontinence, cystocele and prolapse. *Am J Obstet Gynecol* 1961; 81:281.

Burns MW, Watkins SL, Mitchell ME, et al: Treatment of bladder dysfunction in children with end-stage renal disease. *J Ped Surg* 1992; 27, 2:170-174.

Cairns HS, Leaker B, Woodhouse CRJ, et al: Renal transplantation into abnormal lower urinary tract. Lancet 1991; 338:1376.

Camey M: Bladder replacement by ileocystoplasty following radical cystectomy. *World J Urol* 1985; 3:161-166.

Camey M, Richard F, Botto H: Bladder replacement by ileocystoplasty. In King L, Stone AR, Webster GD (eds): *Bladder Reconstruction and Continent Urinary Diversion*. Chicago, Year Book Medical Publishers, 1987; 336-359.

Carone R, Vercelli D, Bertapelle P: Effects of cisapride on anorectal and vesicourethral function in spinal cord injury patients. *Paraplegia* 1993; 31:125-127.

Carroll PR, Presti JC, McAninch JW, et al: Functional characteristics of the continent ileocecal urinary reservoir: Mechanisms of urinary continence. *J Urol* 1989; 142:1032-1036.

Cartwright PC, Snow BW: Bladder autoaugmentation: Early clinical experience. *J Urol* 1989; 142:505-508.

Cartwright PC, Snow BW: Personal communication, 1994.

Casale AJ, Colodny AH, Bauer SB, et al: The use of bowel interposed between proximal and distal ureter in urinary tract reconstruction. *J Urol* 1985; 134:737-740.

Casati E, Boari A: Contributo spermentale alla plastica dull'ureter. Communicazione preventia. Atti Dell Academia delle Scierze Mediche e Naturali in Ferrara. Ano 68, fasc 3. 27 Mai 1894, pp 149-154.

Cecka JM, Terasaki PI: The UNOS Scientific Renal Transplant Registry - 1990. In Terasaki PI (ed): *Clinical Transplants 1990*. Los Angeles, UCLA Tissue Typing Laboratory, 1991, pp 1-10.

Charney EB, Kalichman MA, Snyder HM: Multiple benefits of clean intermittent catheterization for children with myelomeningocele. *Z Kinderchir* 1982; 37:145.

Cher ML, Roehrborn CG: Incorporation of intestinal segments into the urinary tract. In Hohenfellner A, Wammack R (eds): *Continent urinary diversion*. Churchill Livingstone, Edinburg, 1992.

Churchill BM, Aliabadi H, Landon EH, et al: Ureteral bladder augmentation. *J Urol* 1993; 150:716-720.

Churchill BM, Gilmour RF, Willot P: Urodynamics. *Ped Clin N Amer* 1987; 34:1133-57.

Churchill BM, Sheldon CA, McLorie GA, et al: Factors influencing patient and in graft survival in 300 cadaveric pediatric renal transplants. *J Urol* 1988; 140:1129-1133.

Claes H, Stroobants E, van Meerbeek J, et al: Pulmonary migration following periurethral polytetrafluoroethylene injection for urinary incontinence. *J Urol* 1989; 142:321.

Clark SS: Electrolyte disturbance associated with jejunal conduit. *J Urol* 1974; 112:42-47.

Colodny AH: Personal communication, 1980.

Couvelaire R: Le reservoir ileal de substitution apres la cystectomie totale chez l'homme. *J Urol (Paris)* 1951; 57:408.

Creevy CD, Reiser MP: Observations upon the absorption of urinary constituents after ureterosigmoidostomy: The importance of renal damage. *Surg Gynecol Obstet* 1952; 95:589.

Crissey MM, Steele GD, Gittes RF: Rat model for carcinogenesis in ureterosigmoidostomy. *Science* 1980; 207:1079.

Cromie WJ, Barada JH, Weingarten JL: Cecal tubularization: Lengthening technique for creation of catheterizable conduit. *Urology* 1991; 1:41-42.

Cumming J, Woodhouse CR: Role of the kockpouch in adolescent urology. *Prog Ped Surg* 1989; 23:126-134.

Cumming J, Worth PHL, Woodhouse CRJ: The choice of suprapubic continent catheterizable urinary stoma. *Br J Urol* 1987; 60:227-230.

Cunningham J, Bikle DD, Avioli LV: Acute but not chronic metabolic acidosis disturbs 25-hydroxy vitamin D3 metabolism. *Kidney Int* 1984; 25:47-52.

Davis DM: Intubated ureterotomy: a new operation for ureteral and ureteropelvic stricture. *Surg Gynecol Obstet* 1943; 76:514.

deBadiola FIP, Castro-Diaz D, Hart-Austin C, et al: Influence of preoperative bladder capacity and compliance on the outcome of artificial sphincter implantation in patients with neurogenic sphincter incompetence. *J Urol* 1992; 148:1493-1495.

Decter RM, Bauer SB, Mandell J, et al: Small bowel augmentation in children with neurogenic bladder: an initial report of urodynamic findings. *J Urol* 1987; 138:1014.

Dees JE: Congenital epispadias with incontinence. *J Urol* 1949; 62:513.

Diokno AC, Sonda LP: Compatibility of genitourinary prostheses and intermittent self-catheterization. *J Urol* 1981; 125:659.

Dounis A, Gow JG: Bladder augmentation—a long-term review. *Br J Urol* 1979; 51:264-268.

Dretler SP: The pathogenesis of urinary tract calculi occurring after ileal conduit diversion I: Clinical study II: Conduit study, III: Prevention. *J Urol* 1973; 109:204.

Duckett JW, Lotfi AH: Appendicovesicostomy (and variations) in bladder reconstruction. *J Urol* 1993; 149:567-569.

Duckett JW, Raezer DM: Neuromuscular dysfunction of the lower urinary tract. In King L, Kelalis P, Bleman B (eds): *Clinical Pediatric Urology*, Philadelphia, WB Saunders Co, 1976, pp 401-426.

Duckett JW, Snyder HM: Use of the Mitrofanoff principle in urinary reconstruction. *World J Urol* 1985; 3:191-193.

Duckett JW, Snyder HM: Continent urinary diversion: variations on the Mitrofanoff principle. *J Urol* 1986; 135:58-62.

Duckett JW, Snyder HM III: Pediatric Articles-Continent urinary diversion: variations on the Mitrofanoff principle. *J Urol* 1986; 136:58-62.

Durrans D, Wujanto R, Carfrol RN, et al: Bile acid malabsorption: complication of conduit surgery. *Br J Urol* 1989; 64, 485-488.

Dykes EH, Duffy PG, Ransley PG: The use of the Mitrofanoff principle in achieving clean intermittent catheterisation and urinary continence in children. *J Pediatr Surg* 1991; 5:535-538.

Ehrich JHH, Rizzoni G, Brunner FP, et al. Renal replacement therapy for end-stage renal failure before 2 years of age. *Nephrol Dial Transplant* 1992; 7:1171-1177.

Ehrlich O, Brem AS: A prospective comparison of urinary tract infections in patients treated with either clean intermittent catheterization of urinary diverson. Pediatrics 1982; 70:665.

Ehrlich RM, Skinner DG: Complications of transureteroureterostomy. *J Urol* 1975; 113:467.

Elder JS: Periurethral and puboprostatic sling repair for incontinence in patients with myelodysplasia. *J Urol* 1990; 144:434-437.

Elder JS: Continent appendicocolostomy: A variation of the Mitrofanoff principle in pediatric urinary tract reconstruction. *J Urol* 1992; 148:117-119.

Elder JS, Snyder HM, Hulbert WC, et al: Perforation of the augmented bladder in patients undergoing clean intermittent catheterization. *J Urol* 1988; 140:1159-1164.

Elder DD, Moisey CU, Rees RWN: A long-term followup of the colonic conduit operation in children. *Br J Urol* 1979; 51:462.

Ellsworth PI, Merguerian PA, Klein RB: Evaluation and risk factors of latex allergy in spina bifida patients. *J Urol* 1993; 150(2 pt 2):691-693.

Esposti PL: Regeneration of smooth muscle fibers of the ureter following plastic surgery with free flaps of the parietal peritoneum. *Minerva Chir* 1956; 11:1208.

Essig KA, Sheldon CA, Brandt MT, et al: Elevated intravesical pressure causes arterial hypoperfusion in canine colocystoplasty: A fluorometric assessment. *J Urol* 1991; 146:551-553.

Ettenger RB: Children are different: the challenges of pediatric renal transplantation. *Am J Kidney Dis* 1992; 20:668-672.

Ferris DO, Odel HM: Electrolyte pattern of the blood after bilateral ureterosigmoidostomy. *JAMA* 1950; V142:634.

Filmer RB, Spencer JR: Malignancies in bladder, augmentations and intestinal conduits. *J Urol* 1990; 143:671-678.

Firlit CF, Sommer JT, Kaplan WE: Pediatric urinary undiversion. *J Urol* 1980; 123:748-753.

Fisch M, Wammack R, Hohenfellner R: The sigma-rectum pouch (MAINTZ pouch II). In Hohenfellner R and Wammack R (eds): *Continent urinary diversion*. Churchill Livingstone, Edinburg, 1992.

Flocks RH, Culp DA: A modification of technique for anastomosing membranous urethra and bladder neck following total prostatectomy. *J Urol* 1953; 69:411.

Forsythe JLR, Coulthard MG, Taylor PMR, et al: Renal replacement treatment in patients with spina bifida or spinal cord injury. *Br Med J* 300:331-332.

Furlow WL: Implantation of a new semiautomatic artificial genitourinary sphincter: Experience with primary activation and deactivation in 47 patients. *J Urol* 1981; 126:741.

Gearhart JP, Canning DA, Jeffs RD: Failed bladder neck reconstruction: options for management. *J Urol* 1991; 146:1082-1084.

Ghonrim MA: The modified rectal bladder (augmented and valved bladder). In Hohenfellner R, Wammack R (eds): *Continent urinary diversion*. Edinburg, Churchill Livingstone 1992.

Giesy JD, Barry JM, Fuchs EF, et al: Initial experience with the Rosen incontinence device. *J Urol* 1981; 125:794-795.

Gilchrist RK, Merricks JW, Hamlin HH, et al: Construction of substitute bladder and urethra. *Surg Gynecol Obstet* 1950; 90:752.

Gil-Vernet JM Jr: The ileocolic segment in urologic surgery. *J Urol* 1965; 94:418-426.

Gil-Vernet JM: Uretero-vesicoplastie sous-muqueuse: Modification a la technique de Boari. *J Urol Med Chir* 1969; 65:504.

Gil-Vernet JM, Escarpenter JM, Perez-Trujillo G, et al: A functioning artificial bladder: Results of 41 consecutive cases. *J Urol* 1962; 87:825-836.

Gittes RF: Bladder augmentation procedures. In Libertino JA, Zinman L (eds): *Reconstructive urologic surgery: Pediatric and Adult*. Baltimore, Williams & Wilkins Co, 1977, 216-226.

Gittes RF: Carcinogenesis in ureterosigmoidostomy. *Urol Clin N Amer* 1986; 13:201-205.

Gittes RF, Loughlin KR: No incision urethropexy for stress incontinence under local anesthesia (abstract 429). *J Urol* 1988; 139(part 2):270.

Ginsberg D, Huffman JL, Lieskovsky, et al: Urinary tract stones: a complication of the Koch pouch continent urinary diversion. *J Urol* 1991; 145:956-959.

Glass N, Uehling D, Sollinger H, et al: Renal transplantation using ileal conduits in 5 cases. *J Urol* 1985; 133:666-668.

Gleason DM, Gittes RF, Bottaccini MR, et al: Energy balance of voiding after cecal cystoplasty. *J Urol* 1972; 108:259-264.

Gold BD, Bhoopalam PS, Reifen RM, et al: Gastrointestinal complications of gastrocystoplasty. *Arch Dis Child* 1992; 67:1272-1276.

Gold M, Swartz JS, Braude BM: Intraoperative anaphylaxis: an association with latex sensitivity. *J Allergy Clin Immunol*, 1991; 87(3):662-666.

Goldwasser B, Barrett DM, Webster GD, et al: Cystometric properties of ileum and right colon after bladder augmentation, substitution or replacement. *J Urol* 1987; 138:1007.

Goldwasser HR, Webster GD: Augmentation and substitution enterocystoplasty. *J Urol* 1986; 135:215.

Golimbu M, Morales P: Electrolyte disturbances in jejunal urinary diversion, *Urology* 1973; 1:432-438.

Golimbu M, Morales P: Jejunal conduits: technique and complications. *J Urol* 1975; 113:787.

Gonzalez R, Koleilat N, Austin C, et al: The artificial sphincter AS800 in congenital urinary incontinence. *J Urol* 1989; 142:512-515.

Gonzalez R, LaPointe S, Sheldon CA, et al: Undiversion in children with renal failure. *J Pediatr Surg* 1984; 19:632-636.

Gonzalez R, Nguyen DH, Koleilat N, et al: Compatibility of enterocystoplasty and the artificial urinary sphincter. *J Urol* 1989; 142:502-504.

Gonzalez R, Sidi AA: Preoperative prediction of continence after enterocytoplasty or undiversion in children with neurogenic bladder. *J Urol* 1985; 134:705-707.

Goodwin WE, Harris AP, Kaufman JJ, et al: Open, transcolonic ureterointestinal anastomosis: A new approach. *Surg Gynecol Obstet* 1953; 97:295.

Goodwin WE, Winter CC: Techniques of sigmoidocystoplasty. *Surg Gynecol Obstet* 1959; 108:370.

Goodwin WE, Winter CC, Turner RD: Replacement of the ureter by small intestine: Clinical application and results of the 'ileal ureter.' *J Urol* 1959; 81:406.

Gosalbez R, Woodard JR, Broecker BH, et al: Metabolic complications of the use of stomach for urinary reconstruction. *J Urol* 1993; 150:710-712.

Grafter U, Kraut JA, Lee DB, et al: Effect of metabolic acidosis on intestinal absorption of calcium and phosphorus. *Am J Phys* 1980; 239:6480.

Graham SD, Culley CC, Anderson EE: Long-term results with the Kaufman prosthesis. *J Urol* 1982; 128:328.

Gregoir W: Le tratement chirurgical de reflux vesicoureteral congenital. *Acta Chir Belg* 1964; 63:431.

Griffith DP: Urease stones. *Urol Res* 1979; 7:215.

Groenewegen AAM, Sukhal RN, Nauta J, et al: Results of Renal Transplantation in boys treated for posterior urethral valves. *J Urol* 1993; 149:1517-1520.

Guttmann L, Frankel H: Value of intermittent self-catheterization in early management of traumatic paraplegia and tetraplegia. *Paraplegia* 1966; 4:63.

Hadley HR, Zimmern PE, Staskin DR, et al: Transvaginal needle bladder neck suspension. *Urol Clin North Am* 1985; 12:291-303.

Hakelius L, Gieruip J, Grotte G, et al: A new treatment of anal incontinence in children: Free autogenous muscle transplantation. *J Pediatr Surg* 1978; 13:77.

Hall MC, Koch MO, McDougal WS: Metabolic consequences of urinary diversion through intestinal segment. *Urol Clin North Am* 1991; 18:4:725-735.

Halpern GN, King LR, Belman AB: Transureteroureterostomy in children. *J Urol* 1973; 109:504.

Hanna M, Bloiso G: Continence diversion in children: modification of the Kock pouch. *J Urol* 1987; 137:1206-1208.

Harmon WE, Alexander SR, Tejani A, et al: The effect of donor age on graft survival in pediatric cadaver renal transplant recipients: a report of the North American Pediatric Renal Transplant Cooperative Study. *Transplantation* 1992; 54:232-2137.

Harmon WE, Stablein D, Alexander SR, et al: Graft thrombosis in pediatric renal transplant recipients: a report of the North American pediatric renal transplant cooperative study. *Transplantation* 1991; 51:406-412.

Harris SH: Reconstruction of the female urethra. *Surg Gynecol Obstet* 1935; 61:366.

Harrison AR: Clinical and metabolic observations on osteomalacia following ureterosigmoidostomy. *Br J Urol* 1958; 30:455-461.

Hautmann R, Miller K, Steiner U, et al: The ideal neobladder: 6 years of experience with more than 200 patients. *J Urol* 1993; 150:40-45.

Hawthorne NJ, Zincke H, Kelalis PP: Ureterocalicostomy: An alternative to nephrectomy. *J Urol* 1976; 115:583.

Heaney JA, Althausen AF, Parkhurst EC: Ileal conduit undiversion: Experiment with tunneled vesical implantation of tapered conduit. *J Urol* 1980; 124:329-333.

Hendren WH: Reconstruction of previously diverted urinary tracts in children. *J Pediatr Surg* 1973; 8:135-150.

Hendren WH: Urinary tract refunctionalization after prior diversion in children. *Ann Surg* 1974; 180:494.

Hendren WH: Exstrophy of the bladder: alternative method of management. *J Urol* 1976; 115:195-202.

Hendren WH: Reconstruction of the long diverted urinary tract. *Surg Annu* 1976; 8:335-366.

Hendren WH: Some alternatives to urinary diversion in children. *J Urol* 1978a; 119:652-660.

Hendren WH: Tapered bowel segment for ureteral replacement. *Urol Clin North Am* 1978b; 5:607-616.

Hendren WH: Construction of female urethra from vaginal wall and a perineal flap. *J Urol* 1980a; 123:657-664.

Hendren WH: Reoperative ureteral reimplantation: Management of the difficult case. *J Pediatr Surg* 1980b; 15:770.

Hendren WH: Urinary tract refunctionalization after long-term diversion. *Ann Surg* 1990; 212:478-495.

Hendren WH, Hensle TW: Transureteroureterostomy: Experience with 75 cases. *J Urol* 1980; 123:826.

Hendren WH, McLorie GA: Late stricture of intestinal ureter. *J Urol* 1983; 129:584-590.

Henriet MP, Neyra P, Elman B: Kock pouch procedures: continuing experience in evolution in 135 cases. *J Urol* 1991; 145:16-20.

Hensle TW, Burbige KA: Bladder replacement in children and young adults. *J Urol* 1985; 133:1004-1010.

Hensle TW, Connor J, Burbridge KA: Continent urinary diversion in childhood. *J Urol* 1990; 143:981-983.

Herschorn S, Radomski SB: Fascial slings and bladder neck tapering in the treatment of male neurogenic incontinence. *J Urol* 1992; 147:1073-1075.

Hinman F Jr: Selection of intestinal segments for bladder substitution: Physical and physiological characteristics. *J Urol* 1988; 139:519.

Hinman F Jr: Functional classification of conduits for continent diversion. *J Urol* 1990; 144:27-29.

Hinman F, Weyrauch HMJ: A critical study of the different principles of surgery which have been used in ureterointestinal implantation. *Int Abstr Surg* 1937; 64:313.

Hobbs SA, Sexson SB: Cognitive development and learning in the pediatric organ transplant recipient. *J Learning Disabilities* 1993; 26:104-113.

Hodges CV, Barry JM, Fuchs EF, et al: Transureteroureterostomy: Twenty-five year experiences with 100 patients. *J Urol* 1980; 123:834.

Hodges CV, Moore RJ, Lehman TH, et al: Clinical experiences with transuretero-ureterostomy. *J Urol* 1963; 90:552.

Hollowell JG, Hill PD, Duffy PG, et al: Bladder function and dysfunction in exstrophy and epispadias. *Lancet* 1991; 338:926-928.

Hollowell JG, Ransley PG: Surgical management of incontinence in bladder exstrophy. *Br J Urol* 1991; 68:543-548.

Homsy YL, Reid EC: Ileocystoplasty. *Urology* 1974; 4:135.

Horton CE, Politano V: Ureteral reconstruction with split skin grafts: An experimental study. *Plast Reconstr Surg* 1955; 15:261.

Hossain M, MB., BS (Dacca): The osteomalacia syndrome after colocystoplasty; a cure with sodium bicarbonate alone. *J Urol* 1970; 42:243-245.

Hovnanian AP, Javadpour N, Gruhn JG: Reconstruction of the ureter by free autologous bladder mucosa graft. *J Urol* 1956; 93:455.

Hovnanian AP, Kingsley IA: Reconstruction of the ureter by free autologous bladder mucosa graft. *J Urol* 1966; 96:167.

Hradec EA: Bladder substitution: Indications and results in 114 operations. *J Urol* 1965; 94:406.

Husmann DA, Spence HM: Current status of tumor of the bowel following ureterosigmoidostomy: A review. *J Urol* 1990; 144:607-610.

Hutch JA: Vesicoureteral reflux in the paraplegic: Cause and correction. *J Urol* 1952; 68:457.

Ismail-Allouch M, Burke G, Nery J: Kidney transplantation in the pediatric age group: University of Miami Experience. *Transplantation Proceedings,* 1993; 25:2166.

Jacobs SC, Gittes RF: Dissolution of residual renal calculi with hemiacidrin. *J Urol* 1976; 115:2.

Jahnson S, Pedersen J: Cystectomy and urinary diversion during twenty years: complications and metabolic implications. *Eur Urol* 1993; 24:343-349.

Jameson SG, McKinney JS, Rushton JF: Ureterocalycostomy: A new surgical procedure for correction of ureteropelvic stricture associated with an intrarenal pelvis. *J Urol* 1957; 77:135.

Jeffs RD: Analysis of 144 patients with bladder exstrophy treated at The Johns Hopkins Hospital from 1975 to 1985 (abstract 151). AUA Meeting, New York, 1986.

Jeffs RD, Lepor H: Management of the exstrophy/epispadias complex. In Harrison JH, et al. (eds): Campbell's Etiology. 5th ed, Philadelphia, WB Saunders Co, 1986, p 1902.

Jones DA, Holden D, George NJR: Mechanism of upper tract dilatation in patients with thick-walled bladders, chronic retention of urine and associated hydroureteronephrosis. *J Urol* 1988; 140:326-329.

Juma S, Morales A, Emerson L: The mechanisms of continence in the Indiana pouch: A video-urodynamic study. *J Urol* 1990; 143:973-974.

Jumper BM, McLorie GA, Churchill BM, et al: Effects of the artificial urinary sphincter on prostatic development and sexual function in pubertal boys with meningomyelocele. *J Urol* 1990; 144:438-444.

Kabler RI, Cerny JC: Pre-transplant urologic investigation and treatment of end-stage renal disease. *J Urol* 1983; 129:475-479.

Kalble T, Tricker AR, Berger M, et al: Tumor induction in a rat model for ureterosigmoidostomy without evidence of nitrosamine formation. *J Urol* 1991; 146:862-866.

Kaleli A, Ansell JS: The artificial bladder: A historical review. *Urology* 1984; 14:423-428.

Kashi SH, Lodge JPA, Giles GR, et al: Ureteric complications of renal transplantation. *Br J Urol* 1992; 70:139-143.

Kass EJ, Koff SA: Bladder augmentation in the pediatric neuropathic bladder. *J Urol* 1983; 129:552-555.

Kass EJ, McHugh T, Diokno AC: Intermittent catheterization in children less than 6 years old. *J Urol* 1979; 121:792.

Kaufman JJ: A new operation for male incontinence. *Surg Gynecol Obstet* 1970; 131:295.

Kaufman JJ: Surgical treatment of post-prostatectomy incontinence: Use of the penile crura to compress the bulbous urethra. *J Urol* 1972; 107:293.

Kaufman JJ: Treatment of post-prostatectomy incontinence using a silicone-gel prosthesis. *Br J Urol* 1973; 45:646.

Keetch DW, Basler JW, Kavoussi LR: Modification of Mitrofanoff principle for continent urinary diversion. *Urology* 1993; 41:507-510.

Kelami A, Fiedler U, Schmidt V, et al: Replacement of the ureter using the urinary bladder. *Urol Res* 1973; 1:161.

Kelly HA: Incontinence of urine in women. *Urol Cutan Rev* 1913; 19:291.

Kennedy H, Adams M, Mitchell M, et al: Chronic renal failure and bladder augmentation: stomach versus sigmoid colon in canine model. *J Urol* 1988; 140:1138-1140.

Keshin JG, Fitzpatrick TJ: A new technique for urinary diversion using a full thickness skin tube as a conduit. *J Urol* 1962; 88:631.

Kheradpir MH: Neo-ureter made from renal pelvis—a new method for treatment of giant hydronephrosis. *Z Kinderchir* 1983; 38:361-362.

Kim K, Susskind M, King L: Ileocecal ureterosigmoidostomy: an alternative to conventional ureterosigmoidostomy. *J Urol* 1988; 140:1494-1498.

Kim MS, Jabs K, Harmon WE: Long-term patient survival in a pediatric renal transplantation program. *Transplantation* 1991; 51:413-417.

Kinahan TJ, Khoury AE, McLorie G, et al: Imepragal in post-gastrocystoplasty metabolic alkalosia and acidura. *J Urol* 1992; 147:435-437.

King LR: Protection of upper tracts in undiversion. In King LR, Stone AR, Webster GD (eds): *Bladder Reconstruction and Continent Urinary Diversion*. Chicago, Year–Book Medical Publishers, 1987, pp 127-153.

King LR, Robertson CN, Bertram RA: A new technique for the prevention of reflux in those undergoing bladder substitution or undiversion using bowel segments. *World J Urol* 1985; 3:194-196.

Klauber GT, Williams DI: Epispadias with incontinence. *J Urol* 1974; 111:110-113.

Klein EA, Montie JE, Montague D, et al: Jejunal conduit urinary diversion. *J Urol* 1986; 135:244.

Koch MO, McDougal WS: Nicotinic acid: Treatment for the hyperchloremic acidosis following urinary diversion through intestinal segments. *J Urol* 1985; 134:162-164.

Kock NG: Intra-abdominal 'reservoir' in patients with permanent ileostomy: Preliminary observations on a procedure resulting in fecal 'continence' in five ileostomy patients. *Arch Surg* 1969; 99:223.

Kock NG, Ghoneim M, Lyche K: Replacement of the bladder by the urethral Kock pouch: functional results, urodynamics, and radiological features. *J Urol* 1989; 141:1111-1119.

Kock NG, Norlen LJ, Philipson BM: Management of complications after construction of a continent ileal reservoir for urinary diversion. *World J Urol* 1985b; 3:152-154.

Kock NG, Norlen L, Philipson BM, et al: The continent ileal reservoir (Koch pouch) for urinary diversion. *World J Urol* 1985a; 3:146-151.

Koff SA: The abdominal neourethra in children: Technique and long-term results. *J Urol* 1985; 133:244-247.

Koff SA: Guidelines to determine the size and shape of intestinal segments used for reconstruction. *J Urol* 1988; 140:1150-1151.

Koff SA: A technique for bladder neck reconstruction in exstrophy: The Cinch. *J Urol* 1990; 144:546-549.

Koff SA, Lapides J, Piazza DH: Association of urinary tract infection and reflux with uninhibited bladder contractions and voluntary sphincteric obstruction. *J Urol* 1979; 122:373-376.

Koff SA, Murtagh DS: The uninhibited bladder in children: Effect of treatment on recurrence of urinary infection and on vesicoureteral reflux resolution. *J Urol* 1983; 130:1138-1141.

Kramer SA, Kelalis PP: Assessment of urinary continence in epispadias: Review of 94 patients. *J Urol* 1982; 128:290-293.

Krantz KE: The Marshall-Marchetti-Krantz procedure. In Stanton SL, Tanagho EA (eds): *Surgery of Female Incontinence*. New York, Springer-Verlag, 1980.

Kreder KJ, Webster GD: Management of the bladder outlet in patients requiring enterocystoplasty. *J Urol* 1992; 147:38-41.

Kreder KJ, Webster GD, Oakes WJ: Augmentation cystoplasty complicated by postoperative ventriculoperitoneal shunt infection. *J Urol* 1990; 144:955-956.

Kropp KA: Urethral lengthening and reimplantation to create Dryness. In Olsson C (eds): *Surgical Techniques in Urology*. Miles Inc., 1991, pp. 1-8.

Kropp KA, Angwafo FF: Urethral lengthening and reimplantation for neurogenic incontinence in children. *J Urol* 1986; 135:553-536.

Kuss R, Bitker M, Camey M, et al: Indications and early and late results of intestino-cystoplasty: A review of 185 cases. *J Urol* 1970; 103:53.

Kvarstein B, Mathisen W: Sigmoidocystoplasty in adults with enuresis. *Surg Gynecol Obstet* 1981; 153:65-66.

Lapides J: Stricture and function of the internal vesical sphincter. *J Urol* 1958; 80:341-353.

Lapides J, Ajaemian EP, Stewart BH, et al: Further observation on the kinetics of the urethovesical sphincter. *J Urol* 1960; 84:86.

Lapides J, Diokno AC, Gould FR, et al: Further observations on self-catheterization. *J Urol* 1976; 116:169.

Lapides J, Diokno AC, Silber SJ, et al: Clean intermittent self-catheterization in the treatment of urinary tract disease. *J Urol* 1972; 107:458.

Leach GE, O'Donnell P, Raz S: Needle urethral-vesical suspension procedures. In Raz S (ed): *Female Urology*. Philadelphia, WB Saunders Co, 1983.

Leadbetter GW. Urinary incontinence. In Libertino JA Jr, Zinman L (eds): *Reconstructive Urologic Surgery, Pediatric and Adult*. Baltimore, Williams & Wilkins, 1977, p 245.

Leadbetter GW Jr: Surgical correction of total urinary incontinence. *J Urol* 1964; 91:261.

Leadbetter GW Jr: Surgical reconstruction for complete urinary incontinence: a 10- to 22-year follow-up. *J Urol* 1985; 133:205-206.

Leadbetter GW Jr, Zickerman P, Pierce F: Ureterosigmoidostomy and carcinoma of the colon. *J Urol* 1979; 121:5.

Leape LL: Other disorders of the rectum and anus. In Welsh KJ, Randoph JG, Ravitch MM, et al (eds): *Pediatric Surgery*, 4th ed. Yearbook Medical Publishers, 1986, p 1039.

LeDuc A, Camey M, Teillac P: An original antireflux ureteroileal implantation technique: long-term follow-up. *J Urol* 1987; 137:1156-1158.

Lee SW, Russell J, Avioli LV: 25-Hydroxycholecalciferol to 1,25-dihydroxycholecalciferol: conversion impaired by systemic metabolic acidosis. *Science* 1977; V195:994.

Lemann JJ, Litzow JR, Lennon EJ: Studies of the mechanism by which chronic metabolic acidosis augments urinary calcium excretion in man. *J Clin Invest* 1967; 46:1318-1328.

Leong C: Use of the stomach for bladder replacement and urinary diversion. *Ann Roy Coll Surg Engl* 1978; 60:283-289.

Leong C, Ong G: Gastrocytoplasty in dogs. *Aust NZ J Surg* 1972; 41:272-279.

Lepor H, Jeffs RD: Primary bladder closure and bladder neck reconstruction in classical bladder exstrophy. *J Urol* 1983; 130:1142-1145.

Lewis RI, Lockhart JL, Politano VA: Periurethral poly-tetrafluoroethylene injections in incontinent female subjects with neurogenic bladder disease. *J Urol* 1984; 131:459-462.

Light JK: Long-term clinical results using the artificial urinary sphincter around bowel. *Br J Urol* 1989; 64:56-60.

Light JK, Engelmann UH: Reconstruction of the lower urinary tract: Observations on bowel dynamics and the artificial urinary sphincter. *J Urol* 1985; 133:594-597.

Light JK, Engelmann UH: Le Bag: Total replacement of the bladder using a ileocolonic pouch. *J Urol* 1986; 136:27-31.

Light JK, Pietro T: Alternation in detrusor behavior and the effect on renal function following insertion of the artificial urinary sphincter. *J Urol* 1986; 136:632.

Light JK, Scott FB: Treatment of the epispadias-extrophy complex with the AS 792 artificial urinary sphincter. *J Urol* 1983; 129:738.

Light JK, Scott FB: The artificial urinary sphincter in children. *Br J Urol* 1984; 56:54-57.

Lilien OM, Camey M: Twenty-five year experience with replacement of the human bladder (Camey procedure). *J Urol* 1984; 132:886-891.

Liptak GS, Revell GM: Management of bowel dysfunction in children with spinal cord disease or injury by means of the enema continence catheter. *J Pediatr* 1992; 120:190-194.

Lobe TE: Conversion of an ileal conduit into a neourethral enteroplication for urinary continence: Tips in its proper construction. *J Pediatr Surg* 1986; 21:1040.

Lockhart J, Davies R, Cox C, et al: The gastoileal pouch: an alternative continent urinary reservoir for patients with short bowel, acidosis, and/or extensive pelvic radiation. *J Urol* 1993: 150:46-50.

Lome LG, Williams DI: Urinary reconstruction following temporary cutaneous ureterostomy diversion in children. *J Urol* 1972; 108:162.

Lytton B, Schiff M: Interposition of an ileal segment for repair of ureteral injuries. *J Urol* 1981; 125:739.

Mahony JF, Savdie E, Caterson RJ, et al: The natural history of cadaveric renal allografts beyond ten years. *Transplant Proc* 1986; 18:135-137.

Malek RS, Burke EC, Deweerd JH: Ileal conduit urinary diversion in children. *J Urol* 1971; 105:892-900.

Malizia AA, Reiman HM, Myers RP, et al: Migration and granulomatous reaction after periurethral injection of polytef (Teflon). *JAMA* 1984; 251:3277.

Malone PS, Ransley PG, Kiely EM: Preliminary report: the antegrade continence enema. *Lancet* 1990; 336:1217-1218.

Mansson W, Colleen S, Mardh PA: The microbial flora of the continent cecal urinary reservoir, its stoma and the peristomal skin. *J Urol* 1986; 135:247-250.

Mansson W, Colleen S, Sundin T: Continent caecal reservoir in urinary diversion. *Br J Urol* 1984; 56:359-365.

Marshall VG, Marchetti AA, Krantz KE: The correction of stress incontinence by simple vesicourethral suspension. *Surg Gynecol Obstet* 1949; 88:590.

Marshall VG, Whitsell J, McGovern JH, et al: The practicality of renal autotransplantation in humans. *JAMA* 1966; 1966:1154.

Martelli H, Devroede G, Arhan P, et al: Mechanisms of idiopathic constipation: Outlet obstruction. *Gastroenterology* 1978; 75:623.

Martin LW: Use of the appendix to replace a ureter. Case Report. *J Pediatr Surg* 1981; 16:799-800.

Mathew TH: Recurrence of disease following renal transplantation. *Am J Kidney Dis* 1988; 12:85-96.

Mathisen W: Open-loop sigmoido-cystoplasty. *Acta Chir Scand* 1955; 110:227.

McCahill PD, Whittle DI, Jacobs SC: Toxic shock syndrome: A complication of continent urinary diversion. *J Urol* 1992; 147:681-682.

McDermott WV Jr: Diversion of urine to the intestines as a factor in ammoniagenic coma. *N Engl J Med* 1957; 256:460.

McDougal WS: Intestinal ammonium transport by ammonium hydroxide exchange. *J Am Coll Surg* (In press).

McDougal WS: Metabolic complications of urinary intestinal diversion. *J Urol* 1992; 147:1199-1208.

McDougal WS, Koch MO: Effect of sulfate on calcium and magnesium homeostasis following urinary diversion. *Kidney Int* 1989; 35:105.

McDougal WS, Koch MO: Impaired growth and development and urinary intestinal interposition. *Trans Amer Assn Genito-urinary Surg* 1991; 105:3.

McDougal WS, Koch MO, Shands C III, et al: Bony demineralization following urinary intestinal diversion. *J Urol* 1988; 140:853-855.

McEnery PT, Stablein DM, Arbus G, et al: Renal transplantation in children - A report of the North American Pediatric Renal Transplant Cooperative Study. *N Engl J Med* 1992; 326:1727-1732.

McGraw ME, Haka-Ikse K: Neurologic-development sequelae of chronic renal failure in infancy. *J Pediatr* 1983; 106:579.

McGuire EJ: Personal communication, 1986.

McGuire EJ, Wang C, Usitalo H, et al: Modified pubovaginal sling in girls with myelodysplasia. *J Urol* 1986; 135:94-96.

McGuire EJ, Wang S, Appel R, et al: Treatment of urethral incontinence by collagen injection: one-year followup. *J Urol* 1990; 143(2):224A, abstract 142.

McGuire EJ, Woodside JR, Borden TA, et al: Prognostic value of urodynamic testing in myelodysplastic patients. *J Urol* 1981; 126:205-209.

McLeod RS, Fazio VW: Quality of life with the continent ileostomy. *World J Surg* 1984; 8:90-95.

Melnikoff AE: Sur le replacement de l'uretere par une anse isolee de l'intestine grele. *Rev Clin Urol* 1912; 1:601.

Mesrobian HG, Kelalis PP, Kramer SA: Long-term follow-up of 103 patients with bladder exstrophy. *J Urol* 1988; 139:719-722.

Mesrobian HG, Miller CG, Hatchett RL, et al: Modified extravesical ureteral reimplantation in pediatric renal transplantation: 5 years of experience. *J Urol* 1992; 147:1340-1342.

Mevorach RA, Hulbert WC, Merguerian PA, et al: Perforation and intravesical erosion of a ventriculoperitoneal shunt in a child with an augmentation cystoplasty. *J Urol* 1992; 147:433-434.

Middleton AW Jr: Tapered ileum as ureter substitute in severe renal damage: Antireflux technique for bladder implantation. *Urology* 1977; 9:509.

Middleton AW Jr, Hendren WH: Ileal conduits in children at the Massachusetts General Hospital from 1955 to 1970. *J Urol* 1976; 115:591-595.

Millan T: *Retropubic Urinary Surgery*.Baltimore, Williams & Wilkins Co, 1947, p 184.

Mitchell ME: Gastrocystoplasty and bladder replacement with stomach. In Marshall FF (ed): *Operative Urology*. Philadelphia, WB Saunders, 1991, pp 254-255.

Mitchell ME: Use of bowel in undiversion. *Urol Clin North Am* 1986; 13:362.

Mitchell ME, Adams MC, Rink RC: Urethral replacement with ureter. *J Urol* 1988; 139:1282-1285.

Mitchell ME, Piser J: Intestinocytoplasty and total bladder replacement in children and young adults: followup in 129 cases. *J Urol* 1987; 138:579-584.

Mitchell ME, Rink RC: Experience with the artificial urinary sphincter in children and young adults. *J Pediatr Surg* 1983; 18:700-706.

Mitchell ME, Rink RC: Urinary diversion and undiversion. *Urol Clin North Am* 1985; 12:111.

Mitrofanoff P: Cystostomie continente trans-appendiculaire dans le traitement des vessies neurologiques. *Chir Pediatr* 1980; 21:297-305.

Mitrofanoff P, Bonnet O, Annoot MP, et al: Continent urinary diversion using an artificial urinary sphincter. *Br J Urol* 1992; 70:26-29.

Mochon M, Kaiser BA, Dunn S, et al: Urinary tract infections in children with posterior urethral valves after kidney transplantation. *J Urol* 1992; 148:1874-1876.

Mollard P: Bladder reconstruction in exstrophy. *J Urol* 1980; 124:525-529.

Mollard P: Precis D'Urologie de l'Enfant. Paris, Masson Publishing Co. 1984, p. 237.

Mollard P, Jourda R, Valla JS, et al: Colocystoplastie d'agrandissement et de substitution pour vessie neurologique congenitale de l'enfant. *Chir Pediatr* 1983; 24:54.

Monfort G, Guys JN, Lacombe GM: Appendicovesicostomy: An alternative urinary diversion in the child. *Eur Urol* 1984; 10:361-363.

Montague DK: The artificial urinary sphincter (AS800): experience in 166 consecutive patients. *J Urol* 1992; 147:380-382.

Montie JE, MacGregor PS, Fazio VW, et al: Continent ileal urinary reservoir (Koch pouch). *Urol Clin North Am* 1986; 13:251.

Moore EV, Weber R, Woodard ER, et al: Isolated ileal loops for ureteral repair. *Surg Gynecol Obstet* 1956; 102:87.

Mundy AR: A technique for total substitution of the lower urinary tract without the use of a prosthesis. *Br J Urol* 1988; 62:334-338.

Mundy AR: Urethral substitution in women. *Br J Urol* 1989; 63:80-83.

Mundy AR, Nurse DE: Calcium balance, growth and skeletal mineralisation in patients with cystoplasties. *Br J Urol* 1992; 69:257-259.

Najarian JS, Frey DJ, Matas AJ, et al: Successful kidney transplantation in infants. *Transplantation Proceedings* 1991; 23:1382-1383.

Nelson EW, Kessler R, Holman JM: Surgical complications in pediatric renal transplantation. *Transplantation Proceedings* 1989; 21:2006-2007.

Neuwirk K: Implantation of the ureter into the lower calyx of the renal pelvis. In *VII Congres de la Societe Internationale de'Urologie*, part 2. 1947, pp 253-255.

Nguyen DH, Bain M, Salmonson K, et al: The syndrome of dysuria and hematuria in pediatric urinary reconstruction with stomach. *J Urol* 1993; 150:707-709.

Nguyen DH, Burns MW, Shapiro GG, et al: Intraoperative cardiovascular collapse secondary to latex allergy. *J Urol* 1991; 146:571-574.

Noe HN: The role of dysfunctional voiding in failure or complication of ureteral reimplantation for primary reflux. *J Urol* 1985; V134:1172-1175.

Nordling J, Meyhoff HH: Dissociation of urethral and anal sphincter activity in neurogenic bladder dysfunction. *J Urol* 1978; 122:352-356.

Novick AC, Jackson CL, Straffon RA: The role of renal autotransplantation in complex urological reconstruction. *J Urol* 1990; 143:452-457.

Nurse DE, Mundy AR: Metabolic complications of cystoplasty. 1989; 63:165-170.

Ockerblad NF: Reimplantation of the ureter into the bladder by a flap method. *J Urol* 1947; 57:845.

Offner G, Aschendorff C, Hoyer PF, et al: End-stage renal failure 14 years experience of dialysis and renal transplantation. *Arch Dis Child* 1988;63:120-126.

Olsson CA: Cecal reservoirs for continent urinary diversion: Editorial comments: Urinary diversion. *World J Urol* 1985a; 3:197-n-198.

Olsson CA: The Camey procedure: Editorial comments: Urinary diversion. *World J Urol* 1985b; 3:172.

Pagano F, et al: The vesica ileale padovana. In Holenfellner P, Wammack R (eds): *Continent urinary diversion*. Churchill Livingstone Edinburgh, 1992; p 122.

Parra R: A simplified technique for continent urinary diversion: an all-stapled colonic reservoir. *J Urol* 1991; 146:1496-1499.

Pasquariello CA, Lowe DA, Schwartz RE: Experience and reason-briefly recorded. Intraoperative anaphylaxis to latex. *Pediatrics* 1993; 91:983-986.

Peacock EE Jr, Van Winkle W Jr: *Surgery and Biology of Wound Repair*. Philadelphia, WB Saunders Co. 1970, p 601.

Pereyra AJ: A simplified surgical procedure for the correction of stress incontinence in women. *West J Surg* 1959; 65:223.

Perez-Marrero R, Dimmock W, Churchill BM, et al: Clean intermittent catheterization in myelomeningocele children less than 3 years old. *J Urol* 1982; 128:779-781.

Perlmutter AD, Weinstein MD, Reitelman C: Vesical neck reconstruction in patients with epispadias-exstrophy complex. *J Urol* 1991; 146:613-615.

Perry W, Allen LN, Stamp TCB, Walker PG: Vitamin D resistance in osteomalacia after ureterosigmoidostomy. *N Engl J Med* 1977; 297:1110-1112.

Pickrel K, Georgiade N, Richard ER, et al: Gracilis muscle transplant for correction of neurogenic incontinence. *Surg Clin North Am* 1959; 39:1405.

Piser J, Mitchell M, Kulb, et al: Gastrocytoplasty and coloscystoplasty in canines: the metabolic consequences of acute saline and acid loading. *J Urol* 1987; 138:1009-1013.

Pittman T, Williams D, Weber TR: The risk of abdominal operations in children with ventriculoperitoneal shunts. *J Pediatr Surg* 1992; 27:1051-1053.

Polinsky MS, Kaiser BA, Stover JB, et al: Neurologic development of children with severe chronic renal failure from infancy. *Pediatr Nephrol* 1987; 1:157-165.

Politano VA: Periurethral polytetrafluoroethylene injection for urinary incontinence. *J Urol* 1982; 127:439.

Politano VA, Small MP, Harper JM, et al: Periurethral Teflon injection for urinary incontinence. *J Urol* 1974; 111:180.

Potter DE, Najarian J, Belzer F, et al: Long-term results of renal transplantation in children. *Kidney Int* 1991; 40:752-756.

Prout GR Jr, Koontz WW Jr: Partial vesical immobilization: An important adjunct to ureteroneocystostomy. *J Urol* 1970; 103:147.

Quinlan DM, Leonard MP, Brendler CB, et al: Use of the benchekroun hydraulic valve as a catheterizable continence mechanism. *J Urol* 1991; 145:1151-1155.

Raffensperger J: The gracilis sling for fecal incontinence. *J Pediatr Surg* 1979; 14:794.

Raz S, Erlich R, Babiarz J, et al: Gastroplasty without opening the stomach. *J Urol* 1993; 150:713-715.

Reddy P, Lange P, Fraley E: Total bladder replacement using detubularized sigmoid colon: technique and results. *J Urol* 1991; 145:51-55.

Reinberg Y, Gonzalez R, Fryd D, et al: The outcome of renal transplantation in children with posterior urethral valves. *J Urol* 1988; 140:1491-1493.

Reinberg Y, Manivel JC, Froemming C: Perforation of the gastric segment of an augmented bladder secondary to peptic ulcer disease. *J Urol* 1992; 148:369-371.

Reinberg Y, Manivel JC, Fryd D, et al: The outcome of renal transplantation in children with the prune belly syndrome. *J Urol* 1989; 142:1541-1542.

Reisman EM, Preminger GM: Bladder perforation secondary to clean intermittent catheterization. *J Urol* 1989; 142:1316-1317.

Rendleman DF, Anthony JE, Davis C Jr, et al: Reflux pressure studies on the ileocecal valve of dogs and humans. *Surgery* 1958; 44:640-643.

Richie JP, Skinner DG, Waisman J: The effect of reflux on the development of pyelonephritis in urinary diversion: An experimental study. *J Surg Res* 1974; 16:256.

Rittenberg MH, Hulbert WC, Snyder HM III, et al: Protective factors in posterior urethral valves. *J Urol* 1988; 140:993-996.

Robertson GN, King L: Bladder substitution in children. *Urol Clin North Am* 1986; 13:333.

Rosen M: The Rosen inflatable incontinence prosthesis: Symposium on male incontinence. *Urol Clin North Am* 1978; 5:405.

Rosen MA, Light JK: Spontaneous bladder rupture following augmentation enterocystoplasty. *J Urol* 1991; 146:1232-1234.

Rosenberg ML, Dahl GA: Autogenous vein grafts and venous valves in ureteral surgery: An experimental study. *J Urol* 1953; 70:434.

Rotundo A, Nevins T, Lipton M, et al: Progressive encephalopathy in children with chronic renal insufficiency in infancy. *Kidney Intern* 1982; 21:486.

Rowland RG, Bihrle R, Mitchell ME: The Indiana continent urinary reservoir. *J Urol* 1987; 137:1136.

Rowland RG, Mitchell ME, Bihrle R: The cecoileal continent urinary reservoir. *World J Urol* 1985; 3:185-190.

Rowland R, Regan F: The risk of secondary malignancies in urinary reservoirs. In Hohenfellner R, Wammack R (eds): *Continent Urinary Diversion*. New York, Churchill-Livingstone, 1992; pp 299-308.

Rubin SW: The formation of an artificial urinary bladder with perfect continence: An experimental study. *J Urol* 1948; 60:874-906.

Rushton HG, Woodard JR, Parrott TS, et al: Delayed bladder rupture after augmentation enterocystoplasty. *J Urol* 1988; 140:344.

Salahudeen AK, Elliott RW, Ellis HA: Osteomalacia due to ileal replacement of ureters: report of 2 cases. *J Urol* 1984; 131:335-337.

Salisz JA, Diokno AC: The management of injuries to the urethra, bladder or vagina encountered during difficult placement of the artificial urinary sphincter in the female patient. *J Urol* 1992; 148:1528-1530.

Sandoz IL, Pauli DP, MacFarlane CA: Complications with transureteroureterostomy. *J Urol* 1977; 117:39.

Schein CH, Sanders AR, Hurwitt ES: Experimental reconstruction of the ureters. *Arch Surg* 1956; 73:47.

Schmidbauer C, Humberto C, Raz S: The impact of detubularization on ileal reservoirs. *J Urol* 1987; 138:1440-1445.

Schneider KM, Ewing RS, Signer RD: The continent vesicostomy. *J Pediatr Surg* 1975a; 10:221-224.

Schneider KM, Reid RE, Fruchtman B: The continent vesicostomy: Clinical experiences in the adult. *J Urol* 1977; 117:571.

Schneider KM, Reid RE, Fruchtman B, et al: Continent vesicostomy: Surgical technique. *Urology* 1975b; 6:741.

Scholotmeijer RJ, vanMastrigt R: The effect of oxyphenonium bromide and oxygutynin hydrochloride on detrusor contractility and reflux in children with vesicoureteral reflux and detrusor instability. *J Urol* 1991; 146:660-662.

Scott FB, Bradley WE, Timm GW: Treatment of urinary incontinence by an implantable prosthetic urinary sphincter. *J Urol* 1974; 112:75-80.

Sewell WH: Failure of freeze-dried homologous arteries used as arterial grafts. *J Urol* 1955; 74:600.

Sexton GL: Epiurethral suprapubic vaginal suspension. In Slate WG (ed): *Disorders of the Female Urethra and Urinary Incontinence*. Baltimore, Williams & Wilkins Co, 1978, pp 160-173.

Shandling B, Desjardins JG: Anal myomectomy for constipation. *J Pediatr Surg* 1979;4:115.

Shandling B, Gilmour RF: The enema continence catheter in spina bifida: Successful bowel management. *J Pediatr Surg* 1987; 22:271-273.

Shands C III, McDougal WS, Wright EP: Prevention of cancer at the urothelial enteric anastomotic site. *J Urol* 1989; 141:178-181.

Shapiro SR, Lebowitz R, Colondny AH: Fate of 90 children with ileal conduit urinary diversion of a decade later: Analysis of complications, pyelography, renal function and bacteriology. *J Urol* 1975; 114:289.

Sharer K, Gilli G: Growth in children with chronic renal insufficiency, in Fine RN, Grusken AB (eds): *End-Stage Renal Disease in Children*. WB Saunders Co, Philadelphia, 1984, pp 271-290.

Sheiner JR, Kaplan GW: Spontaneous bladder rupture following enterocystoplasty. *J Urol* 1988; 140:1157-1158.

Sheldon CA, Churchill BM, Khoury AE, et al: Complications of surgical significance in pediatric renal transplantation. *J Pediatr Surg* 1992a; 27:485-490.

Sheldon CA, Churchill BM, McLorie GA, et al: Evaluation of factors contributing to mortality in pediatric renal transplant recipients. *J Pediatr Surg* 1992b; 27:629-633.

Sheldon CA, Geary DF, Shely EA, et al: Surgical considerations in childhood end-stage renal disease. *Ped Clin North Am* 1987; 34:1187.

Sheldon CA, Gilbert A: Use of the appendix for urethral reconstruction in children with congenital anomalies of the bladder. *Surgery* 1992; 112:805-812.

Sheldon CA, Gilbert A, Lewis AG, et al: Important surgical implications of genitourinary tract anomalies in the management of the imperforate anus. *J Urol* 1994; 152:196-199.

Sheldon CA, Gilbert A, Wacksman J, et al: Gastrocystoplasty: Technical and metabolic characteristics of the most versatile childhood bladder augmentation modality. *J Ped Surg* 1995: 30:283-288.

Sheldon CA, Gonzalez R, Burns MW, et al. Renal transplantation into the dysfunctional bladder: The role of adjunctive bladder reconstruction. *J Urol* 1994; 152:972-975.

Sheldon CA, Martin L, Churchill B: Surgical perspectives in pediatric renal transplant. In Gillenwater J, Grayhack J, Howard S, et al (eds): *Adult and Pediatric Urology*, 1991 St. Louis, Mosby, pp 2301-2342.

Sheldon CA, McKinley RD, Hartig PR, et al: Carcinoma at the site of ureterosigmoidostomy. *J Dis Colon, Rectum* 1983; 26:55.

Sheldon CA, Reeves D, Lewis AG. Oxybutynin administration diminishes high gastric muscular tone associated with bladder reconstruction. *J Urol* 1995; 153:461-462.

Shirley SW, Mirelman S: Experiences with colocystoplasties, cecocystoplasties and ileocystoplasties in urologic surgery: Forty patients. *J Urol* 1978; 120:165-168.

Shokeir AA, Shamaa MA, Bakr MA, et al: Ileal ureter in renal transplant recipients. *Transplantation Proceedings* 1993; 25:2339-2340.

Sida AA, Sinha B, Gonzalez R: Treatment of urinary incontinence with an artificial sphincter: Further experience with the AS791/792 device. *J Urol* 1984; 131:891.

Siklos P, Davie M, Jung RT, et al: Osteomalacia in ureterosigmoidostomy; healing by correction of the acidosis. *Br J Urol* 1990; 52:61-62.

Sinaiko E: Artificial bladder from gastric pouch. *Surg Gynecol Obstet*, 1960; 111:155-162.

Sinaiko E: Artificial bladder from segment of stomach and study of effect of urine on gastric secretion. *Surg Gynecol Obstet* 1956; 102:433-438.

Skinner DG, Boyd SD, Lieskovsky G: Clinical experience with the Koch continent ileal reservoir for urinary diversion. *J Urol* 1984b: 132:1101-1107.

Skinner DG, Lieskovsky G, Boyd SD: Technique of creation of continent internal ileal reservoir (Koch pouch) for urinary diversion. *Urol Clin North Am* 1984a; 11:741-749.

Skinner DG, Lieskovsky G, Boyd SD: Continuing experience with the continent ileal reservoir (Koch pouch) as an alternative to cutaneous diversion: An update after 250 cases. *J Urol* 1987; 137:1140-1145.

Slater JE: Rubber anaphylaxis. *N Engl J Med* 1989; 320:1126-1130.

Slater JE, Mostello LA, Shaer C: Rubber-specific IgE in children with spina bifida. *J Urol* 1991; 146:578-579.

Smart WR: An evaluation of intubation ureterotomy with description of surgical technique. *J Urol* 1961; 85:512.

Smith RB, Van Cangh P, Skinner DG, et al: Augmentation enterocystoplasty: A critical review. *J Urol* 1977; 118:35-39.

So SKS, Mahan JD, Mauer SM, et al: Hickman catheter for pediatric hemodialysis: A 3-year experience. *Trans Am Soc Artif Intern Organs* 1984; 30:619.

Specht EE: Rickets following ureterosigmoidostomy and chronic hyperchloremia. *J Bone Joint Surg* 1967; 49A:1422-1430.

Spence HM, Hoffman WW, Pate VA: Exstrophy of the bladder: Long-term results in 37 patients treated by ureterosigmoidostomy. *J Urol* 1975; 114:133.

Squire R, Kiely EM, Carr B, et al: The clinical application of the malone antegrade colonic enema. *J Pediatr Surg* 1993; 28:1012-1015.

Stamey TA: Endoscopic suspension of the vesical neck for urinary incontinence. *Surg Gynecol Obstet* 1973; 136:547.

Stamey TA: Endoscopic suspension of the vesical neck for urinary incontinence in females: Report of 203 consecutive patients. *Ann Surg* 1980; 192:465.

Stanton SL, Cardozo L: Results of colposuspension operation for incontinence and prolapse. *Br J Obstet Gynecol* 1979; 86:693.

Starling JR, Uehling DT, Gilchrist KW: Value of colonoscopy after ureterosigmoidostomy. *Surgery* 1984; 96:784.

Steiner MS, Morton RA: Nutritional and gastrointestinal complications of the use of bowel segments in the lower urinary tract. *Urol Clin North Am* 1991; 18:743-754.

Stephens FD: A form of stress incontinence in children: Another method of repair. *Aust N Z J Surg* 1970; 40:125.

Stewart BH, Banowsky LH, Hewitt CB, et al: Renal autotransplantation: Current perspectives. *J Urol* 1977; 118:197.

Stewart M, Macrae A, Williams CB: Neoplasia and ureterosigmoidostomy: a colonoscopy survey. *Br J Surg* 1982; 69:414-416.

Strawbridge LR, Kramer SA, Castillo OA, et al: Augmentation cystoplasty and the artificial genitourinary sphincter. *J Urol* 1989; 142:297-301.

Stribling MD, Cohen MS, Fagan JD, et al: The effect of ascorbic acid on urinary nitrosamines and tumor development in a rat animal model for ureterosigmoidostomy. *J Urol* 1989; 141:304A, abstract 540.

Stockle M, Becht E, Vogers G, et al: Ureterosigmoidostomy: an outdated approach to bladder exstrophy? *J Urol* 1990;143:770-775.

Struthers NW, Scott R: Reconstruction of the upper ureter with colon. *J Urol* 1974; 112:179.

Sullivan H, Gilchrist RK, Merricks JW: Ileocecal substitute bladder: Long-term follow-up. *J Urol* 1973; 109:43-45.

Sumfest JM, Burns MW, Mitchell ME: The Mitrofanoff principle in urinary reconstruction. *J Urol* 1993; 150:1875-1878.

Swenson O, Fisher JH, Cendron J: Megaloureter, investigation as to the cause and report on the results of newer forms of treatment. *Surgery* 1956; 40:223.

Tanagho EA: A case against incorporation of bowel segments into the closed urinary system. *J Urol* 1975; 113:796-802.

Tanagho EA: Bladder neck reconstruction for total urinary incontinence: Ten years of experience. *J Urol* 1981; 125:321-326.

Tanagho EA, Smith DR: The anatomy and function of the bladder neck. *Br J Urol* 1966; 38:54-71.

Tanagho EA, Smith DR, Meyers FH, et al: Mechanism of urinary continence: II. Technique for surgical correction of incontinence. *J Urol* 1969; 101:305.

Tank ES: Clean intermittent self-catheterization in children with bladder-emptying dysfunction. In *Birth Defects: Original Article Series*. New York, Alan R Liss Inc, The National Foundation, 1977, pp 117-121.

Tapper D, Folkman J: Lymphoid depletion in ileal loops: Mechanism and clinical implications. *J Pediatr Surg* 1976; 11:871.

Tejani A, Fine R, Alexander S, et al: Factors predictive of sustained growth in children after renal transplantation. *J Ped* 1993; 122:397-402.

Thomalla JV, Mitchell ME, Leapman SB, et al: Renal transplantation into the reconstructed bladder. *J Urol* 1989; 141:256.

Thompson IM: Repair of ureteropelvic junction and upper ureteral injury with renal capsule flap. *Urol Clin North Am* 1977; 4:45.

Thomsen HS: Pyelorenal backflow. *Danish Med Bull* 1984; 31:348.

Thorne ID, Resnick MI: Use of bowel in urologic surgery: A historical review. *Urol Clin North Am* 1986; 13:179.

Thuroff JW, Alken P, Reidmiller H, et al: The Mainz pouch (mixed augmentation ileum and cecum) for bladder augmentation and continent diversion. *J Urol* 1986; 136:17.

Tobler R, Prader A, Buhlmann A, et al: Rachitis als folge der ureterosigmoidostomie. *Helvet Paediaf Acta* 1957; 12:215-240.

Tosatti E: Relocations of the small and large intestine for substitution of the stomach (and esophagus) and of the urinary bladder (and ureter). *Rass Clin Sci* 1963; 39:233.

Tsulukidze A, Murvanidze D, Davali R, et al: Formation of 'bladder' by a plastic shell after total cystectomy. *Br J Urol* 1964; 36:102.

Turner-Warwick R, Ashken HM: The functional results of partial subtotal and total cystoplasty. *Br J Urol* 1967; 39:3.

Turner-Warwick R, Worth PHH: The psoas bladder-hitch procedure for the replacement of the lower third of the ureter. *Br J Urol* 1969; 41:701.

Vatandaslar F, Reid RE, Freed SZ, et al: Ileal segment replacement of ureter: I. Effects on kidney of refluxing vs nonrefluxing ileovesical anastomosis. *Urology* 1984a; 23:549.

Vatandaslar F, Reid RE, Freed SZ, et al: Ileal segment replacement of ureter: II. Dynamic characteristics of refluxing, nonrefluxing, and totally tapered ileal ureter. *Urology* 1984b; 23:559.

Vinograd I, Merguerian P, Udassin R, et al: An experimental model of a submucosally tunneled valve for the placement of the ileo- cecal valve. *J Pediatr Surg* 1984; 19:726-728.

Wagstaff KE, Woodhouse CJ, Duffy PG, et al: Delayed linear growth in children with enterocystoplasties. *Br J Urol* 1992; 69:314-317.

Wagstaff KE, Woodhouse CJ, Rose GA: Blood and urine analysis in patients with intestinal bladders. *J Urol* 1991; 68:311-316.

Wammack R, et al: The Mainz pouch. In Holenfellner R, Wammack R (eds): *Continent urinary diversion*. Churchill Livingstone Edinburgh, 1992, pp 131-135.

Wan J, McGuire EJ, Blood DA, et al: Stress leak point pressure: A diagnostic tool for incontinence children. *J Urol* 1993; 150:700-702.

Wangensteen OH: Intestinal obstructions, 3rd ed. Springfield, Illinois: Charles C Thomas Publishers, 1955.

Wasnick RJ, Butt KM, Laungani G, et al: Evaluation of anterior extravesical ureteroneocystomy in kidney transplantation. *J Urol* 1981; 126:307.

Waters WB, Whitmore WF, Lage AL, et al: Segmental replacement of the ureter using tapered and nontapered ileum. *Invest Urol* 1981; 18:258.

Wesolowski S: Twenty-year follow-up after uretero-appendico-calicostomy in a solitary kidney. *Eur Urol* 1981; 7:184.

Wespres E, Stone AR, King LR: Ileocaecocystoplasty in urinary tact reconstruction in children. *Br J Urol* 1986; 58:266.

Weston PMT, Morgan JDT, Hussain J, et al: Artificial urinary sphincters around intestinal segments: are they safe? *Br J Urol* 1991; 67:150-154.

White B, Kropp K, Rayport M: Abdominal cerebrospinal fluid pseudocyst: Occurrence after intraperitoneal urological surgery in children with ventriculoperitoneal shunts. *J Urol* 1991; 146:583-587.

Whitehead WE, Parker L, Bosmajian L, et al: Treatment of fecal incontinence in children with spina bifida: Comparison of biofeedback and behavior modification. *Arch Phys Med Rehabil* 1986; 67:218-224.

Whiting SJ, Draper HH: Effects of a chronic acid load as sulfate or sulfur amino acids on bone metabolism in adult rats. *J Nutri* 1981; 111:1721-1726.

Whitmore WF, Gittes RF: Reconstruction of the urinary tract by cecal and ileocecal cystoplasty: Review of a 15-year experience. *J Urol* 1983; 129:494-498.

Williams DI, Snyder HM: Anterior detrusor tube repair for urinary incontinence in children. *Br J Urol* 1976; 48:671-674.

Winter CC, Goodwin WE: Results of sigmoidocystoplasty. *J Urol* 1958; 80:467-472.

Woodard JR, Marshall VF: Reconstruction of the female urethra to reduce posttraumatic incontinence. *Surg Gynecol Obstet* 1961; 113:687.

Woodhouse CRJ: Lower urinary tract reconstruction in young patients. *Br J Urol* 1972; 70:113-120.

Woodhouse CRJ, Malone PR, Cumming J, et al: The Mitrofanoff principle for continent urinary diversion. *Br J Urol* 1989; 63:53-57.

Woodside JR, Borden TA: Suprapubic endoscopic vesical neck suspension for the management of urinary incontinence in myelodysplastic girls. *J Urol* 1986; 135:97.

Yassin MS, Sanyurah S, Lierl MB: Evaluation of latex allergy in patients with meningomyelocele. *Ann-Allergy* 1992; 69(3):207-211.

Young HH: An operation for the cure of incontinence of urine. *Surg Gynecol Obstet* 1919; 28:84.

Young HH: An operation for the cure of incontinence associated with epispadias. *J Urol* 1922; 7:1.

Zabbo H, Kay R: Ureterosigmoidostomy and bladder exstrophy: a long-term follow-up. *J Urol* 1986; 136:396.

Zaragoza MR, Ritchey ML, Bloom DA, et al: Enterocytoplasty in renal transplantation candidates: urodynamic evaluation and outcome. *J Urol* 1993; 1463-1466.

Zincke H, Segura J: Ureterosigmoidostomy: a critical review of 173 cases. *J Urol* 1975; 113:324-327.

Zingg E, Tscholl R: Continent cecoileal conduit: Preliminary report. *J Urol* 1977; 118:724-728.

Zinman L, Libertino JA: The ileo-cecal conduit for temporary and permanent urinary diversion. *J Urol* 1975; 113:417.

Zinman L, Libertino JA: Anti-refluxing ileocecal conduit. *Urol Clin North Am* 1980a; 7:503.

Zinman L, Libertino JA: Technique of augmentation cecocystoplasty. *Urol Clin North Am* 1980b; 60:703.

Zinman L, Libertino JA: Right colocystoplasty for bladder replacement. *Urol Clin North Am* 1986; 13:321.

CHAPTER 51

Urethral Lesions in Infants and Children

Grahame H. H. Smith
John W. Duckett

Anomalies of the urethra include both congenital and acquired lesions. Hypospadias is the commonest congenital urethral lesion and is dealt with in Chapter 55. Obstruction of the urethra is primarily a disease of the male, resulting from lesions such as posterior urethral valves, anterior urethral valves, polyps, and strictures. Urethral strictures in children are often related to previous hypospadias surgery or to trauma; they are also dealt with elsewhere in this text. Lesions causing urethral obstruction in the female are rare and include ureteroceles, hypospadias, and cloacal abnormalities. In the early years of the specialty of pediatric urology, bladder neck contractures, bladder neck stenosis, and urethral stenosis were popular diagnoses. Various procedures were devised to improve urinary flow through the bladder neck and urethra, including Y-V bladder neck plasty and urethral dilatation. These diagnoses have since passed into history and given way to the concepts of dysfunctional voiding and non-neurogenic bladder dysfunction.

Urethral lesions tend to cause nonspecific symptoms including dysuria, frequency, poor stream, incontinence, and terminal hematuria. The gold standard for diagnosis remains the radiographic voiding and retrograde urethrogram. Ultrasound has begun to show some promise in identifying lesions such as posterior urethral valves, polyps, and urethral strictures; however, it is best used to assess the upper urinary tract. Improvements in miniature pediatric endoscopes continue and allow visualization of the lower urinary tract in all except the smallest premature babies.

POSTERIOR URETHRAL VALVES

Historical Perspective

Prior to the 1960s, most patients with posterior urethral valves (PUV) had a very poor prognosis. Placing a cystostomy tube in the bladder was associated with infection, bladder spasms, contractions around the catheter, and obstruction of the ureterovesical junction (Bueschen et al., 1973; Johnson, 1969). Sepsis was difficult to manage and deterioration was rapid. Various treatment modalities were developed for seriously ill infants with valves. In the 1960s, supravesical diversion became the watchword, with low-loop ureterostomies followed later by high-loop ureterostomies with their various modifications (Johnson, 1963). These were usually done in the face of sepsis and an inflamed bladder. After total diversion of urine from the bladder, it contracted and was difficult to rehabilitate. Subsequent reconstructions were prone to failure.

Although vesicostomies were being used for myelomeningocele patients, this technique was not applied to valves except at The Children's Hospital of Philadelphia (Duckett, 1974b). At the time, valve ablation was limited by the instrumentation of the period. None were small enough for the neonatal urethra, and the optics were poor. Primary open resection was the most successful approach. Perineal urethrostomy with direct visualization and ablation of the valves using an otoscope was described by Johnson (1966). Alternatively, it was necessary to wait until babies were much bigger so that larger instruments could be passed transurethrally.

For extreme upper tract dilatation, total immediate reconstruction was advocated by Hardy Hendren in the mid-1960s (Hendren, 1970), with an extensive reconstructive procedure: ablating the valve, tapering the upper tracts, and reimplanting both ureters. His results were quite encouraging.

In the early 1970s, the new Hopkins-Storz lens system became available and miniaturization of endoscopes much more effective. Primary valve ablation was endoscopically feasible, even in neonates. This made possible a program of primary valve ablation alone with observation. At The Children's Hospital of Philadelphia, we started this program in the early 1970s and reported on the progress of the approach (Carpiniello et al., 1977; Duckett, 1974a, 1979b; Hulbert and Duckett, 1988; Smith et al., 1994a, 1994b). Our philosophy has been to ablate the PUV early and then proceed to watchful waiting. Reconstruction with reimplantation of the ureters or ablative surgery is performed later, as needed. The results of this program have been quite satisfactory.

We also showed that vesicostomy was an equally effective method for tubeless drainage of the bladder, allowing a premature baby or sickly baby an opportunity for bladder drainage rather than high ureteral drainage.

In 1980, Krueger and his colleagues in Toronto evaluated their data and concluded that, in the long run, high diversion reduces renal failure and improves somatic growth (Krueger et al., 1980b). Although these data and the conclusions were vigorously debated at the time and have not held up through the years (Reinberg et al., 1992a), this concept in the management of valves found many advocates.

The effect of abnormal bladder function on renal transplantation in PUV patients was discussed by Marshall in 1982. He felt it was not significant. Churchill and associates (1988) disagreed, as did Reinberg and colleagues (1988), when they indicated that voiding dysfunction significantly compromises transplantation success with reduced graft survival. More recent assessment of their results fails to support this conclusion (Hyacinthe et al., 1995).

It has been our impression, after treating over 200 patients with PUV, that very few have persistent severe bladder dysfunction. We feel that this is due to the fact that 80% have had valve ablation alone, without ever having had a urinary diversion. By keeping the bladders intact, we have had little need for bladder augmentation, nor have we seen deterioration of renal function in later life secondary to voiding dysfunction. These same observations have been confirmed by Hendren (1990) and Monford (1994).

Incidence

A posterior urethral valve is the most common structural cause of urinary outflow obstruction in pediatric practice (Atwell, 1983). It is also the most common type of obstructive uropathy leading to childhood renal failure (Warshaw et al., 1980). PUV obstruction is estimated to occur in 1 of every 5000 to 8000 male births (King, 1985) and constitutes about 10% of prenatally diagnosed hydronephrosis (Brown et al., 1987).

Etiology & Embryology

The cause of PUV remains unclear because suitable material at various stages of development is unavailable. It is possible only to study normal embryogenesis and compare this to the fully developed lesion. The similarity of valves to normal submontal folds suggests that the malformation may be seen in a wide spectrum

(Cornil, 1975; Hendren, 1971). The role of genetic factors in PUV is poorly understood. It may occur in twins (Davidsohn and Newberger, 1933; Grajewski and Glassberg, 1983; Kroovand et al., 1977; Williams and Kapila, 1993) and siblings (Borzi et al., 1992; Crankson and Ahmed, 1993; Doraiswamy et al., 1983; Farkas and Skinner, 1976; Thomalla et al., 1989). It may be inherited across successive generations (Hanlon-Lundberg et al., 1994). The exact mechanisms and pattern of inheritance remain unknown. Very few congenital anomalies of the urethro-trigone area have been reported in association with PUV. Apart from pathological changes in the urinary tract secondary to valvular obstruction, associated abnormalities are rare in affected individuals. Krueger and associates (1980a) have reported 12% cryptorchidism in PUV patients, compared to the 2.7% expected incidence.

At about 6 weeks of gestation, the mesonephric ducts open into the cloaca at Müller's tubercle, the midpoint of the cranial and caudal portions of the primitive urogenital sinus. The primitive urogenital sinus becomes separated from the cloaca by the urorectal septum during the seventh week of gestation. The primitive urogenital sinus divides into a cranial portion, giving rise to the bladder and proximal prostatic urethra, and a caudal portion, giving rise to the definitive urogenital sinus. In the female the entire urethra is a short tube extending from the bladder to Müller's tubercle (Arey, 1965), and the definitive urogenital sinus forms the vestibule. In the male, the definitive urogenital sinus forms the lower prostatic urethra, just below Müller's tubercle, and the membranous urethra. The distal mesonephric ducts persist to form the ejaculatory ducts, entering the prostatic urethra (Bennington, 1984). The anterior urethra forms from the tubulized urethral plate, which, unlike the posterior urethra, is 5-α reductase-dependent.

Tolmatschew wrote in 1870 that urethral valves are nothing but a simple enlargement of the folds and ridges that were normally present in area. Bazy (1903) believed that they are the remnants of the incompletely-absorbed urogenital membrane. Lowsley (1914) related valvular formation to defective development of the wolffian and müllerian ducts, noting that these ducts are bound together in a firm sheath as they passed through the prostate. This sheath normally disappears into the floor of the urethra. In the case of PUV, this tissue persists into the urethra to form the PUV leaflets. Watson (1922) postulated that type I valve formation is due to the growth and attachment of the tip of the colliculus seminalis (an oval enlargement on the crista urethralis) to the roof of the urethra at a time of marked epithelial activity, beginning as early as 14 weeks of gestation. Stephens (1955) suggested a similar theory to Lowsley; the inferior urethral crest and the mucosal fins in which it normally terminates are vestiges of the distal ends of the wolffian ducts. He later expanded on this theory to state that PUV develop when the mesonephric ducts enter the cloaca more anteriorly than normal. During infolding and separation of the cloaca, their migration is impeded and they may fuse anterolaterally (Livne et al., 1983; Stephens, 1983).

Bradford Young (1972) has described what we believe to be the most plausible explanation for the formation of type 1 PUV. He believes that the inferior cristal folds arise from the urethrovaginal folds of the urogenital sinus. In the female, these folds form the anterior half of the hymenal ring. He likened the valvular folds to an "imperforate hymen" and felt that PUV form when the ventrolateral folds of the urogenital sinus fail to regress. This later embryogenesis would conform more to the later obstruction seen in PUV, as compared with the early obstruction postulated for prune belly syndrome (Chapter 49).

Classification

Although Hugh Young (1919) described three different morphological types of PUV (Fig. 51-1), much of his original classification is now questioned. Type I PUV is a pair of leaflets passing downward and laterally from the lower border of the verumontanum and extending around the membranous urethra to fuse anteriorly at 12 o'clock (Fig. 51-2). Typically, the leaflets are separated by a slitlike opening. The Young type II PUV are not obstructing, and the type III valve is a congenital urethral membrane, with a pinhole opening, lying above or below the veru (Fig. 51-3) (Gonzales, 1992). Young did not describe any attachment to the veru. This type of valve is typically described as making up 5% of PUV cases and is similar to the "wind sock" lesion of Field and Stephens (1974). Stephens (1983) added a type IV PUV to this classification, in which he described a kinking of the flabby, poorly supported posterior urethra seen in prune belly syndrome.

There is accumulating evidence that a type I PUV may be a partially disrupted type III valve. Presman (1961) reported seven patients who died in infancy. He noted that five had a posterior urethral membrane and suggested that the original classification was incorrect. Robertson and Hayes (1969) reported 20 boys with PUV in 1969, 17 with a membranous obstruction. They performed postmortem examinations, removing the anterior urethral wall without disturbing the obstructing membrane. More recently, Dewan and colleagues (1992) reported 19 boys treated at Great Ormond Street, London. They noted that if endoscopy was performed prior to any other urethral instrumentation, a membrane was seen. The membrane could be converted to a type I valve by passing a catheter through it, or by disrupting it with a Whitaker hook.

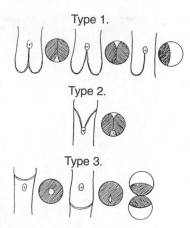

FIG. 51-1
Original diagram of Young's classification of PUV. (From Young HH, Frontz RH, Baldwin TC: *J Urol* 1919; 3:289.)

In view of the fact that the entire valvular concept of Young was questioned, Dewan later proposed a new name for PUV—the congenital obstructing posterior urethral membrane, or COPUM (Dewan, 1992). The only criticism of this new description of PUV is that Young did not describe any attachment of his type III PUV to the veru, and without this attachment, a true Young type III cannot be converted to a type I PUV. Similarly, the congenital urethral membranes described by Stephens (Cobb et al., 1968; Duckett, 1979a; Field and Stephens, 1974; Rosenfeld et al., 1994) do not connect to the veru. It would seem that a type III PUV (or membrane without veru attachment) does exist as a separate rare entity.

Hendren (1971) introduced the concept of grading PUV obstruction into groups from 1 through 4, based largely on the grade of associated reflux. Kurth (1981) has kept this classification. Patients in group 1 had only a partially formed PUV, without fusion at 12 o'clock. The valves may be visible on urethrography, but no other urinary tract changes were present (Fig. 51-4). Groups 2 and 3 had varying degrees of reflux, while group 4 patients had gross secondary changes, with megaureter, hydronephrosis, and uremia. Group 1 patients were later labeled as having "minivalves," and a variety of symptom complexes were attributed to this condition. We do not believe that minivalves have clinical significance (Duckett, 1979b), nor do we subscribe to a classification based on the grade of reflux. We do agree that there is a spectrum of presentations wherein milder obstructions do exist. It is our impression that the thicker and more prominent the leaflet is at 12 o'clock, the more severe the obstruction. A simple grading system is desirable because of the broad clinical spectrum of severity of PUV, but that system has not yet been devised.

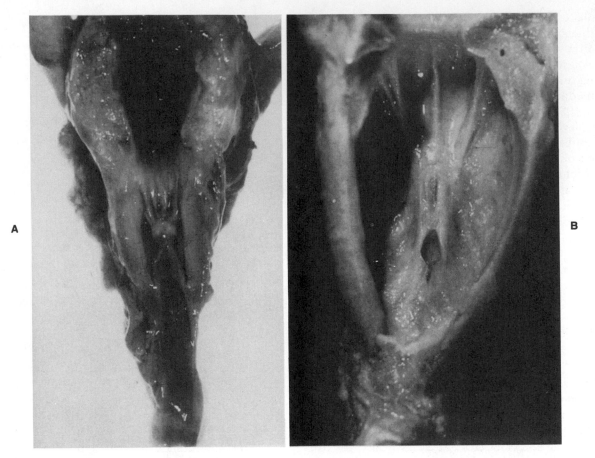

FIG. 51-2
Photographs of two type I PUV. **A,** Posterior urethra opened in the midline; it gives the impression of leaflets. **B,** Posterior urethra unroofed; it gives the impression of a membrane. It is, however, attached to the veru. (From Robertson WB, Hayes JA: *Br J Urol* 1969; 41:592.)

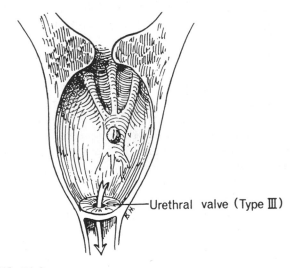

—Urethral valve (Type III)

FIG. 51-3
Diagram of a type III PUV. Note that it is separated from the veru. (From Gonzales ET: Posterior urethral valves and other urethral abnormalities. In Walsh PC, et al (eds): *Campbell's Urology,* ed 6, Philadelphia, WB Saunders, 1992.)

Pathophysiology of Congenital Obstruction

Congenital urethral obstruction develops early in the second trimester, after the remainder of the urinary tract has differentiated normally. The urinary tract, above the membranous urethra, then matures in the face of high intraluminal pressures. This results in a universal injury, involving the posterior urethra, bladder, ureters, and kidneys. The degree of obstruction creates a spectrum of damage that makes the clinical presentation highly variable. Normal fetal urine output into the amniotic fluid is essential for pulmonary development. With severe obstruction, the lack of urine voided into the amniotic cavity leads to oligohydramnios, which in turn makes pulmonary hypoplasia likely.

Renal development may also be impaired. Renal tubular injury results in an inability to concentrate the urine, and glomerular injury results in decreased glomerular filtration rate. Bladder injury results in decreased compliance, reducing storage capacity and delaying urinary continence.

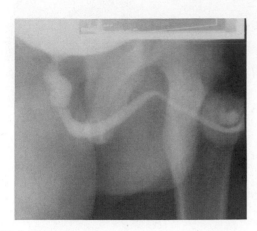

FIG. 51-4
VCUG of a minivalve.

Renal Dysplasia

Dysplasia means very different things to a pediatric urologist and an oncologist. Whereas an oncologist considers dysplasia a premalignant acquired condition, a pediatric urologist defines it as a congenital defect of tissue development, usually without premalignant potential. Renal parenchymal dysplasia is sometimes associated with urethral valves. Although the diagnosis may be suspected on ultrasound, it is a histological diagnosis, made under the microscope.

Dysplasia is characterized by primitive ducts with mesenchymal collars, modest disorganization, and foci of cartilage. It is thought to result from high pelvic pressures during nephrogenesis (Beck, 1971). However, dysplasia has not been consistently demonstrated with in-utero ligation of the lamb ureter (Adzick et al., 1985a; Glick et al., 1983) and is seen in the chick embryo only if the amount of metanephric blastema is reduced (Maizels and Simpson, 1983). Henneberry and Stephens (1980) have suggested that renal dysplasia results from an abnormal position of the metanephric bud. They noted, in a dissection of 11 cases of PUV, that 50% had a laterally ectopic ureteric orifice (D position), and that these kidneys were more dysplastic than kidneys with a normally situated orifice. We have observed that in cases with the VURD syndrome (valves, unilateral reflux, and renal dysplasia), that the ipsilateral kidney is dysplastic or poorly developed, while the contralateral kidney is well preserved (Hoover and Duckett, 1982). However, these cases do not help differentiate whether the dysplasia is caused by a development defect or by high pressures. The unilateral refluxing side effectively acts as a "pop-off" system, protecting the other side (Rittenberg et al., 1988).

Reduced Tubular Function

In experimental obstruction of a mature kidney, the renal medulla bares the brunt of the injury, with tu-bular injury preceding an injury to the glomerulus. Tubular injury results in a reduced ability to concentrate the urine, a reduced ability to acidify the urine, and increased loss of sodium in the urine (Gillenwater, 1992). The effect of PUV obstruction on the fetal renal tubules compared to the glomerulus has not been studied in detail but is probably similar. Parkhouse and Woodhouse (1990) reviewed 24 boys with PUV. Eleven had a GFR <80 ml/1.73 m², and all showed evidence of tubular injury. Thirteen had a GFR >80 ml/1.73 m², and six of these had maximal osmolalities less than 800 mmol, indicating renal tubular injury. We may infer from this study that renal tubular injury probably precedes glomerular injury in PUV.

Renal Failure

There is no precise definition for chronic renal failure (CRF). In children, a serum creatinine two standard deviations above the normal for age is generally accepted. Parkhouse and associates (1988) defined CRF as a plasma creatinine concentration greater than 150 μmol/L. In adults, we have used a creatinine level of 2 mg/dl (Smith et al., 1994a). In contrast, end-stage renal disease (ESRD) is precisely defined as a requirement for dialysis, renal transplantation, or death from renal failure.

There is an ongoing debate about the cause of progression to ESRD in PUV patients. It is very likely a multifactorial problem. There are three situations to consider. First, babies may be born with an inadequate amount of functioning renal tissue. Many of this group die from the associated pulmonary insufficiency. Second, progressive damage may be due to intervening obstruction and infection with delayed diagnosis. Third, although adequate renal tissue is present in childhood, with increasing somatic growth during adolescence, the limited renal reserve is overloaded. This may be accentuated by hyperfiltration, the theory of progressive glomerulosclerosis (Brenner et al., 1982). We can prevent further renal injury with treatment, but there is a definite limit to the amount of renal recovery and growth that will occur after relief of obstruction. Measuring this potential in childhood would be useful for predictive purposes.

End-stage renal disease occurs in 25% to 40% of patients treated for PUV, in two distinct age groups (Scott, 1985; Smith et al., 1994b). Of the group who develop ESRD, about one third do so soon after birth and the remainder during the late teenage years (Fig. 51-5). We believe that infants who develop ESRD soon after birth are born with severe renal dysplasia and do not have enough renal tissue to survive independently. Members of the other group are born with moderately impaired renal function and survive independently during childhood, developing ESRD after puberty. This late ESRD may be due to the

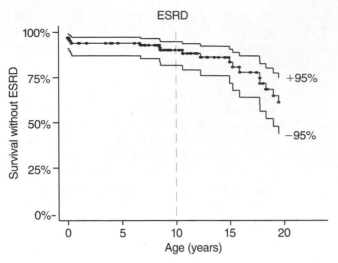

FIG. 51-5
Survival curve of the timing of renal failure in PUV. Note that ESRD occurs in two peaks; the first few months of life, and during the late teenage years. (From Smith GHH, et al: The long-term outcome of posterior urethral valves treated by primary valve ablation and observation, J Urol (in press) 1996.)

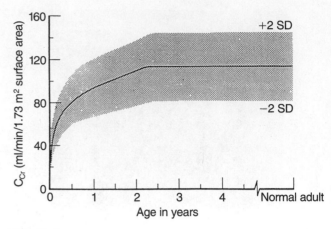

FIG. 51-6
The change in GFR with age. (From McCory WW: *Urol Clin North Am* 1980; 7:243.)

increasing metabolic demands of somatic growth, overloading the poor renal reserve. Parkhouse and colleagues (1988) disagree and feel that late-onset ESRD is due to a combination of hyperfiltration and abnormal bladder function.

In normal babies, the GFR rises rapidly at birth from 25 ml/m/1.73 m² on day 1, increasing to 50 ml/m/1.73 m² by 12 days of life. It then continues to rise to 105 ml/m/1.73 m² at 1 year of age (Fig. 51-6), then more slowly until about age 2 (Aperia et al., 1975). This improvement in GFR begins at birth, both in full-term and premature infants. It is due to an increase in systemic blood pressure with a decrease in intrarenal vascular resistance. This leads to an increase in hydrostatic pressure in the glomerular bed. In addition, an increase in the permeability of the basement membrane of the glomerulus occurs due to an increase in surface area and a change of the permeability constant (Yared and Ichikawa, 1987). This physiological increase in GFR also occurs in kidneys damaged by PUV and is greater in neonates than in later infancy. This is the explanation for the commonly held conception that relief of obstruction in the first few months of life results in a better improvement in renal function than treatment later in life (King et al., 1984).

In normal children, after the initial improvement in renal function in the first year of life, renal function then stabilizes in proportion to body surface area. In other words, as the child grows, renal function increases in direct proportion. In children with PUV, the increase tends to lag behind somewhat; this becomes more obvious around the time of puberty. Somatic growth outstrips renal reserve; with proteinuria

and hypertension, glomerulosclerosis progresses and the patients develop ESRD.

In the face of increasing demands on the kidneys with growth, there are four factors contributing to renal injury and reducing GFR. They are infection, obstruction, high pressure reflux, and hyperfiltration injury. With current treatment, infection and obstruction can be controlled and have very little bearing on ultimate outcome. Untreated, however, infection will rapidly destroy remaining renal function, especially if obstruction remains. Reflux in the absence of abnormal bladder function and infection is probably benign (see later).

Infection and Obstruction.—There is little doubt that recurrent episodes of pyelonephritis will cause renal injury (Schaeffer, 1992), and infection in the presence of obstruction or reflux will more rapidly destroy a kidney. The obstruction need not be anatomical. Abnormal bladder function may result in high resting bladder pressures, which obstruct the ureter at the vesicoureteric junction. McGuire has shown by his work with patients with myelomeningocele that chronic intravesical pressures of greater than 40 cm water are associated with upper-tract deterioration in the majority of patients (McGuire et al., 1981).

Hyperfiltration.—When functional renal mass is reduced, there is a compensatory increase in the single nephron glomerular filtration rate (SNGFR) in the remaining nephrons (Brenner et al., 1982; Ogden, 1967; Suki et al., 1966). No increase in nephron number occurs. Studies in the rat model have demonstrated that at a critical reduction in renal mass, further increases in SNGFR result in focal segmental glomerulosclerosis of the remaining nephrons. This phenomenon has recently been shown to occur in humans (Novick et al., 1991), but it may be more species-specific to the rat. Studies in adult kidney donors, with a follow-up of 15 years, have not shown any ev-

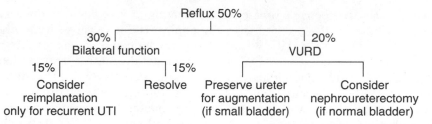

FIG. 51-7
Outcome of vesicoureteral reflux in PUV.

idence of contralateral injury (Suki et al., 1966; Velosa et al., 1983). When Steinhardt and colleagues (1988) examined kidneys removed prior to transplantation in five patients with PUV, with an average age of 1.8 years, they found focal segmental glomerulosclerosis in all, but always associated with an intense interstital and periglomerular inflammation. The conclusion was that it results from an inflammatory response secondary to obstruction, and not hyperfiltration. Lesions were identical to those described by Kimmelstiel and Wilson in 1936 in cases then classified as pyelonephritis but probably representing cases of reflux nephropathy. It follows that deterioration should not be ascribed to a hyperfiltration injury until infection and obstruction have been excluded.

Vesicoureteric Reflux

Vesicoureteric reflux may be primary, due to lateral placement of the ureter, or it may be secondary to abnormal bladder function and elevated intravesical pressures. It is often difficult to differentiate one from the other. Some authors believe that reflux has prognostic significance; however, this has not been our experience (see Prognosis in this chapter).

Reflux has been identified in 50% of PUV patients (Duckett, 1983); however, 20% will have the VURD syndrome (Hoover and Duckett, 1982), leaving only 30% of patients with renal units at risk (Fig. 51-7). Over the 3 years after valve ablation, spontaneous resolution can be expected in over half of these patients (Hulbert and Duckett, 1992). Of the remaining 15%, surgical intervention is reserved for patients with breakthrough urinary tract infections or massive reflux that interferes with adequate bladder function.

Urinary Ascites and Urinomas

Increased renal pelvic pressure leads to pyelorenal backflow and rupture of caliceal fornices (Eklöf et al., 1984; Friedenberg et al., 1983; Krane, 1974). Urine leaks into the renal sinus and may be contained by the renal capsule, leading to a subcapsular urinoma (Fig. 51-8). It may rupture the capsule, leading to a perirenal urinoma, or it may rupture Gerotas fascia and pass into the peritoneal cavity, leading to urinary ascites. It was generally believed in the past that ob-

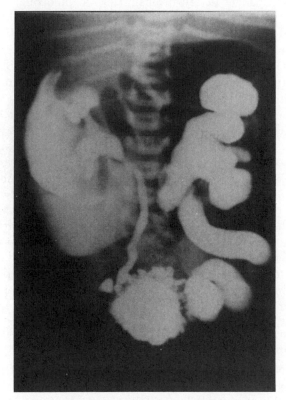

FIG. 51-8
A VCUG of a subcapsular urinoma.

struction severe enough to cause neonatal urinary ascites had an ominous prognosis with a high infant mortality rate. It now seems that the urinoma may act as a "pop-off" mechanism, to relieve pressure on the developing kidney (Rittenberg et al., 1988). Parker (1974) reviewed 27 infants with urinary ascites and noted that 17 survived with good renal reserve. Adzick and colleagues (1985b) noted less than expected renal dysplasia in six patients with fetal urinary tract obstruction associated with urinary ascites, compared to six other patients with obstruction and localized urinomas. They suggested that a localized urinoma provides less decompression than ascites and has a lesser effect on renal preservation. Rittenberg reported six patients, three with urinomas and three with ascites. All did well with serum creatinines at follow-up of less than 1 mg/dl (Rittenberg et al., 1988). We deduced that a localized urinoma was as effective a protective mechanism as urinary ascites.

Detrusor Dysfunction

Congenital bladder outlet obstruction induces hyperplasia and hypertrophy of bladder muscle and collagen. Smooth muscle is infiltrated with increased amounts of type III collagen and elastin (Ewalt et al., 1992). This results in a loss of compliance and the development of a small-capacity, high-pressure bladder. Changes in neurotransmitter receptor concentrations have been demonstrated in obstructed bladders and may lead to hyperreflexia (Elbadawi et al., 1989; Kato et al., 1988; Speakman et al., 1987).

Once obstruction is relieved, these thickened bladders with severe trabeculation can be expected to regain relatively normal function with low voiding pressures and complete emptying. It takes years for the thick bladder wall to regress. For many years it was thought that the thickened bladder wall caused uretero-vesical junction (UVJ) obstruction and persistent upper-tract dilatation. However, Whitaker showed in 1973 that despite appearances, there was usually no mechanical obstruction at the UVJ.

If supravesical diversion is chosen, particularly in the face of active cystitis, valve bladders can be expected to contract down, and rehabilitation later will be difficult. Often bladder augmentation is needed. When diversion is required, vesicostomy is still preferred. This maintains bladder cycling with voiding at low pressure through the abdominal stoma.

Lung Development

Normal pulmonary development depends both on mechanical and chemical factors elaborated by the fetal kidney (Colodny, 1987). Proximal airway branching of the lungs has been completed by the sixteenth week of gestation, before urine contributes to the amniotic fluid volume. However, late oligohydramnios interferes with alveolar development and leads to a high incidence of infant mortality secondary to respiratory failure. Extracorporeal membrane oxygenation (ECMO) has been used successfully in marginal cases. Gibbons reported three survivors with PUV and pulmonary insufficiency after ECMO therapy (Gibbons et al., 1993).

Presenting Symptoms and Signs
Antenatal Diagnosis

Prenatal ultrasound has completely changed the mode of presentation of valves. Most infants with PUV are now identified with bilateral hydronephrosis in utero and are promptly diagnosed after birth with a voiding cystourethrogram.

PUV is the third most commonly prenatally diagnosed urological disorder after ureteropelvic junction obstruction and megaureter (Colodny, 1983). Unfor-

tunately, it is difficult to differentiate bilateral hydronephrosis due to valves from other causes. In a study by Sholder and associates (1988) of 18 fetuses, the antenatal diagnosis corresponded to the postnatal diagnosis in only 66%. The differential diagnosis included prune belly syndrome, gross vesicoureteric reflux, bilateral ureteropelvic junction obstruction, and bilateral vesicoureteric obstruction.

Neonatal Diagnosis

If the diagnosis is not suspected on antenatal ultrasound, then the neonate may have a wide variety of symptoms and signs. Respiratory distress may occur soon after birth due to pulmonary hypoplasia; these infants may never be diagnosed correctly because of the severity of their pulmonary compromise and early mortality. Voiding may be delayed more than 24 hours. There may be a palpable distended bladder, renal mass due to hydronephrosis, or abdominal distention due to ascites. The baby may have a poor stream with voiding. However, a normal stream does not exclude valves; the bladder is often able to compensate for the obstruction. If the baby does not void spontaneously, then we have used bladder massage to assess the stream. This is done by gently kneading the lower abdomen until a bladder contraction commences.

If infection supervenes, the infant may have sepsis and undergo rapid deterioration. If the infant remains uninfected, excessive thirst and polyuria are likely. Otherwise, renal insufficiency and salt wasting may result in failure to thrive or dehydration.

Childhood and Later Diagnosis

Later in childhood, a high index of suspicion is required for diagnosis. Patients with milder obstruction may suffer delayed onset of continence and nocturnal enuresis. They may have polydipsia or a protuberant abdomen. Hematuria with mild trauma or recurrent urinary tract infections may occur. Excessive thirst may be noted by the parent. Gradual renal impairment may be indicated by growth failure or renal osteodystrophy.

Investigation
Ultrasound

Prenatal.—Prenatal ultrasound can reliably identify patients with bilateral hydronephrosis in utero. It has revolutionized the diagnosis of PUV and dramatically altered the clinical presentation.

With the apparent increased frequency of PUV in siblings, antenatal and postnatal ultrasound screening of a proband's siblings is recommended (Borzi et al., 1992).

If ultrasound is limited to a single examination between 17 and 19 weeks of gestation, the majority of nonlethal uropathies will be missed (Helin and Pers-

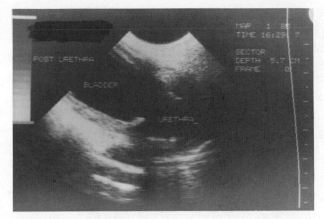

FIG. 51-9
Ultrasound photo of a thick-walled bladder and widened posterior urethra. (From Hulbert WC, Duckett JW: *AUA Update Series* 1992; XI:226.)

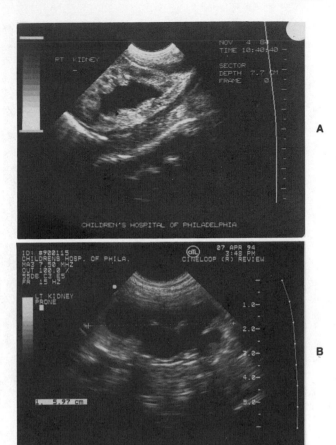

FIG. 51-10
A, Ultrasound showing CMJs. This patient had good renal function. **B,** Ultrasound showing absent CMJs. This patient has CRF and will require transplantation.

son, 1986). In a recent report of 42 patients with PUV, 36 were scanned before 24 weeks gestation, in 33 cases, PUV were not detected (Dinneen et al., 1993). If PUV is detected before 24 weeks of age, the prognosis is bad; in one series, 9 of 17 patients were dead or in chronic renal failure at follow-up (Hutton et al., 1994).

Postnatal.—Ultrasound is best used to evaluate the effect of PUV on the urinary tract, rather than to diagnose PUV. It can assess posterior urethral dilatation, bladder size and wall thickness, ureteral dilatation, hydronephrosis, renal parenchymal thickness, and the corticomedullary junctions. Typically, ultrasound shows a wide prostatic urethra, a thick-walled bladder, and upper tract dilatation (Fig. 51-9) (Cremin, 1986).

Increased echogenicity of the renal parenchyma on ultrasound suggests renal compromise (Sanders et al., 1988). However, the ultrasound appearance of the neonatal kidney differs significantly from that of the adult kidney. In a full-term newborn, the renal cortical echogenicity is isoechoic with the liver, and the medulla is relatively hypoechoic. During the first 6 months of life, there is a decrease in the cellularity of the cortex and a more hypoechoic cortical echogenicity is seen (Haller et al., 1982). We have shown that, in infancy, the single ultrasound feature that correlates with subsequent renal function is the status of the corticomedullary junction (Fig. 51-10) (Hulbert et al., 1992). In 28 infants with PUV, adequate renal function was present in all 17 patients when corticomedullary junctions were visible, whereas only 4 of 11 who had absent corticomedullary junctions maintained adequate function.

VCUG

The voiding cystourethrogram is the gold standard for diagnosing PUV (Fig. 51-11). The study should be delayed if infection is present and should be covered with antibiotics. A cystogram in the presence of a urinary tract infection may precipitate septicemia. The procedure itself may result in seeding the previously uninfected urinary tract with bacteria (Glynn and Gordon, 1970). Typically, the study shows a dilated and elongated posterior urethra with a U-shaped cutoff at the membranous urethra. The valve leaflet arising from the veru may be seen through dilute contrast. There is usually hypertrophy of the posterior bladder neck and interureteric ridge, with a thick-walled sacculated bladder. Reflux of contrast into the seminal vesicals may be seen, and ureteric reflux is present in 50% of patients (Fig. 51-12) (Mohammed, 1988).

If the patient has a normal voiding cystourethrogram, then PUV is excluded. The demonstration of prominent plicae colliculi, without evidence of obstruction, should not be classified as a valve. Care must also be taken not to confuse the appearance of prune belly syndrome with PUV (see Fig. 49-6). In prune belly syndrome, the dilated posterior urethra narrows significantly at the membranous urethra, but

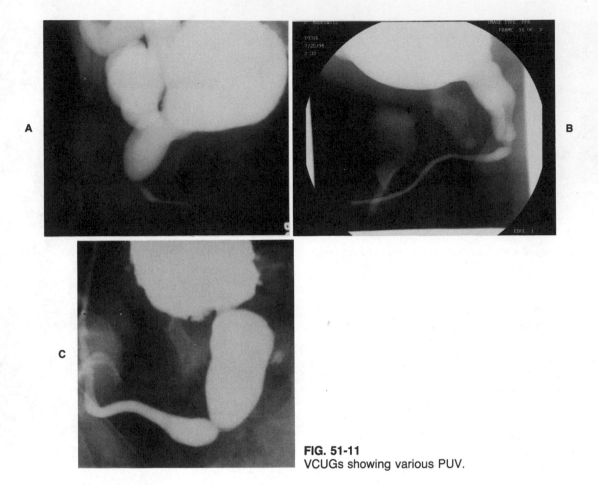

FIG. 51-11
VCUGs showing various PUV.

this is associated with a widely open bladder neck and a large, smooth-walled bladder; a pathognomonic appearance.

Upper Tract Urodynamics

The severely dilated and tortuous ureter in PUV typically demonstrates impaired emptying at the ureterovesical junction. Whitaker (1973) reported 170 boys with PUV and noted 70 ureters that remained grossly dilated at follow-up. In most, anatomic obstruction was excluded by antegrade nephrostograms or retrograde studies. In difficult cases, he drained the bladder and recorded ureteral pressures in the dilated systems under a constant saline infusion of 10 ml per minute. He found that only rarely were the ureters obstructed.

Glassberg performed similar pressure studies on persistently dilated ureters and classified them into three types (Glassberg et al., 1982):

1. Efficient drainage with the bladder empty and full
2. Efficient drainage with the bladder empty but obstructed with the bladder full
3. Obstructed with the bladder empty and full

Type 3 ureters are rarely encountered in our experience. We have seen only 4 in 100 consecutive patients born from 1970 to 1985. All of these patients had had previous ureteric reimplantations, and the obstruction appeared to be secondary to prior surgery. This reflects the danger of ureteric reimplantation into the PUV bladder.

It has also been shown experimentally, using healthy rats, that renal pelvic pressure rises with bladder filling and with increased urine production (Fichtner et al., 1994). This suggests delay at the UVJ also occurs in normal full bladders.

Diuretic Radioisotope Scan

More recently, the invasive Whitaker perfusion test has been replaced by a diuretic radioisotope scan. In most cases, a DTPA or MAG-3 renal scan with Lasix will allow obstruction to be excluded. Apart from excluding obstruction, a diuretic radioisotope scan has the added advantage of assessing split renal function. The amount of isotope taken up by an individual kidney can be measured and the extraction factor calculated. The extraction factor has been shown to be proportional to the GFR (Fig. 51-13) (Heyman and Duckett, 1988), and it allows individual renal function

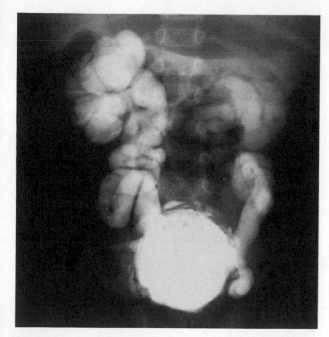

FIG. 51-12
VCUG showing massive reflux.

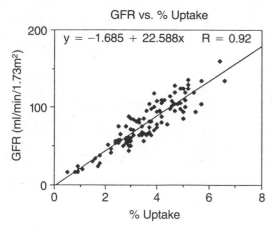

GFR vs. % Uptake

$$y = -1.685 + 22.588x \quad R = 0.92$$

FIG. 51-13
Graph of relationship between % uptake (EF) and GFR.
(From Heyman SH, Duckett JW: *J Urol* 1988; 140:780.)

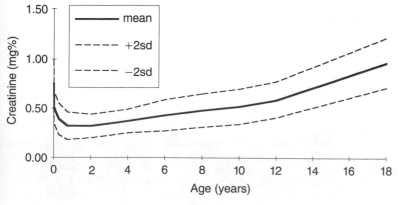

to be monitored. With serial serum sampling the total GFR can be accurately assessed. Any deterioration of renal function needs further assessment.

Serum Creatinine

Immediately after birth, the neonate's serum creatinine reflects the maternal creatinine rather than the neonate's renal function. Over the next 96 hours, the creatinine equilibrates depending on muscle mass and GFR (Chantler and Barratt, 1975; Churchill et al., 1990). The serum creatinine falls slowly over the first year of life as the GFR increases. It rises again after 2 years of age with increasing muscle mass (Fig. 51-14). This complex interaction of muscle mass and GFR must be considered when using serum creatinine (Cr) to calculate the GFR. We use the Schwartz formula (Schwartz et al., 1984):

Infancy:

$$\text{GFR (ml/min/1.73 m}^2) = \frac{0.45 \text{ height (cm)}}{\text{serum Cr (mg/dl)}}$$

Childhood:

$$\text{GFR (ml/min/1.73 m}^2) = \frac{0.55 \text{ Height (cm)}}{\text{serum Cr (mg/dl)}}$$

Serum creatinine is still considered the most practical measurement of renal function (GFR) in the management of valves. The reciprocal (1/Cr) graphed against age offers a prediction of the timing of ESRD (Fig. 51-15). Further, if the nadir creatinine falls below 0.8 mg/dl, then (with up to 8 years follow-up) chronic renal failure and ESRD are unlikely to develop (Duckett, 1983; Hoover and Duckett, 1982; Huebert and Duckett, 1992; Warshaw et al., 1985).

Initial Treatment

Prenatal

Prenatal intervention for PUV is still considered controversial and experimental (Elder and Duckett, 1987; Sholder et al., 1988). The main hurdle for successful intervention at present is that PUV cannot be

FIG. 51-14
Graph of the change in creatinine with age. (Data from Chantler C, Barratt T: Laboratory evaluation. In Holliday MA, Barratt TM, Vernier RL (eds): *Pediatric Nephropathy,* ed 2, Baltimore: Williams and Wilkins, 1975.)

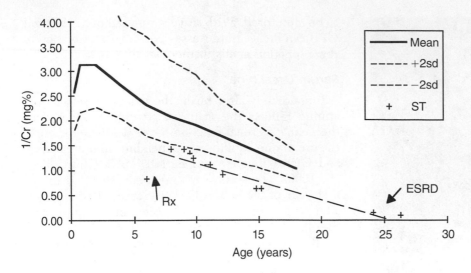

FIG. 51-15
Graph of 1/creatinine changing with age for patient ST. This plot is useful to predict the timing of ESRD.

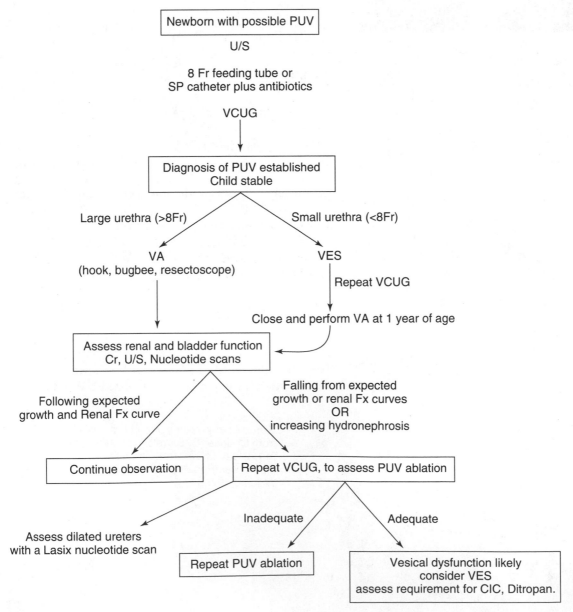

FIG. 51-16
Treatment plan for ▶

reliably differentiated from other causes of bilateral hydronephrosis such as prune belly syndrome. Therefore, prenatal relief of obstruction is reserved for progressive bilateral hydronephrosis with worsening oligohydramnios. The intervention is aimed at improving pulmonary function, rather than attempting to improve renal function. It should be performed at a research fetal treatment center with close collaboration between the treating obstetrician, neonatologist, and urologist. Any antenatal intervention is a procedure on both the fetus and the mother; both fetal and maternal complications can occur. Sholder reported five patients who had shunts placed for PUV. Only two actually had PUV and both died, one in utero from a catheter-related complication, and one after a spontaneous premature delivery (Sholder et al., 1988).

Our experience with seven PUV patients considered for treatment with amniotic shunts reveals a high incidence of shunt failure. It has been difficult to define a survival advantage in the small number of patients successfully shunted (Coplen et al., 1994). At the present time, prenatal intervention is rarely offered (see Chapter 44, Perinatal Urology).

Neonatal

Our treatment plan is outlined in Figure 51-16. Once the diagnosis of PUV is suspected, the treatment consists of stabilizing the baby and providing immediate bladder drainage. Sepsis, acidosis, electrolyte abnormalities, and fluid imbalance need aggressive treatment. Neonates should not be left obstructed under observation because of the risk of sepsis developing. Urinary drainage can be performed with an 8 F feeding tube per urethra or via a suprapubic intracatheter. A Foley catheter may not provide satisfactory drainage (Jordan and Hoover, 1985). These patients can be difficult to catheterize; the catheter may coil in the prostatic urethra because of a prominent bladder neck and yet appear to drain urine. Difficulties with catheterization may be overcome by using a coudé-tipped catheter, straightening the urethra with gentle penile traction and by elevating the prostatic urethra with a finger in the rectum. Icing the feeding tube by placing it in a freezer will make it more rigid and easier to pass. Alternatively, a stainless steel suture can be used (with care) as a catheter guide (Redman, 1993).

Valve Ablation

After stabilization and eradication of infection, and regardless of the severity of the upper-tract dilatation, we recommend primary valve ablation. Cystoscopy is performed with an 8 F endoscope. Most infant urethras may be easily traversed without stricture sequelae (Hulbert and Duckett, 1992). If difficulty is encountered visualizing the valve, then gentle pres-

sure on the full bladder with the cystoscope stopcocks open will create an antegrade flow and balloon the leaflet out.

The valve leaflet is ablated by passing a 3 F Bugbee through or beside the cystoscope (Fig. 51-17, A) (Hendren, 1971; Kogan, 1988). Short bursts of pure cutting current should be used, pushing the leaflet toward the bladder. Alternatively, if the urethra is large enough, an infant resectoscope can be used with the loop bent together to form a hook (Fig. 51-17, B). The valve can be incised at 12 o'clock as advocated by Williams (1973) and Parkkulainen (1977), or at 5 o'clock and 7 o'clock as described by Hendren (1970). Care should be taken not to injure the external sphincter complex lying distal to the veru, although injury has rarely been reported. The use of a resectoscope loop to resect the valve is likely to result in a stricture (Duckett, 1979a; Myers and Walker, 1981) and this should not be attempted.

Alternatively, the valve may be ablated blindly or under fluoroscopic control using a Whitaker diathermy hook (Whitaker and Sherwood, 1986) (Fig. 51-18). The hook is inserted into the bladder and slowly withdrawn, to engage the leaflet. Gentle traction is maintained as a brief cutting current is applied, incising the valve at 12 o'clock. Although the Whitaker hook is no longer manufactured, a similar technique has been described using a cold knife valvulotome under endoscopic or fluoroscopic guidance (Abraham, 1990; Cromie et al., 1994).

There are several other techniques of valve ablation mentioned for completeness. If the urethra is too small to accept an 8 F cystoscope, or one is unavailable, then a perineal urethrotomy can be made and the valve destroyed via an otoscope (Johnson, 1966). The bladder may be punctured suprapubically with a percutaneous sheath and the valve approached in an antegrade fashion (Zaontz and Firlit, 1985). The valve may be ruptured with a Fogarty balloon under fluoroscopic control (Diamond and Ransley, 1987). It may be incised with a neodymium: YAG laser (Ehrlich et al., 1987) or visual cold knife (Tank, 1992).

Vesicostomy

An alternative to primary valve ablation is the creation of a temporary cutaneous vesicostomy (Duckett, 1974b), with delayed valve ablation. This has been shown by Walker to be as effective as primary valve ablation (Walker and Padron, 1990). A 2-cm transverse incision is made halfway between the umbilicus and the pubis. An extraperitoneal dissection, with the bladder filled, is performed to locate the urachus. Gradual decompression of the bladder helps identify the urachus. The dome of the bladder is located and delivered into the wound with traction sutures. A cutaneous-vesical fistula is formed (Fig. 51-19). To pre-

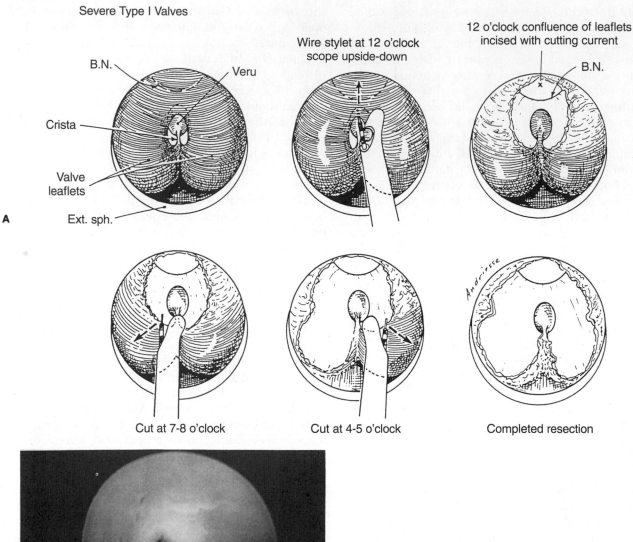

Severe Type I Valves

B.N.

Veru

Crista

Valve
leaflets

Ext. sph.

A

Wire stylet at 12 o'clock
scope upside-down

12 o'clock confluence of leaflets
incised with cutting current

B.N.

Cut at 7-8 o'clock

Cut at 4-5 o'clock

Completed resection

B

FIG. 51-17
A, Demonstration of PUV ablation with a wire stylet and ureteric catheter. **B,** Demonstration of our preferred method of valve ablation—destruction at 12 o'clock. (**A,** From Hendren WH: Urethral valves. In Ashcraft KW, Holder TM (eds): *Pediatric Surgery,* ed 2, Philadelphia: WB Saunders, 1993).

vent prolapse, the fistula should not be larger than 24 F, and the anterior wall of the bladder should not be used. Vesicostomy should not be equated with suprapubic tube drainage of the bladder. Suprapubic cystotomy tubes are associated with infection, bladder inflammation, and continued functional obstruction at the UVJ (Bueschen et al., 1973; Johnson, 1969). With a vesicostomy, the bladder continues to cycle with voiding at low pressures through the stoma.

High Diversion

After valve ablation, there should be a prompt improvement in serum creatinine. Failure to achieve this goal requires reevaluation of the patient. Some authors have set definite criteria for improvement, such as a fall in creatinine by 10% a day to a nadir below 0.8 mg/dl for azotemic postnatally identified patients (Churchill et al., 1990). We have used less rigorous criteria. If there is no obvious improvement in 2 to 3 weeks, then a vesicostomy is performed. If there is still no improvement after 4 to 6 weeks, then high diversion may be considered. We do this mainly for the chance to obtain a renal biopsy, being otherwise unconvinced of its superiority over vesicostomy. Although we have not done so, leaving one side undiverted may be beneficial for bladder function.

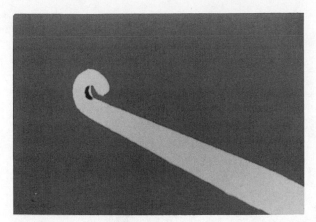

FIG. 51-18
A Whitaker hook. Note the small uninsulated area in the concavity of the hook.

In the group of patients who do not respond to primary valve ablation, high diversion has been advocated by Krueger and associates (1980b) as promoting improved renal function and somatic growth. However, this study was flawed by small patient numbers that combined patient groups treated over a period of 25 years. No statistical evaluation was offered to support their claim. Others have failed to show any benefit for high diversion as an initial treatment (Reinberg et al., 1992b). We believe that high diversion, if ever used, should be reserved until after valve ablation and vesicostomy have failed to show improvement. Others doubt its efficacy over vesicostomy even then (Walker and Padron, 1990). It should be combined with a renal biopsy, since most of these infants will have extensive renal dysplasia. Low loop ureterostomies or end ureterostomies no longer have any place in the treatment of PUV. They are too difficult to reconstruct.

In a consecutive series of 100 patients born prior to 1985, only 9 had initial high diversions (Smith et al., 1994b). Six more had subsequent high diversions after failing to respond to valve ablation or vesicostomy. There was no apparent benefit from these secondary diversions. When the rate of ESRD was compared, using Kaplan-Meier curves, there was no difference between the valve-ablation and diverted groups. High diversions require a second procedure to reconstruct, and this may be associated with further complications (Hendren, 1978). When the number of operative procedures was compared, 44% of the high-diversion group had three or more procedures, compared to only 7% of the valve-ablation group. We found that high diversions were of little benefit.

In the acutely unwell infant, who fails to respond to bladder decompression with a feeding tube and is not thought fit for anesthesia, percutaneous nephrostomies can be inserted using ultrasound guidance.

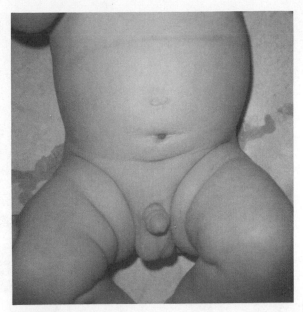

FIG. 51-19
A mature vesicostomy.

Infant and Later

Patients diagnosed after the neonatal period usually have better renal function. Their PUV can usually be incised endoscopically without difficulty. Preoperative urine cultures should be performed, to make sure the urine is sterile. If the valve ablation is straightforward, a urethral catheter is not required postoperatively.

Later Treatment
Correction of Reflux

Vesicoureteric reflux is present in 50% of patients at the time of diagnosis. This seldom requires surgical treatment, and resolution of at least 20% of cases will occur after valve ablation (Duckett, 1983; Connor and Burbige, 1990). Reflux has been demonstrated to resolve up to 3 years after treatment (Hulbert and Duckett, 1992). Prophylactic antibiotics should be continued during the period of watchful waiting. Reflux should be corrected if breakthrough urinary tract infections occur. Renal deterioration in the presence of sterile reflux is an indication of a bladder dysfunction and this should be assessed and treated. If reimplantation is necessary, a postoperative complication rate of 15% to 30% can be expected (Duckett, 1983; Warshaw et al., 1985). Transureteroureterostomy with a unilateral reimplant and psoas hitch may give better results (Hulbert and Duckett, 1992; Hendren, 1993).

VURD Syndrome

Unilateral reflux is a unique situation in valves. Often there is no function on the affected side (Fig. 51-20). A biopsy of this side will show dysplasia. We gave this condition the acronym VURD (*valve, unilateral*

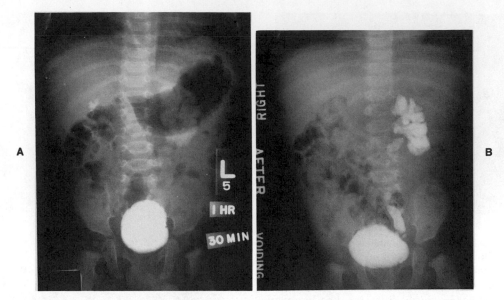

FIG. 51-20
A, An IVP of a VURD showing spurious function on the right side. This kidney did not function on the nucleotide renal scan.
B, A VCUG in the same patient showing reflux into the right system.

reflux, and dysplasia) so it would be recognized early and avoided in reconstructive efforts (Hoover and Duckett, 1982). In our initial review, 85% were on the left side, but subsequently the number approached 70%.

A valve patient with the VURD syndrome has a good prognosis (Rittenberg et al., 1988), apparently due to the pop-off protection given by the affected kidney. The brunt of the in utero pressure is taken by the VURD side, while the contralateral side is less involved.

Reconstruction of the VURD is now controversial. In the past we recommended nephroureterectomy at about 1 year of age. This was so that bladder function would not be hindered by reflux into the large ureteric diverticulum and to prevent infection as a result of stasis. However, it may be beneficial to preserve the protective pop-off mechanism while the bladder recovers normal function. Now there is enthusiasm for using the dilated ureter as an augmentation for ureterocystoplasty (Bellinger, 1993; Churchill et al., 1993; Landau et al., 1994). Our own experience with the rare need for augmentation in valves will not likely make us "preserve" this segment for later use.

Reconstruction

Closing a vesicostomy is a relatively straightforward procedure, and we have encountered few problems. A vesicostomy preserves bladder function because cycling, with filling and emptying, is maintained. Snyder and colleagues (1983) demonstrated that in 16 myelo-

dysplastic children, vesicostomy is reversible without loss of bladder volume; this has been confirmed by others (Khoury et al., 1990; Krahn and Johnson, 1993; Noe and Jerkins, 1985). This is not so with high diversion. In our previously described series of 100 patients, a small-capacity bladder developed in only one. This patient had been treated by high diversion (Smith et al., 1994b). It appears that supravesical diversion leads to reduced bladder capacity. This problem has been noted by others (Lome et al., 1972; Quinn et al., 1994; Tanagho, 1974).

After high diversion, the decompressed bladder should be assessed to see if augmentation is required at the time of reconstruction. Ureteroneocystostomy has a 15% to 30% incidence of complications (as mentioned above); thus it should be avoided if possible. Reflux should not be corrected at the time that urinary continuity is reestablished, since most defunctionalized bladders will reflux initially, and many will stop after bladder function is reinstated. Hendren (1978) has noted that loop ureterostomy is an easy operation to preform but can be followed by serious complications during reconstruction. We agree that loop ureterostomy has been and still is much overused in the treatment of valves.

Urodynamics, Bladder Dysfunction, and Incontinence

Urodynamic studies in children with PUV are technically demanding and difficult to interpret. Ideally, they should be performed using a double-lumen cath-

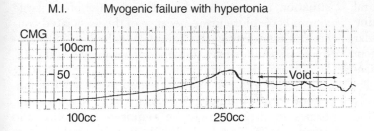

M.I.   Myogenic failure with hypertonia

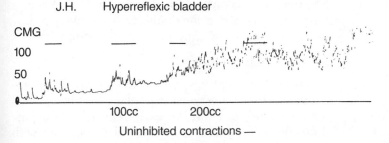

J.H.   Hyperreflexic bladder

Uninhibited contractions —

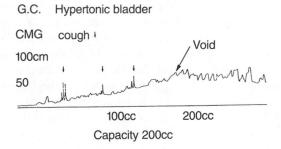

G.C.   Hypertonic bladder

Capacity 200cc

FIG. 51-21
Urodynamic tracings showing the three common types of detrusor dysfunction seen in PUV. (From Peters CA, et al: *J Urol* 1990; 144:122.)

eter inserted suprapubically to allow bladder filling and emptying with simultaneous pressure measurements (Whitaker et al., 1972). A rectal pressure line is required to subtract intra-abdominal pressure. Additionally, in an ideal situation, the study should be performed under fluoroscopic control so that the amount of vesicoureteric reflux can be assessed. We reserve urodynamic studies for patients who are incontinent beyond 6 years of age, or who have demonstrated deterioration of renal function despite adequate PUV resection.

Urinary incontinence is common even when there has been no bladder neck surgery or sphincter damage. Various authors have defined continence differently and many have been vague. Parkhouse and associates (1988) noted that only 55% of 87 patients were dry by day by age 5, although all achieved continence by age 16. Using similar criteria—dry by day and night by age 5—we have noted delayed onset of full continence in 56% of 100 patients (Smith et al., 1994b). All except one were dry by age 20. Incontinence is rarely due to sphincter injury (Walker and

Padron, 1990; Whitaker et al., 1972). It is due to a combination of poor bladder compliance, instability, and polyuria (Parkhouse et al., 1988; Peters et al., 1990).

Peters and colleagues (1990) have demonstrated three types of detrusor dysfunction in 18% of their PUV patients (Fig. 51-21): 7% myogenic failure of the bladder, 5% detrusor hyperreflexia, and 6% poor compliance associated with a small capacity bladder. Myogenic failure is not easily diagnosed; it is common for patients to suffer a degree of "stage fright" during urodynamic testing, with a reduced detrusor contraction. High post-void residuals are often a result of urine being dumped into the bladder from dilated upper tracts after voiding and not from incomplete bladder emptying. Patients with myogenic failure can generate only weak bladder contractions and have elevated post-void residuals. They usually void by the Valsalva maneuver. They should be treated initially with a double or triple voiding regimen. If this fails, then clean intermittent catheterization (CIC) should be commenced. Incomplete emptying may rarely be secondary to incomplete valve ablation or to a urethral stricture, and this should be assessed. It is never due to hypertrophy of the bladder neck, a concept popular many years ago. Bladder neck procedures, done in PUV patients in the past, have led to retrograde ejaculation and delayed continence.

Patients with detrusor hyperreflexia usually empty their bladders adequately but suffer from urgency and urge incontinence due to unstable bladder contractions. They can usually be managed with anticholinergic medication. In 19 urodynamic studies, performed over the last 2 years, we found 6 patients with unstable detrusor contractions during filling. Poor bladder compliance associated with reduced capacity is treated initially with anticholinergic medication. If the bladder capacity does not improve, then bladder augmentation is required.

We believe that high diversion is detrimental to final bladder function. Tanagho (1974) reported 4 of 10 patients developed small contracted bladders after prolonged high diversion. By largely avoiding high diversions, we have avoided further injury to the developing bladder. Thus we have avoided the small-capacity, high-pressure bladders seen by others (Landau et al.,1994; Peters et al., 1990; Quinn et al., 1994).

We feel the most common cause for incontinence in PUV is polyuria. Most patients have a renal concentrating defect that delivers a free-water-loss increase in urine volume of two to four times normal. If the expected bladder volume of a 5-year-old is 200 ml, and he is making 1500 to 2000 ml of urine, he would need to void 8 to 10 times a day to stay dry, clearly a socially difficult task. A PUV bladder may have a diminished capacity due to its thickness and increased collagen, which futher reduces compliance. It should be little surprise that these boys are wet, particularly at night. If they develop some instability, their incontinence increases; and if they use holding maneuvers to control it, we see external sphincter dyssynergia or dysfunctional voiding patterns (Schulman and VanGool, 1993). Patience and understanding are often the best therapeutic approach, rather than drugs and CIC.

Full Valve Bladder Syndrome

In this syndrome (Duckett, 1979a; Duckett and Snow, 1986), upper tract dilatation progresses in older patients in spite of adequate PUV ablation. The sensation of a full bladder is markedly diminished, and elevated intravesical pressures occur at low filling volumes. Typically, the ureterovesical junction obstructs with bladder filling and no more urine enters the bladder. The upper tracts fill with their inherent dilatation. On voiding, the bladder empties; however, it rapidly fills again with drainage from the upper tracts. The situation is exacerbated by the production of large amounts of dilute urine because of the associated concentrating defect of the kidney (Mitchell, 1982). Urodynamic studies may show poor compliance and a delayed sensation of fullness.

The condition should be treated initially with double or triple voiding. If this fails, CIC and anticholinergics medication may be required (McGuire and Weiss, 1975; Mitchell, 1982). Rarely, bladder augmentation may be required. It is often difficult to get a teenager to comply with double voiding during a busy day. We strive for double voiding twice a day, morning and evening, as a reasonable compromise.

Renal Transplantation

There is currently some debate in the literature about the success of renal transplantation in patients with a history of PUV. An early report by Warshaw indicated no reduced graft survival in patients with obstructive uropathy (Warshaw et al., 1980). Churchill and colleagues (1988), however, noted decreased graft survival in PUV patients (30% at 5 years) compared to a group transplanted for reflux nephropathy, Alports syndrome, and medullary cystic disease (70% at 5 years). Reinberg and associates (1988) noted no decrease in graft survival, but there was diminished graft function in the group of PUV patients. The implication was, that if a bladder has been responsible for the destruction of two native kidneys, then it was likely to make short work of a transplanted kidney (Parkhouse and Woodhouse, 1990). Mochon and associates (1992) compared 14 boys transplanted for PUV with 29 boys transplanted for other reasons and noted a significant increase in urinary tract infections in the PUV group. They suggested that this increase was due to the presence of vesicoureteric reflux in the PUV group. Other authors have not noted any decrease in graft survival. Bryant and colleagues (1991) reported a 5-year graft survival of 62% in PUV and 48% in controls; however, they noted a higher creatinine level in the PUV patients. Ross and colleagues (1994) reported 2- and 5-year graft survivals in PUV of 70% and 59% respectively. They did not perform bladder cycling or bladder augmentation prior to transplantation to achieve their good results. A more recent report from Toronto (Hyacinthe et al., 1995) suggests good graft survival in PUV patients treated with cyclosporin (91% at 16 to 60 months).

With the reduction in infant mortality in children with PUV and the availability of dialysis in infancy, there are now more young patients with ESRD requiring renal replacement. It is apparent that the incidence of transplant complications and graft lost rises steeply in younger patients, particularly below the age of 2 (Churchill et al., 1988; Sheldon et al., 1992). These patients will require careful assessment prior to trans-

TABLE 51-1

Incidence of ESRD Reported by Other Authors

Author	Follow-up	ESRD
Parkhouse et al., 1988, GOS, U.K.	11-22 years	33 %
Tejani et al., 1986, Brooklyn, U.S.A.	9 years	44 %
Connor and Burbige, 1990, Columbia, U.S.A.	6.8 years	24 %
Scott, 1985, Newcastle-on-Tyne, U.K.	1-12 years	28 %
Walker and Padron, 1990, Florida, U.S.A.	4.6 years	30 %
Smith et al., 1994b, CHOP, U.S.A.	10 years	10 %
(Kaplan-Meier calculation)	20 years	38 %

plantation and intense surveillance after transplantation.

Complications

End-stage Renal Disease and Growth Failure

The incidence of ESRD varies from 24%, with a 6.8-year follow-up (Connor and Burbige, 1990) to 44% with a 9-year follow-up (Tejani et al., 1986) (Table 51-1). Parkhouse and associates (1988) followed a group of 98 boys for a mean of 15 years and noted the onset of late ESRD in 15%, between the ages of 6 and 14 years. We noted an incidence of ESRD of 10% at 10 years, increasing to 38% at 20 years (Smith et al., 1994b). Ideally, ESRD rates should be reported using Kaplan-Meier curves. The longer the follow-up and the less the mortality, the higher the incidence of ESRD.

Somatic growth retardation occurs in patients with chronic renal failure (Reinberg et al., 1992a). It is characterized by abnormal growth hormone secretion; elevation in plasma aldosterone and glucagon; decreases in serum testosterone, somatomedin, and thyroid hormone; and defective degradation of cortisol and insulin. Impaired bicarbonate reabsorption by the renal tubules leads to acidosis. As a result, carbohydrate and lipid metabolism are disturbed, leading to defective catabolism of structural and enzymatic proteins (Chesney and Avioli, 1992). The worse the renal function, the more severe the growth retardation (McCory, 1980). Growth potential is better in patients who present later in life (Krueger et al., 1980a) and growth improves after treatment. Continued growth increases the demand on the renal reserve. Less severe renal failure does not usually impair childhood growth until the pubertal growth spurt is entered and chronic renal failure ensues (Scott, 1985).

Since the kidney also occupies a pivotal role in the regulation of calcium, derangements of parathyroid function and bone mineralization occur with secondary hyperparathyroidism and renal osteodystrophy. These complications can be minimized by careful nephrological care with correction of acidosis, calcium, and vitamin D supplements.

Sexual Function and Fertility

Impaired sexual function and reduced fertility may be expected in PUV patients. There is an increased incidence of cryptorchidism (Krueger et al., 1980b). Prostatic urethral obstruction is associated with reflux into the ejaculatory ducts and seminal vesicles, which may effect components of the semen. Retrograde ejaculation may occur as a result of unfortunate bladder neck procedures designed to improve voiding. Also, patients with ESRD can be expected to have an increased incidence of impotence and decreased fertility (Barry, 1992).

In a study by Woodhouse and colleagues (1989) of 21 patients with PUV, 2 had impotence, 1 was on dialysis, and 1 had life long impotence. Slow ejaculation was reported by 8 of 11 patients. Viscous, alkaline semen was noted in 5 of 9 patients, and 3 of these had low sperm counts. Only 1 patient was noted to have retrograde ejaculation. In a group of 17 patients followed since 1974 (Smith et al., 1994a), we have noted impotence in 1 recently transplanted patient, and retrograde ejaculation in 1 patient who had a bladder neck incision. Six of the 17 patients have fathered children and are presumably fertile.

Prognosis

Good Factors

Several authors have noted that serum creatinine is a useful prognostic indicator. A 1-month post-treatment nadir Cr <0.8 mg/dl was associated with a normal renal function at follow-up of up to 8 years (Duckett and Norris, 1989; Rittenberg et al., 1988; Warshaw et al., 1985). Connor and Burbidge (1990) noted that a Cr <1 mg/dl at 1 year of age was associated with normal values at follow-up. Since the serum creatinine in normal individuals rises after 1 year of age (see Fig. 51-14), it follows that a serum creatinine <0.8 mg/dl after that time reflects even better renal function. It can be concluded that a Cr <0.8 mg/dl after the age of 1 year makes ESRD less likely.

Rittenberg and associates (1988) have identified three factors that provide a pressure pop-off mechanism in PUV and prevent high intravesical pressures being transmitted to the upper tracts. These are the VURD syndrome, urinary ascites, and a large bladder diverticulum (Fig. 51-22). In a review of 71 patients, 19 had a protective pop-off and, of these, only 1 showed evidence of deterioration of renal function. There was a significant difference in renal function between the two groups (p <.01).

Bad Factors

The age at diagnosis is a well-known prognostic factor. The younger the child is at diagnosis, the worse the prognosis. It was thought that prenatal ultrasound would change this (Churchill et al., 1990). However,

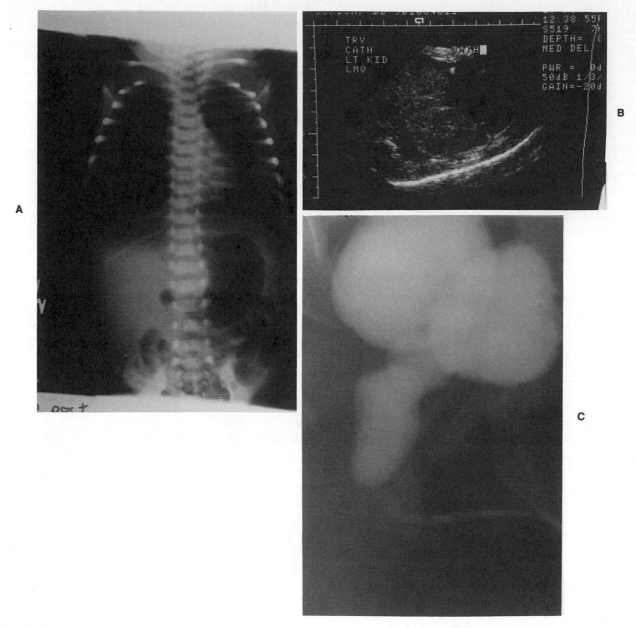

FIG. 51-22
A, Plain X-ray of urinary ascites. **B,** Ultrasound of urinary ascites. **C,** A VCUG of a bladder diverticulum. (**A** and **B,** from T. Ernesto Figueroa and A.I. DuPont.)

prenatal diagnosis is associated with increased morbidity from renal failure and increased mortality from pulmonary hypoplasia (Nakayama et al., 1986; Reinberg et al., 1992b). For PUV to be diagnosed antenatally, it is likely that a higher degree of obstruction producing renal compromise and oligohydramnios is needed (Jee et al., 1993). Nakayama and colleagues (1986) noted a mortality rate of 5 of 11 babies presenting with PUV within the first week of life. They felt that most series of PUV patients were biased be-

cause this group of patients died before coming to a tertiary center for surgery. Tejani and associates (1986) noted that the incidence of ESRD increased if corrective surgery was delayed beyond 2 years of age. This has not been noted by others. Generally, the older the child at diagnosis, the better the prognosis for renal function. Scott (1985) noted that in young infants, a GFR <50% of normal at diagnosis was always associated with continued renal failure.

In a 1971 series, bilateral reflux at diagnosis was

associated with a mortality of 57%, unilateral reflux with a mortality of 17.4%, and no reflux with a mortality of 9.1% (Johnston and Kulatilake, 1971). Persistent vesicoureteric reflux is also reported to be associated with a higher incidence of ESRD (Johnston, 1979; Tejani et al., 1986), but it is not clear if this is due to renal dysplasia secondary to an abnormally situated ureteric bud (Henneberry and Stephens, 1980), renal injury due to high back pressure during in utero development, or continued renal injury from reflux after valve ablation. Our experience with 120 patients seen over 14 years and followed for an average of 5 years showed no correlation between renal function and reflux (Hulbert and Duckett, 1986); nor did Williams (1973) show any such correlation.

The most reliable and useful prognostic indicator of later renal function in the neonate is the presence or absence of corticomedullary junctions on ultrasound (see Fig. 51-10). Bilateral loss of the corticomedullary junction is indicative of renal dysplasia and eventual ESRD (Hulbert et al., 1992).

Delayed urinary continence beyond age 5 is reported by Parkhouse and associates (1988) to be a bad prognostic factor. Connor and Burbige (1990) also noted this association. It has been suggested that this association may be due to continual abnormal bladder function damaging the upper tracts. However, just as the renal injury is due largely to obstruction in the prenatal period, it is likely that bladder injury may be caused by the same mechanism and in the same proportion to renal injury. Thus children born with severely damaged kidneys have severely damaged bladders, too.

Finally, we have noted a morphological subgroup of Type I PUV with a worse prognosis (Fig. 51-23). These cases have the following features: a narrow posterior urethra; a large, smooth-walled bladder; and a thick PUV, making catheterization very difficult. We believe these atypical cases have been mistaken for Type III PUV in the past (Presman, 1961; Rosenfeld et al., 1994).

Conclusion

Over the last two decades, the diagnosis of PUV has been radically altered by the development of ultrasound. Patients now are diagnosed mainly as neonates or infants. Unfortunately, the incidence of ESRD does not seem to have been reduced by in utero intervention or early intervention after delivery, although morbidity and mortality rates have dropped. Endoscopic valve ablation remains the cornerstone of treatment, with vesicostomy reserved for technical failures. The role of high diversion is in question. Increasing numbers of severely affected PUV patients are surviving to require renal transplantation. The out-

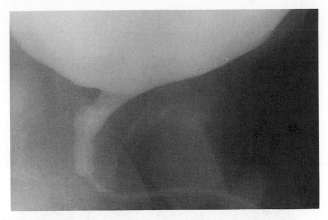

FIG. 51-23
An atypical type I PUV with minimal dilation of the posterior urethra.

look for the majority of patients is good, with high long-term continence and fertility rates.

ANTERIOR URETHRAL VALVES AND/OR DIVERTICULA

Anterior urethral valves are reported to occur seven to eight times less frequently than posterior urethral valves (Firlit et al., 1978; Williams and Retik, 1969). However, Huang and colleagues (1989) noted a ratio of almost 1:1 in a series of 50 patients from Beijing (Belman, 1992). Although posterior urethral valves have received the most attention, anterior urethral valves can be equally obstructing and just as devastating (Firlit et al., 1978). The lesion can be located anywhere along the anterior urethra. They are distributed 40% in the bulbous urethra, 30% at the penoscrotal junction, and 30% in the penile urethra (Golimbu et al., 1978). Rarely, they are reported in the fossa navicularis (Scherz et al., 1987).

The valve mechanism is usually formed by an associated diverticulum. The diverticulum undermines the dilated proximal urethra and forms a ventral lip or obstructing valve (Tank, 1987) (Fig. 51-24). However, isolated valves formed by filamentous cusps or iris-like diaphragms have been reported (Firlit and Burstein, 1985; Golimbu et al., 1978). Surprisingly, in the series of 50 patients from Beijing, Huang and colleagues (1989) reported associated diverticula in only 15. No description of the obstructions were given. Similarly, narrow-necked diverticula not associated with obstruction occasionally occur. It is likely that these two entities represent two ends of a single disease spectrum.

The diverticula may result from incomplete formation of the ventral corpus spongiosum (Colodny, 1991), congenital cystic dilatation of a periurethral gland, or an incomplete urethral duplication. Ac-

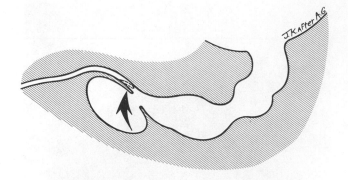

FIG. 51-24
An anterior urethral valve. (Courtesy of Arnold Colodny, MD.)

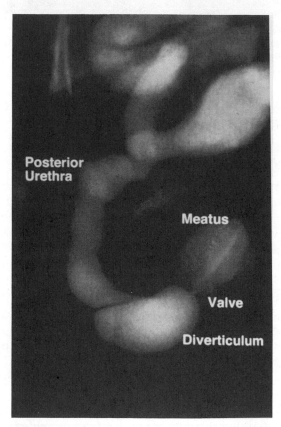

FIG. 51-25
A VCUG of an anterior urethral valve. (From Rushton HG, et al: *J Urol* 1987; 138:107.)

quired diverticula may occur after hypospadias surgery, or after rupture of the membranous urethra treated with a Foley catheter (Williams and Retik, 1969).

Most children with diverticula are diagnosed in infancy with dribbling-type micturition or infection. The dribbling may be due to emptying of the diverticulum or to overflow incontinence (Colodny, 1991). If the obstruction is distal, then ballooning of the urethra may occur with voiding (Scherz et al., 1987). There may be a palpable swelling present at the site of the diverticula.

A voiding cystourethrogram is the key to diagnosis (Fig. 51-25). It is essential to visualize the entire anterior urethra during voiding or the valve may be missed (Rushton et al., 1987; Sarmsin and Cremin, 1984). The characteristic feature is the sharp valvular distal lip of the wide-mouthed diverticulum with an extreme difference in urethral caliber at this level (Williams and Retik, 1969). A retrograde urethrogram may flatten the valve and obscure the diverticulum (Colodny, 1991). Cystoscopy may not be diagnostic for the same reason (Tank, 1987). Vesicoureteric reflux has been reported in 33% of cases (Golimbu et al., 1978). The upper tracts should be screened with ultrasound or IVP. This will reveal some degree of deterioration in up to 47% of cases.

The mainstay of treatment is endoscopic valve ablation. Firlit and associates (1978) reported no complications in a series of 10 cases thus treated. Antegrade flow may be required to demonstrate the valve. The ventral lip of the diverticulum is incised, to destroy the valvular lip. Rushton and colleagues (1987) recommend vesicostomy as the initial form of management in the newborn. They believe subsequent transurethral fulguration of the valve is simplified and that potential complications are reduced. Tank (1987) recommends open urethroplasty for all newborns and reserves endoscopic incision for older children. If a significant diverticulum is present, then open excision with urethroplasty should be performed (Williams and Retik, 1969). Reimplantation of the ureters is occasionally necessary if significant reflux persists.

The prognosis in these patients is determined by the degree of upper-tract damage that occurred prior to treatment.

Congenital Urethral Polyps

Urethral polyps are benign, single, congenital lesions located in the posterior urethra (Downs, 1970), arising from the verumontanum on a 1- to 3-cm stalk. The polyp is covered with transitional epithelium and has a loose fibromuscular stroma. Occurring only in males, there is some evidence that they are similar to

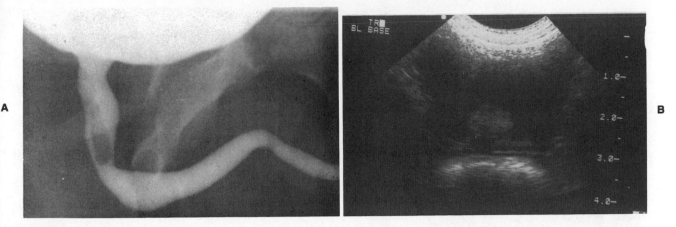

FIG. 51-26
A, A VCUG of a urethral polyp. **B,** An ultrasound view of a urethral polyp, which has prolapsed back into the bladder. (**A,** Courtesy of Arnold Colodny, MD.)

urethral caruncles in females (Klee et al., 1993). Campbell (1954) estimated an incidence of 1%, but this has not been confirmed. Only 48 cases had been reported up to 1979 (Colodny, 1991), although by 1991 over 339 had been reported (Arteaga et al., 1993).

Although most urethral polyps are congenital, they have been reported in late adult life (Perimenis and Panagou, 1992), suggesting that some may be acquired.

Patients may have a history of intermittent obstruction, acute retention, hematuria, dysuria, incontinence, or urinary tract infection. As with other urethral lesions, the most reliable way to diagnose a urethral polyp is with a voiding cystourethrogram (Fig. 51-26a). This will show a filling defect, which may vary in location because of the length of the stalk, from the anterior urethra to the bladder. The polyp may be also be seen on ultrasound (Fig. 51-26b) (Arteaga et al., 1993; DeFilippi et al., 1983).

The treatment of choice is endoscopic resection with either a cold knife or resectoscope loop. The exact base of the stalk must be precisely identified. If the polyp is too large to remove via the urethra, an open cystotomy may have to be performed.

Abnormalities of Cowper's Ducts and Glands in Infants and Children

The bulbourethral or Cowper's glands are two groups of periurethral glands (Fig. 51-27) (Bartone and King, 1986; Moskowitz, 1976). The main, or diaphragmatic, glands are paired and situated in the transverse portion of the urogenital diaphragm. The accessory bulbar glands are multiple and located in the corpus spongiosum along the bulbous urethra. The main glands empty via two ducts, directed forward through the corpus spongiosum to enter the bulbous urethra

with two small flush openings. They are the homologue of Bartholin's glands in the female. The accessory bulbar glands either communicate with the main diaphragmatic ducts or enter the urethra directly. Both sets of glands contribute a clear fluid secretion that acts as a lubricant and coagulation factor for semen during ejaculation (Hart, 1968).

Maizels and colleagues (1982) classified all Cowper's duct abnormalities as syringoceles (Greek; *syringo* = tube + *cele* = swelling) that are either intact, imperforate, perforated, or ruptured. Syringoceles occur in infants and young children and are caused by narrowing of the ductal orifice. Dilated ducts occur secondary to a ruptured syringocele or to a patulous orifice. Edling (1953) reported a series of 24 patients with dilated Cowper's ducts. He divided the lesions into globular and tubular types.

Frequently, abnormalities of Cowper's ducts are asymptomatic. Rarely, they may cause hematuria, urethral obstruction, or post-void dribbling. Occasionally, the dilated duct may appear as a perineal mass (Brock and Kaplan, 1979; Moskowitz, 1976). Retention cysts or reflux in a dilated duct may be seen incidentally on urethrography (Fig. 51-28).

Asymptomatic patients do not require therapy. If symptoms occur, transurethral marsupialization of the dilated duct (Sant and Kaleli, 1985) or fulguration of retention cysts can be performed. Urine infection and hematuria are usually cured, but voiding symptoms may persist (Maizels et al., 1982).

Megalourethra

The condition was first described by Nesbitt (1955). Megalourethra may be thought of as a urethral diverticulum effecting the whole of the penile urethra. It is much less common than saccular diverticula and is

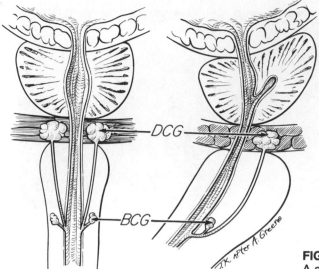

FIG. 51-27
A diagram of Cowper's glands. (Courtesy of Arnold Colodny, MD.)

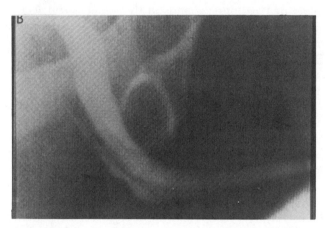

FIG. 51-28
Reflux into a Cowper's duct. (From Bartone F, King LR: Abnormalities of the urethra, penis, and scrotum. In Welch KJ, et al (eds): *Pediatric Surgery,* ed 4. Chicago: Year Book Medical Publishers, 1986.)

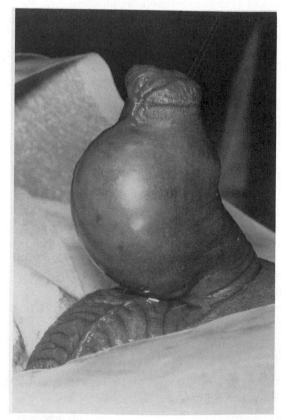

FIG. 51-29
A scaphoid megaloureter during voiding.

usually not associated with obstruction. Less than 50 cases have been reported in the English literature (Sepulveda et al., 1993). Dorairajan (1963) classified the abnormality into scaphoid and fusiform types, with the scaphoid type associated with a localized absence of the corpus spongiosum, and the fusiform type associated with defective corpus cavernosum as well.

In the more common scaphoid megalourethra, the urethra balloons out ventrally with voiding (Fig. 51-29) to assume a boatlike form; hence the name. The rare fusiform type of lesion is more severe. The penile urethra dilates with voiding. The soft penis is elongated with no corporeal bodies palpable and the skin is redundant (Fig. 51-30). Megalourethra is often associated with other severe abnormalities such as prune belly syndrome (Duckett, 1976; Mortensen et al.,

1985), cloacal abnormalities (Stephens, 1963), and the VATER association (Fernbach, 1991).

Stephens and Fortune (1993) have described two aborted fetuses with an epithelial plug obstructing the meatus and an associated fusiform megalourethra. They favor the theory of temporary urethral obstruc-

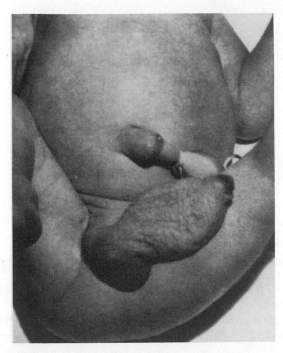

FIG. 51-30
A fusiform megalourethra. (From Belman AB: Hypospadias and other urethral abnormalities. In Kelasis PP, King LR, Belman AB (eds): *Clinical Pediatric Urology,* ed 3. Philadelphia: WB Saunders, 1992.)

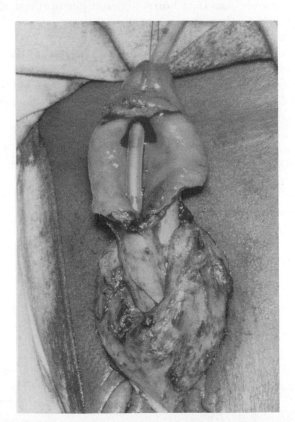

FIG. 51-31
An operative view of the scaphoid megalourethra seen in Fig. 51-29. The urethra has been laid open prior to resection of the mucosa and closure.

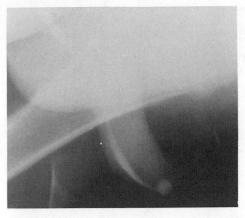

FIG. 51-32
A VCUG of a valve of Guerin. This appearance can be mimicked by a drop of contrast at the meatus.

tion during development. Other reports of megalourethra with in utero hydronephrosis support this contention (Fisk et al., 1990; Sepulveda et al., 1993; Simma et al., 1992). Since megalourethra is associated with a failure of development of the erectile tissue of the penis, some favor a mesenchymal-defect etiology (Reissigl et al., 1991).

The diagnosis is made by the external appearance. A voiding cystourethrogram and ultrasound of the upper tracts should be performed, since the lesion may be associated with other upper-tract abnormalities (Shrom et al., 1981).

The principles of treatment are the same as for hypospadias correction. The scaphoid type of megalourethra can be readily repaired by opening the urethra longitudinally and excising the redundant lateral urethral mucosa (Fig. 51-31). The excess urethral wall should be preserved, to allow a double-breasted closure of the urethra. The fusiform type of lesion is more difficult to correct. There are no erectile elements and most patients do not survive.

The status of the upper tracts and the associated abnormalities determine the ultimate outcome. Combining a literature review with a clinical series of their own, Appel and colleagues (1986) noted an incidence of death or azotemia in 19 of 31 patients with scaphoid megalourethra, and 7 of 10 with fusiform megalourethra.

Valve of Guerin

First described by Guerin (1864), this valve is a dorsal urethral diverticulum or lacuna magna, partially separated from the dorsal glandular urethra by a septum. It can often be seen as a small spherical collection of contrast at the tip of the penis, on a voiding cystourethrogram (Fig. 51-32). Sommer and Stephens (1980) reported this anomaly in 10 of 20 routine postmortems and 6 of 21 boys undergoing routine cystoscopy.

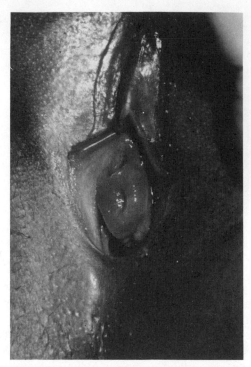

FIG. 51-33
View of a urethral prolapse. (Courtesy of Arnold Colodny, MD.)

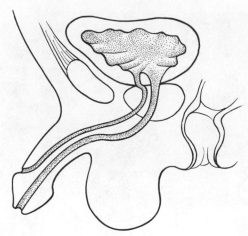

FIG. 51-34
Diagram of a complete urethral duplication. (Courtesy of Arnold Colodny, MD.)

It is thought to be an embryological variant resulting from incomplete fusion between the ingrowing ectoderm at the tip of the penis and the more proximal glandular urethra, formed by fusion of the urethral folds (see Fig. 55-1 in Chapter 55, Hypospadias).

Although the lesion is a common anatomical finding, symptoms are rare. Friedman and King (1993) reported only 10 symptomatic cases collected over a 7-year period. The patients suffered dysuria, gross hematuria, spotting of blood, or hematospermia.

The valve can be located by probing the fossa navicularis with a blunt needle or lacrimal probe or by endoscopic inspection of the distal urethra. Once located, it can be divided with fine scissors.

Urethral Prolapse

The original description of urethral prolapse has been attributed to Solingen in 1732 (Epsteen and Strauss, 1937). This is an uncommon event in young girls, with an estimated incidence of 1 in 3000 (Mitre et al., 1987). It is far more common in black children than white (Jerkins et al., 1984; Lowe et al., 1986; Richardson et al., 1982), and more common in the lower socioeconomic classes (Trotman and Brewster, 1993).

Multiple etiological theories have been proposed, but none has been substantiated. It may be due to excessive urethral mobility, excessive mucosal redundancy, increased abdominal pressure, infection, neuromuscular deficiency, or poor attachment between the muscle layers of the urethra (Lowe et al., 1986).

Vaginal bleeding is often the first symptom, but a vaginal discharge or urinary tract infection may also bring the condition to attention (Fig. 51-33). On examination, there is a characteristic circumferential prolapse of the mucosa. The differential diagnosis includes papilloma, caruncle, urethral polyps, prolapsed ureterocele, sarcoma botryoids, and periurethral abscess. A urethrogram is required if there is a partial or eccentric prolapse.

Conservative treatment can be attempted initially. Resolution has been described with oral antibiotics, estrogen cream, and sitz baths (Richardson et al., 1982; Trotman and Brewster, 1993). Cystoscopy should be performed prior to surgical correction, to confirm the diagnosis. Simple cautery excision should be employed. Infiltration of the lesion with 1% lidocaine and 1:100,000 epinephrine reduces bleeding during the subsequent surgical excision. The redundant mucosa is excised with a catheter in situ and the edges sutured. More radical surgical procedures are not indicated in children, nor is ligation of the redundant mucosa around a catheter (Fernandes et al., 1993).

Urethral Duplications

Duplication of the urethra is a rare anomaly, with only 150 cases described in the literature up until 1986. Several classifications have been devised by different investigators (Das and Brosman, 1977; Effmann et al., 1976; Irmisch and Cook, 1946; Williams and Kenawi, 1975); however, all seem too complex for such a rare condition. A simple description of the lesion suffices (Figs. 51-34, 51-35).

Urethral duplications may originate proximally at the bladder neck or prostatic urethra or more distally from the urethra. They may be either com-

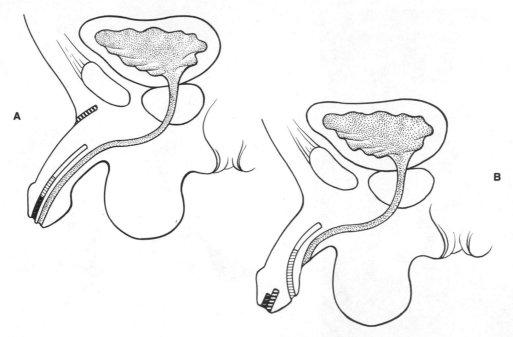

FIG. 51-35
Diagram of various incomplete urethral duplications. (Courtesy of Arnold Colodny, MD.)

plete, venting externally (Fig. 51-36), or incomplete, joining the other urethra (Fig. 51-37). They may be ventral (hypospadiac) or dorsal (epispadiac) to the main urethra, or the two may lie side by side (Kennedy et al., 1988). In most cases, the ventral urethra is the more functional one (Colodny, 1991). Isolated case reports of urethral trification exit (Forgaard and Ansell, 1966; Gulerce et al., 1992; Wirtshafter et al., 1980).

The etiology of the condition is unknown. The malformation varies so widely from case to case that it is unlikely that the same embryological explanation can apply to all cases (Psihramis et al., 1986). Theories suggested include faulty fusion of the genital ridge (Johnson, 1920), and persistence of the urogenital plate during infolding of the genital ridge (Lowsley, 1939). Dorsal duplications may have a widened symphysis and be a variant of epispadias (Effmann et al., 1976). Duplications associated with diphallus or duplicated bladders are probably due to incomplete twinning, with caudal splitting at the stage of development of the primitive streak or notochord (Feins and Cranley, 1986). These cases are often associated with duplications of the lower gastrointestinal tract.

Most patients with incomplete duplications are asymptomatic. Some develop a discharge or infection in the accessory urethra (Sharma et al., 1987). In contrast, most patients with complete duplications are symptomatic. They may have a urinary tract infection, urinary incontinence, obstruction, or a complaint of two urinary streams. Investigations include a voiding

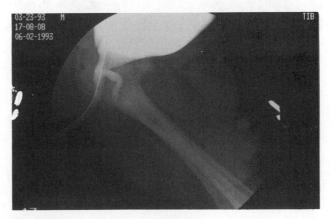

FIG. 51-36
An H-type complete duplication of the urethra. The ventral urethra passes through the rhabdosphincter to open the perineum. The dorsal urethra branches from the prostatic urethra and opens at the tip of the penis.

cystourethrogram and a retrograde urethrogram via both urethras. The upper tracts should be screened with ultrasound.

The treatment of these patients must be individualized. Two thirds of patients with complete duplications will require surgery (Hosomi et al., 1988). A decision must be made regarding which urethra to preserve (usually the ventral one) and the necessity of ablation of the other. Various surgical procedures have been recommended, including complete excision (Effmann et al., 1976), ligation, fulguration, and sclerosis (Das and Brosman, 1977). Hypospadias and epispadias can be treated with standard techniques, including island flaps and buccal mucosal grafts.

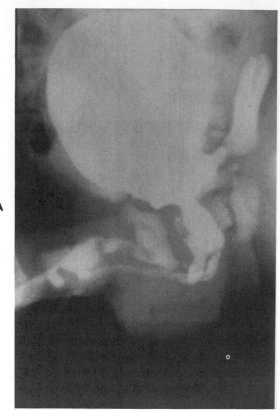

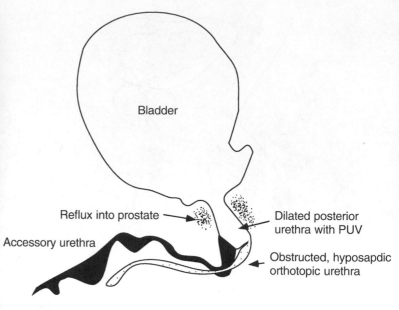

FIG. 51-37
A, A VCUG of an atypical complete duplication. **B,** A diagram of the same. The orthotopic urethra is obstructed by a PUV. The obstruction vents via the accessory urethra. The upper tracts were well preserved.

REFERENCES

Aaronson IA, Cremin BJ: *Clinical Paediatric Uroradiology*. Edinburgh: Churchill Livingstone, 1984.

Abraham MK: Mohan's urethral valvotome: a new instrument. *J Urol* 1990; 144:1196.

Adzick NS, Harrison MR, Flake AW, et al: Urinary extravasation in the fetus with obstructive uropathy. *J Pediatr Surg* 1985a; 20:608.

Adzick NS, Harrison MR, Flake AW, et al: Development of a fetal renal function test using endogenous creatinine clearance. *J Pediatr Surg* 1985b; 20:602.

Aperia A, Broberger O, Thodenius K: Development of renal control of salt and fluid homeostasis during the first year of life. *Acta Paediatr* 1975; 64:393.

Appel RA, Kaplan GW, Brock WA, et al: Megalourethra. *J Urol* 1986; 135:747.

Arey LB: *Developmental Anatomy*. Philadelphia: WB Saunders, 1965.

Arteaga J, Tran-Minh VA, Pracros JP, et al: Sonographic diagnosis of polyp of the prostatic urethra in children. *J Clin Ultrasound* 1993; 21:188.

Atwell JD: Posterior urethral valves in the British Isles: a multicenter B.A.P.S. review. *J Pediatr Surg* 1983; 18:70.

Barry JM: Renal transplantation. In Walsh PC, Retik AB, Stamey TA, et al (eds): *Campbell's Urology*, ed 6. Philadelphia: WB Saunders, 1992, p 2503.

Bartone F, King LR: Abnormalities of the urethra, penis, and scrotum. In Welch KJ, Randolph JG, Ravitch MM, et al (eds): *Pediatric Surgery*, ed 4. Chicago: Year Book Medical Publishers, 1986, p 1318.

Bazy P: Rétrécissement congénital de l'uréthre chez l'homme. *Presse Med* 1903; 19:215.

Beck AD: The effect of intra-uterine urinary obstruction upon the development of the fetal kidney. *J Urol* 1971; 105:784.

Bellinger MF: Ureterocystoplasty: a unique method for vesical augmentation in children. *J Urol* 1993; 149:811.

Belman AB: Hypospadias and other urethral abnormalities. In Kelasis PP, King LR, Belman AB (eds): *Clinical Pediatric Urology*, ed 3. Philadelphia: WB Saunders, 1992, p 619.

Bennington JL: *Perinatal Pathology*. Philadelphia: WB Saunders, 1984.

Borzi PA, Beasley SW, Fowler R: Posterior urethral valves in non-twin siblings. *Br J Urol* 1992; 70:201.

Brenner BM, Meyer TW, Hostetter TH: Dietary protein intake and the progressive nature of kidney disease: the role of hemodynamically mediated glomerular injury in the pathogenesis of progressive glomerular sclerosis in aging, renal ablation, and intrinsic renal disease. *N Engl J Med* 1982; 307:652.

Brock WA, Kaplan GW: Lesions of Cowper's glands in children. *J Urol* 1979; 122:121.

Brown T, Mandell J, Lebowitz RL: Neonatal hydronephrosis in the era of sonography. *Am J Roentgenol* 1987; 148:959.

Bryant JE, Joseph DB, Kohaut EC, et al: Renal transplantation in children with posterior urethral valves. *J Urol* 1991; 146:1585.

Bueschen AJ, Garrett RA, Newman DM: Posterior urethral valves: management. *J Urol* 1973; 110:682.

Campbell MF: *Urology*. Philadelphia: WB Saunders, 1954.

Carpiniello V, Duckett JW, Filmer RB: Posterior urethral valves: a review of 57 cases. *Kimbrough Proceedings* 1977; Annual Proceedings, p. 282.

Chantler C, Barratt T: Laboratory evaluation. In Holliday MA, Barratt TM, Vernier RL (eds): *Pediatric Nephrology*, ed 2. Baltimore: Williams and Wilkins, 1975, p 287.

Chesney RW, Avioli LV: Childhood renal osteodystrophy. In Edelmann CMJ (ed): *Pediatric Kidney Disease*, ed 2. Boston: Little, Brown, 1992, p 647.

Churchill BM, Aliabadi H, Landau EH, et al: Ureteral bladder augmentation. *J Urol* 1993; 150:716.

Churchill BM, McLorie GA, Khoury AE, et al: Emergency treatment and long-term follow-up of posterior urethral valves. *Urol Clin North Am* 1990; 17:343.

Churchill BM, Sheldon CA, McLorie GA, et al: Factors influencing patient and graft survival in 300 cadaveric pediatric renal transplants. *J Urol* 1988; 140:1129.

Cobb BG, Wolf JA, Ansell JS: Congenital stricture of the proximal urethral bulb. *J Urol* 1968; 99:629.

Colodny AH: In utero diagnosis of urological abnormalities. *Dialogues in Pediatric Urology* 1983; 6:11.

Colodny A: Antenatal diagnosis and management of urinary abnormalities. *Pediatr Clin North Am* 1987; 34:1365.

Colodny A: Urethral lesions in infants and children. In Gillenwater, JY, Grayhack JT, Howards SS, et al (eds): *Adult and Pediatric Urology*. St. Louis: Mosby, 1991, p 1995.

Connor JP, Burbige KA: Long-term urinary continence and renal function in neonates with posterior urethral valves. *J Urol* 1990; 144:1209.

Coplen DE, Joanie YH, Zderic S, et al: *Ten-year experience with antenatal in utero intervention*. AAP, Dallas, Texas, 1994.

Cornil C: *Urethral Obstruction in Boys*. Amsterdam: Excerpta Medica, 1975.

Crankson S, Ahmed S: Prenatal diagnosis of posterior urethral valves in siblings. *Aust N Z J Surg* 1993; 63:143.

Cremin BJ: A review of the ultrasound appearances of posterior urethral valve and ureteroceles. *Pediatr Radiol* 1986; 16:359.

Cromie WJ, Cain MP, Bellinger MF, et al: Urethral valve incision using a modified venous valvulotome. *J Urol* 1994; 151:1053.

Das S, Brosman SA: Duplication of the male urethra. *J Urol* 1977; 117:452.

Davidsohn I, Newberger C: Congenital valves of the posterior urethra in twins. *Arch Pathol* 1933; 16:57.

De Filippi G, Derchi LE, Coppi M, et al: Sonographic diagnosis of urethral polyp in a child. *Pediatr Radiol* 1983; 13:351.

Dewan PA: Congenital obstructing urethral membranes (COPUM): further evidence for a common morphological diagnosis. *Pediatr Surg Int* 1992; 8:45.

Dewan PA, Zappala SM, Ransley PG, et al: Endoscopic reappraisal of the morphology of congenital obstruction of the posterior urethra. *Br J Urol* 1992; 70:439.

Diamond DA, Ransley PG: Fogarty balloon catheter ablation of neonatal posterior urethral valves. *J Urol* 1987; 137:1209.

Dinneen MD, Dhillon HK, Ward HC, et al: Antenatal diagnosis of posterior urethral valves. *Br J Urol* 1993; 72:364.

Dorairajan T: Defects of spongy tissue and congenital diverticula of the penile urethra. *Aust N Z J Surg* 1963; 32:209.

Doraiswamy NV, Al Badr MS, Freeman NV: Posterior urethral valves in siblings. *Br J Urol* 1983; 55:448.

Downs RA: Congenital polyps of the prostatic urethra. A review of the literature and report of two cases. *Br J Urol* 1970; 42:76.

Duckett J Jr: Current management of posterior urethral valves. *Urol Clin North Am* 1974a; 1:471.

Duckett JW: Cutaneous vesicostomy in infants and children. *Urol Clin North Am* 1974b; 1:484.

Duckett JW: The prune belly syndrome. In Kelasis P, King LR, Belman AB (eds): *Clinical Pediatric Urology*. Philadelphia: WB Saunders, 1976, p 615.

Duckett JW: Anomalies of the urethra. In Harrison JH, Gittes RF, Perlmutter AD, et al (eds): *Campbell's Urology*. Philadelphia: WB Saunders, 1979a, p 1646.

Duckett JW: Management of posterior urethral valves. *Dialogues in Pediatric Urology* 1979b; 2:7.

Duckett JW: Management of posterior urethral valves. *AUA Update Series* 1983; 2:1.

Duckett JW, Norris M: Management of neonatal valves with advanced hydronephrosis and azotemia. In Carlton CE (ed): *Controversies in Urology*. Chicago: Year Book Medical Publishers, 1989, p 1.

Duckett JW, Snow BW: Disorders of the urethra and penis. In Walsh PC, Gittes RF, Perlmutter AD, et al (eds): *Campbell's Urology*, ed 5. Philadelphia: WB Saunders, 1986, p 2000.

Edling NP: The radiological appearances of diverticula of the male cavernous urethra. *Acta Radiol* 1953; 40:1.

Effmann EL, Lebowit RL, Colodny AH: Duplication of the urethra. *Radiology* 1976; 119:179.

Ehrlich RM, Shanberg A, Fine RN: Neodymium:YAG laser ablation of posterior urethral valves. *J Urol* 1987; 138:959.

Eklöf O, Elle B, Thönell S: Pseudotumour of the kidney secondary to posterior urethral valves: the role of renal backflow and perirenal extravasation. *Pediatr Radiol* 1984; 14:215.

Elbadawi A, Meyer S, Malkowicz SB, et al: Effects of short-term partial bladder outlet obstruction on the rabbit detrusor: an ultrastructural study. *Neurourol Urodyn* 1989; 8:89.

Elder JS, Duckett JW: Intervention for fetal obstructive uropathy: has it been effective? *Lancet* 1987; 2:1007.

Epsteen A, Strauss BP: Prolapse of the female urethra with gangrene. *Amer J Surg* 1937; 35:563.

Ewalt DH, Howard PS, Blyth B, et al: Is lamina propria matrix responsible for normal bladder compliance? *J Urol* 1992; 148:544.

Farkas A, Skinner DG: Posterior urethral valves in siblings. *Br J Urol* 1976; 48:76.

Feins NR, Cranley W: Bladder duplication with one exstrophy and one cloaca. *J Pediatr Surg* 1986; 21:570.

Fernandes ET, Dekermacher S, Sabadin MA, et al: Urethral prolapse in children. *Urology* 1993; 41:240.

Fernbach SK: Urethral abnormalities in male neonates with VATER association. *AJR Am J Roentgenol* 1991; 156:137.

Fichtner J, Boineau FG, Lewy JE, et al: Congenital unilateral hydronephrosis in a rat model: continuous renal pelvic and bladder pressures. *J Urol* 1994; 152:652.

Field PL, Stephens FD: Congenital urethral membranes causing urethral obstruction. *J Urol* 1974; 111:250.

Firlit CF, Burstein JD: Anterior urethra. In Kelalis P, King L, Belman B (eds): *Clinical Pediatric Urology*, ed 2. Philadelphia: WB Saunders, 1985, p 559.

Firlit RS, Firlit CF, King LR: Obstructing anterior urethral valves in children. *J Urol* 1978; 119:819.

Fisk NM, Dhillon HK, Ellis CE, et al: Antenatal diagnosis of megalourethra in a fetus with the prune belly syndrome. *J Clin Ultrasound* 1990; 18:124.

Forgaard DM, Ansell JS: Trification of the anterior urethra: a case report. *J Urol* 1966; 95:785.

Friedenberg RM, Moorehouse H, Gade M: Urinomas secondary to pyelosinus backflow. *Urol Radiol* 1983; 5:23.

Friedman RM, King LR: Valve of Guerin as a cause of dysuria and hematuria in young boys: presentation and difficulties in diagnosis. *J Urol* 1993; 150:159.

Gibbons MD, Horan JJ, Dejter S Jr, et al: Extracorporeal membrane oxygenation: an adjunct in the management of the neonate with severe respiratory distress and congenital urinary tract anomalies. *J Urol* 1993; 150:434.

Gillenwater JY: The pathophysiology of urinary-tract obstruction. In Walsh PC, Retk AB, Stamey TA, et al (eds): *Campbell's Urology*. Philadelphia: WB Saunders, 1992, p 499.

Glassberg KI, Schieder M, Haller JO, et al: Observations on persistently dilated ureter after posterior urethral valve ablation. *Urology* 1982; 20:20.

Glick PL, Harrison MR, Noall RA, et al: Correction of congenital hydronephrosis in utero. II. Early midtrimester ureteral obstruction produces renal dysplasia. *J Pediatr Surg* 1983; 18:681.

Glynn B, Gordon IR: Risk of infection of urinary tract as a result of micturating cystourethrography in children. *Ann Radiol (Paris)* 1970; 13:283.

Golimbu M, Orca M, Al-Askari S, et al: Anterior urethral valves. *Urology* 1978; 12:343.

Gonzales ET: Posterior urethral valves and other urethral anomalies. In Walsh PC, Retik AB, Stamey TA, et al (eds): *Campbell's Urology*, ed 6. Philadelphia: WB Saunders, 1992, p 1872.

Grajewski RS, Glassberg KI: The variable effect of posterior urethral valves as illustrated in identical twins. *J Urol* 1983; 130:1188.

Guerin A: *Elements de Chirurgie Operatorire*. Paris: F Chamerot, 1864.

Gulerce Z, Nazli O, Killi R, et al: Trifurcation of the urethra: a case report. *J Urol* 1992; 148:403.

Haller JO, Berdon WE, Friedman AP: Increased renal cortical echogenicity: a normal finding in neonates and infants. *Radiology* 1982; 142:173.

Hanlon-Lundberg KM, Verp MS, Loy G: Posterior urethral valves in successive generations. *Am J Perinatol* 1994; 11:37.

Hart RG, Greenstein JS: A newly discovered role for Cowper's gland secretion in rodent semen coagulation. *J Reprod Fertil* 1968; 17:87.

Helin I, Persson P: Prenatal diagnosis of urinary tract abnormalities by ultrasound. *J Pediatr* 1986; 78:879.

Hendren WH: A new approach to infants with severe obstructive uropathy: early complete reconstruction. *J Pediatr Surg* 1970; 5:184.

Hendren WH: Posterior urethral valves in boys. A broad clinical spectrum. *J Urol* 1971; 106:298.

Hendren WH: Complications of ureterostomy. *J Urol* 1978; 120:269.

Hendren WH: Urinary tract re-functionalization after long-term diversion. A 20-year experience with 177 patients. *Ann Surg* 1990; 212:478.

Hendren WH: Urethral valves. In Ashcraft KW, Holder TM (eds): *Pediatric Surgery*, ed 2. Philadelphia: WB Saunders, 1993, p 655.

Henneberry MO, Stephens FD: Renal hypoplasia and dysplasia in infants with posterior urethral valves. *J Urol* 1980; 123:912.

Heyman SH, Duckett JW: The extraction factor: an estimate of single kidney function in children during routine radionuclide renography with 99-technetium diethylenetriamine pentaacetic acid. *J Urol* 1988; 140:780.

Hoover DL, Duckett J Jr: Posterior urethral valves, unilateral reflux, and renal dysplasia: a syndrome. *J Urol* 1982; 128:994.

Hosomi M, Ichikawa Y, Takaha M, et al: Complete duplication of male urethra. *Urol Int* 1988; 43:118.

Huang CJ, Bai JW, Liang RX, et al: Congenital anterior urethral valves and diverticula—analysis of 50 cases. *Ann Acad Med Singapore* 1989; 18:665.

Hulbert WC, Duckett JW: Prognostic factors in infants with posterior urethral valves. *J Urol* 1986; 135:121.

Hulbert WC, Duckett JW: Current views on posterior urethral valves. *Pediatr Ann* 1988; 17:31.

Hulbert WC, Duckett JW: Posterior urethral valve obstruction. *AUA Update Series* 1992; XI: Lesson 26.

Hulbert WC, Rosenberg HK, Cartwright PC, et al: The predictive value of ultrasonography in evaluation of infants with posterior urethral valves. *J Urol* 1992; 148:122.

Hutton KA, Thomas DF, Arthur RJ, et al: Prenatally detected posterior urethral valves: is gestational age at detection a predictor of outcome? *J Urol* 1994; 152:698.

Hyacinthe LM, Khoury SE, Churchill BM, et al: Improved outcome of renal transplants in children with posterior urethral valves. *J Urol* 1995; 153:341A.

Irmisch GW, Cook EN: Double and accessory urethra. *Minnestoa Med* 1946; 29:999.

Jee LD, Rickwood AM, Turnock RR: Posterior urethral valves. Does prenatal diagnosis influence prognosis? *Br J Urol* 1993; 72:830.

Jerkins GR, Verheeck K, Noe HN: Treatment of girls with urethral prolapse. *J Urol* 1984; 132:732.

Johnson FP: The later development of the urethra in the male. *J Urol* 1920; 4:447.

Johnston JH: Temporary cutaneous ureterostomy in the management of advanced congenital urinary obstruction. *Arch Dis Child* 1963; 38:161.

Johnston JH: Posterior urethral valves; an operative technique using an electric auriscope. *J Pediatr Surg* 1966; 1:583.

Johnston JH: Posterior urethral valves. In Rickham PP. a. J., J.H. (eds): *Neonatal Surgery*. London: Butterworth, 1969, p 532.

Johnston JH: Vesicoureteric reflux with urethral valves. *Br J Urol* 1979; 51:100.

Johnston JH, Kulatilake AE: The sequelae of posterior urethral valves. *Br J Urol* 1971; 43:743.

Jordan GH, Hoover DL: Inadequate decompression of the upper tracts using a Foley catheter in the valve bladder. *J Urol* 1985; 134:137.

Kato K, Wein AJ, Kitada S, et al: The functional effect of mild outlet obstruction on the rabbit urinary bladder. *J Urol* 1988; 140:880.

Kennedy HA, Steidle CP, Mitchell ME, et al: Collateral urethral duplication in the frontal plane: a spectrum of cases. *J Urol* 1988; 139:332.

Khoury AE, Houle AM, McLorie GA, et al: Cutaneous vesicostomy effect on bladder's eventual function. *Dialog Pediatr Urol* 1990; 13:2-3.

Kimmelstiel P, Wilson C: Inflammatory lesions in the glomeruli in pyelonephritis in relation to hypertension and renal insufficiency. *Amer J Path* 1936; 12:99.

King LR: Posterior urethra. In Kelalis PP, King LR, Belman AB (eds): *Urology*, ed 2. Philadelphia: WB Saunders, 1985, p 527.

King LR, Coughlin PW, Bloch EC, et al: The case for immediate pyeloplasty in the neonate with ureteropelvic junction obstruction. *J Urol* 1984; 132:725.

Klee LW, Rink RC, Gleason PE, et al: Urethral polyp presenting as interlabial mass in young girls. *Urology* 1993; 41:132.

Kogan B: Treatment options for posterior urethral valves in neonates. In King, LR (ed): *Urological Surgery in Neonates and Young Infants*, ed 1. Philadelphia: WB Saunders, 1988, p 244.

Krahn CG, Johnson HW: Cutaneous vesicostomy in the young child: indications and results. *Urology* 1993; 41:558.

Krane RJ: Neonatal perirenal urinary extravasation. *J Urol* 1974; 111:96.

Kroovand RL, Weinberg N, Emami A: Posterior urethral valves in identical twins. *Pediatrics* 1977; 60:748.

Krueger RP, Hardy BE, Churchill BM: Cryptorchidism in boys with posterior urethral valves. *J Urol* 1980a; 124:101.

Krueger RP, Hardy BE, Churchill BM: Growth in boys and posterior urethral valves. Primary valve resection vs upper tract diversion. *Urol Clin North Am* 1980b; 7:265.

Kurth KH, Alleman ER, Schroder FH: Major and minor complications of posterior urethral valves. *J Urol* 1981; 126:517.

Landau EH, Jayanthi VR, Khoury AE, et al: Bladder augmentation: ureterocystoplasty versus ileocystoplasty. *J Urol* 1994; 152:716.

Livne PM, Delaune J, Gonzales E, Jr: Genetic etiology of posterior urethral valves. *J Urol* 1983; 130:781.

Lome LG, Howat JM, Williams DI: The temporarily defunctionalized bladder in children. *J Urol* 1972; 108:469.

Lowe FC, Hill GS, Jeffs RD, et al: Urethral prolapse in children: insights into etiology and management. *J Urol* 1986; 135:100.

Lowsley OS: Congenital malformations of the posterior urethra. *Ann Surg* 1914; 60:733.

Lowsley OS: Accessory urethra: report of two cases with review of literature. *New York State Journal of Medicine* 1939; 39:1022.

Maizels M, Simpson SB: Primitive ducts of renal dysplasia induced by culturing ureteral buds denuded of condensed renal mesenchyme. *Science* 1983; 219:509.

Maizels M, Stephens FD, King LK, et al: Cowper's syringocele: a classification of dilatations of Cowper's gland duct based upon clinical characteristics of 8 boys. *J Urol* 1982; 129:111.

Marshall FF, Smolev JK, Spees EK, et al: The urological evaluation and management of patients with congenital lower urinary tract anomalies prior to renal transportaion. *J Urol* 1982; 127:1078.

McCory WW: Regulation of renal functional development. *Urol Clin North Am* 1980; 7:243.

McGuire EJ, Weiss RM: Secondary bladder neck obstruction in patients with urethral valves: treatment with phenoxybenzamine. *Urology* 1975; 5:756.

McGuire EJ, Woodside JR, Borden TA, et al: Prognostic value of urodynamic testing in myelodysplasic patients. *J Urol* 1981; 126:205.

Mitchell ME: Persistent ureteral dilatation following valve resection. *Dialogues in Pediatr Urol* 1982; 5:8.

Mitre A, Nahas W, Gilbert A, et al: Urethral prolapse in girls: familial case. *J Urol* 1987; 137:115.

Mochon M, Kaiser BA, Dunn S, et al: Urinary tract infections in children with posterior urethral valves after kidney transplantation. *J Urol* 1992; 148:1874.

Mohammed SH: Suprapubic micturition cystourethrography. *Acta Radiol* 1988; 29:165.

Monford G: Posterior urethral valve management; personal communication, Society for Paediatric Urologic Surgeons meeting, Dublin, 1994.

Mortensen PH, Johnson HW, Coleman GU, et al: Megalourethra. *J Urol* 1985; 134:358.

Moskowitz PS, Newton NA, Lebowitz RL: Retention cysts of Cowper's duct. *Radiology* 1976; 120:377.

Myers DA, Walker R 3rd: Prevention of urethral strictures in the management of posterior urethral valves. *J Urol* 1981; 126:655.

Nakayama DK, Harrison MR, and de Lormier A A: Prognosis of posterior urethral valves presenting at birth. *J Pediatr Surg* 1986; 21:43.

Nesbitt TE: Congenital megalourethra. *J Urol* 1955; 73:839.

Noe HN, Jerkins GR: Cutaneous vesicostomy experience in infants and children. *J Urol* 1985; 134:301.

Novick AC, Gephhardt G, Guz B, et al: Long-term follow-up after partial removal of a solitary kidney. *N Engl J Med* 1991; 325:1058.

Ogden DA: Donor and recipient function 2 to 4 years after renal homotransplantation: a paired study of 28 cases. *Ann Intern Med* 1967; 67:998.

Parker RM: Neonatal urinary ascites. A potentially favorable sign in bladder outlet obstruction. *Urology* 1974; 3:589.

Parkhouse HF, Barratt TM, Dillon MJ, et al: Long-term outcome of boys with posterior urethral valves. *Br J Urol* 1988; 62:59.

Parkhouse HF, Woodhouse CR: Long-term status of patients with posterior urethral valves. *Urol Clin North Am* 1990; 17:373.

Parkkulainen KV: Posterior urethral obstruction: valvular or diaphragmatic. Endoscopic diagnosis and treatment. *Birth Defects* 1977; 13:63.

Perimenis P, Panagou A: Re: Acute urinary retention caused by anterior urethral polyp. Letter; comment. *Br J Urol* 1992; 70:695.

Peters CA, Bolkier M, Bauer SB, et al: The urodynamic consequences of posterior urethral valves. *J Urol* 1990; 144:122.

Presman D: Congenital valves of the posterior urethra. *J Urol* 1961; 86:602.

Psihramis KE, Colodny AH, Lebowitz RL, et al: Complete patent duplication of the urethra. *J Urol* 1986; 136:63.

Quinn FMJ, Zadeh K, Duffy PG, et al: *Augmentation cytoplasty in boys with posterior urethral valves.* AAP annual meeting, Dallas, Texas, 1994.

Redman JF: A catheter guide to obviate difficult urethral catheterization in male infants and boys. *J Urol* 1993; 151:1051.

Reinberg Y, de Castano I, Gonzalez R: Influence of initial therapy on progression of renal failure and body growth in children with posterior urethral valves. *J Urol* 1992a; 148:532.

Reinberg Y, de Castano I, Gonzalez R: Prognosis for patients with prenatally diagnosed posterior urethral valves. *J Urol* 1992b; 148:125.

Reinberg Y, Gonzalez R, Fryd D, et al: The outcome of renal transplantation in children with posterior urethral valves. *J Urol* 1988; 140:1491.

Reissigl A, Eberle J, Bartsch G: Megalourethra. *Br J Urol* 1991; 68:435.

Richardson DA, Hajj SN, Herbst AL: Medical treatment of urethral prolapse in children. *Obstet Gynecol* 1982; 59:69.

Rittenberg MH, Hulbert WC, Snyder HM 3rd et al: Protective factors in posterior urethral valves. *J Urol* 1988; 140:993.

Robertson WB, Hayes JA: Congenital diaphragmatic obstruction of the male urethra. *Br J Urol* 1969; 41:592.

Rosenfeld B, Greenfield SP, Springate JE, et al: Type III posterior urethral valves: presentation and management. *J Pediatr Surg* 1994; 29:81.

Ross JH, Kay R, Novick AC, et al: Long-term results of renal transplantation into the valve bladder. *J Urol* 194; 151:1500.

Rushton HG, Parrott TS, Woodard JR, et al: The role of vesicostomy in the management of anterior urethral valves in neonates and infants. *J Urol* 1987; 138:107.

Sanders RC, Nussbaum AR, Solez K: Renal dysplasia: sonographic findings. *Radiology* 1988; 167:623.

Sant GR, Kaleli A: Cowper's syringocele causing incontinence in an adult. *J Urol* 1985; 133:279.

Schaeffer AJ: Infections of the urinary tract. In Walsh PC, Retik AB, Stamey TA, et al (eds): *Campbell's Urology.* Philadelphia: WB Saunders, 1992, p 760.

Scherz HC, Kaplan GW, and Packer MG: Anterior urethral valves in the fossa navicularis in children. *J Urol* 1987; 138:1211.

Schulman SL, VanGool JD: Dyssynergic voiding in PUV. 1993 (personal communication).

Schwartz GJ, Feld LG, Langford DJ: A simple estimation of glomerular filtration rate in full-term infants during the first year of life. *J Pediatr* 1984; 104:849.

Scott JE: Management of congenital posterior urethral valves. *Br J Urol* 1985; 57:71.

Sepulveda W, Berry SM, Romero R, et al: Prenatal diagnosis of congenital megalourethra. *J Ultrasound Med* 1993; 12:761.

Sharma SK, Kapoor R, Kumar A, et al: Incomplete epispadiac urethral duplication with dorsal penile curvature. *J Urol* 1987; 138:585.

Sheldon CA, Churchill BM, McLorie GA, et al: Evaluation of factors contributing to mortality in pediatric renal transplant recipients. *J Pediatr Surg* 1992; 27:629.

Sholder AJ, Maizels M, Depp R, et al: Caution in antenatal intervention. *J Urol* 1988; 139:1026.

Shrom SH, Cromie WJ, Duckett JW: Megalourethra. *Urology* 1981; 17:152.

Simma B, Gabner I, Brezinka C, et al: Complete prenatal urinary tract obstruction caused by congenital megalourethra. *J Clin Ultrasound* 1992; 20:197.

Smith GH, Duckett JW, Canning DA: Posterior urethral valves, a cohort with a 20-year follow-up. *J Urol* 1994a; 151:275.

Smith GHH, Canning DA, Schulman SL, et al: The long-term outcome of posterior urethral valves treated by primary valve ablation and observation. *J Urol* 1996.

Snyder HM, Kalichman MA, Charney E, et al: Vesicostomy for neurogenic bladder with spina bifida: follow-up. *J Urol* 1983; 130:724.

Sommer JT, Stephens FD: Dorsal urethral diverticulum of the fossa navicularis: symptoms, diagnosis, and treatment. *J Urol* 1980; 124:94.

Speakman MJ, Brading AF, Gilpin CJ, et al: Bladder outflow obstruction: a cause of denervation supersensitivity. *J Urol* 1987; 138:1461.

Steinhardt GF, Ramon G, Salinas ML: Glomerulosclerosis in obstructive uropathy. *J Urol* 1988; 140:1316

Stephens FD: Urethral obstruction in childhood: the use of urethrography in diagnosis. *Aust N Z J Surg* 1955; 25:89.

Stephens FD: *Congenital Malformations of the Rectum, Anus, and Genitourinary Tract.* London: E & S Livingston, 1963.

Stephens FD: Congenital intrinsic lesions of the posterior urethra. In Stephens FD (ed): *Congenital Malformations of the Urinary Tract.* New York: Praeger, 1983, p 95.

Stephens FD, Fortune DW: Pathogenesis of megaloure-thra. *J Urol* 1993; 149:1512.

Suki W, Eknoyan G, Rector FC, et al: Patterns of neph-ron perfusion in acute and chronic hydronephrosis. *J Clin Invest* 1966; 45:122.

Tanagho E: Congenitally obstructed bladders: fate after prolonged defunctionalization. *J Urol* 1974; 111:102.

Tank ES: Anterior urethral valves resulting from congeni-tal urethral diverticula. *Urology* 1987; 30:467.

Tank ES: Cold-knife ablation of urethral valves. *Society of Pediatric Urology Newsletter* 1992; 3:2.

Tejani A, Butt K, Glassberg K, et al: Predictors of even-tual end-stage renal disease in children with posterior urethral valves. *J Urol* 1986; 136:857.

Thomalla JV, Mitchell ME, Garett RA: Posterior urethral valves in siblings. *Urology* 1989; 33:291.

Tolmatschew N: Ein Fall von semilunaren Klappen der Harröhre und von vergrösserte Vesicular prostatica. *Virchows Arch (Pathol Anat)* 1870; 49:348.

Trotman MD, Brewster EM: Prolapse of the urethral mu-cosa in prepubertal West Indian girls. *Br J Urol* 1993; 72:503.

Velosa JA, Holley KE, Torres VE, et al: Significance of proteinuria on the outcome of renal function in patients with glomerulosclerosis. *Mayo Clin Proc* 1983; 58:568.

Walker RD, Padron M: The management of posterior urethral valves by initial vesicostomy and delayed valve ablation. *J Urol* 1990; 144:1212.

Warshaw BL, Edelbrock HH, Ettenger RB, et al: Renal transplantation in children with obstructive uropathy. *J Urol* 1980; 123:737.

Warshaw BL, Hymes LC, Trulock TS, et al: Prognostic features in infants with obstructive uropathy due to posterior urethral valves. *J Urol* 1985; 133:240.

Watson EM: The structural basis for congenital valve for-mation in the posterior urethra. *J Urol* 1922; 7:371.

Whitaker RH: The ureter in posterior urethral valves. *Br J Urol* 1973; 45:395.

Whitaker RH, Keeton JE, Williams DI: Posterior ure-thral valves: a study of urinary control after operation. *J Urol* 1972; 108:167.

Whitaker RH, Sherwood T: An improved hook for de-stroying posterior urethral valves. *J Urol* 1986; 135:531.

Williams DI: Urethral valves. *Br J Urol* 1973; 45:200.

Williams DI, Kenawi MM: Urethral duplications in the male. *Eur Urol* 1975; 1:209.

Williams DI, Retik AB: Congenital valves and diverticula of the anterior urethra. *Br J Urol* 1969; 41:228.

Williams N, Kapila L: Posterior urethral valves in twins with mirror image abnormalities. *Br J Urol* 1993; 71:615.

Wirtshafter A, Carrion HM, Morillo G, et al: Complete trification of the urethra. *J Urol* 1980; 123:431.

Woodhouse CR, Reilly JM, Bahadur G: Sexual function and fertility in patients treated for posterior urethral valves. *J Urol* 1989; 142:586.

Yared A, Ichikawa I: Renal blood flow and glomerula fil-tration rate. In Holliday MA, Barratt TM, Vernier RL (eds): *Pediatric Nephrology*, ed 2. Baltimore: Williams and Wilkins, 1987, p 52.

Young BW: *Lower Urinary Tract Obstruction in Child-hood*. Philadelphia: Lea and Febiger, 1972.

Young HH, Frontz RH, Baldwin TC: Congenital obstruc-tion of the posterior urethra. *J Urol* 1919; 3:289.

Zaontz MR, Firlit CF: Percutaneous antegrade ablation of posterior urethral valves in premature or underweight term neonates: an alternative to primary vesicostomy. *J Urol* 1985; 134:139.

CHAPTER 52

Anomalies of the Bladder and Cloaca

Douglas A. Canning
Harry P. Koo
John W. Duckett

BLADDER ABNORMALITIES

Embryology of the Bladder

In contrast to the kidneys and ureter, which are of mesodermal origin, the structures of the lower urinary tract are formed from the endoderm. The development of bladder takes place in two stages, and its development is intimately related to that of the anus, rectum, and the lower reproductive tract.

Division of the Cloaca

At the first stage of development, the *cloaca*, Latin word for "drain," exists. This structure drains both the gastrointestinal and urinary tracts. During the fifth week, the cloaca is separated into two structures, the primitive urogenital sinus and the rectum. Mesoblast between the evolving bladder and the evolving rectum proliferates in all directions, resulting in the formation of the urorectal septum, which actually represents the elongating dorsal wall of the urogenital sinus and the elongating ventral wall of the hindgut. The urinary tract becomes separated from the hindgut when the advancing urorectal septum reaches the cloacal membrane. This separation is unequal, so that most of the cloaca eventually forms the urogenital sinus and, eventually, the bladder. Thus, the cloaca contributes little to the formation of the rectum, which develops mainly from the hindgut (deVries and Friedland, 1974; Forsberg, 1961).

Formation of the Bladder

During the second stage of bladder development, the primitive urogenital sinus becomes differentiated into a bladder portion, a trigonal portion, and a urethral portion. At the same time, the ureteral orifices and the wolffian duct orifices separate.

The bladder portion of the primitive urogenital sinus develops mainly from the cloaca, although the allantois may contribute to the development of the dome. The segment of the wolffian duct between the urogenital sinus and the ureteric bud is termed the *common excretory duct*. The trigonal portion is a composite structure formed partially by the cloaca and partially by the common excretory duct. Because the cloacal epithelium replaces that within the common excretory duct, the new trigonal epithelium is derived from the cloaca and not from the common excretory duct. The ventral portion of the urogenital sinus grows distally, forming the entire urethra in the female and all but the distal end of the urethra in the male (Friedland et al., 1990).

The bladder epithelium originating from the endoderm of the urogenital sinus remains a single layer of epithelium up to the seventh week, then gradually assumes the appearance of transitional epithelium in the third month. The musculature appears as a longitudinal layer, chiefly on the dorsal surface, from the apex to the urethra during the eighth week; circular muscle appears slightly later, beginning at the apex. A third longitudinal layer appears still later, and the adult condition is essentially present during the fourth month (Parrott et al., 1994).

Anomalies of Bladder Formation

Agenesis of the Bladder

Complete agenesis of the bladder is one of the rarest anomalies of the urinary tract with only 44 cases reported in the English literature. Most of the infants with the anomaly are stillborn and have other urogenital tract anomalies, as well as neurologic and orthopedic disorders. All but one of the 15 reported viable newborns were female (Gearhart and Jeffs, 1992). The cause of bladder agenesis remains uncertain. Since the hindgut is usually normal in these infants, it may be assumed that there is normal division of the cloaca by the urorectal septum. Bladder agenesis may be the result of atrophy of the urogenital sinus, perhaps caused by the failure of incorporation of the mesonephric ducts and ureters into the trigone

(Krull et al., 1988). In the absence of a bladder and trigone, the ureteral orifices follow the terminations of the mesonephric ducts, entering into the urethra, vestibule, or Gartner's duct in the female and into the prostatic urethra in the male (Caldamone, 1991). The ureters may remain separate or may form a common channel. The upper urinary tracts are often hydronephrotic or dysplastic from the outset. Treatment in most reported cases of surviving infants historically has included urinary diversion either by ureterosigmoidostomy or external stoma (Glenn, 1959). Now, these children also would be considered for other forms of continent urinary diversion.

Congenital Hypoplasia of the Bladder

Congenital hypoplasia of the bladder results from (1) failure of production or storage of urine or from (2) complete bypass of the bladder. Severe degrees of epispadias, female urogenital sinus abnormalities, bilateral renal agenesis, or severe renal dysplasia are examples of the former situation; bilateral ureteral ectopia with distal urethral or vaginal orifices in the female are examples of the latter. Reconstruction of the bladder neck usually is not successful in these conditions. Most will require reconstruction of the bladder with bowel (Fig. 52-1).

Anomalies of Bladder Compartmentalization

Duplication of the Bladder

Bladder duplication may be complete or incomplete. *Complete bladder duplication* is rare with only 45 cases reported in literature (Kapoor and Saha, 1987). In complete duplication, each bladder receives one or sometimes two ureters and empties into a separate urethra (Fig. 52-2, *A*; Fig. 52-3). This anomaly is observed more commonly in males than in females. In 90% of cases, there is complete duplication of the penis in the male or duplication of the vagina and uterus in the female (Satler and Mossman, 1968). The hindgut is duplicated in 40% to 50% of cases. Spinal duplication and fistulas between rectum, vagina, and urethra are other associated anomalies.

The embryologic factor leading to duplication of the bladder and hindgut may be due to the partial twinning of the tail portion of the embryo (Ravitch and Scott, 1953). However, the skeletal defects are seen less frequently. Some authors have proposed the occurrence of supernumerary urorectal septa that when sagittally oriented could divide the cloaca into two anterior bladders and two hindguts (Muecke, 1986). The Danforth strain of mice unfortunately is now extinct, but it had developed duplication of the body, as well as of the gonads and bladder, and other internal organs (Danforth, 1930).

Treatment is limited usually to procedures for maintaining normal function. No specific recommen-

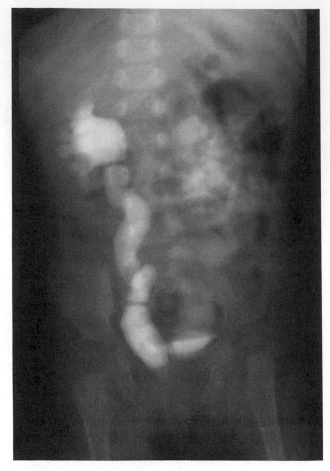

FIG. 52-1
Congenital hyposplasia of bladder. Excretory urogram demonstrating bilateral single system ectopic ureters inserting below the level of symphysis.

dation is possible because of the variations among affected patients. Blind colonic duplications must be anastomosed to provide for emptying. Reconstructive procedures often are required for the genitalia.

Incomplete bladder duplication involves two full-thickness bladders, each with an ipsilateral ureter (Fig. 52-2, *B*). The two bladder units usually communicate and drain into a common urethra (Burns et al., 1947). This anomaly usually does not result in serious sequelae because the upper tracts are often normally developed (Uhlir, 1968). There are no associated genital or anorectal anomalies.

Ischiopagus (i.e., anterior union of the lower trunk) *conjoined twins* is an extremely rare condition that can present with varying combination of bladder, ureteral, and renal anomalies. In the cases of a common, incompletely duplicated bladder, evaluation of trigonal anatomy and bladder neck competence can provide information about each twin's contribution to the shared bladder (Hsu et al., 1995).

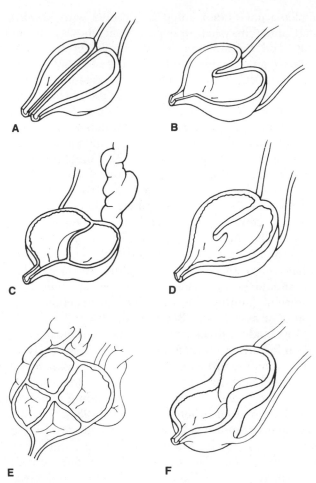

FIG. 52-2
Anomalies of bladder compartmentalization. **A,** Complete duplication. **B,** Incomplete duplication. **C,** Complete sagittal septum. **D,** Incomplete sagittal septum. **E,** Multiloculated bladder. **F,** Hourglass bladder. (Modified from Friedland GW, Devries PA, Nino-Murcia M, et al: Congenital anomalies of the urinary tract. In Pollack HM (ed): *Clinical urography: an atlas and textbook of urological imaging.* Philadelphia, WB Saunders Co, 1990.)

Septation of the Bladder

Septation of the bladder is an unusual anomaly in which a partition composed of either mucosa alone or of muscularis and mucosa divides the bladder completely or incompletely in either the frontal or sagittal plane. A groove on the serosal surface may delineate the site of septation. With a sagittal septation, a ureter enters each compartment. Because there is a single bladder neck and urethra, complete sagittal septation is associated with dysplasia or obstruction (or both) of one unit (Fig. 52-2, *C*). Additionally, it is possible for the obstructed compartment to become distended and result in bladder outlet obstruction and hydronephrosis of the contralateral unit. These septa frequently are difficult to distinguish from large ureteroceles prior to surgery. If however, the septum is

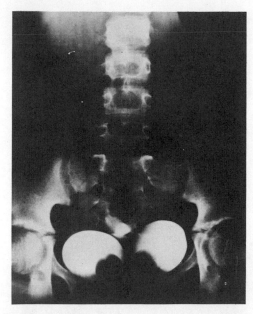

FIG. 52-3
Voiding cystourethrogram showing two separate bladders, each with Foley catheter in place. Note reflux into pelvic kidney. (Courtesy of I.N. Frank, M.D.)

incomplete, each compartment should drain freely (Caldamone, 1991) (Fig. 52-2, *D*). Resection of the redundant mucosal septum by cystotomy is the usual corrective procedure. Nephroureterectomy may be necessary if the obstruction is associated with dysplastic renal segment.

An even rarer form of septation anomaly is the *multiloculated bladder* with only two reported cases (Senger and Santore, 1951). The bladder is compartmentalized into unequal chambers by fibromuscular walls. There is duplication of upper urinary tracts with each ureter entering a separate chamber. Because a single bladder neck and urethra drain only one chamber, the other three bladder segments are obstructed. The renal units communicating into the blind compartments are hydronephrotic and dysplastic (Fig. 52-2, *E*).

Hourglass Bladder

An hourglass configuration of the bladder results when a thick transverse band of muscle incompletely divides the bladder into two unequal segments. The ureters generally open into the lower portion, but may open into the upper portion. This configuration can simulate a large urachal diverticulum or a massively dilated posterior urethra because of posterior urethral valves. Incomplete emptying of the cephalad segment with paradoxical contraction may occur if the constriction is severe. There are no associated anomalies. Patients with hourglass bladders usually present in adult life with a long history of cystitis and frequent, painful micturition. Diagnosis is made by a cystogram. Sur-

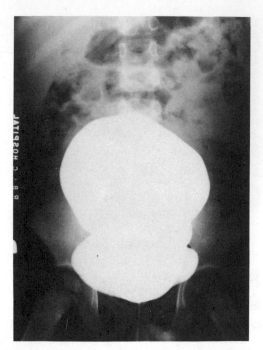

FIG. 52-4
Hourglass bladder visualized on cystogram.

gical removal of the constricting ring is the treatment of choice if symptoms warrant surgical intervention (Fig. 52-2, *F*; 52-4).

Bladder Diverticula

A bladder diverticulum occurs when the bladder mucosa herniates or protrudes through the muscular wall of the bladder. Bladder diverticula may be congenital and primary or may occur secondary to abnormal increases in intravesical pressure from bladder outlet obstruction or neurogenic bladder. The first reported case was in an autopsy of a man in 1614, in whom the diverticulum was noted to be six times larger than the bladder (Caldamone, 1991). Alexander, in 1884, is credited with the first surgical diverticulectomy of the bladder in a 40-year-old woman, who presented with an anterior vaginal mass from a diverticulum containing a calculus.

Congenital Bladder Diverticula

The etiology of congenital bladder diverticula is unknown. The most common location of bladder diverticula in children is lateral and cephalad to the ureteral orifice (Bauer and Retik, 1974; Hutch, 1961). The parahiatal location may occur because of a defect in the development of the fibromuscular meshwork of the vesicoureteral hiatus (Waldeyer's sheath) (Stephens, 1979). A diverticulum also may occur at the dome of the bladder in association with congenital outlet obstruction (posterior urethral valves) or prune belly syndrome. Additionally, congenital bladder di-

verticula have been noted in patients with Menkes' syndrome (kinky hair or copper deficiency syndrome) (Daly and Rabinovitch, 1981; Harcke et al., 1977), Ehlers-Danlos syndrome (Levard et al., 1989; Schippers and Dittler, 1989), and in infants suffering from alcohol embryopathy (Havers et al., 1980). Congenital diverticula are much more common in males, are usually solitary, and do not cause symptoms unless they are complicated by reflux, urinary infection, stones, or neoplasia (Blacklock et al., 1983). Congenital bladder diverticula also have been reported to cause bladder outlet obstruction (Taylor et al., 1979; Verghese and Belman, 1984). In a recent retrospective study of pediatric genitourinary data base of 5084 children, bladder diverticula were found in 1.7%. A significant conclusion from this study was that if a child is found to have more than one diverticulum, further evaluation should be performed to rule out an underlying condition (neurogenic disorder, obstruction, syndrome) or association (Blane et al., 1994).

Most bladder diverticula are diagnosed during evaluation for urinary tract infection. They frequently are not seen on the intravenous urogram (Hernanz-Schulman and Lebowitz, 1985) and are best demonstrated by oblique views taken during the voiding phase of a cystourethrogram (Allen and Atwell, 1980). The solitary diverticulum involving the vesicoureteral hiatus may or may not be associated with ipsilateral vesicoureteral reflux. The occurrence of reflux depends on the extent of involvement of the submucosal ureter by the diverticulum. Those ureteral orifices that lie completely within a diverticulum will reflux, whereas those ureters in which the diverticulum is at some distance from the orifice maintain a competent antiflux mechanism (Brock and Kaplan, 1992). Ultrasound also may demonstrate diverticula, especially if performed with a full and empty bladder. Cystoscopy confirms the diagnosis (Fig. 52-5).

Congenital bladder diverticula must be differentiated from "*bladder ears*," which are transitory bladder pouches projecting anteriorly into the inguinal rings in males under 6 months of age. Bladder ears differ from congenital bladder diverticula because of their anterior position and because there is no obvious neck connecting the pouching sac to the bladder. Bladder diverticula also must be distinguished from an outpouching from the bladder in girls posterolateral to the ureteral orifices. In girls, this is an area of anatomically thin muscle cover, so that the bladder bulges during voiding. Most investigators regard this as a normal anatomical variation (Friedland et al., 1990).

In children with incidentally discovered primary congenital diverticula, no therapy is needed unless the diverticulum involves the vesicoureteral hiatus to the extent that it contributes to the occurrence of

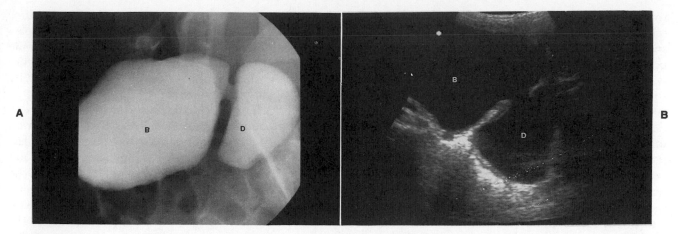

FIG. 52-5
Bladder diverticulum. **A,** Voiding cystourethrogram and **B,** Ultrasound demonstrating bladder diverticulum. *D* = diverticulum; *B* = bladder.

vesicoureteral reflux. In this case, diverticulectomy and simultaneous ureteroneocystostomy are indicated. Large diverticula that are causing infection or obstruction should be excised. The development of carcinoma in bladder diverticula does deserve consideration even though the peak incidence in these patients is approximately 65 years of age and occurs in only 2% to 10 percent of patients with diverticula (Faysal and Freha, 1981; Micic and Illic, 1983). Because of the potential for direct extension beyond the bladder from a carcinoma in a diverticulum, many surgeons would argue for immediate prophylactic diverticular excision.

Acquired Parahiatal Diverticula

Hutch (1952) first described the association of paraureteral diverticula and vesicoureteral reflux in patients with neurogenic bladder. In any condition with elevated intravesical pressures, this area of weakness may give way with a small paraureteral diverticulum. In children, it is seen most commonly with dysfunctional voiding when a cystogram is performed for evaluation of wetting or infection. When the voiding function returns to normal, these diverticula often will regress.

Megacystis

Megacystis means simply "large bladder." Megacystis can be seen in congenital megacystis, the megacystis-megaureter syndrome, the microcolon-hypoperistalsis-megacystis syndrome, and secondarily because of congenital outlet obstruction.

Congenital Megacystis

Congenital megacystis describes a congenitally huge unobstructed bladder (Inamdar et al., 1984). The characteristics include large residual volume, a normal trigone, normal ureteral orifice with no reflux, and a normal upper urinary tract.

Megacystis-Megaureter Syndrome

Megacystis-megaureter syndrome was first described by Williams (1957, 1959), who defined it as a large, smooth bladder with a wide trigone, dilated ureteral orifices, and grossly dilated ureters with reflux. These bladders contract and empty normally, but a significant percentage of their volume goes into the upper urinary tracts. Histologically, there are a normal number of normal-appearing ganglia in the bladder (Leibowitz and Bodian, 1963). The capacious bladder is likely due to the constant recycling or urine between the massively dilated upper urinary tracts and the bladder (Harrow, 1967). The bladder is always overfull and distended, eventually becoming decompensated, dilated, and thin-walled (Burbige et al., 1984).

The key to the diagnosis is observation of the bladder fluoroscopically, ensuring that it contracts and empties normally. Correction of the reflux should lead to normal voiding dynamics. Successful antireflux surgery may be difficult to achieve, however, owing to the thin-walled bladder. A psoas hitch with a long reimplantation and a transureteroureterostomy should be considered as an option if bilateral reimplantations do not appear feasible (Caldamone, 1991). Many of the patients now are being detected in utero as gross reflux. In some, a temporary vesicostomy may be an appropriate early management (Hsu et al., 1995).

Megacystis-Microcolon-Hypoperistalsis Syndrome

Megacystis-microcolon-hypoperistalsis syndrome, also known as *chronic idiopathic intestinal pseudo-obstruction*, represents a functional obstruction of the bladder and intestine caused by an undefined neuropathic process. These patients have a huge bladder, often with reflux, and a dilated upper urinary tract. A small colon and a dilated small bowel exist, and hypoperistalsis is seen throughout the gastrointestinal tract (Berdon et al., 1976). There is also incomplete rotation of bowel and lax abdominal musculature. This syndrome is more common in females and its usually detected in the neonate (Redman et al., 1984). The initial presenting symptom may be urinary tract infection, so the urologist may be the first to detect the serious syndrome. It is usually fatal during the first year of life, although with aggressive parenteral therapy, long-term survivors are seen. The cause is unknown. There is some histologic evidence that the bladders have elastosis with normal muscle bundles (Kirtane et al., 1984).

Urachal Abnormalities

The urachus arises from the anterior bladder wall and extends to the umbilicus. Congenital anomalies of the urachus are rare events that present predominantly in early childhood. There are four types of congenital urachal anomalies (Cullen, 1946): (1) patent urachus, (2) urachal cyst, (3) urachal sinus, and (4) urachal diverticulum (Fig. 52-6). Males are affected twice as often as females. The first description of a patent urachus was by Cabrol, who in 1550 described a young woman who had urinated from a protrusion at her navel all of the life. Cabrol opened the urethra, which had been congenitally occluded, and ligated the umbilical protrusion, effecting a complete cure (Herbst, 1937).

Embryology and Anatomy

During fetal development, as the bladder descends into the pelvis, its apical portion narrows progressively into a fibromuscular strand of urachus, which main-

tains continuity with the allantoic duct. Shortly after the embryonic stage of development, the tract apparently obliterates. In one third of adults, a microscopic communication remains patent (Schubert et al., 1983). However, functionally, it can be considered closed by the last one half of fetal life.

The urachus lies in the space of Retzius between the peritoneum and transversalis fascia and is encased between two layers of umbilicovesical fascia. This fascia extends laterally to each umbilical artery and spreads inferiorly over the dome of the bladder to the hypogastric artery posteriorly and to the pelvic diaphragm anteriorly, thus forming a self-contained space to limit spread of infection and neoplasm (Noe, 1991).

Patent Urachus

Congenital patent urachus is a lesion that is usually recognized in the neonate. Complete failure of obliteration results in a persistent communication between the bladder and the umbilicus that leaks urine. It is a rare anomaly occurring in only three of more than 1 million admissions to a large pediatric center (Nix et al., 1958). The etiology of this condition is unknown. It has been suggested that bladder outlet obstruction may be a contributing factor, however, only 14% of neonates born with a patent urachus have evidence of urinary obstruction (Herbst, 1937). It is unlikely that urinary obstruction is directly related to the development of a patent urachus because even the most severe cases of posterior urethral valves are not associated with this anomaly. Patent urachus has been reported in association with prune belly syndrome, in which there is thought to be transient functional urethral obstruction. Lattimer (1958) found a patent urachus present in 11 of 22 boys with prune belly syndrome. This may suggest that the obstruction in patients with posterior urethral valves occurs later in

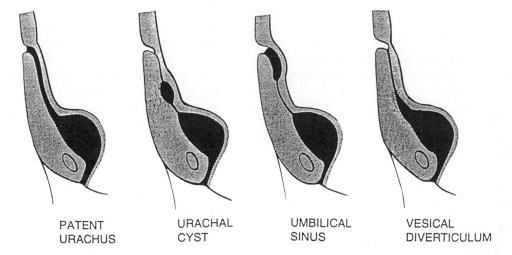

PATENT URACHUS   URACHAL CYST   UMBILICAL SINUS   VESICAL DIVERTICULUM

FIG. 52-6
Congenital urachal anomalies. (Modified from O'Rahilly R, Muller F: *Human embryology and teratology.* New York, Wiley-Liss, 1992.)

gestation than the obstruction that leads to prune belly syndrome.

A patent urachus presents in the neonatal period as a wet umbilicus, often with umbilical granulation. The urinary leakage may be intermittent or continuous and is accentuated when the neonate is in the prone position, straining or voiding. The differential diagnosis of a wet umbilicus in the infant includes patent urachus, omphalitis (an infection of the umbilical stump), simple granulation of a healing umbilical stump, patent vitelline or omphalomesenteric duct (enteroumbilical fistula), infected umbilical vessel, and external urachal sinus. The diagnosis may be confirmed by catheterization or probing of the urachal tract, retrograde fistulography, instillation of methylene blue into the tract or intravesically, or analysis of the discharge fluid for blood urea nitrogen (BUN) and creatinine. A voiding cystourethrogram occasionally demonstrates the communication but is more useful in ruling out other etiologic or associated lower urinary tract anomalies, such as obstruction. Cystoscopy is rarely of any assistance in diagnosis (Fig. 52-7).

Treatment consists of complete extraperitoneal excision of the urachus with an attached cuff or bladder. A probe in the tract permits a complete dissection and excision. Whenever possible the umbilicus should be preserved for cosmetic considerations.

Urachal Cyst

If the urachal lumen only partially obliterates but loses communication with either the bladder or the umbilicus, a urachal cyst may develop. The cyst fills with desquamated epithelial cells and is usually clinically silent during childhood. Symptoms develop because of increased size or secondary infection. The most common organism cultured in the cyst fluid is *Staphylococcus aureus* (MacMillan et al., 1973; Tauber and Bloom, 1951). The fascial layers anterior

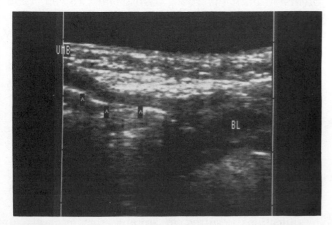

FIG. 52-7
Ultrasound demonstrating patent urachus. *BL* = bladder; *UMB* = umbilicus; *arrows* = patent urachus. (Courtesy of R.D. Bellah, M.D.)

and posterior to the urachus usually confine any infection to the anterior abdominal wall, though intraperitoneal rupture and subsequent peritonitis may occur (Agaststein and Stabile, 1984; Nunn, 1952). A large cyst may lead to urinary retention and azotemia in adults (Stanfield and Shearer, 1981). The cyst also can bleed after relatively minor trauma.

The symptoms and signs of a loculated infected urachal cyst are lower abdominal pain, fever, voiding symptoms, mass, evidence of urinary tract infection. The cyst may be palpable by bimanual abdominal-rectal examination. Urachal cyst should be suspected whenever localized suprapubic pain and tenderness are present with disturbed micturition, even when the urine remains clear. The differential diagnosis includes bladder diverticulum, vitelline cyst, umbilical hernia, and ovarian cyst. Diagnostic evaluation should first be an ultrasound, which is ideal for localizing the mass and defining its limits (Williams and Fisk, 1981). Excretory urography and lateral cystography may demonstrate an external mass compression on the bladder as an incidental finding when evaluating for urinary tract infection. Injection of the cyst in conjunction with a cystogram delineates the relation between the bladder and urachal cyst. Although computed tomographic scan of the abdomen may be helpful in determining the extent of the disease and the possibility of involvement of other organ systems (Berman et al., 1988) it contributes very little to management.

Treatment of a small, uninfected cyst involves extraperitoneal excision, coupled with removal of each end of the urachal remnant. Simple drainage of urachal cyst has been associated with recurrent infections in 30% (Blichert-Toft and Nielsen, 1971). Infected cysts require incision and drainage of the cyst with delayed excision as dictated by the size of the mass (Goldman et al., 1988; Newman et al., 1986). Although adenocarcinoma of the urachus is rare, it has been reported in a patient as young as 15 years old who had a urachal abscess drained 2 years prior to presenting with the tumor (Cornil et al., 1967).

Urachal Sinus

If a small urachal cyst becomes infected, it may drain via a sinus at the umbilicus or into the bladder. One particularly interesting variety is the alternating urachal sinus, in which the drainage shifts alternately between the umbilicus and the bladder (Hinman, 1961). Associated signs and symptoms include periumbilical pain, tenderness, fever, umbilical inflammation with granuloma formation, and persistent umbilical drainage. Since other umbilical remnants may be involved in causing gastrointestinal symptoms, diagnosis may be difficult. If the drainage is at the umbilicus, a fistulogram in the lateral view is preferable.

If the bladder is suspect, a cystogram in the lateral view will better reveal the disease. Cystoscopy also may aid in diagnosis.

Once the acute infection along with any coincidental urinary tract infection is under control, excision of the sinus should be undertaken, keeping in mind the necessity of concomitant removal of any intraperitoneal structures that have become involved if omphalomesenteric duct remnants are present (Bauer and Retik, 1978).

Urachal Diverticulum

Failure of obliteration of the communication between the bladder apex and urachus may result in a vesicourachal diverticulum. This typically is seen in the prune belly syndrome and has been noted with lower urinary tract obstruction. However, an incidental finding of a vesicourachal diverticulum, or "blind internal sinus," is possible. Most small urachal diverticula seen on a routine radiograph of the urinary tract are of no clinical significance and require no treatment. However, if the diverticulum is large, poorly or paradoxically contracting, or has poor emptying attributable to a narrow neck, excision should be undertaken because calculi have been reported to develop (Fig. 52-8) (Ney and Friedenberg, 1968).

BLADDER EXSTROPHY
History

Early descriptions of bladder exstrophy were made in 1595 (Hall et al., 1953) and in 1646 (Connell, 1901). A more complete description followed by Mowat (1747). No attempt was made to surgically correct the defect in these early reports. Initial attempts to control urine soiling and pain resulted in devices designed to collect the urine and protect the exposed bladder from contact with clothing (Fig. 52-9).

In 1850, diversion of urine to the colon in a patient with bladder exstrophy was accomplished by creating a crude anastomosis between the bladder and sigmoid colon. At least one patient treated in this way managed to divert the urine to the rectum by wearing a pad that closed the abdominal opening. By 1853, Richard attempted closure of the bladder, but the patient died of peritonitis (Ashurst, 1871). Another unsuccessful closure was performed in Philadelphia by Pancoast in 1858 at the Clinic of the Jefferson College (The Gross Clinic). Shortly after, Ayres managed a successful closure in a 28-year-old female, who reported marked improvement in pain previously felt from the irritated exposed urothelium (Gross, 1862).

By the beginning of the twentieth century, more modern techniques were used to attempt continent reconstruction. To better approximate the pubic bones, Trendelenburg first attempted sacroiliac osteotomy in 1892 (Fig. 52-10). The first patient became

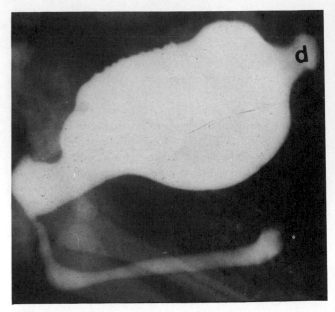

FIG. 52-8
Voiding cystourethrogram in a patient with prune belly syndrome demonstrating urachal diverticulum. *D* = diverticulum.

anemic and died. Trendelenburg then used osteotomy to close three additional patients, one boy and two men, in 1906. Although transient control was achieved in the boy neither of the men improved after the procedure (Trendelenburg, 1906). Few attempts were made to close the bladder during the next 30 to 40 years. Instead, most patients underwent ureterosigmoidostomy combined with cystectomy (Mayo and Hendricks, 1926). In 1942, Young reported a successful bladder closure in one female patient. The bladder neck was later rolled into a tube to provide continence. The patient developed a dry interval of 3 hours. Despite Young's success in this patient, most surgeons continued to utilize cystectomy and urinary diversion until the 1950s (Gross and Cressen, 1952; Higgins, 1962).

Over the past 45 years, the focus has shifted away from urinary diversion to preservation of the bladder. Unfortunately, despite a few early successes (Schultz, 1958) urinary continence has been difficult to achieve for most. Modification of Young's continence procedure (Young, 1922) by Dees (Dees, 1942) to incorporate the prostatic urethra and bladder neck in the rolled urethral strip, resulted in improved urinary control. Later, Leadbetter reimplanted the ureters, moving them cephalad to allow the trigone to be incorporated into the tube to further lengthen the bladder neckplasty (Leadbetter, 1964). Although these modifications resulted in suitable dry intervals for some patients with complete epispadias, continence in exstrophy patients, remained discouraging (Megalli and Lattimer, 1973; Williams and Keeton, 1973).

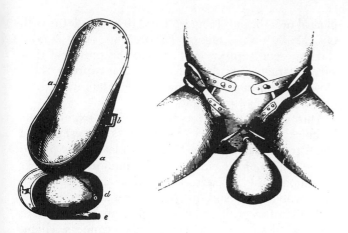

FIG. 52-9
Two examples of urinary collecting devices used in the eighteenth and nineteenth centuries. (From Murphy LJT: *The history of urology.* Springfield Ill, Charles C Thomas, Publisher, 1972, p 333. Used by permission.)

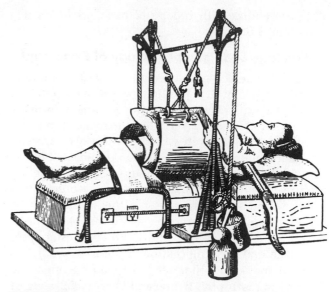

FIG. 52-10
Pelvic sling designed by Trendelenburg to immobilize the pubic symphysis opposition following bilateral sacroiliac osteotomies. (From Murphy LJT: *The history of urology.* Springfield Ill, Charles C Thomas, Publisher, 1972, p 333. Used by permission.)

Thanks in large part to improved anesthesia in newborns, bladder closure in the first days of life is now the norm. Ansell observed that the more mobile infant pelvis made apposition of the pubic bones easier and helped to achieve a better abdominal closure (Ansell, 1971, 1979). The unpleasant symptoms in babies with exposed bladders are minimized with early bladder closure. Epispadias repair prior to bladder neck reconstruction may result in improved bladder volume, which may make bladder neckplasty more successful. It is now possible to preserve renal function by avoiding continence procedures early. Bladder neck reconstruction later can then provide acceptable urinary continence in many patients. Improved genital reconstruction techniques have resulted in better cosmetic appearance and sexual function, especially in males. Most of these contributions come from centers where large numbers of patients are reconstructed each year. The challenge of the next century will be to refine these techniques to simplified steps to allow consistently good results for all surgeons while minimizing hospital stay.

Incidence and Inheritance

Bladder exstrophy is uncommon, being reported every 20,000 to 40,000 live births (Rickham, 1961). In a multicenter retrospective study, pooled data from around the world of nearly 6.3 million births between 1970 and 1975, placed the prevalence at birth of bladder exstrophy at 3.3 per 100,000 births (1 in 30,000) (Systems, 1987). Although the lesion is rare, some families are clearly at higher risk. Of 2500 index cases from another survey (Shapiro et al., 1984), nine affected siblings were found. This projects to an overall risk of a second affected family member of 3.6%. Of 215 children born to parents in this group with ex-

strophy or epispadias, three children inherited bladder exstrophy (one in 70 live births, or 1.4%) (Shapiro et al., 1984). The risk of two affected siblings is about 1% (Carter, 1984).

Epispadias is less common than exstrophy, occurring once in approximately 40,000 live births (Systems, 1987). Earlier reports suggested this number was closer to 1 in 100,000. The increased incidence in recent reports probably reflects increased awareness and more aggressive treatment of milder forms of epispadias rather than actual increased numbers of children presenting.

Although most patients with classic bladder exstrophy have surprisingly few associated defects, exstrophy associated with exomphalos has been recorded in successive pregnancies (Hockey and Bower, 1993). In addition, two patients with bladder exstrophy have developed Wilms' tumor, an exceedingly unlikely event considering the relative incidence of the two conditions. Despite occasional clustering of individuals with the defect, little is known about risk factors for bladder exstrophy. In one study, women less than 20 years of age and high parity (3+) had increased risk for children with exstrophy (Systems, 1987). Maternal use of progestins also has been implicated (Blickstein and Katz, 1991). Despite these occasional reports, most cases are not associated with any particular risk factor.

The male to female ratio for classic bladder exstrophy is between 1.5 and 2:1 (Engel, 1974; Systems, 1987). The ratio generally is quoted higher for complete epispadias with reports of male predominance as high as 3.5:1.

Embryology and Pathophysiology of Exstrophy

Before 2 weeks' gestation, the cloacal membrane occupies a prominent position on the infraumbilical abdominal wall. The membrane is formed from an inner (endodermal) layer. Mesenchyme from the primitive streak migrates between the two layers of the cloacal membrane to reinforce the infraumbilical area while the cloacal membrane regresses. Before rupture of the cloacal membrane, the urorectal fold joins the membrane to separate the cloaca into the urogenital and anal components. Rupture of the membrane at the base of the genital tubercle establishes the urogenital opening (Patton and Barry, 1952).

There are several theories to explain the abnormal anatomy in exstrophy. Patton and Barry (1952) suggest abnormal development of the genital hillocks with fusion in the midline below rather than above the cloacal membrane. This abnormal cephalad migration of the cloaca would result in instability and premature rupture of the cloaca before mesodermal ingrowth occurs. Epispadias would then occur when the genital tubercle is displaced caudally to the point where the urorectal fold divides the cloaca. Later rupture of the cloacal membrane would result in an uncovered dorsal urethra. Further caudal displacement of the tubercle would prevent mesodermal migration to the midline and result in bladder exstrophy. Displacement of the genital primordia even further caudally to the anal portion of the cloacal membrane would result in cloacal exstrophy. Observations on the relative frequencies of the various exstrophy variants suggest that if the exstrophy results from abnormal caudal displacement of the genital tubercle, the defects associated with minimal displacement (epispadias) should be more common than those associated with further displacement (classic bladder exstrophy), but this is not the case. If displacement of the genital tubercle is responsible for the defect, one should expect to see extreme displacement of the phallus to a position off the pubic tubercle at least occasionally, but this condition is never present in exstrophy.

Marshall and Muecke (1962) therefore theorized that the normal mesenchymal migration between the leaflets of the cloacal membrane in exstrophy is truncated, owing to increased thickness of the membrane. Later rupture of the membrane without reinforcement of the mesodermal layer would result in exstrophy. Bladder exstrophy would result if the rupture occurred after completion of the caudal growth of the urorectal septum. Both the bladder and hindgut would be exposed (cloacal exstrophy) if rupture occurred before descent of the urorectal septum. The ultrasound observation of relatively late in utero rupture of the cloacal membrane (Langer et al., 1992) in a fetus with cloacal exstrophy suggests that presence or absence of the urorectal septum, rather than the timing of rupture, characterizes the defect and that rupture of the cloacal membrane can occur relatively late in the second trimester of pregnancy.

This idea is supported by Muecke's experiments in chick embryos. At 48 to 52 hours of gestation, a small triangular piece of Millipore plastic was placed at the region of the cloacal membrane. Several chicks developed the characteristic appearance of exstrophy, probably because the plastic prevented mesodermal migration at this critical stage in development (Muecke, 1964). In a similar set of experiments, Thomalla and Mitchell (1985) found that laser trauma to the cloacal membrane as late as 61 hours (before curling of the tail bud) results in exstrophy in chicks. No data exist to prove that the abnormal thickness of the cloacal membrane itself prevents migration of the mesodermal layer in humans.

A more recent report based on observations of normal development in rat embryos may further refine Muecke's theory. Early in rat development, marked cranial movement of the yolk sac separates the yolk sac from the cloacal membrane. In the region between the yolk sac and the membrane, the genital tubercle proliferates and forces the cloaca into a dorsal caudal position. A thick plate of mesenchymal tissue lies at the base of the genital tubercle. Failure of the cranial progression of the yolk sac in exstrophy would prevent migration of the genital tubercle and posterior displacement of the cloaca. The abdominal wall muscle and genital hillocks (labioscrotal or genital folds) would then fail to meet at the midline. The subsequent superficial cloacal membrane, poorly reinforced with mesoderm, then would be prone to rupture, resulting in exstrophy. This theory, which refines rather than refutes the chick embryo results, may explain the shortened umbilical-anal distance seen in nearly all patients with exstrophy or epispadias, as well as the clinical appearance of several of the exstrophy variants (Mildenberger et al., 1988).

Clinical Presentation

The prenatal sonographic absence of a normal bladder in association with an anterior abdominal mass and low-set umbilicus suggests bladder exstrophy, omphalocele, or gastroschisis (Jaffe et al., 1990). Ultrasonographers can now characterize the changes seen in bladder and cloacal exstrophy as early as the twentieth week of gestation (Barth et al., 1990; Meizner and Bar-Ziv, 1986; Mirk et al., 1986; Richards et al., 1992; Verco et al., 1986).

Unlike patients with cloacal exstrophy and its variants, children with bladder exstrophy or epispadias have few defects in addition to the obvious exposed bladder. The associated abnormalities are confined to the development of the abdomen and perineum, the urinary tract, the genitalia, the spine, and the bony pelvis.

Anatomy

The diamond-shaped area bounded by the umbilicus, the anus, the rectus abdominis muscles, and the skin overlying the puborectal sling houses the defect most apparent in patients with exstrophy or epispadias. The umbilical-anal distance is short, because the umbilicus is more caudally placed than normal and the anus is anterior. The area between the displaced muscles and the margin of the exposed bladder is covered with shiny fibrous tissue. The rectus muscle inserts normally at the pubic tubercle. The displaced pubic bones carry the rectus muscles to a lateral position. This displacement of the rectus muscles widens the internal inguinal canal and places the internal inguinal ring just beneath the external inguinal ring. For this reason, indirect inguinal hernia and incarceration are common, particularly in boys (Connor et al., 1989; Gross and Cressen, 1952; Husmann et al., 1990b; Stringer et al., 1994). The rate of incarceration is higher in children who have the bladder closed than in those who undergo cystectomy plus urinary diversion, probably because of higher abdominal pressure after closure. Because the bladder is not initially located in the pelvis, the peritoneal reflection is deep prior to reconstruction, and a disproportionate percentage of peritoneal contents are located posterior to the bladder at birth.

The bladder size is variable, from a small patch to a larger prolapsing body of 15 to 30 cc capacity. Because the bladder is exposed to air and immediate trauma during delivery and in the nursery, it becomes inflamed. The urothelium often develops a polypoid appearance (Fig. 52-11). Direct contact to salves, diapers, or clothing increases the inflammatory response and worsens the polypoid change. Microscopic changes in the transitional epithelium occur and are present very shortly after birth (Goyanna et al., 1951). In untreated patients, these result eventually in squamous (Culp, 1964) or adenomatous (Mostofi, 1954) metaplasia, which later proceeds to squamous cell carcinoma or adenocarcinoma in patients who live for longer periods (Bunge, 1952; Engel and Wilkinson, 1970). Microvilli within the urothelial cells were noted on transmission electron microscopic views of the epithelium in a biopsy taken from a 1-year-old girl with untreated bladder exstrophy. The presence of microvilli similar to those seen in patients with transitional cell carcinoma suggests that the urothelium in unclosed exstrophy is at a primitive stage and predisposed to malignancy (Clark and O'Connell, 1973).

Since the bladder has normal blood supply and nor-

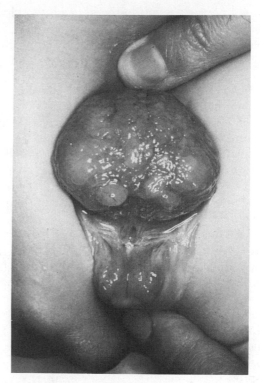

FIG. 52-11
Typical exstrophic bladder in newborn male with polypoid appearance of bladder mucosa.

mal neuromuscular activity, it should be capable of normal function once the bladder is closed (Shapiro et al., 1985). At least two studies, however, have suggested poor detrusor function even in successfully closed bladders (Hollowell et al., 1993; Nisonson and Lattimer, 1972).

Rectal prolapse may develop as long as the bladder is exposed. We know of no cases in which this has occurred in a patient with a closed bladder. Trauma to the bladder surface tends to irritate the epithelium and is painful. Poor support of the displaced anal sling mechanism along with the Valsalva effect of crying in these unhappy children results in rectal prolapse. While no specific surgical treatment is necessary for rectal prolapse other than to reclose the bladder, some advocate fixation of the rectal wall to the sacrum at the time of the closure to prevent reprolapse of the rectum. This is probably advisable and causes no harm and perhaps ensures prevention of rectal prolapse during the initial healing period.

Few renal anomalies occur in patients with bladder exstrophy or epispadias. Duplication of the ureter does occur and must be recognized prior to closure to avoid injury to one of the ureters. A few patients have developed hydronephrosis when the bladder remained exposed for long periods, presumably because of thickening of the wall of the uncovered bladder. This problem is not seen in infancy. Because of the deepened peritoneal cul-de-sac beneath the bladder, particularly in exstrophy but also to a lesser extent in complete epispadias, the ureters course deeply through the bony pelvis to emerge through the bladder muscle with almost no submucosal tunnel. The result is vesicoureteral reflux in nearly all patients who have undergone bladder closure (Nisonson and Lattimer, 1972). Ureteral peristalsis is normal (Maloney and Lattimer, 1965).

The penis in boys with exstrophy is short and wide because of separation of the pubic bones, which prevents the corpora cavernosa from joining at the midline at the usual position near the base of the pubis. Although the protruding portion of the penis is reduced, the deep corporal bodies may be of reasonable length; they are however shortened in absolute length, as measured by cavernosography (Woodhouse and Kellett, 1984). Marked dorsal chordee may be present with a shortened urethral plate. The congenital curvature is compounded by a shorter dorsal tunica albuginea, whereas the ventrum of the corporal tissue is longer. The corpora are nearly always sufficient for reconstruction, although gender reversal rarely may be appropriate in classical bladder exstrophy.

The superficial neurovascular bundles are displaced laterally (Woodhouse and Kellett, 1984). The pudendal nerves innervating the corpora in these patients emerge from the sacral trunk (S2 through S4) and pass posterior to the pelvic floor muscles, medially to the ischial spines, and into Alcock's canal (Schlegel and Gearhart, 1989).

A duplicate urethra has been reported (Slotkin and Mercer, 1953) which may be incorporated into the epispadias repair (Schulze et al., 1985). The urethral meatus in most patients with isolated epispadias is at the penopubic junction. A few have incomplete forms in which the urethral meatus is located partly out on the dorsal penile shaft. Dorsal chordee is present in all but the most mild forms of epispadias, and in all patients with exstrophy.

Following adequate reconstruction, men with bladder exstrophy have fathered children, but fertility rates are decreased (Woodhouse et al., 1983). A tenfold higher than normal incidence of cryptorchidism has been reported in patients with exstrophy or epispadias (Husmann et al., 1990b). However, in our experience, despite testes that appear to be in the inguinal canal at initial examination, most can be manipulated into the scrotum without difficulty following bladder closure. Prior to initial bladder closure, the epididymis (Merksz and Toth, 1990), vas deferens, ejaculatory ducts, and seminal vesicles are normal. This suggests that the undescended testis noted in bladder exstrophy is more an anatomical (or mechanical) problem than an endocrinological problem.

Females with bladder exstrophy have a hemiclitoris on each side. The vaginal orifice may be duplicated, and is located just inferior to the distal extent of the exposed urethra. The vaginal orifice is generally narrowed and is displaced anteriorly (Damario et al., 1994). The uterus may be duplicated. The ovaries and fallopian tubes are usually normal. As in males, the severity of the genital defect is variable. Females with epispadias share some of the abnormalities of those with exstrophy, but generally these are less pronounced. The mons pubis is flattened, with variable separation of the pubic bones, an anterior labial separation, a bifid clitoris, and a urethra that is patulous (Muecke and Marshall, 1968). More minor forms of epispadias in females probably are underreported, which may account for the increased male:female ratio for epispadias compared with classical exstrophy.

In nearly all cases, patients with exstrophy or epispadias have some degree of pubic diastasis. Pelvic growth in length and width is normal (Lascombes et al., 1989). The hips are rotated outward. Despite the rotation, few hip or gait problems result, particularly if closure is performed at an early age. Many patients have a waddling gait in early childhood, which becomes less evident later. Congenital hip dislocation has been reported in only two cases (Thomas and Wilkinson, 1989). Unlike patients with cloacal exstrophy, patients with classic bladder exstrophy have few spinal defects (Loder and Dayioglu, 1990).

Treatment Philosophy

Robert D. Jeffs began his career at the Hospital for Sick Children in Toronto and moved to the Johns Hopkins Hospital in 1975. For 20 years he has refined our understanding of exstrophy by specializing his interest in this difficult anomaly. The authors wish to personally acknowledge his significant contribution to the advances in exstrophy management. Much of what follows has evolved as a result of Jeffs' vast experience.

Modern techniques in exstrophy reconstruction attempt to provide urinary continence while preserving renal function. In males, penile reconstruction should provide an erection straight enough for vaginal penetration and a urethra that allows for upright voiding. Obviously, a good cosmetic appearance is essential in both sexes. With the staged approach to bladder closure and subsequent continence surgery, nearly all patients are candidates for initial bladder closure. Very few patients should undergo primary diversion without an attempt at bladder closure. Even the patient with a very small bladder may develop surprisingly good bladder growth following primary bladder closure and epispadias repair (Canning et al., 1989).

The staged repair begins with closure of the bladder shortly after birth with or without bilateral posterior iliac or anterior innominate osteotomy. The bladder closure is followed by an incontinent period during which the bladder gradually enlarges. Epispadias repair in males is now performed during the incontinent period—usually between 12 and 18 months. No attempt is made to provide continence until 3½ to 5 years of age, when bladder neck plasty is considered. At that time, bladder volume is assessed. Bladder neck reconstruction (BNR) is not attempted until an adequate bladder capacity is obtained. In most cases, a 50 to 60 cc capacity is adequate (Lepor and Jeffs, 1983). Even when the bladder reaches adequate size, the child also must be well motivated to be dry before BNR should be undertaken.

Primary Bladder Closure

Since the bladder is best closed in the first 24 to 48 hours after birth, the infant should be transferred as soon as possible to the tertiary care center where there is a team experienced in newborn exstrophy closure. The exstrophy team is led by the pediatric urologist, but also includes the pediatric anesthesiologist, the pediatric orthopedic surgeon, the neonatologist, and the urology and general pediatric nurses (Lattimer et al., 1979). When transfer requires significant travel, the patient is adequately hydrated initially at the referring hospital and then en route. Gentamicin 2.5 mg/kg and ampicillin 20 mg/kg are started on arrival or at least 1 hour before surgery and maintained for 24 hours after surgery.

Upon arrival, the family is introduced to the members of the exstrophy surgical and support teams. Gender issues are addressed early. The bladder is covered with a square of clear plastic wrap (such as Saran Wrap) in the diaper. Gauze or petroleum jelly is not used since this dressing tends to dry and denude the epithelium. Patients with classic bladder exstrophy have few renal problems; nevertheless, a renal ultrasound should be performed to identify hydronephrosis or duplex kidneys. Reports of older exstrophy patients developing latex allergies have alerted us to the need to prevent exposure to the latex antigen. Children with exstrophy are treated in a latex-free environment throughout the hospital stay and at home.

The goals of the primary bladder closure are as follows: (1) to close the bladder and displace it to a posterior position deep within the pelvis; (2) to provide free urethral and bladder drainage; (3) if needed, to perform initial penile lengthening; and (4) to rotate the innominate bones to approximate the pubic symphysis.

In 1958, Schultz revisited Trendelenburg's (Trendelenburg, 1906) idea of rotating the innominate bones to reduce the pubic diastasis. He reported the use of a bilateral iliac osteotomy, followed 2 weeks later by bladder closure and approximation of the pubic symphysis in a female. The patient reportedly became continent within a week of removing the bladder catheter and remained so. Schultz believed that closer apposition of the pubic bones would better recreate the normal anatomy of the pelvic musculature. Better function of the urogenital diaphragm appeared to provide urinary continence in this one patient (Schultz, 1958). Schultz's initial success led to a strong advocacy for osteotomy. Lattimer and Smith (1966) and Chisholm (1962) each reported a large series of patients using osteotomy at the time of bladder closure. The bladder closure at this time was done with bladder neck tightening to provide continence. The long-term results in these early series were discouraging with low continence rates and upper-tract deterioration being common.

Staged Approach

Jeffs (1977) and associates (1972) and Cendron (1971, 1977) both noticed the protection that a wide open bladder neck provided in the incontinent epispadias patient. They separately proposed a staged approach, first converting exstrophy to incontinent epispadias with an initial bladder closure but no bladder neck reconstruction. Bladder neck reconstruction was postponed until years later. This revolutionized exstrophy management and is the current philosophy today.

Osteotomy

Ansell (1971) showed that within 48 to 72 hours of birth the baby's bones and joints are quite malleable, just like the birth canal in the mother. Taking advantage of this fact makes early newborn closure *without* osteotomy less complicated. The initial goal of approximation of the symphysis pubis is to obtain a solid abdominal wall closure that prevents dehiscence. Even though partial symphyseal separation may be apparent years later, we prefer to approximate the symphysis without osteotomy in infants under 48 hours old and have had only one separation in 22 newborn closures performed without the use of osteotomy (Duckett and Caldamone, 1984).

Today the need for bilateral iliac osteotomy to provide improved pelvic mobility at the time of bladder closure is controversial. Nevertheless, particularly in older patients, osteotomy seems to provide additional mobility of the pelvis, which helps secure a pubic closure with minimal morbidity, and a pubic symphyseal approximation, which may be more permanent. These observations have led some to recommend osteotomy even in infants closed in the first 48 hours (Allen et al., 1992). Proponents of osteotomy have suggested that improved continence rates can be expected following the bladder neck plasty if osteotomy is used at the initial closure. Patients closed after 48 hours of age without osteotomy have not had as much success gaining continence after completing the staged reconstruction (Aadalen et al., 1980; Husmann et al.,

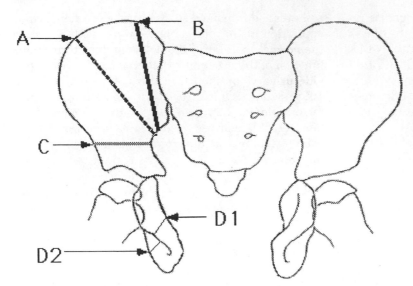

FIG. 52-12
Type of osteotomies. **A,** Anterior diagonal iliac osteotomy (Wedge); **B,** Posterior iliac osteotomy (Schulz); **C,** Anterior transverse (Salter) osteotomy; **D1:** Anterior pubic ramus osteotomy, superior ramus only (Frey); **D1** and **D2:** complete anterior pubic ramus osteotomy (Montagnani). (From McKenna PH, et al: Iliac osteotomy: a model to compare the options in bladder and cloacal exstrophy reconstruction. *J Urol* 1994; 151:182.)

1989). Some even believe penile appearance following epispadias repair is improved if osteotomy is used at the initial closure (McLorie et al., 1991). Osteotomy also may contribute to a lower fistula rate following epispadias (Lepor et al., 1984).

Several techniques have been used: posterior iliac osteotomy, anterior innominate osteotomy, and osteotomy through the superior or superior and inferior pubic rami. To this end, incisions have been as posterior as the sacroiliac ligaments (Lascombes et al., 1988) and as far anterior as the pubic tubercle (Montagnani, 1967, 1982) (Fig. 52-12).

Posterior iliac osteotomy was performed more frequently in the past (Cracchiolo and Hall, 1970; Schultz, 1958). With the patient prone, the iliac bone is exposed lateral to the sacroiliac joint through separate posterior vertical skin incisions. The narrowest part of the ileum is exposed, and the periosteum is incised to the superior edge of the iliac bone. An incision is made through both tables of the ileum, taking care to prevent injury to the sciatic nerve and vessels. A precise fracture will permit the iliac wings to be displaced anteromedially for later fixation of the pubic symphysis. Bone wax controls bone-edge bleeding, and the wounds are closed with drains. The baby is then placed supine and redraped for the bladder closure. A delay of up to 2 weeks may intervene between iliac fracture and bladder closure.

More anterior approaches to the iliac osteotomy permit both procedures in the supine position. Incisions through the superior ramus of the pubic bone (Frey and Cohen, 1989), through both the superior and inferior rami (Montagnani, 1967; Schmidt et al., 1993), with or without bone grafting (Edgerton and Gillenwater, 1986), have been described as quicker and easier to perform than the posterior incisions.

Anterior diagonal iliac osteotomy is currently our preferred method. The anterior approach provides better bone symmetry, brings the lateral soft tissues together more cosmetically, and makes the bladder closure and osteotomy a combined procedure. The incision in bone is made at an oblique angle across the thinnest part of the innominate bone (McKenna et al., 1994). In patients older than 6 months, pins with external fixation are placed across the osteotomy to stabilize the bone fragments.

Bladder Closure

Following the osteotomy, the ureteral orifices are catheterized with small feeding tubes (3.5 F), which are sewn in place with fine chromic suture. These catheters remain in place for 2 to 3 weeks, during which time they are irrigated frequently to assure optimal drainage. Effective external drainage of the upper tracts may reduce the risk of the bladder to dehisce (Husmann et al., 1989). An incision made (Fig. 52-13, *A*) along the lateral edge of the exposed urothelium extends from superior to the umbilicus to the base of the bladder. This incision removes the umbilicus. If the umbilicus remains, the necrotic tissue serves as a source for infection, which can result in dehiscence. Although others have preserved the umbilicus, we think it is better to fashion a new umbilicus in a more normal position, 2 to 3 cm superior to the original location, at the level of the anterior-superior iliac crest. Creation of the umbilicus is postponed until the conclusion of the bladder closure with placement of the suprapubic tube through the neoumbilicus.

Following the skin incision, the retroperitoneal space is entered superior to the umbilicus, and the bladder is widely mobilized from the rectus fascia. The peritoneum is separated from the posterior wall of the bladder and elevated to allow the bladder to

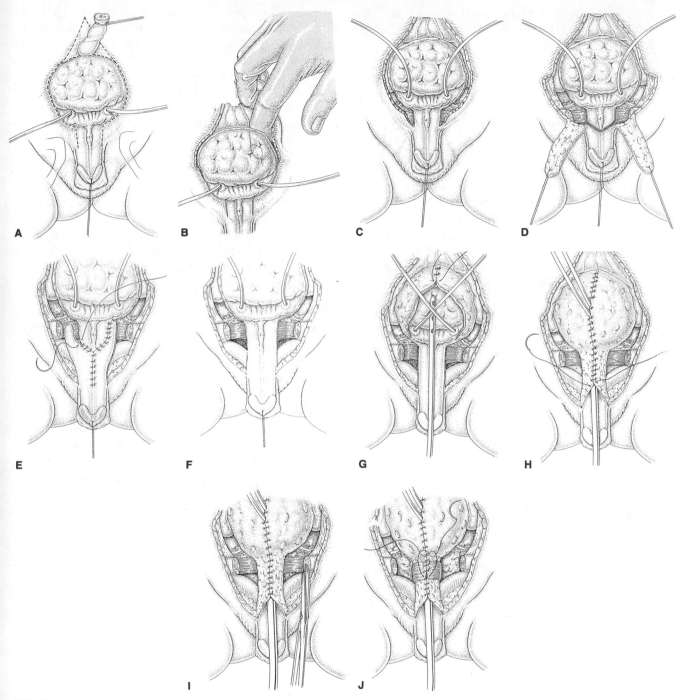

FIG. 52-13

Bladder Closure: **A,** Incision. After placement of ureteral catheters, the umbilicus is removed and the incision is carried well distal to the verumontanum. Care is taken to prevent incorporation of the squamous tissue lateral to the bladder. **B,** The bladder is mobilized off of the peritoneum superiorly and inferolaterally. **C,** The dissection is carried inferior to the pubis. **D-E,** Paraexstrophy flaps can be used to import additional tissue to assure a wide open bladder neck when the bladder and proximal urethra are closed. If flaps are used, they should be made no longer than 3:1 length to width. These are drawn too long in this figure. **F,** The corporal bodies are freed from the urethral tissue, and the prostatic urethra is mobilized from the intersymphyseal band to allow the urethra and bladder neck to recess posteriorly deep within the pelvis. The dissection of the corpora is taken along the inferior margin of the pubis but not beyond. In this diagram the urethral plate is too narrow to allow for safe closure. **G-H,** The bladder is closed with two layers of PGA suture. The urethra is closed. **I-J,** The tissue inferolateral to the pubic arch is freed further (and the urethral incision extended) to allow more posterior displacement into the pelvis. Closure of the intrasymphyseal tissue over the urethra as depicted in **J** is not always possible and probably not necessary as long as the lateral dissection is adequate enough to allow posterior displacement. (From Ransley PG, Duffy PG: Bladder exstrophy closure and epispadias repair. In Spitz L, Coran AG (eds): *Rob and Smith's Operative Surgery: pediatric surgery,* Chapman and Hall, ed 5. London, 1995.)

drop deeper into the retroperitoneum. The dissection is carried inferior to the pubis. The fibromuscular attachments of the corporal bodies to the pubis bilaterally are dissected away from the bone in a subperiosteal plane, taking care to prevent injury to the neurovascular bundle, which is lateral (Fig. 52-13, *B, C*).

The next step is controversial. The "standard" was to divide the urethral plate distal to the prostate, separate the corporal bodies from the intercrural prostate and deliver the bladder and prostatic urethra back into the pelvis, untethering it from the distal urethra and penis (Duckett, 1977). To bridge the gap of the separation, paraexstrophy skin flaps (PEF) were developed from the adjacent shiny skin and brought together in the midline (Fig. 52-13, *D, E*). The distal flaps were sutured to the prostatic urethra and the bladder neck to widen the prostatic urethra. This assures a wide open bladder neck when the bladder and proximal urethra are closed. Penile lengthening is accomplished by incising the anterior attachments of the corporal bodies to the pubis. The paraexstrophy flaps are tubularized as a urethral extension distally to the abdominal wall closure while the distal epispadias remains for later reconstruction.

Now that experience with the Cantwell-Ransley-Epispadias Procedure (CREP) has proven so successful as a cosmetic and functional penile reconstruction, the PEF concept is under siege. The CREP, by design, leaves the entire urethral plate intact so it may be tubularized and transposed ventrally (Fig. 52-13, *F-H*). In addition, Gearhart and colleagues (1993a) in their exstrophy experience have seen 40 patients referred with strictures at the prostatic urethra where the PEFs have been placed. As a result, surgeons from Johns Hopkins and the Great Ormond Street hospitals are no longer using the PEF concept *except* in very short epispadias cases where closure will be jeopardized. Nevertheless, properly deployed, PEF will not lead to stricture if the details of the technique are followed (Duckett, 1993). As an alternative to a formal paraexstrophy flap, a Z plasty of paraexstrophy skin can be interposed along the cut edges of the prostatic urethral plate. Although this modification does not provide as much length as a paraexstrophy flap, it may prove suitable in many cases and may lessen the risk of prostatic urethral stricture.

It has been surmised that the intersymphyseal band of tissue that traverses the bladder neck area has in it the rudimentary urogenital diaphragm (external sphincter) muscle complex. Therefore, lateral dissection frees this band from the pubis; a wrap-around of the bladder neck is often depicted in the diagrams (Fig. 52-13, *I, J*). In execution, however, this may not be so clear cut, nor physiologically sound. Dissection inferiolateral to the pubic arch will free the levators

for more posterior displacement into the pelvis when the prostatic urethra is released from its intercrural position. This dissection does not jeopardize the blood supply to the bladder since the blood supply to the exstrophied bladder comes from deep in the pelvis and runs with the prostate and ureters. This posterior displacement of the bladder neck and posterior urethra that is accomplished with extensive inferolateral dissection is essential to a successful closure. Following mobilization of the urethral plate, the bladder and proximal urethra are closed in two layers with fine, absorbable suture. The bladder is closed with a vertical suture line in an attempt to draw the bladder dome superiorly and thereby minimize risk of prolapse through the bladder neck after closure. The bladder neck is closed to 12 F caliber. This size seems wide enough to provide good drainage but is usually small enough to prevent bladder prolapse.

Herniorrhaphy

Because of a relative lack of shutter mechanism in the inguinal canal, boys and girls with bladder exstrophy have an increased risk of incarcerated hernia. In one study, 56% of boys and 15% of girls developed inguinal hernias over a follow-up period of 10 years; 46% of the boys presented with incarceration requiring emergent management (Husmann et al., 1990b). Another retrospective review of 70 consecutive patients with bladder exstrophy noted that 42 (86%) boys and three (15%) girls developed inguinal hernias, bilateral in 78% of the cases. No recurrence following correction occurred in females, whereas 17% of boys developed a recurrence (Stringer et al., 1994). Although a hernia rarely is observed prior to bladder closure, we recommend bilateral herniorrhaphy at the time of bladder closure to prevent incarcerated hernia, which is more common after closure than before. A preperitoneal approach through the abdominal incision obviates an additional inguinal incision (Husmann et al., 1990b). Orchiopexy is performed later if the testes are truly cryptorchid. Usually, however, the testes only appear high because of the laterally displaced rectus muscle.

Umbilicoplasty

Various types of umbilicoplasties have been described (Hanna and Ansong, 1984; Sumfest and Mitchell, 1994). We prefer creation of a circular flap surrounding the suprapubic tube. A latex Malecot catheter is avoided now because of the allergy risk. In newborns, we currently are using 12 F silastic tubing with additional side holes to improve drainage. The tube is sutured in place at the skin with permanent suture and to the bladder mucosa with a fine chromic suture to ensure that it will function for 3 to 4 weeks. In older patients, either larger shunt tubing or a silastic Foley catheter is used. No urethral catheters are placed because these may cause erosion of the pubic suture into the urethra. Drains anterior to the bladder are unnecessary since the suprapubic tube effectively drains the subcutaneous space.

Pelvic Immobilization

After bladder and urethral closure in the newborn, an assistant manually rotates the greater trochanter on each side to approximate the pubic bones. A heavy nylon horizontal mattress suture is placed, tied with the knot anterior to prevent erosion into the urethra. The rectus muscles are brought together with fascial sutures for a solid abdominal wall closure. The urethral meatus opens at the base of the epispadias.

Current techniques of pelvic immobilization seek to simplify nursing care and shorten hospital stay. In the newborn, a gentle "mermaid" dressing keeps the legs internally rotated with foam pads at the knees and ankles to avoid pressure necrosis. If urine leaks despite the ureteral and suprapubic tubes, a circular diaper is placed, avoiding any pads between the legs. Velcro foam straps permit frequent cleansing of feces. This nursing care is taught to the parents so that the mermaid position is maintained for 4 to 6 weeks at home.

Scherz and co-workers (1990) have advocated a fascia lata strip, which is sutured across the pubic bones at the time of closure to provide additional stability. Jeffs (1987) has advocated modified Bryant's traction in infants, which seeks to lift the buttocks just off the bed with minimal weight. Allen and associates (1992) believe that infants closed earlier than 48 hours with osteotomy may not require fixation at all. In older patients, we prefer external fixation with pins. If an external fixation device is used, care must be taken to prevent over zealous compression on the device. Too much medial rotation of the pelvis results in tension on the sciatic nerve with resulting transient weakness or reflex-induced vasoconstriction and hypertension (Heij et al., 1993; Husmann et al., 1993).

The suprapubic tube and, if possible, ureteral catheter are maintained during the period of traction. These are irrigated gently as needed. Prior to removal of the suprapubic tube, patency of the urethra is assessed by measuring residual urine in the bladder. If bladder neck resistance prevents drainage, gentle dilation of the urethra may be accomplished with sounds either in the operating room with light general anesthetic or at the bedside. The bladder drainage tube must not be removed before ensuring adequate urethral drainage. Broad-spectrum antibiotics are continued for 24 hours to prevent osteomyelitis at the pin sites or at the site of the pubic suture. Oral antibiotic prophylaxis is then started, which is maintained throughout the incontinent interval.

Incontinent Period

For the next 3 to 5 years following bladder closure, the bladder gradually increases capacity awaiting bladder neck reconstruction (BNR). During this period, the bladder must not be permitted to develop high pressures, yet the bladder outlet should have enough resistance to allow "accommodation" of urine to stimulate bladder growth increasing volume.

To better define the pressures associated with increased bladder capacity, as well as those associated with renal damage, Hollowell and co-workers (1992) reviewed a series of patients following initial closure. A leak pressure of greater than 40 cm H_2O or end-fill pressure of greater than 10 cm H_2O was associated with increased bladder capacity, but also was associated with renal damage. Since preservation of renal function is essential in exstrophy reconstruction, extreme vigilance, particularly in the first year following closure, is essential.

Bladder and renal ultrasound are obtained every 3 months in the first year to detect hydronephrosis. If increased pressure is suspected with recurrent urinary tract infections or residual urine volumes, the bladder outlet should be examined under a general anesthetic. Aggressive action to resolve hydronephrosis should be taken. This may require initiation of clean intermittent catheterization, urethral dilation, or even as a last resort, vesicostomy. Some have proceeded with early bladder augmentation with bowel or ureter in this situation. We do not advocate this in general.

Because all patients with exstrophy have vesicoureteral reflux, after bladder closure, urinary tract infection will result in renal scarring, particularly if bladder pressure is high. Husmann and associates (1990a), in a review from the Hospital for Sick Children in Toronto, noted febrile urinary tract infection, poor compliance with prophylactic antibiotics, and elevated residual urines all were associated with renal scarring in patients following bladder closure. Good bladder emptying and prevention of urinary tract infections throughout the incontinent period with prophylactic antibiotics are essential.

The increased urethral length following epispadias repair seems to stimulate bladder growth by providing additional resistance without obstructing the bladder neck. This can result in as much as 50% to 70% increase in bladder capacity during the incontinent period (Gearhart and Jeffs, 1989a). The bladder must be at least 60 ml in volume before bladder neck reconstruction is undertaken. If bladder volume is still a problem after epispadias repair, injection of collagen at the bladder neck can be tried. Caione and co-workers (1993) have reported increases in bladder capacity in males as much as 47%, whereas improvement in females is much less. Collagen injection in this setting is intended to provide just enough additional resistance to the bladder neck to stimulate bladder growth without resulting in increased intravesical pressure. In our limited experience, we have found the technique difficult to perfect because of scarring in the bladder neck, which makes injection of large enough volumes of the implant difficult. We doubt that this will develop into a significant contribution to staged reconstruction of exstrophy.

Epispadias Repair

The epispadias repair should lengthen and straighten the penis to a dependent position and provide a urethra adequate for normal voiding and for smooth catheter passage, if needed. Several different techniques have been described to correct epispadias. Since penile lengthening (separation of the corporal attachments to the pubic rami) often is performed during the initial bladder closure, a dorsal tubularization of the urethral plate or a modification of the Young urethroplasty is adequate, in some cases. In many cases, however, the urethra is still ventral after initial penile lengthening and a modification of the Cantwell Ransley epispadias procedure (CREP) is a better choice. The CREP adds a unique corporal rotation and curvature correction by a corporocorporrhaphy. The ability to detach the urethra from the corporal bodies without disruption of the urethral plate to allow the urethra to drop ventrally may result in lower fistula rates in epispadias (Perovic et al., 1992). It is this concept that makes the CREP procedure successful.

Cantwell-Ransley Epispadias Repair

With the CREP procedure, after placement of a glans-holding suture, a Heineke-Mikulicz advancement of the urethral plate is performed at the tip of the spade-like glans to advance the new meatus to a more ventral position. A 15-mm wide strip is marked along the urethral plate from the tip of the glans to the base of the penis around the urethral meatus. The penile shaft skin is separated from the corpora. Tissue lateral to the incised urethral plate is widely mobilized with care taken to prevent injury to the paired neurovascular bundles. The corpora are mobilized again from the pubis if not adequately separated at the initial closure (Fig. 52-14, A). Careful dissection separates the urethral plate completely from the corporal bodies along the length of the shaft from just distal to the prostate to the glanular urethra. Glanular wedges are excised to facilitate approximation of glans wings over the tubularized glanular urethra. The urethra is closed over a soft Silastic tube with fine, running PGA suture (Fig. 52-14, B).

Separate tourniquets are placed on each corpora and separate injections with saline are made to determine the concavity of the location of maximal curvature. The corpora will be rotated medially to a dorsal po-

sition that will correct most of the curvature. However, in many cases, transverse incisions into each tunica albuginea at the point of maximal bend will be needed to further lengthen the corpora. These incisions are converted to diamond-shaped defects (Fig. 52-14, C). When these two diamonds are approximated with dorsomedial rotation, the curvature will be greatly improved and a dependent penis will result. This also places the urethra beneath the corpora and the neurovascular bundles at the dorsal midline (Fig. 52-14, D) for dorsal skin coverage. The ventral prepuce may then be used to form an island flap for dorsal skin coverage (Fig. 52-14, E). If insufficient urethral length is present following mobilization of the corpora, free preputial skin grafts, buccal mucosa grafts, or transverse island flaps may be utilized to lengthen the urethra (Ransley, 1988).

Mitchell Epispadias Procedure

Recent experience with preservation of the urethral plate in severe hypospadias (Baskin and Duckett, 1994; Mollard et al., 1991; Perovic and Vukadinovic, 1994) may be extrapolated to even more aggressive epispadias reconstructions. For instance, in epispadias, Hendren (1979), Mollard and co-workers (1986), and recently Mitchell and Bägli (1995), have dissected the thick urethral plate distally and based a long flap of urethra proximally on the prostatic blood supply. The Mitchell epispadias procedure (MEP) (Fig. 52-15) has modified the CREP by extending the urethral plate dissection into the glans edge where it is freed into a long flap. The glans is split in the midline so that each corporal body and hemiglans is free. This separates the phallus into three components: the urethral plate and two hemiglanulocorporal bodies, which are completely separated in the midline. The glans blood supply is dependent on preservation of the lateral neurovascular bundles. The urethral plate is rolled into a tube. The penis is reconstructed with ventral placement of the urethra and dorsal rotation of the corpora. According to Mitchell, in most cases this ventrally placed neourethra is sufficiently long to reach the glans. The corpora are freely rotated to completely correct dorsal curvature. It is sometimes necessary to correct dorsoventral length discrepancies by suturing together adjacent corporotomies, as in the CREP repair (Ransley, 1988). The urethra is positioned in the ventral groove between the corporal bodies and sutured to the glans halves distally to produce an orthotopic urethral meatus.

Mitchell and Bägli (1995) report successful results with their repair in two cases where paraexstrophy flaps have been used in the initial exstrophy closure. Of 10 cases so far, excellent cosmetic results have been obtained.

As with all reconstructive problems, no one procedure is effective for all patients. The "tumble tube" epispadias repair (Snyder, 1990), a modified Young repair, or urethral reconstruction using a ventral preputial island flap (Thomalla and Mitchell, 1984) also are used occasionally with good results.

Following epispadias repair, a dressing similar to that employed in hypospadias repair is left for 3 to 5 days. A 7 F to 10 F silastic urethral stent is placed and allowed to drain into the diaper. If the patient is older, a nonlatex Foley catheter is used. This arrangement eliminates the cumbersome gravity drainage tubes. The tube is removed in 14 days.

A urethrocutaneous fistula develops about 20% of the time in epispadias repair (Lepor et al., 1984). These are found most commonly at sites where tissue is scarce. As a result, in the Young repair, fistulas usually occur at the corona. Because the urethra at the level of the corona is more effectively covered in the CREP, a fistula is more common at the base of the penis (Perovic et al., 1992). This location has the least skin available to cover the neourethra and is under the most tension after closure. If a fistula occurs, a second procedure to close the fistula is done with the BNR. Complex strictures that recur generally are due to poor blood supply at the fistula site, and these may be corrected with buccal mucosa free grafts. We have been impressed with the versatility of buccal mucosa and find it easier to harvest and more easily handled than bladder mucosa (Duckett et al., 1995).

Continence Surgery — Bladder Neck Reconstruction

Reconstruction of the open bladder neck endeavors to provide voluntary voiding with continence without jeopardizing renal function. Before BNR, the child must be motivated to be dry and old enough to cooperate with both parents and physicians. Considerable time and effort are required to train the child to recognize the feeling of a full bladder and to faithfully urinate when the bladder feels full. The family must be committed to a period of training, during which frequent telephone calls and occasional office visits to the medical center, monitoring with urinalysis, intermittent catheterization, and periodic cystoscopy may be necessary.

Several factors need to be considered prior to plan-

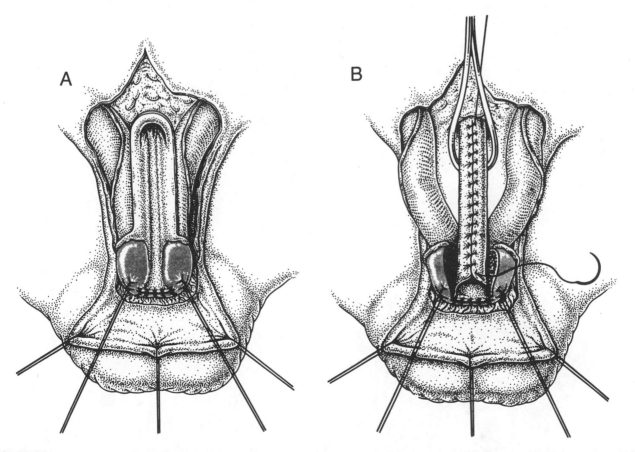

FIG. 52-14
Cantwell-Ransley Epispadias Repair (CREP). **A,** Glans-holding sutures have been placed and the Heineke-Mikulicz advancement has been performed to move the urethral meatus ventrally. The urethral strip has been mobilized and the penile shaft skin has been separated from the corpora. **B,** Careful dissection separates the urethral plate from the corporal bodies. The dissection extends from prostatic to glanular urethra. Glanular wedges facilitate approximation of glans wings over the tubularized glanular urethra.

Continued

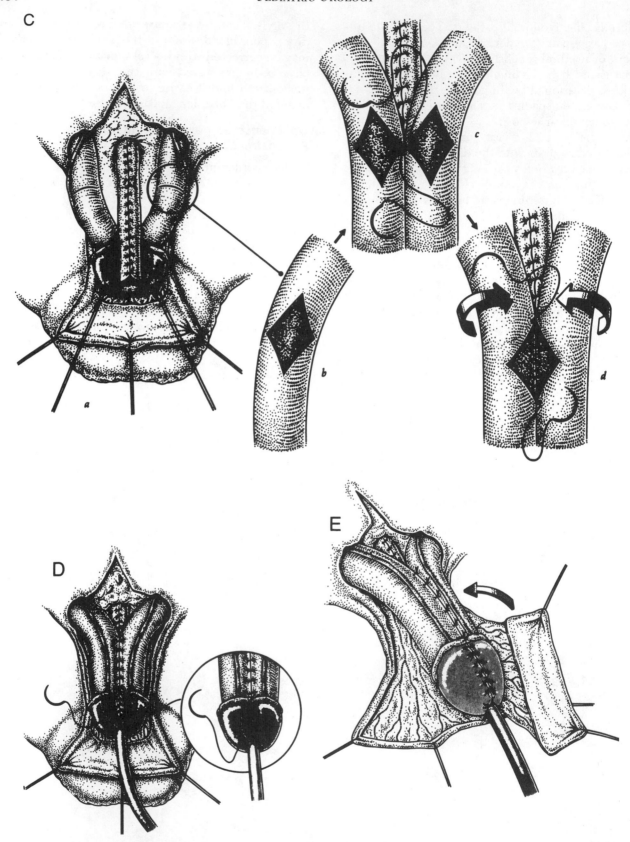

FIG. 52-14 (cont.).
C, If necessary to correct corporal curvature, dorsal incisions at the point of maximal curvature are made. These are joined as the corpora are rotated. **D,** A series of interrupted sutures approximates the corpora. The glans is brought together in layers. **E,** The inner prepuce is isolated on a vascular pedicle and brought to the dorsum for skin coverage. The ventrum is covered with the outer prepuce. (From Snyder HM III: The surgery of bladder exstrophy and epispadias. In Frank JD, Johnston JH (eds): *Operative Paediatric Urology.* Edinburgh, Churchill-Livingstone Inc, 1990.)

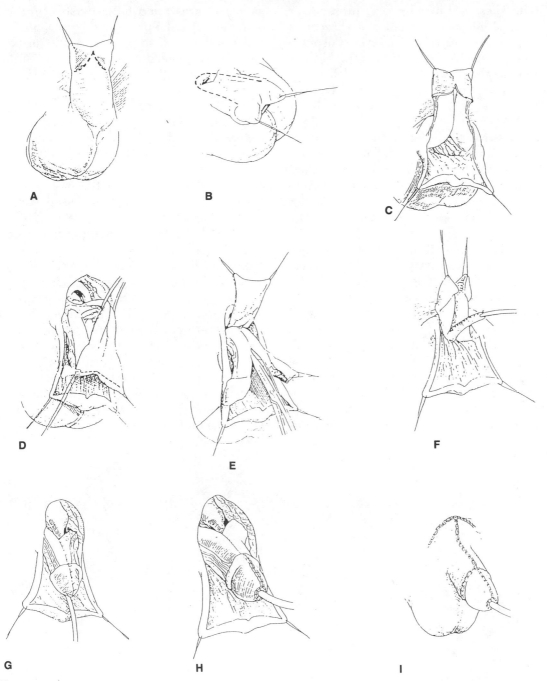

FIG. 52-15

The Mitchell Epispadias Repair (MEP). **A,** Traction sutures are placed into each hemiglans, oriented horizontally (these stay sutures will become vertical in orientation following later corporal rotation). **B,** A circumcising incision is made ventrally and the urethral plate is outlined dorsally to allow later tubularization. **C,** The remainder of the penile shaft skin is dissected off the lateral and ventral aspects of the paired corporal bodies. The neurovascular bundles, which run lateral on the corpora, should be carefully avoided during the degloving of the shaft skin. **D,** The urethral plate is then dissected off the corporal bodies. **E,** The entire plate based on its proximal blood supply is lifted off the glans and corporal tissues. The two hemiglanular corporal bodies are separated completely in the midline by a vertical incision, which begins distally and extends through the glans. The glans is divided into two halves, each supplied by the vessels of the paired lateral neurovascular bundles. **F,** The urethral plate is tubularized and positioned ventral to the entire length of the corporal bodies. **G,** The corpora are freely rotated to correct dorsal chordee. **H,** The corpora cavernosa are sutured together with fine nonabsorbable suture on the dorsum. The urethra is positioned in the ventral groove between the corpora cavernosa and sutured to each glans half distally to produce an orthotopic urethral meatus. If the tubularized urethra is too short, it can be matured onto the ventral aspect of the penis to form a hypospadias, which can be corrected with a second staged procedure. **I,** Final appearance after skin coverage. (From Mitchel ME, Bägli DJ: Complete penile disassembly for epispadias repair: Mitchell technique. Personal communication, Jan 1955.)

ning the BNR. These are bladder size, presence or absence of chronic infection, presence or absence of hydronephrosis or renal scarring, and severity of pubic diastasis. In some cases augmentation of the bladder should be done as the next step (Kajbafzadeh et al., in press). Because a portion of the bladder wall is used during bladder neck plasty, the bladder size is always reduced after BNR.

If the bladder is too small before the repair, compliance will be markedly reduced following surgery and the child will be at risk for chronic high bladder pressures and hydronephrosis. Attempted reconstruction of the bladder neck before adequate bladder growth usually fails (Kramer and Kelalis, 1982). The bladder should be at least 60 ml in volume (Jeffs, 1983). Prior to planning BNR in the past, static cystogram studies using anesthesia were obtained to measure bladder volumes estimating the volume of urine that is refluxing. A better estimate of separate bladder and reflux volumes and combined volume can be made using the nuclear cystogram.

If bladder size is sufficient, if the kidneys are not hydronephrotic or scarred, and if the pubis is well approximated, BNR without augmentation is appropriate. If the pubis is still markedly widened, repeat osteotomy may be helpful to place the urethra within the pelvic ring and achieve voluntary control of uri-

nation (Gearhart and Jeffs, 1989b). Urethral support with the striated muscles of the urogenital diaphragm and bladder neck suspension results in better continence rates. An effective osteotomy is felt to optimize this advantange (Lepor and Jeffs, 1983).

Young-Dees-Leadbetter-Jeffs Procedure

With the Young-Dees-Leadbetter-Jeffs (YDLJ) procedure the bladder is opened through a low, transverse incision placed near the bladder neck with a vertical extension. The ureteral orifices are identified and stents are placed. In the past, a cross-trigonal reimplantation technique was used (Cohen, 1975). The reimplanted ureters also may be directed in a cephalad direction with success (Canning et al., 1993), since the path of the distal ureter in exstrophy is nearly cephalad after coursing deeply in the true pelvis (Fig. 52-16, *A-C*). The new reimplant allows a greater proportion of the trigone to be safely incorporated into the bladder neck repair. The Young-Dees portion of the bladder neckplasty is created after the reimplantation is done. A 30 × 14 mm wide strip is outlined in the posterior urethra and into the trigone. This strip begins at the penile urethra and extends superior to the trigone. After a solution of epinephrine (1:100,000) is injected beneath the mucosa, the epithelium is removed adjacent to the strip. The detrusor is notched

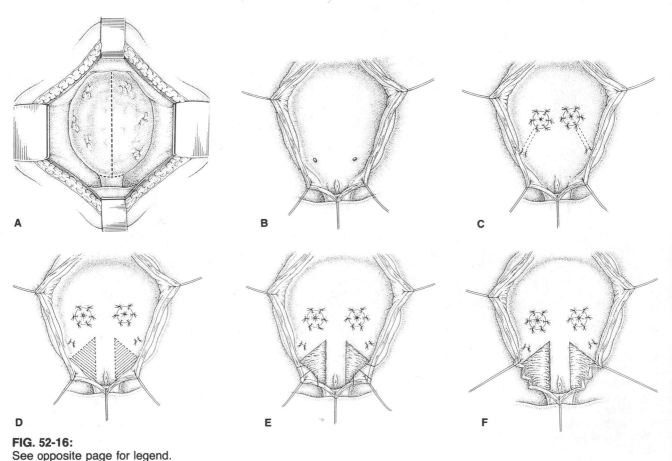

FIG. 52-16:
See opposite page for legend.

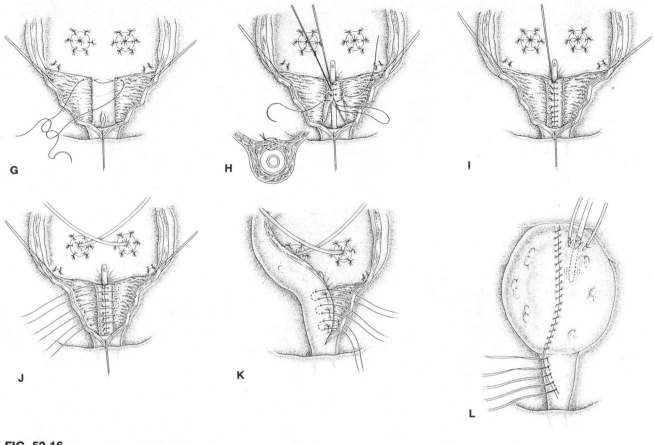

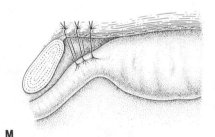

FIG. 52-16

Young-Dees-Leadbetter-Jeffs Bladder Neck Reconstruction (BNR) **A,** After mobilization of the bladder neck and proximal urethra, a low transverse incision is extended vertically exposing the ureteral orifices and the entire trigone and proximal urethra. **B,** The bladder muscle lateral to the mucosal strip is denuded by sharp dissection. **C,** Ureteral reimplantation is performed using either a cross-trigonal technique or a cephalotrigonal technique to provide additional trigonal tissue for the repair. **D,** A strip of mucosa approximately 15 to 20 mm in width by 30 mm in length that extends from the midtrigone to the prostatic or posterior urethra is outlined. **E-F,** Multiple, small incisions into the bladder muscle in the area of the denuded lateral triangles allow lengthening of the bladder neck area and allow the bladder to retract into a more cephalad position. **G-H,** The bladder neck is closed, beginning with a suture that incorporates detrusor muscle and urothelium. Each suture is placed on traction to draw up more of the strip to allow for easier subsequent placement of the more distal sutures. **I,** The completed mucosal layer of the repair. **J,** Ureteral stents, which will be left for 10 to 14 days, are placed and sutured. The first layer of the double-breasted bladder neckplasty are placed. **K,** The second layer of horizontal mattress sutures are placed. **L,** The bladder is closed after placement of a suprapubic catheter, which will remain in place for 3 weeks. **M,** The outer layer of the vest-over-pants repair is brought anteriorly as a Marshall-Marchetti-Krantz bladder neck suspension. (From Gearhart JP: Bladder neck reconstruction in the incontinent child. In Frank J, Johnston, JH (eds): *Operative Paediatric Urology.* Edinburgh, Churchill Livingstone, 1990.)

in a series of Z-plasties to lengthen the bladder neck with minimal reduction of bladder volume (Fig. 52-16, *D-F*). The strip is rolled into a tube over an 8 F stent. The de-epithelialized detrusor is closed over the tube in double-breasted fashion to provide three functional layers (Fig. 52-16, *G-L*).

The urethra and bladder are separated from the pubis to allow mobilization of the urethra deep beneath the pelvic ring. This maneuver allows placement of bladder neck sutures designed to adequately elevate the bladder neck and fix the lengthened urethra (Fig. 52-16, *M*) (Toguri et al., 1978a). Intraoperative urethral pressure is usually greater than 60 cm of H_2O after closure (Gearhart et al., 1986). A two-layer midline closure of the low transverse incision further narrows and elongates the bladder neck. A silastic suprapubic catheter is left in place for 3 weeks. Ureteral stents are left to drain for 10 days. No stents or catheters remain through the urethra.

The urethra is undisturbed for at least 3 weeks. At that time, an 8 F catheter is passed through the urethra. Gentle dilation may be necessary. Occasionally, urethroscopy helps to define the anatomy. The urethra must be catheterized without difficulty before removal of the suprapubic catheter. The catheter is clamped and the child is allowed to void. Once the child can void without difficulty, the kidneys and ureters are viewed with sonography or intravenous pyelography to identify hydronephrosis if present. If hydronephrosis is no greater than that noted on the static cystogram before ureteroneocystostomy, the suprapubic tube is removed.

Careful monitoring of the patient continues while the bladder increases in capacity. If infections occur, sonography, radiography, or cystoscopy is performed to rule out a stone or a suture that may have migrated into the repair.

Other BNR Procedures

Duckett and Caldamone (1985) used an "eccentric detrusor tube" neourethra from the bladder strip, lateral to the ureteral hiatus. De-epithelialized detrusor from the opposite side was wrapped around the bladder neck leaving a retort configuration similar to Jeffs Marshall-Marchetti-Krantz (MMK). Continence was successful but catheterization often was required, which was difficult at times. This procedure has been abandoned.

Mollard (1980) also has modified the repair to include a longitudinal muscle flap of the paraurethral strip to wrap around the new bladder neck creating a "reverse retort." The opposite detrusor muscle folds over the urethral strip transversely (Fig. 52-17). Continence of 60% is reported.

Koff (1990) made a wide anterior bladder flap to accentuate the muscular bladder neck. This procedure (Fig. 52-18) provided good continence; however, because a large segment of bladder neck and urethra is used, the postoperative bladder capacity is reduced even more than with the YDLJ repair.

Kelley (Kelley, 1994) has reported verbally a radical periosteal dissection of the entire levator complex in the exstrophic pelvis with reconfiguring of the normal anatomy. Early results are excellent but the details of the procedure have not been formally reported.

Jones and colleagues (1993) have substantially modified the BNR from the more traditional YDLJ procedure. The distal extent of the dilated prostatic urethra is incised transversely as in the YDLJ (Fig. 52-19, *A*). Instead of extending the transverse incision

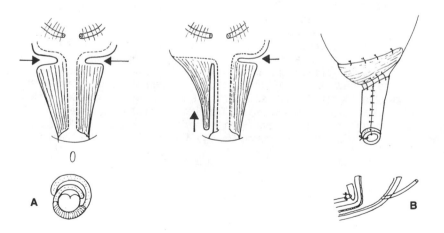

FIG. 52-17
The Young-Dees-Leadbetter Bladder Neckplasty Compared with the Mollard Bladder Neck plasty. **A,** The Young-Dees-Leadbetter Bladder Neck plasty. **B,** Mollard's modification shows an eccentric triangle mobilized and brought around the bladder neck after mucosal closure and ureteral reimplant. This draws the bladder neck posteriorly, forming a "reverse retort," which is central to the success of this procedure. (From Mollard P: Exstrophies et epispades. In *Preces D'urologie de l'enfant*. Paris, Masson Publishing Co, 1984, pp 226-255.)

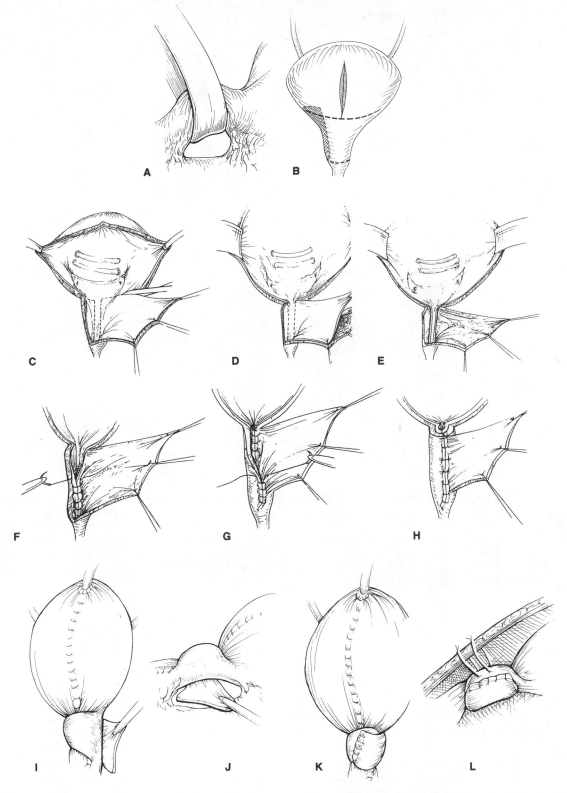

FIG. 52-18
Koff Bladder Neckplasty. **A,** Formation of dissection plane posterior to bladder neck and proximal urethra. **B,** Bladder incisions required to create bladder flap. **C-E,** Mobilization of strip following cross-trigonal reimplant includes removal of mucosa along the dashed lines. **F-H,** The mucosal layer is closed with interrupted absorbable sutures. Detrusor flap is then closed in double breasted fashion. **I-K,** The flap is then brought around the bladder neck and proximal urethra and sutured to itself. **L,** Bladder neck is then suspended into the anterior abdominal wall. (From Koff SA: A technique for bladder neck reconstruction in exstrophy: the cinch. *J Urol* 1990; 144:546.)

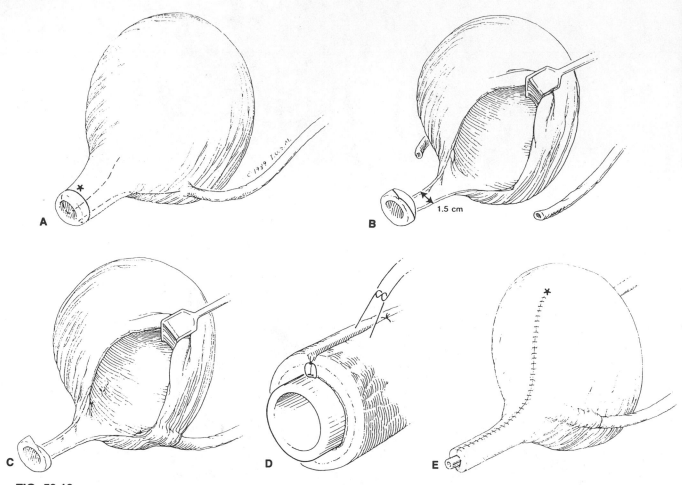

FIG. 52-19
Mitchell Bladder Neckplasty: **A,** A transverse incision is made distal to the original bladder neck area. Note the location of the asterisk relative to the incision. **B,** The incision is extended laterally, posteriorly, and then cephalad towards the ipsilateral ureteric orifice on each side. **C,** The ureters are dissected free from the bladder and reimplanted cephalad in the posterior bladder wall. **D,** The resultant posterior strip of bladder is tubularized in two layers. **E,** The bladder is closed longitudinally as an extension of the bladder neck closure. Note the site of the original bladder neck marked by the asterisk, which is now near the dome. (From Jones J, Mitchell M, Rink R: Improved results using a modification of the Young-Dees-Leadbetter bladder neck repair. *Br J Urol* 1993; 71(5):555.)

vertically, a V flap of bladder neck is incised anteriorly leaving a strip of urethra and bladder neck posteriorly approximately 15 mm wide (Fig. 52-19, *B*). After ureteral reimplantation, the urethra, bladder neck, and trigone are tubularized over an 8 F to 10 F stent for a distance of 3 to 4 cm while the anterior bladder is closed vertically (Fig. 52-19, *C, D*). The point of the V ends at the superior extent of the closure (Fig. 52-19, *E*). In this way, the bladder neck is narrowed without loss of bladder volume. This repair does *not* buttress the bladder neck area with extra layers of de-epithelialized detrusor. Mitchell does not add the MMK fixation to the abdominal wall as reported in the YDLJ. Continence results with this procedure are reported as high as 80% in exstrophy patients with follow-up of 5 years (Mitchell, 1995).

Results of Reconstruction Stages
Results Following Bladder Closure

Although the bladder is closed successfully in most patients, dehiscence, stone formation, and hydronephrosis requiring urethral dilation or vesicostomy can occur. Of 75 patients completing staged repair, some for the second time at Johns Hopkins Hospital, 52 had successful closure. Sixteen (21.3%) developed a major complication, such as prolapse, dehiscence, or hydronephrosis, which required a repeat closure. Seven had minor complications, such as bladder stone, pubic suture infection, or squamous metaplasia along the suture line at the dome of the closed bladder (Canning et al., 1989). Even though we believe that bilateral osteotomy makes the initial closure easier, no study has been able to associate use of osteotomy with decreased dehiscence rates following the initial closure. Dehiscence of the bladder closure in one report seemed to be related more to loss of ureteral diversion stents prior to the seventh postoperative day, abdominal distention, and bladder prolapse through an enlarged urethra (Husmann et al., 1989).

Results Following Epispadias Repair

In one series from the Mayo Clinic, two groups of patients were followed into adulthood following epispadias repair. One group included 44 patients with classic bladder exstrophy (Mesrobian et al., 1988). Another group of 42 patients had complete epispadias (Kramer et al., 1986). Fifty-five percent of the exstrophy patients had a straight penis compared with 67% of the epispadias patients. In another series of 18 boys with exstrophy who had completed epispadias repair, the flaccid penis was directed horizontally or downward in all but three (Lepor et al., 1984). Despite extensive dissection during epispadias repair, most patients are potent following reconstruction of the penis.

A recent review from Mainz (Stein et al., 1994) of 28 male patients treated primarily with ureterosigmoidostomy reported a discouraging outlook for male sexual function if their genitalia were reconstructed. Forty percent still had penile curvature, which was distressing in only three. Epididymitis was present in 33%, necessitating two orchiectomies and three vasectomies. No patient could ejaculate normally or father children. All five patients who did not undergo genital reconstruction had normal ejaculation and two had fathered children.

Better ejaculatory function was reported in diverted patients in the Mayo Clinic series (Mesrobian et al., 1986). In their group of 53 patients 25 could be evaluated for ejaculatory function; 16 of these (64%) had antegrade ejaculation and nine (36%) were an ejaculatory. All had been diverted to ureterosigmoidostomy. These authors note the difficulty of preserving a patent urethra for transport of ejaculate in patients who have had urinary diversion. They believe that the "dry" urethra in these patients is prone to scarring. If fertility is desired, they recommend a short neourethra that may not extend to the tip of the glans but is advantageous for transport or collection of semen. Even with this consideration, only 5 of 12 married patients had fathered children.

Results with the Cantwell-Ransley (CREP) repair in short-term follow-up suggest that this technique may reduce the fistula rate by one third while preserving excellent cosmetic results. In one report 13 boys with either complete epispadias or classic bladder exstrophy underwent the procedure. All had excellent initial results with only one patient needing revision of the proximal anastomosis (Borzi and

Thomas, 1994). Perovic and co-workers (1992) in a larger series of 40 patients undergoing the CREP in most cases, report a 15% complication rate. These recent reports can be compared with an earlier study of 24 patients from Johns Hopkins in which the majority of patients had a modified Young epispadias repair (Lepor et al., 1984). In this group, 22% developed a fistula that required subsequent repair. Results with the MEP (Mitchell and Bägli, 1995) are too early for comparison; however, in the preliminary report, results look most encouraging.

Results Following BNR

Despite major advances, continence in exstrophy patients is far from perfect. Even in centers with large exstrophy populations, less than 50% of patients are truly dry and voiding. Most require intermittent catheterization or bladder augmentation with bowel to achieve suitable dry intervals.

It is impossible to predict which patients will be able to volitionally void. Some studies suggest very good voiding ability (Toguri et al., 1978b), with normal gas cystometrography and normoreflexic bladders. Others report large numbers of patients requiring intermittent catheterization to provide dry intervals and good emptying (Hollowell et al., 1991). The resistance added at the bladder neck to provide continence frequently results in incomplete emptying or involuntary contractions (hypertonicity), requiring close follow-up to prevent upper-tract damage (Hollowell et al., 1993).

Other reports suggest results can be better. In 75 exstrophy patients completing staged reconstruction at Johns Hopkins between 1976 and 1988, a total of 51 (68%) of the exstrophy patients are dry for 3 or more hours; 43 of these 51 (84%) void spontaneously, and eight (16%) patients empty with intermittent catheterization. Fifty-seven percent of those who void are dry. Of the 75 exstrophy patients, 68% of 55 males are dry compared with 80% of 20 females. During the same period, 17 patients with complete epispadias completed staged repair. Fourteen of 17 (82%) of the epispadias patients are continent; all but two void spontaneously. Males and females were equally continent in the epispadias group. All patients in this study underwent intravenous urography or renal sonography to assess the status of the kidneys from 6 months to 10 years following BNR. Only two patients developed significant hydronephrosis, which required revision of the bladder neckplasty and bladder augmentation. A total of 23 complications developed in 20 exstrophy patients following the bladder neck reconstruction, including bladder outlet obstruction requiring intermittent catheterization or prolonged suprapubic drainage in 16 patients, hydronephrosis in two patients, bladder stones in two patients, and epididymitis in three patients (Canning et al., 1989).

Identifying factors that correlate with success from retrospective reviews is difficult. Nevertheless, two observations seem worthy of mention. First, patients who had a successful initial bladder closure more frequently become continent following bladder neck reconstruction than patients who require a second bladder closure. Only 7 of 18 (39%) patients who failed initial closure were dry for more than 3 hours after completing reconstruction, compared with 43 of 57 (75%) patients who had successful initial closure (Canning et al., 1989). This suggests that an early, successful closure may begin to stimulate bladder growth so that capacity and fibrosis are minimized, leading to better compliance at the time of bladder neckplasty.

Secondly, even though bilateral iliac osteotomy has not been proven to reduce dehiscence rates at the time of the initial closure, it does seem to contribute to improved continence rates in patients closed later than the first 72 hours of life. In the same study, 49 of 67 (73%) who underwent closure before 72 hours of age or closure with osteotomy were continent, compared with only two of eight (25%) who had closure without osteotomy after 72 hours of age (Canning et al., 1989). Husmann and associates' (1989) study from the Hospital for Sick Children in Toronto supports this and even suggests no advantage to early closure, as long as osteotomy is performed.

Some believe that marginal continence may improve with time following bladder neck reconstruction. Most patients go through a "training period" during which continence seems to improve. Bladder capacity may increase, or the child who has never before had the sensation of a full bladder may simply improve his or her awareness of the need to void when the bladder increases in volume. Of 34 patients selected from a group of 92 patients with exstrophy or complete epispadias completing staged reconstruction at Johns Hopkins examined at 6-month intervals to identify the length of time needed to achieve maximal continence, all but four (88%) became continent during the second year following BNR. Most had not yet reached puberty. In the few that entered puberty following BNR, continence did not improve dramatically (Canning et al., 1989). Others have reported a pronounced increase in continence in males at puberty, presumably because of prostate enlargement and increased resistance at the bladder outlet (Ritchey et al., 1988). Gearhart and colleagues' (1993b) study seems to refute the theory that prostatic growth results in improved continence at puberty. In MRI studies, their group found that the urethra in exstrophy remains anterior to the prostate after closure. Prostatic hypertrophy would then result in anterior displacement of the urethra rather than increased bladder outlet resistance. We believe that if the patient is wet

within 2 years of the bladder neck reconstruction, reoperation to improve continence is warranted despite the patient's age.

Despite good results with the staged repair at some centers (Connor et al., 1989; Mesrobian et al., 1988; Mollard, 1980; Ritchey et al., 1988), others have been less encouraging. In most centers, overall continence rates following reconstruction of the native bladder have been depressing (Table 52-1). This has resulted in a turn away from the staged approach to one relying ultimately on augmentation or diversion as a means of achieving continence and preserving renal function with exstrophy at some centers (de la Hunt and O'Donnell, 1989; Kajbafzadeh et al., 1995; Mansi and Ahmed, 1993). If the results with the staged approach are so abysmal that the child suffers six or more major surgical procedures with the final result augmentation and catheterization, one can readily see the temptation to proceed with immediate diversion or augmentation at the time of BNR. However, the complications of this approach with stones, hydronephrosis, renal scarring, and development of tumors within the augmented intestinal segment may prove to be higher than in patients undergoing the staged approach with the native bladder. The algorithm for this decision tree is the most difficult dilemma facing the pediatric urologist today. We will not resolve it in this chapter.

Management of Complications
Bladder Prolapse or Dehiscence:

Once bladder prolapse begins, usually with a minor appearance of urothelium at the inferior margin of the repair, complete dehiscence is a near certainty. There is nothing one can do to reverse this process. A second attempt at closure should be delayed at least 6 months. A formal osteotomy using external fixation will be required. Even with a successful second closure, continence without augmentation is rare. In 38 patients referred to Johns Hopkins Hospital with a failed closure, one third have completed repeat bladder neckplasties with augmentations and all are dry on intermittent catheterization. All had preservation of the upper tracts (Gearhart, 1991). None of the patients who had a failed first stage developed bladder capacities enabling them to void on their own.

Small Capacity Bladder/Failed BNR

Despite successful bladder closure, a group of patients will fail to gain suitable bladder capacity for bladder neck reconstruction. If epispadias repair has not yet been performed, urethroplasty may add enough passive resistance to the urinary outlet to increase bladder capacity further (Gearhart and Jeffs, 1989a). In some cases, even with adequate bladder volumes prior to BNR, acceptable postoperative continence does not occur. If these patients undergo an-

TABLE 52-1

Results of Bladder Neck Continence Surgery

Reference	Good	Fair	Poor
Johnston and Kogan, 1974	21.9	78.1	
Williams and Keeton, 1973	32	68	
Fisher and Retik, 1969	23	77	
Cendron and Petit, 1971	50	50	
Marshall and Muecke, 1970	25	25	50
Jeffs et al., 1982	60	16	23
Rickham and Stauffer, 1984	31	31	38
Duckett and Caldamone, 1984	60	20	20
Cumulative result	38	—	—

other BNR, the success is no better than 35% (Husmann et al., 1989).

The decision to proceed with repeat BNR should be individualized. Many exstrophy patients do not seem to initiate a good detrusor contraction after bladder neck repair. At the Great Ormond Street Hospital of London, Hollowell and co-workers (1993) studied the 21 nonaugmented patients and found only six who could initiate a sustained detrusor contraction for voiding. These data are dissimilar to the Hopkins experience where a significant number of patients (57%) void. The reasons why remain elusive. If after careful analysis of bladder compliance, capacity, and detrusor effectiveness with urodynamic studies, compliance and bladder capacity are low, the decision to augment the bladder should be made.

Artificial Sphincter

Placement of an artificial sphincter has been attempted in cases of failed BNR (Hanna, 1981; Mitchell and Rink, 1983). However, since failed staged reconstructions most commonly are caused by poorly compliant small bladders, placement of an artificial sphincter may result in progressive hydronephrosis in these cases (Light and Scott, 1983). These patients frequently develop erosion and infection of the artificial sphincter cuff even after delayed activation. Although initial success has been quoted to be as high as 70%, the later erosion rate is high, and virtually all will need reoperation (Decter et al., 1988). Attempts have been made to protect the bladder neck area at the time of initial bladder neck closure by wrapping a silastic sheath around the repair. These too ultimately failed. Others reported some success with an inactivated sphincter cuff sandwiched between a two-layer wrap of omentum (Duffy and Ransley, 1988). Long-term results with this approach have been unsuccessful. A few adolescents or adults with exstrophy may be candidates for placement of artificial sphincters but they must have adequate bladder capacities or have undergone bladder augmentation before or during placement of the device (Decter et al., 1988).

Clean Intermittent Catheterization

Often intermittent catheterization is required to drain a bladder that will not empty with a detrusor contraction. This may be difficult to perform through a newly rolled urethra after epispadias repair, or the patient may not cooperate if the catheterization is uncomfortable or difficult. A bladder neck with several previous attempts at continence may become so scarred that it is appropriate to transect the bladder proximal to the verumontanum and close the bladder outlet to keep it from leaking (Leonard et al., 1990). In this case, a continent abdominal stoma should be created. When the bladder neck is closed, care must be taken to preserve ejaculatory function. Since the verumontanum is close to the field of dissection when closing the bladder neck, this is easily damaged; this is perhaps the reason for the poor sexual function in the long-term Mainz series (Stein et al., 1994).

Augmentation Cystoplasty

Nearly all patients can be made dry by augmenting the bladder and emptying with intermittent catheterization. Large series from several centers report better than 90% of the patients dry (Gearhart and Jeffs, 1988; Kajbafzadeh et al., in press; Kramer, 1989). Procedures employing the Mitrofanoff principle provide consistent, durable continence and have become the preferred approach (Duckett and Snyder, 1986; Sumfest et al., 1993). If the appendix is not available, a tapered segment of small bowel can be used in place of the appendix (Duckett and Lofti, 1993). Techniques that use intussusception of the ileum as a nipple (Hendren, 1986) have not resulted in reliable long-term continence mechanisms in our experience. The Benchekroun procedure (Benchekroun et al., 1989; Leonard et al., 1990), a reversed intussuscepted loop of ileum, has likewise been ineffective in the long term.

In some cases, there is so little bladder available that a complete urinary pouch from bowel is better than trying to preserve the small bladder. The small bladder is left in place for seminal secretions in the male (Duckett and Snyder, 1986). The gastroileal reservoir as an alternative to the colonic or ileal pouch has been reported to provide fewer metabolic complications, no stones, and excellent patient tolerance. Since the pouch incorporates mostly ileum with a small stomach patch, it is more time consuming to construct and is more complicated to configure. The addition of acid-secreting gastric mucosa to the alkaline-secreting ileal mucosa may provide better electrolyte balance (Lockhart et al., 1993) and reduce the risk of chronic urinary tract infection and stone formation.

Bladder stones occur in all types of reservoirs, especially those infected with *Proteus mirabilis* (Blyth et al., 1992; Duckett and Lofti, 1993). Patients with exstrophy have a higher risk of stone formation when intestinal mucosa has been added to the urinary tract (Lebowitz and Vargas, 1987). To avoid stones, we have our patients irrigate with 300 cc of tap water each night to clear mucus. Bushman and Howards (1994) have recently reported the effectiveness of nightly irrigation with a urea solution to prevent stones in augmented patients. If stones develop, they should be removed without fragmentation through a small incision. Fragmentation to facilitate endoscopic removal only results in difficulty rendering the patient stone free.

Perforation is perhaps the most concerning risk in patients with an augmented bladder or a continent pouch. Chronic infection and chronic distension are the common denominators that lead to perforation. Even though patients with exstrophy have normal sensation and should feel a distended pouch, unlike the myelomeningocele population, the rupture rate is still high in this group of patients. Any patient who experiences abdominal discomfort, especially with associated fever, should be treated as an emergency and undergo laparotomy urgently. Ultrasound and cystography will sometimes show evidence of extravasation on the drainage film. Perforations, however, are often not detectable with radiologic study. Failure to recognize and treat bladder perforation promptly results in significant morbidity (Elder et al., 1988), and even death (Braverman and Lebowitz, 1991).

Ureterosigmoidostomy

Ureterosigmoidostomy is the oldest form of urinary diversion to provide continence for patients with exstrophy. The concept is simple: the ureters are tunneled into the tinea of the sigmoid colon, and the urine and feces mix. The anus provides the continence mechanism for both urine and feces. When a successful antirefluxing ureterocolonic anastomosis is made, few upper-tract problems occur. This procedure generally has been well tolerated, and anal continence usually is achieved (Duckett and Gazak, 1983). It may be the best alternative for patients with exstrophy living in developing countries where the day to day management of more complicated composite bladders is difficult to achieve (Bagchi, 1990).

Ureterosigmoidostomy has not been successful as a fall back in patients with hydroureteronephrosis who fail exstrophy reconstruction. In a review by Husmann and Spence (1990) of 103 patients undergoing various types of reconstruction for bladder exstrophy, they noted that patients with ureterosigmoidostomy had the highest continence rate but also had the highest incidence of renal deterioration with 10% dying of renal failure and 23% with loss of one kidney. These results, however, reflect the high rate of colon-ureteral reflux present in earlier cases.

In addition to risks of renal scarring and stones, patients who have had ureterosigmoidostomy are at a high risk for colon cancer. The lifelong risk of tumor in these patients is about 10% (Husmann and Spence, 1990). Deaths have occurred in some of those who get malignancies. Late detection is the reason for this poor outcome. Tumors that develop within the colon are thought to be dependent on the presence of urine, feces, urothelium, and colonic epithelium in close apposition at a healing suture line. In Gittes' (1986) study, certain strains of rats that have undergone uretero-sigmoidostomy developed colon carcinoma that appeared similar in histology to tumors seen in humans. Other strains of rat did not. Tumors in humans tend to occur along the anastomotic site between the ureter and colon, but have occurred elsewhere in the colon (Strachan and Woodhouse, 1991) and have even occurred after defunctionalization of the ureterosigmoidostomy (Krishnamsetty et al., 1988). Similar tumors have been found in patients who have had variations of ureterosigmoidostomy, such as trigonosigmoidostomy, and also in other types of urinary diversion (Husmann and Spence, 1990; Kliment et al., 1993; Mortensen et al., 1990).

Because of the reports of tumor, urologists feel compelled to recommend conversion of the ureterosigmoidostomy to a continent catheterizable pouch in hopes of reducing the long-term risk. However, many patients when offered the opportunity to convert to an alternative form of diversion, are reluctant. Even when confronted with risk of cancer, many patients are pleased enough with the lifestyle afforded by ureterosigmoidostomy and refuse conversion to a continent pouch. Few desire to trade to a diversion that, in most cases, requires an abdominal stoma and a lifelong commitment to intermittent catheterization. Because tumors also have been reported in other forms of augmentation, therefore rendering no form of continent pouch absolutely safe, use of ureterosigmoidostomy has regained favor in some circles.

Continence rates with ureterosigmoidostomy have been reported as high as 80% to 90% (Duckett and Gazak, 1983; Stockle et al., 1990). Unfortunately, leakage of the mixture of stool and urine, if it occurs, is very unpleasant. Daytime wetness in some younger patients with ureterosigmoidostomy may be improved with behavioral biofeedback (Purcell et al., 1987). Modifications of the distal colon with an internal pouch (Mainz II) has been most successful in breaking the peristaltic contraction that leads to the incontinence (Fisch et al., 1993). The technique splits the antimesenteric surface of the sigmoid colon at the rectosigmoid junction to reconfigure the sigmoid into a capacious reservoir. This vastly improves continence without impairing passage of stool or urine.

A more complicated modification, also designed to reduce rectal pressure without compromising emptying, was described by Kock (Kock et al., 1988). The ureterosigmoidostomy is diverted to a rectal pouch, which is augmented with ileum for urine storage. An intussuscepted colostomy is created to prevent reflux of urine back into the colon, and the ureters are protected from higher pressures. In this way, rectal pressure is kept low, and in limited experience, continence has improved (Mahran et al., 1994).

Other modifications of the ureterosigmoidostomy have included proximal colon diversion to separate the fecal stream from the urine. The Boyce-Vest procedure, trigonosigmoidostomy with diverting colostomy offers acceptable long-term continence with minimal upper-tract deterioration (Kroovand and Boyce, 1988). The Gersuny or Heinz-Boyer-Hovelacque rectal pouch, constructed from ureters reimplanted into the colon and separated from the fecal stream, has not been effective in the long term (Bracci and Laurenti, 1979; Cromie and Duckett, 1980; Tacciuoli et al., 1977). This modification has been associated with malignancy as well (Phillips et al., 1991).

Ureteroileal colonic sigmoidostomy (Kim et al., 1988), an alternative to ureterosigmoidostomy, separates the ureteral anastomosis from the colonic stream. This technique was developed in response to Gittes' (1986) studies that suggested interposition of ileum between the ureter and colon would result in reduced numbers of carcinomas. No long-term results have been recorded. Hendren (1976) supports this theory in proposing a two-stage procedure: a colon conduit is made to the skin and later intussuscepted into the rectum.

Complications of the Epispadias Repair

Despite better suture material available today and careful technique, urethral strictures and urethrocutaneous fistulas are still common following epispadias repair. Most of the small fistulas can be closed with a secondary procedure with good results. There are still a few patients, however, that will require extensive reconstruction or replacement of the urethra.

In some cases, urethral replacement using a segment of ureter based on an internal iliac pedicle (Mitchell et al., 1988) as a flap can be effective. Long-term follow-up suggests that durability is good and stricture rate is low. Unfortunately, few patients can donate a segment of ureter. Full-thickness skin grafts generally give poor results (Vincent et al., 1988). Bladder mucosal grafts likewise have been unsatisfactory in long-term follow-up (Keating et al., 1990). Our free graft of choice today is buccal mucosa (Duckett et al., 1995). Buccal mucosa is easy to harvest, and it has a thicker epithelium and an excellent vascular bed in the lamina propria for a durable take. Results are much better in re-do urethral reconstruction. In patients with exstrophy and recurrent fistulas at the penopubic junction and prostatic urethra, flaps of rectus abdom-inis muscle and fascia can be incorporated to reduce fistula recurrence rate and improve appearance of the mons (Horton et al., 1988).

Monsplasty:

Successful close approximation of the pelvis results in better approximation of the mons tissue and with a better cosmetic approximation of the genitalia. Older patients who have wide pubic diastasis and a laterally placed escutcheon may benefit from rotational flaps to relocate the mons tissue and improve the appearance of the escutcheon. Secondary reconstructive surgery to improve the abdominal appearance and remove the unsightly scars may be of benefit in these patients (Cocke, 1993). Tissue expanders have been used to obtain additional nonscarred skin and subcutaneous tissue to improve the final cosmetic appearance.

Vaginoplasty

Surgical enlargement of the introitus is frequently required for coitus. An aggressive vaginoplasty, however, usually results in uterine prolapse, which is particularly common in patients who have poor approximation of the pelvic floor (Damario et al., 1994). Uterine suspension may be required (Kennedy et al., 1993).

Sexual Function

As children born with exstrophy mature, issues of sexual performance and fertility assume particular importance. Males with exstrophy and epispadias seem to do well despite what appears to be a severe sexual handicap. At least 70% of males with repaired epispadias followed into adulthood achieved satisfactory erections for sexual intercourse; however, despite adequate sexual function, Woodhouse and co-workers (1983), in a long-term follow-up of 27 reconstructed boys with exstrophy, noted only six who successfully fathered children. Lattimer and colleagues (1978b) reported decreased sperm counts in seven of nine reconstructed exstrophy patients. Most other reports are even more discouraging (Stein et al., 1994). Two main problems contribute to decreased fertility: an incompetent bladder neck with retrograde ejaculation, and scarring of the ampulla of the vas. In cases of retrograde ejaculation, artificial insemination may be successful by retrieving sperm from the urine or by passing a catheter into the often dilated retrourethral space. Patients with scarring at the ampulla of the vas, which leads to vasal obstruction, are not without hope (Duel et al., 1994). Harvesting sperm from the ampulla, the vas, or even the epididymal head might be accomplished in these patients.

Females, in general, have few problems with sexual intercourse. Many develop uterine prolapse and some require unique positioning for successful and comfortable coitus. Fertility in reconstructed females is much more common than in males. A survey of 2500 exstrophy patients identified only 38 males who had fathered children. Yet, 132 females had given birth to 156 children (Shapiro et al., 1984). In another report of 29 girls with exstrophy, eight had borne 11 children (Woodhouse et al., 1983).

In general, exstrophy patients should deliver through a Cesarean section. In one report (Kennedy et al., 1993), four patients, each with an augmented bladder and an orthotopic urethra, carried a healthy child to term. Mild to severe hydronephrosis occurred and persisted through the pregnancy but resolved spontaneously in all cases after delivery. A few patients had progressive difficulty with urethral catheterization and ultimately required indwelling catheters. Those who diverted to abdominal stomas who had delivered vaginally developed postpartum uterine prolapse 75% of the time. It can be concluded now that C-section should be advised in all pregnant patients with exstrophy and that vaginal delivery should be vigorously avoided. Because of the risk of uterine prolapse, consideration for uterine suspension at the time of initial bladder closure should be considered. At the same time, given the difficulty experienced with catheterization of the orthotopic urethra in late pregnancy, consideration also should be made for abdominal appendicovesicostomy rather than orthotopic reconstruction in females at the time of bladder reconstruction.

Bladder Cancer

Adenocarcinoma of the bladder occurs in patients with exstrophy approximately 400 times more commonly than in the normal population and accounts for about 90% of bladder tumors in these patients (Kandzari et al., 1974; Krishnamsetty et al., 1988). Adenocarcinoma is the most commonly reported tumor in untreated cases of bladder exstrophy (Davillas et al., 1991). It also occasionally occurs in adults who have had bladder closure after infancy (Facchini et al., 1987), but has not yet been reported in a patient whose bladder was successfully closed at birth. Chronic irritation of the exposed bladder is thought to cause metaplastic transformation of the urothelium to cystitis glandularis, with later malignant degeneration to carcinoma (Mostofi, 1954). A more recent description likened the histochemical and immunohistochemical appearance to colorectal carcinoma (Witters and Baert-Van Damme, 1987).

Although adenocarcinoma is most common, squamous carcinoma, rhabdomyosarcoma (Semerdjian et al., 1972), and undifferentiated urothelial carcinoma also are reported in patients with bladder exstrophy (Krishnamsetty et al., 1988). Until a large number of patients who have completed modern staged reconstruction are followed into adulthood, it is difficult to quantify the risk of tumors in patients closed in infancy. As a result, long-term monitoring with cytologic evaluation is recommended.

Now that patients who have undergone modern exstrophy treatment techniques have been followed into adulthood, it is gratifying to see the successful lives many of them enjoy. Many of these treated patients have become scholars, business people, athletes, and happily married parents (Lattimer et al., 1978a; Macfarlane et al., 1979; Woodhouse et al., 1983). Progress in continence procedures and in techniques to enlarge and safely catheterize the bladder are largely responsible. Nevertheless, this complex problem remains a challenge, and room exists for greater advances in the future.

CLOACAL EXSTROPHY

Cloacal exstrophy remains the most devastating of genitourinary anomalies offering a great challenge to reconstructive ingenuity. Also called vesicointestinal fissure, cloacal exstrophy is exceedingly rare (1 in 200,000 births), five to six times less common than classic exstrophy of the bladder. The sex ratio is equal. First described by Meckel (1812), this condition resulted in misery for most infants who suffered a prolonged death from malnutrition because of the forshortened gut. In 1960, Rickham made a poignant plea for aggressive surgical reconstruction with preservation of the intestinal segment and end colostomy of the short microcolon. This opened the modern era of management of cloacal exstrophy, which we will summarize.

Anatomy

The defect occurs when an abnormally large cloacal membrane perforates early in development prior to division of the cloaca by the urorectum septum. The defect produced has two halves of the exstrophied bladder separated by an exstrophied ileocecal bowel area (Fig. 52-20, A). On the superior side of the bowel, the ileum prolapses as a long proboscis. On the inferior side, a small orifice goes to a blind-ending, short colonic segment (Fig. 52-20, B). Imperforate anus is always associated. The colon may be duplicated as are the broad appendiceal stumps. In some patients, the bladder halves are surprisingly large. Hurwitz and coworkers (1987) reported on 34 patients with cloacal exstrophy. They found three patterns in the classic type: (1) hemibladder confluent cranial to the bowel, (2) hemibladder lateral to the bowel, and (3) hemibladder confluent caudal to the bowel. In the male, the penis is quite rudimentary and frequently duplicated. Females are likely to have a bifid vagina and uterine abnormalities. Upper urinary tract anomalies are common and were seen in 66% of Hurwitz's (1987)

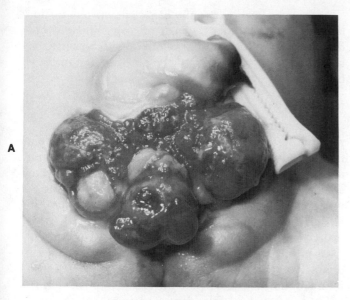

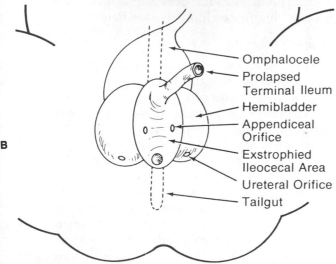

FIG. 52-20
A, Classic cloacal exstrophy with centrally located prolapsed ileocecal segment flanked bilaterally by bladder halves, confluent cranially. **B,** Diagram of classic cloacal exstrophy. Bladder may be confluent at the superior margin of the exstrophied ileoceceal plate as in **A,** or separate as illustrated here. (From Hurwitz R, et al: Cloacal exstrophy: a report of 34 cases. *J Urol* 1987, 138:1060.)

report. These include hydronephrosis, megaureter, pelvic kidneys (25%), and unilateral (20%) and bilateral (5%) renal agenesis. They also noted a high percentage of vertebral (48%) and lower limb deformities (26%). Over 50% of the children have myelomeningoceles or lipomeningoceles. A large omphalocele usually is present, which may contain liver and a large portion of the intestine. Survival can now be expected in these patients, with Hurwitz and colleagues (1978) reporting a 90% survival rate and Howell and associates (1983) reporting an 86% survival rate in 15 patients.

Surgical Reconstruction
Omphalocele

Although closure of the omphalocele is the final portion of the newborn reconstruction, the size of the omphalocele and its content must be considered early when assessing the chances of getting a complete fascial closure. If the omphalocele is small, this is not a major issue. However, most of the time the omphalocele is large enough to require staging the abdominal wall closure. If staged closure is required, it is best to leave the halves of the exstrophied bladder together on the lower abdomen to use as abdominal wall tissue. Sometimes, as in the case of ruptured omphaloceles, a silastic silo may be required, which gradually is reduced over several weeks to achieve closure. Rickham (1960) first used this technique in his third patient, using a nylon sheath sutured to the skin.

Exstrophied Ileocecal Bowel

Rickham (1960) emphasized the need to salvage the hind gut in infants with cloacal exstrophy to prevent the problems of ileostomy management and the short bowel syndrome, which is potentially life threatening. The two halves of the bladder are separated from the ileocecal area. The bowel plate is folded on itself like a book, approximating the lumen of the colon and the ileum after the prolapse is reduced. The distal end of the microcolon can be brought out the perineum as a perineal colostomy. Alternatively, it may be sited on the side of the abdomen far lateral so that it will not contaminate the abdominal wall closure later in the procedure. The colon may be so tiny as to tempt one to remove it. However, its potential is vital for the patient's immediate well being, and later, in proper bowel function for these babies. It is likely that the "short gut syndrome" is not due to deficiency of a length of small bowel, but more to the ravages of an ileostomy in a frail newborn child.

Although some authors previously recommended ileostomy with long-term hyperalimentation and parenteral feedings, we would strongly discourage this approach today (Sukarochana and Sieber, 1978; Tank and Lindenauer, 1970; Welch, 1979). In our experience at Children's Hospital of Philadelphia (Howell et al., 1983), three of our 15 patients had been managed with ileostomy, resulting in poor nutritional status and failure to thrive. Conversion to an end colostomy by salvage of the distal colonic segment resulted in immediate improvement in their nutritional status. Other GI tract anomalies include malrotation, duplication, duodenal atresia, and Meckel's diverticulum (Hurwitz et al., 1987).

Urinary Tract

If the abdominal wall is broad enough to allow primary reapproximation of the two bladder halves with closure and internalization, this is the preferred new-born approach. In their review of 12 patients, Diamond and Jeffs (1985) attempted this in four cases. Two patients died in the newborn period. Of four patients in their series with functional bladder closures, three are continent with intervals of 3 to 4 hours; however, only one can void to completion; the others catheterize.

After the colon is turned in, the two hemibladders are approximated in the midline and assessment of abdominal contents is made. If it appears that the lateral incisions of the bladder will permit fascial closure, the two halves are approximated and the bladder is closed. No attempt is made to tighten the bladder neck. This brought to the perineum as a short urethra under the approximated symphysis.

Approximation of the Symphysis Pubis

Although in the newborn, it may be possible to bring the two pubic bones together, in patients with cloacal exstrophy it is appropriate to do bilateral iliac osteotomies or innominate osteotomies to achieve a good pelvic closure. Osteotomy is particularly helpful if the bladder has not been closed in the newborn period. A tight abdominal wall closure will lead to the devastating complications of sepsis and abdominal wound separation in the infant. Attempting to get the bladder inside and the symphysis approximated in the newborn with large omphalocele is unwise. A later bladder closure with the help of the osteotomy is often safer and more effective.

Genitalia

In 1970, Tank and Lindenauer in their review of 97 cases strongly recommended that males with cloacal exstrophy be converted to females because of the almost uniform disappointment in trying to reconstruct inadequate genitalia into a workable male phenotype. Of the three genetic males in our series who were reconstructed as males, all have inadequate genitalia, and one probably took his life as a result. There are opinions to the contrary (Jeffs, 1978; Sukarochana and Sieber, 1978; Welch, 1979). It is most appropriate to make a gender conversion in the newborn period, indicating to the family that gender was unfinished and a female reconstruction will commence. It is unnecessary to get chromosomes as part of the record. In our six genetic females, five were found to have bifid uterus, one a double vagina, three an exstrophic vagina, and two with a covered vaginal opening.

Later Reconstructions

A satisfactory abdominal wall closure without respiratory distress is essential for survival in the newborn period. Use of a silastic silo may be required to gradually reduce the omphalocele, as it was in three of our 15 cases.

An externalized exstrophy causes few problems for these babies. At about 1 year of age, sufficient abdominal wall laxity should allow one to reconstruct and close the bladder with the help of iliac, innominate osteotomies, or both.

Neurological Anomalies

Myelomeningoceles and lipomeningoceles are common in these children. Closure of a myelomeningocele must be done in the newborn period and it is often appropriate to do this prior to the abdominal reconstruction, waiting 1 week or so for healing. Unfortunately, cerebrospinal fluid leaks are quite common in cloacal exstrophy back reconstructions. This is especially so with lipomeningoceles, which should not be excised until a much later date. Because of the sacral anomalies, there is little chance for fecal continence following an anorectal pull through, nor is it appropriate to predict that bladder function might be normal in these children with severe sacral anomalies.

Stomal Therapy

In the past, many of these children relied on an ileal conduit for urinary drainage and maintained a colostomy on the opposite side. One cannot expect the colostomy to become manageable through an enema program; the stool remains loose in cloacal exstrophy patients. Elimination of one draining stoma is a relief to these patients. When the child becomes concerned about incontinence and becomes more independent, a catheterizable pouch can be created. If bladder is present, it can be augmented. Because many of these children have marginal nutrition attributable to limited intestinal length, it is appropriate to use stomach for this augmentation (Sumfest and Mitchell, 1994). Unless there is a generous amount of colon remaining, colonic augmentation is discouraged. It is possible to use short segments of ileum as a composite reservoir with stomach (Lockhart, 1993). If the appendices are too broad and short to use as catheterizable tracts, in several of our patients we have utilized distal ureteral segments for the catheterizable port (Duckett and Snyder, 1986).

Vaginal Reconstruction

Although relocation of large segments of the gastrointestinal tract for urinary reconstruction is unwise, a smaller segment may be used for vaginal reconstruction. For adequate width, the colon is more appropriate than the ileum. If ileum is used, it should be opened and folded on itself to add volume to the vaginoplasty. We initially used ileum for vaginoplasty in younger patients. Unfortunately, when these children became adolescents, we were unable to dilate the reconstructed vagina satisfactorily. A secondary reconstruction was required. In one colon vaginoplasty, the sacrum interferes with coitus with resulting dyspareunia. This patient will require revision in the near future.

Conclusion

The reconstructive aspects of cloacal exstrophy challenge the most innovative of pediatric urologists. With a team approach to this multifaceted disorder, the children can achieve a quite acceptable adult lifestyle.

CLOACAL ANOMALIES

A cloaca exists when the rectum, vagina, and urinary tract meet and fuse into a single common channel. This group of defects appears in the female as a separate spectrum of malformations of anal-rectal anomalies.

Anatomy

The length of the common channel varies from 1 to 12 cm. If a short channel exists (<3 cm), a well-developed sacrum and good sphincters will likely be present. A longer channel, however, indicates a more complex defect with a poor sphincter mechanism and an abnormal sacrum. The rectum and vagina share a common wall, as do the vagina and urethra (Fig. 52-21). In more than 50% of these cases, the vagina is partially obstructed and filled with mucous secretions (hydrocolpos). About 50% of the time there is a duplicated vagina and didelphis. This may be manifest by just a septum between the two vaginas or two completely separated structures. A distended vagina will often compress the trigone and lead to hydroureteronephrosis (Peña, 1995).

Associated Defects

In persistent cloaca, there is a 90% frequency of associated urogenital defects (Rich et al., 1988). Hydronephrosis, urosepsis, and metabolic acidosis with poor renal function represent the main sources of mortality in neonates with anorectal malformations. Other malformations include esophageal atresia, duodenal atresia, and cardiovascular defects, especially Tetralogy of Fallot. The sacral anomalies correlate with the degree of functional prognosis. More than two absent sacral vertebra represent a poor prognostic sign.

The presence of a single perineal orifice is pathognomic of a cloaca. These patients have a typically phallic looking structure with flattened labioscrotal folds. The proboscis of tissue has no erectile bodies present. The single opening of the cloaca may be at the base of the phallus or can be channeled to the tip. There may be some rudimentary glans tissue. Rarely, these children inappropriately are designated males at birth. A feminizing genitoplasty is required later.

Once the cloacal diagnosis is made, abdominal ultrasound is carried out. This will likely show hydroureteronephrosis, and a catheter is passed with coude tip into the bladder for a cystogram. The catheter often

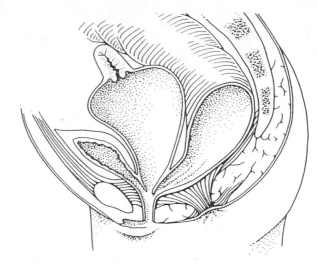

FIG. 52-21
Usual anatomy in patients with persistent cloaca. (From Peña A: Anorectal anomalies. In Spitz L, Coran A (eds): *Rob and Smith's operative surgery*, ed 5, London, 1995, Chapman & Hall, pp 423-451.)

will be directed into one of the dilated hydrocolpos and give a false impression of a bladder. Double contrast studies, such as iodinated contrast in the bladder with air in the vaginas, will often delineate the two chambers well.

Surgical Correction
Colostomy

A colostomy must be performed after the GU evaluation. When there are significant urologic problems, a divided colostomy is more appropriate than a loop colostomy (Fig. 52-22). This prevents contamination into the urinary tract with feces spilling into the distal limb of the colon. Cystoscopic evaluation of the urogenital sinus with dilatation of the vaginal openings into the urogenital sinus may provide adequate drainage of the mucus in the hydrocolpos. Urine may be voided from the bladder into the vaginas with stasis and lead to urinary infection. A urethral sound passed posteriorly often will dilate the membrane that deflects the urine into the vaginas. It may be appropriate to do a vesicostomy at the time of the colostomy in order to drain the urinary tract appropriately.

Recovery after colostomy and appropriate urinary diversion is usually uneventful. The final repair of this defect is a posterior sagittal anorectovaginourethroplasty and is usually carried out at about 6 months of age.

Before the definitive repair, a distal colostography is carried out with water soluble contrast. This identifies the precise site of the rectourinary fistula located in the most distal part of the rectum. Sometimes, considerable hydrostatic pressure will be required to fill out the distal colon and locate the fistula. This may be done with a Foley catheter, inflating the balloon

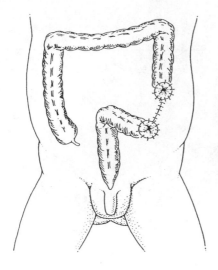

FIG. 52-22
The colostomy: the proximal stoma is placed at the supero-lateral margin of the wound. The mucous fistula is opened minimally to prevent prolapse and taken to the inferomedial margin of the wound. (From Peña A: Anorectal anomalies. In Spitz L, Coran A (eds): *Rob and Smith's operative surgery,* ed 5, London, 1995, Chapman & Hall, pp 423-451.)

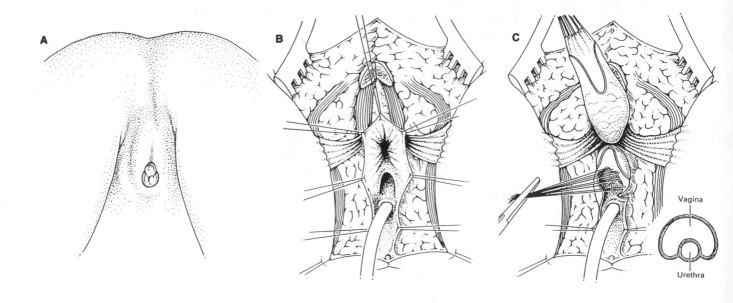

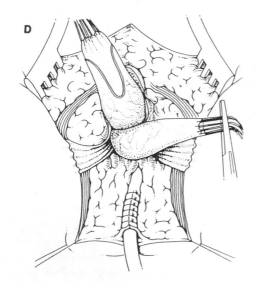

FIG. 52-23
A, Usual positioning for PSARP. **B,** Muscles have been separated carefully at the midline using electrostimulation to identify the appropriate incision line. Carefully placed sutures help separate the opened rectum from the sinus. The plane must be initially made in the common wall between the rectum and vagina, there is no definite line of dissection at this level. Catheter is in the urethra. **C,** The vagina surrounds the urethra for a variable distance. If the vagina is high and the channel is longer than 3 cm, vaginal elongation will be necessary to prevent injury to the vagina or urethra from overzealous dissection. **D,** In cases of common channels of less than 3 cm, the urethra is reconstructed using the whole common channel. (From Peña A: Anorectal anomalies. In Spitz L, Coran A (eds): *Rob and Smith's operative surgery.* ed 5, London, 1995, Chapman & Hall, pp 423-451.)

and applying distal pressure. This will overcome the muscle tone of the striated muscles surrounding the rectum (Peña, 1995).

Posterior Sagittal Anorectal Plasty

In posterior sagittal anorectalplasty (PSARP) the patient is placed in the prone position with the pelvis elevated (Fig. 52-23, A). Electric stimulation elicits muscle contractions throughout the operation so that no paralysis is used with anesthesia. A long incision starting at the midportion of the sacrum extends anteriorly to the single perineal orifice. The anatomic relationship of the rectum to the genitourinary structures is complex. When all muscle structures have been divided in the midline, the rectum can be seen, as can the sphincter fibers of the external anal sphincter. Separation of the rectum represents the most risky part of the procedure.

The urogenital sinus is incised posteriorly up to the confluence of rectum/vagina. Traction sutures are carefully placed on the rectal wall and lifted superiorly so that the three openings can be identified. A catheter is in the bladder (Fig. 52-23, B). The rectal wall is separated from the vaginas, and the vagina is separated from the bladder neck area and urethra (Fig. 52-23, C). The urethra can be extended out to the perineum by rolling a tube of the urogenital sinus (Fig. 52-23, D).

The vagina surrounds the urethra and the bladder neck for approximately 2 to 3 cm of the dissection (Fig. 52-23, C insert). This dissection must be carried cranial enough to mobilize the vagina to reach the perineum without devascularization. For a urogenital sinus longer than 3 cm, some form of vaginal elongation or replacement should be chosen, otherwise overzealous dissection may result in devascularization and urethral injury. Vaginal replacement can be done with a segment of small intestine with preservation of its mesentery. After the end-to-end anastomosis of the small intestines, the upper segment of a small bowel segment is connected to the upper vagina while the lower part comes to the perineal skin (Fig. 52-24).

Two large hemivaginas divided by a midline septum may provide enough vaginal wall to reach the perineum. This can be done by removing the rudimentary uterus on one side and rotating the vagina from that side down into the perineum, dividing the septum in between.

The perineum is reconstructed in such a way that there is a perineal body between the vagina and the new anus. The rectum is tapered so as to locate it into the internal and external sphincter complexes, which can be readily seen from the careful posterior sagittal dissection. The incision is closed carefully to reapproximate the sphincter muscles.

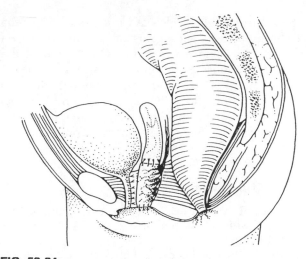

FIG. 52-24
In cases where a long channel exists, a segment of intestine is used to bridge the defect from the high vagina and the perineum. (From Peña A: Anorectal anomalies. In Spitz L, Coran A (eds): *Rob and Smith's operative surgery,* ed 5, London, 1995, Chapman & Hall, pp 423-451.)

Postoperative Bowel Management

Two weeks after the procedure, anal dilatations are started twice daily by the parents. Once the desired rectal size is reached, the colostomy is closed. For a period of time, frequent bowel movements are a problem, but this pattern improves by 6 months after closure of the colostomy. If the baby has one to three bowel movements each day and remains clean in between, this indicates that there is feeling during the defecation process and, in general, a good functional prognosis. On the other hand, if stool is passed constantly, colonic irrigations must be instituted for cleansing purposes. Constipation may become the major postoperative problem.

Antegrade Continence Enema (ACE)

Some of these cloacal patients will benefit from the ACE. A cecal attachment to the skin, either through the appendix or through a tubularized portion of cecum, permits the patient to catheterize the stoma and irrigate the colon. This situation is much preferred by the patient to a high rectal colonic irrigation (Griffiths and Malone, 1995; Malone et al., 1990).

Neurogenic Bladder

If sacral anomalies occur or if the urogenital sinus is greater than 3 cm in length, it is likely that bladder function may be impaired also. A plastic catheter can be used for intermittent catheterization in the postoperative period to manage urinary drainage intermittently. A coude tip may be helpful.

The clinical results in cloacas were reported by Peña in 1989 in 19 cases with a normal sacrum and seven cases with an abnormal sacrum. Only three of the seven with abnormal sacrum had voluntary bowel movements, whereas all but one of the patients with a normal sacrum did. Five of the seven abnormal sacrums had urinary incontinence, whereas five of the normal sacrum patients had urinary incontinence.

REFERENCES

Bladder Abnormalities

Agaststein EH, Stabile BE: Peritonitis due to intraperitoneal perforation of infected urachal cyst. *Arch Surg* 1984; 119:1269.

Alexander W: Interesting cases of bladder disease. *Liverpool Med Chir J* 1884; 4:245.

Allen NH, Atwell JD: The paraureteric diverticulum in childhood. *Br J Urol* 1980; 52:269.

Bauer SB, Retik AB: Bladder diverticula in infants and children. *Urology* 1974; 3:712.

Bauer SB, Retik AB: Urachal and related umbilical disorders. *Urol Clin North Am* 1978; 5:195.

Berdon WE, Baker DH, Blanc WA, et al: Megacystis microcolon-intestinal hypoperistalsis syndrome: a new cause of intestinal obstruction in the newborn. Report of radiologic findings in five newborn girls. *AJR* 1976; 126:957.

Berman SM, Tolia BM, Laor E, et al: Urachal remnants in adults. *Urology* 1988; 31:17.

Blacklock ARE, Geddes JR, Shaw RE: The treatment of large bladder diverticula. *Br J Urol* 1983; 55:17.

Blane CE, Zerin JM, Bloom DA: Bladder diverticula in children. *Radiology* 1994; 190:695.

Blichert-Toft M, Nielsen CW: Congenital patent urachus and acquired variants. *Acta Chir Scand* 1971; 137:807.

Brock WA, Kaplan GW: Abnormalities of the lower urinary tract. In *Pediatric Kidney Disease*. ed 2, Boston, Little, Brown, & Co, 1992, p 2037.

Burbige KA, Lebowitz RL, Colodny AH, et al: The megacystis-megaureter syndrome. *J Urol* 1984; 131:1133.

Burns E, Cummins H, Hyman J: Incomplete reduplication of the bladder. *J Urol* 1947; 57:257.

Caldamone AA: Anomalies of the bladder and cloaca. In Gillenwater JY, Grayhack JT, Howards SS, et al (eds): *Adult and Pediatric Urology*, ed 2. St Louis, Mosby, 1991, pp 2023-2053.

Cornil C, Reynolds CT, Kickham CJE: Carcinoma of the urachus. *J Urol* 1967; 98:93.

Cullen TS: *Embryology, Anatomy and Diseases of the Umbilicus Together with Diseases of the Urachus*. Philadelphia, WB Saunders Co, 1946.

Daly WJ, Rabinovitch HH: Urologic abnormalities in Menkes' syndrome. *J Urol* 1981; 126:262.

Danforth CH: Development anomalies in a special strain of mice. *Am J Anat* 1930; 45:275.

deVries PA, Friedland GW: The staged sequential development of the anus and rectum in human embryos and fetuses. *J Pediatr Surg* 1974; 9:755.

Faysal MH, Freha FS: Primary neoplasm in vesical diverticula: a report of 12 cases. *Br J Urol* 1981; 53:141.

Forsberg J: On the development of the cloaca and the perineum and the formation of the urethral plate in female rat embryos. *J Anat* 1961; 95:423.

Friedland GW, DeVries PA, Nino-Murcia M, et al: Congenital anomalies of the urinary tract. In Pollack HM (ed): *Clinical Urography: An Atlas and Textbook of Urological Imaging*. Philadelphia, WB Saunders Co, 1990, pp 559-736.

Gearhart JP, Jeffs RD: Exstrophy of the bladder, epispadias, and other bladder anomalies. In Walsh PC, Retik AB, Stamey TA, et al (eds): *Campbell's Urology*, ed 6. Philadelphia, WB Saunders Co, 1992, pp 1772-1821.

Glenn JF: Agenesis of the bladder. *JAMA* 1959; 169:2016.

Goldman IL, Caldamone AA, Gauderrer M, et al: Infected urachal cysts: a review of 10 cases. *J Urol* 1988; 140:373.

Harcke HT, Capitanio MA, Grover WD, et al: Bladder diverticula and Menkes' syndrome. *Radiology* 1977; 124:459.

Harrow BR: The myth of the megacystis syndrome. *J Urol* 1967; 98:205.

Havers W, Majewski F, Obling H, et al: Anomalies of the kidneys and genitourinary tract in alcohol embryopathy. *J Urol* 1980; 124:108.

Herbst WP: Patent urachus. *South Med J* 1937; 30:711.

Hernanz-Schulman M, Lebowitz RL: The elusiveness and importance of bladder diverticula in children. *Pediatr Radiol* 1985; 15:399.

Hinman F Jr: Surgical disorders of the bladder and umbilicus of urachal origin. *Surg Gynecol Obstet* 1961; 113:604.

Hsu HS, Duckett JW, Templeton JM, et al: Experience with urogenital reconstruction of ischiopagus conjoined twins. *J Urol* 1995; 154:563.

Hutch JA: Vesicoureteral reflux in the paraplegic; cause and correction. *J Urol* 1952; 68:457.

Hutch JA: Saccule formation at the ureterovesical junction in smooth-walled bladders. *J Urol* 1961; 86:390.

Inamdar S, Mallouh C, Ganguly R: Vesical gigantism or congenital megacystis. *Urology* 1984; 24:601.

Kapoor R, Saha MM: Complete duplication of the bladder, common urethra and external genitalia in the neonate: a case report. *J Urol* 1987; 137:1243.

Kirtane J, Talwalker V, Dastar DK: Megacystis-microcolon-intestinal hypoperistalsis syndrome: possible pathogenesis. *Pediatr Surg* 1984; 19:206.

Krull CL, Hanes DF, DeKlerk DP: Agenesis of the bladder and urethra: a case report. *J Urol* 1988; 140:793.

Lattimer JK: Congenital deficiency of the abdominal musculature and associated genitourinary anomalies: a report of 22 cases. *J Urol* 1958; 79:264.

Leibowitz S, Bodian M: A study of the vesical ganglia in children and the relationship to the mega-ureter megacystis syndrome and Hirschsprung's disease. *J Clin Pathol* 1963; 16:342.

Levard G, Aigrain Y, Ferkadji L, et al: Urinary bladder diverticula and the Ehlers-Danlos syndrome in children. *J Pediatr Surg* 1989; 24:1184.

MacMillan RW, Schulinger JN, Santulli VT: Pyourachus: an unusual surgical problem. *J Pediatr Surg* 1973; 8:87.

Micic S, Illic V: Incidence of neoplasm in vesical diverticula. *J Urol* 1983; 129:734.

Meucke EC: Exstrophy, epispadias, and other anomalies of the bladder. In Walsh PC, Gittes RF, Perlmutter AD, et al (eds): *Campbell's Urology*, ed 5. Philadelphia, WB Saunders Co, 1986, pp 1856-1880.

Newman BM, Karp MP, Jewett TC, et al: Advances in the management of infected urachal cysts. *J Pediatr Surg* 1986; 21:1051.

Ney C, Friedenberg RM: Radiographic findings in the anomalies of the urachus. *J Urol* 1968; 99:288.

Nix JT, Menville JG, Albert M, et al: Congenital patent urachus. *J Urol* 1959; 79:264.

Noe HN: Urachal anomalies and related umbilical disorders. In Glenn JF (ed): *Urologic Surgery*, ed 4. Philadelphia, JB Lippincott Co, 1991.

Nunn LL: Urachal cysts and their complications. *Am J Surg* 1952; 84:252.

O'Rahilly R, Muller F: *Human Embryology and Teratology*. New York, Wiley-Liss, 1992.

Parrott TS, Gray SW, Skandalakis JE: The bladder and urethra. In Skandalakis JE, Gray SW (eds): *Embryology for Surgeons*, ed 2. Baltimore, Williams and Wilkins, 1994, pp 671-717.

Ravitch MM, Scott WW: Duplication of the entire colon, bladder and urethra. *Surgery* 1953; 34:843.

Redman JF, Jimenez JF, Golladay ES, et al: Megacystis-microcolon-intestinal hypoperistalsis syndrome: case report and review of the literature. *J Urol* 1984; 131:981.

Satler EJ, Mossman HW: A case report of a double bladder and double urethra in the female child. *J Urol* 1968; 79:274.

Schippers E, Dittler HJ: Multiple hollow organ dysplasia in Ehlers-Danlos syndrome in children. *J Pediatr Surg* 1989; 24:1181.

Schubert GE, Pavkovic MB, Bethke-Bedurftig BA: Tubular urachal remnants in adult bladders. *J Urol* 1983; 127:40.

Senger TL, Santore VJ: Congenital multilocular bladder. *Trans Am Assoc Genitourin Surg* 1951; 43:114.

Stanfield NJ, Shearer RJ: Prostatism, obstructive uropathy and uraemia associated with urachal cyst. *Br J Urol* 1981; 53:482.

Stephens FD: The vesicoureteral hiatus and paraureteral diverticula. *J Urol* 1979; 121:786.

Tauber J, Bloom B: Infected urachal cyst. *J Urol* 1951; 66:692.

Taylor WN, Alton D, Toguri A, et al: Bladder diverticula causing posterior urethral obstruction in children. *J Urol* 1979; 122:415.

Uhlir K: Rare malformations of the bladder. *J Urol* 1968; 99:53.

Verghese M, Belman AB: Urinary retention secondary to congenital bladder diverticula in infants. *J Urol* 1984; 132:1186.

Williams BD, Fisk JD: Sonographic diagnosis of giant urachal cyst in the adult. *AJR* 1981; 136:417.

Williams DI: Congenital bladder neck obstruction and megaureter. *Br J Urol* 1957; 29:389.

Williams DI: Megacystis and megaureter in children. *Bull NY Acad Med* 1959; 35:317.

Ziylan O, Duckett JW: Uses and abuses of vesicostomy. *AUA Update* 1995; 14:130.

Bladder Exstrophy

Aadalen RJ, O'Phelan EH, Chisholm TC, et al: Exstrophy of the bladder: long-term results of bilateral posterior iliac osteotomies and two-stage anatomic repair. *Clin Orthop* 1980; 151:193.

Allen TD, Husmann DA, Bucholz RW: Exstrophy of the bladder: primary closure after iliac osteotomies without external or internal fixation. *J Urol* 1992; 147(2):438.

Ansell JS: Primary closure of exstrophy in the newborn: a preliminary report. *Northwest Med* 1971; 70(12):842.

Ansell JS: Surgical treatment of exstrophy of the bladder with emphasis on neonatal primary closure: personal experience with 28 consecutive cases treated at the University of Washington hospitals from 1962 to 1977: techniques and results. *J Urol* 1979; 121(5):650.

Ashurst J: Exstroversion or exstrophy of the bladder successfully treated by means of a plastic operation after Wood's method. *Am J Med Sci* 1871; 42:70.

Bagchi AG: Seven years' experience of ureterosigmoidostomy in surgically failed exstrophy of the bladder. *J Indian Med Assoc* 1990; 88(9):255.

Barth RA, Filly RA, Sondheimer FK: Prenatal sonographic findings in bladder exstrophy. *J Ultrasound Med* 1990; 9(6):359.

Baskin L, Duckett J: Dorsal tunica albugenia plication (TAP) for hypospadias curvature. *J Urol* 1994; 151:1668.

Benchekroun A, Esskall HN, Faik M, et al: Urostomie continente. Douze annees d'experience avec la vessie ileocecale continente. *Ann Urol* 1989; 23:188.

Blickstein I, Katz Z: Possible relationship of bladder exstrophy and epispadias with progestins taken during early pregnancy. *Br J Urol* 1991; 68(1):105.

Blyth B, Ewalt D, Duckett J et al: Lithogenic properties of enterocystoplasty. *J Urol* 1992; 148(2):457.

Borzi PA, Thomas DF: Cantwell-Ransley epispadias repair in male epispadias and bladder exstrophy. *J Urol* 1994; 151(2):457.

Bracci U, Laurenti C: Rectal bladder in the treatment of bladder exstrophy. *Eur Urol* 1979; 5(3):161.

Braverman RM, Lebowitz RL: Perforation of the augmented urinary bladder in nine children and adolescents: importance of cystography. *Am J Roentgenol* 1991; 157(5):1059.

Bunge R: Podophyllin in treatment of human adenocarcinoma of the bladder. *J Urol* 1952; 68:475.

Bushman W, Howards S: The use of urea for dissolution of urinary mucus in urinary tract reconstruction. *J Urol* 1994; 151(4):1036.

Caione P, Capozza N, Lais A, et al: Female genito-urethroplasty and submucosal periurethral collagen injection as adjunctive procedures for continence in the exstrophy-epispadias complex. Preliminary results. *Br J Urol* 1993; 71(3):350.

Canning DA, Gearhart JP, Peppas DS, et al: The cephalo-trigonal reimplant in bladder neck reconstruction for patients with exstrophy or epispadias. *J Urol* 1993; 150(1):156.

Canning D, Oesterling J, Gearhart J, et al: A computerized review of exstrophy patients managed during the past thirteen years. *J Urol* 1989; 141:224A.

Carter CO: The genetics of urinary tract malformations. *J Genet Hum* 1984; 32(1):23.

Cendron J: La reconstruction vesicale. *Ann Chir Infant* 1971; 12:371.

Cendron J: Bladder exstrophy from an external to an internal diversion. *Birth Defects* 1977; 13(5):197.

Cendron J, Petit P: Symposium on treatment of complete exstrophy of the urinary bladder. *Ann Chir Infant* 1971; 6:359.

Chisholm T: Exstrophy of the urinary bladder. In Welch K (ed): *Pediatric Surgery*. Chicago, Year Book Medical Publishers, 1962, p 933.

Clark M, O'Connell, K: Scanning and transmission electron microscopic studies of an exstrophic human bladder. *J Urol* 1973; 110:481.

Cocke W Jr: Secondary reconstruction of abdominal wall defects associated with exstrophy of the bladder. *Ann Plast Surg* 1993; 31(5):459.

Cohen S: Ureterozystoneostomie eine neue Antireflux-technik. *Aktuel Urol* 1975; 6:1.

Connell FG: Exstropy of the bladder. *JAMA* 1901; 36:637.

Connor JP, Hensle TW, Lattimer JK, et al: Long-term follow-up of 207 patients with bladder exstrophy: an evolution in treatment. *J Urol* 1989; 142(3):793.

Cracchiolo A, Hall C: Bilateral iliac osteotomy: the first stage in repair of exstrophy of the bladder. *Clin Orthop Rel Res* 1970; 68:156.

Cromie W, Duckett J: Urinary diversion in children — past and present. *Monogr Urol* 1980; 1:26.

Culp D: The histology of the exstrophied bladder. *J Urol* 1964; 91:538.

Damario MA, Carpenter SE, Jones H Jr, et al: Reconstruction of the external genitalia in females with bladder exstrophy. *Int J Gynaecol Obstet* 1994; 44(3):245.

Davillas N, Thanos A, Liakatas J, et al: Bladder exstrophy complicated by adenocarcinoma. *Br J Urol* 1991; 68(1):107.

de la Hunt MH, O'Donnell B: Current management of bladder exstrophy: a BAPS collective review from eight centers of 81 patients born between 1975 and 1985. *J Pediatr Surg* 1989; 24(6):584.

Decter RM, Roth DR, Fishman IJ, et al: Use of the AS800 device in exstrophy and epispadias. *J Urol* 1988; 140(5 Pt 2):1202.

Dees JE: Epispadias with incontinence in the male. *Surgery* 1942; 12:621.

Duckett JW: Use of paraexstrophy skin pedicle grafts for correction of exstrophy and epispadias repair *Birth Defects* 1977; 13(5):175.

Duckett JW: Editorial comment to "Complications of paraexstrophy skin flaps in the reconstruction of classical bladder exstrophy. *J Urol* 1993; 150(2 Pt 2):630.

Duckett JW, Caldamone A: Bladder exstrophy. *AUA Update Series* III 1984; (13):1.

Duckett JW, Caldamone A: Congenital disorders of the bladder. In Hendry W, Whitfield H (eds): *Textbook of Genitourinary Surgery*. London, Churchill-Livingston, 1985, p 192.

Duckett JW, Coplen D, Ewalt D, et al: Buccal mucosal urethral replacement. *J Urol* 1995; 153:1660.

Duckett JW, Gazak J: Complications of ureterosigmoidostomy. *Urol Clin North Am* 1983; 10:473.

Duckett JW, Lofti A: Appendicovesicostomy (and variations) in bladder reconstruction. *J Urol* 1993; 149:567.

Duckett JW, Snyder H: Continent urinary diversion: variations on the Mitrofanoff principle. *J Urol* 1986; 136:58.

Duel B, Retik A, Atala A, et al: Prostatic fistulae in male bladder exstrophy patients: an emerging problem. In *American Academy of Pediatrics Urology Section*. (Abstract 125). Dallas, 1994.

Duffy P, Ransley P: Personal communication, 1988.

Edgerton MT, Gillenwater JY: A new surgical technique for phalloplasty in patients with exstrophy of the bladder. *Plast Reconstr Surg* 1986; 78(3):399.

Elder JS, Snyder HM, Hulbert WC, et al: Perforation of the augmented bladder in patients undergoing clean intermittent catheterization. *J Urol* 1988; 140(5 Pt 2):1159.

Engel RM: Exstrophy of the bladder and associated anomalies. *Birth Defects* 1974; 10(4):146.

Engel RM, Wilkinson HA: Bladder exstrophy. *J Urol* 1970; 104(5):699.

Facchini V, Gadducci A, Colombi L, et al: Carcinoma developing in bladder exstrophy. Case report. *Br J Obstet Gynaecol* 1987; 94(8):795.

Fisch M, Wammack R, Steinbach F, et al: Sigma-rectum pouch (Mainz pouch II). *Urol Clin North Am* 1993; 20(3):561.

Fisher JH, Retik AB: Exstrophy of the bladder. *J Pediatr Surg* 1969; 4:620.

Frey P, Cohen SJ: Anterior pelvic osteotomy. A new operative technique facilitating primary bladder exstrophy closure. *Br J Urol* 1989; 64(6):641.

Gearhart JP: Bladder neck reconstruction in the incontinent child. In Frank JD, Johnston JH: (eds): *Operative Paediatric Urology*. Edinburgh, Churchill Livingstone, 1990.

Gearhart JP: Failed bladder exstrophy repair. Evaluation and management. *Urol Clin North Am* 1991; 18(4):687.

Gearhart JP, Jeffs RD: Augmentation cystoplasty in the failed exstrophy reconstruction. *J Urol* 1988; 139(4):790.

Gearhart JP, Jeffs RD: Bladder exstrophy: increase in capacity following epispadias repair. *J Urol* 1989a; 142(2 Pt 2):525.

Gearhart JP, Jeffs RD: State-of-the-art reconstructive surgery for bladder exstrophy at the Johns Hopkins Hospital. *Am J Dis Child* 1989b; 143(12):1475.

Gearhart JP, Peppas DS, Jeffs RD: Complications of paraexstrophy skin flaps in the reconstruction of classical bladder exstrophy. *J Urol* 1993a; 150(2 Pt 2):627.

Gearhart JP, Williams K, Jeffs R: Urethral pressure profilometry as a adjunct to bladder neck reconstruction for patients with exstrophy or epispadias. *J Urol* 1986; 136:1055.

Gearhart JP, Yang A, Leonard MP, et al: Prostate size and configuration in adults with bladder exstrophy. *J Urol* 1993b; 149(2):308.

Gittes RF: Carcinogenesis in ureterosigmoidostomy. *Urol Clin North Am* 1986; 13(2):201.

Goyanna R, Emmett J, McDonald J: Exstrophy of the bladder complicated by adenocarcinoma. *J Urol* 1951; 65:391.

Gross RE, Cressen SL: Exstrophy of the bladder: observations from 80 cases. *JAMA* 1952; 149:1640.

Gross SD: Diseases and injuries of the urinary bladder. In Gross SD (ed): *System of Surgery: Pathological, Diagnostic, Therapeutic and Operative*, Philadelphia, Blanchard and Lea, 1862, pp 270-272.

Hall EG, McCandless AE, Rickham PP: Vesico-intestinal fissure with diphallus. *Br J Urol* 1953; 25:219.

Hanna MK: Artificial urinary sphincter for incontinent children. *Urology* 1981; 18(4):370.

Hanna MK, Ansong K: Reconstruction of umbilicus in bladder exstrophy. *Urology* 1984; 24(4):324.

Heij HA, Ekkelkamp S, Vos A: Hypertension associated with skeletal traction in children (letter; comment). *J Pediatr Surg* 1993; 28(11):1524.

Hendren WH: Exstrophy of the bladder—an alternative method of management. *J Urol* 1976; 115(2):195.

Hendren WH: Penile lengthening after previous repair of epispadias. *J Urol* 1979; 121(4):527.

Hendren W: Urinary tract undiversion. In Welch K, Randolph J, Ravitch M, et al: *Pediatric Surgery*. Chicago, Year Book Medical Publishers, 1986, p 1281.

Higgins C: Exstrophy of the bladder: report of 158 cases. *Am J Surg* 1962; 28:99.

Hockey A, Bower C: Bladder exstrophy and exomphalos in successive pregnancies. *Birth Defects* 1993; 29(1):211.

Hollowell JG, Hill PD, Duffy PG, et al: Bladder function and dysfunction in exstrophy and epispadias. *Lancet* 1991; 338(8772):926.

Hollowell JG, Hill PD, Duffy PG, et al: Lower urinary tract function after exstrophy closure. *Pediatr Nephrol* 1992; 6(5):428.

Hollowell JG, Hill PD, Duffy PG, et al: Evaluation and treatment of incontinence after bladder neck reconstruction in exstrophy and epispadias. *Br J Urol* 1993; 71(6):743.

Horton CE, Sadove RC, Jordan GH, et al: Use of the rectus abdominis muscle and fascia flap in reconstruction of epispadias/exstrophy. *Clin Plast Surg* 1988; 15:(3):393.

Hurwitz RS, Manzoni GA, Ransley PG, et al: Cloacal exstrophy: A report of 34 cases. *J Urol* 1987; 138:1060.

Husmann DA, McLorie GA, Churchill BM: Closure of the exstrophic bladder: an evaluation of the factors leading to its success and its importance on urinary continence. *J Urol* 1989; 142(2 Pt 2):522.

Husmann DA, McLorie GA, Churchill BM: Factors predisposing to renal scarring: following staged reconstruction of classical bladder exstrophy. *J Pediatr Surg* 1990a 25(5):500.

Husmann DA, McLorie GA, Churchill BM, et al: Inguinal pathology and its association with classical bladder exstrophy. *J Pediatr Surg* 1990b; 25(3):332.

Husmann DA, McLorie GA, Churchill BM: Hypertension following primary bladder closure for fesical exstrophy (see comments) *J Pediatr Surg* 1993; 28(2):239.

Husmann DA, Spence HM: Current status of tumor of the bowel following ureterosigmoidostomy: a review. *J Urol* 1990; 144(3):607.

Jaffe R, Schoenfeld A, Ovadia J: Sonographic findings in the prenatal diagnosis of bladder exstrophy. *Am J Obstet Gynecol* 1990; 162(3):675.

Jeffs RD: Functional closure of bladder exstrophy. *Birth Defects* 1977; 13(5):171.

Jeffs RD: Complications of exstrophy surgery. *Urol Clin North Am* 1983; 10(3):509.

Jeffs RD: Exstrophy, epispadias, and cloacal and urogenital sinus abnormalities. *Pediatr Clin North Am* 1987; 34(5):1233.

Jeffs RD, Guice SL, Oesch I: The factors in successful exstrophy closure. *J Urol* 1982; 127:974.

Jeffs R, Charrios R, Many M, et al: Primary closure of the exstrophied bladder. In Scott R (ed): *Current controversies in Urologic Management*. Philadelphia, WB Saunders, 1972, p 235.

Johnston JH, Kogan SJ: The exstrophic anomalies and their surgical reconstruction. *Curr Probl Surg* 1974; 1:3.

Jones J, Mitchell M, Rink R: Improved results using a modification of the Young-Dees-Leadbetter bladder neck repair. *Br J Urol* 1993; 71(5):555.

Kajbafzadeh A, Quinn G, Ransley P: Single-stage repair in the management of the exstrophy-epispadias complex. *J Urol* (in press).

Kandzari SJ, Majid A, Orteza AM, et al: Exstrophy of urinary bladder complicated by adenocarcinoma. *Urology* 1974; 3(4):496.

Keating MA, Cartwright PC, Duckett JW: Bladder mucosa in urethral reconstructions. *J Urol* 1990; 144(4):827.

Kelley J: Bladder neck reconstruction in exstrophy. Personal communication, 1994.

Kennedy W II, Hensle TW, Reiley EA, et al: Pregnancy after orthotopic continent urinary diversion. *Surg Gynecol Obstet* 1993; 177(4):405.

Kim KS, Susskind MR, King LR: Ileocecal ureterosigmoidostomy: an alternative to conventional ureterosigmoidostomy. *J Urol* 1988; 140(6):1494.

Kliment J, Luptak J, Lofaj M et al: Carcinoma of the colon after ureterosigmoidostomy and trigonosigmoidostomy for exstrophy of the bladder. *Int Urol Nephrol* 1993; 25(4):339.

Kock NG, Ghoneim MA, Lycke KG, et al: Urinary diversion to the augmented and valved rectum: preliminary results with a novel surgical procedure. *J Urol* 1988; 140(6):1375.

Koff SA: A technique for bladder neck reconstruction in exstrophy: the cinch. *J Urol* 1990; 144(2 Pt 2):546.

Kramer SA: Augmentation cystoplasty in patients with exstrophy-epispadias. *J Pediatr Surg* 1989; 24(12):1293.

Kramer S, Kelalis P: Assessment of urinary continence in epispadias: a review of 94 patients. *J Urol* 1982; 128:290.

Kramer S, Mesrobian H, Kelalis P: Long-term follow-up of cosmetic appearance and genital function in male epispadias. *J Urol* 1986; 135:543.

Krishnamsetty RM, Rao MK, Hines CR, et al: Adenocarcinoma in exstrophy and defunctional ureterosigmoidostomy. *J Ky Med Assoc* 1988; 86(8):409.

Kroovand RL, Boyce WH: Isolated vesicorectal internal urinary diversion: a 37-year review of the Boyce-Vest procedure. *J Urol* 1988; 140(3):572.

Langer JC, Brennan B, Lappalainen RE, et al: Cloacal exstrophy: prenatal diagnosis before rupture of the cloacal membrane. *J Pediatr Surg* 1992; 27(10):1352.

Lascombes P, Dautel G, Grosdidier G: Anatomical basis of pelvic growth in bladder exstrophy. *Surg Radiol Anat* 1989; 11(2):85.

Lascombes P, Dautel G, Grosdidier G, et al: Anatomic basis for the orthopedic treatment of bladder exstrophy: anatomic study of the sacrosciatic ligaments in the newborn. *Surg Radiol Anat* 1988; 10(2):97.

Lattimer JK, Beck L, Yeaw S, et al: Long-term follow-up after exstrophy closure: late improvement and good quality of life. *J Urol* 1978a; 119(5):664.

Lattimer JK, Hensle TW, MacFarlane MT, et al: The exstrophy support team: a new concept in the care of the exstrophy patient. *J Urol* 1979; 121(4):472.

Lattimer JK, MacFarlane MT, Puchner PJ: Male exstrophy patients: a preliminary report on the reproductive capability. *Trans Am Assoc Genitourin Surg* 1978b; 70:42.

Lattimer JK, Smith MJ: Exstrophy closure: a follow-up on 70 cases. *J Urol* 1966; 95(3):356.

Leadbetter GWJ: Surgical correction of total urinary incontinence. *J Urol* 1964; 7:1.

Lebowitz RL, Vargas B: Stones in the urinary bladder in children and young adults. *Am J Roentgenol* 1987; 148(3):491.

Leonard MP, Gearhart JP, Jeffs RD: Continent urinary reservoirs in pediatric urological practice. *J Urol* 1990; 144(2 Pt 1):330.

Lepor H, Jeffs RD: Primary bladder closure and bladder neck reconstruction in classical bladder exstrophy. *J Urol* 1983; 130(6):1142.

Lepor H, Shapiro E, Jeffs RD: Urethral reconstruction in boys with classical bladder exstrophy. *J Urol* 1984; 131(3):512.

Light JK, Scott FB: Treatment of the epispadias-exstrophy complex with the AS792 artificial urinary sphincter. *J Urol* 1983; 129(4):738.

Lockhart JL, Davies R, Cox C, et al: The gastroileoileal pouch: an alternative continent urinary reservoir for patients with short bowel, acidosis and/or extensive pelvic radiation. *J Urol* 1993; 150(1):46.

Loder RT, Dayioglu MM: Association of congenital vertebral malformations with bladder and cloacal exstrophy. *J Pediatr Orthop* 1990; 10(3):389.

Macfarlane MT, Lattimer JK, Hensle TW: Improved life expectancy for children with exstrophy of the bladder. *JAMA* 1979; 242(5):442.

Mahran M, Ghaly A, Sheir K, et al: The modified rectal bladder (the augmente and valved rectum) for urine diversion in children. *Urology* 1994; 44(5):737.

Maloney PJ, DM G, Lattimer J: Ureteral physiology and exstrophy of the bladder. *J Urol*, 1965; 93:588.

Mansi M, Ahmed S: Young-Dees-Leadbetter bladder neck reconstruction for sphincteric urinary incontinence: the value of augmentation cystoplasty. *Scand J Urol Nephrol* 1993; 27(4):509.

Marshall VF, Muecke EC: Variations in exstrophy of the bladder. *J Urol* 1962; 88:766.

Marshall VF, Muecke EC: Functional closure of typical exstrophy of the bladder. *J Urol* 1970; 104:205.

Mayo CH, Hendricks WA: Exstrophy of the bladder. *Surg Gynecol Obstet* 1926; 43:129.

McKenna PH, Khoury AE, McLorie GA, et al: Iliac osteotomy: a model to compare the options in bladder and cloacal exstrophy reconstruction. *J Urol* 1994; 151(1):182.

McLorie GA, Bellemore MC, Salter RB: Penile deformity in bladder exstrophy: correlation with closure of pelvic defect (see comments). *J Pediatr Surg* 1991; 26(2):201.

Megalli M, Lattimer JK: Review of the management of 140 cases of exstrophy of the bladder. *J Urol* 1973; 109(2):246.

Meizner I, Bar-Ziv J: Prenatal ultrasonic diagnosis of anterior abdominal wall defects. *Eur J Obstet Gynecol Reprod Biol* 1986; 22(4):217.

Merksz M, Toth J: The state of the testicle and the epididymis associated with exstrophy of the bladder in undescended testes. *Acta Chir Hung* 1990; 31(4):297.

Mesrobian H, Kelalis P, Kramer S: Long-term follow-up of cosmetic appearance and genital function in boys with exstrophy: review of patients. *J Urol* 1986; 136:256.

Mesrobian HG, Kelalis PP, Kramer SA: Long-term follow-up of 103 patients with bladder exstrophy. *J Urol* 1988; 139(4):719.

Mildenberger H, Kluth D, Dziuba M: Embryology of bladder exstrophy. *J Pediatr Surg* 1988; 23(2):166.

Mirk P, Calisti A, Fileni A: Prenatal sonographic diagnosis of bladder extrophy. *J Ultrasound Med* 1986; 5(5):291.

Mitchell M: Personal communication, 1995.

Mitchell ME, Adams MC, Rink RC: Urethral replacement with ureter. *J Urol* 1988; 139(6):1282.

Mitchell M, Bägli D: Complete penile disassembly for epispadias repair: Mitchell Technique. Personal communication, Jan 1995.

Mitchell M, Rink R: Experience with the artificial urinary sphincter in children and young adults. *J Pediatr Surg* 1983; 18:700.

Mollard P: Bladder reconstruction in exstrophy. *J Urol* 1980; 124(4):525.

Mollard P: Extrophies et epispades. In Mollard P (ed): *Preces D'urologie de l'enfant*. Paris, Masson Publishing Co, 1984, pp 226-225.

Mollard P, Basset T, Deseubis M, et al: Resultats de la reconstruction vesicale et uretrale pour exstrophie. *Chirurgie Pediatrique* 1986; 27(1):27.

Mollard P, Mouriquand P, Felfela T: Application of the onlay island flap urethroplasty to penile hypospadias with severe chordee. *Br J Urol* 1991; 68:317.

Montagnani CA: Innominate osteotomy in reconstructive surgery for exstrophy of the bladder. *J Pediatr Surg* 1967; 2(6):583.

Montagnani CA: One-stage functional reconstruction of exstrophied bladder: report of two cases with six-year follow-up. *Z Kinderchir* 1982; 37(1):23.

Mortensen PB, Jensen KE, Nielsen K: Adenocarcinoma development in the trigone 34 years after trigonoclonic urinary diversion for exstrophy of the bladder. *J Urol* 1990; 144(4):980.

Mostofi F: Postentialities of bladder epithelium. *J Urol* 1954; 71:705.

Mowat J: An account of a child born with the urinary and genital organs preteranaturally formed. *Medical Essays and Observations* 1747; 3:220.

Muecke EC: The role of the cloacal membrane in exstrophy: the first successful experimental study. *J Urol* 1964; 92:659.

Muecke E, Marshall V: Subsymphyseal epispadias in the female patient. *J Urol* 1968; 99:622.

Murphy LJT: *The History of Urology*. Springfield, Ill, Charles C Thomas, Publisher, 1972, p 333.

Nisonson I, Lattimer J: How well can the exstrophied bladder work? *J Urol* 1972; 107:664.

Patton BM, Barry A: The genesis of exstrophy of the bladder and epispadias. *Am J Anat* 1952; 90:35.

Perovic S, Scepanovic D, Sremcevic D, et al: Epispadias surgery—Belgrade experience. *Br J Urol* 1992; 70(6):674.

Perovic S, Vukadinovic V: Onlay island flap urethroplasty for severe hypospadias: a variant of the technique. *J Urol* 1994; 151(3):711.

Phillips TH, Ritchey ML, Dunn CD, et al: Complications of the Heitz-Boyer urinary diversion: case report of late development of malignancy. *J Urol* 1991; 146(1):159.

Purcell MH, Duckro PN, Schultz K, et al: Follow-up of ureterosigmoidostomy diversion for bladder exstrophy—behavioral biofeedback as an alternative treatment for fecal-urinary incontinence: a case report. *J Urol* 1987; 137(5):945.

Ransley P: Epispadias repair. In Dudley H, Carter D, Russell R, (eds): *Operative Surgery*. London, Butterworth, 1988, pp 627-632.

Richards DS, Langham M Jr, Mahaffey SM: The prenatal ultrasonographic diagnosis of cloacal exstrophy. *J Ultrasound Med* 1992; 11(9):507.

Rickham PP: The incidence and treatment of ectopia vesicae. *Proceeds R Soc Med* 1961; 54:389.

Rickham PP, Stauffer UG: Exstrophy of the bladder. Progress of management during the last 25 years. *Prog Pediatr Surg* 1984; 17:169.

Ritchey ML, Kramer SA, Kelalis PP: Vesical neck reconstruction in patients with episodias-exstrophy. *J Urol* 1988; 139(6):1278.

Scherz HC, Kaplan GW, Sutherland DH, et al: Fascia lata and early spica casting as adjuncts in closure of bladder exstrophy. *J Urol* 1990; 144(2 Pt 2):550.

Schlegel PN, Gearhart JP: Neuroanatomy of the pelvis in an infant with cloacal exstrophy: a detailed microdissection with histology. *J Urol* 1989; 141(3):583.

Schmidt AH, Keenen TL, Tank ES, et al: Pelvic osteotomy for bladder exstrophy. *J Pediatr Orthop* 1993; 13(2):214.

Schultz WG: Plastic repair of exstrophy of bladder combined with bilateral osteotomy of the ilia. *J Urol* 1958; 79:453.

Schulze K, Pfister R, Ransley P: Urethral duplication and complete bladder exstrophy. *J Urol* 1985; 133:276.

Semerdjian HS, Texter J Jr, Yawn DH: Rhabdomyosarcoma occurring in repaired exstrophied bladder: a case report. *J Urol* 1972; 108(2):354.

Shapiro E, Jeffs R, Gearhart J, et al: Muscarinic cholinergic receptors in bladder exstrophy: insights into surgical management. *J Urol* 1985; 134:308.

Shapiro E, Lepor H, Jeffs RD: The inheritance of the exstrophy-epispadias complex. *J Urol* 1984; 132(2):308.

Slotkin E, Mercer A: Case of epispadias with a double urethra. *J Urol* 1953; 70:743.

Snyder HM III: The surgery of bladder exstrophy and epispadias. In Frank J, Johnston J (eds): *Operative Paediatric Urology*. Edinburgh, Churchill Livingstone Inc, 1990, pp 153-185.

Stein R, Stockle M, Fisch M, et al: The fate of the adult exstrophy patient. *J Urol* 1994; 152:1413.

Stockle M, Becht E, Voges G, et al: Ureterosigmoidostomy: an outdated approach to bladder exstrophy? *J Urol* 1990; 143(4):770.

Strachan JR, Woodhouse CR: Malignancy following ureterosigmoidostomy in patients with exstrophy. *Br J Surg* 1991; 78(10):1216.

Stringer MD, Duffy PG, Ransley PG: Inguinal hernias associated with bladder exstrophy. *Br J Urol* 1994; 73(3):308.

Sumfest JM, Burns MW, Mitchell ME: The Mitrofanoff principle in urinary reconstruction. *J Urol* 1993; 150(6):1875.

Sumfest JM, Mitchell ME: Reconstruction of the umbilicus in exstrophy. *J Urol* 1994; 151(2):453.

Systems, International Clearinghouse for Birth Defects Monitoring: Epidemiology of bladder exstrophy and epispadias: a communication from the International Clearinghouse for Birth Defects Monitoring Systems. *Teratology* 1987; 36(2):221.

Tacciuoli M, Laurenti C, Racheli T: Sixteen years' experience with the Heitz Boyer-Hovalacque procedure for exstrophy of the bladder. *Br J Urol* 1977; 49(5):385.

Thomalla JV, Mitchell ME: Ventral preputial island flap technique for the repair of epispadias with or without exstrophy. *J Urol* 1984; 132(5):985.

Thomalla J, Rudolph R, Rink R, et al: Induction of cloacal exstrophy in the chick embryo using the CO2 Laser. *J Urol* 1985; 134(5):991.

Thomas WG, Wilkinson JA: Ectopia vesicae and congenital hip dislocation: brief report. *J Bone Joint Surg (Br)* 1989; 71(2):328.

Toguri AG, Churchill BM, Schillinger JF, et al: Continence in cases of bladder exstrophy. *J Urol* 1978a; 119(4):538.

Toguri AG, Churchill BM, Schillinger JF, et al: Gas cystometry in cases of continent bladder exstrophy. *J Urol* 1978b; 119(4):536.

Trendelenburg F: Treatment of ectopia vesicae. *Ann Surg* 1906; 44:281.

Verco PW, Khor BH, Barbary J, et al: Ectopia vesicae in utero. *Australas Radiol* 1986; 30(2):117.

Vincent MP, Horton CE, Devine CJ Jr: An evaluation of skin grafts for reconstruction of the penis and scrotum. *Clin Plast Surg* 1988; 15(3):411.

Welch KJ, Benson CD, et al (eds): Pediatric Surgery. Chicago: Year Book Medical Publishers, 1979; pp 802-808.

Williams DI, Keeton JE: Further progress with reconstruction of the exstrophied bladder. *Br J Surg* 1973; 60(3):203.

Witters S, Baert-Van Damme L: (1987). Bladder exstrophy complicated by adenocarcinoma. *Eur Urol* 1987; 13(6):415.

Woodhouse C, Kellett M: Anatomy of the penis and its deformities in exstrophy and epispadias. *J Urol* 1984; 132:1122.

Woodhouse C, Ransley P, Williams D: The patient with exstrophy in adult life. *Br J Urol* 1983; 55:632.

Young HH: An operation for the cure of incontinence associated with epispadias. *J Urol* 1922; 79:453.

Young HH: Exstrophy of the bladder: the first case in which a normal bladder and urinary control have been obtained by plastic operations. *Surg Gynecol Obstet* 1942; 74:729.

Cloacal Exstrophy

Diamond DA, Jeffs RD: Cloacal exstrophy: a 22-year experience. *J Urol* 1985; 133:779.

Duckett JW, Snyder HM: Continent urinary diversion: variations on the Mitrofanoff principle. *J Urol* 1986; 136:58.

Howell C, Caldamone A, Snyder H, et al: Optimal management of cloacal exstrophy. *J Pediatr Surg* 1983; 18:365.

Hurwitz RS, Manzoni GAM, Ransley PG, et al: Cloacal exstrophy: a report of 34 cases. *J Urol* 1987; 138:1060.

Jeffs RD: Exstrophy and cloacal exstrophy. *Urol Clin North Am* 1978b; 5:127.

Lockhart JL, Davies R, Cox C, et al: The gastroileoileal pouch: an alternative continent urinary reservoir for patients with short bowel, acidosis and/or extensive pelvic radiation. *J Urol* 1993; 150(1):46.

Rickham PP: Vesico-intestinal fissure. *Arch Dis Child* 1960; 35:97.

Sukarochana K, Sieber WK: Vesicointestinal fissure revisited. *J Pediatr Surg* 1978; 13:713.

Sumfest JM, Mitchell ME: Gastrocystoplasty in children. *Eur Urol* 1994; 25:89.

Tank ES, Lindenaur SM: Principles of management of exstrophy of the cloaca. *Am J Surg* 1970; 119:95.

Welch KJ: Cloacal exstrophy. In Ravitch MM, Welch KJ, Bowson CG, et al (eds): *Pediatric Surgery*. Chicago, Year Book Medical Publishers, 1979, pp 802-808.

Cloacal Anomalies

Griffiths D, Malone PS: The Malone antegrade continence enema. *J Ped Surg* 1995; 30:68.

Malone PS, Ransley PG, Kiely EM: Preliminary report: the antegrade continence enema. *Lancet* 1990; 336:1217.

Peña A: The surgical management of persistent cloaca: results in 54 patients treated with a posterior sagittal approach. *J Pediatr Surg* 1989; 24:590.

Peña A: Current management of anorectal anomalies. *Surg Clin North Am* 1992; 72:1393.

Peña A: Anorectal malformations in paediatric surgery. Spitz L, Coran A (eds): *Rob and Smith's Operative Surgery*. Chapman and Hall Medical, London, 1995.

Rich MA, Brock WA, Peña A: Spectrum of genitourinary malformations in patients with imperforate anus. *Pediatr Surg Int* 1988; 3:110.

CHAPTER 53

Myelomeningocele and Neuropathic Bladder

Mark F. Bellinger

In its normal state, the lower urinary tract functions through the balanced activity of many interrelated neural and muscular structures. Normal bladder function, a result of coordinated reflex activity of the detrusor and intrinsic and extrinsic periurethral striated musculature, results in both low-pressure storage of urine and voluntary micturition with complete bladder emptying. The sensation of bladder fullness acts as both a trigger to voluntary micturition and a protective mechanism against vesical overdistension and upper-tract damage. Neurologic, infectious, structural, and psychological processes that alter normal bladder activity may both jeopardize renal function and become the source of common clinical problems. In addition, the congenital and developmental aspects unique to pediatric neurovesical dysfunction challenge urologists to prevent the development of hydronephrosis and vesicoureteric reflux (VUR), preserve renal function, and provide for urinary continence.

NEUROVESICAL DYSFUNCTION IN CHILDREN

The Development of Normal Bladder Control

The lower urinary tract provides low-pressure storage and voluntary elimination of urine, functions that are regulated by somatic, sacral parasympathetic, and thoracolumbar sympathetic nerves (DeGroat et al., 1988). Coordinated neuromuscular activity in the resting state results in increased urethral pressure and a negligible rise in intravesical pressure during bladder filling. The normal sequence of outlet relaxation followed by detrusor contraction results in micturition. In the infant, neural pathways involved in micturition are incompletely developed. Thus micturition is the end result of an involuntary spinal reflex; as detrusor and sphincter act in a coordinated fashion, voiding occurs frequently, and the bladder is completely emptied (Klimberg, 1988). This phase of bladder development has been termed detrusor micturition

(Muellner, 1960). Maturation of the central and peripheral nervous systems gradually brings the act of micturition under voluntary control, the first conscious awareness of bladder function usually occurring between 1 and 2 years of age (Klimberg, 1988). During the second year of life, normal development enables most children to sense bladder fullness, communicate that fact, and hold increasing volumes of urine for longer periods of time. Micturition therefore occurs less frequently. Between 15 and 24 months of age, most infants become fully aware of voiding, and toileting habits begin to develop with parental encouragement. During this first phase of maturation, reflex micturition ceases as the child begins to exert conscious control, first evident as a voluntary tightening of the bladder outlet in response to the sensation of bladder fullness. Although this brief phase of discoordinated micturition rapidly gives way to the normal adult mechanism of suppressing detrusor activity to maintain continence, pathological persistence of the earlier stage may be seen in dysfunctional voiding of minor degrees, and is most severe in the Hinman-Allen syndrome (non-neurogenic neurogenic bladder) (Hinman, 1986). Increased neuromuscular coordination involving the pelvic floor, abdominal muscles, and diaphragm allows voluntary initiation or interruption of micturition to take place at any stage of bladder filling. This final phase of maturation usually occurs between 3 and 4½ years. During this period, nocturnal dryness is achieved in most children, although persistent enuresis is common (Hellstrom et al., 1990; MacKeith et al., 1973). Bloom and colleagues (1993) surveyed the development of bladder control in 1192 children. They found that toilet training was achieved at 9 months to 5.25 years (mean 2.4 ± 0.6 years).

Bladder capacity increases gradually with age, playing an important role in the development of urinary continence. Rather than being a primary cause of bladder development, however, increased capacity likely is a reflection of both maturation of the nervous system and gradual developmental and behavioral adaptation. During childhood, bladder capacity increases approximately 30 cc per year (Klimberg, 1988). Muellner (1960) documented a rapid increase in voided volume from 2 to 4½ years, with a further gradual increase through childhood. Several authors have offered guidelines for estimation of appropriate bladder capacity in children. Berger and associates (1983) estimated bladder capacity in childhood as "age in years plus 2 equals bladder capacity in ounces." Houle and associates (1993) reviewed 923 urodynamic studies in children, using as an end point for bladder filling desire to void, sensation of fullness, discomfort, or leak. They defined the minimal acceptable bladder capacity for age as "16 (age in years) + 70 ml" (Fig. 53-1).

The development of normal continence is a complex process involving neurologic, developmental, maturational, and social factors. It has also been shown that emotional and psychological disturbances may influence the normal maturation process (Douglas, 1973). As a result, many considerations arise when the question is asked whether bladder function is normal in the infant or young child. It is during the period of transition from reflex infant bladder to conscious control that the assessment of bladder function is most difficult. The urologist must be prepared to make use of all available methods of clinical assessment to determine whether bladder function is normal or abnormal.

The Classification of Neurovesical Dysfunction

Dysfunction of the lower urinary tract may result from congenital or acquired lesions, and may be expressed clinically as urinary retention, frequency, urgency, interrupted urination, incontinence, or urinary tract infection. Lower-tract dysfunction may alter ureterovesical dynamics and impair ureteral motility. Hydronephrosis or vesicoureteric reflux may result. The complexity and heterogeneity of neurovesical dysfunction has led to the description of several clinically useful classification schemes, several of which are described below.

Lapides (1970) outlined a classic description of neuropathic bladder dysfunction that includes five categories: sensory paralytic bladder, motor paralytic bladder, autonomous bladder, reflex bladder, and uninhibited bladder. This simplistic classification scheme has been replaced by many other systems of categorization and is outmoded by newer nomenclature based on functional derangement; however, it remains familiar to most urologists. In 1971, Bors and Comarr classified neurological lesions affecting bladder function into sensory or motor, complete or incomplete, and location above or below the level of the sacral reflex arc.

A *sensory paralytic bladder* describes intact motor function without normal sensation. The absence of sensation may result in chronic overdistention to the point of decompensation, but bladder rehabilitation by timed voiding can restore normal detrusor function. This type of neuropathic dysfunction is uncommon in childhood. A *motor paralytic bladder* results from loss of motor fibers while sensation remains intact. Causes are trauma, poliomyelitis, and lumbar disc disease. *Autonomous bladder* dysfunction results from loss of both sensory and motor innervation. A large-capacity bladder with absent detrusor contraction results. Causes are trauma below the cauda equina, radical pelvic surgery, and meningomyelocele

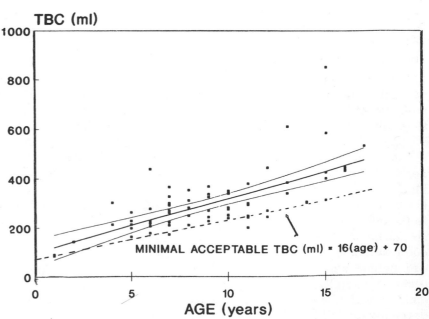

FIG. 53-1
Linear regression between age (years) and total bladder capacity (TBC [ml]) with 95% confidence interval for regression. Dashed line represents minimal acceptable total bladder capacity (ml) equals 16(age) + 70. (From Houle A, Gilmour RF, Churchill BM, Gaumond M, Bissonnette B: *J Urol* 1993; 149:561.

or sacral agenesis. A *reflex bladder* results from complete injury above the level of the sacral reflex arc, commonly from spinal cord injury, tumor, or transverse myelitis. Unchecked sacral reflex activity results in a hypertonic bladder with uninhibited contractions. Sensation is absent. *Uninhibited neuropathic bladder* dysfunction reflects incomplete inhibition of reflex activity by suprasacral inhibitory centers, and may be caused by central nervous system lesions (vascular, tumor, degenerative, traumatic). Sensation is present, extreme urgency is seen, and urge incontinence may result from uninhibited detrusor contractions.

Although the Lapides classification is descriptive, few patients fall into a single category, and in clinical practice most demonstrate mixed lesions with various degrees of severity. For these reasons, urodynamic classification systems as described by Krane and Siroky (1984) (detrusor: hyperreflexic, normoreflexic, or hyporeflexic; sphincter: coordinated, dyssynergic, or nonrelaxing) and the International Continence Society (1981) (detrusor: normal, overactive, underactive; urethra: normal, overactive, incompetent; sensation: normal, hypersensitive, hyposensitive) have appeal. For practical purposes, the end result of neurovesical dysfunction may be classified as either *failure to store* or *failure to empty* (Duckett and Raezer, 1976).

The Clinical Presentation of Neurovesical Dysfunction in Childhood

Dysfunction of the lower urinary tract may result from congenital or acquired lesions, and may be expressed clinically as urinary dribbling or retention, interrupted urinary stream, hesitancy, frequency, urgency, incontinence, urinary tract infection, or renal failure. Many children with congenital causes of neurovesical dysfunction simply never gain normal urinary control. Urinary tract infection, typically recurrent, is a frequent reason for urological consultation. Constipation or fecal soiling is common. Hydronephrosis or vesicoureteric reflux are common radiological findings.

Evaluation of a Child with Suspected Neurovesical Dysfunction
History

Urologists are frequently called upon to evaluate children with known, suspected, or unrecognized neurovesical dysfunction. When neurovesical dysfunction is suspected, it is extremely important to review the child's medical and developmental history to determine whether the dysfunctional pattern is acute or chronic, stable or progressive, and primary or secondary to a period of normal urinary control. It should be noted whether other symptoms that frequently accompany neurovesical dysfunction are present, such as changes in bowel habit or gait, back or leg pain, seizures or neurological complaints, and erectile dysfunction in the older child. It is important to review a history of the prior management of urinary symptoms, including medical and surgical interventions.

Incontinence is a common presentation of urological disease in childhood, and an accurate history is perhaps the most important aspect of its differential diagnosis. Incontinence should be categorized as primary or secondary, continuous dribbling or occasional leakage (large or small volume), stress or urge, pre-void or post-void, and nocturnal or diurnal. Is the urinary stream weak or strong? Is there sensation of fullness or any sensation of voiding, or is the wetness noticed only after voiding occurs? Is voiding spontaneous, or merely associated with Valsalva? Hinman (1974), Allen (1977), Galdston and Perlmutter (1973), and others have documented that psychological, psychosocial, and behavioral disturbances can seriously alter voiding dynamics. A brief review of social history should therefore assess family dynamics and stress, school performance, and peer relationships. This assessment can usually be accomplished superficially with a few probing but nonthreatening questions. It is particularly important in cases of secondary incontinence, or in the face of what appears clinically to be neurovesical dysfunction but without signs of an obvious neurological cause. It is important to note parent-child interaction during the interview and examination, since strained relationships and affective disorders may suggest social problems in the home, a possible additional factor in the development of dysfunctional voiding.

Physical Examination

A complete physical examination should include an assessment of gait, balance, muscular symmetry, and general neurologic status. Reflexes should be tested for symmetry. The back should be examined for skin tags or dimples, hemangiomas, overlying hair patches, or other signs of dysraphism (Albright et al., 1991; Hall et al., 1981) (Fig. 53-2). Examination of the abdomen is performed to assess kidney size and detect bladder distention or a colon filled with stool. The ability to either stimulate bladder emptying by gentle bladder "massage" or to express urine by suprapubic compression should be noted. The genitalia are examined for skin excoriation (as a result of incontinence), hypospadias or meatal stenosis, cryptorchidism, and labial, introital, or anal anomalies. Rectal examination should assess perianal sensation and tone, the presence of hard stool (indicating possible bowel dysfunction), and the presence of a normal sacrum. The bulbocavernosus reflex can be elicited by squeez-

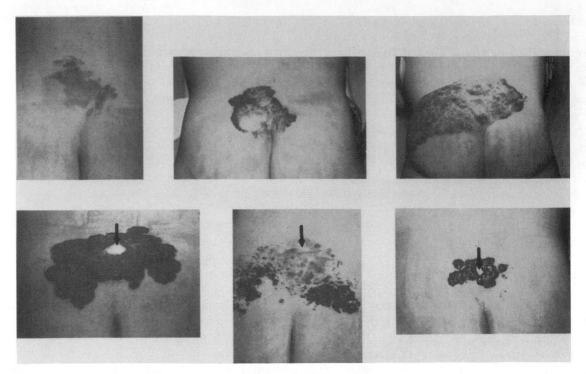

FIG. 53-2
Lumbar cutaneous hemangiomas associated with tethered spinal cords. Arrows point to transparent membranes. (From Albright AL, Gartner JC, Wiener ES: *Pediatrics* 1989; 83:977.

ing the glans penis or clitoris and evaluating the anal wink produced, an indication of an intact sacral reflex arc.

Laboratory Examination

Urinalysis is an important part of the initial examination of all children with suspected urinary tract disease. In the infant, urine can be obtained by a bag technique, and occasionally by stimulating the voiding reflex by gentle suprapubic massage, in which case a midstream specimen may be obtained from both boys and girls. In older children, clean-catch specimens are generally reliable for culture when proper instruction is provided to the child and parents. When contamination is a problem, suprapubic or catheter specimens may be obtained. All urines with abnormal sediment suggestive of infection should be plated for culture and sensitivity.

Once neurovesical dysfunction has been documented, serum creatinine should be measured. If either elevated serum creatinine or renal scarring is present, glomerular filtration rate (GFR) should be determined by measurement of creatinine clearance. Infants and children who are incontinent may have GFR determination by radionuclide clearance techniques that do not require urine collection (Tauxe et al., 1982), or estimated using the method described by Schwartz and associates (1976). (See Chapter 44, Perinatal Urology). If proteinuria is documented, urinary protein excretion should be quantified.

Radiologic Examination

Radiologic examination of the urinary tract is an integral part of the evaluation of children with neurovesical dysfunction, since abnormal bladder function is known to be a cause of upper urinary tract deterioration from hydronephrosis and VUR (Wang et al., 1988). The plain abdominal film should be examined for bony abnormalities (spina bifida occulta, sacral agenesis, widened interpedicular distance), to document severe constipation, and to rule out calculus disease (Fig. 53-3).

The upper urinary tract may be imaged by ultrasound, intravenous pyelography (IVP), or radionuclide scan, depending upon the age of the child, a knowledge of preexisting renal pathology, the information desired, and the expertise of the radiologist. Most children are adequately screened with diagnostic ultrasound, which may assess renal size, upper-tract dilatation, gross renal scarring, bladder capacity, bladder wall thickness, and post-void residual urine volume (Erickson et al., 1989). When abnormal findings are documented by ultrasound, follow-up urography or radionuclide studies may be indicated. Although IVP is used less commonly for routine imaging in children with neurovesical dysfunction since the advent of diagnostic ultrasound, it may be particularly useful in specific instances and can be tailored to fit the needs of the urologist and to minimize radiation exposure to the patient. Evaluation of a child with severe kyphoscoliosis in whom ultrasound imaging of

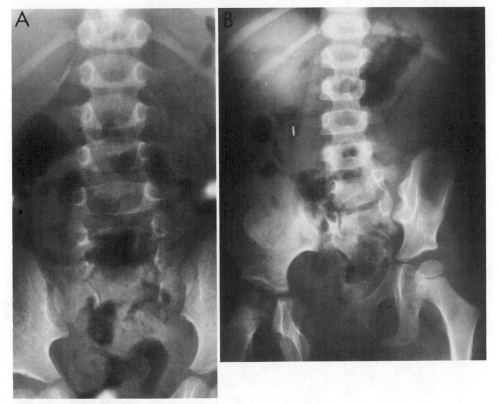

FIG. 53-3
Lumbosacral anomalies associated with neurovesical dysfunction.

the kidney is technically difficult, anatomic delineation of ureteral and cayceal anatomy in patients with calculus disease, evaluation of patients with urinary diversion, and delineation of the renal anatomy in children with rotational or fusion anomalies of the kidneys are common indications for the use of intravenous urography.

Radionuclide renal imaging has assumed an ever-increasing role in the evaluation of children with neurovesical dysfunction. Because a multitude of radionuclides are currently in use, the urologist who orders or interprets radionuclide images must understand something about both the characteristics of the radionuclide and the important technical aspects of patient preparation and handling during the imaging process (Velchik, 1985). Thus each study should be tailored to answer the clinical questions being asked.

Diuresis renography is usually performed to confirm or exclude the diagnosis of supravesical obstructive uropathy, and is most helpful in the assessment of chronic hydronephrosis or hydroureteronephrosis when the question of dilation versus true obstruction arises (Fig. 53-4) (Conway, 1989). Technetium-99m-diethylenetriamine pentaacetic acid (DTPA) (O'Reilly, 1986) or technetium-99m-mercaptoacetlytriglycine (MAG3) (Conway and Maizels, 1993) are most frequently used for these studies since they offer rapid renal clearance and tubular excretion. The renogram

is performed after oral hydration, and frequently after a period of intravenous hydration as well. This aspect of the study is critical because furosemide acts on the ascending limb of the loop of Henle to promote diuresis, and the results may be invalid if the patient is dehydrated or renal function is poor. The bladder should be drained continuously by an indwelling feeding tube to ensure complete bladder drainage during the study. This is most important in patients with neurovesical dysfunction or other causes of poor bladder compliance such as posterior urethral valves, because a bladder even partially full may hinder upper-tract drainage and cause a false impression of obstruction (Maizels et al., 1986). The patient is usually imaged in the supine position, and once the collecting system is seen to be full of radionuclide, furosemide is injected and imaging continued. The images are analyzed by computer after selecting appropriate regions of interest. The final study should offer information about differential renal function and upper-tract drainage. Diuresis renography is one of the most technically demanding imaging studies both to perform and analyze, and many pitfalls exist (Conway, 1992). The Society for Fetal Urology and the Pediatric Nuclear Medicine Council have described a "well-tempered" renogram that attempts to standardize the many aspects of this study (Conway and Maizels, 1993).

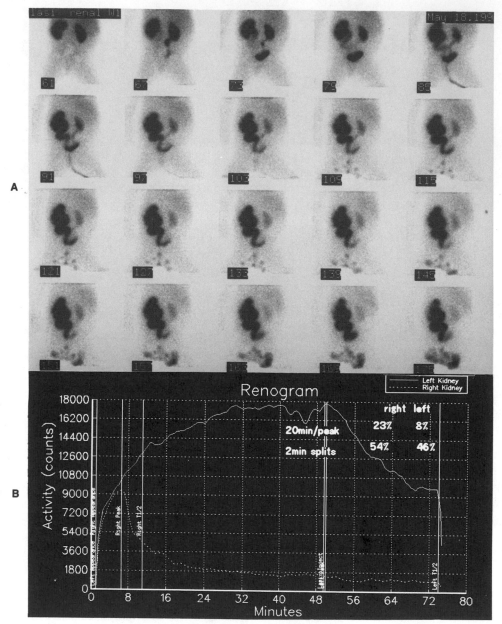

FIG. 53-4
A, Diuresis renogram images. Right kidney drains well, left kidney slowly. **B,** Washout curves from diuresis renogram of same patient. Right kidney drains readily, while left kidney takes longer to accumulate radionuclide and drains slowly after Lasix administration.

Static renal imaging using technetium-99m-dimer-captosuccinic acid (DMSA) has played an increasingly important role in several clinical scenarios. DMSA provides information about differential renal size and function in children with disordered renal anatomy, and delineates renal parenchymal scarring in children (Rushton and Majd, 1992) (Fig. 53-5, *B*). DMSA imaging has also proven to be most helpful in the delineation of the acute parenchymal inflammation of pyelonephritis (Fig. 53-5, *B*) (Jakobbsen et al., 1992). This diagnosis is not always easy to make on clinical grounds alone, especially when a child who is managed

by intermittent catheterization and who has chronic bacteriuria has a fever and no other symptoms. Urinary tract infection is frequently considered the source of fever, even though the differential diagnosis may include a viral syndrome. A positive DMSA scan, confirming pyelonephritis, allows the physician to begin appropriate treatment, while a negative scan may prevent unnecessary treatment and even hospitalization. A high degree of interobserver agreement has been found when the reliability interpretation of DMSA scans was examined (Patel et al., 1993).

The voiding cystourethrogram (VCU) plays an im-

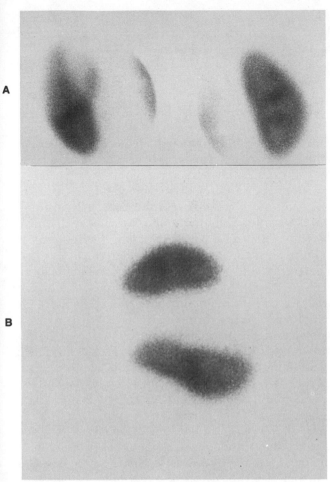

FIG. 53-5
A, DMSA scan showing acute pyelonephritis of upper pole of left kidney. Right kidney appears normal. **B,** DMSA scan six months later showing scar in upper pole of left kidney.

portant role in the evaluation of children with neurovesical dysfunction and should always be performed in infants and patients with newly diagnosed neurovesical dysfunction, and when upper-tract imaging documents the new onset of hydronephrosis or renal scarring. Likewise, pyelonephritis occurring in a child without known VUR demands that a VCU be performed, preferably after infection has been eradicated and the child given suppressive antibacterial therapy for several weeks. Voiding cystourethrography is easily performed with a small catheter (8 F feeding tube in most infants). The bladder is filled with room-temperature contrast until voiding occurs. Bladder capacity and configuration, bladder neck and external sphincter competence, and urethral anatomy should be documented, in addition to the presence and grade of VUR. VUR should be graded using the standard criteria of the International Reflux Study in Children (International Reflux Committee, 1981). A carefully performed VCU may offer, in addition to anatomic detail, a gross assessment of bladder capacity, void-

ing dynamics, and detrusor-sphincter coordination. The radionuclide VCU is preferred as a follow-up study when the presence or absence of reflux is to be evaluated in children with normal bladder function (Lebowitz, 1992), but the contrast VCU offers a great deal of anatomic, structural, and functional information in the child with neurovesical dysfunction and is generally preferred even for follow-up study. The VCU and urodynamic evaluation are frequently combined in a videourodynamic evaluation.

Urodynamic Evaluation

Urodynamic assessment of children with proven or suspected neurovesical dysfunction must be tailored to fit both the ability of the patient to understand and cooperate, and the information desired, including the assessment of bladder capacity, detrusor function, bladder neck and urethral dynamics, detrusor-pelvic floor coordination, and voiding dynamics (Bauer, 1983). Complex urodynamic studies are invasive and require extraordinary cooperation that may be achieved only by adults or very cooperative children. However, more limited studies designed to elicit specific information about bladder function are often successful. Although urodynamic studies may be performed frequently on infants with neurologic deficits, many children presenting for evaluation are grossly neurologically intact and require even more intense preparation for catheterization, because discomfort will be associated with testing. These children, especially, must be approached gradually, in a friendly and nonthreatening manner, so that an atmosphere of trust is created. It is critical to the success of each study that, prior to the procedure, the parents and child understand the reason for study, the nature of the testing, and the fact that all attempts will be made to minimize discomfort and anxiety. Although children may be sedated for urodynamic evaluation, little more than basic cystometry can be achieved in a sedated child. In many cases, urodynamic testing is best abandoned if the child is unable to cooperate. The state of bladder function must then be inferred from other available data (VCU, post-void residual volume, voiding or catheterization diary). In this context, it is important to realize that not all children with presumed or documented neurovesical dysfunction require urodynamic evaluation, and that not every urodynamic study will yield useful data.

Meaningful urodynamic data can rarely be obtained until several visits with a child have taken place. This allows the physician to make an assessment of the potential for patient cooperation, and a realistic determination of which urodynamic studies may be best suited for the individual problem in question. Since many children referred for urodynamic study will have had previous radiologic, endoscopic, or surgical procedures, the physician should try to assess the child's reaction to and cooperation with this testing. Urodynamic studies in children are best performed and interpreted by the physician or an extremely well-trained and experienced observer who is able to assess the child's response to testing, to separate fact from artifact, and to modify the procedure to suit the cooperation of the child and the needs of the examiner. After 5 years of age, many children are cooperative enough to provide reliable urodynamic data if they are well prepared prior to the procedure.

Noninvasive urodynamic tests include uroflowmetry and electromyographic/uroflow studies (Churchill et al., 1987). Uroflow studies are the most noninvasive of urodynamic studies and allow the examiner to assess the flow rate and character of the urinary stream. An adequate volume of urine must be voided to permit an accurate assessment of urinary flow rate. We have used a simple flowmeter designed by Drake (1954) in some situations to evaluate voided volume, peak urinary flow rate, and the character of the voided urinary stream. Micturition studies combined with pelvic floor electromyography (EMG) are aimed at assessing the function of the periurethral striated musculature during voiding (Firlit et al., 1978; Maizels and Firlit, 1979). Anal plug and urethral catheter electrodes can be used, but are liable to introduce artifact. Direct measurement of periurethral striated muscle activity can be achieved by the insertion of small needle or wire electrodes into the periurethral area in girls and into the prostatic apex in boys. Bauer (1985) has demonstrated the usefulness of the oscilloscope in recording action potentials from the sphincter musculature, thus aiding optimal electrode positioning. Electrodes may be inserted under anesthesia with testing performed later, or may be inserted using local or cutaneous anesthesia in a cooperative child. Insertion of a small trocar cystostomy catheter may facilitate bladder refilling for repetitive urodynamic study, especially if biofeedback training is desired. However, even small cystostomy catheters may introduce a considerable amount of discomfort and artifact in many children.

In an effort to achieve noninvasive monitoring of pelvic floor activity, Maizels and associates (1979) described the use of skin patch electrodes. These nonspecific electrodes require skin preparation with alcohol or acetone and tincture of benzoin adhesive to achieve good contact and prevent dislodgment. They are associated with more artifact than is seen when needle electrodes are used. During normal voiding, internal sphincter, pelvic floor, and external urethral musculature relax to allow satisfactory bladder emptying. Detrusor-pelvic floor dyssynergia is documented when pelvic floor musculature fails to relax and EMG activity persists during detrusor contraction

(Maizels et al., 1979). Such activity is particularly difficult to separate from artifact generated by abdominal straining. The use of abdominal EMG patch electrodes to detect abdominal straining (Koff and Kass, 1982) or a rectal balloon to subtract abdominal pressure may be important so that the diagnosis of dyssynergia is not made inappropriately (Koff, 1983).

The performance of cystometry in children requires patience, understanding, and adequate patient preparation. Patient assessment is important, since a child who balks at catheterization is unlikely to be cooperative enough to provide meaningful data. Sedation is usually not beneficial, but lidocaine jelly instilled into the urethra prior to catheterization may diminish discomfort and improve cooperation. If cystometry is to be performed, it is best done after voiding so that a determination of post-void residual volume can be made. A small 7 F or 8 F double- or triple-lumen urodynamic catheter or microtip transducer catheter will prove to be appropriate for most studies. A small balloon catheter placed into the rectum is used to subtract abdominal pressure and negate artifact produced by straining. It is important to avoid latex catheters and balloons in all patients with spina bifida, and especially those with proven latex allergy (Schneck and Bellinger, 1993). If pelvic floor electromyography is to be performed, catheterization should take place after the micturition urodynamic study is completed. Cystometry may be performed using water or gas. Gas cystometry, although quicker and more convenient, is less physiologic and perhaps less accurate than studies using water (Gleason et al., 1977). Slow-fill cystometry using body-temperature water is preferred for most pediatric studies. Bladder filling should be approximately 10% to 15% of expected bladder capacity per minute (bladder capacity in ounces = age in years + 2) (Berger, 1983). During bladder filling, EMG activity may be monitored. In cooperative children, documentation of bladder capacity, sensation, and uninhibited bladder activity can be expected to be obtained. The pressure and volume at which urine leaks around the catheter during filling should be noted. If the child is capable of spontaneous voiding, the pressure generated in the bladder (voiding pressure) is measured. Cystometry and voiding cystourethrography may be combined in videourodynamic studies, since it has been shown that contrast medium, when used as a medium for cystography, does not adversely influence urodynamic findings (Joseph, 1993).

Static urethral pressure profilometry measures the passive resistance of the urethra along its length. The side-hole catheter may be positioned at any location in the urethra that requires study, but the measurement has little practical use in children with neurovesical dysfunction unless the efficacy of an artificial urinary sphincter cuff, bladder neck sling, or reconstructed bladder neck is being evaluated. Urethral pressure may vary at the same position in the urethra and is affected by bladder volume, the characteristics of the catheter itself, and infusion parameters (Bauer, 1985).

Pediatric urodynamic data are extremely valuable when thoughtfully and carefully obtained. The data are useful in diagnosis and for providing prognostic information, and may be used in biofeedback training, particularly in children with non-neuropathic voiding dysfunction (Maizels et al., 1979).

CONGENITAL NEUROSPINAL DYSRAPHISMS

Spina Bifida

The term spina bifida includes a group of developmental anomalies that result from defects in neural tube closure (Strassburg, 1982a). Lesions may include spina bifida occulta, a generally incidental finding in which only a bony defect is present; meningocele, with a meningeal sac but intact neural elements; spina bifida cystica (myelomeningocele), with a skin-covered intact sac containing neural elements; or spina bifida aperta, in which the sac is open. Myelomeningocele is by far the most common defect seen, and the most devastating. Spina bifida is a disease of variable prevalence, ranging from 4.5 per 1000 births in Belfast to 0.12 per 1000 births in Singapore (Strassburg, 1982b). In the United States, the prevalence is estimated at 1 per 1000 births but varies geographically, being more common in the eastern states. Stein (1982) reported a steady decline in incidence in all ethnic groups in the northeastern United States from 1930 to 1980, and a progressive decrease in incidence in the United States as a whole from 1970 to 1980, while a significant decline was noted in Liverpool, England, between 1974 and 1979 (Owens, 1981).

The etiology of neural tube defects appears to be multifactoral (Strassburg, 1982a, 1982b). Epidemiologic data incriminate environmental factors because the birth prevalence has varied over time and by geographical location, and epidemics of neural defects appear to have taken place at different times and in different locations worldwide (Oakley, 1993). Genetic factors are incriminated by studies showing female preponderance, ethnic variability, and increased familial tendencies. Sibling incidence has varied from 1.4% to 6.0%, and when two siblings are affected, the risk rises from 4.8% to 12% (Toriello, 1982). Neural tube defects likewise are associated with Meckel's syndrome (autosomal recessive), trisomies 13 and 18, and cloacal exstrophy (possibly on a local developmental basis) (Toriello, 1982).

Growing evidence over the past several decades that periconceptual supplementation with multivita-

mins might diminish the risk of neural tube defects correlates with the higher incidence of these anomalies found in areas with lower socioeconomic levels (Mulinare et al., 1988; MRC, 1991). A decade of debate has been resolved by two recent multicenter randomized controlled studies. The first found a 72% reduction in the recurrence of neural tube defects among women who received a 4-mg daily supplement of folic acid in the periconceptual period (MRC, 1991). This study led the United States Public Health Service to recommend in 1992 that all women of childbearing age consume 0.4 mg of folic acid daily. These data were given further significance by a second randomized controlled trial that found the risk of the occurrence of first-time neural tube defects to be reduced by 60% by the use of periconceptual folic acid supplementation (Werler et al., 1993). The Food and Drug Administration is reportedly considering the fortification of a food staple with folic acid to further diminish risk to the general population (Oakley, 1993).

Spina bifida is a significant disease that has dramatic impact on involved children and families. Lessons learned from management of the urologic consequences of spina bifida have provided urologists with a markedly expanded armamentarium with which to treat neuropathic bladder dysfunction of all causes. Goals of management for the patient with neurovesical dysfunction are to preserve or stabilize renal function, prevent complications of urinary tract infection, and provide socially acceptable continence. The perception of what constitutes acceptable continence may vary among parent, child, caretakers, and peers. A child's age, mental and physical abilities, and socioeconomic status will also influence this perception, and normal developmental processes, schooling, and peer pressure may gradually alter his or her personal concept of what represents an acceptable bladder regimen. When continence and social acceptance (rather than medical concerns) become the main goals of urologic therapy in a child with neurovesical dysfunction, particular care must be taken to individualize treatment to fit the needs of the child and not to treat merely for treatment's sake. It is imperative that urologists have an appreciation for other related problems that may occur as a result of spina bifida (orthopedic, neurosurgical, neurologic, psychologic, social, developmental, endocrinologic, sexual) because these may impact on or be altered by urologic management (Meyer and Landau, 1984).

Perinatal Evaluation

Spinal dysraphism is usually found unexpectedly at birth but may be detected during prenatal ultrasound examination (Hobbins et al., 1979). A detailed examination of the entire spine by an experienced ultrasonographer is necessary to rule out neural tube defects, and even in ideal situations errors may be made (Watson et al., 1991). Antenatal detection of neural tube defects is suggested when amniocentesis reveals an elevated level of α-fetoprotein (Brock and Sutcliffe, 1972). However, controversy surrounds the use of maternal serum screening for α-fetoprotein, due to the fact that both false positive and false negative determinations have been reported, and the distribution of normal values of maternal serum α-fetoprotein overlaps values seen in the presence of neural tube defects (Watson et al., 1991).

Optimal perinatal management of a fetus with myelomeningocele remains the subject of debate. Elective cesarean section has been thought to be beneficial in diminishing trauma to neural elements (Chervenak et al., 1984). This conclusion, however, was based upon a review of older series of deliveries and has been called into question. Benson and associates (1988) reviewed the route of delivery and outcome of 75 babies and concluded that there was no difference in outcome no matter which route of delivery was chosen. These data also have been called into question, and the final answer awaits a more controlled study (Hogge et al., 1990).

Neonate

The initial examination of a neonate with spina bifida should proceed along guidelines noted earlier for a child with suspected neurovesical dysfunction. Since back closure and ventriculoperitoneal shunt placement may have been performed prior to initial urologic evaluation, the child's general neurologic status should be documented. Abdominal wall tone, lower extremity function, anal sphincter tone, and function of the sacral reflex arc (bulbocavernosus reflex) should be assessed. It is important to note that the level of the bony defect will not determine the functional cord level, which may be altered by the degree of involvement of the spinal cord and nerve roots, CNS anomalies (hydrocephalus, Arnold-Chiari malformation), and perhaps the surgical trauma of sac closure (Kroovand et al., 1990). Each child has a unique neurologic status, and each therefore requires a complete urologic evaluation. Nurses' observations of spontaneous voiding, continuous dribbling, or a forceful stream provide valuable information about bladder capacity and function that, when added to the radiographic appearance of the bladder, may provide data similar to that provided by the cystometrogram. Abdominal examination is performed to assess renal size, detect bladder distention, and assess the efficacy of bladder massage or the Credé maneuver to induce bladder emptying. The Credé maneuver, which has been routinely taught in the neonatal period to many parents of children with spina bifida, is extremely limited in both effectiveness and applicability, and is

best avoided since most infants will spontaneously void enough to provide adequate bladder emptying. Barbalias and associates (1983) documented that Credé actually produced increased urethral resistance in 98% of patients studied; thus the maneuver may significantly elevate intravesical pressure. Credé is particularly contraindicated when outlet resistance is high or VUR is present, because the increased hydrostatic pressure will be transmitted directly to the renal parenchyma.

All neonates with spina bifida should have a complete urological evaluation performed during the neonatal period. Urinary tract ultrasonography is performed to document the state of the upper tracts and assess bladder-wall thickness. Post-void sonography can also assess the completeness of spontaneous voiding. Although fewer than 10% of neonates with spina bifida exhibit hydronephrosis, Stafford and colleagues (1983) studied 10 consecutive neonates of whom 6 had hydronephrosis. Gaum and associates (1982) studied 68 neonates with IV urography and found abnormal upper tracts in 13 (19%); 7 bilateral hydronephrosis, 3 ureterectasis, 1 pyelectasis, 1 dysplastic kidney, and 1 horseshoe kidney. Of the group with normal urography, 69% had an abnormal VCU; of the group with abnormal urography, 92.3% had an abnormal VCU. Cystographic abnormalities included reflux (16%), diverticula of the bladder (23.5%), and subjective abnormalities of bladder-wall thickness or bladder shape seen in the majority of patients. Given these data, it is mandatory that voiding cystourethrography and urodynamic evaluation be performed as part of the initial evaluation of all infants. Studies should be repeated whenever new-onset hydronephrosis is detected by sonography, or when there is a significant change in bladder habits or continence.

Once a complete urological evaluation has been performed, an appropriate bladder regimen is designed for each individual patient. For many infants, spontaneous voiding into diapers represents optimal care. The Credé maneuver should generally be avoided. Transient urinary retention or elevated residual urine volumes immediately after back closure may require at least temporary management by intermittent catheterization. If prolonged catheterization is necessary, cystourethrography should be performed to determine the presence or absence of VUR. All neonates started on intermittent catheterization should be placed on prophylactic antibacterials at least until the absence of VUR is documented.

Urodynamic Assessment of the Neonate.—Urodynamic evaluation of children with spina bifida traditionally has been carried out in the late preschool or early school-age years in conjunction with the initiation of a bladder training program, the studies serving as a guide to bladder management and pharmacologic manipulation (Raezer et al., 1977). McGuire and associates (1981) evaluated urodynamic findings in 42 children studied over a 7-year period and found urodynamic testing to be of prognostic value in determining which patients were at risk for upper-tract deterioration. In the low-intravesical-pressure group (intravesical pressure 40 cm H_2O or less at the time of urethral leakage), no patient had VUR, and only 2 of 22 had ureteral dilatation. In the high-intravesical-pressure group, however, 68% showed VUR, and 81% had ureteral dilatation. More recently, Bauer and colleagues (1984) studied 36 neonates with spina bifida soon after sac closure and in follow-up for 18 to 48 months. In the group demonstrating detrusor-external sphincter dyssynergy, 72% had or developed hydronephrosis during the period of study, whereas only 22% with synergy and 11% with absent sphincter activity showed upper-tract deterioration. In a subsequent study, hydronephrosis developed in less than 10% of infants at risk for upper-tract deterioration who were placed on a program of prophylactic intermittent catheterization and anticholinergic therapy. These data confirm that early urodynamic evaluation is helpful for both guiding therapy and determining which infants are in need of more closely spaced follow-up studies, or aggressive bladder management regimens such as intermittent catheterization, urethral dilation, or cutaneous vesicostomy. Urodynamic findings are also helpful when counseling parents about the long-term prognosis for both upper-tract preservation and the management of urinary continence.

It is important to remember that a great deal of artifact can be introduced into urodynamic studies when they are performed in infants and children, and that voiding cystourethrography and a voiding or catheterization diary can provide a great deal of information about bladder function. This adjunctive information should not be overlooked when urodynamic testing is not available. Adjunctive data should be compared with urodynamic studies when both are available so that any discrepancy between the two can be reconciled when a plan for bladder management is formulated.

General Principles of Management

One of the most important aspects of the urologic care of patients with neurovesical dysfunction is periodic re-evaluation. A well-designed lifelong plan for follow-up should begin in infancy. If neonatal sonography demonstrates normal upper tracts, urodynamic studies are favorable, urine is sterile, and bladder emptying adequate, the infant may be discharged to be managed in diapers by spontaneous voiding. Parents must be counseled that close urologic follow-up is necessary both to prevent renal damage and to provide for periodic reassessment of the efficacy of the child's bladder program. When initial urodynamic and radiographic findings are favorable (good bladder compliance, absence of reflux and hydronephrosis), appropriate follow-up may necessitate sonography only in 3 to 4 months, at 1 year, and at yearly intervals thereafter. If hydronephrosis or urinary infection is documented, a VCU and urodynamic evaluation should be performed as soon as infection is cleared, as part of the evaluation of the efficacy of the current bladder management regimen. When hydronephrosis, urinary retention, vesicoureteric reflux, poor bladder compliance, or detrusor-sphincter dyssynergia is documented in infancy, a plan of action other than spontaneous voiding must be formulated. Intermittent catheterization with or without pharmacotherapy, urethral dilation (Bloom et al., 1990; Wang et al., 1989), or temporary cutaneous vesicostomy (Duckett, 1974) may be appropriate in specific settings for any of these medical indications.

In the face of stable bladder function and normal upper tracts, close urological surveillance is appropriate until a formal bladder management program is instituted for social reasons. Since this group of children will have bladder manipulation performed for social indications only, determination of the most appropriate time for initiation of bladder manipulation must be made based not on chronologic age, but on factors such as the child's desire for continence and manual dexterity, and family dynamics, support, and resources. Not all children or families share the same concept of dryness, and motivation may play a large part in the success or failure of any proposed regimen of bladder management. For practical purposes, therapy for incontinence may be aimed at either failure of the bladder to store urine or failure to empty, most patients demonstrating a deficit in both functions.

Failure of adequate urine storage may be a result of diminished detrusor compliance or hyperactivity, inadequate outlet resistance, detrusor-outlet dyssynergy, or a combination of factors. In some instances, these causes of incontinence result in minimal problems with infection and upper-tract deterioration, primarily presenting social and psychologic concerns for the family and patient. This is especially true when outlet resistance is also diminished. However, incontinence secondary to either diminished vesical compliance and elevated intravesical pressures at small bladder volumes, or detrusor hypertrophy secondary to detrusor-sphincter dyssynergy, is a common cause of upper-tract deterioration (McGuire et al., 1981).

The management of failure to empty must be aimed at the source of dysfunction. Detrusor hyperactivity may be managed with anticholinergic agents or by diminishing smooth muscle tone (Table 53-1). Combination therapy may prove beneficial. Transurethral electrical stimulation has demonstrated some promise

TABLE 53-1

Common Pharmacotherapy of Pediatric Neurovesical Dysfunction

Action	Drug	Maximum Dose	Frequency
Cholinergic	Bethanechol	0.6 mg/kg/day	3-4 times daily
Anticholinergic	Propantheline	1.5 mg/kg/day	3-4 times daily
	Oxybutynin	0.2 mg/kg/dose	2-4 times daily
	Dicyclomine	5-10 mg/dose	3-4 times daily
Sympathomimetic	Ephedrine sulfate	1 mg/kg/dose	3-4 times daily
	Phenylpropanolamine (in combination drugs)	2.5 mg/kg/dose	2-3 times daily
Miscellaneous	Imipramine	0.7 mg/kg/dose	2-3 times daily

for increasing bladder capacity, but the effect is only transient in many cases (Lyne and Bellinger, 1993). Failure of pharmacologic therapy may necessitate a consideration of sacral rhizotomy therapy (Toczek et al., 1975) or bladder denervation therapy (Staskin et al., 1981), both of which have been performed rarely in children with spina bifida. Augmentation cystoplasty (Mitchell, 1981) may be required in severe cases with markedly diminished bladder capacity or compliance. These bladders will thus be converted to the failure-to-empty category and managed as such. Insufficient bladder outlet resistance may be managed by pharmacologic agents that stimulate alpha-sympathetic receptors in the bladder neck and posterior urethra (Table 53-1). Surgical reconstruction or compression of the bladder neck may be necessary in severe cases. The newest approach to intrinsic sphincter deficiency involves transurethral or periurethral injection of bulking materials such as Teflon or collagen (Kaplan, 1991; Wan et al., 1992).

Failure of bladder emptying may result from inadequate detrusor function. Since it is generally considered that bethanechol is inactive on a long-term basis, pharmacologic agents are rarely useful in clinical practice to improve detrusor function (Wein, 1979). Electrical stimulation (bladder pacemaker) has proved to be of very limited usefulness, particularly in the pediatric population (Wheatley et al., 1982). Transurethral electrostimulation has appeared to be beneficial in some children, although conflicting data have been reported (Boone et al., 1992; Decter, 1994; Kaplan and Richards, 1988; Lyne and Bellinger, 1993). Myogenic failure may result from chronic overdistention, and, in this scenario, intermittent catheterization may improve detrusor tone.

Outlet resistance of the bladder neck and proximal urethra may be diminished pharmacologically by α-sympatholytic agents. Striated-muscle relaxants may lower outlet resistance at the level of the pelvic floor (dantrolene, baclofen), but side effects related to generalized striated-muscle relaxation (generalized weakness, dizziness, drowsiness) are common and have severely limited the usefulness of these agents (Wein,

TABLE 53-2

Therapeutic Options for the Management of Neurovesical Dysfunction

Failure to store
  Detrusor
    Pharmacologic therapy
      Anticholinergic
      Smooth-muscle relaxant
      Imipramine
    Neurologic therapy
      Sacral rhizotomy
      Bladder denervation
    Bladder augmentation
  Bladder outlet
    Pharmacologic therapy
      α-Sympathomimetic
      Imipramine
    (Urinary diversion)
Failure to empty
  Detrusor
    Pharmacologic therapy
      Cholinergic
    Electrical stimulation
    Intermittent catheterization
  Bladder outlet
    Pharmacologic therapy
      α-Sympatholytic
      Smooth=muscle relaxant
    Neurologic therapy
    Dilatation
    Surgical
      YV-plasty of the bladder neck
      Transurethral incision of bladder neck
      External sphincterotomy
    Mechanical
      Valsalva
      Credé
    Intermittent catheterization
    Urinary diversion

1979). Pharmacological interruption of nerves responsible for increased outlet resistance (pudendal block) has been used infrequently in children (Raz et al., 1971). Johnston and Kathel (1971) and Shochat and Perlmutter (1972) described overdilatation of the bladder outlet in females, therapy that has been reintroduced by Bloom (Bloom et al., 1990; Wan, 1992).

Surgical destruction of outlet resistance may be accomplished by transurethral incision of the bladder neck, or external sphincter, YV-plasty of the bladder neck, or bladder flap urethroplasty. These procedures result in incontinence that is reversible only by surgical means (see Table 53-2).

Mechanical bladder emptying may be produced by the Valsalva or Credé maneuvers. It has been demonstrated that the Credé maneuver may simultaneously increase outlet resistance and intravesical pressure, and may produce harmful effects on the upper urinary tract (Barbalias et al., 1983). Intermittent catheterization is of proven benefit in managing incontinence in conjunction with pharmacotherapy or appropriate surgical intervention. Although temporary diversion frequently has proven beneficial in the management of children with renal deterioration due to neurovesical dysfunction (Snyder et al., 1983), permanent urinary diversion has been allotted a position of last resort (Cass et al., 1984; Wammack et al., 1992). It must be kept in mind that incontinence associated with sterile urine and normal upper tracts may be best managed conservatively in small children, older children unconcerned with wetness, and in social situations where diminished functional capacity or noncompliance to pharmacologic and catheterization regimens is a problem.

Specific Options for The Management of Neurovesical Dysfunction

Clean Intermittent Catheterization

Although indwelling catheterization has been used to manage neurovesical dysfunction, many adverse sequelae of long-term indwelling catheterization have been reported, particularly in boys. In 1966, Guttman and Frankel introduced sterile intermittent catheterization to the care of patients with neurovesical dysfunction. The subsequent popularization of nonsterile clean intermittent catheterization (CIC) by Lapides (Lapides et al., 1972) has allowed this technique to become the mainstay of management for neurovesical dysfunction in both children and adults, its popularity aided by the poor experience with bladder management by both the Credé maneuver and long-term indwelling catheterization. Cass (1976) documented a 72% incidence of chronic infection, upper-tract dilation in 45%, and incontinence in 100% of children managed by Credé. When managed with long-term indwelling catheterization, 100% of children were infected and 57% showed upper-tract dilation. In contrast, Plunkett and Braren (1979) described stable upper tracts in 82% and improved upper tracts in 15% on intermittent catheterization, with 6% incidence of pyelonephritis. Cass (1976) documented an 87.5% incidence of stable upper tracts, improvement in 12.5%, stable or improved VUR in 75%, and persistently ster-

ile urine in 90% of patients. Nonsterile self-intermittent catherization, especially in children who may be less concerned about cleanliness in performance of catheterization, is associated with a significant incidence of bacteriuria. Although Cass (1976) achieved a 90% incidence of persistently sterile urine on suppressive antibiotic therapy, Plunkett and Braren (1979) documented persistent infection in 80%, yet pyelonephritis occurred in only 6%, each in a patient with significant VUR. Crooks and Enrile (1983) documented that asymptomatic bacteriuria in children on a CIC program was not a problem unless VUR was present, data confirmed by Lewis and associates (1984).

Nonsterile intermittent catheterization may be initiated to manage VUR, upper-tract deterioration, urinary tract infection, or incontinence. The aim of an intermittent catheterization program is to provide periodic, complete bladder emptying. The success of the program depends highly on the compliance and motivation of the parents or caretakers, the child, and the professionals caring for the child. When self-catheterization is instituted, a great deal of responsibility is thrust on the child. This responsibility is best undertaken when the individual displays interest in personal hygiene and self-image, a stage that coincides with the acknowledgment of peer pressure and social interaction. This stage in growth and development cannot be measured in years and may vary tremendously with the child's individual needs and abilities. Nor can it be assumed that all children will be able to quickly master the techniques of catheterization; in fact, some may be physically unable because of motor deficits, incoordination, skeletal deformity, or orthotic appliances. Time invested in bladder training at the outset will prove to be invaluable in helping both parents and child cope with setbacks and occasional or persistent wetness, especially when repeated urodynamic assessments and alterations in pharmacologic therapy are necessary. If self-catheterization proves unsuccessful, interaction with school personnel, caretakers, and other family members may be necessary to devise an adequate catheterization program. Each child successfully enrolled in a self-catheterization program will eventually come to design a personalized program that allows an unobtrusive catheterization schedule and technique. Catheters are carried in a small plastic bag and reused. They are simply rinsed under running water before and after use. Many girls can manipulate short plastic or stainless steel catheters more easily than catheters of standard length. Catheterization can be performed while standing at or sitting on the toilet, and micturition will appear close to normal as far as others are concerned.

The likelihood of achieving total continence using a program of intermittent catheterization and pharmacologic therapy depends greatly upon bladder storage characteristics and patient compliance and motivation. Wolraich and colleagues (1983) achieved 49% total daytime continence with CIC and pharmacotherapy. Cass (1976) documented 17% slight dampness but only 34% dryness, while Purcell and Gregory (1984) reported 24% total dryness, 33% wetness primarily due to poor patient compliance, and 30% wetness in spite of total patient compliance. Knoll and Madersbacher (1993) found an overall continence rate of 40%, but this was as high as 55% in the group whose detrusor hyperreflexia was controlled by pharmacotherapy in association with a competent bladder outlet. These data must be taken into consideration when goals of a CIC program are discussed with patients and family. Adjuncts to CIC and pharmacotherapy should be considered when adequate continence is not achieved.

Pharmacologic Therapy of the Child With Neurovesical Dysfunction

Drug therapy may effectively alter bladder or outlet function and provide continence in milder cases of neurovesical dysfunction. More commonly, however, drugs are used as an adjunct to intermittent catheterization to modify the function of the detrusor or bladder outlet in an effort to provide both adequate storage capacity and adequate emptying. In children, the dosage and side effects of pharmacologic agents must be monitored carefully. Medication is best prescribed per kilogram of body weight. It is common practice to begin with a single agent at a low dose. As efficacy is monitored, dosages are increased and drugs combined in a stepwise fashion in order to achieve a desired clinical effect while minimizing adverse side effects (see Table 53-1).

Urethral Dilation

Johnston and Kathel (1971) were the first to report that urethral dilation could improve both bladder emptying and hydronephrosis in patients with myelomeningocele, a finding confirmed in a small series by Schochat and Perlmutter (1972). Little attention was paid to this technique until the report by Bloom (1990) that detailed the urodynamic and radiographic effects of urethral dilation in 18 children with meningomyelocele and high vesical pressures who underwent dilation as an alternative to cutaneous vesicostomy. The urodynamic effect of dilation in this group of patients resulted in a decreased leak-point pressure from an average of 55.75 cm water to 31 cm water soon after dilation, and 19.3 cm water at later evaluation. Longitudinal studies demonstrated a persistent improvement in bladder compliance after dilation, and suggest that the ability to diminish adverse compliance at an early age by any technique may have a salutary effect on long-term bladder function. Dilation may be performed in girls using urethral dilators and in boys using balloon dilation under fluoroscopic control. General anesthesia is used in most children, but may be performed at the bedside in girls who have little or no urethral and perineal sensation.

Cutaneous Vesicostomy

Clean intermittent catheterization (CIC) is the most widely used intervention for the management of vesical dysfunction. Intermittent catheterization may be instituted as part of a bladder management program to treat incontinence, or to manage hydronephrosis, vesicoureteric reflux, or recurrent urinary tract infection resulting from poor bladder compliance or inadequate bladder emptying. Although catheterization can be performed safely even in infants, Blocksom's technique for cutaneous vesicostomy, popularized by Duckett (1974) has become an effective alternative for dealing with the poorly emptying neuropathic bladder and its secondary effects on the urinary tract, particularly in infants. The Blocksom technique utilizes a small transverse skin incision placed halfway between the pubic symphysis and umbilicus; exposure and isolation of the bladder dome from peritoneum, urachus, and umbilical vessel remnants; and creation of a small stoma after resection of a button of detrusor. The vesicostomy in effect acts as a pop-off valve, lowering intravesical volume and pressure, while allowing the bladder to maintain some urine storage, and in many instances to allow voiding per urethra. The decision as to whether vesicostomy drainage will provide satisfactory bladder and upper-tract decompression can be made by visualizing marked improvement of the radiographic appearance of the upper urinary tracts after bladder catheterization (a vesicostomy equivalent) (Fig. 53-6). The decision to perform a cutaneous vesicostomy in preference to intermittent catheterization, or when catheterization fails to effectively decompress the upper urinary tract, must be made on clinical grounds and seems most warranted in the infant or small child with moderate or severe hydronephrosis or reflux and worrisome urodynamic parameters. Management is simple with routine diapering, and the demands of a catheterization program are not imposed on caretakers (Cohen et al., 1978). The vesicostomy can be managed in children with orthoses, even those with orthoplast jackets or braces with pelvic bands, if minor orthotic adjustments are made. Adequate continence without diapers may be achieved with a pad and belt combination in older children if urethral leakage does not occur, and routine stomal appliances may be used effectively, although occasional leakage may be problematic since the vesicostomy is located in an area of skin that may crease when the child sits.

Vesicostomy and intermittent catheterization have been equated in terms of upper-tract preservation

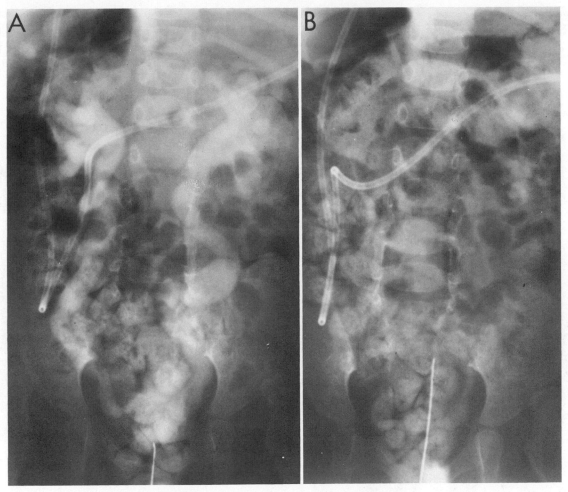

FIG. 53-6
IVP with full bladder and after bladder catheterization.

(Bruce and Gonzales, 1980). Plunkett and Braren (1979) described stable upper tracts in 82% and improved upper tracts in 15% of patients managed by intermittent catheterization, with 6% incidence of pyelonephritis. Cass (1976) documented an 87.5% incidence of stable upper tracts, improvement in 12.5%, stable or improved VUR in 75%, and persistently sterile urine in 90% of patients on intermittent catheterization. However, Duckett (personal communication) reported that 54% of patients on a regimen of CIC developed upper-tract deterioration (most by 3 years of age), while 85% of patients managed with vesicostomy had complete resolution of hydronephrosis and the remainder were stabilized. No patient with a functioning vesicostomy showed upper-tract changes. It is likely that the failure of CIC in many cases is a failure of patient, parents, or caretakers to comply with the rigorous schedule that catheterization demands, especially when it must be performed on a strict schedule in order to prevent upper-tract deterioration. Finding a caretaker to provide these services in school or when the parents work may be an additional source

of stress for a family struggling already with the demands of a handicapped infant.

Complications of vesicostomy are not uncommon but are generally minor and easily managed (Horwitz and Ehrlich, 1983). Snyder (1983) reported 3 patients with bladder calculi, 6 patients who required reoperation for stenosis or prolapse, and 1 patient requiring stomal catheterization for stenosis among a group of 48 patients. Severe prolapse is extremely rare, but minor mucosal prolapse requiring no revision occurs frequently, whereas stomal stenosis, even to a severe degree, usually continues to allow adequate urinary tract decompression, with revision being unnecessary. Unless the vesicostomy is created during an acute episode of cystitis, bladder capacity is maintained during the period of diversion (Snyder, 1983). Vesicostomy closure combined with ureteral reimplantation if necessary, timed to coincide with institution of a planned self-catheterization program, is the outlook for most patients who undergo cutaneous vesicostomy. Long-term vesicostomy drainage has been used in patients unable to perform self-catheterization, usually

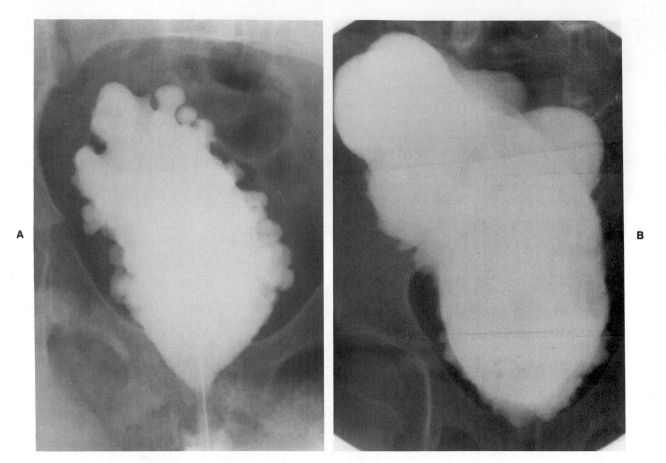

FIG. 53-7
A, Cystogram pre-enterocystoplasty. **B,** Cystogram post-enterocystoplasty.

severely handicapped individuals with poor bowel control who must be managed in diapers. In these individuals, a vesicostomy, although not providing continence, may provide upper-tract stability and ease of management without the need for catheterization.

Bladder Augmentation

Enterocystoplasty

Children with hydronephrosis, reflux, or incontinence due to diminished vesical compliance and/or capacity may fail to improve continence or stabilize upper tracts in spite of an optimal trial of intermittent catheterization and pharmacotherapy. Treatment options include bladder augmentation (with or without continent diversion, with or without bladder neck revision, with or without ureteral reimplantation) or cutaneous urinary diversion (Fig. 53-7). When bladder augmentation is being considered, several prerequisites are important. Urodynamic studies should confirm diminished capacity and/or compliance. If hydronephrosis or reflux is thought to be due to bladder dysfunction, catheter drainage should improve the appearance of the upper-tract fullness. The function and adequacy of the bladder outlet should be assessed. An adequate intermittent catheterization program should

be in place (Mitchell et al., 1986). Finally, the patient should have adequate bowel length and function to permit exclusion of a segment long enough to satisfy the need for increased bladder capacity. Small bowel, colon, and stomach have been the material of choice for bladder augmentation, which gained popularity for the treatment of neurovesical dysfunction after the introduction of intermittent catheterization eliminated concerns about bladder emptying (Raezer et al., 1985; Smith et al., 1977). Although the choice of bowel segment remains controversial, it is imperative that the native bladder is either widely bisected from just above the bladder neck to trigone or is resected to a level just above the trigone, and that enough bowel is used to provide adequate capacity and low intravesical pressure. Failure to prepare the bladder base in this manner prior to augmentation may cause the intestinal segment to act as a diverticulum of the bladder, minimizing the effectiveness of the procedure. Making optimal use of the shortest bowel segment that will be adequate for the patient's specific needs not only ensures a successful augmentation, but also reduces the potential for malabsorption and electrolyte disturbances. Detubularization of bowel segments produces geometrical changes that alter capacity, ac-

TABLE 53-3

Ultimate Augmentation Volume of Small Bladders Enlarged with Bowel Segments of Different Dimensions

Bladder Volume (cc)	+ Bowel Length (cm)	Bowel Radius (cm)	= Augmentation Volume (cc)
50	20	1	250
50	30	1	382
50	40	1	532
50	50	1	697
50	60	1	877
50	10	1	250
50	20	2	532
50	30	2	877
100	10	1	203
100	20	1	327
100	30	1	470
100	40	1	630
100	50	1	804
100	10	2	327
100	20	2	630
100	30	2	992
150	10	1	380
150	20	1	530
150	30	1	695
150	40	1	875
150	10	2	530
150	20	2	875

From Koff SA: *J Urol* 1988, 130:1150.

commodation, and compliance of the bladder reservoir in a manner that improves both its storage characteristics and effect on the upper tracts. The geometrical advantage of detubularization is dependent upon the geometry of the volume of a cylinder ($\pi r^2 \times$ length) (McDougal, 1987) compared to the volume of a sphere ($\frac{4}{3} \pi r^3$) (Koff, 1988). Koff has tabulated the theoretical increase in bladder volume that can be expected when various lengths of small and large bowel are detubularized prior to augmentation (Table 53-3).

Detubularization produces other beneficial effects for the bladder reservoir. Hinman (1988) has shown that accommodation, compliance, and contractility are also altered. Accommodation (increase in bladder volume without a significant increase in pressure) is related to the radius of the reservoir, and, at any given pressure, a reservoir with a larger radius will accommodate more volume. Compliance (the ratio of change in volume to change in pressure) is an important facet of bladder augmentation in most cases. Compliance is related to the viscoelastic properties of the reservoir wall, and thus may change over time as the wall stretches and relaxes. Peristaltic activity of intestinal smooth muscle is both phasic and tonic, and is thought to be a cause of incontinence after intestinocystoplasty in some patients (King et al., 1984). Detubularization effectively interrupts the normally coordinated activity of the intestinal musculature. The more complicated the folding process that is carried out, the more disorganized and blunted the bowel contractions become. Sidi and associates (1986) compared the clinical and urodynamic results of enterocystoplasty in patients with tubular-sigmoid, intact-ileocecal, and sigmoid-cup-patch augmentations, and found better continence and lower pressures in the cup-patch (detubularized) group, a finding confirmed by others using ileum.

disorganized and blunted the bowel contractions become. Sidi and associates (1986) compared the clinical and urodynamic results of enterocystoplasty in patients with tubular-sigmoid, intact-ileocecal, and sigmoid-cup-patch augmentations, and found better continence and lower pressures in the cup-patch (detubularized) group, a finding confirmed by others using ileum.

Persistent incontinence secondary to peristaltic activity of the bowel segment may be treated with anticholinergic medication or smooth-muscle relaxants. In severe cases, enteroplasty, using a second bowel segment as a patch to interrupt the peristaltic activity of the primary bowel reservoir segment, can be considered.

Gastrocystoplasty has been advocated as an alternative form of enterocystoplasty to minimize electrolyte imbalance and urea reabsorption, especially in patients with chronic renal failure (Adams et al., 1988). The net excretion of hydrogen and chloride into the urine from gastric segments is beneficial in the face of metabolic acidosis due to renal failure, which may be worsened by the use of small or large bowel segments which absorb hydrogen and chloride ions. Gastrocystoplasty, however, is not free from complications. Gosalbez and colleagues (1993) reported two patients with severe intractable hypochloremic hypokelemic metabolic alkalosis, one with an intractable seizure disorder, and one with respiratory depression and alteration in mental status. Hypergastrinemia has been reported in other patients (Tiffany et al., 1986). Nguyen and associates (1993) described the syndrome of dysuria and hematuria in 36% of 57 patients after gastrocystoplasty. The syndrome is defined as one or more of the following symptoms: bladder spasm or suprapubic, penile, or periurethral pain; coffee-colored or red urine without infection; skin irritation or excoriation and dysuria without infection. Patients particularly at risk are those with diminished renal function and those with incontinence. Treatments have included observation, baking soda, and omeprazole, an inhibitor of the hydrogen-potassium ion adenosine triphosphate (ATP) pump (Nguyen et al., 1993).

Mucus production, alteration of bowel function, diarrhea, electrolyte imbalance, the formation of bladder calculi, spontaneous bladder rupture, and malignancy are other reported complications of enterocystoplasty, the incidence varying with the intestinal segment used. Mucus production, generally considered to be a minor nuisance, has been linked to outlet obstruction and spontaneous bladder perforation (Haupt et al., 1990). Daily irrigation with saline is usually sufficient to prevent complications, although acetylcysteine has been administered orally (700 mg, 4 times daily) and intravesically (30 cc of a 20% solution) (Benderev, 1988), and urea has been used (30 cc of a 40% solution left indwelling overnight) with success (Bushman and Howards, 1994). Diarrhea may be a transient effect of enterocystoplasty, engendered by both the removal of absorptive surface and the bowel preparation prior to surgery. In patients with neuropathic bowel dysfunction, the function of the ileocecal valve is particularly important, since intractable diarrhea has been reported after ileocecal cystoplasty. The use of this segment should be avoided in these patients.

Urinary calculus formation is reported in 30% to 52.5% of patients after enterocystoplasty, most stones occurring in the bladder. Risk factors appear to be urinary tract infection, mucus formation, and the use of both absorbable and nonabsorbable staples (Haupt et al., 1990). Palmer and colleagues (1993) have implicated hypocitraturia as a contributing factor, and, in a preliminary statement, suggest that oral citrate supplementation has diminished the risk of new and recurrent stone formation. Bladder stones have been managed by bladder irrigation, and transurethral and open surgical techniques. Some authors feel that the open surgical technique lessens the risk of recurrent stone formation from stone fragments (Blyth et al., 1992).

Although bladder perforation secondary to intermittent catheterization has been reported, incidents are rare in the nonaugmented bladder. However, a growing body of literature has documented delayed "spontaneous" bladder rupture after enterocystoplasty (Elder et al., 1988). Bauer and colleagues (1992) reported 15 spontaneous perforations in 12 of 264 children who underwent enterocystoplasty using small bowel, large bowel, and stomach. All sites of rupture were located in the bowel itself, at or near the junction of the bladder and the enteral patch. Ischemic necrosis is thought to play a role in the mechanism of rupture, and suture granulomas were found in the reservoir wall near the site of rupture. Rosen and Light (1991) reported similar findings and concluded that a common factor was a high outlet resistance. Crane and colleagues (1991) postulated that chronic overdistension leads to vascular compromise and ischemia. The lack of sensation of bladder filling, mucus plugs, and noncompliance with routine catheterization schedules may contribute to spontaneous rupture. A significant percentage of patients suffering spontaneous rupture have died. Recommendations for prevention include daily bladder irrigation and prevention of overdistension, especially in patients who have a competent bladder outlet or who have under-

gone a surgical procedure to increase outlet resistance. Spontaneous bladder rupture should be part of the differential diagnosis of the acute abdomen in all patients after enterocystoplasty. Differential diagnosis may be difficult because of abnormal abdominal and visceral sensation. Sonography may demonstrate increased peritoneal fluid. Although cystography should be performed, a normal cystogram, even when the bladder is filled with considerable pressure, does not rule out rupture. If spontaneous rupture is suspected as a cause of an acute abdominal catastrophe, prompt laparotomy is indicated.

The occurrence of neoplasia at the ureterocolonic anastomosis is a recognized risk of ureterosigmoidostomy (Stewart et al., 1982). A report of malignancy after bladder augmentation has raised concern about the long-term outlook for children after enterocystoplasty. (Grainger et al., 1988) Filmer and Spencer (1990) tabulated 14 cases of malignancy arising between 5 and 29 years after augmentation. Patient ages were from 42 to 69 years at the time of tumor discovery. Tumor types were transitional cell carcinoma (3), adenocarcinoma (8), signet ring carcinoma (1), sarcoma (1), and oat cell carcinoma (1). The pathogenesis of these lesions is likely multifactorial, and surveillance cystoscopy appears to be warranted, beginning approximately 10 years after augmentation.

Two clinical concerns face the urologist considering bladder augmentation in patients with neurovesical dysfunction: assessment of the bladder outlet, and treatment of vesicoureteric reflux. Assessment of the bladder outlet is particularly important in patients with myelodysplasia who commonly display bladder neck incompetence (Gonzalez and Sidi, 1985). If bladder augmentation is to be performed in these children, preoperative assessment is important to determine whether a simultaneous continence procedure should be carried out at the bladder neck. Appropriate evaluation of bladder neck competence can be made by fluoroscopic examination of the bladder neck during videocystography or videourodynamic evaluation with the patient in the upright or semi-upright position (Fig. 53-8) (Kreder and Webster, 1982). Valsalva and Credé should be used as a provocative maneuver if the bladder neck is closed during filling. An open bladder neck indicates the need for a simultaneous continence procedure. Cher and Allen (1993) prefer to assess the need for bladder neck revision urodynamically, and have found that a bladder outlet resistance that exceeds 25 to 30 cm H_2O will be sufficient to prevent postoperative incontinence after enterocystoplasty. Vesicoureteric reflux that occurs as a result of poor bladder compliance may be refractory to intermittent catheterization and pharmacotherapy, and is seen in many patients who become candidates for bladder augmentation.

The decision whether or not to perform simultaneous ureteral reimplantation is an important one, because reimplantation can be technically difficult in abnormal bladders, and yet may resolve spontaneously after bladder augmentation. Historical data are important, because reflux that develops secondary to abnormal bladder function can be expected to reverse following augmentation (Nasrallah and Aliabadi, 1991). When historical data document primary reflux; when cystoscopy or operative examination reveals disordered ureterovesical anatomy, parautereric weak-

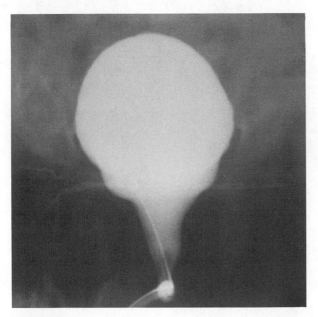

FIG. 53-8
Voiding cystourethrogram in a boy with myelomeningocele demonstrates an incompetent bladder neck (intrinsic sphincter deficiency).

ness, or nonexistent submucosal tunnels; and when indications for reimplantation are marginal, simultaneous reimplantation should be performed.

When enterocystoplasty has been performed in childhood, long-term follow-up is important. A concern has been the effect of such surgery on pregnant females and how this might alter the management of pregnancy and delivery. Hill and Kramer (1990) surveyed 15 pregnancies after enterocystoplasty. Urinary tract infection or pyelonephritis occurred in 60%, independent of the presence of reflux. Four patients experienced pre-term labor. No incontinence occurred in patients who were delivered vaginally if there had been no prior bladder neck incontinence procedure. It is recommended that cesarean section be performed on patients with a prior bladder neck reconstruction, but vaginal delivery appears generally safe if only enterocystoplasty was performed.

Autoaugmentation and Ureterocystoplasty

The reported complications of enterocystoplasty have led researchers and clinicians to continue to search for viable alternative means of increasing bladder capacity and compliance. Although patches of peritoneum, skeletal muscle, de-epithelialized bowel, bowel adventitia, and others have been reported, only autoaugmentation (Cartwright and Snow, 1989) and ureterocystoplasty (Bellinger, 1993; Churchill et al., 1993) have had reproducible clinical success. Autoaugmentation (detrusor myotomy) is best suited for bladders with reasonable capacity that require a modest improvement in capacity and compliance (Fig. 53-9). The procedure can be performed extraperitoneally, and involves using cautery and sharp and blunt dis-

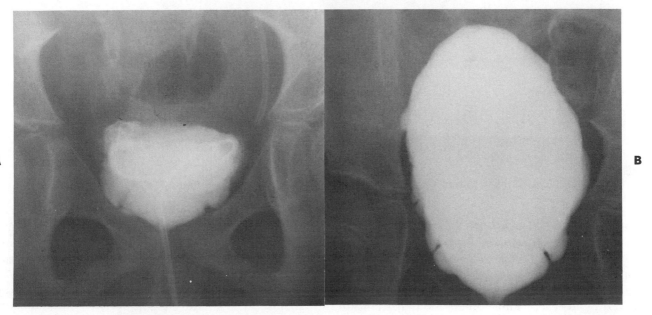

A   B

FIG. 53-9
A, Cystogram pre-autoaugmentation. **B,** Cystogram post-autoaugmentation.

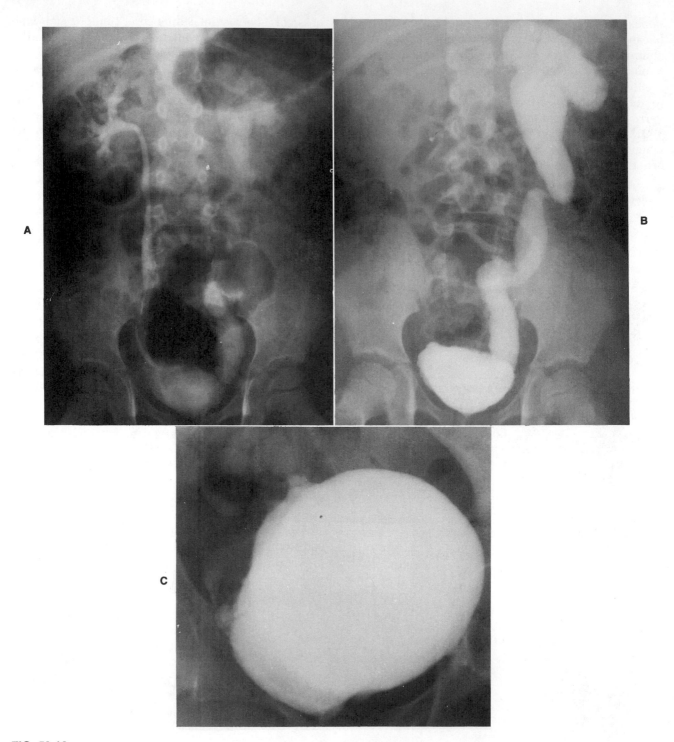

FIG. 53-10
A, IVP pre-ureterocystoplasty: poorly functioning left kidney. **B,** Cystogram pre-ureterocystoplasty. **C,** Cystogram post-ureterocystoplasty.

section to tease muscle fibers from the mucosa. Surgery is performed with a bladder catheter in place, varying the degree of bladder filling to assist dissection. When half to two thirds of the detrusor has been teased off, the muscle is excised. Although not successful in all cases, autoaugmentation does not interfere with subsequent enterocystoplasty if this subsequently proves necessary. Thus it seems to be a

sensible procedure to attempt if there is reasonable consideration that it will improve bladder dynamics. Autoaugmentation has been performed laparoscopically in a small number of patients.

Ureterocystoplasty is a newly described procedure that by its very nature is appropriate for only a limited number of patients (Bellinger, 1993; Churchill et al., 1993). Prerequisites are either a dilated ureter with a significant volume that is estimated to provide a significant additional increment to bladder capacity, or a refluxing megaureter that has already proven its ability to serve as a pop-off mechanism to protect the contralateral kidney from development of hydronephrosis or reflux (Fig. 53-10). The technique may include nephrectomy if the refluxing kidney has poor function, or transureteroureterostomy if function is salvageable. The donor ureter (and renal pelvis if it is large) is mobilized carefully, preserving all adventitial and collateral vessels. The ureter is then divided along its antimesenteric border, the incision taken through the ureteral orifice and continuing to bisect the bladder in the midline or diagonally, as in enterocystoplasty. The detubularized ureter is folded upon itself and sewn into the bladder defect as in enterocystoplasty. Simultaneous procedures such as contralateral ureteral reimplantation or appendicovesicostomy may be performed. As with autoaugmentation, the main advantage of the procedure is the ability to avoid incorporating extra-urinary mucosa into the urinary tract.

Treatment of Detrusor Hyperreflexia
Sacral Rhizotomy

Selective sacral rhizotomy as a treatment for detrusor hyperreflexia was developed after early experience with bilateral rhizotomy resulted in an unacceptable incidence of impotence and bowel dysfunction. Selective dorsal rhizotomy has received little attention in the daily management of detrusor hyperreflexia, but several centers have developed expertise, and long-term data are becoming available. Gasparini and colleagues (1992) reported follow-up over a mean of 32 months in patients with cervical and thoracic spinal cord injury. They found no adverse effects, and a 94% improvement in continence. Storrs (1987) combined untethering of the cord with selective posterior rhizotomy in two children with myelomeningocele and reported success in both. There is still uncertainty as to the place of sacral rhizotomy in the treatment of detrusor hyperreflexia.

Intrathecal Baclofen

Oral therapy for spasticity resulting from neurological disease has proven unsuccessful in large part because the systemic actions of the medications produce generalized weakness but are unable to sufficiently diminish spasticity. Intrathecal baclofen has been used successfully for patients with cerebral palsy or spinal cord injury (Albright et al., 1991). Investigators have been encouraged by this experience, and some data is available on the effect of intrathecal Baclofen on bladder and sphincter function. Nanninga and associates (1989) studied seven patients with spasticity secondary to spinal cord injury, and found a decrease in sphincter activity that paralleled a general decrease

in spasticity. Six of the seven patients demonstrated an increased bladder capacity, and an improved continence was seen in the majority.

Incontinence: Increasing Outlet Resistance

Diminished outlet resistance is a common problem for patients with neurovesical dysfunction, especially in cases of myelodysplasia. Appropriate evaluation of bladder neck competence can be made by upright fluoroscopic examination of the bladder neck during cystography or videourodynamic evaluation (Gonzalez and Sidi, 1985). Valsalva and Credé should be used as a provocative maneuver if the bladder neck is closed during filling. Electromyographic studies can also be used to assess neuromuscular activity of the pelvic floor and periurethral musculature. An open bladder neck may indicate that intrinsic sphincter weakness is the cause of incontinence, but bladder compliance and capacity must also be taken into consideration, because bladder augmentation may be indicated.

When outlet resistance is diminished, pharmacotherapy should be initiated prior to considering surgical intervention (see Table 53-1). Ephedrine, propanolamine, and imipramine are the most common agents used in the pediatric age group, and they are commonly administered in conjunction with anticholinergic or smooth-muscle relaxing agents in order to achieve continence with a program of intermittent catheterization. The catheterization trial affords the urologist a period of time prior to surgical intervention to ensure that the child and family are committed to a rigorous program of catheterization.

When surgical intervention is chosen to correct an incompetent urethral sphincter, many options are available. These can be grouped into procedures for urethral lengthening, urethral suspension, and urethral compression. Within each category, many alternatives and modifications exist (Table 53-3). The sheer number and variety of procedures that have been proposed, each with its proponents and detractors, attests to the fact that a perfect continence mechanism has yet to be described. It is important to recognize that detrusor behavior is frequently altered after bladder neck reconstruction, the detrusor displaying diminished compliance and instability that may result in upper-tract deterioration (Murray et al., 1988). Preoperative urodynamic evaluation in all patients should include a provocative cystometrogram. Woodside and McGuire (1982) described the use of a balloon catheter to occlude the vesical neck during the preoperative cystometrogram if urethral leakage occurs. After performing a routine cystometrogram, the study is repeated using a balloon catheter inflated at the bladder neck to simulate increased outlet resistance. Increased detrusor pressure or instability is worrisome and raises the question of whether pharmacological (anticholinergic) or surgical (bladder augmentation) intervention to improve detrusor compliance will be necessary in conjunction with or subsequent to the bladder neck procedure.

Urethral lengthening procedures in common use have been described by Young (1922), Dees (1949), Leadbetter (1964) and, more recently, by Kropp and Angwafo (1986). The Young-Dees-Leadbetter procedure incorporates proximal reimplantation of the ureters and tubularization of the trigone to afford additional urethral length. A urethral length of 3 to 4 cm should be obtained, and the mucosa tubularized over a small 5 F or 8 F catheter with a pants-over vest or modified closure of the muscularis. Jones and colleagues (1993) reported a 9% continence failure rate and a 27% reoperation rate after using a modification of this technique. Kropp and Angwafo (1986) described a novel procedure using a detrusor tube reimplanted into a submucosal trigonal tunnel. They reported continence in 20 of 24 (80%) of patients. Belman and Kaplan (1989) reported a 78% success rate with this technique. The most common postoperative problem in this group was difficult urethral catheterization. Bladder neck suspension procedures are frequently performed in conjunction with urethral lengthening.

Urethral suspension for outlet deficiency is routinely performed for incontinence of many types, including neurovesical dysfunction. Common techniques include suprapubic suspension (Gearhart and Jeffs, 1988; Raz et al., 1988) and variations of the periurethral and puboprostatic fascial sling. Bauer and colleagues (1989) reported dryness in 72% of girls after a sling procedure, and Elder (1990) achieved dryness in 9 of 10 girls and 4 of 4 boys after a combined sling and augmentation procedure. Decter (1993) found 90% immediate postoperative dryness, but some increased wetness with time. There was no difference in success whether rectus fascia or fascia lata was used. Three patients had difficulty catheterizing postoperatively, and three required bladder augmentation because of postoperative upper-tract deterioration.

Urethral compression for incontinence is most often achieved by artificial sphincter implantation or submucosal injection therapy. The artificial urinary sphincter has proved valuable in achieving continence in a highly select group of children with neurovesical dysfunction. Before sphincter placement is considered, it is mandatory to have a low-pressure, compliant bladder. This may be achieved by pharmacologic therapy or may require augmentation cystoplasty (Murray et al., 1988). Gonzalez and Sheldon (1982) implanted sphincters in 10 boys and 5 girls aged 5 to 17 years. Nine boys achieved continence over an average of 51 months, but only one girl was continent.

Erosions occurred in girls whose bladder necks were violated during surgery. Kroovand (1983) noted that 37 of 44 (84%) of his patients were dry, 5 of 44 (11%) had stress incontinence, and 3 of 44 (7%) developed erosions. In this group, 20 sphincter replacements were necessary because of mechanical failure, and the 44 patients underwent a total of 99 surgical procedures during the period of study. Bosco and colleagues (1991) followed 36 consecutive children for at least 5 years after artificial sphincter implantation and found 75% of the sphincters still functioning. The most common complication requiring reoperation was leakage of fluid from the sphincter mechanism. The overall continence rate was 84% at 2 years and 62% at 5 years. The success rate was best with the newest model sphincters. Jumper and associates (1991) found no evidence that the artificial sphincter cuff interfered with sexual development or function, or with prostate growth or morphology in the growing child with myelodysplasia. Barrett and colleagues (1991) demonstrated that particle shedding from implanted silicone devices does occur, with foreign-body granuloma formation seen in local tissues and regional lymph nodes. Reinberg and associates (1993) studied six children after artificial sphincter implantation and found silicone particles in the peri-sphincteric tissue but not in the regional lymph nodes. The clinical significance of this phenomenon is uncertain.

Endoscopic submucosal injection therapy is a relatively new approach to the treatment of intrinsic sphincter deficiency. The purpose of injection therapy is to provide a mechanism for coaptation of the bladder neck and proximal urethra in patients whose open proximal urethra allows increases in intra-abdominal pressure to be transmitted directly to the urethra and external sphincter. Polytetrafluoroethylene (Teflon paste), collagen, and autologous fat have been utilized. Teflon is an inert substance that cannot be broken down by the body. Vorstman and associates (1985) reported on 11 children who were treated with one or more periurethral or transperineal injections of Teflon paste. Four girls had neurovesical dysfunction, and two became dry on intermittent catheterization after injection therapy. In this series, large volumes of Teflon paste (5 to 21 ml) were used. Other series have found similar results, but the use of Teflon in children has come into disfavor because of the local inflammatory reaction at the injection site, and migration of Teflon particles to distant organs. Brown and colleagues (1991) carried out histological examination of 32 ureters that were subjected to ureteral reimplantation after submucosal injection of Teflon paste to treat VUR. Four ureters were subsequently found to have granulomatous polyps at the site of injection. When the Teflon was injected into the proper submucosal plane, it remained encapsulated and incited a minimal foreign-body reaction; however, this was the case in only 3 of 27 ureters that had persistence of VUR, while the remainder were found to have diffuse localization of the Teflon and an increased inflammatory reaction. Malizia and colleagues (1984) injected Teflon paste periurethrally in female dogs and male monkeys. At pathological examination 10½ months later, Teflon particles were found at the injection site and in lymph nodes, lungs, kidney, and brain. The pathological findings at these sites were characterized as a pronounced chronic inflammatory reaction with giant cells. Based on these data, the authors advised against use of this material in children, a point of view held by many urologists in this country.

Glutaraldehyde cross-linked collagen has been released for the treatment of intrinsic sphincter deficiency. Animal experiments have shown that the collagen becomes integrated with the surrounding tissue and produces no foreign-body reaction. Wan and associates (1992) reported on 8 children treated with collagen, 6 of whom had neurovesical dysfunction. A total of 17 injections were required (average 2.1 injections per patient) at an average volume per treatment of 10.9 ml. Continence was produced in 63% of patients, and another 25% improved. Similar improvement was seen by Shortliffe and colleagues (1989), but no long-term data are yet available. Collagen seems to be a safer material in terms of migration, but sensitivity to the material is reported, and all patients must undergo skin testing one month prior to injection therapy. If the skin test is reactive, implant placement is contraindicated.

Santarosa and Blaivas (1994) reported on the use of autologous fat for injection in adults with intrinsic sphincter deficiency. No data are yet available on long-term results of the use of this procedure in children.

Continence Alternatives

Although intermittent catheterization has become the primary mode of bladder management for many children with neurovesical dysfunction, institution of a bladder catheterization program provides dryness in only 24% to 49% of reported series (Cass et al., 1985; Purcell and Gregory, 1984; Wolraich et al., 1983). Modern urological management has provided an excellent outlook for renal function in most children, and social acceptance and freedom from odor, wetness, and embarrassment have become realistic goals for most children and their families, with an overall social continence of 80% (McLone, 1992; Myers et al., 1981). Lindehall and associates (1994) found that, even when complete dryness was not achieved, adolescents and young adults were encouraged by diminished wetness and less likelihood of embarrassing incontinence. Individualized and sometimes innovative continence alternatives have become part of the urologic arma-

mentarium, and it is extremely important that urologists separate medical and social indications for bladder manipulation, particularly when major surgical procedures will be involved.

Diapering is the usual management for infants and may be appropriate for incontinent older children who are severely handicapped and unable to provide self care, especially if effective bowel control is lacking. Institutionalized children are frequently managed in this way. Older children who are incontinent in spite of an intermittent catheterization program may prefer changing diapers to catheterizing and still being wet, or to surgical intervention and catheterization. As long as normal upper tracts are maintained, spontaneous voiding is a reasonable alternative if wetness can be managed to the satisfaction of the child and caretakers. The only contraindication to this management scheme is children with an elevated leak-point pressure and poor vesical compliance who might develop upper tract deterioration if a catheterization regimen is altered or stopped.

Aggressive management of urinary incontinence requires that a satisfactory program for bowel continence be established prior to bladder training. The development of an effective bowel regimen is not an overnight process, and should be started at a young age in all children with neurovesical dysfunction. Once established, however, an effective bowel program may provide encouragement for bladder training in children.

The definition of what comprises an appropriate program for management of urinary continence will depend upon the desires, social awareness, and individual concerns of each patient and caretakers. For many children, diapering is appropriate. Children on a catheterization program with minimal dampness between catheterizations should be encouraged to discard diapers. Occasional dampness may be managed by underwear and a sanitary napkin worn in case of accidents, avoiding the use of a bulky diaper. Condom urinary drainage is feasible in boys with adequate penile length and diameter and may provide socially acceptable continence when bladder emptying is adequate and bowels are well-managed. Skin irritations and major penile trauma may occur, and the caretaker and child must be admonished against tight application or prolonged application of condom devices without skin examination (Jayachandran et al., 1985). Ideally, the condom should be changed daily. For small boys with persistent incontinence who do not want immediate surgical intervention, we have devised a modified condom drainage that has been successful using stomal adhesive at the base of the penis. External sphincterotomy has been used in conjunction with condom urinary drainage in boys with spina bifida, but this procedure creates a permanent incontinence that can be corrected only surgically, so it is rarely used in children (Koontz et al., 1972). External urinary collection devices have been designed for females, although satisfactory dryness has been achieved in a small number of adult patients in a few clinical series. Data for children are anecdotal.

The creation of a continent vesicostomy using detrusor tubes as catheterizable stomas never achieved a significant degree of success in adults or children. Appendicovesicostomy, as described by Mitrofanoff (1980), and its subsequent popularization by several authors (Dykes et al., 1991; Sumfest et al., 1993), however, has made continent urinary diversion immediately applicable to the care of many children with neurovesical dysfunction. The Mitrofanoff principle, using a small-caliber conduit such as the appendix or a distal ureter in an antireflux fashion to provide a tiny catheterizable stoma, has been applied to the native bladder and to bladder replacement reservoirs (Elder, 1992; Sumfest et al., 1993). This technique was originally used in conjunction with surgical closure of the bladder neck, but in most cases is offered as an alternative to urethral catheterization when catheterization of the urethra is painful or difficult because of urethral stricture, introital anatomy, or physical handicap that makes access to the urethral meatus difficult. Many other applications of continent urinary diversion have been applied to the pediatric population (Hensle et al., 1990; Quinlan et al., 1991).

Urinary Diversion and Undiversion

Permanent cutaneous urinary diversion has become a therapy of last resort in the management of children with neurovesical dysfunction. Ileal conduit diversion, once considered a panacea to salvage kidneys from reflux and infection, has proved hazardous over time. Schwarz and Jeffs (1975) followed up 96 patients 2 to 16 years after diversion, finding that radiographic evidence of deterioration correlated with the span of diversion, and that stomal stenosis, excessive conduit length, and ureteroileal obstruction contributed to more rapid deterioration. Cass (1976) noted upper-tract deterioration in 16.5% of 50 children followed up longer than 10 years. Crooks and Enrile (1983) found transient upper-tract improvement after ileal diversion with later deterioration in 80% of patients, compared with stabilization or improvement in upper-tract appearance in children managed by intermittent catheterization. Nonrefluxing colon conduit diversion has been proposed to prevent the long-term effects seen with ileal conduits, although the hazards of operation are greater. Hill and Ransley (1983) reported stomal stenosis in 34%, upper-tract dilatation in 36%, and an overall complication rate of 81% in 47 children with colon conduit diversion. Husman and colleagues (1989) found an acceptable rate of upper-tract pres-

ervation, but voiced concern about the long-term effects of chronic bacteriuria. Clearly, permanent cutaneous diversion should be considered a therapy of last resort when dealing with children with neurovesical dysfunction.

Urinary undiversion was made possible by the application of bladder augmentation and reconstructive principles to urinary tracts previously subjected to either temporary or permanent urinary diversions (Hendren, 1976). The evaluation of a child for undiversion may include urography, cystography, retrograde or loopogram studies, determination of creatinine clearance, and urodynamic studies (Menon et al., 1982). However, the single most important aspect of evaluation, above and beyond that of bladder function, is that of the child's and family's expectations and motivation (Jeter, 1983).

Bladder storage may be assessed prior to undiversion by suprapubic or urethral catheter bladder cycling. An intermittent catheterization trial carried out at home for several weeks or months allows the urologist to assess not only the child's technical ability, but also his or her motivation to persist with this procedure for lifelong bladder management. To proceed with undiversion without this skill and motivation may commit the child to lifelong incontinence or to rediversion, since the bladder has simply been put back into its prediversion state. The unique psychosocial stresses that bring children to consider undiversion, and the expectations they hold, must also be weighed strongly before proceeding with surgery. Urinary undiversion or reconstruction may be carried out in carefully selected patients as preparation for renal transplantation when diversion has been previously performed for complications of neurovesical dysfunction (Gonzalez et al., 1984).

Transurethral Electrical Bladder Stimulation (TEBS)

In 1958, Katona first used transurethral electrical bladder stimulation (TEBS) for the treatment of neurovesical dysfunction secondary to spinal cord injury (Katona et al., 1975). He and his associates reported the results of TEBS therapy in a group of 100 children with myelodysplasia; 71% had attained day and night continence. TEBS has been popularized in the United States by Kaplan and Richards (1988) for neurovesical dysfunction in the pediatric myelomeningocele group. It is postulated that TEBS stimulates mural receptors that have remained dormant due to a lack of afferent innervation. Activation of the receptors triggers small detrusor contractions. Vegetative afferentation progresses, efferent pathways are facilitated, and both motor and sensory functions improve. Biofeedback training is then used to link sensation to detrusor contraction as micturition is learned. Reported beneficial

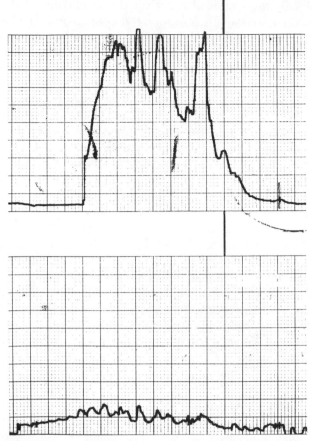

FIG. 53-11
Bladder pressure tracing demonstrating a detrusor contraction in response to transurethral intravesical bladder stimulation (upper tracing). Lower tracing reflects intra-abdominal (rectal) pressure.

effects have included improvement of bladder sensation, stimulation of detrusor contraction, increase in bladder capacity, and the establishment of urinary continence. Ebner and associates (1992) studied TEBS in a neurologically intact animal model and found that stimulation involved direct activation of mechanoreceptor afferents, which in turn elicited detrusor contractions.

TEBS therapy is very time consuming, necessitating daily 90-minute sessions. At least 30 sessions are needed to determine whether the patient might respond to therapy, and many patients have received over 100 stimulation sessions to achieve maximal results. Therapy is initiated after performing a baseline urodynamic evaluation and an initial test stimulation. Stimulation is performed after filling the bladder to one-half capacity with saline via a special electrode catheter. Electrical impulses are passed through the saline. Frequency, intensity, duration, and waveform of the impulse are varied over multiple sessions to produce an optimal result (detrusor contraction) (see Fig. 53-11).

Clinical experience with TEBS has been limited to a small group of patients at a few centers, and the results of therapy were initially encouraging. Lyne and Bellinger (1993) reported on a series of 17 patients who had undergone a total of 618 sessions of transurethral electrical bladder stimulation. All patients demonstrated detrusor contraction, and 88% had some degree of sensation of the contractions. Six patients showed a significant (14 to 58%) increase in bladder capacity during therapy, but in half of these a return to near-baseline capacity was noted after therapy was completed. No patient achieved voluntary micturition after therapy, but 29% experienced some improvement in bladder parameters, and one patient has had continued improvement in fecal continence. Decter and colleagues (1992) reported a similar experience in 21 patients with neurovesical dysfunction, finding limited encouraging results, but in a later report Decter has indicated that he has abandoned offering this therapy to patients due to lack of significant improvement in bladder function (Decter, 1994). Boone and associates (1992) carried out a prospective randomized clinical trial in 36 children over a 3-week period. They found no statistically significant increase in bladder capacity, detrusor activity, or bladder sensation during this short trial period. The discrepancy of reported results using this mode of therapy implies that further clinical trials are indicated.

The Management of Vesicoureteric Reflux

Vesicoureteric reflux (VUR) is found in 3% to 5% of neonates with myelomeningocele, and may develop in as many as 30% to 40% by 5 years of age secondary to high intravesical pressures and detrusor-sphincter dyssynergia. Bauer (1984) has shown that reflux is rarely seen in neonates unless abnormal bladder dynamics are found. Although Levitt and Sandler (1975) found no VUR in infants under 6 weeks of age, Stafford (1983) found reflux in 3 of 10 neonates studied. Gaum and colleagues (1982) studied 68 consecutive neonates. Of 55 patients with normal urograms, 14.5% had VUR; when urography was abnormal, 23% were found to have VUR. These data support the view that urography and sonography are insufficient to screen for VUR in the neonate with neurovesical dysfunction. Cass and associates (1985) followed 210 children over 15 years. Although 21% initially had reflux, in follow-up studies 38% were found to reflux eventually, pointing out the importance of periodic reevaluation. Reflux should always be considered when new-onset hydronephrosis is found. Although nuclear cystography is used for the follow-up evaluation of VUR in most cases, the anatomic detail offered by a routine contrast VCU makes it more applicable to patients with neurovesical dysfunction, even in follow-up. The VCU can be combined with urodynamic study in a fluorourodynamic study (video cystometrogram).

The management of VUR in neurologically intact children includes antimicrobial prophylaxis, repeated urine cultures, periodic reevaluation, and occasional surgical intervention. Management in children with neurovesical dysfunction must include appropriate attention to abnormal bladder and urethral dynamics that may promote secondary reflux. Although elevated intravesical pressures generated in the neuropathic bladder may be transmitted to the kidney in the presence of VUR, infection is the primary mediator of renal damage in the face of moderate VUR (Ransley and Risdon, 1978). All children with VUR must be maintained on long-term suppressive antibiotic therapy (Edwards et al., 1978; Lenaghan et al., 1978). In young children with minimal reflux, adequate bladder emptying, and persistently sterile urine, only urinary suppression and close surveillance are necessary. Moderate VUR (grades 2-3, International System) (International Reflux Committee, 1981) in young or older children with neurovesical dysfunction demands aggressive therapy. Urodynamic evaluation is important to assess whether pharmacotherapy is needed to improve vesical compliance, and CIC begun. If the social stiuation prohibits an effective catheterization program, or if catheterization fails to decompress the bladder adequately, cutaneous vesicostomy is performed. Kass and associates (1981) documented spontaneous resolution of VUR in 31% of ureters once CIC was instituted (100% in nondilated ureters and 0% in dilated ureters). Kaplan and Firlit (1983) found resolution of VUR in 62% of 200 children when CIC was instituted. Close bacteriologic surveillance and periodic radiologic follow-up are necessary in this group.

The surgical management of VUR in children with neurovesical dysfunction demands adequate bladder capacity, compliance, and emptying. The poor results of reimplantation in many early series (Hirsch et al., 1978; Johnston et al., 1976) have improved dramatically once bladder rehabilitation with antibiotics, pharmacologic therapy, intermittent catheterization, and bladder augmentation, if necessary, have been achieved. In severe cases with massive reflux, temporary vesicostomy may prove extremely valuable. Subsequent closure combined with ureteral reimplantation may be necessary if VUR persists. In general, indications for reimplantation are alike in normal and neuropathic bladders: persistent VUR in spite of adequate pharmacotherapy and intermittent catheterization, persistent infection (which may be a significant problem for a child on CIC), and upper-tract deterioration. Technically, any reimplantation technique may be used, but the technique of Cohen (1975) has been advocated, because a long tunnel can be achieved and dissection is on the trigone, which is usually less trabeculated than the remainder of the bladder. However, postoperative obstruction may be difficult to deal with if the Cohen technique is used (Lamesch, 1981). Suprapubic diversion and ureteral stents are routinely used when performing reimplantation in thickened neurogenic bladders. Using careful bladder management, Jeffs and colleagues (1976) corrected reflux in 33 of 37 children (89%) using the Paquin or Cohen technique. Kaplan and Firlit (1983) achieved 96% success in 40 ureters, and Woodard and associates (1981) accomplished successful reimplantation in 76% (83% in nontapered ureters and 33% in tapered ureters). Clearly, optimal bladder management contributes to success in reimplantation. On occasion, bladder augmentation may be a necessary adjunct to reimplantation in high-pressure, noncompliant bladders.

Submucosal injection therapy was introduced by O'Donnell and Puri in 1986, and was subsequently applied to children with neurovesical dysfunction by Puri (Puri and Guiney, 1986) and Kaplan (1991), who reported a success rate of 84% after one injection and 87% after two injections. Although Kaplan found no evidence of microscopic migration of Teflon particles to lymph nodes sampled at open surgery after Teflon injection, concern has been raised in animal studies (Malizia et al., 1984) (see previous section, Incontinence), and many authors have abandoned the use of this material for injection in children (Burns and Mitchell, 1991). Cendron and associates (1991) reported an overall success rate at 1 year of 65%, using cross-linked bovine dermal collagen injection for reflux. Although this material is currently available for the treatment of intrinsic sphincter deficiency, it has not been released for the treatment of VUR. The long-term efficacy and reactivity of collagen implant therapy is still to be determined.

Urinary Tract Infection

Although close surveillance of urinary tract infections is an important part of the management of children with vesicoureteric reflux, there is conflicting data regarding the utility of chronic antibacterial prophylaxis in children without VUR who are maintained on nonsterile intermittent catheterization. Bakke and Vollset (1993) studied 262 patients on intermittent catheterization and found persistently sterile urine in 28%, occasional bacteriuria in 44%, and chronic bacteriuria in 28%. Among those using chronic antibacterial prophylaxis, fewer episodes of bacteriuria but a greater number of clinical urinary tract infections were noted. Factors related to the presence of bacteriuria included high catheterization volumes and a low frequency of catheterization. Johnson and colleagues (1994) studied the efficacy of short-term nitrofurantion prophylaxis in 56 children during a 24-week double-blinded placebo-controlled crossover study. They found a diminished incidence of urinary tract infection in the treated group, but only a 76.9% compliance with medication usage and a 6% incidence of symptomatic urinary tract infection. It appears that routine antimicrobial prophylaxis is not indicated in patients managed with intermittent catheterization in the absence of VUR.

Associated Concerns

Bowel Incontinence

Bowel and urinary incontinence together present a tremendous handicap to normal social interaction for children with spina bifida. Although a great deal of effort is commonly expended to provide adequate urinary control, failure to provide a good bowel program may leave a child diaper-dependent. The purpose of establishing a bowel routine is to provide a method of periodic, effective bowel evacuation while preventing accidental soiling. An effective program must combine diet, controlled evacuation, and a well-regimented schedule (Chapman et al., 1979).

Diet is extremely important for management of fecal incontinence. Although infants generally have loose or soft stools, the addition of table foods to the diet commonly results in hard stools. In general, a high-fiber diet is successful in preventing hard stools, and this diet should be started in early childhood to encourage a lifetime dietary regimen. When necessary, medications may be added to provide increased stool water.

Manual stimulation, reflex stimulation by suppositories, or mechanical stimulation by enemas may provide the impetus for evacuation of the colon. Each child is an individual, and, as with bladder function, trial and error may be necessary to design an effective bowel program. For many children, saline or soapsuds expansion enemas given via a rubber ear syringe are remarkably effective, simple, and inexpensive (Chapman et al., 1979). Blair and colleagues (1992) have described the use of a new continence catheter. Whatever program is used for evacuation, it is important to start early, when the child can sit on the potty chair. Successful evacuation may be timed to occur after meals at the same time each day, in an unhurried atmosphere. Anorectal manometry has been described as a method of assessing the effect of neuromuscular dysfunction on the lower bowel and sphincters, and biofeedback training has been used with some success in myelodysplastic children (McLone, 1992; Wald, 1981). Malone and associates (1990) have reported on an innovative modification of the Mitrofanoff principle to provide a nonrefluxing catheterizable stoma for antegrade colonic enemas (ACE).

Sexuality

Normal sexual development may be altered in children with hydrocephalus. Meyer and Landau (1984), using hormonal data to document true isosexual precosity, have recognized that precocious puberty may occur in both male and female patients. Although the endocrinologic mechanisms are poorly understood, both parents and child will benefit from early discussion of normal adolescent development and menarche. Data on sexual function in spina bifida are poorly documented, much having been inferred from the spinal cord injury literature (Robin, 1980). Shurtleff (1983) described 80% erectile ability and 40% ejaculation in a survey of older spina bifida males. Eighty percent of women were sexually active, all describing satisfactory orgasms. In another series, 12 of 17 women having intercourse had become pregnant (Cass et al., 1986). Sexual counseling for preadolescents and adolescents is a valuable part of any total rehabilitation program, and children should be encouraged to attend regular sex education courses in school, from which they may otherwise be excluded because of the mistaken impression that all handicapped children are nonfunctional or sterile. Girls in particular must realize that their fertility is normal and that normal sexual function is possible. Thus knowledge of effective birth control is essential. Routine gynecologic examination should be encouraged in all girls, beginning at puberty.

Miscellaneous Urologic Concerns

Circumcision offers two significant advantages for many boys with neurovesical dysfunction: diminished risk of urinary tract infection and increased ease of performing catheterization. Fussell and colleagues (1988) have shown that human foreskin shows a propensity for adherence and colonization by pathogenic bacteria. Wiswell and Hachey (1993) confirmed the significance of bacterial adherence in boys, finding a tenfold increased incidence of urinary tract infections in uncircumcised boys in a group of 209,399 infants. They also reviewed the findings of other authors, who showed a risk of urinary tract infections in uncircumcised boys that ranged from 5 to 89 times greater than the risk for circumcised boys (Wiswell and Hachey, 1993). Removal of the foreskin thus not only exposes the meatus for technically easier catheterization, it also removes a contiguous source of periurethral skin colonization.

Cryptorchidism in spina bifida males is not uncommon (Kropp and Voeller, 1981). The management of these children should not differ from treatment plans for other boys.

Inguinal hernias (communicating hydroceles) may appear or worsen soon after ventriculoperitoneal

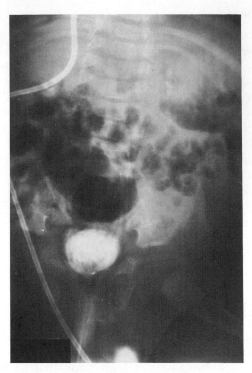

FIG. 53-12
Three-month-old boy with large communicating hydroceles.
At surgery, shunt tubing was found in the processus vaginalis.

shunting in infants. Kaufman and Carmel (1981) noted hydroceles in 7% of girls and 23% of boys younger than 1 year of age with shunts. They postulated that a combination of increased abdominal fluid and pressure, alteration in peritoneal membrane characteristics, and proximity of the shunt tubing to the inguinal canal influenced hydrocele formation. In some instances, the shunt tubing may migrate into the scrotum. (Fig. 53-12). Surgical repair is indicated in these children, and bilateral exploration should always be carried out in young children. Rarely, spinal fluid pseudocysts may be seen as abdominal masses and may cause urinary tract obstruction (Piercy et al., 1984).

The Tethered Spinal Cord

Normal growth of a child with spina bifida may produce alterations in gait, lower extremity strength and function, and bowel and bladder control, and may result in orthopedic deformities due to neuromuscular imbalance. This tethered cord syndrome may progress silently (Rigel, 1983). The cord, fixed abnormally by deformity and postsurgical scarring, may be placed on stretch with growth and activity, causing neurologic damage (Fig. 53-13). Cord tethering may also be seen with diastematomyelia, intraspinal lipomas, and dermoid tumors. Changes in bowel pattern, incontinence between catheterizations, or unexpected changes in

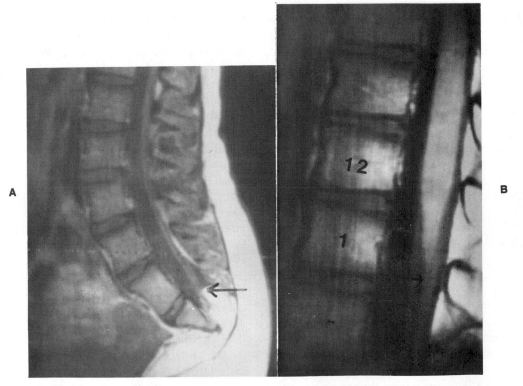

FIG. 53-13
A, MRI of normal lumbosacral spine. Conus *(arrow)* ends at L1. **B,** MRI of patient with tethered cord and partial sacral agenesis. Conus *(arrow)* ends at L5.

urinary control or bladder function should raise concern about cord tethering. Urodynamic studies should be performed to document change, and neurosurgical consultation should be requested to document other neurologic changes and consider whether imaging and surgical repair are indicated (Lais et al., 1993). Several series have shown that surgical correction of a tethered spinal cord may result in increased bladder capacity in some patients, while other patients show no change in bladder function, and some deteriorate. In many cases, postoperative urodynamic changes prove to be transitory (Kaplan et al., 1998).

Latex Allergy

IgE-mediated immediate hypersensitivity to latex is now a well-documented phenomenon that has been reported most often in children with myelodysplasia during surgery or other exposures to latex. Although delayed (type IV) hypersensitivity may be manifest as an eczematous contact dermatitis, immediate hypersensitivity to a yet undefined component of latex has ranged in severity from rhinitis and conjunctivitis to bronchospasm, anaphylaxis, and cardiovascular collapse (Gonzalez, 1992). The almost epidemic reporting of latex reactions in children with myelomeningocele is not readily explained; Schneck and Bellinger (1993) found 45% of patients tested to have hypersensitivity. It appears likely that previous allergic or cardiovascular episodes were attributed to other allergens or unknown causes, and that physicians are now attuned to the probability of latex hypersensitivity; thus many children now undergo prophylactic skin testing. It is assumed that recurrent exposure to latex-containing gloves, catheters, and other medical devices (Table 53-4) during multiple medical and surgical procedures sensitizes children at an early age, although many non-myelomeningocele children are exposed to latex via baby bottle nipples and pacifiers and have an apparently much lower incidence of hypersensitivity. It is speculated that exposure of peritoneal and mucosal surfaces as well as direct tissue exposure during surgery may heighten the development of hypersensitivity.

In the absence of a confirmed negative latex allergy test, all patients with myelomeningocele or other forms of spina bifida should be considered to have the potential for latex hypersensitivity. A high index of suspicion is important, and the identification of patients at risk begins with their medical history, including a history of urticarial reactions to common latex-containing products such as crib pads, rubber balls, and balloons. Patients at risk should undergo further definitive testing. Skin testing using colloidal suspensions of rubber particles is sensitive, but severe anaphylactic reactions may result. RAST (radioallergosorbent) testing, which measures the binding of IgE antibodies, has been used in many series. RAST testing has sensitivity ranging from 53% to 86%, with specificity of 76% (Slater, 1992). Schneck and Bellinger (1993) found reactivity to 3-antigen radioimmunoassay (RIA) latex-specific IgE to be a more sensitive test.

The identification of patients at risk, prophylactic avoidance of latex-containing products, and prompt treatment of hypersensitivity reactions are important to avoid life-threatening complications of latex allergy. When possible, children with spina bifida or other congenital anomalies who will be required to undergo multiple surgical procedures should be placed on a protocol of latex avoidance from birth. When latex hypersensitivity is documented, avoidance of latex-containing material should be practiced, and special precautions should be taken during medical and surgical procedures. If early signs of latex allergy are detected, removal of the latex device should occur immediately and systemic treatment of anaphylaxis begun (Kolski, 1988).

The Team Approach to Spina Bifida

The consequences of spina bifida may be medical, social, psychological, economic, and educational in scope (Dorner, 1973; Leonard, 1983). The medical consequences concern growth, developmental, general pediatric, neurologic, orthopedic, and urologic concerns, to name only the most basic. With such major concerns, the interdisciplinary approach to the child and family has advantages, the most practical being that one area will not be neglected inadvertently by the family, resulting in a major handicap for the child. Although the interdisciplinary concept has detractors (Pearson, 1983), it offers the urologist the nursing skills necessary to initiate and manage a bowel and bladder program, and to integrate this program

TABLE 53-4

Common Latex-containing Medical Devices
_____

- Electrocardiogram pads
- Tape
- Foley catheters
- Dilating catheters
- Surgical drains
- Nasogastric tubes
- Surgical/examination gloves
- Reservoir bags
- Blood pressure cuffs
- Tourniquets
- Face masks
- Ventilators, hoses, and bellows
- Injection ports of IV tubing and IV bags
- Stoppers in medication vials and syringes
- Floating disc valves on some IV burette chambers

From Pasquariello CA, Lowe DA, Schwartz RE: *Pediatrics* 1993, 91:985

with care of the child's other neurologic and orthopedic disabilities both at home and in school.

SACRAL AGENESIS

Complete or partial sacral agenesis is a rare anomaly that may occur as an isolated lesion or in conjunction with imperforate anus, cloacal anomalies, and the syndromes of caudal regression (Braren and Jones, 1983; Passarge and Lenz, 1966). Maternal diabetes mellitus is found in 12% to 18% of cases of sacral agenesis, and 1% of diabetic mothers have infants with sacral agenesis (Guzman et al., 1983). Although affected children are usually evident as neonates, Guzman and associates found only 50% in the newborn period, and it is not unusual for children to present at later ages with a lifelong history of urinary incontinence and encopresis.

Physical findings may include an absent gluteal cleft and abnormal contour to the buttocks. Sacral agenesis may be confirmed by anteroposterior and lateral spine films (Fig. 53-14), but the neurologic deficit may not correlate well with the bony defects noted. Many patients with isolated sacral agenesis have symptoms related only to bladder and bowel control. The high incidence of hydronephrosis or reflux in cases presenting late in childhood demands an early and complete uroradiologic and urodynamic evaluation of all children with documented sacral deformity (Braren and Jones, 1983). Urodynamic findings are extremely variable. Guzman and associates (1983) studied 16 patients, finding detrusor areflexia in 7 and hyperreflexia in 9, whereas sphincter EMG showed considerable variation in activity and variable dyssynergia. Therapy is based on clinical and urodynamic findings.

OCCULT SPINAL DYSRAPHISM

Anterior meningocele, lipoma, lipomeningocele, diastematomyelia, ligamentous bands, dermoid cysts, and congenital anomalies of the spinal cord itself may produce variable neurologic deficits, many primarily of neurovesical dysfunction (Borzyskowski and Neville, 1981). Such lesions should be considered when plain films display abnormal lumbosacral anatomy. Conversely, it is mandatory that the spine be examined carefully on radiographs of all children studied for incontinence or urinary tract infection. The physical examination of all children with urinary disorders should include a search of the lower back for skin tags, abnormal tufts of hair, lipomas, dermal sinuses, or pigmented lesions that may be associated with underlying pathologic conditions (Albright et al., 1989; Hall et al., 1981). Urodynamic studies may be necessary to document neurovesical dysfunction, because other neurologic tests may be completely normal. Foster found abnormal urodynamic findings to be the only sign of spinal cord tethering in 42% of 31 patients with lipomeningocele (Foster et al., 1990). If surgery is performed, postoperative urodynamic follow-up is important to document functional improvement or deterioration from the neurosurgical procedure itself. Gross and colleagues (1993) found an increase in bladder capacity in 10 of 17 patients, overall improvement

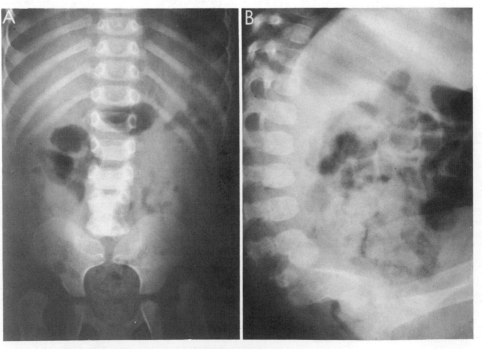

FIG. 53-14
Sacral agenesis.

in bladder function in 13, no change in 5, and deterioration in 3. In Rigel's series, after release of cord tethering, 3 patients originally thought to have permanent neurologic deficit improved, 5 of 9 with recent loss of bladder function recovered, and 17% lost bladder function after cord untethering (Rigel, 1983). Khoury and associates (1990) reported on a controversial group of 31 patients with secondary urinary incontinence who had resection of a thickened filum terminale. Incontinence resolved in 72%, urodynamic evidence of detrusor hyperreflexia improved in 59%, and bladder compliance improved in 66% after surgery, but the indications for surgical intervention were unclear. Clearly, appropriate urologic and urodynamic evaluation is extremely important in children with incontinence, and neurosurgical evaluation may be appropriate if urologic findings indicate the possibility of neurovesical dysfunction.

SPINAL CORD INJURY/TRANSVERSE MYELITIS

Transverse myelitis and traumatic spinal cord injuries are causes of neurovesical dysfunction that are uncommon in infants and small children, but not rare in adolescents. Infants may suffer spinal cord injury during traumatic delivery, and most other spinal cord injuries are secondary to automobile accidents, gunshot wounds, and diving accidents.

A child with an acute spinal cord injury commonly displays urinary retention, which may be a transient phenomenon, may persist for weeks or months, or may be permanent. Since most spinal cord trauma occurs above the level of the sacral reflex arc, urinary retention is frequently temporary. An indwelling bladder catheter is placed in most patients with spinal cord injury soon after the injury, but this should be replaced by intermittent catheterization as soon as the patient has been medically and surgically stabilized, and urine output is at a level at which intermittent catheterization can safely be performed frequently enough to prevent bladder overdistension and thus an additional myogenic component of urinary retention. McGuire and Savastano (1984) have shown that long-term intermittent catheterization in patients with spinal cord injury is effective in preservation of the upper urinary tract and prevention of pyelonephritis, while allowing an ongoing assessment of the efficacy of spontaneous detrusor contractions in spontaneous voiding, and of residual urine volumes. Since detrusor hyperreflexia and detrusor-sphincter dyssynergia are common findings after spinal cord injury, urodynamic and radiographic studies should be carried out as a baseline and in follow-up of all patients. Evaluation and management of these children parallels that of children with spina bifida and other causes of neurovesical dysfunction.

HEAD TRAUMA

Trauma to the spinal cord is a leading cause of neurovesical dysfunction and morbidity (Webb et al., 1984). Head trauma may result in minor degrees of neurovesical dysfunction that may be an added aggravation during the rehabilitation process. Incontinence, urinary frequency, and urgency are common symptoms in this group of patients. Urinary tract infection, urethral stricture from prolonged catheterization during the acute phase of management, and bladder calculi from indwelling catheters should be considered as possible etiologies for bladder dysfunction, and appropriately evaluated. Uninhibited bladder contractions may be discovered on urodynamic evaluation. Treatment must be individualized to meet the needs and functional abilities of the child.

CEREBRAL PALSY AND MISCELLANEOUS NEUROLOGICAL DISEASES

Cerebral palsy and many nonspecific stable and progressive neurological disorders may be causes of bladder dysfunction and urinary incontinence with or without urinary tract infection (McNeal et al., 1983). In many cases, generalized spasticity is a common finding, and often the child may be unable to communicate much or any information about the sensation or type of incontinence present. History and physical examination are extremely important in these cases, and typically one must seek information from the child's caretakers about frequency of urination, force of the urinary stream, bowel habits, and other aspects of history that may be important in terms of differential diagnosis and aspects of management.

Evaluation should begin with history and physical examination and include whatever testing seems appropriate for the level of concern that has arisen. If urinary tract infection is a concern, renal sonography, VCUG, and urodynamic evaluation are appropriate. If incontinence is the sole problem, evaluation should begin with a renal and post-void ultrasound to determine the efficacy of bladder emptying. Urodynamic studies are indicated in many children with incontinence, and in many cases detrusor hyperreflexia will be found. Anticholinergic therapy may prove beneficial, but intermittent catheterization may be required if a large post-void residual urine volume is a cause of incontinence.

NON-NEUROPATHIC VOIDING DYSFUNCTION AND THE HINMAN-ALLEN SYNDROME

Voiding dysfunction in the neurologically intact child includes a group of children with a wide spectrum of abnormal voiding pattern, ranging from frequency to enuresis to severe incontinence, and with radiographic and urodynamic findings from mild detrusor hyperreflexia to severely disordered bladder function, reflux, hydronephrosis, and renal failure. Many of the more severely afflicted children share various clinical, radiologic, urodynamic, and psychosocial characteristics (non-neurogenic neurogenic bladder, occult neurologic bladder, subclinical neurogenic bladder, the Hinman-Allen syndrome) (Allen, 1977; Dorfman et al., 1969; Hinman, 1974, 1986; Hinman and Bauman, 1973; Koff et al., 1979; Martin et al., 1971). Although most researchers originally thought these disorders represented true neurovesical dysfunction related to occult spinal dysraphism, it has been accepted that acquired behavioral and psychosocial disorders may be reflected in bladder and bowel dysfunction, mimicking neurologic disease.

The symptom complex associated with dysfunctional voiding varies from mild dampness to severe daytime frequency (the frequency syndrome of childhood) (Zoubek and Bloom, 1990) to day and nighttime enuresis, encopresis, and constipation; recurrent urinary tract infection, hydronephrosis, reflux, and renal failure. Bladder and bowel dysfunction are usually preceded by the development of continence and a recognized period of normal bladder renal bowel control, as opposed to neurovesical dysfunction in which urinary continence may have never developed. When seen by a urologist; many of the most severely dysfunctional children have a history of recurrent urinary tract infection and may have undergone endoscopy or failed urologic surgery for reflux or hydronephrosis.

The initial consideration of dysfunctional voiding is usually raised by the past medical, urological, and social developmental history. Prior urinary tract infections should be noted, as dysfunctional voiding may trigger or be triggered by acute and chronic cystitis. A thorough evaluation of the child's voiding pattern and social history, both present and during the period of toilet training, must be obtained. Geist and Antolak (1970) noted a high incidence of emotional problems in children with symptoms of interstitial cystitis. Galdston and Perlmutter (1973) have shown that anxiety in children may be manifested by alterations in urinary frequency and voiding characteristics. Hinman and Baumann (1973) likewise noted shyness, timidity, and an attitude of failure, with some children displaying hyperactivity and general anxiety. Family and social histories frequently reveal strained relationships, separation, or divorce. The child who wets may have been punished repeatedly or ridiculed both at home and at school. Peer interaction is frequently strained, and many children dislike school, performing poorly. Parent-child interaction during the interview and examination may prove important clues to social problems in the home. Physical examination is generally normal, although a distended bladder may be palpable, and impacted stool may be noted on rectal and abdominal examination. Post-void bladder ultrasound studies may reveal a large post-void residual urine volume. Neurologic examination is normal. Many children with severe dysfunctional voiding are withdrawn and uncooperative to examination.

The level of concern raised by dysfunctional voiding and the intensity of evaluation it deserves should be related less to the severity of symptoms than to the clinical, radiographic, and urodynamic findings that result. Likewise, the intensity of therapy should be related to the degree of dysfunction and the severity of bladder and upper-tract dysfunction that results.

Daytime Urinary Frequency

The frequency syndrome of childhood is an increasingly common complaint that brings children to urological evaluation (Watemberg and Shalev, 1994). The typical symptoms of this disorder are daytime frequency out of proportion to what may be perfect nocturnal dryness, occasional nocturia, and, rarely, an episode of enuresis. Children hardly ever complain of symptoms, but parents, teachers, and caretakers are commonly quite distressed by the voiding pattern. Urinary tract infection is not present and radiographic findings are normal. Zoubek and Bloom (1990) found that the average length of symptoms in this group was 7 months, that pharmacological therapy did not improve symptoms in the majority of cases, and that observation, lack of intervention, and benign neglect were the most effective means of assuring resolution. Screening sonography will rule out significant bladder wall thickness or hydronephrosis, and reassurance can be given that resolution will occur in the majority of cases.

Moderate dysfunctional voiding is frequently associated with urinary tract infection in either a cause or effect relationship. Moderate voiding dysfunction is frequently classified clinically as the small-capacity bladder, hyperreflexic bladder, and lazy bladder syndromes. Urinary frequency, incontinence, urinary tract infection, and constipation are seen in varying degrees in these syndromes. Renal ultrasonography, voiding cystourethrography, and, occasionally, urodynamic evaluation are important to characterize the nature of voiding dysfunction and document whether or not VUR or hydronephrosis is present. Reflux, in particular, may be a worrisome finding and requires close observation. Koff and Murtagh (1983) first related abnormal vesical function to VUR in 1979. They studied 53 neurologically intact children with urinary tract infections, urinary frequency, urgency, and/or nocturnal enuresis. All children demonstrated uninhibited detrusor contractions, and 50% were found to have VUR. Taylor and associates (1982) confirmed the correlation between the unstable bladder and VUR. Koff and Murtagh (1983), in a later prospective study,

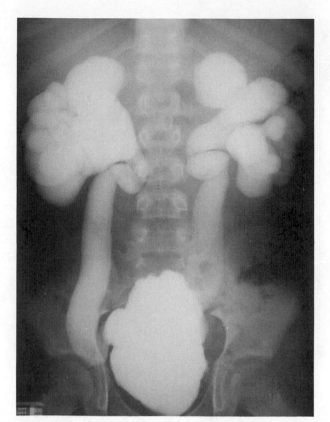

FIG. 53-15
Cystogram of 13-year-old boy with Hinman-Allen syndrome.

documented that anticholinergic therapy, when added to a complete program of nonsurgical management of VUR, resulted in a tripled rate of spontaneous resolution of VUR when compared with controls. Treating urinary tract infection with antibiotic prophylaxis results in some cases in resolution of both the dysfunctional voiding and reflux, while improvement in the dysfunctional pattern of voiding may conversely diminish the risk of urinary tract infection. This appears to be the result of improving the typical pattern of stop-and-start micturition seen with bladder hyperreflexia that allows milk-back of urethral contents into the bladder. Anticholinergic therapy is beneficial in many cases, and timed voiding regimens, treatment of constipation, and attention to stress-related factors are important aspects of therapy.

The Hinman-Allen syndrome (non-neurogenic neurogenic bladder) represents the most severe end of the spectrum of voiding dysfunction. Uroradiographic studies are generally abnormal. Hydronephrosis (generally bilateral) is found in 66% to 70% of patients, with significant VUR in 50% to 57%. Vesicoureteric reflux may have been absent in prior studies, and there may be evidence that VUR was acquired secondary to abnormal voiding mechanics. (Allen, 1977; Hinman, 1974). The bladder may appear large in capacity and may be smooth or trabeculated. A signifi-

cant post-void residual may be seen (Fig. 53-15 and 53-16). Voiding films may demonstrate persistent narrowing at the level of the external sphincter, mimicking posterior urethral valvular obstruction. The urinary stream may be intermittent, associated with intermittent closure of the external sphincter during voiding. Voiding may be seen to be produced by abdominal straining. Ochoa (1992) has described a distinctive urofacial syndrome (the Ochoa syndrome) seen in children with non-neurogenic vesical dysfunction who display a unique facial inversion or grimace during the act of smiling. He postulates the existence of a lesion somewhere in the reticular formation of the brain-stem to account for both aspects of neurological dysfunction.

Both VCU and urodynamic evaluation may be extremely difficult to carry out in children with non-neuropathic voiding dysfunction because of a lack of patient cooperation. In some instances, insertion of a small trocar cystostomy and external sphincter electrodes or patches must be carried out under anesthesia, with urodynamic study after recovery. This technique is especially helpful when repeated study or biodfeedback training is anticipated, although some children tolerate even small urodynamic catheters poorly, and a great deal of artifact may result. Urodynamic findings may reveal increased bladder capacity and resting pressure, occasionally with uninhibited detrusor activity during filling (McGuire and Savastano, 1984). It is imperative to detect straining to void with abdominal EMG or intra-abdominal pressure monitors. During voiding, the external urethral sphincter fails to relax and may show increased activity (detrusor-sphincter dyssynergy). These abnormal urodynamic findings appear to represent learned disorders of micturition, either as persistence of habits acquired during transition from the infantile bladder to normal continence, or as a response to social or psychologic stress. Once wetness occurs, the child may further strain to tighten pelvic floor muscles and prevent leakage, a habit that may be difficult to unlearn.

Treatment for children with dysfunctional voiding must be highly individualized. As in any functional disorder, therapy must be aimed not only at the bladder dysfunction and improved bladder emptying, but also at the psychosocial stresses contributing to the dysfunction. In this context, psychotherapy, behavior modification, and biofeedback training may be extremely important, and the urologist must work closely with a child psychologist or psychiatrist who fully understands the nature and significance of non-neuropathic voiding dysfunction. In some cases, hypnosis has been used successfully. Biofeedback training can be extremely rewarding if the child will cooperate, and learned responses may markedly diminish external sphincter contraction during voiding (Maizels et

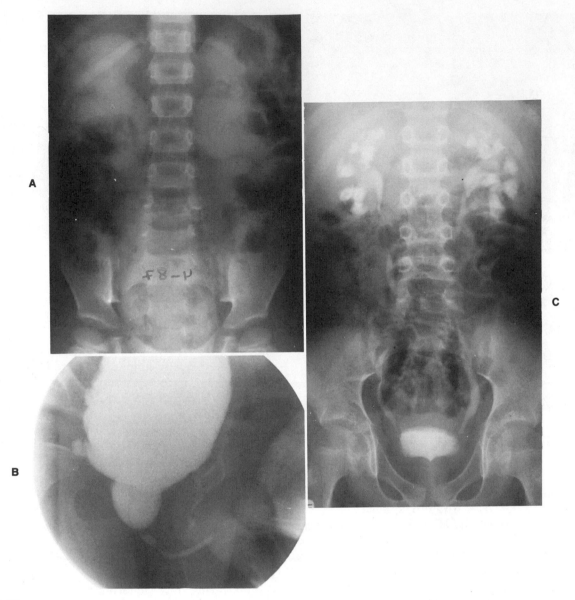

FIG. 53-16
A, IVP of 10-year-old boy with Hinman-Allen syndrome. **B,** Voiding cystourethrogram of same boy mimics posterior urethral valves. **C,** IVP of same boy 3 years later, after cutaneous vesicostomy, psychotherapy, family counselling, and vesicostomy closure.

al., 1979). Double and triple voiding may help reduce residual bladder urine. The child with severe hydronephrosis or reflux may benefit from intermittent catheterization to provide bladder drainage while psychotherapy is in process, but many children are so uncooperative that catheterization is impossible. In such severe circumstances, temporary urinary diversion (cutaneous vesicostomy) may be necessary to ensure against further renal damage. In severe cases with end-stage bladder dysfunction and fibrosis, bladder augmentation and even continent urinary diversion may be necessary. Whatever treatment plan is chosen, family counseling and stress reduction are of paramount importance. Long-term follow-up and periodic reassessment are mandatory (Hinman, 1986).

REFERENCES

Adams MC, Mitchell ME, Rink RC: Gastrocystoplasty: an alternative solution to the problem of urological reconstruction in the severely compromised patient. *J Urol* 1988; 140:1152.

Albright AL, Cervi A, Singletary J: Intrathecal baclofen for spasticity in cerebral palsy. *JAMA* 1991; 265:1418.

Albright AL, Gartner JC, Wiener ES: Lumbar cutaneous hemangiomas as indicators of tethered spinal cords. *Pediatrics* 1989; 83:977.

Allen TD: The non-neurogenic neurogenic bladder. *J Urol* 1977; 117:232.

Bakke A, Vollset SE: Risk factors for bacteriuria and clinical urinary tract infection in patients treated with clean intermittent catheterization. *J Urol* 1993; 149:527.

Barbalias GA, Klauber GT, Blaivas JG: Critical evaluation of the Credé maneuver: a urodynamic study of 207 patients. *J Urol* 1983; 130:720.

Barrett DM, O'Sullivan DC, Malizia A, et al: Particle shedding and migration from silicone genitourinary prosthetic devices. *J Urol* 1991; 146:319.

Bauer SB: Urodynamics in children; indications and methods. In Barrett DM, Wein AJ (eds): *Controversies in Neuro-Urology*. New York, Churchill-Livingstone, 1983.

Bauer SB: Vesicoureteral reflux in children with neurogenic bladder dysfunction. In Johnston JH (ed): *Management of Vesicoureteric Reflux*. Baltimore, Williams and Wilkins, 1984.

Bauer SB: Urodynamic evaluation and neuromuscular dysfunction. In Kelalis PP, King LR, Belman AB (eds): *Clinical Pediatric Urology*, ed 2, Philadelphia, WB Saunders, 1985.

Bauer SB, Hallett M, Khoshbin S, et al: Predictive value of urodynamic evaluation in newborns with myelodysplasia. *JAMA* 1984; 252:650.

Bauer SB, Peters CA, Colodny A, et al: The use of rectus fascia to manage urinary incontinence. *J Urol* 1989; 142:516.

Bauer SB, Hendren WH, Kozakewich H, et al: Perforation of the augmented bladder. *J Urol* 1992; 148(2):699.

Bellinger MF: Ureterocystoplasty: a unique method for vesical augmentation in children. *J Urol* 1993; 149:811.

Belman AB, Kaplan GW: Experience with the Kropp anti-incontinence procedure. *J Urol* 1989; 141:1160.

Benderev TV: Acetylcysteine for urinary tract mucolysis. *J Urol* 1988; 139:353.

Benson JT, Dillard RG, Burton BK: Open spina bifida: does caesarian section improve prognosis? *Obstet Gynecol* 1988; 71:532.

Berger RM, Maizels M, Moran GC, et al: Bladder capacity (ounces) equals age (years) plus 2 predicts normal bladder capacity, aids in diagnosis of abnormal voiding patterns. *J Urol* 1983; 129:327.

Blair GK, Djonlic K, Fraser GC, et al: The bowel management tube: an effective means for controlling fecal incontinence. *J Pediatr Surg* 1992; 27:1269.

Bloom DA, Knechtel JM, McGuire EJ: Urethral dilation improves bladder compliance in children with myelomeningocele and high leak-point pressures. *J Urol* 1990; 144:430.

Bloom DA, Seeley WW, Ritchey ML, et al: Toilet habits and continence in children: an opportunity sampling in search of normal parameters. *J Urol* 1993; 149:1087.

Blyth B, Ewalt DH, Duckett JW, et al: Lithogenic properties of enterocystoplasty. *J Urol* 1992; 148(2):575.

Boone TB, Roehrborn CG, Hurt G: Transurethral intravesical electrotherapy for neurogenic bladder dysfunction in children with myelodysplasia: a prospective, randomized clinical trial. *J Urol* 1992; 148:550.

Bors E, Comarr AE: *Neurological Urology*. Baltimore, University Park Press, 1971.

Borzyskowski M, Neville GBR: Neuropathic bladder and spinal dysraphism. *Arch Dis Child* 1981; 65:176.

Bosco PJ, Bauer SB, Colodny AH, et al: The long-term results of artificial sphincters in children. *J Urol* 1991; 146:396.

Braren V, Jones W: Sacral agenesis: diagnosis, treatment, and follow-up of urological complications. *J Urol* 1983; 121:543.

Brock DJH, Sutcliffe RG: Alpha fetoprotein in the antenatal diagnosis of anencephaly and spina bifida. *Lancet* 1972; 2:197.

Brown S, Stewart RJ, O'Hara MD, et al: Histological changes following submucosal Teflon injection of the bladder. *J Pediatr Surg* 1991; 26:546.

Bruce RR, Gonzales ET Jr: Cutaneous vesicostomy: a useful form of temporary urinary diversion in children. *J Urol* 1980; 123:927.

Burns MW, Mitchell ME: Why we've abandoned polytef injection for VUR. *Contemporary Urology* December 1991; 12:43.

Bushman W, Howards SS: The use of urea for dissolution of urinary mucus in urinary tract reconstruction. *J Urol* 1994; 151:1036.

Cartwright PC, Snow BW: Bladder autoaugmentation: early clinical experience. *J Urol* 1989; 142(2):505.

Cass AS: Urinary tract complications in myelomeningocele patients. *J Urol* 1976; 115:102.

Cass AS, Luxenberg M, Gleich P, et al: A 22-year follow-up of ileal conduits in children with a neurogenic bladder. *J Urol* 1984; 132:529.

Cass AS, Luxenberg M, Johnson CF, et al: Incidence of urinary tract complications with myelomeningocele. *Urology* 1985; 25:374.

Cass AS, Bloom BA, Luxenberg M: Sexual function in adults with myelomeningocele. *J Urol* 1986; 136:425.

Cendren M, Leonard MP, Gearhart JP, et al: Endoscopic treatment of vesicoureteric reflux using cross-linked bovine dermal collagen. *Pediatr Surg Int* 1991; 6:295.

Chapman W, Hill M, Shurtleff DB: *Management of the Neurogenic Bowel and Bladder*. Oak Brook, Ill, Eterna Press, 1979.

Cher ML, Allen TD: Continence in the myelodysplastic patient following enterocystoplasty. *J Urol* 1993; 149:1103.

Chervenak FA, Duncan C, Ment LR, et al: Perinatal management of myelomeningocele. *Obstet Gynecol* 1984; 63:376.

Churchill BM, Gilmour RF, Williot P: Urodynamics. *Pediatr Clin North Am* 1987; 34:1133.

Churchill BM, Aliabadi H, Landau EH, et al: Ureteral bladder augmentation. *J Urol* 1993; 150:716.

Cohen SJ, Harbach LB, Kaplan GW: Cutaneous vesicostomy for temporary urinary diversion in infants with neurogenic bladder dysfunction. *J Urol* 1978; 119:120.

Cohen SJ: Ureterozystoneostomie; eine neue antireflux technik. *Aktuel Urol* 1975; 6:1.

Conway JJ: The principles and technical aspects of diuresis renography. *J Nucl Med Technol* 1989; 17:208.

Conway JJ: "Well-tempered" diuresis renography: its historical development, physiological and technical pitfalls, and standardized technique protocol. *Semin Nucl Med* 1992; 22:74.

Conway JJ, Maizels M: The "well-tempered" diuretic renogram: a standard method to examine the asymptomatic neonate with hydronephrosis or hydroreteronephrosis. A report from the combined meetings of The Society for Fetal Urology and members of The Pediatric Nuclear Medicine Council—The Society of Nuclear Medicine. *J Nucl Med* 1993; 34:1029.

Crane JM, Scherz HS, Billman GF, et al: Ischemic necrosis: a hypothesis to explain the pathogenesis of spontaneously ruptured enterocystoplasty. *J Urol* 1991; 146:141.

Crooks KK, Enrile BG: Comparison of the ileal conduit and clean intermittent catheterization for myelomeningocele. *Pediatrics* 1983; 72:203.

Decter RM: Use of the fascial sling for neurogenic incontinence: lessons learned. *J Urol* 1993; 150:683.

Decter RM: Transurethral electrical bladder stimulation: a follow-up report. *J Urol* 1994; 152:812.

Decter RM, Snyder P, Rosvanis TK: Transurethral electrical bladder stimulation: initial results. *J Urol* 1992; 148:651.

Dees JL: Congenital epispadias with incontinence. *J Urol* 1949; 62:513.

DeGroat WC, Booth AM, Yoshimura Y: Neurophysiology of micturition and its modification in animal models of human disease. In Maggi CA (ed): *Autonomic Nervous System*, vol 3. Cher, Switzerland, Harwood Academic Publishers, 1993.

Dorfman LE, Bailey J, Smith JP: Subclinical neurogenic bladder in children. *J Urol* 1969; 101:48.

Dorner S: Psychological and social problems of families of adolescent spina bifida patients: a preliminary report. *Dev Med Child Neurol* (Suppl) 1973; 15:24.

Douglas JWB: Early disturbing events and late enuresis. In Colvin I, MacKeith RC, Meadow SR (eds): *Bladder Control and Enuresis*. Philadelphia, JB Lippincott, 1973.

Drake WM Jr: The uroflowmeter in the study of bladder neck obstruction. *JAMA* 1954; 156:1079.

Duckett JW: Cutaneous vesicostomy in childhood. *Urol Clin North Am* 1974; 1:485.

Duckett JW: Personal communication.

Duckett JW Jr, Raezer DM: Neuromuscular dysfunction of the lower urinary tract. In Kelalis PP, King LR, Belman AB (eds): *Clinical Pediatric Urology*, vol 1. Philadelphia, WB Saunders, 1976.

Dykes EH, Duffy PG, Ransley PG: The use of the Mitrofanoff principle in achieving clean intermittent catheterization and urinary continence in children. *J Pediatr Surg* 1991; 26:535.

Ebner A, Jiang C, Lindstrom S: Intravesical electrical stimulation—an experimental analysis of the mechanism of action. *J Urol* 1992; 148:920.

Edwards D, Normand ICS, Prescod N, et al: Disappearance of vesicoureteric reflux during long-term prophylaxis of urinary tract infection in children. *Br Med J (Clin Res)* 1978; 2:285.

Elder JS: Periurethral and puboprostatic sling repair for incontinence in patients with myelodysplasia. *J Urol* 1990; 144:434.

Elder JS: Continent appendicocolostomy: a variation of the Mitrofanoff principle in pediatric urinary tract reconstruction. *J Urol* 1992; 148:117.

Elder JS, Snyder HM, Hulbert WC, et al: Perforation of the augmented bladder in patients undergoing clean intermittent catheterization. *J Urol* 1988; 140:1159.

Erickson D, Bartholomew T, Marlin A: Sonographic evaluation and conservative management of newborns with myelomeningocele and hydronephrosis. *J Urol* 1989; 142:592.

Filmer RB, Spencer JR: Malignancies in bladder augmentations and intestinal conduits. *J Urol* 1990; 143:671.

Firlit CF, Smey P, King LR: Micturition urodynamic flow studies in children. *J Urol* 1978; 119:250.

Foster LS, Kogan BA, Cogen PH, et al: Bladder function in patients with lipomeningocele. *J Urol* 1990; 143:984.

Fussell EN, Kaack MB, Cherry R, et al: Adherence of bacteria to human foreskins. *J Urol* 1988; 140:997.

Galdston R, Perlmutter AD: The urinary manifestations of anxiety in child. *Pediatrics* 1973; 52:818.

Gasparini ME, Schmidt RA, Tanagho EA: Selective sacral rhizotomy in the management of the reflex neuropathic bladder: a report of 17 patients with long-term follow-up. *J Urol* 1992; 148:1207.

Gaum LD, Wese FX, Alton DJ, et al: Radiologic investigation of the urinary tract in the neonate with myelomeningocele. *J Urol* 1982; 127:510.

Gearhart JP, Jeffs RD: Suprapubic bladder neck suspension for the management of urinary incontinence in the myelodysplastic girl. *J Urol* 1988; 140:1296.

Geist RW, Antolak SJ Jr: Interstitial cystitis. *J Urol* 1970; 104:922.

Gleason DM, Bottaccini MR, Reilly RJ: Comparison of cystometrograms and urethral profiles with gas and water media. *Urology* 1977; 9:155.

Gonzalez E: Latex hypersensitivity: a new and unexpected problem. *Hosp Prac* 1992; Feb:103.

Gonzalez R, LaPointe S, Sheldon CA: Undiversion in children with renal failure. *J Pediatr Surg* 1984; 19:632.

Gonzalez R, Sheldon CA: Artificial sphincter in children with neurogenic bladders; long-term results. *J Urol* 1982; 128:1270.

Gonzalez R, Sidi AA: Preoperative prediction of continence after enterocystoplasty or undiversion of children with neurogenic bladder. *J Urol* 1985; 134:705.

Gosalbez R Jr, Woodard JR, Broecker BH, et al: Metabolic complications of use of stomach for urinary reconstruction. *J Urol* 1993; 150(2):710.

Grainger R, Kenny A, Walsh A: Adenocarcinoma of the caecum occurring in a caecocystoplasy. *Br J Urol* 1988; 61:164.

Gross AJ, Michael T, Godeman F, et al: Urological findings in patients with neurosurgically treated tethered spinal cord. *J Urol* 1993; 149:1510.

Guttmann L, Frankel H: The value of intermittent self-catheterization in the early management of traumatic paraplegia and tetraplegia. *Paraplegia* 1966; 4:63.

Guzman L, Bauer SB, Hallett M, et al: Evaluation and management of children with sacral agenesis. *Urology* 1983; 22:506.

Hall DE, Udvarhelyi GB, Altman J: Lumbosacral skin lesions as markers of occult spinal dysraphism. *JAMA* 1981; 246:2606.

Haupt G, Pannek J, Knopf HJ, et al: Rupture of ileal neobladder due to urethral obstruction by mucous plug. *J Urol* 1990; 144:740.

Hellstrom AL, Hanson E, Hansson S, et al: Micturition habits and incontinence in 7-year old Swedish school entrants. *Eur J Pediatr* 1990; 149:434.

Hendren WH: Reconstruction ("undiversion") of the diverted urinary tract. *Hosp Pract* 1976; Jan:70.

Hensle TW, Connor JP, Burbidge KA: Continent urinary diversion in childhood. *J Urol* 1990; 143:981.

Hill DE, Kramer SA: Management of pregnancy after augmentation cystoplasty. *J Urol* 1990; 144:457.

Hill JT, Ransley PG: The colonic conduit: a better method of urinary diversion? *Br J Urol* 1983; 44:629.

Hinman F: Urinary tract damage in children who wet. *Pediatrics* 1974; 54:142.

Hinman F Jr: Selection of intestinal segments for bladder substitution: physical and physiological characteristics. *J Urol* 1988; 139:519.

Hinman F Jr: Non-neurogenic neurogenic bladder (the Hinman syndrome)—15 years later. *J Urol* 1986; 136:769.

Hinman F, Baumann FW: Vesical and ureteral damage from voiding dysfunction in boys without neurologic or obstructive disease. *J Urol* 1973; 109:727.

Hirsch S, Carrion H, Gordon J: Ureteroneocystostomy in the treatment of reflux in neurogenic bladders. *J Urol* 1978; 120:552.

Hobbins JC, Grannum PAT, Berkowitz RL, et al: Ultrasound in the diagnosis of congenital anomalies. *Am J Obstet Gynecol* 1979; 134:331.

Hogge WA, Dungan JS, Brooks MP, et al: Diagnosis and management of prenatally detected myelomeningocele: a preliminary report. *Am J Obstet Gyencol* 1990; 163:1061.

Houle A, Gilmour RF, Churchill BM, et al: What volume can a child normally store in the bladder at a safe pressure? *J Urol* 1993; 149:561.

Hurwitz RS, Ehrlich RM: Complications of cutaneous vesicostomy in children. *Urol Clin North Am* 1983; 10:503.

Husman DA, McLorie GA, Churchill BM: Nonrefluxing colon conduits: a long-term life-table analysis. *J Urol* 1989; 142:1201.

Huttenlocher PR: Cerebral palsy. In Vaughan VC, McKay RJ, Behrman RE (eds): *Textbook of Pediatrics*, ed 11. Philadelphia, WB Saunders, 1979.

International Continence Society Standardization Committee: Fourth report on the standardization of terminology of lower urinary tract infection. *Br J Urol* 1981; 53:333.

International Reflux Committee: Medical versus surgical treatment of primary vesicoureteric reflux. *Pediatrics* 1981; 67:392.

Jakobbsen B, et al: 99m-technetium-dimercaptosuccinic acid scan in the diagnosis of acute pyelonephritis in children: relation to clinical and radiological findings. *Pediatr Nephrol* 1992; 6:328.

Jayachandran S, Mooppan UM, Kim H: Complications from external (condom) urinary drainage devices. *Urology* 1985; 25:31.

Jeffs RD, Jonas P, Schillinger JF: Surgical correction of vesicoureteral reflux in children with neurogenic bladder. *J Urol* 1976; 115:449.

Jeter KF (ed): Psychosocial issues in CIC, urinary diversion, and undiversion. *Dialogues in Pediatric Urology* 1983; 6:3.

Johnson HW, Anderson JD, Chambers GK, et al: A short-term study of nitrofurantoin prophylaxis in children managed with clean intermittent catheterization. *Pediatrics* 1994; 93:752.

Johnston JH, Kathel BL: The obstructed neurogenic bladder in the newborn. *Brit J Urol* 1971; 43:206.

Johnston JH, Shapiro SR, Thomas GG: Anti-reflux surgery in the congenital neuropathic bladder. *Br J Urol* 1976; 48:639.

Jones JA, Mitchell ME, Rink RC: Improved results using a modification of the Young-Dees-Leadbetter bladder neck repair. *Br J Urol* 1993; 71:555.

Joseph DB: The use of iothalamate meglumine 17.2% as an effective testing medium in lower urinary tract urodynamic assessment of children. *J Urol* 1993; 149:92.

Jumper BM, McLorie GA, Churchill BM, et al: Effects of the artificial urinary sphincter on prostatic development and sexual function in boys with meningomyelocele. *J Urol* 1990; 144:438.

Kaplan WE: Endoscopic injection of Teflon: a US perspective. *Dialogues in Pediatric Urology* 1991; 14:3.

Kaplan W, Firlit CF: Management of reflux in the myelodysplastic child. *J Urol* 1983; 129:1195.

Kaplan WE, McLone DG, Richards I: The urological manifestations of the tethered spinal cord. *J Urol* 1988; 140:1285.

Kaplan WE, Richards I: Intravesical bladder stimulation in myelodysplasia. *J Urol* 1988; 140:1282.

Kass EJ, Koff SA, Diokno AC: Fate of vesicoureteral reflux in children with neuropathic bladders managed by intermittent catheterization. *J Urol* 1981; 125:63.

Katona F, Berenyi M: Intravesical transurethral electrotherapy in myelomeningocele patients. *Acta Paediatrica Hungary* 1975; 16:363.

Kaufman HH, Carmel PW: Hydrocele after ventriculoperitoneal shunting. *Am J Dis Child* 1981; 135:359.

Khoury AE, Hendrick EB, McLorie GA, et al: Occult spinal dysraphism: clinical and urodynamic outcome after division of the filum terminale. *J Urol* 1990; 144:426.

King LR, Webster GD, El-Marouky A: The non-compliant cecum: a cause for incontinence after bladder substitution (cecocystoplasty) or bladder replacement. Presented at the Urology Section, The American Academy of Pediatrics, Chicago, September 1984.

Klimberg I: The development of voiding control. *AUA Update Series*, vol 7, lesson 21, 1988.

Knoll M, Madersbacher H: The chances of a spina bifida patient becoming continent/socially dry by conservative therapy. *Paraplegia* 1993; 31:22.

Koff SA: Interpretation of dyssynergia in children. *Dialogues in Pediatric Urology* 1983; 6:7.

Koff SA: Guidelines to determine the size and shape of intestinal segments used for reconstruction. *J Urol* 1988; 140:1150.

Koff SA, Kass EJ: Abdominal wall electromyography: a noninvasive technique to improve pediatric urodynamic accuracy. *J Urol* 1982; 127:736.

Koff SA, Lapides J, Piazza DH: Association of urinary tract infection and reflux with uninhibited bladder contractions and voluntary sphincteric obstruction. *J Urol* 1979; 122:373.

Koff SA, Murtagh DS: The uninhibited bladder in children: effect of treatment on recurrence of urinary infection and on vesicoureteral reflux resolution. *J Urol* 1983; 130:1138.

Kolski GB: Allergic emergencies: In *Textbook of Pediatric Emergency Medicine*. Baltimore, Williams and Wilkins, 1988.

Koontz WW, Smith MJV, Currie RJ: External sphincterotomy in boys with meningomyelocele. *J Urol* 1972; 108:649.

Krane RJ, Siroky MB: Classification of voiding dysfunction: value of classification systems. In Barrett DM, Wein AJ (eds): *Controversies in Neuro-Urology*. New York, Churchill-Livingstone, 1984.

Kreder KJ, Webster GD: Management of the bladder outlet in patients requiring enterocystoplasty. *J Urol* 1982; 147:38.

Kroovand RL: The artificial urinary sphincter for urinary incontinence. *Dev Med Child Neurol* 1983; 25:520.

Kroovand RL, Bell W, Hart LJ, et al; The effect of back closure on detrusor function in neonates with myelomeningocele. *J Urol* 1990; 144:423.

Kropp KA, Angwafo FF: Urethral lengthening and reimplantation for neurogenic incontinence in children. *J Urol* 1986; 135:533.

Kropp KA, Voeller KKS: Cryptorchidism in meningomyelocele. *J Pediatr* 1981; 99:110.

Lais A, Kasabian GN, Dyro FM, et al: The neurosurgical implications of continuous neurosurgical surveillance of children with myelodysplasia. *J Urol* 1993; 150:1879.

Lamesch AJ: Retrograde catheterization of the ureter after antireflux plasty by the Cohen technique of transverse advancement. *J Urol* 1981; 125:73.

Lapides J: Neuromuscular, vesical, and ureteral dysfunction. In Campbell MF, Harrison JH (eds): *Urology*. Philadelphia, WB Saunders, 1970.

Lapides J, Diokno AC, Silber SJ, et al: Clean, intermittent self-catheterization in the treatment of urinary tract disease. *J Urol* 1972; 107:458.

Leadbetter GW: Surgical correction of total urinary incontinence. *J Urol* 1964; 91:261.

Lebowitz RL: The detection and characterization of vesicoureteric reflux in the child. *J Urol* 1992; 145(2): 1640.

Lenaghan D, Whitaker JG, Jensen F, et al: The natural history of reflux and long-term effects of reflux on the kidney. *J Urol* 1978; 115:728.

Leonard CO: Counseling parents of a child with myelomeningocele. *Pediatr Rev* 1983; 4:317.

Levitt SB, Sandler HJ: The absence of vesicoureteral reflux in the neonate with myelodysplasia. *J Urol* 1975; 114:118.

Lewis RI, Canion HM, Lockhart JL, et al: Significance of asymptomatic bacteriuria in neurogenic bladder disease. *Urology* 1984; 23:343.

Lindehall B, Moller A, Hjalmas K, et al: Long-term intermittent catheterization: the experience of teenagers and young adults with myelomeningocele. *J Urol* 1994; 152:187.

Lyne CJ, Bellinger MF: Early experience with transurethral electrical bladder stimulation. *J Urol* 1993; 150:697.

MacKeith R, Meadow SR, Turner RK: How children become dry. In Colvin I, MacKeith RC, Meadow SR (eds): *Bladder Control and Enuresis*. Philadelphia, JB Lippincott, 1973.

Maizels M, Firlit CF: Pediatric urodynamics: clinical comparison of surface versus needle pelvic floor/external sphincter electromyography. *J Urol* 1979; 122:518.

Maizels M, King LR, Firlit CF: Urodynamic biofeedback: a new approach to treat vesical sphincter dyssynergia. *J Urol* 1979; 122:205.

Maizels M, Firlit CF, Conway JJ, et al: Troubleshooting the diuresis renogram. *Urology* 1986; 28:355.

Malizia A, Reiman H, Myers R: Migration and granulomatous reaction after periurethral injection of Polytef (Teflon). *JAMA* 1984; 251:3277.

Malone PS, Ransley PG, Kiely EM: Preliminary report: the antegrade continence enema. *Lancet* 1990; 336:1217.

Martin DC, Datta NS, Schweitz B: The occult neurological bladder. *J Urol* 1971; 105;733.

McDougal WS: Mechanics and neurophysiology of intestinal segments as bowel substitutes: an editorial comment. *J Urol* 1987; 138:1438.

McGuire EJ, Savastano JA: Urodynamic studies in enuresis and the non-neurogenic neurogenic bladder. *J Urol* 1984; 132:299.

McGuire EJ, Woodside JR, Borden TA, et al: Prognostic value of urodynamic testing in myelodysplastic patients. *J Urol* 1981; 126:205.

McLone DG: Continuing concepts in the management of spina bifida. *Pediatr Neurosurg* 1992; 18:254.

McNeal DM, Hawtrey CE, Wolraich ML, et al: Symptomatic neurogenic bladder in a cerebral-palsied population. *Dev Med Child Neurol* 1983; 25:612.

Menon M, Elder JS, Manley CB, et al: Undiverting the ileal conduit. *J Urol* 1982; 128:998.

Meyer S, Landau H: Precious puberty in myelomeningocele patients. *J Pediatr Orthop* 1984; 4:28.

Mitchell ME: The role of bladder augmentation in undiversion. *J Pediatr Surg* 1981; 16:790.

Mitchell ME, Kulb TB, Backes DJ: Intestinocystoplasty in combination with clean intermittent catheterization in the management of vesical dysfunction. *J Urol* 1986; 136:288.

Mitrofanoff P: Cystostomie continente trans-appendiculaire dans le traitement des vessies neurologiques. *Chir Pediatr* 1980; 21:297.

MRC Vitamin Study Research Group: Prevention of neural tube defects: results of the Medical Research Council Vitamin Study. *Lancet* 1991; 338:131.

Muellner SR: Development of urinary control in children. *JAMA* 1960; 172:1256.

Mulinare J, Cordero JF, Erickson JD, et al: Periconceptional use of multivitamins and the occurrence of neural tube defects. *JAMA* 1988; 260:3141.

Murray KHA, Nurse DE, Mundy AR: Detrusor behavior following implantation of the Brantley Scott artificial urinary sphincter for neuropathic incontinence. *Br J Urol* 1988; 61:122.

Myers GJ, Cerone SB, Olson AL: *A Guide for Helping the Child With Spina Bifida*. Springfield, Ill, Charles C Thomas, 1981.

Nanningia JB, Frost F, Penn R: Effect of intrathecal baclofen on bladder and sphincter function. *J Urol* 1989; 142:101.

Nasrallah PF, Aliabadi HA: Bladder augmentation in patients with neurogenic bladder and vesicoureteric reflux. *J Urol* 1991; 146:563.

Nguyen DH, Bain MA, Salmonson KL, et al: The syndrome of dysuria and hematuria in pediatric urinary reconstruction with stomach. *J Urol* 1993; 150(2):707.

Oakley GP: Folic acid-preventable spina bifida and anencephaly. *JAMA* 1993; 269:1292.

Ochoa B: The urofacial (Ochoa) syndrome revisited. *J Urol* 1992; 148:580.

O'Donnell B, Puri P: Endoscopic correction of primary vesicoureteric reflux. *Br J Urol* 1986; 58:601.

O'Reilly PH: Diuresis renography 8 years later: an update. *J Urol* 1986; 136:993.

Owens JR, McAllister A, Harris F, et al: Nineteen-year incidence of neural tube defects in area under constant surveillance. *Lancet* 1981; 2:1032.

Palmer LS, Franco I, Kogan SJ, et al: Urolithiasis in children following cystoplasty. *J Urol* 1993; 150(2):726.

Passarge E, Lenz K: Syndrome of caudal regression in infants of diabetic mothers: observation of further cases. *Pediatrics* 1966; 37:672.

Patel K, Charron M, Hoberman A, et al: Intra- and interobserver variability in interpretation of DMSA scans using a set of standardized criteria. *Pediatr Radiol* 1993; 23:506.

Pearson PH: The interdisciplinary team process, or the professionals' Tower of Babel. *Dev Med Child Neurol* 1983; 25:390.

Piercy SL, Gregory JG, Young PH: Ventriculo-peritoneal shunt pseudocyst causing ureteropelvic junction obstruction in a child with myelomeningocele and retrocaval ureter. *J Urol* 1984; 132:345.

Plunkett JM, Braren V: Clean intermittent catheterization in children. *J Urol* 1979; 121:469.

Purcell MH, Gregory JG: Intermittent catheterization: evaluation of complete dryness and independence in children with myelomeningocele. *J Urol* 1984; 132:518.

Puri P, Guiney EL: Endoscopic correction of vesicoureteric reflux secondary to neuropathic bladder. *Br J Urol* 1986; 58:504.

Quinlan DM, Leonard MP, Brendler CB, et al: Use of the Benchekroun hydraulic valve as a catheterizable continence mechanism. *J Urol* 1991; 145:1151.

Rabin BJ: *The Sensuous Wheeler*. San Francisco, Multi-Media Resource Center, 1980.

Raezer DM, Evans RJ, Shrom SH: Augmentation ileocystoplasty in neuropathic bladder. *Urology* 1985; 25:26.

Raezer DM, Benson GS, Wein AJ, et al: The functional approach to the pediatric neuropathic bladder: a clinical study. *J Urol* 1977; 117:649.

Ransley PG, Risdon RA: Reflux and renal scarring. *Br J Radiol* 1978; (suppl 14):1.

Raz S, Magora F, Caine M: The evaluation of pudendal nerve block by measurements of urethral pressure profile. *Surg Gynecol Obstet* 1971; 133:453.

Raz S, Ehrlich RM, Zeidman EJ, et al: Surgical treatment of the incontinent female patient with myelomeningocele. *J Urol* 1988; 139:524.

Reinberg Y, Manivel JC, Gonzalez R: Silicone shedding from artificial urinary sphincter in children. *J Urol* 1993; 150:694.

Rigel DH: Tethered spinal cord. *Concepts Pediatr Neurosurg* 1983; 4:142.

Rosen MA, Light JK: Spontaneous bladder rupture following enterocystoplasty. *J Urol* 1991; 146:1232.

Rushton HG, Majd M: Dimercaptosuccinic acid renal scintigraphy for the evaluation of pyelonephritis and scarring: a review of experimental and clinical studies. *J Urol* 1992; 148:1726.

Santarosa RP, Blaivas JG: Periurethral infection of autologous fat for the treatment of sphincteric incontinence. *J Urol* 1994; 151:607.

Schneck FX, Bellinger MF: The "innocent" cough or sneeze: a harbinger of serious latex allergy in children during bladder stimulation and urodynamic testing. *J Urol* 1993; 150:687.

Schwartz GR, Jeffs RD: Ileal conduit urinary diversion in children: computer analysis of follow-up from 2 to 16 years. *J Urol* 1975; 114:285.

Schwartz GJ, Feld LG, Langford DJ, et al: A simple estimate of glomerular filtration rate in children derived from body length and plasma creatinine. *Pediatrics* 1976; 58:259.

Shochat SJ, Perlmutter AD: Myelodysplasia with severe neonatal hydronephrosis: the value of urethral dilatation. *J Urol* 1972; 107:146.

Shortliffe LMD, Freiha FS, Kessler R, et al; Treatment of urinary incontinence by the periurethral implantation of glutaraldehyde cross-linked collagen. *J Urol* 1989; 141:538.

Shurtleff DB: What are the medical concerns of adults with spina bifida? *Spina Bifida Insights* 1983; 11(3):3.

Sidi AA, Reinberg Y, Gonzalez R: Influence of intestinal segment and configuration on the outcome of augmentation enterocystoplasty. *J Urol* 1986; 136:1201.

Slater JE: Allergic reactions to natural rubber. *Ann Allergy* 1992; 68:203.

Smith RB, van Cangh P, Skinner DG, et al: Augmentation enterocystoplasty: a critical review. *J Urol* 1977; 118:35.

Snyder HM, Kalichman MA, Charney E, et al: Vesicostomy for neurogenic bladder with spina bifida: follow-up. *J Urol* 1983; 130:724.

Stafford SJ, Fried FA, Sackett CK, et al: Hydronephrosis in the asymptomatic neonate with myelodysplasia. *J Urol* 1983; 129:340.

Staskin DR, Parsons KF, Levin RM, et al: Bladder transection—functional, neurophysiological, neuropharmacological, and neuroanatomical study. *Br J Urol* 1981; 53:552.

Stein SC, Feldman JG, Friedlander M, et al: Is myelomeningocele a disappearing disease? *Pediatrics* 1982; 69:511.

Stewart M, Macrae FA, Williams CB: Neoplasia and utererosigmoidostomy: a colonoscopy survey. *Brit J Surg* 1982; 69:414.

Storrs BB: Selective posterior rhizotomy for treatment of progressive spasticity in patients with myelomeningocele. *Pediatr Neurosci* 1987; 13:135.

Strassburg M: The epidemiology of anencephalus and spina bifida: a review. Part I: Introduction, embryology, classification, and epidemiological terms. *Spina Bifida Therapy* 1982a; 4(2):53.

Strassburg M: The epidemiology of anencephalus and spina bifida: a review. Part II: Geographical variations, secular trends, seasonality, time-place interactions. *Spina Bifida Therapy* 1982b; 4(4):181.

Sumfest JM, Burns MW, Mitchell ME: The Mitrofanoff principle in urinary reconstruction. *J Urol* 1993; 150:1875.

Tauxe WN, Dubovsky EV, Kidd T: New formulae for the calculation of effective renal plasma flow by a single-sample method. *Eur J Nucl Med* 1982; 7:51.

Taylor CM, Corkery JJ, White RHR: Micturition symptoms and unstable bladder activity in girls with primary vesicoureteric reflux. *Br J Urol* 1982; 54:494.

Tiffany P, Vaughan ED, Marion D, et al: Hypergastrinemia following antral gastrocystoplasty. *J Urol* 1986; 136:692.

Toczek SK, McCullough DL, Garfour GW, et al: Selective sacral rootlet rhizotomies for hypertensive neurogenic bladder. *J Neurosurg* 1975; 42:567.

Toriello HV: Periconceptual vitamin supplementation for the prevention of NTD: a review. *Spina Bifida Therapy* 1982; 4(2):59.

Velchik MG: Radionuclide imaging of the urinary tract. *Urol Clin North Am* 1985; 12(4):603.

Vorstman B, Lockhart J, Kaufman MR, et al: Polytetrafluoroethylene injection for urinary incontinence in children. *J Urol* 1985; 133:248.

Wald A: Use of biofeedback in treatment of fecal incontinence in patients with meningomyelocele. *Pediatrics* 1981; 68:45.

Wammack R, Fisch M, Hohenfellner R: Pediatric urinary diversion: review and own experience. *Eur Urol* 1992; 22:177.

Wan J, McGuire EJ, Bloom DA, et al: The treatment of urinary incontinence in children using glutaraldehyde cross-linked collagen. *J Urol* 1992; 148:127.

Wang SC, McGuire EJ, Bloom DM: A bladder pressure management system for myelodysplasia-clinical outcome. *J Urol* 1988; 140:1499.

Wang SC, McGuire EJ, Bloom DM: Urethral dilation in the mangement of urological complications of myelodysplasia. *J Urol* 1989; 142:1054.

Watemberg N, Shalev H: Daytime urinary frequency in children. *Clinical Pediatrics* 1994; January:50.

Watson WJ, Chescheir NC, Katz VL, et al: The role of ultrasound in the evaluation of patients with elevated maternal serum alpha-fetoprotein: a review. *Obstet Gynecol* 1991; 78:123.

Webb DR, Fitzpatrick JM, O'Flynn JD: A 15-year follow-up of 406 consecutive spinal cord injuries. *Br J Urol* 1984; 56:614.

Wein AJ: Pharmacologic approaches to the management of neurogenic bladder dysfunction. *J Contin Ed Urol* 1979; 18(5):17.

Werler MM, Shapiro S, Mitchell AA: Periconceptual folic acid exposure and risk of occurrent neural tube defects. *JAMA* 1993; 269:1257.

Wheatley JK, Woodard JR, Parrott TS: Electronic bladder stimulation in the management of children with myelomeningocele. *J Urol* 1982; 127:283.

Wiswell TE, Hachey WE: Urinary tract infections and the uncircumcised state: an update. *Clinical Pediatrics* 1993; March:130.

Wolraich ML, Hawtrey C, Mapel J, et al: Results of clean intermittent catheterization for children with neurogenic bladders. *Urology* 1983; 22:479.

Woodard JR, Anderson AM, Parrott TS: Ureteral reimplantation in myelodysplasia children. *J Urol* 1981; 126:387.

Woodside JR, McGuire EJ: Technique for detection of detrusor hypertonia in the presence of urethral sphincteric incompetence. *J Urol* 1982; 127:740.

Young HH: An operation for the cure of incontinence associated with epispadias. *J Urol* 1922; 7:1.

Zoubek J, Bloom DA: Extraordinary urinary frequency. *Pediatrics* 1990: 85:1112.

CHAPTER 54

Genital Anomalies

Terry W. Hensle

GENITAL ANOMALIES—MALE

Embryology

The critical period for genital differentiation in the human is between 10 and 16 weeks of gestation. Even though the genetic sex of the human embryo is determined at conception, the gonads of the male and female are indistinguishable until nearly 40 days of embryonic life (Federman, 1967; Jirasek, 1971). In the male, transformation of the indifferent gonad into a testis occurs between 6 and 7 weeks of gestation (Simpson, 1976). Differentiation is due to the induction of the primitive gonad on the genital ridge by genetic information carried on the Y chromosome. The presence of the Y chromosome and the cascade of factors it directs are crucial for the bipotential undifferentiated gonad to differentiate as a testis. Appreciation of the role of the Y chromosome has progressed since the late 1950s when it was first shown (Jacobs and Strong, 1959) that the Y chromosome was essential for male determination. The sex-specific region of the Y chromosome has been identified as a transcript of 35 kilobases containing a single copy gene (SRY) that encodes a protein that is presumably involved in initiating differentiation of the gonad into the testis (Berta et al., 1990; Jager et al., 1990). In the female, development of the indifferent gonad into an ovary occurs very slowly compared with the development of the testis and can be considered a passive event (Federman, 1967).

Beginning at 8 weeks of gestation, genital development occurs in two distinct areas: internal duct structures and, external genitalia. Development of internal duct structures in both male and female is dependent on the presence or absence of a fetal testis (Fig. 54-1). In the presence of a fetal testis, there will be production of androgen (testosterone) as well as müllerian-inhibiting subtance (MIS). Secretion of fetal androgen stimulates the wolffian duct to differentiate into the vas deferens, seminal vesicle, and epididymis. At the same time, the fetal testis secrets a nonsteroidal subtance (MIS) that prevents development of müllerian duct structures into the fallopian tube, uterus, and upper third of the vagina. The development of the female internal duct system does not depend on hormonal induction and occurs normally in the absence of MIS, whereas the wolffian duct structures will regress in the absence of high levels of fetal androgen (Jost, 1971).

Differentiation of the external genitalia occurs somewhat later, probably between 12 and 16 weeks of gestation (see Fig. 54-1). The process requires not only the fetal testis and adequate amounts of fetal androgen, but also the ability of the target organ to respond to the circulating androgen. Testosterone exerts its effect on the target organ in several ways, the most important of which is the conversion of testosterone to dihydrotestosterone (DHT) under the enzymatic influence of 5 α-reductase (Anderson and Liao, 1968; Bruchovsky and Wilson, 1968). This conversion takes place within the tissue of the common genital anlage, where DHT combines with a cytosol receptor that is coded for by one or more X-linked genes (Amrhein et al., 1976; Meyer et al., 1975). These androgen receptor complexes are then activated and moved to nuclear acceptors. Subsequently, DNA-dependent RNA preliminase activity increases, followed by enhanced production of protein. These serve as the initial steps for differentiation of the common genital anlage (Imperato-McGinley et al., 1979). Under the influence of DHT, the genital tubercle will differentiate into the glans penis, the genital folds become the shaft of the penis, and genital swellings become the scrotum. If there is a deficiency in production of fetal testosterone, failure of conversion of testosterone to DHT, or insensitivity in the target organ to DHT, the genital tubercle will passively develop into the clitoris, the genital folds will become labia minora, and the genital swellings will become labia majora (Griffin and Wilson, 1980).

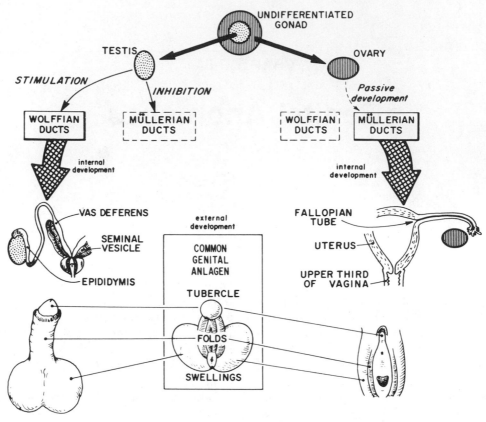

FIG. 54-1
Normal sexual development in the male and female. (Adapted from Federman DD: *Abnormal Sexual Development: A Genetic and Endocrine Approach to Differential Diagnosis.* Philadelphia, WB Saunders, 1967.)

DEVELOPMENTAL ANOMALIES

Penile Agenesis

Congenital absence of the penis is a rare condition that probably results from a failure of the genital tubercle to develop. The incidence is thought to be somewhere between 1 in 10 million and 1 in 30 million live births (Kessler and McLaughlin, 1973). In most cases there is a fully formed scrotum (Fig. 54-2); total agenesis of the penis and scrotum is even less common (Fig. 54-3). In penile agenesis alone, the testes are normally descended, and the urethral opening is usually in the perineum close to the anus. Associated genitourinary anomalies are found in more than 50% of patients with penile agenesis, the most common of which is cryptorchidism, followed by renal aplasia or dysplasia (Kessler and McLaughlin, 1973). Anomalies of the gastrointestinal (GI) tract such as imperforate anus and rectovesical fistula are also common. Penile agenesis has also been reported by Robinow (Vera-Roman, 1973) in association with vertebral anomalies and a dwarfing syndrome, which includes orbital hypertelorism, widened palpebral fissures, and dental malalignment (Robinow's syndrome).

Endocrine testicular function in patients with penile agenesis has been shown to be normal as judged by a normal response to gonadotropin stimulation (Gau-

tier et al., 1981). Recommended treatment should be early gender reassignment and gonadectomy. The urethra should be transposed anteriorly away from the anal verge, and the scrotal skin should be preserved to aid later vaginal construction.

Penile Duplication

Duplication of the penis is another rare anomaly, probably resulting from incomplete fusion of the genital tubercle. The anomaly appears in two basic forms, the first and more common being the bifid penis, which is often associated with the exstrophy-epispadias complex (Fig. 54-4) and is present in almost every male with cloacal exstrophy. In these cases, the bifid penis consists of a single corporal body on each side associated with a hemiglans penis (Johnston, 1975).

The other form of penile duplication is true diphallia. This is an extremely rare condition in which there is a duplication of all or part of the penis (Rodriguez, 1965). The deformity exists in a spectrum that ranges from duplication of glans alone, arising from the single shaft (Fig. 54-5), to complete duplication with two separate scrotums. With complete duplication, each penis has a complete urethra, which is associated with an independent bladder or at times with a bifid bladder. The urethral opening can be in the

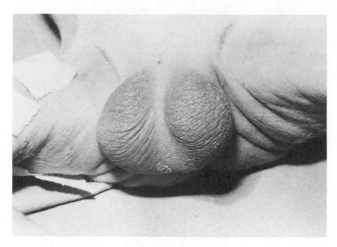

FIG. 54-2
Penile agenesis.

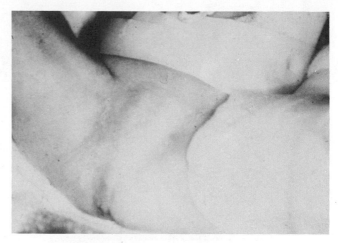

FIG. 54-3
Agenesis of the penis and scrotum.

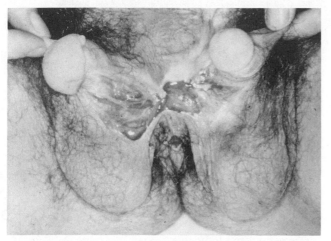

FIG. 54-4
Penile duplication in a patient with bladder exstrophy.

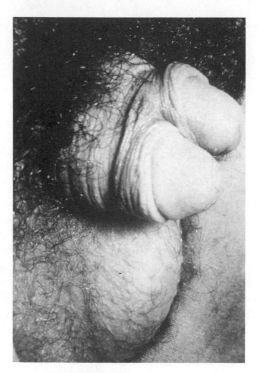

FIG. 54-5
Complete penile duplication.

normal position or either hypospadiac or epispadiac. When there is bladder duplication associated with penile duplication, both erection and urination can occur synchronously or asynchronously.

Treatment of penile duplication varies depending on whether other congenital anomalies are present. If the bifid penis is associated with cloacal exstrophy, penile reconstruction is usually not technically possible, and gender reassignment is recommended. One of the bifid phalluses can be removed, retaining the other to act as a clitoris. In true diphallia, the decision of which penis should be removed and which salvaged should be based on not only the physical appearance of both structures, but also on the size of the bladder associated with each segment, and the erectile function of each unit. Patients with true diphallia should also be thoroughly evaluated for other genitourinary or GI tract anomalies, since the association of other anomalies with this defect is abnormally high.

Microphallus

Microphallus can best be defined as a normally formed penis (Fig. 54-6) whose length is more than 2.5 SD below the norm for age (Table 54-1) (Feldman and Smith, 1975; Schonfeld and Beebe, 1942). In the neonatal period, the penis should measure at least 2 cm from pubis to tip when fully stretched (Lee et al., 1980). The term microphallus by definition excludes hypospadias and ambiguous genitalia.

In general, the etiology of microphallus can be thought of as either inadequate androgen stimulation of the target organ or an insensitivity of the target organ to available androgen. Inadequate amounts of

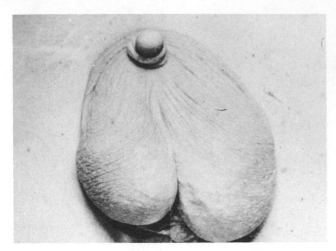

FIG. 54-6
True microphallus.

TABLE 54-1

Stretched Penile Length in Normal Males

Age	Mean ± SD cm	Mean − 2.5 SD cm
Newborn, 30 wk	2.5 ± 0.4	1.5
Newborn, 34 wk	3.0 ± 0.4	2.0
Newborn, term	3.5 ± 0.4	2.4
0-5 mo	3.9 ± 0.8	1.9
6-12 mo	4.3 ± 0.8	2.3
1-2 yr	4.7 ± 0.8	2.6
2-3 yr	5.1 ± 0.9	2.9
3-4 yr	5.5 ± 0.9	3.3
4-5 yr	5.7 ± 0.9	3.5
5-6 yr	6.0 ± 0.9	3.8
6-7 yr	6.1 ± 0.9	3.9
7-8 yr	6.2 ± 1.0	3.7
8-9 yr	6.3 ± 1.0	3.8
9-10 yr	6.3 ± 1.0	3.8
10-11 yr	6.4 ± 1.1	3.7
Adult	13.3 ± 1.6	9.3

Adapted from Feldman KW, Smith DW: *J Pediatr* 1975; 86:395.

androgen reaching the target organ can be on the basis of either poor Leydig's cell stimulation, thus suggesting a problem in the hypothalamic-pituitary axis, or a failure of the conversion of testosterone to DHT by 5 α-reductase.

The nature of the defect can be determined by the individual's response to gonadotropin stimulation. In most infants with microphallus, the ability to secrete luteinizing hormone (LH) and follicle-stimulating hormone (FSH) in response to gonadotropin-releasing hormone (GnRH) is present, and the testis is able to respond to LH by secreting testosterone. In addition, androgen-sensitive target organs such as the penis generally respond to testosterone administered locally or parenterally. Thus it seems that in the majority of infants with microphallus, the hypothalamic-pituitary-end organ axis distal to the hypothalamus is intact, implicating the hypothalamus as the site of the primary defect (Lee et al., 1980). Additional evidence for this is seen in several associated disorders, such as Kallman's syndrome and the Prader-Willi syndrome. Other endocrine disturbances, such as abnormal levels of adrenocorticotropic hormone (ACTH), thyroid-stimulating hormone (TSH), and growth hormone can be seen frequently in patients with microphallus.

The treatment of microphallus should begin early (Guthrie et al., 1973). In those rare individuals with identifiable androgen insensitivity syndromes and associated microphallus, gonadectomy and gender conversion to female is best done at an early stage. In the majority of patients with true microphallus, male gender assessment can be maintained, and androgen stimulation should begin in the first year of life. Monthly injections of testosterone enanthate are given for 3 months in doses of 25 to 50 mg delivered parenterally (Burstein et al., 1979). Application of 3% testosterone cream locally is also a reasonable way to deliver androgen; however, the absorption is variable, and the

dose is not as easily controlled (Klugo and Cerny, 1978). In most instances of true microphallus, an increase of phallic growth of approximately 2 cm in the first year of treatment can be expected. When this early stimulation is stopped, the penis does not usually revert to its previous proportions. Multiple courses of androgen stimulation can be used, and if significant growth does not occur, gender conversion can be considered (Money et al., 1969).

The long-term outlook for patients with true microphallus has recently been reviewed by Reiley and Woodhouse (1989). In 12 postpubertal patients, who had carried the diagnosis since childhood, they found the prospect for long-term sexual activity to be hopeful. Eleven of their patients experienced ejaculation, and nine were sexually active, all reporting vaginal penetration. All of the patients in their series had been stimulated with human chorionic gonadotropin, testosterone, or cortisone during childhood.

Penile Torsion

Rotational defects of the penis, or penile torsion (Fig. 54-7), can occur in either a clockwise or counterclockwise position, with or without other associated defects such as hypospadias (Pomerantz et al., 1978). The defect usually has more cosmetic than functional significance. Mild degrees of torsion are not associated with either erectile or voiding dysfunction, and the surgical correction of penile torsion is usually not indicated for children with a rotation of less than 90 degrees from the midline. Surgical correction of mild penile torsion usually involves nothing more than simply degloving the penis and reorienting the median raphe to its normal position (Pomerantz et al., 1978).

In cases of more significant penile torsion, there can be a defect in the position of the glans penis on the corporal bodies. In the treatment of patients with ex-

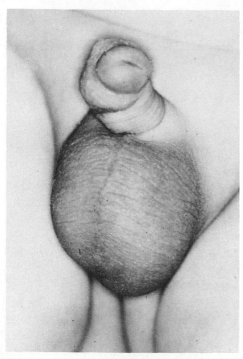

FIG. 54-7
Penile torsion. (Courtesy of A. Barry Belman, M.D.)

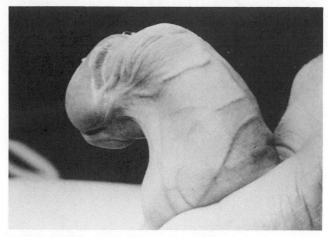

FIG. 54-8
Curvature of the penis secondary to unilateral corporal overgrowth. (Courtesy of John Duckett, M.D.)

treme torsion, usually the glans must be mobilized to some degree and rotated on the corpora to achieve derotation. This is a significant surgical undertaking and should not be considered in mild forms of penile torsion.

Lateral Curvature of the Penis

Lateral penile curvature is rarely recognized in infancy but certainly can be noted in early childhood and must be differentiated from chordee without hypospadias (Fig. 54-8). Lateral curvature is usually caused by an overgrowth of one corporal body, or concomitant hypoplasia of the contralateral corpora (Fitzpatrick, 1976). The defect can be associated with corporal injury, but in most instances there is no history of trauma.

Surgical correction of corporal discrepancies should be considered only when the discrepancy significantly interferes with erection. The procedure of choice in most instances was described by Nesbit and involves excising elipses of the tunica albuginea from the dominant corpora in the area of maximum curvature to reduce the apparent defect (Gravell, 1974). When corporal discrepancies are the result of trauma, there is often a scar on the contralateral (shorter) corpora, which can be excised and grafted with either tunica vaginalis or some other form of genitourinary tissue.

Penile Lymphedema

Primary lymphedema (Fig. 54-9) of the foreskin and penile shaft is a chronic condition seen in children

with either abnormal penile lymphatics or a decreased number of lymph channels draining the foreskin (Buckley, 1962). The condition is frequently seen after circumcision; however, it may be seen in uncircumcised newborn children as well as in adolescents. When it is seen in the uncircumcised newborn, elective circumcision should be avoided, because this generally escalates the process of poor lymph drainage and makes the situation worse than it would be if left alone.

In most instances, a reduction of the excess skin and subcutaneous tissue will give a reasonable cosmetic result. When the problem is extensive, the edema may involve the entire shaft and scrotum. Feins (1980) has suggested extensive resection of the subcutaneous and lymphatic tissue to deal with the problem in its more severe form.

Penoscrotal Transposition

Complete transposition of the penis and scrotum (Fig. 54-10) is a rare anomaly that is often associated with other congenital anomalies, many of which are incompatible with life. The embryologic defect is probably the abnormal positioning of the genital tubercle in relation to the genital swellings, and this abnormality has also been referred to as a prepenile scrotum (Cohen-Addad et al., 1985).

Scrotal transposition has been reported with both a normal penis and with bifid scrotum and various penile deformities. Surgical correction of the scrotal transposition is advocated for cosmetic and psychologic reasons, although urinary and erectile function are not always impeded by this anatomic inversion. There is at least one case report of a patient with complete penile scrotal transposition who has produced four children (Appleby, 1923). Surgical correction can be achieved either by completely dividing the scrotum

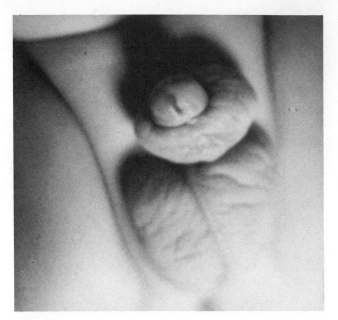

FIG. 54-9
Lymphedema of the foreskin following newborn circumcision.

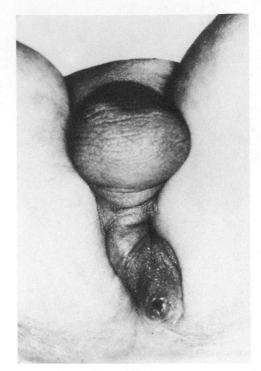

FIG. 54-10
Penoscrotal transposition. (Courtesy of A. Barry Belman, M.D.)

and transposing the penis upward, or by tunneling the penis to a midline position.

Bifid Scrotum

Bifid scrotum is usually seen in conjunction with severe degrees of hypospadias such as penoscrotal or perineal hypospadias (Fig. 54-11). It is usually associated with significant skin chordee, where the skin of the lateral surface of the penis is firmly attached to the midline between the two hemiscrotums. Surgical correction of the bifid scrotum involves release of skin anteriorly to be rotated down to the midline, with realignment of the two scrotal halves in the midline. The most severe form of bifid scrotum is scrotal transposition in which the scrotum appears to be transposed above the penis. This is not true penile-scrotal transposition as described earlier.

Scrotal Ectopia

Scrotal ectopia is a rare condition occasionally seen in boys with otherwise normal genitalia (Lamm and Kaplan, 1977). The ectopic scrotum is usually found somewhere near the external inguinal ring but can be found anywhere along the inner thigh or buttocks (Fig. 54-12). The testis on the side of the scrotal ectopia can be normal or dysplastic, and treatment should be based on the amount of ectopic scrotum present and the condition of the testes. If there is a significant amount of scrotum and reasonable testes, an attempt should be made to bring the testes down along with the ectopic scrotal tissue. If there is only a small, rudimentary amount of ectopic scrotal tissue or dysplastic testes, one or both should be removed.

Scrotal Hypoplasia

Scrotal hypoplasia can be either unilateral or bilateral and is usually associated with the absence of a testis on one or both sides (Fig. 54-13). If there is monorchia or anorchia, the scrotum is typically flat and nonrugated on the affected side. Usually the placement of a testicular prosthesis along with the application of local testosterone cream will improve the cosmetic situation to a significant degree.

Scrotal Hemangioma

Hemangiomas of the scrotum are rare lesions first reported by Robert in 1851. Hemangiomas are common and occur in 10% of all infants less than 1 year old. They may involve any area of the body and are not uncommon in the urogenital tract. However, hemangiomas of the external genitalia compose only 1% of all cutaneous hemangiomas and are more common in females than males. Currently there are fewer than 45 cases of scrotal hemangiomas reported in the literature (Ray and Clark, 1976). Hemangiomas of the scrotum generally are seen in the first 20 years of life but may occur at any age; the youngest case reported is a 1-month-old infant. There are no reports of a complete involution of this lesion; rather, a progressive enlargement is commonly noted.

On physical examination, the scrotal hemangioma is a soft, spongy compressible mass that has a "bag of worms" sensation somewhat similar to a variocele of

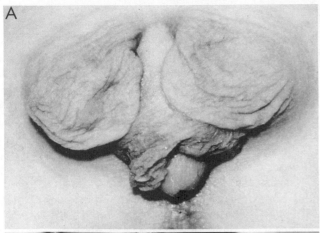

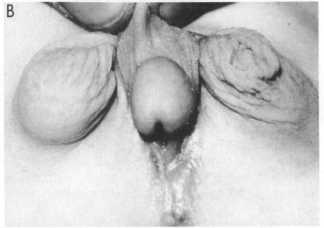

FIG. 54-11
Bifid scrotum in a patient with perineal hypospadias.

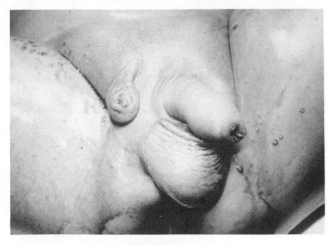

FIG. 54-12
Scrotal ectopia.

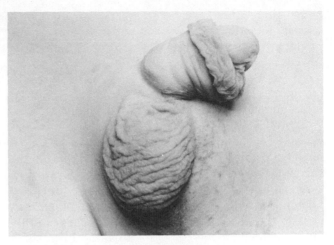

FIG. 54-13
Unilateral scrotal hypoplasia (left hemiscrotum is absent).

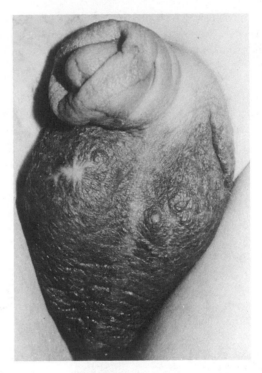

FIG. 54-14
Scrotal hemangioma.

the cord. There is no pulsation or bruit associated with the mass. The overlying skin can have a normal color or a pinkish, bluish, or purplish tinge. Often the skin is thinned in some areas due to the pressure of the tumor, and thickened in other regions (Fig. 54-14). The testes, epididymides, and vas deferens are gen-

erally normal on palpation. The mass remains distended without visible decrease in size when the patient in supine with the scrotum elevated. The lesion occurs with equal frequency on the right and left sides, unlike a varicocele. Scrotal hemangioma can also occur bilaterally, and cases have been reported in association with bladder tumors and Klippel-Trenaunay syndrome (Lindenauer, 1965).

The scrotal hemangioma is usually painless and nontender, although the mass can be associated with a feeling of heaviness and a dragging sensation. Angiography generally shows a capillary or venous (or both) hemangioma that may be supplied by a number of vessels, including the internal pudendal and the testicular artery among others. Microscopic examination reveals a benign unencapsulated lesion made up of a large number of cavernous vascular spaces supported by the subcutaneous tissue, with reduced cells and intraluminal thrombi present in the vascular spaces.

Complications of scrotal hemangioma include thrombosis, phlebitis, massive hemorrhage, and infertility. Eastridge and colleagues (1979) reported that this lesion has no effect on potency or fertility. However, Gotoh and associates (1983) reported a case of bilateral testicular damage, with absence of germinal cells in the seminiferous tubules and changes in the Sertoli cells, in a 16-year-old with a largely left-sided lesion. The authors postulated that the azoospermia was related to the high temperature of the hemangioma.

The treatment of choice is wide local excision of the tumor with the overlying skin, if possible. Other modalities that have been used include subcutaneous ligation, electrofulguration, intravenous (IV) prednisolone, solid carbon dioxide, and hemiscrotectomy and orchiectomy. Hemiscrotectomy and orchiectomy appear unnecessary, because no testicular involvement or malignant changes within the lesion have been reported. Because of their natural involution, hemangiomas of other areas of the skin normally require no treatment (Ray and Clark, 1976).

Splenogonadal Fusion

Splenogonadal fusion is an unusual malformation consisting of an abnormal connection between the spleen and the gonad. The entity was first described in 1883 (Bostrom, 1883). Since that time, 110 cases have been reported to date (Guarin et al., 1975). The majority of cases present as a scrotal mass or scrotal tenderness (Fig. 54-15). Some are found as an inci-

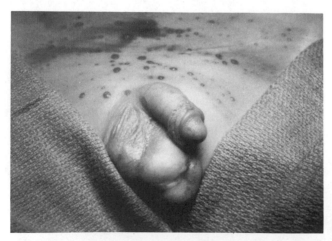

FIG. 54-15
Left hemiscrotal mass is consistent with splenogonadal fusion.

dental finding at the time of herniorrhaphy or orchidopexy, and about 25% are found at autopsy. There have been four cases reported in females (Halvorsen and Stray, 1978), and the abnormality has been seen from newborn to old age. About one half of the cases are reported in children, and there has been only one case of splenogonadal fusion reported on the right side (Putschar and Manion, 1956). The most common preoperative diagnosis is testicular neoplasm, which is reasonable because these splenic nodules are firm and do not transilluminate.

Two forms of the malformation have been presented clinically: continuous and discontinuous splenogonadal fusion (Tsingoglou and Wilkinson, 1976). In continuous splenogonadal fusion, the main spleen remains connected to the left gonad by a strand of tissue. This cord may be completely splenic, fibrous, or beaded with multiple nodules of splenic tissue. With discontinuous splenogonadal fusion, there is no connecting cord between the spleen proper and the left gonad. The ectopic splenic tissue is usually a distinct and encapsulated mass. About 25% of the reported cases of continuous splenogonadal fusion will have other anomalies, including micrognathia, anal atresia, asymmetry of the skull, or abnormal fissures of the lung and liver. None of the reported cases of discontinuous splenogonadal fusion has demonstrated any other malformations.

The evaluation of splenogonadal fusion usually takes place in the operating room. In theory, a technetium-99 colloid liver spleen scan could easily identify splenic tissue in the scrotum (Tudor, 1988); however, this is not usually done as a preoperative event. Scrotal ultrasound has not been helpful.

The treatment of splenogonadal fusion usually involves removal of both the testis and the adjoining mass (Fig. 54-16). If one were able to make a diagnosis of ectopic splenic tissue before surgery, a simple excision of the splenic nodule would suffice in virtually all cases of discontinuous splenogonadal fusion. In cases of continuous splenogonadal fusion, exploratory laparotomy is usually necessary to properly identify any anatomy involved and to deal with the continuous cord usually present.

GENITAL ANOMALIES—FEMALE
Embryology

The female reproductive system is derived primarily from the müllerian or paramesonephric ducts. In the absence of a fetal testis, there is no elaboration of androgen or MIS, so that the wolffian system regresses and the müllerian system is free to differentiate. Between the sixth and eighth weeks of gestation, the paired müllerian ducts develop lateral to the wolffian ducts and then cross medially to fuse in the midline. The fused müllerian ducts then join the urogenital sinus at the müllerian tubercle, and by the tenth week of gestation form a single tube called the uterovaginal canal.

The lateral aspect of the müllerian ducts, which remains separate, will ultimately become the fallopian tubes, and the fused portion of the ducts, which thickens, will become the fundus, body, and cervix of the uterus.

The exact embryologic origin of the vagina is somewhat uncertain. Koff (1933) suggested that the upper four fifths of the vagina is formed from the müllerian duct and lower fifth from the urogenital sinus. The major body of evidence supports the dual nature of the vagina, but the exact contribution from each source is still uncertain. At the twelfth week of gestation, vaginal development begins at the müllerian tubercle, where the uterovaginal canal joins the urogenital sinus. Bilateral endodermal invaginations called sinovaginal bulbs form in the area of the müllerian tubercle. As the bulbs grow, the müllerian tubercle regresses, and the distance between the uterovaginal lumen and the urogenital sinus increases. The sinovaginal bulb completes its growth by the fifteenth or sixteenth week of gestation and is called the primitive vaginal plate. Canalization of this cord of cells beings at the urogenital sinus and progresses cephalad, so that by the fifth month of embryonic growth, vaginal development is complete (Fig. 54-17).

Differentiation of the external genitalia of the female occurs between 12 and 16 weeks of gestation. In the absence of fetal androgen, particularly dihydrotestosterone, the common genital anlage develops passively into external genitalia of the female. The general tubercle enlongates slightly and becomes the clitoris, the urethral folds do not fuse and form labia minora, and the genital swellings form labia majora. The urogenital groove remains open and forms the vestibule of the vagina (Jost, 1971).

Vaginal Agenesis (Mayer-Rokitansky Syndrome)

Complete absence or agenesis of the vagina probably results from a disorder of the ureterovaginal canal or the vaginal plate (Fig. 54-18). Mayer (1829) first reported vaginal agenesis in stillborn infants with multiple birth defects. Kuster (1910) and Rokitansky (1928) described the entity and recognized that there was also usually a rudimentary uterus with normal ovaries and normal external genitalia (Fig. 54-19). Hauser and colleagues (1961) reported the frequent association of renal and skeletal anomalies. The incidence of this syndrome has been reported to vary from 1 in 4000 to 1 in 5000 live female births (Bryan et al., 1949); the patients are typically 46, XX females with normal secondary sex characteristics who most commonly have primary amenorrhea (Ross and Vande Wiele, 1974). The uterus in these patients may vary from normal to the more characteristic finding of a rudimentary bicornuate structure without a lumen. The association between congenital absence of the vagina and anomalies of the urogenital system is very common, approximately one third (34%) of these patients having renal abnormalities (Fore et al., 1975; Griffin et al., 1976). The most common abnormality is agenesis of one kidney or ectopia of one or both kidneys. Fusion abnormalities such as horseshoe kidney and crossed renal ectopia are also very common.

Skeletal anomalies have been reported in 12% of these patients, which would make such anomalies about one half as common as the renal anomalies seen (Griffin et al., 1976). Two thirds of the patients with skeletal anomalies have spine, limb, or rib anomalies.

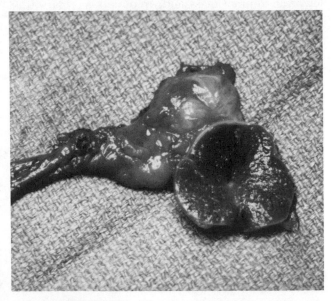

FIG. 54-16
Splenic tissue open adjacent to gonad.

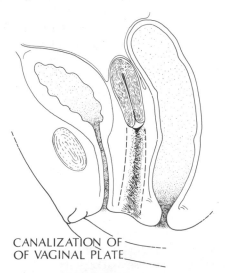

CANALIZATION OF
OF VAGINAL PLATE

FIG. 54-17
Vaginal development.

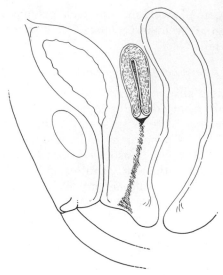

FIG. 54-18
Vaginal agenesis resulting from a failure of canalization of the vaginal plate.

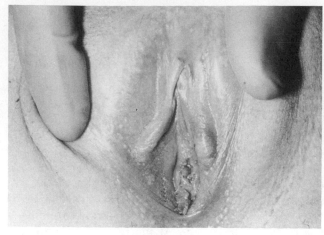

FIG. 54-19
External genitalia of a 13-year-old girl with vaginal agenesis.

Six percent of the skeletal malformations were of the Klippel-Feil type, which reflects an aberration in cervical thoracic somite development (Gunderson et al., 1967). Duncan and associates (1979) have recently recognized the frequency of these associated events and suggested that this combination of malformations be termed the MURCS association, an acronym for *Müllerian* duct aplasia, *r*enal aplasia, and *c*ervicothoracic *s*omite association.

The diagnosis of vaginal agenesis, although made most frequently at the time of puberty in association with amenorrhea, can be made occasionally in the neonatal period in an infant with an abdominal mass. In older patients, pelvic ultrasonography, computed axial tomography (CAT) scanning, and laparoscopy are the best means of making an accurate diagnosis.

Treatment of vaginal agenesis is predicted on the anatomy present. If there is a uterus and the vaginal remnant is too short to reach the perineum, construction of a vagina that will communicate with the uterus should be undertaken before the onset of menses (Counseller and Flor, 1957). This is usually accomplished using a free split-thickness skin graft as advocated by McIndoe (1959) or an isolated intestinal segment (Markland Hastings, 1974). If only the distal portion of the vagina is absent, posterior and lateral skin flaps can be mobilized and rotated into the proximal portion of the vagina to provide an introitus; however, in most isntances this is difficult to accomplish, and the long-term results vary. If no uterus is present, construction of a vagina should be undertaken just before the initiation of sexual activity. A split-thickness skin graft or an isolated intestinal segment is most often used for vaginal construction.

Congenital Vaginal Obstruction (Hydrocolpos and Hydrometrocolpos)

Congenital vaginal occlusions are probably the result of an incomplete canalization of the vagina that occurs during the fifth month of gestation. An imperforate hymen can result in gross distention of the vagina, which is termed hydrocolpos, or in distention of both the vagina and uterus, which is called hydrometrocolpos. Congenital vaginal obstruction is most commonly due to a simple imperforate hymen (Tompkins, 1939) (Fig. 54-20, *A*) and less commonly to more proximal lesions such as a high transverse vaginal septum (Bowman and Scott, 1954) (Fig. 54-20, *B*). A high transverse vaginal septum can also be associated with partial anterior vaginal agenesis, as well as with persistence of a common urogenital sinus.

The newborn with vaginal obstruction will have a lower abdominal mass and, frequently, urinary tract obstruction. The abdominal mass is the distended vagina, which results from excessive secretion of the cervical glands in response to maternal estrogen. Abdominal utrasonography will reveal a large midline sonolucent mass displacing the bladder forward and the rectum posteriorly. Percutaneous needle aspiration and injection of contrast material may aid in the diagnosis and can be done either through the perineum or the anterior abdominal wall (Fig. 54-21). If no abdominal mass is present at birth, the condition is often not detected until early adolescence, at which time symptoms may include amenorrhea, cyclic abdominal pain, and an abdominal mass secondary to hematocolpos (Fig. 54-22).

The treatment of vaginal obstruction depends on the anatomy. An imperforate hymen in the newborn that bulges at the introitus can be incised easily without anesthesia. It is important to identify the anatomy at the time of the drainage procedure to be certain that there is neither a common urogenital sinus nor

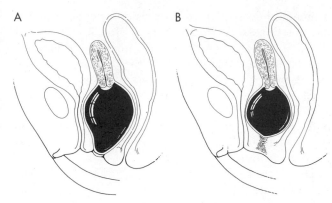

FIG. 54-20
Congenital vaginal obstruction. **A,** Imperforate hymen. **B,** High transverse septum.

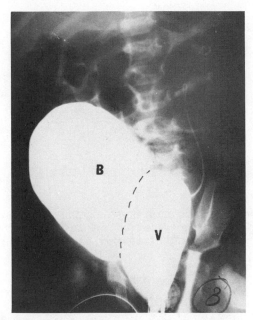

FIG. 54-21
Percutaneous injection of obstructed vagina (*V*) in newborn, with simultaneous cystogram (*B*) and retrograde catheterization of solitary left ureter and kidney.

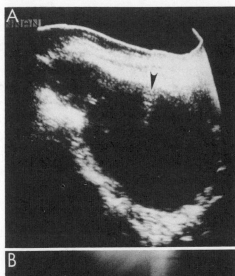

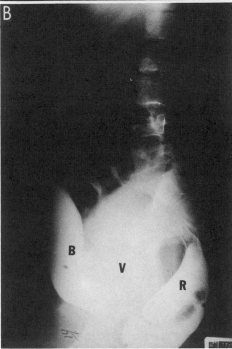

FIG. 54-22
A, 13-year-old girl with sonolucent midline mass. Note cervical impression *(arrow)*. **B,** Lateral view of same patient with midline mass pushing bladder (*B*) forward and rectum (*R*) posteriorly. *V* indicates vagina.

other urinary anomaly associated with the lower vaginal obstruction. Obstruction due to a high transverse vaginal septum or a partial agenesis of the anterior portion of the vagina can be more difficult to correct. These children must be investigated thoroughly before treatment. The high transverse vaginal septum with or without a common urogenital sinus is probably best treated by draining the vagina anteriorly with a simultaneous perineal vaginal pull-through. However, if the rectum and anus are displaced anteriorly, it may be difficult to perform a definite vaginoplasty in the infant. In this situation, it may be more appropriate simply to drain the obstructed vagina through the common urogenital sinus and delay the vaginal reconstruction until a later date, when it can be done in conjunction with a posterior anoplasty.

Fusion and Duplication Anomalies

Disorders of embryogenesis that produce duplication anomalies of the vagina and uterus occur at approximately 9 weeks of gestation and involve progression of the uterovaginal septum. These anomalies, which are very common, can include two uteri and two cervices fused with a single vagina or two separate vaginas, and two uteri fused with a single cervix and a single vagina (Dewhurst, 1968) (Fig. 54-23).

If there is complete vaginal duplication, one vagina can be obstructed and the other patent, so that the external genitalia will appear normal (Bowman and

Scott, 1954; Tompkins, 1939) (Fig. 54-24). The diagnosis of uterus didelphys and a unilateral obstructed vagina should be entertained as part of the differential diagnosis in a newborn with a sonolucent abdominal mass. Classically, the mass will push the bladder forward and the normal vagina posteriorly (Fig. 54-25). Vaginoscopy may reveal a bulging mass high in the vaginal sidewall. If technically possible, simple incision of the obstructing septum will provide adequate drainage; however, further division of the septum is usually necessary (Burbige and Hensle, 1984). At times, a formal laparotomy is required to provide adequate drainage and to confirm the diagnosis. Careful attention to the anatomy is essential to avoid an unnecessary ablative procedure. Simple division of the vaginal septum is all that is warranted in most of these patients, since successful term pregnancies have been reported in both uterine horns, suggesting that fertility is not impaired.

This condition should also be considered in pubertal girls who, despite having menses, present with cyclic pelvic discomfort and a mass. By ultrasound, the mass will either be sonolucent or have some scattered internal echoes. A vaginogram will once again show the

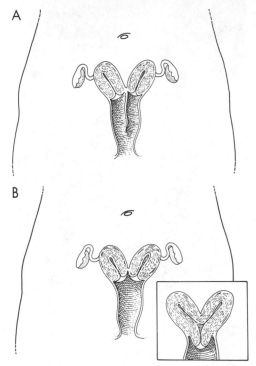

FIG. 54-23
A and **B,** Fusion anomalies of uterus and vagina.

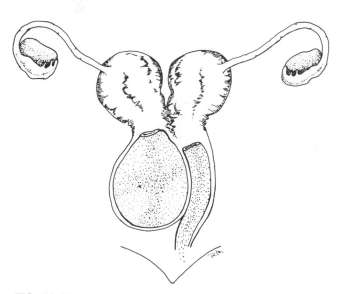

FIG. 54-24
Unilateral obstruction of duplex vagina in patient with uterus didelphys.

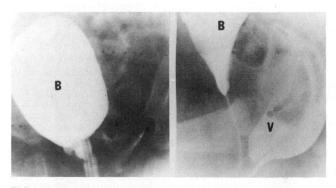

FIG. 54-25
Simultaneous cystogram and vaginogram in a patient with uterus didelphys and unilateral obstruction of a duplex vagina, showing separation of the bladder (B) and normal vagina (V).

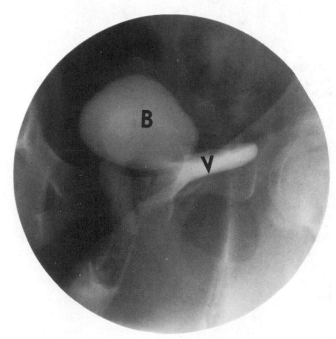

FIG. 54-26
Separation of the bladder (B) and normal vagina (V) by a distended obstructed hemivagina.

bladder and normal vagina pushed apart by the mass (Fig. 54-26). Pelvic magnetic resonance imaging (MRI) will typically show a normal uterine horn above a dilated blood-filled vagina. The blood gives off a very bright signal on the T1-weighted image (Fig. 54-27). Treatment of pubertal girls is identical to that for younger patients and can most frequently be done vaginally.

Urogenital Sinus Anomalies

Urogenital sinus is defined as a common channel into which both the urinary and genital tracts open. There is a wide spectrum of urogenital anomalies caused by a lack of development of the urogenital sinus and its derivatives. The common urogenital sinus is a normal stage of embryonic development in both sexes. In the normal female, an arrest in development of the müllerian ducts at 9 weeks of gestation, after they have fused with the urogenital sinus, could be manifested as a urovaginal confluence or common urogenital sinus (Fig. 54-28) (Witschi, 1970). An arrest of vaginal differentiation at a slightly later date can lead to the varying degrees of the urogenital sinus anomaly seen clinically (Fig. 54-29). A long urogenital sinus with a short vagina and a high urethral opening will result if the defect occurs at an early stage. A short urogenital sinus with an almost normal vaginal vestibule and low urethral orifice will occur if the arrest is late in development (Marshall et al., 1979). Early defects with a high insertion of the vagina and urethra into the urogenital sinus are also frequently associated with an anteriorly placed anus. This would indicate that there is also poor formation of the urorectal septum in these patients.

The diagnostic approach to the urogenital sinus is based on adequately defining the anatomy present. Retrograde contrast material injection into the urogenital sinus will help delineate the length of the common channel and identify the anatomic relationship of the vagina and urethra (Hendren and Crawford, 1969) (Fig. 54-30).

Once the anatomy of the defect has been clearly identified, the various treatment options can be considered. If the urogenital sinus is low, with a short common channel, a simple U-flap vaginoplasty will be effective (Hendren, 1977). Unfortunately, the urogenital sinus is frequently associated with an anteriorly placed anus, which may require posterior relocation to accomplish a skin-flap vaginoplasty from the perineum (Hendren and Donahoe, 1980). If the vagina enters the urogenital sinus too far proximally, a division of the vaginal moiety from the urogenital sinus will be necessary in conjunction with a pull-through vaginoplasty. In the most difficult form, there is a confluence of both the bladder and vagina high in the urogenital sinus. This defect requires not only a pull-through vaginoplasty, but often the creation of a neourethra from the anterior vaginal wall (Hendren, 1980b).

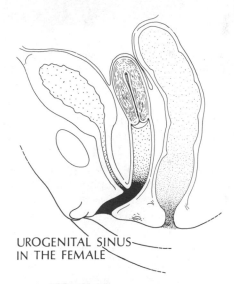

UROGENITAL SINUS IN THE FEMALE

FIG. 54-28
Urogenital sinus anomaly.

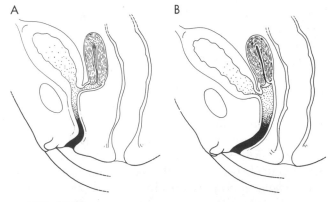

FIG. 54-29
A and **B,** variations of the urogenital sinus anomaly.

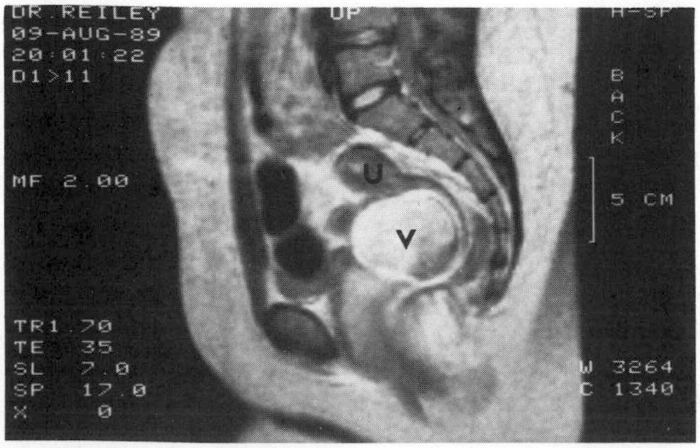

FIG. 54-27
U = uterus; *V* = vagina.

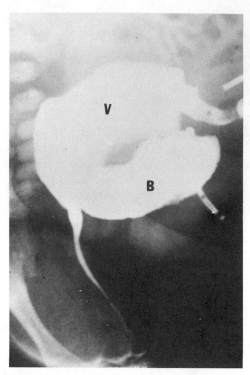

FIG. 54-30
Sinogram of urogenital sinus showing high confluence of bladder *(B)* and vagina *(V)* into a long urogenital sinus.

Cloacal Anomalies

The combination of a urogenital sinus and an anorectal anomaly is usually referred to as a cloacal malformation (Gough, 1959). In the early embryo, there is a cloacal stage during which there is confluence of the allantois and hindgut (Stephens and Smith, 1971). At 4 to 6 weeks of gestation, the urorectal septum should divide the allantois from the hindgut; however, if this separation does not take place, a common cloaca will result. These infants generally are born with abdominal distention and an abnormal perineum. There is usually no anus or vagina, and a single perineal opening is found. Frequently there is a hooded appearance to the phallus-like structure, which gives an initial masculinized gender appearance (Fig. 54-31). The bladder may enter the common urogenital sinus either just inside the perineal opening or very high. The insertion of the bladder may be associated with a relatively normal length of urethra or occur very close to the bladder neck. The entrance of the rectum into the cloaca can similarly be either high or low, near the perineum (Johnson et al., 1972) (Fig. 54-32). Vaginal abnormalities are common in patients with a cloacal anomaly, and vaginal duplication is the most common of the abnormalities seen. There also may be significant obstruction at the perineum in these patients, causing both hydrocolpos and obstructive uropathy (Fig. 54-33).

The diagnosis of a cloacal anomaly is confirmed by

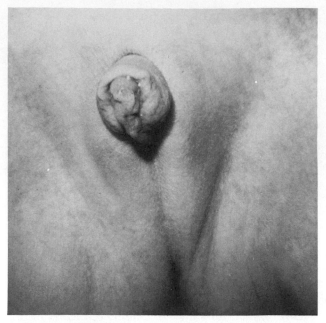

FIG. 54-31
Perineum of a patient with a cloacal anomaly.

retrograde contrast studies through the single perineal opening. Frequently, there is a confluence of the genitourinary and the GI systems. Often, however, all the components of the anomaly will not fill on a retrograde study; thus, it is not until an open procedure is performed that the exact anatomy can be defined.

Treatment of the various forms of cloacal anomalies is complex and presents one of the more difficult problems for pediatric surgeons and pediatric urologists. The first principle of treatment is to completely identify the anatomy involved (Kay and Tank, 1977). Clearly, the GI tract must be dealt with initially, and if the opening of the rectum into the urogenital sinus is low, a simple cutback anoplasty in the perineum may be possible (Hendren, 1980a). More frequently, however, a supralevator opening is present, and a primary colostomy is necessary, followed by a later pull-through procedure. If there is no significant urinary obstruction, specific treatment may not be necessary in the immediate perinatal period. If, however, urinary obstruction exists, a simple cutback of the urogenital sinus may afford adequate egress of urine to relieve obstruction.

Complete reconstruction of a cloacal anomaly is technically easier in later infancy and should be delayed until after 1 year of age, if possible (Raffensperger and Ramenofsky, 1973). Reconstruction should be performed in one stage, if feasible. When a cutback anoplasty or pull-through is done, it is important to be certain that the anus is placed far enough posteriorly to allow enough perineum for an adequate vaginal introitus and urethra. Once detachment of the rectum has been accomplished, the op-

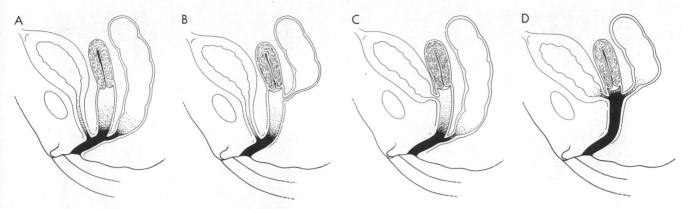

FIG. 54-32
A-D, Various forms of the cloacal anomaly.

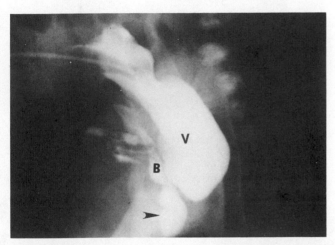

FIG. 54-33
Antegrade study of the bladder *(B)* and vagina *(V)* in a patient with a cloacal anomaly, demonstrating a dilated urogenital sinus *(arrow)* and relative obstruction at the perineal outlet.

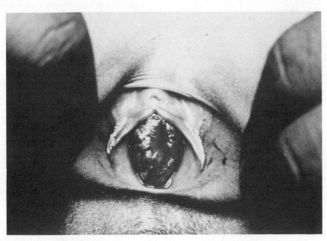

FIG. 54-34
Prolapsed urethra in a 9-year-old black girl.

erative approach to the anterior portion of the cloacal anomaly is very similar to that of a straightforward urogenital sinus (Hendren, 1977).

Masses of the Introitus

A mass at the introitus between the labia is often a diagnostic dilemma. The differential diagnosis includes prolapse of the urethra, prolapsed ectopic ureterocele, or prolapsed rhabdomyosarcoma. It is important to recognize each of these entities and to understand the diagnostic criteria for each.

Prolapse of the urethra (Fig. 54-34) occurs almost exclusively in black girls between the ages of 3 and 9 years. The child frequently has blood spotting on the underwear and a necrotic mass at the introitus, which represents a prolapsed and infarcted portion of the anterior urethra (Owens and Morse, 1968). The etiology of this lesion is unclear, although the histology closely resembles the capillary hemangioma pattern of a urethral caruncle in an adult. An accurate diagnosis depends on recognition of the entity. No diagnostic studies are needed, and the treatment usually involves simple excision of the prolapsed segment with suturing of the normal urethra to the meatus (Redman, 1982). Complications are virtually nonexistent except mild degrees of meatal stenosis following excision of the prolapsed segment and primary repair.

A prolapsed ectopic ureterocele can present as an intralabial introital mass (Mandell et al., 1980) (Fig. 54-35). This is usually a smooth white or slightly edematous lesion that extrudes from the urethral meatus. The urethral meatus can usually be seen above the lesion. The diagnosis can often be made on IV urography, which will demonstrate a lower pole collecting system, which is pushed laterally and inferiorly (drooping lily sign) with displacement of the ureter away from the midline on the affected side, and a filling defect in the bladder (Fig. 54-36) (Nussbaum and Lebowitz, 1983). Direct injection of the prolapsed segment is possible and may demonstrate the anatomy involved; however, this is often difficult to do, especially in newborns in whom this lesion is frequent.

Sarcoma botryoides, or rhabdomyosarcoma of the bladder or vagina, is the most common malignancy of

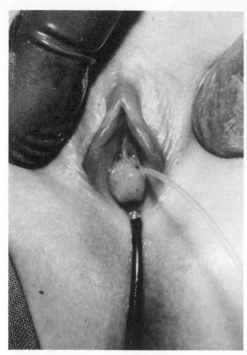

FIG. 54-35
Prolapsed ureterocele in a 3-year-old girl.

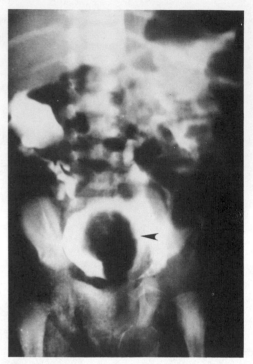

FIG. 54-36
Intravenous urogram in a patient with an ectopic ureterocele, demonstrating a right lower pole collecting system being pushed laterally and inferiorly (drooping lily sign) along with a filling defect in the bladder *(arrow)*.

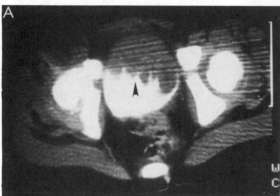
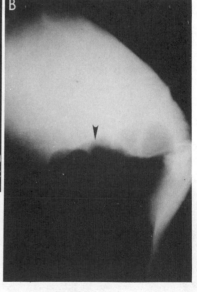

FIG. 54-37
CT scan **(A)** and cystourethrogram **(B)** in a patient with a bladder rhabdomyosarcoma, demonstrating a filling defect in the anterior portion of the bladder *(arrow)*.

lower genitourinary system seem in infancy (Hilgers et al., 1970). It commonly presents with blood spotting on the underwear, and the lesion appears as a lobulated, grapelike mass. The diagnosis can be made by direct biopsy, but the extent of the lesion is best determined by pelvic ultrasonography and CAT scan (Middleton et al., 1981) (Fig. 54-37).

Other lesions that can appear as intralabial masses include a low simple imperforate hymen, which can present as a bulging intralabial mass in newborn girls (Reed and Griscom, 1973) (Fig. 54-38). This is often simply an imperforate hymen with some degree of hydrocolpos due to maternal estrogen stimulation. These lesions are easily recognized and need incision

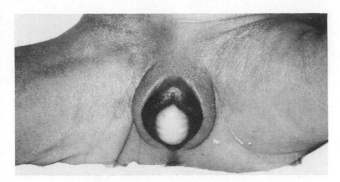

FIG. 54-38
Bulging hymen in a newborn girl.

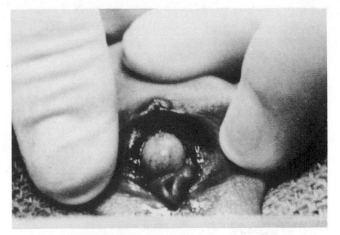

FIG. 54-39
Paraurethral cyst in a 1-year-old girl.

A

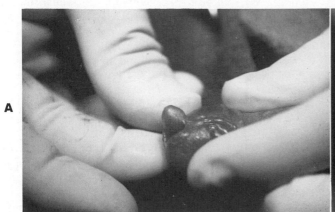

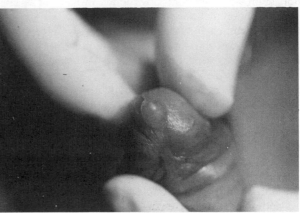

B

FIG. 54-40
A and **B**, Parameatal cyst in a 3-year-old boy.

and drainage; rarely do they require further therapy.

Parauretheral cysts (Blaivas et al., 1976) also present as interlabial masses in female infants. They tend to displace the urethral meatus to one side, and a normal urethra and vaginal introitus can usually be identified (Fig. 54-39). These cysts seem to be embryologic remnants of Skene's glands or Gartner's duct. Most of these cysts will rupture spontaneously, but they may have to be incised and drained.

Cystic lesions of the meatus can also occur in males (Fig. 54-40). Parameatal urethral cysts were first reported in the English literature in 1956 (Thompson and Lantin, 1956) and scattered reports have appeared since. Most recently, 41 cases were reviewed from Japan (Koga, et al., 1990) and, in that review, although the patients ranged in age from 9 months to 43 years, almost 50% presented at less than 15 years of age. The mass was totally asymptomatic in 75% of the cases, and dysuria was the presentation in the other 25%.

Although the etiology of these cysts is unclear, we feel that they are most likely related to some obstruc-

tion of one of the paired parameatal glands, which we have previously described (Gilhooley and Hensle, 1984). Histologic features include a cyst wall lining that can vary from columnar to transitional to cuboidal epithelial. The most common lining is columnar. Treatment of these parameatal urethral cysts usually consists of simple unroofing. In a very small number of patients, the cyst may recur, and, in this situation, total excision of the lining is required.

REFERENCES

Allan N, Cowan LE: Uterus didelphys with unilateral imperforate vagina: report of 4 cases. *Obstet Gynecol* 1963; 22:442.

Amrhein JA, Meyer WJ, Jones HW, et al: Androgen insensitivity in man: evidence for genetic heterogeneity. *Proc Natl Acad Sci USA* 1976; 73:891.

Anderson KM, Liao S: Selective retention of dihydrotestosterone by prostatic nuclei. *Nature* 1968; 219:277.

Appleby LH: Synchronous rupture of bilateral ectopics. *Can Med Assoc J* 1923; 13:514.

Berta P, Hawkins JR, Sinclair AH, et al: Genetic evidence equating SRY and the testis-determining factor. *Nature* 1990; 348:448.

Blaivas JG, Pais VM, Retik AB: Paraurethral cysts in female neonates. *Urology* 1976; 7:504.

Bostrom: *Gesellschaft Deutscher naturforscher und Aezte Verdnadlungen der 56 Versamming*. Frieburg, 1883, p 149.

Bowman, J Scott R: Transverse vaginal septum. *Obstet Gynecol* 1954; 3:441.

Bruchovsky N, Wilson JD: The conversion of testosterone to 5α-androstane-17b-ol-3-one by rat prostate in vivo and in vitro. *J Biol Chem* 1968; 243:2012.

Bryan AL, Nigro JA, Counseller VS: One hundred cases of congenital absence of the vagina. *Surg Gynecol Obstet* 1949; 88:79.

Buckley GT: Scrotal and penile lymphedema. *J Urol* 1962; 87:422.

Burbige KA, Hensle TW: Uterus didelphys and vaginal duplication with unilateral obstruction presenting as a newborn abdominal mass. J Urol 1984; 132:1195.

Burstein S, Grumbach MM, Kaplan SL: Early determination of androgen-responsiveness is important in the management of microphallus. *Lancet* 1979; 2:983.

Cohen-Addad N, Zarafu IW, Hanna MK: Complete penoscrotal transposition. *Urology* 1985; 26:149.

Counseller VS, Flor FS: Congenital absence of the vagina: further results of treatment and a new technique. *Surg Clin North Am* 1957; 37:1107.

Dewhurst CJ: Congenital malformations of the genital tract in childhood. *Br J Obstet Gynaecol* 1968; 75:377.

Duncan PA, Shapiro LR, Stangel JJ, et al: The MURCS association: müllerian duct aplasia, renal aplasia, and cervicothoracic somite dysplasia. *J Pediatr* 1979; 95:399.

Eastridge RR, Carrion HM, Politano VA: Hemangioma of scrotum, perineum, and buttocks. *Urology* 1979; 14:61.

Federman DD: *Abnormal Sexual Development: A Genetic and Endocrine Approach to Differential Diagnosis*. Philadelphia, WB Saunders, 1967.

Feins NR: A new surgical technique for lymphedema of the penis and scrotum. *J Pediatr Surg* 1980; 15:787.

Feldman KW, Smith DW: Fetal phallic growth and penile standards for newborn male infants. *J Pediatr* 1975; 86:395.

Fitzpatrick TJ: Hemihypertrophy of the human corpus cavernosum. *J Urol* 1976; 115:560.

Fore SR, Hammond CB, Parker RT, et al: Urologic and genital anomalies in patients with congenital absence of the vagina. *Obstet Gynecol* 1975; 46:410.

Gautier T, Salient J, Pena S, et al: Testicular function in 2 cases of penile agenesis. *J Urol* 1981; 126:556.

Gilhooly P, Hensle TW: Parameatal ducts of glans penis; structure, symptoms, and treatment of the uncommon focus of infection. *Urology* 1984; 24(4):375.

Gotoh M, Tsai S, Sugiyama T, et al: Giant scrotal hemangioma with azoospermia. *Urology* 1983; 22:637.

Gough MH: Anorectal agenesis with persistence of cloaca. *Proc R Soc Med* 1959; 52:886.

Gravell CJ: Congenital curvature of the penis. *J Urol* 1974; 112:489.

Griffin JE, Edwards C, Madden JD, et al: Congenital absence of the vagina. *Ann Intern Med* 1976; 85:224.

Griffin JE, Wilson JD: The syndromes of androgen resistance. *N Engl J Med* 1980; 302:198.

Guarin U, Dimitrieva Z, Ashley S: Splenogonadal fusion—a rare congenital anomaly demonstrated by ^{99m}Tc-sulfur colloid imaging. *J Nucl Med* 1975; 16:922.

Gunderson CH, Greenspan RH, Glaser GH, et al: The Klippel-Feil syndrome: genetic and clinical reevaluation of cervical fusion. *Medicine (Baltimore)* 1967; 46:491.

Guthrie RD, Smith DW, Graham CR: Testosterone treatment for micropenis during early childhood. *J Pediatr* 1973; 83:247.

Halvorsen JF, Stray O: Splenogonadal fusion. *Acta Paediatr Scand* 1978; 67:379.

Hauser GA, Keller M, Koller T, et al: Das Rokitansky-Kuster syndrome: uterus bipartitus solidus rudimentarius cum vagina solida. *Gynaecologia* 1961; 151:111.

Hendren WH: Surgical management of urogenital sinus abnormalities. *J Pediatr Surg* 1977; 12:339.

Hendren WH: Construction of female urethra from vaginal wall and a perineal flap. *J Urol* 1980a; 123:657.

Hendren WH: Urogenital sinus and anorectal malformation: experience with 22 cases. *J Pediatr Surg* 1980b; 15:628.

Hendren WH, Crawford JD: Adrenogenital syndrome: the anatomy of the anomaly and its repair: some new concepts. *J Pediatr Surg* 1969; 4:49.

Hendren WH, Donahoe PK: Correction of congenital abnormalities of the vagina and perineum. *J Pediatr Surg* 1980; 15:751.

Hilgers RD, Malkasian GD Jr, Soule EH: Embryonal rhabdomyosarcoma (botyroid type) of the vagina. *Am J Obstet Gynecol* 1970; 107:484.

Imperato-McGinley J, Peterson RE, Gautier T, et al: Androgens and the evolution of male-gender identity among male pseudohermaphrodites with 5 α-reductase deficiency. *N Engl J Med* 1979; 300:1233.

Jacobs PA, Strong JA: A case of human intersexuality having a possible XXY sex-determining mechanism. *Nature* 1959; 183:302.

Jager RJ, Anvert M, Hall K, et al: A human XY female with a frame shift mutation in the candidate testis-determining gene SRY. *Nature* 1990; 348:452.

Jirasek JE: *Development of the Genital System and Male Pseudohermaphroditism*. Baltimore, Johns Hopkins Press, 1971, pp 3-4.

Johnson RJ, Palken M, Derrick W, et a: The embryology of high anorectal and associated genitourinary anomalies in the female. *Surg Gynecol Obstet* 1972; 135:759.

Johnston JH: The genital aspects of exstrophy. *J Urol* 1975; 113:701.

Josso N: Permeability of membranes to the müllerian-inhibiting substance synthesized by the human fetal testis in vitro: a clue to its biochemical nature. *J Clin Endocrinal Metab* 1972; 34:265.

Jost A: Embryonic sexual differentiation. In Jones HW Jr, Scott WW (eds): *Hermaphroditism, Genital Anomalies, and Related Endocrine Disorders*, ed 2. Baltimore, Williams and Wilkins, 1971.

Kay R, Tank ES: Principles of management of the persistent cloaca in the female newborn. *J Urol* 1977; 117:102.

Kessler WO, McLaughlin AP: Agenesis of penis: embryology and management. *Urology* 1973; 1:226.

Klugo RC, Cerny JC: Response of micropenis to topical testosterone and gonadotropin. *J Urol* 1978; 119:667.

Koff AK: Development of the vagina in the human fetus. *Contemp Embryol* 1933; 24:61.

Koga S, Arakaki Y, Matsuoka M, et al: Parameatal cysts of the glans penis. *Br J Urol* 1990; 65:101.

Kuster H: Uterus bipartitus solidus rudimentarius cum vagina solida. *Z Geburtshilfe Perinatol* 1910; 67:692.

Lamm DL, Kaplan GW: Accessory and ectopic scrotum. *Urology* 1977; 9:149.

Lee PA, Mazur T, Danish R, et al: Micropenis: 1. Criteria, etiologies, and classification. *Johns Hopkins Medical Journal* 1980; 146:156.

Lindenauer SM: The Klippel-Trenaunay-Weber syndrome: varicosity, hypertrophy, and hemangioma with no arteriovenous fistula. *Ann Surg* 1965; 162:303.

Mandell J, Colodny AH, Lebowitz RL, et al: Ureteroceles in infants and children. *J Urol* 1980; 123:921.

Markland C, Hastings D: Vaginal reconstruction using cecal and sigmoid bowel segments in transsexual patients. *J Urol* 1974; 111:217.

Marshall FF, Jeffs RD, Sarafyan WK: Urogenital sinus abnormalities in the female patient. *J Urol* 1979; 122:568.

Mayer CAJ: Uber Verdoppelungen des Uterus und ihre Arten, nebst Bemerkungen uber Hasenscharte und Wolfsrachen. *J Chir Auger* 1829; 13:525.

McIndoe A: Discussion on treatment of congenital absence of vagina with emphasis on long-term results. *Proc R Soc Med* 1959; 52:952.

Meyer WJ, Migeon BR, Migeon CJ: Locus on human X chromosome for dihydrotestosterone receptor and androgen insensitivity. *Proc Natl Acad Sci USA* 1975; 72:1469.

Middleton AW, Elman AJ, Stewart JR, et al: Combined modality therapy with conservation of organ function in childhood genitourinary rhabdomyosarcoma. *Urology* 1981; 18:42.

Money J, Potter R, Stall CS: Sex reannouncement in hereditary sex deformity: psychology and sociology of habilitation. *Soc Sci Med* 1969; 3:207.

Nussbaum AR, Lebowitz RL: Interlabial masses in little girls. *AJR* 1983; 141:65.

Owens SB, Morse WH: Prolapse of the female urethra in children. *J Urol* 1968; 100:171.

Pomerantz P, Hanna M, Levitt S, et al: Isolated torsion of penis—report of 6 cases. *Urology* 1978; 11:37.

Putschar WG, Manion WC: Splenic-gonadal fusion. *Am J Pathol* 1956; 32:15.

Raffensperger JG, Ramenofsky ML: The management of a cloaca. *J Pediatr Surg* 1973; 8:647.

Ray B, Clark SS: Hemangioma of scrotum. *Urology* 1976; 8:502.

Redman JF: Conservative management of urethral prolapse in female children. *Urology* 1982; 19:509.

Reed MH, Griscom WT: Hydrometrocolpos in infancy. *AJR* 1973; 118:1.

Reiley JM, Woodhouse CRJ: *J Urol* 1989; 142:569.

Robert: *Bull Soc Anat Paris* 1851; 26:194.

Rodriguez C: Report of a case of diphallus. *J Urol* 1965; 94:436.

Rokitansky K: Uber die sogenannten Verdoppelungen Des Uterus. *Med Jb Ost Staat* 1928; 26:39.

Ross GT, Vande Wiele R:l The ovaries. In Williams RH (ed): *Textbook of Endocrinology*. ed 5, Philadelphia, WB Saunders, 1974, p 368.

Schonfeld WA, Beebe GW: Normal growth and variation in the male genitalia from birth to maturity. *J Urol* 1942; 48:759.

Simpson JL: *Disorders of Sexual Differentiation: Etiology and Clinical Delineation*. New York, Academic Press, 1976, pp 51-110, 183-224.

Stephens FD, Smith ED: *Anorectal Malformations in Children*. Year Book Medical Publishers, 1971.

Thompson IM, Lantin PM: Parameatal cysts of the glans penis. *J Urol* 1956; 76:753.

Tompkins P: Imperforate hymen and hematocolpos. *JAMA* 1939; 113:913.

Tsingoglou S, Wilkinson AW: Splenogonadal fusion. *Br J Surg* 1976; 63:297.

Tudor RB: Splenogonadal fusion: 110 cases. In *Childhood Disease Registry*. Bismarck, N.Dak., Q&R Clinic, report no. 4, 1988.

Vera-Roman JM: Robinow dwarfing syndrome accompanied by penile agenesis and hemivertebrae. *Am J Dis Child* 1973; 126:206.

Witschi F: Development and differentiation of the uterus. In Mack HC (ed): *Prenatal Life*. Detroit, Wayne State University Press, 1970, p 11.

CHAPTER 55

Hypospadias

John W. Duckett
Laurence S. Baskin

The term hypospadias is derived from the Greek language and refers to a rent (spadon) on the ventrum of the penis, whereas epispadias is a rent on the dorsum of the penis. Hypospadias is a congenital defect of the penis resulting in incomplete development of the anterior urethra. The abnormal urethral opening may be any place along the shaft of the penis or may open onto the scrotum or perineum. As the position of the meatus becomes more proximal, ventral shortening and curvature during erection are more likely.

The normal anatomy of the penis consists of paired corpora cavernosa covered by thick elastic tunica albuginea with a midline septum. The urethra traverses the penis within the corpus spongiosum, which lies in a ventral position in the groove between the two corporal bodies. The urethra emerges at the distal end of the conical glans penis, which is the distal aspect of the spongiosum. The spermatic fascia, or dartos fascia, is the loose layer of connective tissue immediately beneath the skin. Superficial lymphatics and the dorsal veins of the penis are located in this fascia. Beneath the dartos fascia is Buck's fascia, which surrounds the corpora cavernosa and splits to contain the corpus spongiosum in a separate compartment. The neurovascular bundle lies deep to Buck's fascia dorsally in the groove between the corpora cavernosa. Hypospadias results in various degrees of deficiency of the urethra, corpus spongiosum, and corpora cavernosa. The skin on the ventral surface may be thin, and the prepuce is deficient ventrally and forms a dorsal hood over the glans.

As a rule, dystopia of the meatus does not cause significant obstructive urinary symptoms, although ventral deflection of the stream may occur. When the meatus is more proximal, the stream flows straight downward or backward, requiring these males to urinate "ad modum feminarum." The curvature of the penis is alleged to cause painful erections and, if uncorrected, may result in obviously severe psychologic consequences (Kelami, 1983).

Sexually, the dystopia of the meatus may cause *impotentia generandi*, which is illustrated from the following historic note concerning Henry II of France.

Henry II was known to have hypospadias, as recorded by his physician Fernal. His marriage with Catherine the Medici was infertile until Fenral "advised his patient that in such cases *coitus more ferarum* permitted him to overcome the difficulty" (Ombredanne, as quoted by Van der Muelen, 1964). Henry II then proceeded to sire three kings of France, along with seven other children.

Throughout Greek culture, there was high appreciation for the goddess Hermaphrodite, half man, half woman. Many statues reflect hypospadiac genitalia, perhaps indicative of admiration for this condition. It is, therefore, understandable why it was not until the first and second centuries A.D. that the Alexandrian surgeons Heliodorus and Antyllus are given credit for the first attempted correction of this anomaly by amputation of the distal curved portion (DeVries, 1986; Rogers, 1973).

CLASSIFICATION

Anatomic classification of hypospadias recognizes the level of the meatus without taking into account curvature. The *first degree* identifies the meatus from the corona to the distal shaft, the *second degree* locates the meatus from the distal shaft of the penoscrotal junction, and the *third degree* is from the penoscrotal junction to the perineum (Smith, 1938). Schaeffer and Erbes (1950) classified the location as *glanular* from the subcorona out, *penile* from the corona to the penoscrotal junction, and *perineal* from there down. The system of Browne (1936) was more specific, with *subcoronal, penile, penoscrotal, scrotal,* and *perineal* varieties. Unforunately, these classifications do not allow one to determine in a given series whether the common subcoronal lesions were present or whether a severe curvature was associated with a subcoronal meatus. Therefore, we prefer the classification relat-

TABLE 55-1

Classification of Hypospadias According to Meatal Location After Release of Curvature

Anterior hypospadias (50% of cases) (Figs. 55-5 and 55-8)
  Glanular (meatus situated on the inferior surface of the glans)
  Coronal (meatus situated in the balanopenile furrow)
  Anterior penile (meatus situated in the distal third of the shaft)
Middle hypospadias (20% of cases) (Figs. 55-2 and 55-6)
  Middle penile (meatus situated in the middle third of the shaft)
Posterior hypospadias (30% of cases) (Figs. 55-9 and 55-10)
  Posterior penile (meatus situated in the posterior third of the shaft)
  Penoscrotal (meatus situated at the base of the shaft in front of the scrotum)
  Scrotal (meatus situated on the scrotum or between the genital swellings)
  Perineal (meatus situated behind the scrotum or behind the genital swellings)

ing the new location of the meatus after the curvature has been released (Barcat, 1973) (Table 55-1).

Welch (1979) collected more than 1000 cases of hypospadias from seven separate reports and estimated that 62% of the openings were subcoronal or penile, 22% were at the penoscrotal angle, and 16% opened in the scrotum or perineum. Out of 1286 cases over 5 years at Children's Hospital of Philadelphia, 49% were anterior, 21% were middle, and 30% were in a posterior location (Fig. 55-1). Juskiewenski and colleagues (1983) reported a study of 536 patients with hypospadias. Anterior hypospadias comprised 71%, middle 16%, and posterior 13%. He subdivided the hypospadias of the anterior group of 383 patients into 13% balanitic, 43% subcoronal, 38% distal shaft, and 6% with prepuce intact.

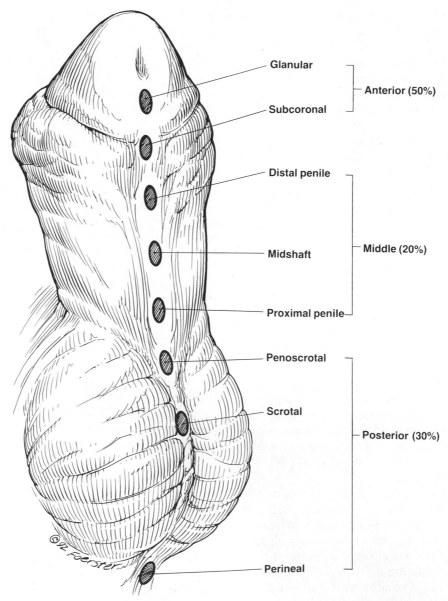

FIG. 55-1
Classification of hypospadias. (From Duckett JW: Hypospadias. In *Contemporary Urology* April, 1992. Used by permission.)

INCIDENCE AND GENETICS

The incidence of hypospadias has been calculated to be 3.2 in 1000 live male births, or about 1 in every 300 male children (Sweet et al., 1974). Another survey in the United States in which particular attention was given to minor degrees of hypospadias estimated the incidence at 1 in 125 live male births (Chung and Myrianthopoulos, 1968). Sorenson (1953) estimated 1 in 300 live births, and Avellan (1975) determined the incidence in Sweden to be approximately 1 in 300. These figures mean that approximately 1,848,500 male birth in the United States in 1986, there were about 6200 cases of hypospadias.

The diagnosis of all but the most minor forms of hypospadias is self-evident on examination of newborn males. The incomplete formation of the prepuce with the excess dorsal hood leads to an immediate recognition of the urethral defect. More recently, we have been able to make the diagnosis of hypospadias with prenatal ultrasound. The classic findings are a wide distal end of the penis that correlates with the excess dorsal prepuce (Fig. 55-2).

Familial tendencies have been identified. Fathers have been found to have hypospadias in 8% of the patients. Fourteen percent of the male siblings of an index child have hypospadias, and if two members of the family have hypospadias, the risk of a subsequent child having hypospadias is 21% (Bauer et al., 1981).

The cause of hypospadias is still unknown. It is probably polygenic because of the higher familial incidence. The condition is more common in whites than in blacks, and is most common in Italians and Jews (Welch, 1979). The incidence of hypospadias among monozygotic twins is 8.5 times higher than in singletons (Roberts and Lloyd, 1973). It might be explained by the demand of two male fetuses on the placental production of human chorionic gonadotropin (HCG) in phase 3 organogenesis. It is also possible that with monozygotic twins, one placenta may not be able to meet the HCG requirements for masculinization of two male fetuses. In addition, there may be a higher incidence of hypospadias in winter conceptions, perhaps reflecting the effect of daylight on maternal, and hence fetal, pituitary function (Roberts and Lloyd, 1973). In a larger study, however, comparing the incidence of hypospadias between the Northern and Southern hemispheres, no differences in seasonal variation were noted (Castilla et al., 1990).

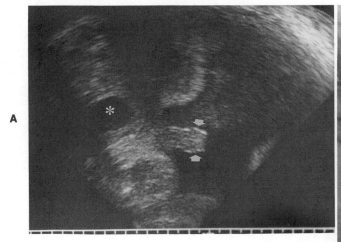

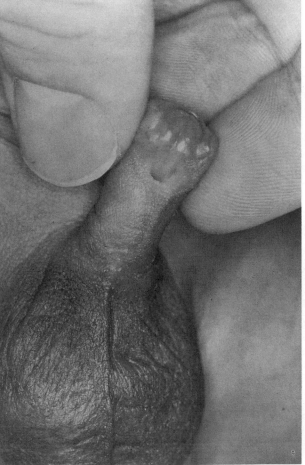

FIG. 55-2
A, Prenatal fetal sonogram at 31 weeks gestation revealing a wide distal end of the penis *(white arrows)* which correlates with the excess dorsal prepuce and the diagnosis of hypospadias *(fetal bladder marked by white asterisks)* **B,** Postnatal photograph of same patient showing midshaft hypospadias with excess dorsal prepuce.

EMBRYOLOGY

By the end of the first month of gestation, the hindgut and future urogenital system reach the surface of the embryo at the cloacal membrane on the ventral surface. The cloacal membrane is divided by a septum into a posterior, or anal, half, and an anterior half, the urogenital membrane. Three protuberances appear around the latter. The most cephalad is the genital tubercle. The other two, the genital swellings, flank the urogenital membrane on each side (Fig. 55-3, A). Up to this point, the male and female genitalia are essentially indistinguishable. Under the influence of

testosterone in response to a surge of luteinizing hormone from the pituitary, masculinization of the external genitalia takes place. One of the first signs of masculinization is an increase in the distance between the anus and the genital structures, followed by elongation of the phallus, formation of the penile urethra from the urethral groove, and development of the prepuce (Hinman, 1993; Jirasek, 1968).

There are three separate portions of the male urethra. The portion above the wolffian duct opening forms the urethra down to and including the verumonatanum, utricle, and urogenital sinus. The second

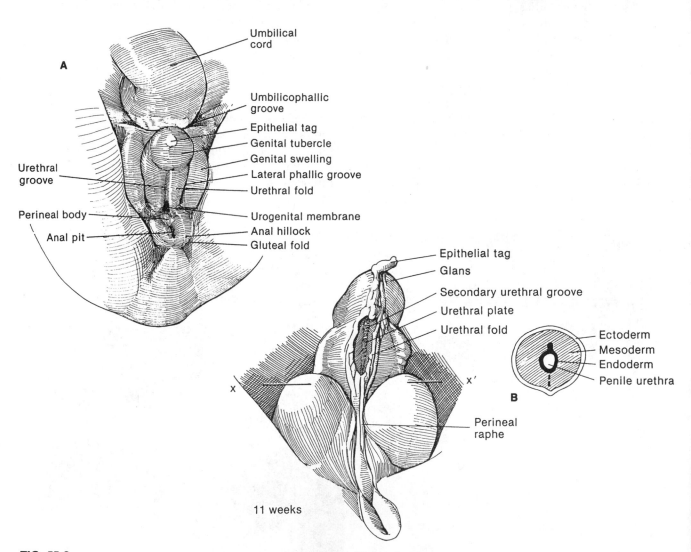

FIG. 55-3

Development of penis and urethra. **A,** Indifferent stage ~ 8 weeks. Note that the primitive urethral groove forms on the caudal slope of the genital tubercle. Paired genital (labioscrotal) swellings arise on either side of the urogenital membrane above the anal pit and the perineal body. **B,** Enclosure of the urethra at 11 weeks. Beginning near the anus, the adjacent ectodermal urethral folds fuse over the urethral plate to form the penile urethra, with the distal urethra at the coronal sulcus being the last to close. **C,** Formation of the glanular urethra and fossa navicularis occurs late in gestation. A plug of ectoderm from the tip of the glans invades the mesenchyme as an ectodermal intrusion. The floor of the ectodermal intrusion makes contact with the end of the urethral plate that forms the roof of the advancing urethra, and the intervening double wall breaks down. **D,** The prepuce forms by the differentiation of the epithelial cells of the glanular lamella, which forms a groove between the preputial folds and the glans. (From Hinman F Jr: *Surgical Anatomy of the Genitourinary Tract.* Philadelphia, WB Saunders 1994, pp 418-470. Used by permission.)

anlage forms the segment extending from the veru to the base of the glans. The glans segment is formed separately. There is an endodermal lining down to the bulbar enlargement of the urogenital sinus. Beyond this point, the urethra is lined by ectoderm. The urogenital sinus begins at the openings of the wolffian and müllerian ducts and extends to the urogenital membrane, which separates it from the cloacal fossa above. The elongation of this sinus accompanies growth of the genital tubercle. On its underside, a longitudinal groove appears, which is the first indication of the second portion of the urethra. The urethral gutter closes by infolding of its margins, while the urogenital membrane of the cloacal fossa closes from behind, forming a urethral tube that is open to the bladder and to the exposed gutter. The epithelial outpocketings of the proximal urethra subsequently form the lobes of the prostate gland. At about the same time, the abdominal wall is closing anteriorly, and the total ventral fusion process is completed by the twelfth week (first trimester). At this time, the labioscrotal folds are evident, and their fusion in the midline creates the perineal median raphe (Fig. 55-3, B), which extends from the region of the anus through the midline of the scrotum to the level of the glans.

Meanwhile, the glans develops into a recognizable structure, and the third segment of the urethra develops from a urethral plate. The mesenchyme within the urethral folds forms the corps spongiosum after their fusion. Ultimately, the main endodermal urethral channel joins the ectoderm as it invades more deeply into the glans (Fig. 55-3, C). Because it is the last step in formation of the completed urethra, there is a higher incidence of hypospadias with the meatal opening at the subcoronal region. The abortive urethral depression seen at the normal meatal site in hypospadias may be explained by abnormalities of ectodermal intrusion.

At about 8 weeks gestation, low preputial folds appear on both sides of the penile shaft, which join dor-

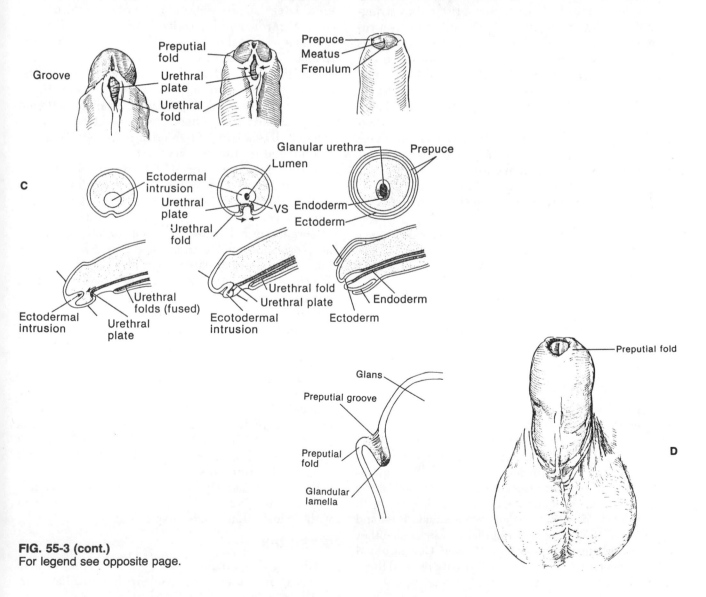

FIG. 55-3 (cont.)
For legend see opposite page.

sally to form a flat ridge at the proximal edge of the corona (Fig. 55-3, *C*). The ridge does not entirely encircle the glans because it is blocked on the ventrum by incomplete development of the glandular urethra. Thus the preputial fold is transported distally by active growth of the mesenchyme between it and the glandular lamella (Fig. 55-3, *D*). The process continues until the preputial fold covers all of the glans. The fusion is usually present at birth, but subsequent desquamation of the epithelial fusion allows the prepuce to retract. If the genital folds fail to fuse, the preputial tissues do not form ventrally; consequently, in hypospadias, preputial tissue is absent on the ventrum, and it is excessive dorsally.

Chordee

The abnormal ventral curvature of the penis associated with hypospadias is poorly understood. It has been labeled chordee; however, this term implies a strand of connective tissue stretched like a cord between the meatus and glans, giving rise to bowstringing. According to Mettauer (1842), this cord is a rudiment of the urethral corpus spongiosum. This hypothesis, however, is untenable, because the corpus spongiosum is formed in the periurethral tissue only at the end of the fourth month. The chordee tissue that fans out on the ventrum of the penis is probably the rudimentary vestige of the urethral plate, as suggested by Paul and Kanagasuntheram (1956). This strand, or chordee, which in the past has been depicted beautifully by medical illustrators, rarely causes curvature of the penis (Van der Meulen, 1964).

There are other explanations for the chordee tissue:

1. The mesenchyme distal to the hypospadic meatus condenses to form chordee tissue (Kaplan and Brock, 1981; Kaplan and Lamm, 1975).
2. Abnormal disintegration of the urethral plate in the absence of mesenchymal ingrowth gives rise to the fibrous chordee tissue.
3. There is growth differential between the normally formed dorsal phallic tissue and the abnormal ventral urethral plate (Bellinger, 1981).

Associated Anomalies

Undescended testis and inguinal hernia are the most common associated anomalies with hypospadias. In one series, 9.3% of hypospadias patients had an undescended testis (Khuri et al., 1981). Posterior hypospadias had a 32% incidence, middle 6%, and anterior 5%. Khuri and associates (1981) also found the overall incidence of inguinal hernia to be 9%, with 17% associated with posterior hypospadias. Ross and colleagues (1959) reported a similar incidence of either cryptorchidism or hernia in 16%, and Cerasaro and co-workers (1986) found 18% of 301 patients had these anomalies.

A utriculus masculinus (utricle) is found in a high percentage of the more severe cases. For example, Devine and associates (1980) found that of 44 patients whose meatus was posterior, 6 (14%) had a utricle. Of seven with perineal hypospadias, four (57%) had a utricle, compared with 2 of 20 (10%) with a penoscrotal meatus. None of the 17 patients with penile hypospadias had a utricle. Shima and colleagues (1979) found a utricle in 1 of 29 glandular, 3 of 74 penile, 11 of 122 penoscrotal, and 10 of 29 scrotal-perineal hypospadias cases. Thus the incidence is 14% in 151 penoscrotal or perineal hypospadias cases. If both studies are combined, there is an 11% incidence of a utricle in severe hypospadias.

Usually there are no complications from the presence of a utricle except for infection and difficulty passing a catheter. Ritchey and co-workers (1988) have reviewed some late problems.

It is not surprising that urinary tract anomalies are infrequent, because the external genitalia are formed much later than the supravesical portion of the urinary tract. McArdle and Lebowitz (1975) found only 6 genitourinary anomalies among 200 patients with hypospadias (3%). Cerasaro and associates (1986) found 1.7% (4 of 233) patients with significant anomalies. Avellan (1975) found only 1% renal anomalies in his Swedish patients with hypospadias, whereas he found 7% of patients with other systems involved. In a review of 169 patients, Shelton and Noe (1985) do not recommend routine urinary tract evaluation.

Khuri and co-workers (1981) reviewed 1076 patients, and their data are presented in Tables 55-2 and 55-3. Urinary tract anomalies considered to be significant were ureteropelvic junction obstruction, severe reflux, renal agenesis, Wilms' tumor, pelvic kidney, crossed renal ectopia, and horseshoe kidney. They conclude that patients with hypospadias and an associated inguinal hernia or undescended testis need not have further urinary tract evaluation. However, patients who have hypospadias in association with other organ system anomalies should undergo an upper urinary tract screening with an abdominal ultrasound.

Henderson and associates (1976) studied urogenital abnormalities in 500 sons of women treated with diethylstilbestrol (DES). He found 2% had hypospadias, and 4.4% had abnormalities of the penile urethra (Goldman, 1977). Gupta and Goldman (1986) implicated metabolic disturbances of the arachidonic acid cascade in midline fusion defects, such as cleft palate and hypospadias. Hypospadias occurs in association with a number of well-known syndromes as well as with Wilms' tumor (see Chapter 60).

INTERSEX

Hypospadias is considered by some to be a form of intersex. In patients with severe hypospadias, cer-

TABLE 55-2

Influence of Undescended Testicle and Other System Anomalies on the Incidence of Significant Anomalies of the Upper Tract in Patients With Hypospadias of Any Degree

	Total No. of Patients	Available IV Pyelograms*	Incidence (%) of Significant Anomalies of the Upper Urinary Tract
Isolated hypospadias (no undescended testicle, no other system anomalies)	799	274	15 (5.5)
Hypospadias with undescended testis and no other associated anomalies (± inguinal hernia)	75	51	3 (5.9)
Hypospadias + 1 other system anomaly ± undescended testis ± inguinal hernia	129	74	9 (12.2)
Hypospadias + 2 other system anomalies ± undescended testis ± inguinal hernia	30	24	4 (16.7)
Hypospadias + 3 or more other system anomalies ± undescended testicle ± inguinal hernia	24	18	9 (50.0)
Hypospadias + imperforate anus ± other anomalies	13	13	6 (46.2)
Hypospadias + meningomyelocele, tethered cord, or sacral agenesis ± any other anomalies	6	6	2 (33.3)
Total	1076	460	48 (10.4)†

From Khuri FJ, Hardy BE, Churchill BM: *Urol Clin North Am* 1981; 8:565-571. Used by permission.
*IV = intravenous.
†Overall rate of occurrence.

TABLE 55-3

Significant Anomalies of the Upper Urinary Tract Noted on 48 Urograms in Patients With Hypospadias

Renal agenesis	10
Ureteropelvic junction obstruction	8
Grade IIB to III reflux	18
Bilateral Wilms' tumor	1
Bilateral cystic disease	1
Severe renal dysplasia	1
Bilateral hydroureteronephrosis + megacystis ? valves	1
Crossed renal ectopia	1
Horseshoe kidney	4
Pelvic kidney	3
Total	48

From Khuri FJ, Hardy BE, Churchill BM: *Urol Clin North Am* 1981; 8:565-571. Used by permission.

tainly intersex should be investigated, but in the majority of hypospadias patients with normally descended testes, the presence of an intersex condition is unlikely.

Patients with anterior or middle hypospadias and normally descended testes do not need an evaluation for ambiguous genitalia. However, patients with more severe hypospadias, or hypospadias in association with a nonpalpable undescended testis, should have a karyotype performed to evaluate intersex states (Fig. 55-4). The most common type is *mixed gonadal dysgenesis*. These patients have hypospadias, a testis on one side, and a streak gonad on the other. They usually have fallopian tubes, a uterus or vagina, and a negative chromatin pattern with a mosaic karyotype of 45, XO, 46, XY (Davidoff and Federman, 1973). Most of these patients (60%) are undervirilized, have short stature, and are reared as females. However, those assigned a male gender may not be diagnosed until their hy-

pospadias is repaired. They usually have a testis in the inguinal or scrotal position and no testis on the opposite side (see Chapter 56).

Allen and Griffin (1984) have suggested that hypospadias is not only a dysmorphic phenomenon but also a local manifestation of a systemic endocrinopathy. In their series, 11 of 15 patients were found to have an endocrine abnormality. Nearly one half of their patients had a substandard response to HCG, although four of these patients eventually had an improved response. Shima and colleagues (1986) found luteinizing hormone (LH) response to luteinizing hormone-releasing hormone (LHRH) stimulation significantly impaired in 98 boys with hypospadias. They also noted that the testosterone response to HCG stimulation was significantly depressed. Gearhart and associates (1988) could not find any androgen receptor level or 5 α-reductase deficiencies in their study of preputial skin from hypospadias boys.

ELEMENTS OF THE HYPOSPADIAS ANOMALY

Meatus

Hypospadias is characterized primarily by dystopia of the meatus. As the opening of the urethral defect develops more proximally, it is associated with a series of changes determining the morphology of each anomaly (Figs. 55-5 through 55-10). The penis curves and the base of the somewhat reduced penis shows caudal displacement. There may be penoscrotal transposition of a bifid scrotum. This configuration is analogous to the normal female anatomy with severe curvature of the clitoris that is caudally located between the labia.

The urethral meatus may be only slightly ventrally placed just below a blind dimple at the normal meatal

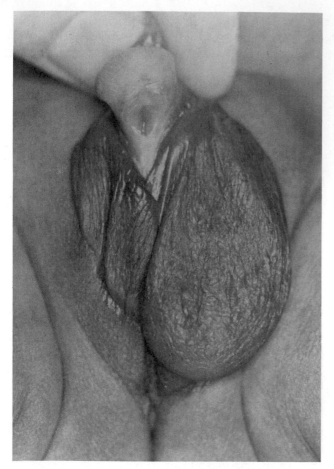

FIG. 55-4
Ambiguous genitalia. Proximal hypospadias with a unilateral nonpalpable testicle.

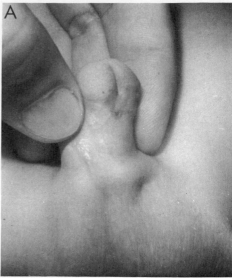

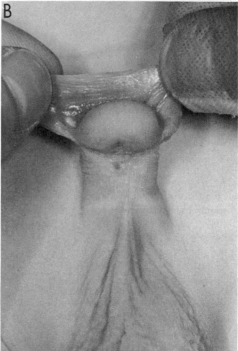

FIG. 55-5
A and **B,** Anterior hypospadias, subcorneal meatus. It is the most common presentation and is the most suitable for the MAGPI procedure. (**A** and **B** are different patients.)

opening on the glans (an intranavicular hypospadias). On the other hand, the urethra may be so far back in the perineum that it appears as a "vaginal hypospadias" (Young, 1937). Most patients have the meatus in one of the many transitional forms. The meatus is encountered in a variety of configurations in form, diameter, elasticity, and rigidity. It can be fissural in both transverse and longitudinal directions or can be covered with delicate skin at times. The more distal locations in particular are often associated with a stenotic meatus. In the case of the megameatus intact prepuce, the distal urethral is enlarged, tapering to a normal caliber in the penile shaft (Fig. 55-7).

Often, there is an orifice of a *periurethral duct*, located distal to the meatus, that courses dorsal to the urethral channel for a short distance. It is blind ending and does not communicate in any way with the urinary stream. The periurethral duct corresponds with Guérin's sinus or Morgagni's lacunae (Sommer and Stephens, 1980; Van der Meulen, 1961).

Skin

The skin of the penis is radically changed as a result of the disturbance in the formation of the urethra.

Distal to the meatus, the normal skin shows a V-shaped defect, referred to by Van der Meulen (1964) as the *urethral delta*. The edges of this defect gradually merge into the reverted fold of the divided prepuce. The frenulum is always absent. Vestiges of a frenulum are sometimes found inserting on either side of the open navicular fossa.

Lateral to the penis, two *raphes* obliquely extend from the edge of the urethral delta on a dorsal course to end in paramedian dog ears on the dorsum, spaced about 1 cm apart. Depending on the location of the meatus and the degree of penile curvature, these

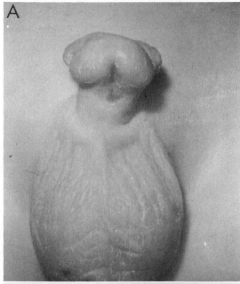

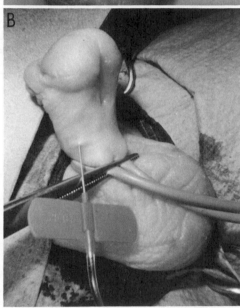

FIG. 55-6
Middle hypospadias. **A,** Patient with midshaft meatus. **B,** Same patient with artificial erection. After skin drop-back, no significant curvature exists. It is most suitable for an onlay island-flap procedure.

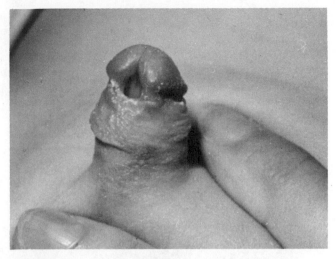

FIG. 55-7
Megameatus, anterior hypospadias with intact prepuce (MIP). Circumcision was inadvertently performed on this patient.

oblique raphes may take either a distal or proximal course. Each line ends at the apex of a small skin cone or peaks of a cowl-shaped monk's hood. They are sometimes called *cobra eyes*.

An explanation of these findings may be based on the conclusions reached by Glenister (1954) that the ectoderm-lined edges of the urethral groove do not participate in the formation of the urethra proximal to the corona. When these edges fail to come together due to the disturbance of the urethral plate, they split off and obliquely go around the dorsal prepuce.

The skin proximal to the urethral meatus may be extremely thin, so much so that a catheter or probe

passed proximally is readily apparent through a tissue-paper thickness of skin. When thin skin is present, it abrogates the use of perimeatal skin flaps in repairs (Fig. 55-8).

The *urethral plate*, extending from the meatus to the glanular groove, may be well developed. Even with a meatus quite proximal on the shaft, this normal urethral plate is very elastic and nontethering. Artificial erection demonstrates no ventral curvature in these situations. A normal urethral plate may be incorporated into the surgical repair. However, if the urethral plate is underdeveloped, it will act as a tethering fibrous band that bends the penis ventrally during artificial erection. When this fibrous chordee tissue is divided, the penis will frequently straighten out with this maneuver alone.

The *corpus spongiosum* surrounding the normal proximal urethra is partially developed distally and then splays out in a V onto the lateral penile shaft in a rudimentary fashion. It is best to discard the thin unsupported urethra distal to the normal spongiosum and use only the urethra with good spongiosal tissue.

Curvature

Curvature of the penis is caused by deficiency of the normal structures on the ventral side of the penis. It can be found as a skin deficiency, a dartos fascial deficiency, a true fibrous chordee with tethering of the ventral shaft, or deficiency of the corpora cavernosa on the concave side of the penis.

The role played by *skin deficiency* in the formation of curvature seems especially striking in the manipulation of the penis without an artificial erection. It is very easy to pull the skin downward and create considerable ventral curvature. However, with release of the skin, the penis will be quite straight on artificial erection. Infrequently, there exists a skin component

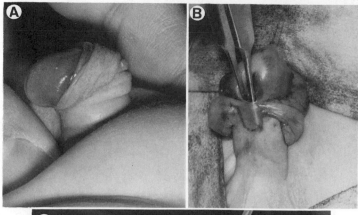

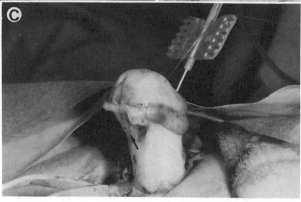

FIG. 55-8
A, Coronal hypospadias with penile curvature. **B,** The thin ventral skin is not suitable for a parameatal-type procedure. **C,** After release of the skin and dartos fascia (straightening the penis), the meatus *(arrow)* is cut back to remove thin urethral skin in preparation for an onlay island-flap urethroplasty. (From Baskin LS, et al: Changing concepts of hypospadias curvature lead to more onlay island-flap procedures. *J Urol* 1994; 151:191. Used by permission.)

to the ventral curvature that is resolved when the ventral skin attachments are dissected free of the parameatal area.

The *dartos fascia* may have varying degrees of fibrous development. Release of the dartos fascia fibrosis likewise will straighten the apparent bend to the penis, and even stretch out obvious curvature with artificial erection prior to its resection.

True *fibrous chordee* is considered a deficiency or fibrous replacement of of the normally elastic urethral plate. This tissue must be divided transversely in a broad extent to release the tethering of distal penile shaft. This resection of the fibrous chordee must be carried proximally elevating the urethra off the tunica albuginea along with its rudimentary spongiosum back to good normal urethra surrounded by corpus spongiosum. This fibrous chordee is most often seen when the penis is fixed between the bifid scrotum with the glans near the perineal meatus.

Finally, the most difficult situation to correct, the *corpora cavernosa deficiency* itself, may be present after all of the fibrous tissue is resected from the ventrum of the penis. The penis will still have a corporal disproportion that leads to ventral curvature (Udald, 1980). Various techniques have been proposed for this release, including a vertical incision between the two corporal bodies, allowing an outward rotation (Koff and Eakins, 1984); dorsal plication of the tunica albuginea (Baskin and Duckett, 1994); a transverse in-

cision of the tunica albuginea, and insertion of an elastic graft such as tunica vaginalis (Das, 1980); dermal graft (Horton and Devine, 1973); or lyophilized dura mater (Kelami et al., 1975). The latter is presently unavailable for use.

Penoscrotal Transposition and the Bifid Scrotum

Normally, the genital tubercle should develop in a craniad position above the two genital swellings. The penis may be caught between the two scrotal halves and become engulfed with fusion of the penoscrotal area. The boundary between the penis and the scrotum may be formed by two oblique raphes that extend from the very proximal meatus to the dorsal side of the penis. An extreme example of penoscrotal transposition is the prepenile scrotum, which is a rare congenital anomaly (Forashall and Rickham, 1956; Paramo et al., 1981) (Fig. 55-10).

Hypoplasia of the penis may be associated with hypospadias to such a degree that micropenis should be declared and gender conversion considered at birth. Fortunately, these rudimentary penises are quite uncommon with hypospadias, and a very careful examination of the suprapubic fat pad will usually determine a respectable shaft buried beneath the skin. One of the parents' most disheartening moments occurs when the specialist examines the hypospadic penis and fails to demonstrate its potential when repaired.

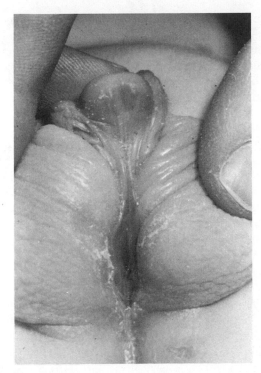

FIG. 55-9
Posterior hypospadias, scrotoperineal meatus, and severe chordee.

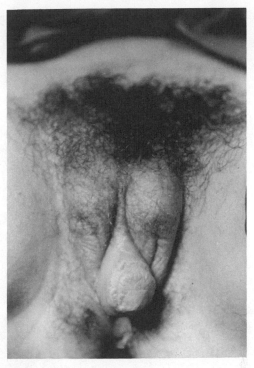

FIG. 55-10
Prepenile scrotum. An extreme example of penoscrotal transposition.

Finally, an *enlarged prostatic utricle* is not uncommon with more severe forms of hypospadias (Howard, 1948). Devine and colleagues (1980) and Shima and coworkers (1979) found an enlarged prostatic utricle in about 11% of patients with severe hypospadias. These generally cause little problem except when a catheter is passed into the bladder and the tip is deflected into the utricle. Removal of prostatic utricles is rarely necessary in hypospadias surgery, nor do they cause incontinence or lead to infection. Utricular enlargement in itself does not indicate intersexuality but reflects the lack of hormone effect on the urogenital sinus and the urethral groove (Devine et al., 1980). When removal is required, the transtrigonal approach is used.

CHORDEE WITHOUT HYPOSPADIAS

There are occasional reports of other penile anomalies that represent variations of the embryologic defect causing hypospadias. They can be characterized as a defect in the course of the urethra (congenital urethral fistula), and there is a group characterized by curvature of the penis (chordee) without hypospadias.

Congenital urethral fistula occurs when the formation of the urethra is disrupted by transient disturbance. The urethra can show an opening (Fig. 55-11) as well as a blind end, or there can be a secondary fusion of the edges of the urethral groove (Ritchey et al., 1994; Van der Meulen, 1964).

Congenital curvature of the penis with hypospadias is quite rare. Much more common in adults are the secondary curvatures associated with Peyronie's disease, or periurethral sclerosis associated with urethral stricture. There are two kinds of primary curvatures: those associated with a normal urethral spongiosum, and those with a hypoplastic urethra.

Primary curvature with a normal corpus spongiosum comprises two thirds of congenital curvatures (Daskalopoulos et al., 1993). When flaccid, the penis looks normal with a circular prepuce. However, during erection, the penis is usually curved ventrally, although there may be lateral curvature of as much as 90 degrees. A dorsal curvature (without epispadias) is exceptional (Udald, 1980). This deformity becomes noticeable to the adolescent or young adult. However, few with this condition have difficulty with intercourse. The lateral deviation seen in about one third of patients is almost always to the left. With erection, disproportion of the corpora cavernosa is usually apparent.

Physiologic ventral curvature of the penis in the fetus has been documented at different stages of fetal development (Kaplan and Brock, 1981; Kaplan and Lamm, 1975). It usually disappears by birth, yet it may be found more commonly in premature infants. Within the first several years of life, it slowly disappears (Cendron and Melin, 1981).

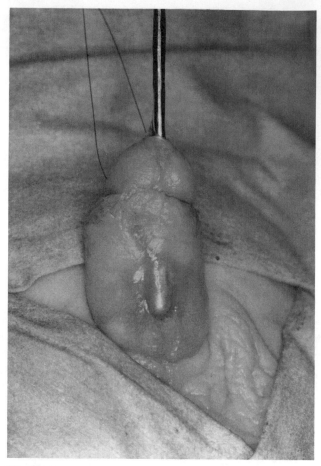

FIG. 55-11
Congenital urethral fistula.

Treatment

With patients in whom the urethra is normal, treatment depends on the direction of the deviation and whether one believes that true chordee tissue is responsible for the ventral bend (Devine and Horton, 1975). Devine and Horton (1975) reported good results with resection of fibrous dartos fascia beneath and beside the mobilized normal urethra. However, this rather extensive dissection does not offer consistent results (Kramer et al., 1982). More accepted has been the concept Nesbit has described (1965) of taking tucks or plicating the disproportionately large tunica albuginea. This technique was first described by Syng Physick, the father of American surgery, in the early nineteenth century. He treated chordee by shortening the dorsal tunica albuginea (Pancoast, 1844). When the arc of maximum curvature is identified during artificial erection, wedges of tunica albuginea are excised in a permanent stepwise fashion. These diamond wedges are closed transversely with permanent suture until the penis is straight. We have modified Nesbit's technique of dorsal tunica albuginea plication (TAP) for the correction of penile curvature in the setting of corporeal disproportion (Fig. 55-12) (Baskin and Duckett, 1994). It is also possible to plicate the fascia without cutting the tunica by placing several rows of sutures at the site of maximum convexity. Nesbit (1966), however, reported his long-term follow-up with this method as disappointing. Exposure for the surgical approach is achieved by retracting the penile skin toward the base as a sleeve.

The age at which chordee without hypospadias should be corrected is important. Cendron and Melin (1981) believe it should not be done too early for two reasons: the curvature may improve spontaneously with age, and there is risk of disturbing the growth of the phallus by altering the tunica of the corpora. When curvature is pronounced, we have corrected it with the TAP procedure in the first year.

Primary curvature with a hypoplastic urethra comprises about one third of these congenital curvature cases (Cendron and Melin, 1981; Daskalopoulos et al., 1994). In this type, the urethral meatus is well situated on the glans, but the foreskin is incomplete, and the ventral penis is not normal (Fig. 55-13). The skin covering the urethra is very thin, and there is no spongiosal tissue for a long portion. Chordee is present with erection. Lengthening the frenulum and eliminating the penoscrotal web does not alter the curvature. Since the segment of urethra is hypoplastic, it may be considered a *concealed hypospadias*. *Congenitally short urethra* may be a variant of this condition.

Treatment for the hypoplastic urethra or short urethra variant of congenital curvature requires a chordee release with division of the midportion of the hypoplastic urethra (Hendren and Caesar, 1992; Kramer et al., 1982). Urethroplasty using the same techniques applicable to the usual hypospadias anomaly will follow. We prefer to replace the midurethral segment with an island flap from the dorsal prepuce, making two oblique anastomoses with the remaining healthy proximal and distal urethral segments, leaving the meatus naturally on the glans (Daskalopoulos et al., 1994).

TREATMENT OF HYPOSPADIAS

The object of therapy is to reconstruct a straight penis with a meatus as close as possible to the normal site to allow a forward-directed stream and normal coitus. Culp and McRoberts (1968) stated, "It is the basic right of every hypospadiac patient to write his name legibly in the snow." Culp (1959) also stated, "It is the inalienable right of every boy to be a pointer instead of a sitter by the time he starts school." In 1968, Culp and McRoberts reviewed more than 50 techniques of chordee correction, and more than 150 reputed original methods of urethral reconstruction. Another 100 must have been added since that time; thus it is clear that the ideal procedure to produce

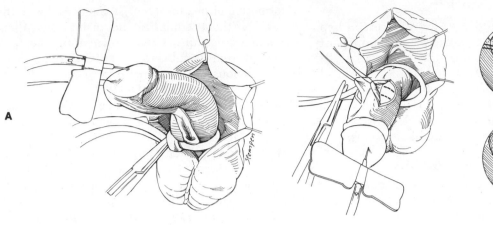

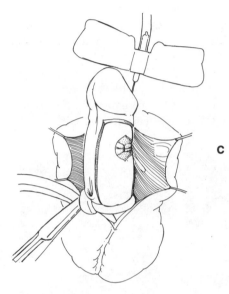

FIG. 55-12
Tunica albuginea plication. **A,** Penoscrotal hypospadias with penile curvature after surgical release of the skin and dartos fascia to the penoscrotal junction. Note preservation of the urethral plate. **B,** With penis erect, Buck's fascia is elevated at point of maximum curvature on either side of the midline at 10 and 2 o'clock positions to avoid damage to the neurovascular bundle. Parallel incisions 4 to 6 mm apart and about 8 mm long are made through tunica albuginea. Outer edges of incisions are approximated with permanent sutures (5-0 polypropylene in infants) in a way that buries the knot. **C,** Straight penis is confirmed by repeat intraoperative artificial erection. (From Baskin LS, Duckett JW: Dorsal tunica albuginea plication for hypospadias curvature. *J Urol* 1994; 151:1668. Used by permission.)

maximum correction with a minimum of possible complications is still in its developmental stage.

Since "hypospadiology" is liberally sprinkled with eponyms, each representing a symbol for a technique or principle, it seems appropriate to continue this descriptive method so entrenched in surgery today. There are still those who, appropriately, try to eliminate the use of eponyms, and to them we apologize.

T. Twistington Higgins wrote a forward to a one-stage operation described by Humby (1941):

> Hypospadias is a grievous deformity which must ever move us to the highest surgical endeavor. The refashioning of the urethra offers a problem as formidable as any in the wide field of our art. The fruits of success are beyond rubies—the gratitude of a boy has to be experienced to be believed.
>
> Those of us who could not evade the responsibility of attempting to deal faithfully with these patients, received a lively encouragement from the work of Edmunds. The three-stage operation, so skillfully evolved and successfully practiced by him was a notable advance for which all owe him a grateful tribute.
>
> If, however, one could succeed in remodeling the urethra in one operation, the gain would be manifest.

> The operation here described is designed to achieve this. It has been my privilege to be associated with Mr. Humby in the treatment of some of these cases. The results have appeared to demand the publication of details, to justify the hope that the wider employment of this ingenious procedure may prove that a further landmark in the treatment of hypospadias has been reached.

Others have arrived at perfection, and yet their success was not accepted or at least transferable to colleagues. D.M. Davis (1951) wrote:

> I would like to say that I believe the time has arrived to state that the surgical repair of hypospadias is no longer dubious, unreliable, or even extremely difficult. If tried and proven methods are scrupulously followed, a good result should be obtained in every case. Anything less than this suggests that the surgeon is not temperamentally fitted for this kind of surgery.

So much depends on experience, but even more so on familiarity with all the options available. Indeed, with this familiarity as a prerequisite, *hypospadiology* would be an appropriate term for this discipline (Duckett, 1981a).

Elements of Surgical Repair

There are five basic phases for a successful hypospadias outcome: (1) meatoplasty and glanuloplasty, (2) orthoplasty (straightening), (3) urethroplasty, (4) skin cover, and (5) scrotoplasty. These various elements of surgical technique can be applied either sequentially or in various combinations to achieve a surgical success. We first discuss these elements and then combine them as to specific clinical situations.

Meatoplasty and Glanuloplasty

For many years, the two-stage techniques left the meatus just beneath the glans in the subcoronal area. More recently, an effort has been made to move the meatus to the apex of the glans, particularly in the more extensive one-stage repairs. Even in patients with relatively minor defects, we have attempted to achieve the same goal.

Mills and co-workers (1981) reviewed 23 cases of distal hypospadias repaired by the Devine-Horton flip-flap procedure or the Ombredanne flip-flap technique and found a 25% complication rate, with fistula

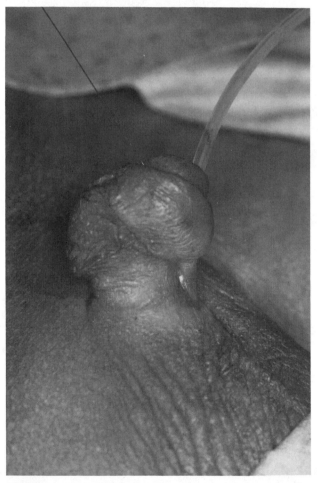

FIG. 55-13
Chordee without hypospadias. Note abnormal urethral spongiosum.

formation or meatal stenosis. Compared with their 11 cases without complications using the Allen and Spence procedure (1968), in which the meatus is not moved from its subcoronal position, their conclusion was obvious—at what price perfection. The MAGPI procedure (Fig. 55-14) (Duckett, 1981b; Duckett and Snyder, 1991) has come under considerable scrutiny in this regard, but has emerged with a favorable review. McMillan and colleagues (1985), using electronic video photography, recorded high-speed pictures of urinary streams after the MAGPI repair and concluded, "With the advent of the MAGPI repair, which virtually guarantees perfect cosmetic results and fully preserves micturitional function, all boys with distal hypospadias should be offered early surgical correction" (Fig. 55-15). Bloom has come to the same conclusion with his review (Faerber et al., 1994).

There are several different techniques to achieve an apical meatus, depending on the variations of the proximal meatus (Gibbons and Gonzalez, 1983). The *triangularized glans* (Devine and Horton, 1961) achieves a flap meatoplasty and avoids a circumferential meatal closure. Although it may prevent meatal stenosis, the glans is flattened and distorted from the normal conical configuration (Klimberg and Walker, 1985).

Extension of the meatus onto the ventral glans may be effected with either a meatal-based flap (Mathieu, 1932) or an onlay vascularized flap (Baskin et al., 1994; Elder et al., 1987); as described later. The glans filet described by Cronin and Guthrie (1973) and Turner-Warwick (1979) is a two-staged procedure that lays preputial skin onto the ventrum of the "kippered" glans. The meatus may later be tubularized, and the glans can be closed over it to achieve a normal-appearing glans with an apical meatus. This technique is more applicable to the adult penis.

The *glans split* has been used in various reports to move the meatus to the apex. Beck (1971) and Barcat (1973) are the usual names associated. The balanic groove technique of Barcat is a more extensive Mathieu procedure whereby the glanular strip is mobilized and a glans split is made to further advance the urethra into the middle of the glans. Redman (1987) has reported good cosmetic results with this method in 105 patients, with a 15% complication rate, and Koff and associates (1994) have also obtained good results. Hodgson (1986) currently favors the glans split for his inner preputial tangential tube.

The *glans channel technique* to deliver the urethra to the apex is another method that has been used for many years (Russell, 1900). Bevan (1917) reported a technique that created a proximal penile flap that was converted into a urethral tube and was pulled through a tunnel in the glans. Mustarde (1965) later popularized the procedure and included a dorsal V-flap with

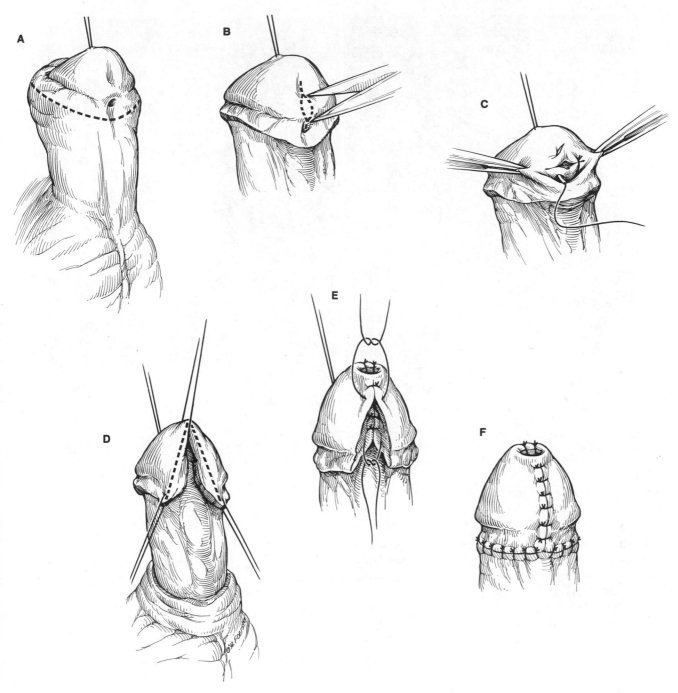

FIG. 55-14
The MAGPI procedure. **A,** Subcoronal meatus. **B-C,** Circumferential subcoronal incision 8 mm proximal to meatus and corona; excision of bridge of tissue between meatus and granular groove. Note the transverse Heineke-Mikulicz closure of dorsal meatal edge to distal glanular groove. **D,** Three traction sutures placed at apex of ventral meatus and lateral glans where foreskin stops; glans edges are pulled together ventrally in V fashion, and redundant edges excised. **E,** A two-layer closure of the glans edges reconfigures a clonical glans. **F,** Sleeve reapproximation for skin coverage. (Rotational flap closure is used if a ventral skin defect exists.) (From Duckett JW: Hypospadias. In *Contemporary Urology* 1992. Used by permission.)

the glans channel. Mays (1951) employed a staged technique that straightened the penis, bringing the prepuce over the glans to cover the ventral defect and constructing a glanular urethra that was carried through a tunnel to the tip of the glans. Davis (1940), Ricketson (1958), and Hendren (1981) have channeled

a full-thickness skin tube through the glans. Hinderer (1971) uses a trochar to tunnel, entering the glans at the tip and emerging a few millimeters below the coronal sulcus through a trap-door flap of albuginea.

We have combined the glans channel technique with the creation of a vascularized island flap neo-

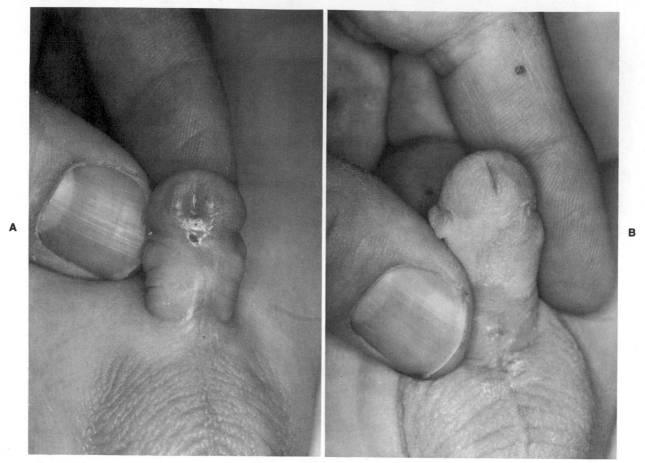

FIG. 55-15
A and **B,** Preoperative and postoperative views of anterior hypospadias amenable to the MAGPI.

urethra (Duckett, 1980b). This procedure requires a generous channel through the glans tissue, allowing the vascularized skin flap to be placed through the glans without compression of the blood supply. Because the rigid tissue of the glans may predispose to stricture formation, the glans channel technique must avoid too timid a channel. We have not thought a V-flap meatoplasty to be necessary.

In analyzing the hypospadias glans, it has been noted that the glans configuration may be a reliable indicator for technique selection (Elder, 1992; Snyder, 1991). Patients with a conical-shaped glans tend to have a fibrous urethral plate that is best managed with division of the urethral plate, a transverse preputial island tube, and a tunneling glansplasty. In contrast, patients with a flat glans tend to have a normal urethral plate that is amenable to an onlay island flap and a glans-wing-wrap glansplasty. A broad approximation of glans tissue around a generous glans urethra will avoid meatal stenosis. If the new meatus does not have adequate glans support, breakdown of the glansplasty is more likely, which results in an unacceptable retrusive meatus.

Orthoplasty

Orthoplasty is the logical designation for the plastic procedure to straighten the penis: the Greek root for straight is *orthos*. Release of chordee is currently the more common term; however, it implies that the bend is caused by a fibrous band, which is not always the case. The concept of chordee remains debatable, so the term is interchangeable with any bend to the penis. A discussion of the various surgical methods to accomplish an orthoplasty follows.

Artificial erection, introduced by Gittes and McLaughlin (1974) has been a very significant contribution to orthoplasty. A tourniquet is placed at the base of the penis, and a corpus cavernosum is injected with saline. Both corporal bodies fill so that it is possible to determine the extent of curvature and the success after resection of the fibrous tissue. The assurance of complete correction is essential to proceed to further urethroplasty and one-stage repair. There have been no reports of damage to the cavernous tissue with this technique as long as care is taken to ensure that injectable saline/epinephrine is used. Penile necrosis has occurred when 50% saline was injected inadvertently.

In about 10% of hypospadias cases, the ventral curvature is attributable to a true fibrous band or fan-shaped area of fibrosis tethering the penis ventrally. When this tissue is excised, the penis straightens. This simplified explanation is not altogether applicable to the variety of expressions of hypospadias. Certainly, the concept of a bowstring tethering that requires a simple excision is not true (Mettauer, 1842). Kaplan and Lamm (1975) put forth a convincing case that chordee may be an arrest of normal embryologic development analogous to failure of testicular descent. In reality, all penises have chordee during development. Thus it is no surprise that fibrosis is conspicuously absent in some clinical cases of ventral curvature. Curvature may also result from different growth of the dorsal and ventral aspect of the corpora (Bellinger, 1981), which is best corrected by shortening the dorsal tunica albuginea.

Some have suggested that occasional adherence of skin to the distal hypoplastic urethra is the element that causes chordee and, that correction of the bend may be achieved by simply freeing the skin attachments; so-called skin chordee. It may be so, rarely, associated with a marked skin deficiency in the ventrum (Allen and Spence, 1968). Devine and Horton (1973) have offered a classification of chordee. In their view, type III is a deficiency of dartos fascia that may contribute to penile curvature similar to skin chordee.

For *true fibrous chordee*, the penis is curved ventrally, with only a short distance between the location of the meatus and the glans. An incision is made in a circumferential manner around the corona and is carried well below the glans cap, just distal to the urethral meatus and down to the tunica albuginea of the corpora cavernosa. Proximal dissection is then achieved, freeing the fibrous plaque of tissue closely adherent to the tunica albuginea. Sharp scissor dissection is used, moving from side to side and proximally as the ventral curvature is released. The urethra is elevated from the corpora in this en bloc dissection. In most cases, the fibrous tissue surrounds the urethral meatus and extends proximal along the urethra for a distance. This tissue should be freed completely down to the penoscrotal junction and often into the scrotal or perineal area. Once this urethral mobilization is accomplished, the shaft of the penis should be stripped of any fibrous tissue, extending out to the lateral aspect of the penis. Careful tangential cuts are made with the convex curve of iris scissors. Artificial erection is used to check the success of this excision.

Several further maneuvers have been offered for releasing the last bit of bend. Lateral incisions of the outer tunica albuginea in the groove between the dorsal corpora and the ventral segment of corpora in a stepwise manner may be effective. Corporal rotation as described by Koff and Eakins (1984) for epispadias may be useful in hypospadias curvature also (Kass,

1993; Snow, 1989). Theoretical concern with this method for hypospadias arises from the fact that the permanent suture may impinge on the neurovascular bundle, causing pressure necrosis and/or subsequent erectile dysfunction. Unlike epispadias, where the neurovascular bundle is lateral and out of harm's way, in hypospadias the neurovascular bundle lies in an unstrategic position directly under the plication sutures. A midline incision along the septum between the two corpora cavernosa has been effective in some cases (Devine, 1983).

If, after adequate excision of all abnormal fibrous tissue, artificial erection continues to demonstrate curvature, corporal disproportion may be the cause. This should be corrected by a modification of Nesbit's dorsal plication, taking out wedges of tunica albuginea in an ellipse and closing this with permanent suture (Nesbit, 1965). As previously described, we use tunica albuginea plication (TAP) for the correction of penile curvature, a modification of Nesbit's original procedure (Baskin and Duckett, 1994). A glans tilt may be removed by permanent sutures on the dorsum, but care must be taken to avoid the neurovascular structures supplying the glans (Hodgson, 1981; Juskiewenski et al., 1982).

In rare cases, there is so much deficiency of the tunica albuginea on the ventrum that excision of the tunica is required with replacement by an elastic graft of tunica vaginalis (Das, 1980, Perlmutter et al., 1985), dermal graft (Horton and Devine, 1973), or lyophilized dura (Kelami et al., 1975) (dura is not available today). The tunica vaginalis patch is the one we prefer and is obtained by exposing the testis and removing a patch of tunica from around the testis.

Once the curvature has been straightened, a urethroplasty may proceed in the one-stage repair (Hendren and Caesar, 1992). Some still prefer to resurface the ventrum of the penis with preputial skin to await a second-stage urethroplasty (Retik et al., 1994). There are several disadvantages to this approach, and the one-stage techniques are much preferred today.

Urethroplasty

Urethroplasty techniques for the more difficult 50% of hypospadias cases with the proximal meatus midshaft or below fall into three basic categories: (1) adjacent skin flaps, (2) free skin grafts, and (3) mobilized vascularized flaps.

Skin adjacent to the meatus may be rotated or tubularized for the neourethra as performed by Mathieu (1932) (Fig. 55-16), Broadbent and colleagues (1961), and DesPrez and associates (1961) in their one-stage procedures. Transfer of dorsal skin to the ventrum in a previous stage will also provide skin that is adjacent to the meatus for urethroplasty. Less than optimum vascularity to these thin ventral rotational flaps makes

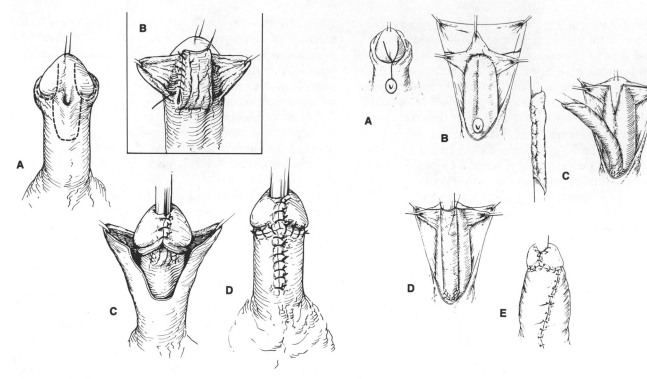

FIG. 55-16
Mathieu procedure. **A,** The dotted lines outline the skin flaps.
B, The proximal flap is rotated, and the lateral glans flaps
are developed. **C,** The glans flaps cover around the neourethra, and preputial skin is moved if necessary. **D,** completed
repair. (From Duckett JW: Hypospadias. In Walsh PC, Gittes
RF, Perlmutter AD, et al [eds]: *Campbell's Urology,* ed 5.
Philadelphia, WB Saunders, 1986, pp 1969-1999. Used by
permission).

FIG. 55-17
Devine-Horton free graft. **A,** Glans V incision and chordee
resection after mobilization of penile skin. **B,** Triangularized
glans wings developed, ventral preputial skin used for full-
thickness free graft, and free graft formed into neourethra
over stent. **C,** Proximal anastomosis, middle glans dart fixed
to corpora, and suture line of tube against corpora. **D,** Meatoplasty with dorsal glans dart. **E,** Completed repair. (From
Devine CJ Jr: Chordee and hypospadias. In Glenn JF, Boyce
WH [ed]: *Urologic Surgery,* ed 3. Philadelphia, JB Lippincott
1983, p 788. Used by permission.)

results with these methods more prone to complications.

Free skin grafts should be full thickness rather than
split thickness. Devine (1983) has had successful experience for more than 25 years using the inner preputial skin detached and defatted as a thin, full-thickness graft to form the neourethra (Fig. 55-17). His
good results have not been reproducible in a uniform
manner in the hands of others, however (Filmer et
al., 1977; Redman, 1983; Rober et al., 1990; Vugas et
al., 1987; Woodard and Cleveland, 1982). Since the
free graft must be revascularized, the key element to
success is a perfect skin cover of the graft with
well-vascularized dorsal, preputial, and penile skin.
Humby (1941) described use of a full-thickness of graft
taken from the inner surface of the arm the groin as
a urethroplasty and done as a one-stage procedure.
For some reason, this method did not catch on at that
time, despite Higgins's advocacy (see earlier discussion).

Vascularized flaps of the preputial or penile skin
may be mobilized to the ventrum for urethroplasty
either by leaving them attached to the outer surface
of the prepuce or as an island flap unrestricted by

the limitations of the skin of the outer face. Hodgson
(1970) used the inner-face prepuce in a vertical
orientation with the tumble flap technique he first
described (Hodgson I technique). He later added the
vertical-oriented dorsal penile skin neourethra (Hodgson II and III techniques), which was transposed to
the ventrum with a buttonhole maneuver (Hodgson,
1972, 1975). Asopa and co-workers (1971) used a
vascularized flap attached to the outer prepuce. In
the Asopa technique, the ventral preputial skin is
used for the new urethra, but it is left attached to
the penile skin and spiraled around to the ventrum.
The final result is often asymmetric and bulky. A
similar procedure is now preferred by Hodgson,
which he calls "an inner preputial tangential tube"
(Hodgson, 1978, 1981). Standoli (1979, 1982) has
reported an island flap procedure using outer preputial skin to form the neourethra. Healing of these
neourethras is more assured than with the free-graft
techniques.

We prefer the *transverse preputial island flap*
(TPIF) neourethra with a glans channel positioning

for the meatus (Duckett, 1980a). This technique has been developed over the last 18 years as a modification of the Hodgson II and Asopa procedures, and as an alternative to the Devine-Horton free full-thickness skin graft. We have concluded that a vascularized urethral tube is preferable for the construction of the neourethra. However, it seems inappropriate to use the penile skin on the dorsum for the new urethra, as Hodgson and Standoli have done, while discarding the delicate ventral preputial skin or using it as skin cover.

The blood supply to the hypospadias preputial tissue is reliable and easily delineated (Fig. 55-18) (Hinman, 1991; Juskiewenski, 1982). The abundance of cutaneous tissue to the dorsum of the penis is vascularized in a longitudinal fashion (Quartey, 1983). This tissue may be dissected from the penile skin, creating an island flap from the inner layer of the prepuce. The blood supply to the dorsal skin of the foreskin and the penile skin comes from the broad base of the penis and is not dependent on subcutaneous tissue except at the remote edges of the dorsal preputial skin. The tips of the distal portion of the penile skin flaps are excised and not used in the repair.

In plastic surgical principles, an *island flap* is an isolated segment of skin, the viability of which is maintained by an inner vascular pedicle. Certainly, the transverse ventral preputial rectangle of skin that has been isolated with its own vascular pedicle qualifies as an island flap (DeSy and Oosterlinck, 1981; DeVries, 1986; Duckett, 1980a, 1980b, 1980c, 1981c; Standoli, 1979, 1982). The viability of an arterialized island flap may be tested by systemically injecting 15 to 20 mg kg of fluorescein and then evaluating the fluorescence of the flap with an ultraviolet light in a dark room 10 to 15 minutes later. The intensity of the skin fluorescence is a function of the amount of extracellular or interstitial deposition of fluorescein and is dependent on the functional microcirculation (McCraw et al., 1977). We have used this technique to demonstrate viability of the preputial island flap and the dorsal penile skin from which the underlying subcutaneous tissue is mobilized for the island flap. In 35 patients in whom fluorescein was used, all island flaps demonstrated excellent microcirculation (Duckett, 1981c). In contrast, rotational skin flaps are based on the intrinsic blood supply of the skin, which is random. To ensure viability, the length to width ratio of a skin flap should not exceed 2:1.

Viability of the neourethral flap is further demonstrated in practice in situations in which ventral skin loss has occurred without development of urethral fistulas or the formation of strictures. In these cases, secondary epithelialization has occurred without scar formation.

Skin Cover

After orthoplasty and urethroplasty, the penis must be resurfaced with skin. Because of the abundant dorsal foreskin, coverage may be achieved by mobilizing the penile and preputial skin to the ventrum in most cases. The skin may be transferred by one of several techniques.

The preputial tissue may be transposed by opening a small *buttonhole* in the midline, spreading the vasculature laterally, and bringing the glans penis through the buttonhole. The well-vascularized dorsal preputial tissue will resurface the ventrum. The major drawback is the lateral edges that are difficult to fashion without leaving bulky wedges of skin. One must be cautious not to trim these lateral pedicles too much at this stage and risk devascularizing the flap. A secondary procedure may be required to remove these extra bits of skin. Transposition in this manner is first credited to Thiersch (1869). However, Ombredanne (1932) and Nesbit (1941) also used this method (cited in Horton et al., 1973). We have abandoned its use entirely.

The prepuce may be *split vertically*, taking care not to disturb the vertically oriented vessels. The bipedicled preputial skin may be brought around to the ventrum for resurfacing. If it is done in a symmetric fashion as the first stage of a two-stage procedure (as in the Blair-Byars technique), redundant preputial skin is relocated on the distal shaft and glans (Smith, 1981). We use this technique to cover an island flap in a one-stage technique almost exclusively. The "bear hug" arrangement of the two flaps on the ventrum above and below each other may avoid midline suturing (Devine, 1983), but the cosmetic result is not acceptable. Likewise, an eccentric preputial split transposed to the ventrum may avoid a midline suture line, as described by King (1981) or Marberger and Pauer (1981).

We use this dorsal preputial midline split, allowing the shaft skin to retract proximally. The lateral wings of skin will join in the midline ventrally for a vertical skin closure. The coronal closure is fashioned by trimming the preputial skin obliquely (see Fig. 55-17, *C* and 55-17, *D*).

Ventral skin cover may also be achieved by rotation of the entire penile and preputial skin in a spiral method around to the ventrum. Van der Muelen (1971, 1982), Asopa and colleagues (1971), and Hodgson (1981) use this technique. In the Hodgson technique and the Asopa technique, the neourethra is attached to the dorsal preputial or penile skin.

Fortunately, healing of the penile skin and preputial layers is generally quite satisfactory without unsightly scarring or hypertrophic thickening. The scars usually blend in with the coloring of the penile skin and are quite unnoticeable. It is possible, as Browne (1953)

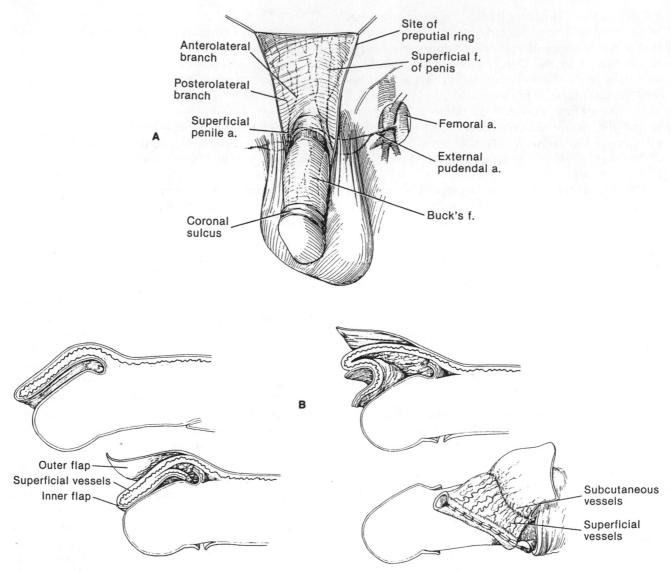

FIG. 55-18
Preputial blood supply. **A,** The prepuce is supplied by two branches from the inferior external pudendal arteries, the superficial penile arteries. These arteries divide into anterolateral and posterolateral branches. On reaching the preputial ring, the branches become tortuous and minute, and the terminal arteries turn circumferentially before ending at the coronal sulcus. **B,** Single-faced island flap. If the vessels within the superficial fascia are carefully dissected, an island flap will remain viable. The island flap, typically based on the anterolateral superficial vessels on one side, is rolled into a tube for construction of a neourethra. Although the principal arterial support has been diverted away from the outer skin flap, sufficient circulation usually remains from the subcutaneous vessels for skin coverage. (From Hinman F Jr: *Surgical Anatomy of the Genitourinary Tract.* Philadelphia, WB Saunders, 1994, pp 418–470. Used by permission.)

has demonstrated, to incise the dorsal penile skin down the midline, relaxing the tension on the ventral skin. It will epithelialize with very little scarring. Although this technique is rarely needed, the results from its use have been helpful in understanding penile scarring. There is no need to skin graft such a defect.

When an inner preputial island flap is developed, the lateral tips of the outer preputial skin may be devascularized to a certain degree. Although the edges of these flaps are discarded in most cases, sometimes the poor vascularization extends further than anticipated. There may be a slough of this ventrally positioned preputial skin. When slough has occurred in our experience, the neourethra is well vascularized and does not suffer. When the eschar is removed, this area epithelializes similar to the Browne (1953) experience on the dorsum.

Using the *double-faced preputial island flap technique* (Duckett, 1986) provides symmetric skin cover. The outer preputial skin rectangle is left attached to the joint blood supply to the inner prepuce. Thus, when transposed to the ventrum, the thicker outer preputial skin serves as a skin cover of the ventral midportion of the penile shaft, and the dorsal penile skin covers the rest. Our results using the double-faced island flap have not been as satisfactory as the standard island flap. Perhaps the extra skin attached to the inner preputial tube taxes the blood supply to both with deficient healing quality. We do not use this technique now.

Either the inner or outer preputial surfaces may be used as an island flap (Standoli, 1982) for ventral skin coverage in cases of chordee without hypospadias when urethroplasty is not needed.

Scrotoplasty

The final element to complete hypospadias repair is needed only rarely. When the penis is buried between the two scrotal halves and becomes engulfed, this *penoscrotal transposition* must be corrected. We usually stage the scrotoplasty after the orthoplasty and urethroplasty have healed adequately. Rearrangement of the prepenile scrotal halves to a more normal position beneath the penis is accomplished by rotational flaps (Ehrlich and Scardino, 1982; Marshall et al, 1979; Nonomura et al., 1988). At times, a *bifid scrotum* is so pronounced that shinny nonscrotal skin intervenes between the two scrota. Excision of this skin accomplishes a more normal appearance.

Modern History of Surgical Procedures

The following brief history of the development of hypospadiology is offered to give identity to the eponyms commonly used in discussing principles of various procedures. Horton and colleagues (1973) present a more thorough history with diagrams. Creevy (1958) also gives a good historic review.

In 1838, Dieffenbach pierced the glans to the normal urethral meatus, allowing a cannula to remain in position until the channel became lined with epithelium, an unsuccessful procedure. In 1842, Mettauer, to straighten the bend, suggested that the "organ be liberated by multiple subcutaneous incisions." In 1861, Bouisson was the first to suggest a transverse incision at the point of greatest curvature. He also reported the use of scrotal tissue to reconstruct the urethra. In 1869, Thiersch described the use of local tissue flaps to repair epispadias, a technique he later used in hypospadias. He suggested that perineal urinary diversion be done to divert the urine away from the urethral reconstruction temporarily. He also did the first buttonhole flap in the prepuce to allow the ventrum of the penis to be resurfaced with the prepuce.

In 1874, Duplay used Bouisson's technique to release chordee. At a later stage, he formed a central flap, which was tubed and covered with lateral penile skin flaps. He also stated that it did not matter if the central tube was incompletely formed, because he believed epithelialization would occur to form a channel if the tube was buried under lateral flaps, as was later popularized by Browne in 1953 (Horton et al., 1973). In 1875, Wood described a meatal-based flap to form the urethral channel and combined with the Thiersch-type buttonhole flap to cover the raw surface, a technique quite similar to Ombredanne's (1932) and Mathieu's (1932).

Rosenberger in 1891, Landerer in 1891, Bidder in 1892, and Bucknall in 1907 used scrotal tissue for urethroplasty and decribed burying the penis in the scrotum to obtain skin coverage, similar to the technique used by Leveuf in 1936 and by Cecil-Culp in 1951 (Horton et al., 1973).

In 1896, Hook described a vascularized preputial flap for urethroplasty, similar to the procedure Davis used in 1950 (Horton et al., 1973). Hook further suggested the use of a lateral oblique flap from the side of the penis, which was later popularized by Broadbent and colleagues (1961) and Koyanagi and associates (1991).

In 1897, Beck and Hacker undermined and advanced the urethra onto the glans for subcoronal cases (Horton et al., 1973), similar to the technique used by Waterhouse and colleagues (1981). Beck in 1897 and White and Martin in 1917 used adjacent rotation flaps from the scrotum for resurfacing after a Duplay-type urethroplasty (Horton et al., 1973), similar to the procedure by Turner-Warwick (1979) and Marberger and Pauer (1981). In 1897 and again in 1914, Nove-Josserand reported attempts to repair hypospadias with split-thickness grafts similar to the technique used by McIndoe in 1937 (Horton et al, 1973). In 1899, Rochet used a large distally based scrotal flap for urethroplasty and buried it in a tunnel on the ventral surface of the penis (Horton et al., 1973). In 1913, Edmunds was the first to transfer the skin of the prepuce to the ventral surface of the penis at the time of chordee release (Horton et al., 1973). This abundant ventral skin was then used in a Duplay-type urethroplasty at a later site, similar to what Blair accomplished in 1933 and, later, Byars (1955). In 1917, Bevan used a urethral meatal-based flap, channeled through the glans for distal repair, similar to that used by Mustarde in 1965 (Horton et al., 1973).

Multistage Repairs

In the standard two-stage repair, the chordee release (orthoplasty) was accomplished by dividing the urethral plate distal to the meatus, straightening the penis, and allowing the meatus to retract to a more proximal position. Skin cover of the ventrum was achieved by mobilizing the dorsal preputial and penile skin around to the ventrum to be used in a later urethroplasty. Since the technique of artificial erection (Gittes and McLaughlin, 1974) was not used, residual chordee was not an unusual result of this orthoplasty.

Secondary chordee releases were required before moving to form the urethra, which was the main argument used before the last decade to oppose one-stage hypospadias repair.

Browne (1953) was very influential in promoting his "buried strip" principle for hypospadias repair. A ventral strip of skin was covered by generous mobilized skin flaps brought together in the midline with "beads and stops." The channel under the skin flaps would epithelialize around a stenting catheter that was left for 3 to 6 weeks. Results were never very satisfactory until Van der Meulen (1964) demonstrated that a rotated skin cover from the dorsum with an eccentric suture line would offer more successful healing. In fact, he uses no stenting or diversion of urine and has the patient void through the repair, leaving only subcutaneous drains for several days. His results are dramatic, with no fistulas (Van der Meulen, 1982).

Byars (1955) further developed the two-stage method by extending the foreskin onto the glans in the first stage and rolling a complete tube in the second. Smith (1981) refined the Byars approach by denuding the epithelium on one skin edge to allow a double breasting of raw surfaces. His review of 285 repairs with only a 3% incidence of fistulas is commendable. Retik and associates (1994) have renewed this procedure with good results in rare severe cases.

In 1955, Belt devised a technique that he never published (Duckett, 1986), but that gained acclaim after Fuqua (1971) published his series. Hendren (1981) had the largest series, with excellent results. This has been renewed recently by Greenfield and colleagues (1994).

Numerous more modern methods have been introduced to repair hypospadias. Creevy (1958) and Backus and DeFelice (1960) provide excellent reviews of the multistaged procedures performed up to 1960. All of these methods must be studied in the field of hypospadiology to understand the pitfalls of this difficult surgery. However, emphasis in this chapter is placed on the one-stage methods that are currently popular.

One-Stage Repairs

Urethroplasty immediately following orthoplasty in a combined one-stage repair met with little acceptance in the early years, although several procedures received notice. In 1900, Russell described a procedure for one-stage repair of hypospadias using a urethral tube constructed from a flap that was developed on the ventral surface of the penis. This flap extended around the entire circumference of the corona to include a cuff of the prepuce. This new urethra was placed through a tunnel in the glans and secured to the tip of the glans. Koyanagi and colleagues describe a similar repair (1991).

In 1941, Humby reported a one-stage reconstruction using a free full-thickness skin graft from the groin or arm. The initial report was thought by Higgins to introduce a new era for hypospadias repair, but the method failed to receive general acceptance. In 1947, Memmelaar described a one-stage repair using a free graft of bladder mucosa for the urethroplasty. This technique has recently been revived for use in secondary cases (Keating et al., 1990).

The modern era of one-stage surgery began slowly in the late 1950s when surgeons were more confident of their ability to straighten the penis and proceed with urethroplasty. Broadbent and associates (1961) created a urethral tube from the skin of the penis and prepuce and laid this tube into the split glans. DesPrez and colleagues (1961) developed a one-stage procedure similar to that of Broadbent and colleagues. McCormack (1954) reported a two-stage procedure in which a full-thickness tube graft urethroplasty was placed at the first procedure, but the proximal anastomosis closure was delayed. In 1955, Devine and Horton (1961) developed this technique further by using a free graft of preputial skin to replace the urethra after release of chordee, and completed the proximal anastomosis in one stage (see Fig. 55-17). In 1970 and 1972, Hodgson described three different procedures that used vascularized flaps from the dorsal prepuce as well as penile skin. This neourethral flap was brought to the ventral aspect with a buttonhole transposition (Hodgson, 1975).

One-stage hypospadias repair has had the test of time, supporting the feasibility of this type of surgery. Besides the desirability of completing the reconstruction in one operation, a one-stage procedure has the additional advantage of using skin that is unscarred from previous surgical procedures, the normal blood supply of which has not been disrupted. The main impediment to the success of this procedure—inadequate chordee release—has been nearly eliminated since the introduction of the artificial erection technique (Gittes and McLaughlin, 1974) and dorsal plication maneuvers for orthoplasty (Baskin and Duckett, 1994) (see Fig. 55-12).

Specific Techniques for Surgical Repair
Methods for Anterior Hypospadias Without Chordee

Meatal Advancement and Glanuloplasty Incorporated (MAGPI) Procedure.—This procedure has been described by Duckett (1981b) and Duckett and Snyder (1991). A circumferential incision is made around the corona proximal to the meatus (see Fig. 55-14, *A*). The exact placement of this circumferential incision is not important at this stage because excess skin will be trimmed as the glanuloplasty develops. The penile skin is mobilized as a sleeve back to the penoscrotal junction, thus freeing any tethering fibers of the skin and subdartos fascia, particularly on the ventrum. This is the most probable cause for the ventral tilt of the glans frequently seen in these cases. Penile torsion will also be corrected in many cases if the dissection is carried back to the base of the penis. The straightness of the penis is then checked with an artificial erection. The rare case of curvature is usually caused by corporal disproportion, and fibrous tissue involving the dorsal urethra.

The meatal advancement of the dorsal urethral wall is accomplished by a Heineke-Mikulicz vertical incision and horizontal closure (see Fig. 55-14, *B*). More commonly, a wedge of glanular tissue that includes the glanular meatal wall is removed. The horizontal closure flattens out the glanular bridge and permits the dorsal urethra to be advanced out onto the glans tissue to the apex of the glanular groove, where it is sutured with interrupted 7-0 Vicryl (see Fig. 55-14, *C*). This flattens the deflecting ridge of the glans and permits the stream to be directed forward.

The glansplasty is made by reconfiguring the flattened glans into a conical shape (see Fig. 55-14, *D*). By rotating the lateral wings around to the midline proximal to the meatus, a proper conical glans shape can be re-created. There will be skin adjacent to the glanular edges that must be excised in a precise angle to reapproximate the glanular wings together in the midline on the ventrum. The deep glanular tissue is brought together with interrupted 6-0 Vicryl, and the superficial epithelial edges are closed with 7-0 chromic suture (see Fig. 55-14, *E*). In this way, mesenchymal glans tissue heals to glans tissue between the epithelial layers of the urethra and the outer epithelium of the glans, which prevents meatal retraction. This rotation of the glans wings reconfigures a nearly normal glanular appearance. A bougie-à-boule is used to calibrate the meatus and ensure that the glanuloplasty has not compromised the lumen of the distal glanular urethra.

A sleeve reapproximation of the penile skin usually is sufficient for skin cover (see Fig. 55-14, *E*). When a ventral skin deficiency exists, dorsal preputial skin can be transposed in Byars' flap fashion to the ventrum. No stents or catheters are required for diversion. The MAGPI procedures are done in the day surgical unit.

In 1986, we reported 500 MAGPI procedures with 2 fistulas and 11 cases of meatal advancement breakdown. Failure to recognize the occasional epithelialized channel dorsal to the meatus may be the cause for the meatal breakdown. If this channel is not removed or incorporated into the meatal advancement, healing may be compromised. Since that time, we have a complication rate of 1%, doing 130 to 150 MAGPI procedures per year (Duckett and Snyder, 1991). Preservation of the foreskin is requested by

parents more commonly, especially Europeans. Preservation is possible in combination with the MAGPI procedure. Polus and Lotte (1965) also demonstrated foreskin preservation in a combined procedure similar to Mathieu's.

Arap Modification of the MAGPI Procedure.—The ARAP procedure (Arap et al., 1984) is a variation of the MAGPI operation whereby two holding sutures are placed on the ventral skin edge and pulled forward to form an M configuration. The medial edges are sutured, which extends the floor of the urethra. The lateral edges of the M are approximated to complete the glanuloplasty.

In practice, however, patients with distal hypospadias tend *not* to have a dorsal lip of tissue in the glanular groove that lends itself to the classic Heineke-Mikulicz rearrangement that is performed in the MAGPI repair. These patients typically have a flat urethral plate that is more amenable to an onlay island flap, or if the distance is short, a parameatal-based flap. Furthermore, in distal hypospadias the ventral skin along the urethra is often quite thin, necessitating resection to healthy urethral spongiosum, leaving a gap too great for the ARAP procedure to bridge.

The Glans Approximation Procedure.—The GAP procedure (Zaontz, 1989) may be applicable in a small subset of patients with a glanular hypospadias with a wide and deep glanular groove. A noncompliant or fish-mouth meatus may be present in patients who do not have the bridge of glanular tissue that typically deflects the urinary stream ventrally. Ventral glanular tilt, meatal retraction, and splaying of the urinary stream can result from the inappropriate use of the MAGPI technique in these circumstances.

Another method of dealing with the subcoronal meatus is urethral mobilization. Reported as far back as Beck and Hacker (1897) and Beck (1917), urethral mobilization was more recently revived by Belman (1977), Waterhouse and Glassberg (1981), Koff (1981), Nasrallah and Minott (1984), and DeSy and Oosterlinck (1985). This technique offers very little advantage over the MAGPI technique and requires a more extensive procedure to mobilize the penile urethra. The meatal stenosis rate is significant.

In cases where preservation of the foreskin is requested, glanular, coronal, and mild coronal hypospadias can be repaired by the GRAP repair (glanular reconstruction and preputioplasty) (Gilpin et al., 1993). This technique is another modification of the King procedure (1970) with the added benefit of prepuce preservation.

Perimeatal-based Flap (Mathieu's Procedure).—When the meatus is too proximal on the shaft to achieve a MAGPI procedure and there is no chordee by artificial erection, the meatus may be advanced onto the glans as described by Mathieu (1932), and

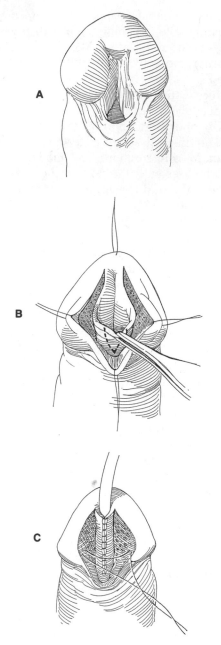

FIG. 55-19
Pyramid procedure. **A,** Megameatus-intact prepuce variant in a patient who has been circumcised. **B,** Periurethral dissection to apex of imaginary inverted pyramid, with ventral urethral reduction by removing a wedge of tissue. **C,** Closure of neourethra and glans.

reported by Hoffman and Hall (1973), Kim and Hendren (1981), Wacksman (1981), Gonzales and colleagues (1983), Devine (1983), and Brueziere (1987) (see Fig. 55-16). A flap of perimeatal skin is raised from tissue proximal and adjacent to the meatus, taking care to preserve the vascular subcutaneous tissue. Parallel incisions are made on either side of the glanular groove, developing the lateral glans as wings. The proximal flap closes into the glans groove as leaves of a book, and two suture closures are made on either

side of the flap, extending the meatus to the tip of the glans. Preserving the vasculature to the flap is important. The lateral glans wings will come together for closure over the urethral advancement. Appropriate skin cover is achieved. Urinary diversion is used for 5 to 7 days. Our recent experience with the Mathieu method resulted in 1 fistula in 56 cases (Elder et al., 1987). Others have shown that no diversion is needed (Rabinowitz, 1987).

Redman (1987) has recently revived the Barcat (1973) modification of the Mathieu procedure by mobilizing a glans flap in addition to the perimeatal-based flap, and splitting the glans dorsally to bury the urethral extension further to the apex of the glans. Koff and colleagues (1994) have had extensive experience with this technique with excellent results.

Megameatus Intact Prepuce (MIP), or Pyramid, Procedure.—In 6% of anterior hypospadias, the prepuce is intact, and a megameatus exists under the normal foreskin with a wide glanular defect and no penile curvature (see Fig. 55-7). These anomalies may be recognized only after circumcision is performed. Correction is therefore more complex. We describe a procedure (Duckett and Keating, 1989) that we designated the "pyramid technique" (Fig. 55-19). The enormous distal urethra is carefully dissected down the shaft of the glans and distal penis by way of a four-quadrant exposure (hence the pyramid designation). The urethra is tapered and buried into the glans very similar to an epispadias repair.

Techniques for Penile Shaft Hypospadias with and without Penile Curvature

Onlay Island Flap Urethral Extension (Baskin et al., 1994; Duckett, 1980c, 1986; Elder et al., 1987; Hollowell et al., 1990) (Fig. 55-20).—If the meatus is too proximal for an anterior procedure (MAGPI) or a parameatal procedure (Mathieu), or the ventral skin is too thin to use (see Fig. 55-8), a procedure to replace the ventral urethra is required. The urethral plate in this situation may be left intact. A strip of urethral plate skin onto the glans will serve as the dorsal urethral wall, and the ventral urethral wall is created by a vascularized island flap of tissue from the inner prepuce. A U-shaped closure extends the meatus to the glans tip. The glanular tissue is wrapped around the new urethral tube in such a way that a suitable conical glans will be attained. Initially this technique was applied to middle and distal hypospadias repairs without penile curvature, but more recently we have found it successful for more proximal hypospadias. Correction of penile curvature by tunica albuginea plication (TAP) is used when necessary (Fig. 55-20) (Baskin and Duckett et al., 1994).

Our recent results with this onlay island flap technique have been satisfactory, with a secondary surgical

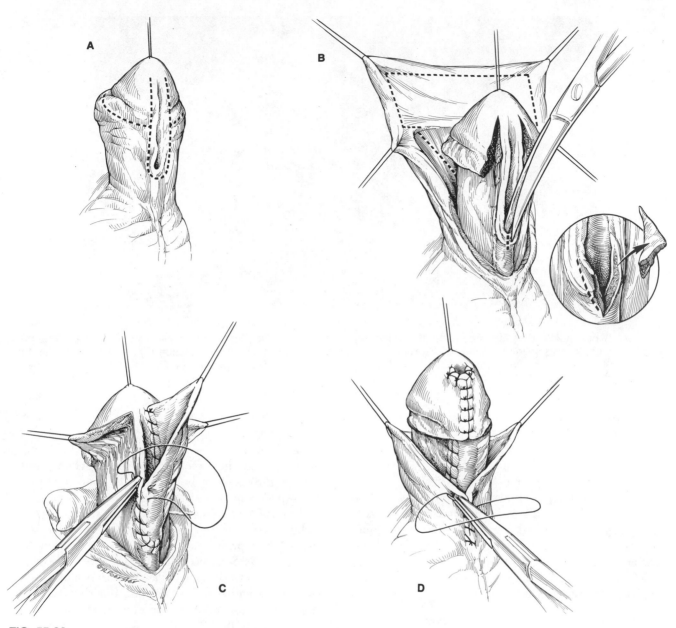

FIG. 55-20
Onlay island flap. **A,** For proximal, middle, or distal shaft meatus with and without penile curvature. Urethral plate is left intact. **B,** Parallel incision is made on glans from dorsal urethral strip 8 mm wide. Island flap is outlined from inner prepuce 8 to 10 mm wide. Proximal urethra is cut back to the spongiosum. **C,** Onlay flap is sutured with running 7-0 polyglycolic suture to urethral plate. Flap is trimmed to appropriate size. **D,** Glans wings are closed with deep mesenchymal sutures, forming an apical meatus. The dorsal prepuce is split down the midline and rotated to the ventrum for skin cover. (From Duckett JW: Hypospadias. In *Contemporary Urology* 1992. Used by permission.)

rate of 5% to 6%. Others have extended the indications of the onlay island flap to include more severe hypospadias with and without penile curvature (Baskin et al., 1994; Mollard et al., 1991; Perovic and Vukadinovic, 1994). Such a technique will cover a rather long strip on the ventrum if the proximal urethra is deficient. Even though the proximal meatus may be located near the corona, the urethra should be opened back to good spongiosum tissue, discarding the thin ventral urethra (Fig. 55-8 and 55-20). With the popularity of the onlay island flap for the more proximal

meatus, some have felt the need to dissect under the urethral plate to remove fibrous tissue, yet leave the skin strip intact attached to the glans and proximal meatus. We feel strongly that this is unnecessary and alters the better results associated with the extended onlay flap. If curvature correction is required, tunica albuginea plication should be done. Dissection under the urethral plate will not correct the curvature (Fig. 55-21). Other techniques to extend the distal meatus with hypospadias include tubularization of the distal urethral plate into a full tube with skin coverage by

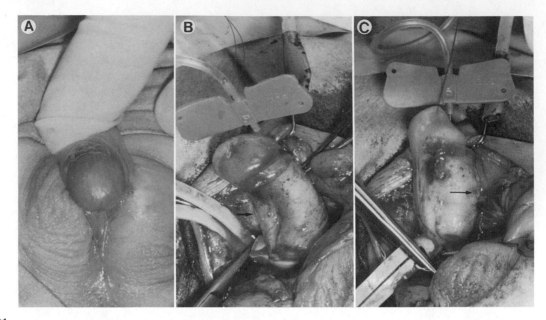

FIG. 55-21
A, Scrotal hypospadias. **B,** Artificial erection after releasing the skin and dartos fascia with preservation of the urethral plate *(arrow)* demonstrates penile curvature. **C,** Straight penis after dorsal tunica albuginea plication (TAP) *(arrow)* with urethral plate ready for onlay island-flap urethroplasty. (From Baskin LS, Duckett JW: Dorsal tunica albuginea plication for hypospadias curvature. *J Urol* 1994; 151:1668. Used by permission.)

tensive rearrangements. Tunica plication for correction of curvature was used in 13% of the cases, and various means (Nesbit, 1966). Others have also described this method (Belman and King, 1979; King 1970, 1981; Perlmutter and Vatz, 1975).

When the concept of "bowstring chordee" was prevalent, an incision dividing the urethral plate distal to the meatus was deemed important. Two techniques have been described to handle the situations of a 1- to 2-cm gap: the Devine-Horton flip-flap procedure (1977), and the Mustarde procedure (1965). Today these are of historical interest only.

Techniques for Posterior Hypospadias

Posterior hypospadias represents approximately 30% of all hypospadias. This is certainly the most challenging hypospadias to repair, and reconstructive procedures have a higher complication rate compared with correction of less severe forms. The techniques used for posterior hypospadias repair are (1) adjacent skin flaps, (2) vascularized flaps, and (3) free skin, bladder, or buccal mucosa grafts.

Adjacent Skin Flaps.—In one-stage repairs, skin adjacent to the meatus in the axis of the shaft of the penis has been tubularized to form a neourethra (Broadbent et al., 1961; DesPrez et al., 1961; Hinderer, 1971; Koyanagi et al., 1984, 1991; Snow, 1991).

In the first stage of two-stage posterior hypospadias repairs, following chordee release, dorsal skin is transferred to the ventrum so that there will be skin adjacent to the meatus for the urethroplasty in the sec-

ond stage (Creevy, 1958; Greenfield et al., 1994; Retik et al., 1994).

Free Skin Grafts.—A free full-thickness skin graft should be used in preference to split-thickness grafts because they have a better growth characteristic in children (Young and Benjamin, 1949). Devine and Horton (1961) and Devine (1983) have shown that full-thickness skin grafts can be used successfully (see Fig. 55-17). Their preference is to use the inner preputial skin after it is defatted to form a neourethra. Devine and Horton (1961) as well as Hendren and Horton (1988) have had excellent results, but they have not been transferable to other surgeons in a uniform manner (Filmer et al., 1977; Redman, 1983; Rober et al., 1990; Vyas et al., 1987; Woodard and Cleveland, 1982). It must be kept in mind that the free graft requires a revascularization. Great care should be taken to obtain an excellent skin cover to allow the graft a well-vascularized bed.

Vascularized Flaps.—Preputial or penile skin may be mobilized on a vascular pedicle attached to overlying skin, or mobilized as an island flap unrestricted by skin attachments and brought to the ventrum to form a neourethra. Hodgson (1970) used the inner aspect of the prepuce in a vertical orientation with a tumble-flap technique (Hodgson I). He subsequently used vertically oriented dorsal penile skin as a neourethra, which he transferred to the ventrum with a buttonhole maneuver using the Hodgson II and III procedures (Hodgson, 1972, 1975). Asopa and co-workers (1971) used a vascularized flap attached to the foreskin. The ventral preputial skin was used to create a new urethra that stayed attached to the penile skin as it was spiraled to the ventrum. This procedure, unfortunately, left an asymmetric and bulky result. Hodgson (1981) now prefers a similar technique called an *inner preputial tangential tube*. Standoli (1979, 1982) used the outer preputial skin to form a neourethra, which leaves the inner prepuce intact for the uncircumcised look. The outer prepuce may be stretched for a longer length to bridge longer gaps (Carmignani et al., 1982; Passerini et al., 1986).

Hinderer (1978) modified his adjacent-skin-flap vascularized tube to an island-flap method. The flap is based on vertically oriented skin from the penis onto the inner prepuce. He used a trochar to make a generous glans channel.

Since the blood supply of these vascularized pedicle flaps is more certain than that with free grafts, the healing of these neourethras is more reliable. Our experience over 20 years with the transverse preputial island flap neourethra, with a glans channel to position the meatus at the tip of the glans (Duckett, 1980b), has been consistently acceptable, with a secondary surgery rate of 10% to 15%. Others have reproduced these results (Kass and Bolong, 1990; Monfort et al., 1983; Parsons and Abercrombie, 1982). The long-term follow-up into puberty has also been satisfactory.

Technique for Transverse Preputial Island Flap (Duckett, 1980a).—A circumferential incision is made well proximal to the corona so that a generous cuff of ventral glanular tissue is preserved (Fig. 55-22, *A*). The penile skin with the attached prepuce is dissected free of the penis at the level of Buck's fascia in a cylindrical fashion. The meatus, urethra, and fibrous tissue are all dissected together with the cylinder of skin from the corpora cavernosa as proximal as needed to release all the ventral bend (Fig. 55-22, *B*). The fibrous tissue frequently extends around the lateral aspects of the shaft of the penis and distally beneath the glans. Mobilization of the proximal urethra is generally required to resect the fibrous tissue completely. This mobilization will drop the meatus back to the penoscrotal junction or into the scrotum. Adequate resection of the tissue causing the penile curvature is tested by the artificial erection technique. Residual penile curvature is straightened by the TAP procedure (see Fig. 55-12) (Baskin and Duckett, 1994). The meatus is circumcised to free the urethra from the overlying skin. The distal urethra and meatus are trimmed back to good spongiosum, and the cutaneous edges are removed. The proximal spatulated meatus and urethra are fixed to the corpora in a splayed-out fashion to receive the proximal end of the obliqued neourethra. If the proximal urethra lies in the perineum with a bifid scrotum, the periurethral tissue may be tubularized for a short distance to join the island-flap urethra (Fig. 55-23).

The neourethra is created by placing the ventral surface of the prepuce (the shiny undersurface) on tension with holding sutures in the skin of the dorsal prepuce (see Fig 55-22, *B*). The measured urethra is outlined with a marking pencil, usually 3 to 4 cm long and 12 to 15 mm wide in a 1-year-old. A neourethra as long as 6 cm has been created with this technique in a 2-year-old. In a severe case, the foreskin is allocated in a horseshoe fashion, permitting a long island flap always adequate to bridge the gap. The outlined inner preputial tube is incised, and a plane is developed between the dorsal skin and the island flap. Mobilization is achieved about two thirds of the way down the dorsal skin. A generous pedicle to the skin of the new urethra remains so that the neourethra may be rotated around the ventrum without distorting the penile skin or creating torsion of the penis. Careful dissection is required to preserve the pedicle to the flap, yet leave enough vascularization of the penile skin.

The rectangle of inner prepuce is rolled into a tube over an 8 F or 10 F catheter (see Fig. 55-22, *C*), used as a guide rather than a template. The caliber of the new urethra should be 12 F to 14 F when completed. Polyglycolic 7-0 sutures are used with a cutting needle. Interrupted sutures are used on the ends so that excess length may be excised.

The flap is usually rotated so that the right side is attached to the proximal urethra. An oblique anastomosis is made, freshening up the proximal urethra so that good tissue along with spongiosum is sutured to the tube (see Fig. 55-22, *D*). Excessive epithelium is excised. The suture line of the neourethra lies against the corporal groove. The neourethra is gently pulled distally toward the glans to avoid redundancy of the tube and kinking of the proximal anastomosis. We had this problem as a complication early in our experience and now avoid it by fixing the proximal anastomosis to the tunica albuginea of the corpora. Leakage of the tube and proximal anastomosis is checked with an 8 F tube by irrigating saline and obstructing the perineal urethra with a finger.

The glans channel is created with fine plastic scissors flat against the corpora cavernosa and snipping into the glanular tissue in the plane between the cap of the glans and the corpora (see Fig. 55-22, *E*). This plane is readily identified. The points of the scissors are taken up to the apex of the glans just above to the dimple of the blind-ending fossa. A button of glans epithelium is excised. Glanular tissue may need to be excised within this new channel to make a generous lumen. The channel should not be simply dilated because it will later constrict. Once a free channel that will calibrate at 16 F to 18 F is created, the distal portion of the flap with its pedicle may be delivered through the channel. It is pulled up so that the suture line of the neourethra lies adjacent to the corporal

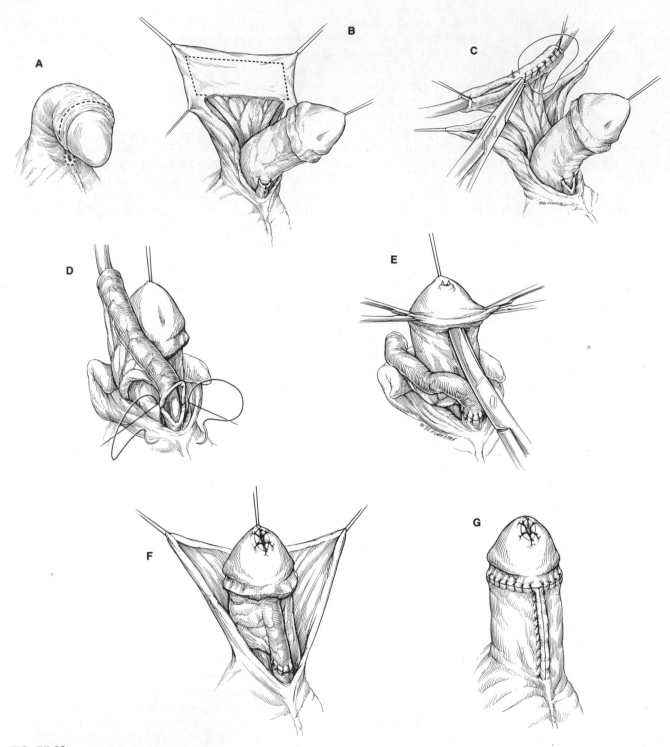

FIG. 55-22

Transverse preputial island flap with glans channel hypospadias repair. **A,** Release of penile curvature by surgical release of the skin and dartos fascia, and ancillary straightening procedures as needed. **B,** Development of island flap by dissecting subcutaneous tissue from dorsal penile skin. **C,** The transverse preputial island flap is developed and tubularized to 12 F, which is monitored by a bougie-á-boule. The distal edges of the tube are sewn with interrupted sutures so that the edges can be trimmed to fashion the appropriate length. **D,** Rotation to the ventrum must avoid torsion of the shaft by freeing the base of the flap adequately. A proximal oblique anastomosis is made, fixing the urethroplasty to the tunica albuginea along its posterior anastomosis. **E,** A wide glans channel is made underneath the glans cap against the corporal bodies by removing glans tissue within the channel. **F,** To avoid redundancy, the neourethra is tailored to fit the gap; it is then trimmed for a meatoplasty at the apex of the glans. **G,** Lateral transposition of Byars' flaps of dorsal penile skin to midline, and excision of the tips. The repair is stented with a 6 F catheter. (From Duckett JW: Hypospadias. In *Contemporary Urology* April, 1992. Used by permission.)

tissue. The excess tip of the flap is excised so that no redundancy exists. Interrupted fine chromic sutures used circumferentially fix the edge of the tube to the glanular tissue. No glanular darts are necessary. The proximal anastomosis is covered with subcutaneous pedicle tissue.

The dorsal penile skin is fanned out, and a vertical incision is made in the midline down to the point where the dorsal skin of the penis can be drawn comfortably up to the subcoronal incision (see Fig. 55-22, *F*). The remaining shaft skin is retracted proximally so that the lateral preputial wings will join in the midline ventrally with a vertical skin closure. The coronal closure is fashioned by trimming the preputial skin obliquely (see Fig. 55-22, *G*).

Technique for Scrotal Hypospadias

It has been our experience that, even with a meatus in the deep scrotum or perineum, we have always been able to achieve a long transverse preputial tube urethroplasty as depicted in Fig. 55-23. The concept that only a rectangle of skin may be taken from the inner prepuce is incorrect. If one thinks of the foreskin deployment as a horse-shoe going from the scrotum, around the top of the penis, and back to the scrotum, the inner skin margin may be taken as a flap as long as 6 to 7 cm. Since it is so broad at the base, the pedicle is transposed ventrally as a bipedicled flap. The cosmetic and functional results with these long flaps have been quite satisfactory. There currently is no need to return to two-stage procedures (Retik et al., 1994).

Techniques of Complex (Redo) Hypospadias

There are patients who have had multiple hypospadias repairs that have failed; they have been categorized as hypospadias cripples. This term should be abandoned for the patients' sake. These unfortunate outcomes occur even in skilled hypospadias surgeon's hands. It if often necessary in these patients to discard the problem-plagued urethra created previously and start anew. The penis must be straightened if needed. It is not at all inappropriate to stage these patients. In the past, bladder mucosa has been used for the neourethra (Coleman et al., 1981; Keating et al., 1990; Li et al., 1981; Memmelaar, 1947) because the long-term results with free skin grafts have not been as successful as previously reported (Burbige et al., 1984; Hendren and Crooks, 1980; Rober et al., 1990; Rogers, 1973). More recently, we have been pleased with buccal mucosa grafts as a urethral replacement for these difficult patients (Duckett et al., 1995).

An excellent review of 177 cases should be studied in this regard (Secrest et al., 1993). Fifty percent of the 177 patients were considered "cripples," 7% simple fistulas, 17% mild rearrangements, and 27% ex-

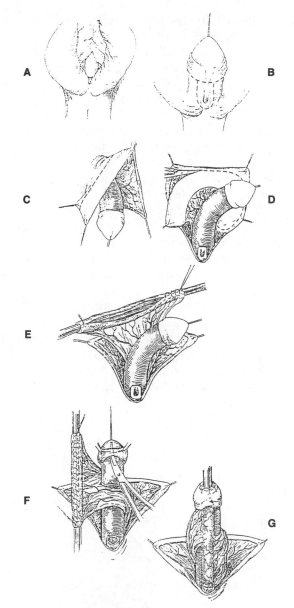

FIG. 55-23

Scrotal hypospadias. **A,** In severe cases in which the glans is tethered with a short urethral plate to a scrotal or perineal meatus, a more extended preputial tubed urethroplasty is preferred over a two-stage procedure. **B,** Lines of incision dividing the short urethral plate tethered to the scrotal meatus. **C,** Mobilization of the penile and preputial skin noting the elongated preputial area in the form of a "horseshoe." **D,** Consider the deployment of the preputial skin as a "horseshoe" permitting a 5 to 7 cm vascularized inner preputial flap. **E,** Tubularization of the lengthy flap maintaining vascularity to each end. Interrupted sutures on the ends of the tube permit excisions to tailor length. **F,** A buttonhole of the pedicle in the midline permits transposition to the ventrum with a bipedicle flap. The urethra should be stretched so that no redundancy exists. Both ends should be trimmed to fit perfectly. A glans channel is depicted. **G,** Note bipedicled flap for long urethroplasty. It is important to calibrate the width of the tubed urethra to no more than 10 to 12 F so that a diverticulum is avoided due to redundancy. Skin closure is done by rotating dorsal penile skin around to the ventrum (Byars' flaps). A urethral "drip" stent is used for two weeks.

dermal grafts in 21%. The remainder had scar excision alone to correct penile curvature. Simple fistulas had a 10% recurrence rate. Full-thickness extragenital skin grafts had only a 70% success, while secondary flip-flap procedures only a 53% success. Flap procedures with penile or scrotal skin or dorsal preputial flaps were 90% to 100% successful. Bladder mucosa grafts were used rarely (11 cases) and the results were poor. Twenty-three percent had staged redos using meshed split-thickness grafts.

Bladder Mucosa Grafts.—Memmelaar (1947) first described using bladder mucosa as a one-stage hypospadias repair. Marshall and Spellman (1955) were initially enthusiastic about using bladder mucosa but found it necessary to stage the procedure as McCormack (1954) had done with the full-thickness skin graft. The method was revived by Coleman and associates (1981) and Li and co-workers (1981). Aside from cystotomy—the extra procedure required to harvest the graft—the method initially met with some success (Hendren and Reda, 1986; Koyle and Ehrlich, 1987; Ramsley et al., 1987; Song et al., 1982). However, a review of 268 reported cases by Keating and associates (1990) was not as encouraging

as initially thought. In this report, bladder mucosa was used mainly in secondary cases of both hypospadias and epispadias, especially in postpubertal patients. The main complications were meatal problems. Eversion of the bladder mucosa at the meatus and stenosis made up 30% of the complications. Meatal dilatation on a daily basis could avoid this problem. Further enthusiasm for the use of bladder mucosa grafts has been tempered by similar complications reported in long-term follow-up by Kinkead and colleagues (1994).

Buccal Mucosa.—In patients with a paucity of adjacent well-vascularized skin for flap procedures, we have recently turned to buccal mucosa as a free graft for urethral replacement (Duckett et al., 1994) (Fig. 55-24). From a graft biology viewpoint, buccal mucosa is an ideal material. In comparison to both skin and bladder mucosa grafts, the epithelial layer is four times thicker, while the relatively thin lamina propria allows efficient transfer of nutrients by diffusion (imbibition) from the recipient site to the new graft. The extensive vascularity in the lamina propria also allows new capillaries to grow into the graft (inosculation). This may explain the excellent take of buccal free grafts. Buccal

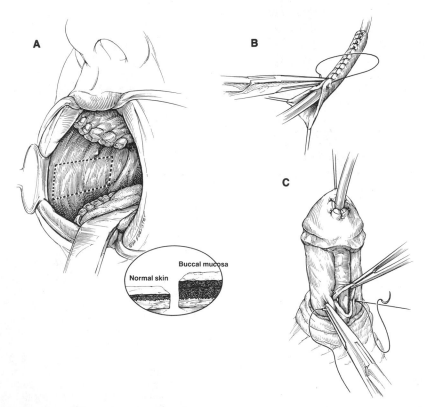

FIG. 55-24
Buccal mucosal graft for secondary hypospadias procedures when no penile skin is available for a flap procedure. **A,** The inner-cheek mucosa is harvested, avoiding Stenson's duct, to make an appropriate urethral replacement for age. (Inset: The difference in thickness between buccal mucosa and normal skin—an even thinner bladder mucosa-is apparent.) **B,** The urethral graft is formed appropriate for age and **C,** Channeled to the tip of the glans. The proximal oblique anastomosis is fixed to the tunica albuginea. Adequate skin cover is critical for revascularization of the graft. (From Duckett JW: Hypospadias. In *Contemporary Urology* April, 1992. Used by permission.)

mucosa grafts do not have the same tendency to shrink like bladder mucosa grafts, which need to be harvested approximately 25% to 35% larger than their final caliber. Harvesting of a buccal mucosa graft from both the inner cheek (Burger et al., 1992; Ewalt et al., 1992) and the inner surface of the lip (Dessanti et al., 1992) is reliable and easily performed by the urologist. The morbidity from this procedure is surprisingly minimal, and the scar well hidden. In comparison, harvesting of a bladder mucosa graft requires a separate cystotomy incision.

Humby (1941) is credited with the first use of buccal mucosa for urethral reconstruction. This was before the antibiotic era, which may account for the failure that caused Humby to settle on bladder mucosa as the ideal urethral substitution. In 1986, we successfully used a buccal graft to replace a urethra in an adult with exstrophy/epispadias (Duckett et al., 1994). Buccal mucosa free graft has also been used as a patch graft for the repair of complicated urethral strictures (el-Kasaby et al., 1993).

In the future, it may be possible to treat difficult cases of hypospadias with autologous grafts of cultured urethral epithelium (Romagnoli et al., 1990, 1993). Finding the ideal supporting matrix to scaffold the urothelial cells may make this technique widely applicable.

Technical Considerations
Instruments

The principles of hypospadiology have been enhanced over the years by the precise delicate-tissue handling taught by plastic surgeons using delicate instruments and fine suture material. Instruments may be borrowed from the ophthalmologic or plastic surgery cabinets. Sharp-pointed iris scissors and delicate-toothed forceps are the principal tools. Castroviejo needle holders and 0.5-mm forceps are useful for the very delicate maneuvers with 7-0 sutures. As the procedure progresses, bougie-à-boule probes are most useful for calibrating the sizes of tubes and the anastomoses as well as the meatus. Fine lacrimal duct probes are useful for identifying fistulas and periurethral ducts.

Suture Material

Absorbable material (chromic catgut) is favored for the skin because it absorbs rapidly in 10 to 20 days. Polyglycolic acid (Dexon) or polyglactin 910 (Vicryl) will stay in the tissues longer and have a little better tensile strength than their same-size chromic sutures. We use these sutures on the inner layer for the neourethra but prefer chromic sutures for the skin. Polydioxanone (PDS) remains much longer than either of the other two sutures, and it is not advised for hypospadias surgery (Bickerton and Duckett, 1984).

Pull-out permanent sutures such as nylon or Prolene are less reactive and may be used to close the urethra and the skin suture lines in several layers (Belman, 1982). In the future, it may be possible to use laser welding systems to solder tissue (Merguerian et al., 1992).

Magnification

Optical magnification is essential. The more expensive loupes are generally supplied in 2.5 to 6.5 power. They give a narrow field of vision; however, when one is familiar with their use, they are indispensable. We prefer an Optivisor #2, which allows a broader field of vision but lower magnification at 1.5 to 2.5 power. Focal length is 35 to 50 cm (14 to 20 in.), which is quite satisfactory for this type of surgery. Some operating microscopes will go down to 3.5 power, but most of those in standard operating rooms are 10 power, which is too great a magnification. The justification for purchasing one's own operating microscope for hypospadias surgery depends on the volume at the institution, clearly a limiting factor. The individual preference for magnification is broad, and the microscopists are currently passionate about their improved results using this instrument (Wacksman, 1987).

Hemostasis

Control of bleeding from the very vascular penis and glans may be achieved in a number of ways. Placing a tourniquet at the base of the penis is simplest (Ossandon and Ransley, 1982; Redman, 1987). Recommended lengths of tourniquet time vary from 20 minutes to 1 hour. We prefer the injection of 1/100,000 of epinephrine in 1% xylocaine (lidocaine) using a 26-gauge needle. Infiltration around the urethra and into the glans for developing glans wings is helpful. Usually, only 1.5 to 2.0 ml is required. There is a wide range of safety before epinephrine will sensitize the myocardium to arrhythmias with inhalational anesthetics (Karl et al., 1983). The safety dose is 1 ml/kg of a 1/100,000 solution. We have never believed that epinephrine compromised the vascularity of the flaps. Various methods of coagulation have been recommended; we prefer a low-current electrocautery (Bovie). Bipolar electrodes stick to the tissues too much.

Analgesia

In anticipation of postoperative discomfort, a supplemental local block with 3 ml of 0.5% bupivacaine (Marcaine) is placed just beneath the symphysis to infiltrate the dorsal penile nerve bundle (Jensen, 1981; Yeoman, 1983). It is placed before the surgical procedure and lasts for nearly 12 hours. It also reduces the anesthetic needs and erections that are sometimes very bothersome and cause extra bleeding. Penile blocks seem a better choice for hypospadias surgery than caudal blocks, although some believe that bleeding is less with caudal (Gunter et al., 1990).

Dressings

The main purpose of a proper dressing is to provide immobilization with prevention of hematoma and edema. Protection of the suture lines from contamination is less important. It is unlikely that dressings contribute to skin slough or subsequent fistula formation (Cromie and Bellinger, 1981). Preference for the dressing is as varied as the other fetishes of hypospadias surgery.

For distal hypospadias performed without urinary diversion, our current dressing is a Tegaderm wrap. We have the parents remove the dressing at home in 24 to 48 hours. For hypospadias with urinary diversion our current favorite sandwich dressing allows more diffuse pressure to be applied by placing the penis onto the abdominal wall for compression. A layer of Telfa. a 4-by-4-in. gauze is folded three times on the ventrum of the penis and secured with a medium Tegaderm sheet of sticky plastic. The dressing is removed after 72 hours at home.

Diversions

Bladder spasms caused by irritation of the trigone with a catheter remain the most aggravating complication. The other problem relates to the connections of tubing to a drainage bag. We avoid a Foley catheter except in adults and prefer a "dripping stent" in patients age 6 to 18 months. Kendall makes a 6 F hypospadias catheter prepackaged. It is sutured to the glans with a 5-0 polypropylene noncutting needle. We have had quite good success with this technique, which allows all cases of hypospadias now to be done on an outpatient basis (Baskin et al., 1994).

Bladder spasms are most aggravating to the patient and family. We have used methantheline bromide (Banthine) and opium suppositories (B & O) cut into thirds for several days although the pediatric dosage of opium suppositories has never been verified. Oral oxybutynin chloride may also help. As long as the meatus is kept open from crusting, occasional passage of urine with a spasm through the newly repaired urethra should not be harmful.

Age for Repair

Hypospadias repair is being performed at progressively younger ages. Schultz and colleagues (1983) pointed out that an ideal window might be age 6 to 18 months to minimize the emotional effect of this traumatic experience. We now prefer to do surgery between 3 and 9 months and believe that the penis is of sufficient size to achieve success equal to that of surgery performed at ages 2 to 5 years which was

previously popular (Devine, 1983). Kaplan and associates (1989) studied 69 middle-childhood boys (ages 6 to 10 years) who had hypospadias repair done in infancy and could not find any increase of significant psychopathology during childhood.

In addition, improved optical magnification and fine instruments have made surgical correction at an earlier age more successful (Manley and Epstein, 1981). Since the majority of hypospadias repairs can be managed as a day surgical procedure, management of younger infants at home is much easier (Clair and Caldamone, 1988).

Testosterone Stimulation

Enlargement of the infant penis is possible by testosterone stimulation. A 5% testosterone cream rubbed on the genitals daily for 3 weeks works by local absorption. Blood levels of testosterone reach pubertal levels quickly. Dihydrotestosterone (DHT) is also used (Monfort and Lucas, 1982). Equally effective is 25 mg of testosterone proprionate given intramuscularly once per week for 3 weeks (Gearhart and Jeffs, 1987). The intramuscular dosage is better controlled and is preferable to the aesthetically displeasing request made of the parents to rub cream on the penis to make it bigger. We have not found the use of testosterone stimulation to be beneficial, and there is a suggestion that it may be harmful on the later maturation of prostatic tissue (Nasland and Coffee, 1985) as well as penile growth (Hussman and Cain, 1994).

Outpatient Surgery

Because the postoperative management of hypospadias surgery is concerned mainly with the difficulties associated with diversion and dressings, minimization of side effects and complications of these two factors can make outpatient surgery possible. It obligates the surgeon to coordinate postoperative care by adequate preoperative education, simplification of instructions, and ready accessibility to the telephone to accomplish outpatient care (Clair and Caldamone, 1988).

Psychosocial Support

The surgeon or a well-trained nurse must alleviate parental guilt that frequently accompanies this genital anomaly. Unexpressed anxieties as to the cause of hypospadias and later sexual capabilities must be anticipated and discussed. The child's future positive body image may well depend on his parents' thorough understanding of his condition. The surgeon must be certain that these issues are made clear to the parents.

Follow-up Care

Dressing changes, catheter or tube removal, wound care, and infection control depend on the complexity of the procedure required. All of these can be done in the office or outpatient clinic without the need for general anesthetic support. Bougienage of the meatus or urethroplasty may be accomplished deftly and with minimal discomfort if small-caliber straight sounds or bougie-à-boules are used. Care should be taken not to force through a narrowing. A kink at the proximal anastomosis is more likely than a stricture in the early postoperative period. Urethral diversions are used for 7 to 14 days. We schedule follow-up visits at 3 and 6 weeks and at 3- to 6-month intervals as needed thereafter. Observation of the voided stream or uroflowmetry are preferred to sounding the urethra as the child grows.

Early Complications
Infection

Every effort should be made to prevent wound infections. Separation of the foreskin adherent to the glans and removal of desquamated epithelial debris should be done under anesthesia prior to skin preparation. When the patient is postpubertal, skin preparation should be undertaken several days before surgery with thrice-daily cleansing. Prophylactic antibiotics are of little value in avoiding wound infections in hypospadias surgery. However, postoperatively, trimethoprim-sulfa or nitrofurantoin suppression may be helpful to prevent cystitis, particularly if the tube is left to open drainage in the diaper (Montagnino et al., 1988; Sugar and Firlit, 1989). In general, drains are not used except when a skin graft or buccal mucosal graft is used. In such cases, a vacuum suction drain is created by placing a scalp vein needle into the vacuum tube while the tubing from the needle is placed under the skin. This helps keep the graft adherent to the overlying skin. Drains should be removed promptly when one believes their purpose has been served, in order to keep the skin in continuity with the graft (24 to 48 hours).

Meatal Stenosis

The meatus can become stenotic by crusting, edema, or synechia. A stent left in place usually avoids all three of these complications. If a stent is not left in place, sitz baths twice daily, after which the parents place an ophthalmic ointment tube nozzle into the urethral meatus, will suffice. Gentle bougienage with a straight sound in initial follow-up visits also assists in meatal patency.

Loss of Skin Flaps

Poor wound healing is due primarily to ischemic flaps. If care is taken during the procedure, this problem should be avoided. If skin-flap loss occurs over a well-vascularized island-flap neourethra, healing can occur after the sloughed skin is gone. If a free-graft technique has been used, a sloughed skin flap over the neourethra will jeopardize the entire procedure.

Edema

Edema occurs after most hypospadias repairs and can be diminished by a compression dressing. Edema within the urethra may compromise healing if a urethral stent is too large. A compressible stent is described by Mitchell and Kulb (1986).

Hemorrhage

Intraoperative hemorrhage can be controlled by a tourniquet or epinephrine infiltration. Cautery is used sparingly intraoperatively for bleeding points. Postoperative bleeding is controlled by the application of a compressive dressing. Evacuation of a hematoma is not usually necessary unless a free graft is used.

Erections

In the postpubertal patient, postoperative erections can be a significant problem. Various medications and procedures have been tried with little success. The best of these is amyl nitrite pulvules.

Late Complications
Urethrocutaneous Fistulas

Urethrocutaneous fistulas are the most common late complication of hypospadias repair, and their incidence has been used to evaluate the effectiveness of the surgical procedure (Retik et al., 1988).

An expected fistula rate is between 10% and 15% for most one-stage hypospadias surgery. Often, distal obstruction is related to persistent fistulas. Once a fistula has matured, subsequent fistula closure procedures have a discouraging recurrence rate. Therefore, some have suggested repairing urethrocutaneous fistulas with wide mobilization, adjacent skin flaps, multilayered closures, and the use of urinary diversion (Belman, 1988; Horton et al., 1980; Turner-Warwick, 1972; Walker, 1981).

We recommend using magnification and delicate instruments for fistula repair. A lacrimal duct probe is placed through the fistulous track to help identify its epithelial lining. Dissection is carried down to the urethra, and a 7-0 polyglycolic suture is used to close the urethral edges in an inverting fashion. Watertight closure is assured by irrigating the urethra with proximal compression. Two layers of closure are obtained, and "super glue" is used as a wound sealant. No urinary diversion is used. The patient is allowed to void through his urethra and goes home on the same day.

We reviewed 32 fistula closures over a 3.5-year period (Duckett et al., 1982). Twenty-nine fistulas were repaired by this technique, with three recurrences (10%). They were successfully closed with a second similar procedure. Three fistulas were large and were closed with suprapubic urinary diversion for added safety. We concluded from this experience that for pinpoint or moderate-sized fistulas, urinary diversion and extensive flap mobilization are not necessary. Se-

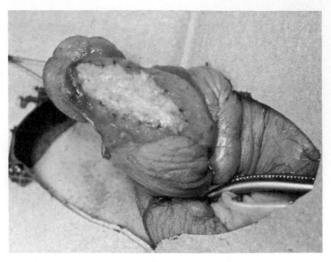

FIG. 55-25
Dermal graft replacement of ventral tunica albuginea.

crest and colleagues (1993) report a similar 10% recurrence with fistula repair.

It is extremely important to recognize a concomitant urethral stricture or diverticulum at the time of fistula closure. They should be repaired to ensure success of the fistula closure. Occasionally, a meatoplasty may be necessary at the time of fistula repair.

A fistula near the glans is best repaired by opening the bridge between meatus and fistula, mobilizing inner urethral edges, and closing in two layers with good glans approximation.

Meatoplasty

A narrowing of the meatus may be alleviated by simply elevating a glans flap, excising the scar beneath, and interdigitating the skin flap. More extensive scarring of the glanular urethra and meatus may be due to poor vascularization of a perimeatal flap (the Mathieu or Mustarde procedure). A more extensive glanulomeatoplasty, such as that described by Brannen (1976) and modified by DeSy (1984), may be required. A ventral flap is developed and folded into the split glans. This method is also useful for a coronal fistula and meatal stenosis combination.

Residual Curvature

Before the use of the artificial erection, residual curvature was much more common. This problem is corrected by mobilizing a sleeve of urethra and overlying skin down to the penoscrotal junction. Any residual scar tissue is resected until the artificial erection shows a straight penis. There are occasions when extension of the urethroplasty will be possible by mobilizing a skin flap on the ventrum similar to a Mustarde procedure. A glans channel may be used to place the meatus at the tip of the penis. Other innovative techniques for more extensive urethroplasty may be required (Stecker et al., 1981). Slight ventral chordee

can be repaired with dorsal suture plication with a permanent suture (Baskin and Duckett, 1994; Livne et al., 1984; Secrest et al., 1993).

Rarely, extensive scarring of the ventrum of the penis requires excision of the tunica albuginea with replacement grafts of dermis (Devine and Horton, 1975), tunica vaginalis (Duckett et al., 1980d), or venous graft (Fournier et al., 1993). If dermal grafts are to be used, care should be taken to be certain that all epidermal elements are removed; otherwise, dermal cysts can develop. Hendren and Keating (1988) demonstrated that using a dermal graft in conjunction with a free urethral graft was successful in revascularizing the graft. We prefer using tunica vaginalis (Fig. 55-25).

Once the penis is straight, an additional length of neourethra will likely be required to extend the urethra to the glans tip. Preferably, adjacent penile skin is used as a flap. Otherwise, a free graft will be required. Our current preference is for buccal mucosa.

Stricture

Strictures after hypospadias repair result from technical problems at the initial repair. Proximal anastomotic strictures may result from either a luminal calibration miscalculation resulting in a narrow neourethral or an anastomotic overlap. The overlap problem can be avoided by lateral fixation of the oblique anastomoses to the tunica albuginea. In the late case, a meatal stricture results from chronic balanitis xerotica obliterans (BXO) (Garat et al., 1986). This reaction is located at the meatus or may extend into the more proximal urethroplasty. We feel this may be due to a poorly vascularized meatoplasty, especially the Mathieu procedure. The most likely cause for meatal stenosis is vascular compromise of the urethra at the apex of the meatus. It may be secondary to an inadequate glans channel that compresses the vascularity of the pedicle. Once a stricture has developed, it may be repaired by excision and reanastomosis, a patch graft, or a vascularized pedicle graft (Scherz et al., 1988). We have had little success treating strictures secondary to hypospadias surgery with optical internal urethrotomy (Lofti, Snyder, and Duckett, 1991).

Diverticulum

A *fusiform urethral diverticulum* may form because the neourethra was made too wide, and meatal stenosis allowed ballooning of the proximal urethra (Aigen et al., 1987). Reduction of a diverticulum may be necessary and should be done in a longitudinal fashion. Most often, a circumcising incision is used, and the penile skin is dropped to the penoscrotal junction, which allows for the longitudinal repair of the diverticulum without overlying suture lines. Care must be taken to evaluate the neourethra for an associated fistula as well. A discrete diverticulum may

DesPrez JD, Persky L, Kiehn CL: A one-stage repair of hypospadias by island-flap technique. *Plast Reconstr Surg* 1961; 28:405.

Dessanti A, Rigamonti W, Merulla V, et al: Autologous buccal mucosa graft for hypospadias repair: an initial report. *J Urol* 1992; 147:1081.

DeSy WA: Aesthetic repair of meatal stricture. *J Urol* 1984; 132:678.

DeSy WA, Oosterlinck W: One-stage hypospadias repair by free full-thickness skin graft and island-flap techniques. *Urol Clin North Am* 1981; 8:491.

DeSy WA, Oosterlinck W: *Urethral Advancement for Hypospadias Repair*. Film presented at the International Congress of Urology, Vienna, 1985.

Devine CJ Jr: Chordee and hypospadias. In Glenn JF, Boyce WH (eds): *Urologic Surgery*, ed 3. Philadelphia, JB Lippincott, 1983, pp 775-797.

Devine CJ, Gonzales-Serva L, Stecker JF Jr, et al: Utricular configuration in hypospadias and intersex. *J Urol* 1980; 123:407.

Devine CJ Jr, Horton CE: A one-stage hypospadias repair. *J Urol* 1961; 85:166.

Devine CJ Jr, Horton CE: Chordee without hypospadias. *J Urol* 1973; 110:264.

Devine CJ Jr, Horton CE: Use of dermal graft to correct chordee. *J Urol* 1975; 113:56.

Devine CJ Jr, Horton CE: Hypospadias repair. *J Urol* 1977; 118:188.

DeVries JDM: *Hypospadias Repair With the Transverse Inner Preputial Island-Flap Technique*. Nijmegen, The Netherlands, 1986.

Duckett JW: Transverse preputial island-flap technique for repair of severe hypospadias. *Urol Clin North Am* 1980a; 7:423.

Duckett JW: Hypospadias. *Clin Plast Surg* 1980b; 7:149.

Duckett JW: Repair of hypospadias. In Hendry WF (ed): *Recent Advances in Urology/Andrology*. New York, Churchill-Livingstone, 1980c, vol 3, pp 279-290.

Duckett JW: Foreword. Symposium on Hypospadias. *Urol Clin North Am* 1981a; 8:371.

Duckett JW: MAGPI (meatal advancement and glanuloplasty): a procedure for subcoronal hypospadias. *Urol Clin North Am* 1981b; 8:513.

Duckett JW: The island-flap technique for hypospadias repair. *Urol Clin North Am* 1981c; 8:503.

Duckett JW: Hypospadias. In Walsh PC, Gittes RF, Permutter AD, et al (eds): *Campbell's Urology*, ed 5. Philadelphia, WB Saunders, 1986, pp 1969-1999.

Duckett JW, Caldamone AA, Snyder HM: Hypospadias fistula repair without diversion. Abstract 11. AAP Annual Meeting, New York, Oct 23-28, 1982.

Duckett JW, Coplen DA, Ewalt DH, et al: Buccal mucosal urethral replacement. *J Urol* 1995; 153:1660.

Duckett JW, Kaplan GW, Woodard JR, et al: Panel: Complications of hypospadias repair. *Urol Clin North Am* 1980d; 7:443.

Duckett JW, Keating MA: Technical challenge of the megameatus intact prepuce hypospadias (MIP) variant: the pyramid procedure. *J Urol* 1989; 141:1407.

Duckett JW, Snyder H III: The MAGPI hypospadias repair in 1111 patients. *Ann Surg* 1991; 213:620.

Eberle J, Uberreiter S, Radmoyr C, et al: Posterior hypospadias: long-term follow-up after reconstructive surgery in the male direction. *J Urol* 1993; 150:1474.

Ehrlich RM, Scardino PT: Surgical correction of scrotal transposition and perineal hypospadias. *J Pediatr Surg* 1982; 17:175.

Elder JE: Influence of glans morphology on choice of island-flap technique in children with proximal hypospadias. *J Urol* 1992; part 2: AUA Abstract #417.

Elder JS, Duckett JW, Snyder HM: Onlay island flap in the repair of mid- and distal penile hypospadias without chordee. *J Urol* 1987; 138:376.

el-Kasaby AW, Fath-Alla M, Noweir AM, et al: The use of buccal mucosa patch graft in the management of anterior urethral strictures. *J Urol* 1993; 149:276.

Ewalt DH, Baskin LS, Duckett JW: Buccal mucosa: rationale for use as urethral graft material. Abstract Section on Urology, American Academy of Pediatrics. San Francisco, 1992.

Faerber GJ, Park JM, Bloom DA: Long-term outcome with the MAGPI hypospadias repair. *J Urol* 1995; 153:1655.

Filmer RB, Duckett JW, Sowden R: One-stage correction of hypospadias/chordee. *Birth Defects* 1977; 13:267.

Forashall I, Rickham PP: Transposition of the penis and scrotum. *Br J Urol* 1956; 28:250.

Fournier GR, Lue TF, Tanagho EA: Peyronie's plaque: surgical treatment with the CO_2 laser and a deep dorsal vein patch graft. *J Urol* 1993; 149:1321.

Fuqua F: Renaissance of a urethroplasty: the Belt technique of hypospadias repair. *J Urol* 1971; 106:782.

Garat JM, Chechile G, Algaba F, et al: Balanitis xerotica obliterans in children. *J Urol* 1986; 136:436.

Gearhart JP, Donohou PA, Brown TR, et al: Endocrine evaluation of adults with mild hypospadias. *J Urol* 1990; 143:274.

Gearhart JP, Jeffs RD: The use of parenteral testosterone therapy in genital reconstructive surgery. *J Urol* 1987; 138:1077.

Gearhart JP, Linhard HR, Berkovitz GD, et al: Androgen receptor levels and 5 alpha-reductase activities in preputial skin and chordee tissue of boys with isolated hypospadias. *J Urol* 1988; 140:1243.

Gibbons AD, Gonzales ET Jr: The subcoronal meatus. *J Urol* 1983; 130:739.

Gilpin D, Clements WD, Boston VE: GRAP repair: single-stage reconstruction of hypospadias as an outpatient procedure. *Br J Urol* 1993; 71:226.

Gittes RF, McLaughlin AP III: Injection technique to induce penile erection. *Urology* 1974; 4:473.

Glenister TW: The origin and fate of the urethral plate in man. *J Anat* 1954; 288:413.

Goldman AS: Abnormal organogenesis in the reproductive system. In Wilson JG, Fraser FC (eds): *Handbook of Teratology*, New York, Plenum Press, 1977, vol 2, pp 391-419.

Gonzales ET Jr, Veeraraghavan KA, Delaune J: The management of distal hypospadias with meatal-based, vascularized flaps. *J Urol* 1983; 129:119.

Greenfield SP, Sadler BT, Wan J: Two-stage repair for severe hypospadias. *J Urol* 1994; 152:488.

Gunter JB, Forestner JE, Manley CB: Caudal epidural anesthesia reduces blood loss during hypospadias repair. *J Urol* 1990; 144:517.

Gupta C, Goldman A: Arachidonic acid cascade is involved in the masculinization of embryonic external genitalia in mice. *Proc Natl Acad Sci USA* 1986; 83:4346.

Henderson BE, Benton R, Cosgrove M, et al: Urogenital tract abnormalities in sons of women treated with diethylstilbestrol. *Pediatrics* 1976; 58:505.

Hendren WH: The Belt-Fuqua for repair of hypospadias. *Urol Clin North Am* 1981; 8:431.

Hendren WH, Crooks KK: Tubed free-skin graft for construction of male urethra. *J Urol* 1980; 123:858.

Hendren WH, Caesar RE: Chordee without hypospadias: experience with 33 cases. *J Urol* 1992; 147:107.

Hendren WH, Horton CE Jr: Experience with one-stage repair of hypospadias and chordee using free graft of prepuce. *J Urol* 1988; 140:1259.

Hendren WH, Keating MA: Use of dermal graft and free urethral graft in penile reconstruction. *J Urol* 1988; 140:1265.

Hendren WH, Reda EF: Bladder mucosa graft for construction of male urethra. *J Pediatr Surg* 1986; 21:189.

Hinderer U: New one-stage repair of hypospadias (technique of penis tunnelization). In Hueston JT (ed): *Transactions of the 5th International Congress of Plastic and Reconstructive Surgery*. Stoneham, Mass., Butterworth, 1971, pp 283-305.

Hinderer U: Hypospadias repair in long-term results. In Goldwyn RM (ed): *Plastic and Reconstructive Surgery*. Boston, Little, Brown, 1978, pp 378-410.

Hinman F Jr: The blood supply to prepartial island flaps. *J Urol* 1991; 145:1232.

Hinman F Jr: Penis and male urethral. In Hinman F Jr: *Urosurgical Anatomy*. Philadelphia, WB Saunders, 1993, pp 418-470.

Hodgson NB: A one-stage hypospadias repair. *J Urol* 1970; 104:281.

Hodgson NB: In defense of the one-stage hypospadias repair. In Scott R Jr, Gordon HL, Scott FB, et al (eds): *Current Controversies in Urologic Management*. Philadelphia, WB Saunders, 1972, pp 263-271.

Hodgson NB: Hypospadias. In Glenn JF, Boyce WH (eds): *Urologic Surgery*, ed 2. New York, Harper & Row, 1975, pp 656-667.

Hodgson NB: Hypospadias and urethral duplication. In Harrison JH (ed): *Campbell's Urology*, ed 4. Philadelphia, WB Saunders, 1978, pp 1566-1595.

Hodgson NB: Use of vascularized flaps in hypospadias repair. *Urol Clin North Am* 1981; 8:471.

Hodgson NB: Personal communication, 1986.

Hoffman WW, Hall WV: A modification of Spence's hood for one-stage surgical correction of distal shaft penile hypospadias. *J Urol* 1973; 109:1017.

Hollowell JG, Keating MA, Snyder HM, et al: Preservation of urethral plate in hypospadias repair: extended applications and further experience with the onlay island-flap urethroplasty. *J Urol* 1990; 143:98.

Horton CE, Devine CJ: Peyronies' disease. *Plast Reconst Surg* 1973; 52:503.

Horton CE, Devine CJ, Baran N: Pictorial history of hypospadias repair techniques. In Horton CE (ed): *Plastic and Reconstructive Surgery of the Genital Area*. Boston, Little, Brown, 1973, pp 237-248.

Horton CE, Devine CJ, Graham JK: Fistulas of the penile urethra. *Plast Reconstr Surg* 1980; 66:407.

Howard FS: Hypospadias with enlargement of the prostatic utricle. *Surg Gynecol Obstet* 1948; 86:307.

Humby G: A one-stage operation for hypospadias. *Br J Surg* 1941; 29:84.

Hussman DA, Cain MP: Microphallus: eventual phallic size is dependent on the timing of androgen administration. *J Urol* 1994; 152:734.

Jensen BH: Caudal block for postoperative pain relief in children after genital operations. A comparison between bupivacaine and morphine. *Acta Anesthesiol Scand* 1981; 25:373.

Jirasék JE, Raboch J, Uher J: The relationship between the development of gonads and external genitals in human fetuses. *Am J Obstet Gynecol* 1968; 101:830.

Juskiewenski S, Vaysse P, Guitard J, et al: Traitement des hypospadias anterieurs. *Chir Pediatr* 1983; 24:75.

Juskiewenski S, Vaysse P, Moscovici J, et al: A study of the arterial blood supply to the penis. *Anat Clin* 1982; 4:101.

Kaplan GW: Repair of proximal hypospadias using a preputial free graft for neourethral construction and a preputial pedicle flap for ventral skin coverage. *J Urol* 1988; 140:1270.

Kaplan GW, Brock WA: The etiology of chordee. *Urol Clin North Am* 1981; 8:383.

Kaplan GW Lamm DL: Embryogenesis of chordee. *J Urol* 1975; 114:769.

Kaplan SD, Hensle TW, Burbige KA, et al: Hypospadias: associated behavior problems and male gender role development. *J Urol* 1989; 141:45 (abstract 11).

Karl GW, Swedlon DB, Lee KW, et al: Epinephrine-halothane interaction in children. *Anesthesiology* 1983; 58:142.

Kass EJ: Dorsal corporeal rotation: an alternative technique for the management of severe chordee. *J Urol* 1993; 150(2):635.

Kass EJ, Bolong D: Single-stage hypospadias reconstruction without fistula. *J Urol* 1990; 144:520.

Keating MA, Cartwright PC, Duckett JW: Bladder mucosa in urethral reconstructions. *J Urol* 1990; 144:827.

Kelami A: Classification of congenital and acquired penile deviation. *Urol Int* 1983; 38:229.

Kelami A, Gross U, Fieldler U, et al: Replacement of tunica albuginea of corpus cavernosum penis using human dura. *Urology* 1975; 6:464.

Kenawi MM: Sexual function in hypospadias. *Br J Urol* 1975; 47:883.

Khuri FJ, Hardy BE, Churchill BM: Urologic anomalies associated with hypospadias. *Urol Clin North Am* 1981; 8:565.

Kim SH, Hendren WH: Repair of mild hypospadias. *J Pediatr Surg* 1981; 16:806.

King LR: One-stage repair without skin graft based on a new principle: chordee is sometimes produced by skin alone. *J Urol* 1970; 103:660.

King LR: Cutaneous chordee and its implications in hypospadias repair. *Urol Clin North Am* 1981; 8:397.

Kinkead TM, Borzi PA, Duffy PG, et al: Long-term follow-up of bladder mucosa graft for male urethral reconstruction. *J Urol* 1994; 151:1056.

Klimberg I, Walker RD: A comparison of the Mustarde and Horton-Devine flip-flap techniques of hypospadias repair. *J Urol* 1985; 134:103.

Koff SA: Mobilization of the urethra in the surgical treatment of hypospadias. *J Urol* 1981; 125:394.

Koff SA, Brinkman J, Ulrich J, et al: Extensive mobilization of the urethral plate and urethra for repair of hypospadias: the modified Barcat technique. *J Urol* 1994; 151(2):466.

Koff SA, Eakins M: The treatment of penile chordee using corporal rotation. *J Urol* 1984; 131:931.

Koyanagi T, Nonomura K, Asano Y, et al: Onlay urethroplasty with parameatal foreskin flap for distal hypospadias. *Eur Urol* 1991; 19(3):221.

Koyanagi T, Nonomura K, Gotoh T, et al: One-stage repair of perineal hypospadias and scrotal transposition. *Eur Urol* 1984; 10:364.

Koyle MA, Ehrlich RM: The bladder mucosal graft for urethral reconstruction. *J Urol* 1987; 138:1093.

Kramer SA, Aydin G, Kelalis PP: Chordee without hypospadias in children. *J Urol* 1982; 128:559.

Kumar S: Hypospadias with normal prepuce. *J Urol* 1986; 136:1056.

Li ZC, Zheng ZH, Shen YX, et al: One-stage urethroplasty for hypospadias using a tube constructed with bladder mucosa—a new procedure. *Urol Clin North Am* 1981; 8:463.

Livne PM, Gibbons MD, Gonzales ET: Meatal advancement and glanuloplasty. An operation for distal hypospadias. *J Urol* 1984; 131:95.

Lofti AH, Snyder HM, Duckett JW: The treatment of urethral strictures: the contribution of clean intermittent catheterization to direct vision urethrotomy. *J Urol* 1991; 145:810A.

Manley CB, Epstein ES: Early hypospadias repair. *J Urol* 1981; 125:698.

Marberger H, Pauer W: Experience in hypospadias repair. *Urol Clin North Am* 1981; 8:403.

Marshall M, Johnson SH, Price SE, et al: Cecil urethroplasty with concurrent scrotoplasty for repair of hypospadias. *J Urol* 1979; 121:335.

Marshall VF, Spellman RM: Construction of urethra in hypospadias using vesical mucosal graft. *J Urol* 1955; 73:335.

Mathieu P: Traitement en un temps de l'hypospadias balaniqué et juxta-balanique. *J Chir (Paris)* 1932; 39:481.

Mays HB: Hypospadias: a concept of treatment. *J Urol* 1951; 65:279.

McArdle F, Lebowitz R: Uncomplicated hypospadias and anomalies of upper urinary tract. Need for screening? *Urology* 1975; 5:712.

McCormack RM: Simultaneous chordee repair and urethral reconstruction for hypospadias. *Plast Reconst Surg* 1954; 13:257.

McCraw JB, Myers B, Shanklin KD: The value of fluorescein in predicting the viability of arterialized flaps. *Plast Reconstr Surg* 1977; 60:710.

McMillan RDH, Churchill BM, Gilmore RF: Assessment of urinary stream after repair of anterior hypospadias by meatoplasty and glanuloplasty. *J Urol* 1985; 134:100.

Memmelaar J: Use of bladder mucosa in a one-stage repair of hypospadias. *J Urol* 1947; 58:68.

Merguerian PA, Seremetis G, Becher MW: Hypospadias using laser welding of ventral skin flap in rabbits. Comparison with sutured repair. *J Urol* 1992; 148:667.

Mettauer JP: Practical observations on those malformations of the male urethra and penis, termed hypospadias and epispadias, with an anomalous case. *Am J Med Sci* 1842; 4:43.

Mills C, McGovern J, Mininberg D, et al: An analysis of different techniques for distal hypospadias repair: the price of perfection. *J Urol* 1981; 125:701.

Mitchell ME, Kulb TB: Hypospadias repair without a bladder drainage catheter. *J Urol* 1986; 135:321.

Mollard P, Mouriquand P, Felfela T: Application of the onlay island-flap urethroplasty to penile hypospadias with severe chordee. *Br J Urol* 1991; 68:317.

Monfort G, Jean P, Lacoste M: One-stage correction of posterior hypospadias using a trasverse pedicle flap (Duckett's operation). *Chir Pediat* 1983; 24:71.

Monfort G, Lucas C: Dihydrotestosterone penile stimulation in hypospadias surgery. *Eur Urol* 1982; 8:201.

Montagnino BA, Gonzales ET Jr, Roth DR: Open catheter drainage after urethral surgery. *J Urol* 1988; 140:1250.

Mustarde JC: One-stage correction of distal hypospadias and other people's fistulae. *Br J Plast Surg* 1965; 18:413.

Myrianthopoulos NC, Chung CS: Congenital malformations in singletons: epidemiologic survey. *Birth Defects* 1974; 10(11):1.

Nasland MJ, Coffee DS: The hormonal imprinting of the prostate and the regulation of stem cells in prostate growth. In Proceedings of the 2nd NIADDK Symposium on the Study of Benign Prostatic Hyperplasia. Washington, D.C., U.S. Government Printing Office, May 1985.

Nasrallah PF, Minott HB: Distal hypospadias repair. *J Urol* 1984; 131:928.

Nesbit RM: Plastic procedure for correction of hypospadias. *J Urol* 1941; 45:699.

Nesbit RM: Congenital curvature of the phallus: report of three cases with description of corrective operation. *J Urol* 1965; 93:230.

Nesbit RM: Operation for correction of distal penile ventral curvature with and without hypospadias. *Trans Am Assoc Genitourin Surg* 1966; 58:12.

Noe HN: Management of severe hypospadias with 2-stage repair. *J Urol* 1994; 152:751 (editorial comment).

Nonomura K, Koyanagi T, Imanaka K, et al: One-stage total repair of severe hypospadias with scrotal transposition: experience in 18 cases. *J Pediatr Surg* 1988; 23:177.

Ombredanne L: *Precis clinique et operation de chirurgie infantile*. Paris, Masson, 1932, p 851.

Ossandon F, Ransley PG: Lasso tourniquet for artificial erection in hypospadias. *Urology* 1982; 19:656.

Pancoast JA: *Treatise on Operative Surgery*. Philadelphia, Carrey and Hart, 1844, pp 317-318.

Paramo PG, Hinderer U, San Antonio J, et al: Prepenile scrotum. *Eur Urol* 1981; 7:246.

Parsons KF, Abercrombie GF: Transverse preputial island-flap neourethroplasty. *Br J Urol* 1982; 54:745.

Passerini G, Maio G, Cisternino A, et al: One-stage repair of severe hypospadias. Abstract presented at the International Congress of Pediatric Urology, Florence, Italy, 1986.

Paul M, Kanagasuntheram R: The congenital anomalies of the lower urinary tract. *Br J Urol* 1956; 28:118.

Pegoraro V, Dal Poz R, Zattoni F, et al: Controllo a lungo termine dell'pospadico operato. *Estratto Urol* 1979; 46:1.

Perlmutter AD, Montgomery BT, Steinhardt GF: Tunica vaginalis free graft for the correction of chordee. *J Urol* 1985; 134:311.

Perlmutter AD, Vatz AD: Meatal advancement for distal hypospadias without chordee. *J Urol* 1975; 113:850.

Perovic S, Vukadinovic V: Onlay island-flap urethroplasty for severe hypospadias: a variant of the technique. *J Urol* 1994; 151(3):711.

Polus J, Lotte S: Chirurgie de hypospades. Une nouvelle technique esthetique et fonctionnelle. *Ann Chir Plast Esthet* 1965; 10:3.

Quartey JKM: One-stage penile/preputial cutaneous island-flap urethroplasty for urethral stricture: a preliminary report. *J Urol* 1983; 129:284.

Rabinowitz R: Outpatient catheterless modified Mathieu hypospadias repair. *J Urol* 1987; 138:1074.

Ransley PG, Duffy PG, Oesch IL, et al: The use of bladder mucosa and combined bladder mucosa/preputial skin grafts for urethral reconstruction. *J Urol* 1987; 138:1096.

Redman JF: Experience with 60 consecutive hypospadias repairs using the Horton-Devine techniques. *J Urol* 1983; 129:115.

Redman JF: The balanic groove technique of Barcat. *J Urol* 1987; 137:83.

Retik AB, Bauer SB, Mandell J, et al: Management of severe hypospadias with two-stage repair. *J Urol* 1994; 152:749.

Retik AB, Keating M, Mandel J: Complications of hypospadias repair. *Urol Clin North Am* 1988; 15:223.

Rich MA, Keating MA, Snyder HM, et al: "Hinging" the urethral plate in hypospadias meatoplasty *J Urol* 1989; 142:1551.

Ricketson G: A method of repair for hypospadias. *Am J Surg* 1958; 95:279.

Ritchey ML, Benson RC Jr, Kramer SA, et al: Management of müllerian duct remnants in the male patient. *J Urol* 1988; 140:795.

Ritchey ML, Sinha A, Argueso L: Congenital fistula of the penile urethra. *J Urol* 1994; 151:1061.

Rober PE, Perlmutter AD, Reitelman C: Experience with 81 one-stage hypospadias/chordee repairs using free-graft urethroplasties. *J Urol* 1990; 144:526.

Roberts CJ, Lloyd S: Observations on the epidemiology of simple hypospadias. *BMJ* 1973; 1:768.

Rogers BO: History of external genital surgery. In Horton CE (ed): *Plastic and Reconstructive Surgery of the Genital Area*. Boston, Little, Brown, 1973, pp 3-47.

Romagnoli G, De LM, Faranda F, et al: One-step treatment of proximal hypospadias by the autologous graft of cultured urethral epithelium. *N Engl J Med* 1990; 323:527.

Romagnoli G, De LM, Faranda F, et al: One-step treatment of proximal hypospadias by the autologous graft of cultured urethral epithelium. *J Urol* 1993; 150:1204.

Ross F, Farmer AW, Lindsay WK: Hypospadias—a review of 230 cases. *Plast Reconst Surg* 1959; 24:357.

Russell RH: Operation for severe hypospadias. *BMJ* 1900; 2:1432.

Sauvage P, Rougeron G, Bientz J, et al: Use of the pedicled transverse preputial flap in the surgery of hypospadias. Apropos of 100 cases. *Chir Pediatr* 1987; 28:220.

Schaeffer DD, Erbes J: Hypospadias. *Am J Surg* 1950; 80:183.

Scherz HC, Kaplan GW, Packer MG, et al: Post-hypospadias repair of urethral strictures: a review of 30 cases. *J Urol* 1988; 140:1253.

Schultz JR, Klykylo WM, Wacksman J: Timing of elective hypospadias repair in children. *Pediatrics* 1983; 71:342.

Secrest CL, Jordan GH, Winslow BH, et al: Repair of complications of hypospadias surgery. *J Urol* 1993; 150:1415.

Shelton TB, Noe HN: The role of excretory urography in patients with hypospadias. *J Urol* 1985; 135:97.

Shima H, Ikoma F, Terakawa T, et al: Developmental anomalies associated with hypospadias. *J Urol* 1979; 122:619.

Shima H, Ikoma F, Yahumoto H, et al: Gonadotropin and testosterone response in prepubertal boys with hypospadias. *J Urol* 1986; 135:539.

Smith CK: Surgical procedures for correction of hypospadias. *J Urol* 1938; 40:239.

Smith ED: A de-epithelialized overlap flap technique in the repair of hypospadias. *Br J Plast Surg* 1973; 26:106.

Smith ED: Durham-Smith repair of hypospadias. *Urol Clin North Am* 1981; 8:451.

Snow BW: Transverse corporeal plication for persistent chordee. *Urology* 1989; 34:360.

Snow BW: Yoke hypospadias repair. AAP, Urology Section, October 1991.

Snyder HM: Does glans configuration indicate the type of chordee present in hypospadias. *Society for Pediatric Urology Newsletter* 1991; 5/24:38.

Sommer JT, Stephens FD: Dorsal ureteral diverticulum of the fossa navicularis: symptoms, diagnosis, and treatment. *J Urol* 1980; 124:94.

Song R, Wang X, Zuo Z: Hypospadias repair. *Clin Plast Surg* 1982; 9:91.

Sorenson R: Hypospadias with special reference to etiology. *Op Dom Biol Hered Hum* 1953; 31:1.

Standoli L: Correzione Dell'ipospadias in tempo unico: technica dell'ipospadias con tempo ad isola prepuziale. *Rass Italia Chir Pediatr* 1979; 21:82.

Standoli L: One-stage repair of hypospadias: Preputial island-flap technique. *Ann Plast Surg* 1982; 9:81.

Stecker JF, Horton CE, Devine CJ, et al: Hypospadias cripples. *Urol Clin North Am* 1981; 8:539.

Sugar EC, Firlit CF: Urinary prophylaxis and postoperative care of children at home with an indwelling catheter after hypospadias repair. *Urology* 1989; 32:418.

Svensson J, Berg R: Micturition studies and sexual function in operated hypospadiacs. *Br J Urol* 1983; 55:422.

Sweet RA, Schrott HG, Kurland R, et al: Study of the incidence of hypospadias in Rochester, Minnesota, 1940-1970, and a case control comparison of possible etiologic factors. *Mayo Clin Proc* 1974; 49:52.

Tessier J, Carr M, Gassior B, et al: Scrotal venous leak: impotence following hypospadias repair. *J Urol* 1989; 141:45 (abstract 9).

Thiersch C: Ueber die Entstehungsweise und operative Behandlung der epispadie. *Arch Heitkunde* 1869; 10:20.

Turner-Warwick R: The use of pedicle grafts in the repair of urinary tract fistulae. *Br J Urol* 1972; 44:644.

Turner-Warwick R: Observations upon techniques for reconstruction of the urethral meatus, the hypospadiac glans deformity, and the penile urethra. *Urol Clin North Am* 1979; 7:643.

Udald A: Correction of three types of congenital curvatures of the penis including the first reported case of dorsal curvature. *J Urol* 1980; 124:50.

Van der Meulen JC: *Hypospadias Monograph*. Leiden, The Netherlands, AG Stenfert, Kroese, NV, 1964.

Van der Meulen JC: Hypospadias and cryptospadias. *Br J Plast Surg* 1971; 24:101.

Van der Meulen JC: Correction of hypospadias, types I and II. *Ann Plast Surg* 1982; 8:403.

Vordermark JS: Adhesive membrane: a new dressing for hypospadias. *Urology* 1982; 20:86.

Vyas PR, Roth DR, Perlmutter AD: Experience with free grafts in urethral reconstruction. *J Urol* 1987; 137:471.

Wacksman J: Modification of the one-stage flip-flap procedure to repair distal penile hypospadias. *Urol Clin North Am* 1981; 8:527.

Wacksman J: Repair of hypospadias using new mouth-controlled microscope. *Urology* 1987; 29:276.

Walker RD: Outpatient repair of urethral fistulae. *Urol Clin North Am* 1981; 8:582.

Waterhouse K, Glassberg KI: Mobilization of the anterior urethra as an aid in the one-stage repair of hypospadias. *Urol Clin North Am* 1981; 8:521.

Welch KJ: Hypospadias. In Ravitch MM, Welch KJ, Benson CD, et al (eds): *Pediatric Surgery*, ed 3. Chicago, Year Book Medical Publishers, 1979, pp 1353-1376.

Winslow BH, Vorstman B, Devine CJ Jr: Urethroplasty using diverticular tissue. *J Urol* 1985; 134:552.

Woodard JR, Cleveland R: Application of Horton-Devine principles to the repair of hypospadias. *J Urol* 1982; 127:1155.

Yeoman DM, Cooke R, Hain WR: Penile block for circumcision? A comparison with caudal block. *Anesthesia* 1983; 38:862.

Young F, Benjamin W: Preschool-age repair of hypospadias with free inlay skin grafts. *Surgery* 1949; 26:384.

Young HH: *Genital Abnormalities, Hermaphroditism, and Related Adrenal Diseases*, Baltimore, Williams and Wilkins, 1937.

Zaontz MR: The GAP (glans approximation procedure) for glanular/coronal hypospadias. *J Urol* 1989; 141:359.

CHAPTER 56

Intersex

Bruce Blyth
Bernard M. Churchill

BASIC PRINCIPLES IN SEXUAL DIFFERENTIATION

General Principles

Sexual determination and differentiation is a sequential process that begins at the moment of fertilization, with the determination of chromosomal sex. Before 7 weeks of life and the development of the gonadal ridge, the fetus is phenotypically indifferent, with female and male embryos having common primordia. Subsequently the gonadal sex sequentially directs the development of the internal genital ducts, the urogenital sinus, and the external genitalia, constituting the phenotypic expression of a male or female gender. Each step in the development pathway is dependent on the preceding event. Without the continued expression of the Y chromosome, and subsequently the testis, the gonadal and phenotypic development defaults to a normal female pathway, which does not appear to be hormonally directed. The sequence of development is outlined in Figure 56-1. Note that active masculinization of the primordia precedes the formation of the normal female derivatives.

Basic Factors in Sexual Development

The major characteristics that determine sexual development and later sexual identity are represented schematically in Figure 56-2. This forms a framework for the analysis and understanding of normal and abnormal sexual development and a basis for diagnosing clinical problems and implementing therapy.

Determination of Chromosomal Sex

Chromosomal sex is determined at fertilization. The fertilizing sperm provides either an X chromosome, resulting in a 46,XX zygote (female genotype), or a Y chromosome, resulting in a 46,XY zygote (male genotype). The chromosomal composition can be determined from a karyotype, which is an array of the chromosomes from a single cell in metaphase (Hammerton et al., 1973). The presence of an X chromosome can also be determined in some cases from a buccal smear. Barr and Bertram (1949) noted the presence of a stainable chromatin mass at the periphery of the nucleus in most mammalian peripheral female cells. In patients with a single X chromosome (e.g., normal XY male) no Barr body can be identified, whereas in those patients with two or more X chromosomes, the number of Barr bodies present is one less than the total number of X chromosomes (Barr and Bertram, 1949). The usefulness of a buccal smear, however, is limited in the neonatal assessment of sexual ambiguity, as it is present in only 20% of infant female cells.

The genetic material necessary for the development of normal testes is carried on the short arm of the Y chromosome. Also found here are many common sequences of DNA present also in the X chromosome (Allen, 1985; de la Chapelle et al., 1986). Genes necessary for normal male development are also carried on the X chromosome, and for the full phenotypic development of both males and females, genes from the autosomes are also necessary. At least 19 genes are involved in sex determination in humans (Wilson and Goldstein, 1975).

Individuals who have an XXY, XXXY, XXXXY, or XXXX + Y karyotype develop along masculine lines that, although imperfect, are not ambiguous. This clinical observation demonstrates that the presence of the Y chromosome provides the signal for testicular development, which is not inhibited by the presence of two or more X chromosomes. In these individuals, however, testicular development is imperfect, with seminiferous tubular dysgenesis and azospermia the rule. Other associated anomalies include tall stature, disproportionately long legs, and gynecomastia, with an increasing incidence of mental retardation as the number of additional X chromosomes increases.

In addition to chromosomal anomalies represented by the presence of supernumerary sex chromosomes,

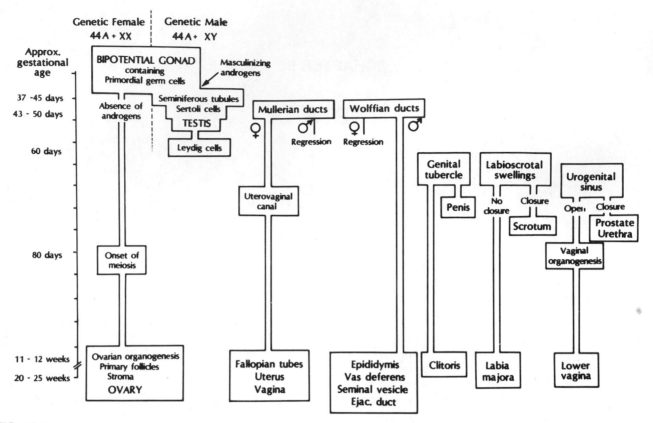

FIG. 56-1
Schematic sequence of sexual differentiation in the human. Note that testicular differentiation in the presence of masculinizing androgens precedes all other forms of differentiation.

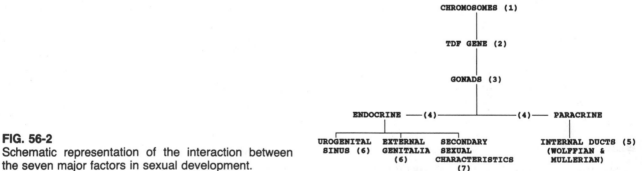

FIG. 56-2
Schematic representation of the interaction between the seven major factors in sexual development.

other defects of chromosomal division include non-disjunction, deletion, breakage, rearrangement, and translocation of genetic material (Donohoe and Hendren, 1980). Nondisjunction is of particular importance. It consists of an incomplete division of the chromosomes during meiosis, or the chromatids during mitosis. Nondisjunction resulting in the loss of either the X or Y chromosome prior to conception produces an XO karyotype, characterized by an infant with streak gonads and the stigmata of Turner's syndrome.

Without the second X chromosome ovarian organogenesis is incomplete, and short stature occurs without a second (either X or Y) sex chromosome. Nondisjunction prior to conception producing a YO karyotype is not compatible with life (Grumbach and Conte, 1981). Nondisjunction occurring after conception can result in mosaicism, which is the presence of two or more different chromosomal cell lines in the same zygote. This occurs in mixed gonadal dysgenesis (45,X/46,XY mosaic karyotype), present in 40% of true hermaphrodites, and in some cases of pure gonadal dysgenesis and Klinefelter's syndrome. Of these, only mixed gonadal dysgenesis and true hermaphrodites display sexual ambiguity in the neonatal period.

Testis Determining Factor Gene

The testis determining factor (TDF) gene is the segment of DNA that provides the signal for differentiation of the gonad into a testis. This genetic locus has been identified on a distal portion of the short arm of the Y chromosome (Goodfellow, 1987). This segment of DNA has now been cloned, with the TDF gene localized to a 35-kilobase segment of DNA (Palmer et al., 1989). This gene has been termed the SRY (sex-determining region of the Y chromosome) gene and has been found in a wide range of mammals. Its role as the TDF gene was supported when transgenic mice containing normal female XX chromosomes, plus 14 kilobases of the Y chromosome bearing the SRY gene, were born, with some of these chromosomal female mice developing into males with normal testes (Koopman et al., 1990).

An earlier candidate gene for the TDF gene, called ZFY, had been identified just proximal to SRY on the short arm (Page et al., 1987), within the 160-kilobase segment of DNA immediately adjacent to the pseudoautosomal region. This gene coded for a protein that contains a series of zinc fingers, a motif characteristic of proteins that bind DNA or RNA. This was later found to be a non–sex chromosome gene in marsupials, and it was absent in some 46,XX males (Palmer et al., 1989). In the past the TDF gene was considered one and the same with the gene coding for the H-Y antigen. The H-Y antigen was described as a cell membrane component in inbred mice (Eishwald and Silmser, 1955); as a minor histocompatibility antigen, it triggered uniform rejection of male donor grafts to female recipients but allowed female-to-male acceptance. Further support for the role of the H-Y antigen as the testis-determining factor came from the work of Ohno and co-workers (Ohno et al., 1978, 1979; Ohno and Stapleton, 1981), who studied the effect of anti–H-Y serum on dissociated single-cell suspensions of newborn mice or rat testes. Those treated with the anti–H-Y serum formed primordial ovarian follicles, whereas those untreated reaggregated to form seminiferous tubules. Conversely, free cell suspensions of undifferentiated bovine XX embryonic ovary that were treated with human H-Y antigen began to form of seminiferous tubules; untreated suspensions continued as undifferentiated ovary (Nagai et al., 1979; Ohno et al., 1979; Zenzes et al., 1978a). This work led to support for the role of the H-Y antigen in determining the differentiation of the gonad, but it is now recognized that the low-titre antibodies were not

specific for the H-Y antigen, but included antisera to the TDF locus (called Tdy in mice). It has been shown convincingly using cytotoxic T-cell assays that the Tdy and H-Y antigen can be separated by mutation in the mouse, and in the human TDF and H-Y can be mapped to very different regions of the Y chromosome (Wolfe, 1987). Reference to the presence of H-Y antigen will be used throughout this chapter in discussing the distinguishing criteria of different forms of intersex, as this usage is still widespread in the literature. It must be recognized that a positive recognition for H-Y antigen reflects the presence of a DNA sequence on the long arm of the Y chromosome that does not necessarily correlate with the presence of the TDF gene on the short arm of the Y chromosome, which regulates the formation of the testis.

The SRY gene appears to be the initial trigger mechanism for testicular differentiation. The SRY gene contains an 80-amino-acid domain resembling other proteins that act by binding to DNA to regulate gene transcription. It probably acts directly or indirectly by regulating the transcription of a cascade of genes necessary for testicular determination and differentiation. Proteins other than SRY are also required for proper gonadogenesis, as evidenced by disorders of gonadal differentiation that are autosomal or X-linked, and therefore not due to defects in SRY.

The SRY protein belongs to a family of DNA-binding proteins called high-mobility-group (HMG) proteins. These proteins contain an 80-amino-acid domain resembling the HMG box from the nuclear chromosomal nonhistone proteins HMG_1 and HMG_2 (Moore and Grumbach, 1992). Within the family of HMG proteins are those with a highly conserved HMG box, and a second group, including SRY, where the HMG box amino acids are more divergent. Those that are more divergent bind to sequences of DNA implicated in transcriptional regulation. Their action, however, is unlike that of traditional transcription regulators, which directly increase transcription; rather, they bend or kink DNA, possibly facilitating an interaction between proteins bound on either side, which then alters transcription (Moore and Grumbach, 1992).

It is recognized that even if SRY is the master switch, sex determination depends on more than simply a single switch. Not all transgenic XX mice containing SRY sequences developed as phenotypic males; some were phenotypic females (Koopman et al., 1990). In 46 patients (from different series) with gonadal dysgenesis with SRY present, only 7 demonstrated mutations in the SRY sequence, implying that other genes are responsible for most cases of gonadal dysgenesis. In addition, the majority of 46,XX hermaphrodites are lacking in SRY, ZFY, or other Y chromosomal sequences of DNA (Hawkins et al., 1992; Tho et al., 1992).

A number of mutations within the amino acid structure of the HMG box binding domain of the SRY gene have now been determined. As a result of these mutations in nucleotide sequence, different amino acids are formed that affect the final tertiary configuration of the protein, or that may even insert a stop codon or create a frame shift, which prevents transcription of the DNA. As a result of this, the action of the SRY gene can be impeded, resulting in an intersex condition.

The TDF gene acts on the somatic mesenchymal cells of the developing gonad, and not on the germ cells that have migrated from the yolk sac. XY germ cells can undergo oogenesis, and XO germ cells can reach the early stages of spermatogenesis. These results suggest that germ cells are irrelevant to sex determination and that germ cells themselves respond to environmental signals (McLaren, 1985).

Within the fetal gonad, the first male-specific cells to differentiate are the Sertoli cells. Experimental mouse chimeras made by aggregating an XX and an XY embryo usually develop as males. When the tissues of such chimeras are examined, equal numbers of XX cells and XY cells are found in the total cell population of every tissue type except the Sertoli cells (Burgoyne et al., 1988). The Sertoli cell population in these XX/XY chimeras is composed entirely of XY cells; thus in this group of cells the TDF gene is binding to DNA or RNA to exert its switch function. The next step in unraveling the expression of the TDF gene is to find the gene it is regulating, which is most likely present on another chromosome. One very plausible theory of the action of the TDF gene is that it is regulating

the rate of growth of the somatic cells in the gonadal ridge. In the presence of the TDF gene, the cells divide more rapidly (Mittwoch, 1986).

Differentiation of the Testis and Ovary

The gonad develops as the genital ridge, a thickening along the ventral cranial area of the mesonephros and from the migration of the primordial germ cells (Fig. 56-3). The somatic elements of the gonad are derived from mesonephric cells that migrate into the area of the genital ridge very early in development, from the mesenchyme, and from the coelomic epithelium, although the role of the epithelium is considered minor (Byskov, 1986).

The genital ridge is initially devoid of germ cells, which are first identified on the dorsal endoderm of the yolk sac at 24 days of gestation (Witschi, 1948). The primordial germ cells migrate by amoeboid action to the gonadal ridge via the mesenchyme of the mesentery (Fig. 56-3) and appear to be attracted to the gonadal area by a chemotactic factor (Rogulska et al., 1971). In addition, there is a close association between the primordial germ cells and fibronectin and other components of the extracellular matrix during the migration (Fujimoto et al., 1988). Soon after reaching the gonad, the primordial germ cells are enclosed in specific germ cell compartments where their proliferation and differentiation are regulated by the surrounding somatic cells.

The gonad is indifferent until approximately 45 days of gestation, when in the male the TDF triggers differentiation, which is characterized by three consecutive events. Initially the germ cells and Sertoli cells become enclosed as testicular cords. Next, differentiation of the steroid-producing Leydig cells occurs in the extracordal compartment, and finally the testis becomes rounded. The primitive testicular cords appear first as platelike structures of tightly packed germ cells and somatic cells (future Sertoli cells), which throughout differentiation remain in contact with the basal portion of the mesonephric cell mass. This cell mass, which gradually transforms into the rete testis, together with the testicular cords is derived from the preexisting gonadal mesonephric tissue (Zamboni et al., 1981). The testicular cords lose their connection with the coelomic epithelium and become surrounded by the tunica albuginea derived from the loose mesenchymal tissue (Wartenberg, 1983). The Leydig cells differentiate into typical steroid-producing cells shortly after the testicular cords have formed. The trigger for this step is unknown, but in rabbits it is thought to be due to extragonadal influences (Byskow, 1986). Certainly the presence of the testicular cords is required for Leydig cell development, and later in fetal life the Leydig cell steroid production is regulated by gonadotrophins (Winter et al., 1977).

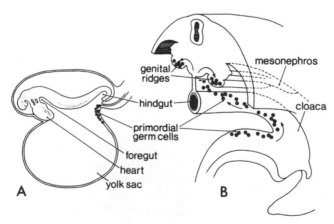

FIG. 56-3
A, Schematic drawing showing the site of origin of the germ cells in the wall of the yolk sac in a 3-week-old embryo. **B,** Migratory path of the primordial germ cells along the wall of the yolk sac and dorsal mesentery and into the genital ridge. (After Langman J: *Medical Embryology: Human Development—Normal and Abnormal,* ed 4. Baltimore, Williams and Wilkins, 1986. Used by permission.)

The last important event in the early stages of testicular organogenesis is the rounding of the testis itself. This results in attenuation of the connection of the testis with the mesonephros, stopping the further migration of mesonephric cells to the testis (Byskov, 1986). Without this attenuation, the mesonephros exerts a feminizing influence upon the testicular cords, inducing meiosis.

Differentiation of the ovary occurs significantly later than that of the testis (see Fig. 56-1), at around 80 days. Three events occur in the early stages of ovarian development. The first event observed is the initiation of meiotic prophase. Much later the diplotene oocyte becomes enclosed in the germ cell compartment, the follicle. Finally, steroid-producing cells in the extrafollicular compartment are differentiated.

The characteristic sign of a differentiating ovary is the presence of germ cells entering meiotic prophase, but in many species there is a delay in the time between the formation of germ cell cords and the onset of meiosis (Byskov, 1979). In humans this delay is around 10 days, with the germ cells having poorly defined outlines compared with the testis. The first meiotic cells appear in the central part of the developing ovary close to the connection with the mesonephros. It is believed that the mesonephros secretes a meiosis-inducing substance (Fajer et al., 1979), but other factors are also involved in the induction of meiosis by the gonad (Byskov, 1986). Whether the initiation of meiotic prophase is triggered by humoral substances, by somatic cell–germ cell contact, or by a preprogrammed event is still not known.

The process of oogenesis continues until the oocytes are arrested in the last phase of meiotic prophase, the diplotene stage. The oocyte is then enclosed by granulosa cells and a basal lamina to form a follicle. This is the counterpart to the testicular cord, where the germ cells are enclosed and separated from their surroundings. The development of the basal lamina separates the follicles from the intraovarian rete cords. The production of hormones from the differentiating ovary occurs at the same time as the onset of testosterone synthesis in the male (George et al., 1978b), although the production of estrogen plays no known role in the phenotypic development.

Determination of Phenotypic Sex

The development of phenotypic sex is governed by the action or absence of testicular secretions. This was determined by the classic experiments of Jost (1960, 1972), who demonstrated that the removal of the gonads from embryo rabbits prior to the onset of phenotypic differentiation resulted in the development of the female phenotype. When testicular secretions are present, a male phenotype is induced, whereas female differentiation is not dependent on the presence of an ovary and therefore does not require secretions from the embryonic gonad. Jost (1971) also deduced that two types of secretions of the fetal testis are involved in male development, a müllerian-inhibiting substance and androgen.

Antimüllerian Hormone.—Antimüllerian hormone (AMH), also known as müllerian-inhibiting substance or factor, is a peptide hormone that acts in the male to induce regression of the paramesonephric (müllerian) ducts. It is formed by the embryonic testis soon after the onset of differentiation of the spermatic tubules and is the first secretory function of the testis. The inhibiting substance is a glycoprotein (MW 70,000) and is formed by the spermatogenic tubules (Blanchard and Josso, 1974; Donahoe et al., 1977). The hormone has now been purified (Picard and Josso, 1987), cloned (Picard et al., 1986), and mapped to the tip of the short arm of chromosome 19 (Cohen-Haguenauer et al., 1987).

AMH may prove to be the key in the expression of the TDF gene. When added to fetal rat ovaries explanted in organ culture, AMH induces gonadal morphological masculinization through differentiation of seminiferous cordlike structures (Vigier et al., 1987). The hormonal effects of AMH are fairly well known, but the morphogenic actions are still to be unraveled. The gene for AMH has been incorporated into the genome in transgenic mice, and some interesting observations have been made. In the females, who would not normally express any AMH activity, the fallopian tubes and uterus degenerate, as expected. In the majority of the adult females, however, there were no ovaries (Behringer et al., 1990). When AMH is added to tissue cultures of fetal rat ovaries, the germ cells are depleted, and this occurs at the stage when the cells are entering meiosis (Vigier et al., 1987). If a germ cell does enter meiosis, it is an oocyte and it induces the surrounding supporting cells to differentiate as follicle cells rather than as Sertoli cells. If the oocyte disappears, then so do the follicles, and the supporting cells are transformed into structures that resemble testicular cords (Taketo et al., 1993). One of the physiologic actions, then, of AMH may be to mop up any cells that are entering meiosis, so that the only germ cells that remain are enclosed and protected within the testicular cords. Potentially, it is the lack of this action in true hermaphrodites that allows the persistence of both an ovary and a testis.

AMH has also been shown to inhibit the aromatase activity in fetal rat ovaries, thus dramatically decreasing the conversion of testosterone to estradiol (Vigier et al., 1989). The release of testosterone that results when AMH is added to the explants of rat ovarian tissue induces the formation of the seminiferous cordlike structures. Because normal testicular differentiation can still occur with isolated defects in AMH biosynthesis, AMH is not the only factor involved in the differentiation of the testis. AMH can be detected in human testicular tissue up to the age of 6 years and may continue to play a trophic role in the differentiation of the testis beyond its initial formation (Tran et al., 1987).

Single-gene defects have been detected in which there is persistence of the müllerian duct, a condition where genetic and phenotypic men have persisting fallopian tubes and uteri together with wolffian duct structures (Sloan and Walsh, 1976). Thus AMH acts in an active manner to promote regression of the paramesonephric duct, and this is mediated between 62 and 77 days of gestation. There is a period of maximum sensitivity during the early phase, and delays in the timing of this action can result in the persistence of remnants of müllerian ducts.

Androgen Secretion.—The second substance secreted by the fetal testis was identified by Jost as an androgen, later deduced to be testosterone (Wilson and Siiteri, 1973). Testosterone production by the fetal testis commences shortly after the differentiation of the spermatogenic tubules and concomitant with the histological differentiation of the Leydig cells of the testis (Wilson and Siiteri, 1973). Testosterone acts both within the fetal testis, where it has a role in promoting maturation of the spermatogonia, and beyond the testis, where its paracrine and endocrine actions play an essential role in the development of the male phenotype.

There are at least five separate genetic defects in the human known to cause inadequate testosterone synthesis, incomplete virilization of the male embryo during embryogenesis (Wilson, 1978), and other defects of steroid synthesis that result in an excess of androgens. A knowledge, therefore, of steroid synthesis is pertinent to the understanding of intersex anomalies. An outline is shown in Figure 56-4. Al-

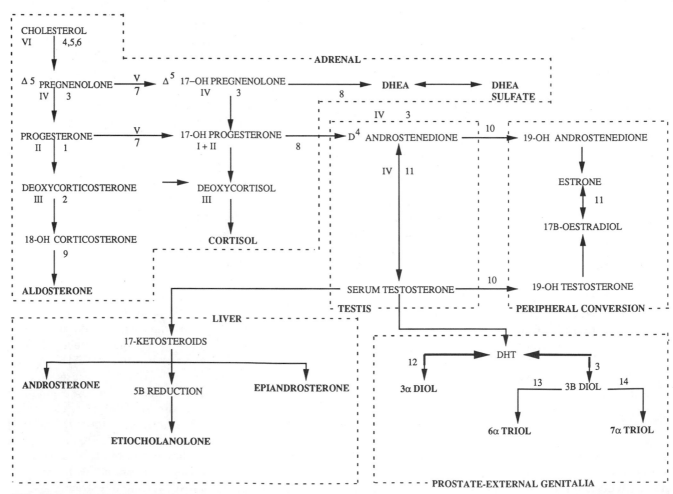

FIG. 56-4

A diagrammatic representation of the steroid biosynthetic pathways in the adrenal, gonads, liver, and external genitalia. *I* to *VI* correspond to enzymes whose deficiency results in congenital hyperplasia. *1* to *14* correspond to the different enzymes implicated in the cascade. *1*, 21-hydroxylase; *2*, 11-hydroxylase; *3*, 3β-hydroxydehydrogenase; *4*, 20α-hydroxylase; *5*, 20,22-desmolase; *6*, 22α-hydroxylase; *7*, 17α-hydroxylase; *8*, 17,20-desmolase; *9*, 18-hydroxylase; *10*, 19-hydroxylase (aromatase); *11*, 17α-keto-reductase; *12*, 3α-hydroxydehydrogenase; *13*, 6α-hydroxylase; *14*, 17α-hydroxylase.

though the differentiated testis and ovary possess the enzymatic pathways necessary to produce steroid hormones, the adrenal gland is often responsible for the production of excess androgens and mineralocorticoids in genetic defects of cortisol synthesis (see Fig. 56-4 for specific enzyme defects). With the failure of production of cortisol, the increased secretion of ACTH by the pituitary stimulates the adrenal gland with the overproduction of all precursors in the steroid synthetic pathway.

The cellular mechanism for androgen action in target tissues is summarized in Figure 56-5. The response of the urogenital sinus and external genitalia to androgen requires the conversion of testosterone to dihydrotestosterone (DHT). Testosterone enters the cell by passive diffusion and in the cytoplasm is converted to dihydrotestosterone by the enzyme 5α-reductase. Testosterone or DHT is then bound to the same high-affinity androgen receptor *(R)* in the cytosol. The hormone-receptor complexes move into the nucleus, where they bind to chromatin receptor sites composed of DNA and protein. Transcription RNA polymerase allows transcription of DNA to messenger RNA, and subsequently new proteins are synthesized. The testosterone-receptor complex is responsible for regulation of gonadotropin secretion by the hypothalamic-pituitary axis, for regulation of spermatogenesis and for virilization of the mesonephric (wolffian) duct during embryogenesis, whereas the DHT-R complex induces virilization of the urogenital sinus and external genitalia during embryogenesis and is responsible in large part for the maturational events at male puberty. The affinity of the receptor is four times greater for DHT than for testosterone; in addition, the testosterone-receptor complexes that do form do not bind as long as the DHT-R complexes (Wilson, 1992).

The Androgen Receptor.—The androgen receptor belongs to the thyroid/steroid family of receptors and has now been cloned. The androgen receptor mRNA is approximately 10 kilobases in length and encodes a 110,000 MW protein containing 920 amino acid residues, the androgen receptor. The receptor contains four domains: a hormone-binding region, a hinge region, a DNA-binding domain, and an N-terminal domain. The DNA-binding domain is the part of the receptor that interacts with the regulating genes. The

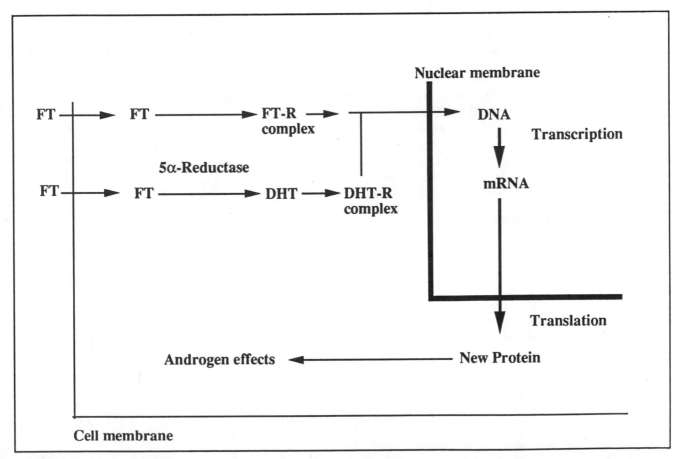

FIG. 56-5
Diagrammatic representation of the mechanism of action of testosterone at the target organ. *FT,* free testosterone; *DHT,* dihydrotestosterone; *R,* receptor.

nucleotide sequence within the DNA binding region is highly conserved and is similar not just across species, but also within the family of steroid hormone receptors (Janne and Shan, 1992).

The gene for the androgen receptor is located on the X chromosome, close to the centromere on the long arm, and is approximately 100 kilobases in size. The androgen receptor gene is composed of eight exons, the segments of DNA in the polypeptide chain that code for the amino acid sequence (Janne and Shan, 1992). There are two DNA-binding exons, and these code for two zinc fingers, typical structures for this class of receptor. The DNA-binding portions of the androgen receptor code for a protein that contains multiple cysteine residues. These cysteine residues form domains that bind one zinc ion, resulting in a structural configuration, known as a zinc finger, that allows the receptor to bind with DNA (Feldman, 1992).

Androgen receptor abnormalities may occur as a result of a mutation that alters the structure of the androgen receptor mRNA or the androgen receptor protein. Also possible are mutations that affect the concentration of either the androgen receptor mRNA or the androgen receptor protein. Examples of all but the last category of mutations have been demonstrated in patients and experimentally in mice. A few patients have demonstrated large-scale alterations within the androgen receptor gene, with consequent severe aberrations in the mRNA transcribed. More often, single nucleotide substitutions have occurred, with resultant alteration in the protein transcribed (McPhaul et al., 1991). The substitution of a proline amino acid for an arginine can result in a significant structural alteration in one of the zinc finger–binding domains, which can render it ineffective in binding to DNA, resulting in complete androgen insensitivity (Feldman, 1992).

Development of the Genital Ducts

The internal genital ducts in both sexes are derived from the mesonephric kidney system. The mesonephric (wolffian) duct drains the mesonephric kidney, which develops during the fourth week of gestation and empties into the primitive urogenital sinus. It is from this duct that the ureteric bud arises to induce differentiation of the metanephric kidney. The paramesonephric (müllerian) duct develops at 6 weeks of gestation as an evagination in the coelomic epithelium just lateral to the mesonephros proper, and then forms into a tube, the caudal end of which becomes closely attached to the mesonephric duct (Gruenwald, 1941). Thus at 7 weeks of intrauterine life the fetus has both mesonephric and paramesonephric primordia, which are capable of forming male and female genital ducts (Fig. 56-1 and 56-6).

At 7 weeks the secretion of AMH from the fetal testis promotes the involution of the paramesonephric

ducts, whereas in the absence of this substance the paramesonephric duct persists. In the male all of the paramesonephric duct is reabsorbed except the cranial portion, termed the appendix testis, and the extreme lower end, which contributes to the prostatic utricle (Glenister, 1962). Shortly after the secretion of anti-müllerian hormone the testis also secretes testosterone, which acts to stabilize the mesonephric duct. Both of these hormone actions of the fetal testis occur through a paracrine mechanism, in which the steroids move from their site of action to the target tissue by local diffusion through the extracellular space. The response, therefore, of the mesonephric and paramesonephric ducts depends on the function of the ipsilateral testis.

Under the influence of testosterone the mesonephric duct differentiates into the epididymis, the vas deferens, the ejaculatory ducts, and the seminal vesicles (Fig. 56-6, Table 56-1). In the absence of the influence of testosterone the mesonephric duct involutes and the paramesonephric duct develops into the oviduct, uterus, cervix, and upper vagina (Grumbach and Conte, 1981).

Development of the Urogenital Sinus and External Genitalia

The development of the external genitalia and the urogenital sinus occurs following division of the cloaca and the formation of the tail fold in the embryo. After

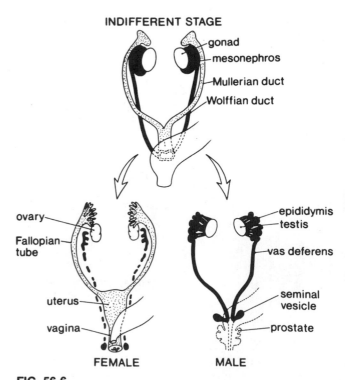

FIG. 56-6
Contribution of the wolffian and müllerian ducts and the urogenital tract. (From Walsh PC, Gittes RF, Perlmutter AD, et al (eds): *Campbell's Urology*, ed 5. Philadelphia, WB Saunders, 1986. Used by permission.)

tail fold formation the cloacal membrane lies in a depression between the umbilicus and the primitive streak, from which proliferating mesoderm streams in all directions. The migration of mesenchymal cells around the cloacal membrane in the third week of development forms a pair of slightly elevated folds, the cloacal folds. Directly cranial to the cloacal membrane, the folds unite to form the genital tubercle. The genital tubercle elongates as a phallus, and simultaneously the cloacal depression extends on to the caudal aspect of the phallus as a urethral groove. This is bounded by the genital folds, which have meanwhile formed separately from the lateral swellings. The ectoderm of the floor of the urethral groove is in contact with the endoderm of the urethral plate, an outgrowth of the endodermal sinus along the phallus. As the urorectal septum, dividing the cloaca, reaches the cloacal membrane, the membrane breaks down and provides an external opening for the urogenital sinus. This disintegration of the cloacal membrane extends

forward into the floor of the urethral groove, thus deepening it and exposing the endodermal urethral plate. With the formation of the perineal body from downgrowth of the urorectal septum, the genital folds meet in the midline, anterior to the anus. These events represent the indifferent stage of development, which occurs by 60 days of gestation.

At this time the portion of the primitive urogenital sinus cranial to the mesonephric ducts is the vesicourethral canal, and that caudal to the mesonephric ducts is the definitive urogenital sinus (Hamilton and Mossman, 1976). The portion of the sinus near the bladder is narrow (pelvic urethra), and the portion near the urogenital membrane is expanded (phallic urethra). In the male, under the influence of dihydrotestosterone the phallic portion of the urogenital sinus develops into the bulbar and penile urethra. This occurs at 60 to 70 days of gestation, while in the female development does not occur until much later, near 140 days of gestation. In the presence of dihydrotes-

TABLE 56-1

Derivation of Reproductive Tract Structures from Wolffian and Müllerian Primordia

Male Vestigial Structure	Primordia	Female Vestigial Structure
	Genital Ridges	
Testis		Ovary
Seminiferous tubules		Pfluger's tubules
Rete testis		Rete ovarii
Gubernaculum testis		Round ligament of the uterus
	Wolffian Derivatives	
Ductuli efferentes	Mesonephric tubules	Epoöphoron
Ductuli aberrantes		Ductuli aberrantes
Paradidymis		Paroöphoron
Ureter, pelvis, and collecting tubules of the kidney	Mesonephric ducts	Ureter, pelvis, and collecting tubules of the kidney
Trigone of the bladder		Trigone of bladder
Ductus epididymis		Gartner's duct
Ductus deferens		Duct of epoöphoron
Ejaculatory duct		
Seminal vesicle		
Appendix epididymis		Appendix vesiculosa
	Müllerian Derivatives	
		Oviduct
		Uterus
Prostatic utricle		Cervix and upper portion of the vagina
Colliculus seminalis		
Appendix testis		?Hymen
		Hydratid of Morgagni
	Urogenital Sinus Derivatives	
Bladder		Bladder
Posterior urethra		Urethra
Anterior urethra		
Membranous urethra		Lower portion of the vagina and the vestibule
Cavernous urethra		
Cowper's glands		Bartholin's glands
Prostate gland		Paraurethral glands of Skene
	External Genitalia	
Glans penis		Glans clitoris
Floor of the penile urethra		Labia minora
Scrotum		Labia majora

tosterone the pelvic urethra forms the neck of the primitive bladder and prostatic urethra as far as the utricle, where the müllerian tubercle becomes the seminal colliculus. The glandular part of the prostate develops from endodermal buds from the pelvic urethra (Kellklumpu-Lehtinen, 1985). Beyond the prostatic utricle, the pelvic part of the urogenital sinus forms the rest of the prostatic urethra and the membranous urethra.

As the genital folds close over the phallic portion of the sinus and the urethral groove, proximal to distal, the opening of the urogenital sinus migrates forward along the ventral aspect of the phallus. The genital swellings also meet and fuse to form the scrotum. Meanwhile, under the influence of dihydrotestosterone the genital tubercle elongates cylindrically to become the penis. The endodermal edges of the urethral groove fuse to tubularize the penile urethra while ectoderm grows in from the glans as a plug that meets the penile urethra and later cavitates as the glanular urethra. When formation of the male urethra is complete, at 80 days, the size of the male phallus is not substantially different from that of the female, but under the continued influence of androgens the external male genitalia grows progressively during pregnancy and at term is much larger than the female phallus.

In the absence of dihydrostestosterone the vesicourethral canal elongates to form the majority of the urethra while the pelvic part of the urogenital sinus develops into the distal portion of the urethra and the vagina. Epithelial tubules originate from the primitive urethra after 80 days and become the paraurethral glands, the female homologues of the prostate (Hamilton and Mossman, 1976). The vagina begins development with the formation of a solid mass of cells (the uterovaginal plate) between the caudal buds of the paramesonephric ducts and the posterior wall of the urogenital sinus. The relative contributions of the mesonephric and paramesonephric ducts to the development of the vagina is still being debated, with some attributing the origin of the epithelial lining of the vagina to the dorsal wall of the urogenital sinus (Bulmer, 1957) and others claiming that it is formed only from downgrowth of the mesonephric and paramesonephric ducts (Mauch et al., 1985). The cells of the vaginal plate proliferate until around 80 days of gestation, and then the plate becomes canalized by the extension of the uterovaginal canal from above and by the formation of a lumen from below. By 20 weeks of gestation the vagina is completely canalized but remains separated from the urogenital sinus by a thin membrane of mesenchymal tissue, the hymen. In the female the presence of androgenic stimuli after formation of the vaginal opening will not result in posterior fusion of the genital swellings, but only in hypertrophy of the clitoris. The urethral folds do not fuse but form the labia minora, and the genital swellings enlarge to form the labia majora.

The Development of Secondary Sex Characteristics

The appearance of secondary sex characteristics at puberty is entirely under the control of the endocrine system. In chronological order, the female development consists of pubarche, the development of pubic and axillary hair; thelarche, with breast enlargement and redistribution of fat; and finally menses, or menarche. Pubarche is secondary to an increase in the adrenal production of DHEA-S (see Fig. 56-4), which stimulates the pilosebaceous apparatus. Ovarian secretion of estrogen, under the influence of LH from the pituitary, stimulates breast development and the redistribution of fat. Menarche is controlled also by ovarian secretion under the cyclic influence of LH and FSH.

In the male, secondary sex characteristics include the appearance of pubic and axillary hair, deepening of the voice, the development of facial hair, and increases in muscle mass, testicular size, and penile length. Testosterone and dihydrotestosterone effect all these changes except pubarche, which occurs under the influence of DHEA-S from the adrenal.

CLINICAL APPROACH TO PROBLEMS OF SEXUAL DIFFERENTIATION

Classification

To reach a diagnosis in a neonate with a sexual ambiguity is to unravel the developmental process that led to the presenting phenotype. At birth the child presents a summary of its sexual development, but the defect can occur at any step in the path of differentiation. The classification of such disorders can therefore be organized according to the gonadal defect resulting in inadequate or inappropriate effects on the internal genital ducts and external genitalia, or according to extragonadal influences, such as the virilization of a female fetus secondary to congenital adrenal hyperplasia or maternal ingestion of androgenic hormones. The classification also has to encompass the result of end organ failure, as seen in the 5α-reductase deficiency, where there is no response to appropriate levels of androgenic stimuli. However, it is impossible to incorporate all clinical conditions into a simple classification. The most widely accepted classification is based on the histology of the gonad, with subclassification according to the etiology, as proposed by Allen (1976). This gonadal classification includes five major categories:

I. Ovary only: female pseudohermaphrodite
II. Testis only: male pseudohermaphrodite

TABLE 56-2
Usual Characteristics of the Classic Intersex States

Diagnosis	Karyotype	Gonad	Internal Ducts	External Ducts	Pubertal Change	Fertility	Gonadal Malignancy	Sex Assignment	Comment
Female									
Pseudohermaphrodite									
3β-ol-Dehydrogenase deficiency	XX	Ovary	Müllerian	Mildly ambiguous	Feminization (if treated)	Yes (if treated)	No	Female	Severe salt wasting
11β-Hydroxylase deficiency	XX	Ovary	Müllerian	Ambiguous	Feminization (if treated)	Yes (if treated)	No	Female	Hypertension
21-Hydroxylase deficiency	XX	Ovary	Müllerian	Ambiguous	Feminization (if treated)	Yes (if treated)	No	Female	Frequent salt wasting
Secondary to maternal androgens	XX	Ovary	Müllerian	Ambiguous	Feminization	Yes	No	Female	
True hermaphrodite	XX, XY, XX/XY, etc.	Ovary and testis	Müllerian and wolffian	Ambiguous	Tendency to virilization; gynecomastia	No	Rare*	Variable	
Male									
Pseudohermaphrodite									
Herni uteri inguinalis	XY	Testis	Müllerian and wolffian	Cryptorchid male	Virilization	Rare	Rare*	Male	
20α-Hydroxylase deficiency	XY	Testis	Wolffian	Female	Unknown	No	No*	Female	Severe salt wasting
3β-ol-Dehydrogenase deficiency	XY	Testis	Wolffian	Hypospadiac male	Partial virilization with gynecomastia	No	No*	Usually male	Severe salt wasting
17α-Hydroxylase deficiency	XY	Testis	Wolffian	Female	Usually eunuchoid	No	No*	Female	Hypertension
17,20-Desmolase deficiency	XY	Testis	Wolffian	Ambiguous	Unknown	No	No*	Uncertain	
17-Ketosteroid reductase deficiency	XY	Testis	Wolffian	Female	Partial virilization with gynecomastia	No	No*	Female	
Lubs' syndrome	XY	Testis	Wolffian	Ambiguous (feminization)	Feminization	No	No*	Female	Elevated testosterone and LH levels
Gilbert-Dreyfus syndrome	XY	Testis	Wolffian	Ambiguous	Partial virilization with gynecomastia	No	No*	Variable	Elevated testosterone and LH levels
Reifenstein's syndrome	XY	Testis	Wolffian	Hypospadiac male	Virilization with gynecomastia	No	No*	Usually male	Elevated testosterone and LH levels
Testicular feminization syndrome	XY	Testis	Wolffian	Female	Feminization	No	Yes	Female	Elevated testosterone and LH levels
Pseudovaginal perineoscrotal hypospadias	XY	Testis	Wolffian	Female	Virilization	No	No*	Female	
Dysgenetic testes	XO/XY, etc.	Testis	Wolffian and müllerian	Ambiguous	Virilization	No	Yes	Variable	
Mixed gonadal dysgenesis	XXY, XX, etc. / XO/XY, etc.	Testis and streak	Wolffian / Wolffian and müllerian	Variable / Ambiguous	Partial virilization / Usually virilization	No / No	No / Yes	Variable / Variable	
Gonadal dysgenesis Turner's syndrome	XO, etc.	Streak	Immature müllerian	Female	Eunuchoid	No†	Usually no	Female	Webbed neck, shield chest, etc.
Pure gonadal dysgenesis									
XX type	XX	Streak	Immature müllerian	Female	Eunuchoid	No	Usually no	Female	
XY type	XY	Streak	Immature müllerian	Female	Eunuchoid	No	Yes	Female	

From Allen TD: Disorder of sexual differentiation. *Urology* 1976; 7 (suppl):20–21. Used by permission.
*All patients with cryptorchid testes have an increased incidence of gonadal malignancy.
†One exception.

III. Ovary plus testis: true hermaphrodite
IV. Testis plus streak: mixed gonadal dysgenesis
 V. Streak plus streak: pure gonadal dysgenesis

The usual features of the classic intersex states are detailed in Table 56-2.

In children the presentation of ambiguous genitalia occurs typically in the neonatal period. A different group presents later in life with a functional failure of the assigned gender role. In this chapter the presentation in the neonatal period is therefore considered separately from that in later life. The stepwise evaluation and diagnostic algorithms are considered later.

Clinical Presentation

Ambiguous Genitalia in the Neonatal Period

Female Pseudohermaphrodites.—Female pseudohermaphrodites are the most important group as they constitute 60% to 70% of all intersex cases in the neonatal period. These patients have a 46,XX karyotype, are chromatin positive, are H-Y antigen and TDF gene negative, and have exclusively ovarian tissue. The müllerian system develops into fallopian tubes, uterus, and upper vagina, and the wolffian system regresses. Clinically, the virilization of external genitalia varies from minimal phallic enlargement to almost complete masculinization. At birth there is usually hypertrophy of the clitoris with severe chordee, a variable degree of labioscrotal fold fusion, and, in the more masculinized cases, a glanular urethra. The labioscrotal folds are bulbous and rugated, giving the general appearance of a male with bilateral cryptorchidism and hypospadias. As a result of the increase in ACTH drive, they have hyperpigmented skin over their external genitalia and their nipples. Female pseudohermaphrodites can be divided into two groups: those in whom the abnormal masculinization results from the presence of an inappropriate androgen, and those affected by a nonsteroidal mechanism.

Nonsteroidal female pseudohermaphrodites are always associated with significant cloacal or urogenital sinus problems. In a patient with a 46,XX karyotype, the presence of two ovaries and associated urogenital or cloacal abnormalities is diagnostic of this rare condition.

Cases resulting from abnormal androgens constitute the vast majority of female pseudohermaphrodites. The masculinization is limited to the external genitalia and clitoral hypertrophy if the androgenic stimulus is received after 12 weeks of gestation. If the stimulus is received earlier, clitoral hypertrophy still occurs, along with retention of the urogenital sinus and labioscrotal fusion. These patients must be correctly diagnosed, as they should be raised as females. The prognosis of such patients raised as females is excellent for pubertal development and the attainment of normal female characteristics, sexual activity, and reproduction.

Abnormal androgen may result from fetal biosynthetic anomalies (representing the vast majority of cases) or from a maternal source, either endogenous or exogenous. Fortunately, cases of maternal androgen origin are now very rare.

Congenital adrenal hyperplasia (CAH) encompasses the vast majority of female pseudohermaphrodites (Allen et al., 1982). There are six types of adrenogenital syndromes, all characterized by a defect in the production of cortisol, with secondary increases in the secretion of ACTH and consequent hyperplasia of the adrenals (Conte and Grumbach, 1984). Only types I through IV are virilizing and cause female pseudohermaphroditism (see Fig. 56-4).

The adrenal cortex is histologically divided into three zones: the zona granulosa (outer), the zona fasciculata, and the zona reticulata (inner) (mnemotechnic term GFR). The zona granulosa is responsible for the biosynthesis of the mineralocorticoids (mainly aldosterone), the zona fasciculata the glucocorticoids (mainly cortisol), and the zona reticulata the sex steroids. The secretion of the adrenal steroids is regulated by the hypothalamus and pituitary secretion of ACTH, and by negative feedback the plasma concentration of cortisol regulates the hypothalamic and hypophyseal release of ACTH. Thus any enzymatic defect that impedes the formation of cortisol will lead to an increase in ACTH release and stimulation of adrenal synthesis. With this in mind, it is easier to appreciate the biochemical abnormalities found in each type of congenital adrenal hyperplasia (see Fig. 56-4).

In type I abnormality, the defect of C-21-hydroxylation is localized in the zona fasciculata but not in the zona granulosa. This results in increased production of 17-hydroxyprogesterone and blockage of cortisol production. The concentration of 17-hydroxyprogesterone is of great clinical importance in making the diagnosis. The overproduction of androgens resulting from the blockage causes the inappropriate masculinizing effect on the urogenital sinus and external genitalia. Cortisol deficiency and the resulting continued ACTH stimulation with secondary hyperpigmentation are other important downstream effects of the defect in C-21-hydroxylation (see Fig. 56-7).

In type II CAH, the 21-hydroxylase deficiency involves the zona granulosa as well. The effects on the 17-hydroxyprogesterone (increase), androgens (increase), cortisol (decrease), and ACTH (increase) are similar, but there is also a deficiency of biologically active mineralocorticoid (see Figs. 56-4 and 56-8). The latter results in electrolyte imbalance with salt and water loss, usually requiring treatment.

In type III CAH, the enzymatic block occurs at the 11-hydroxylase level (Figs. 56-4 and 56-9). Again, two

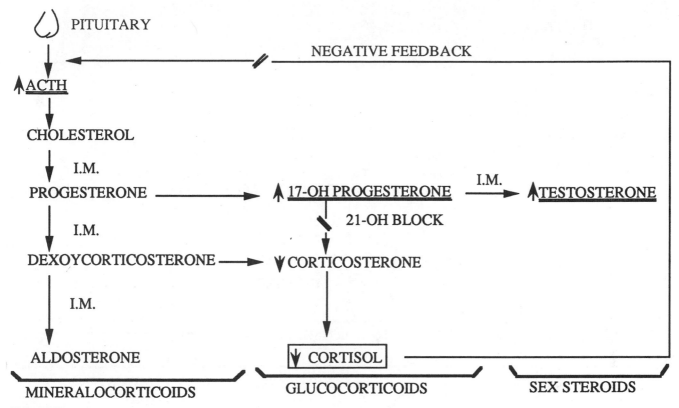

FIG. 56-7
CAH type I: Schematic diagram with emphasis on clinically important metabolites. *I.M.* signifies intermediate metabolites of lesser clinical importance.

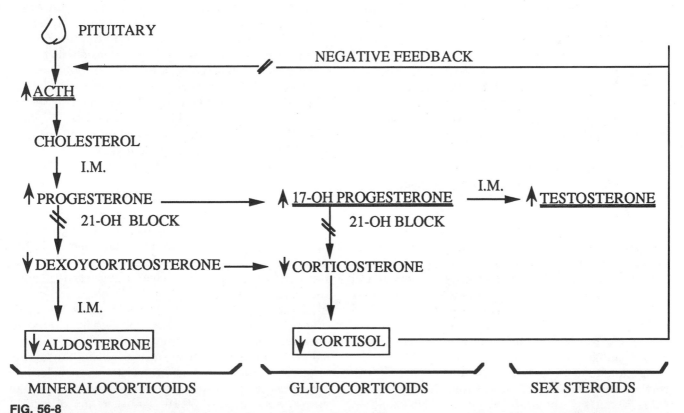

FIG. 56-8
CAH type II: Schematic diagram with emphasis on clinically important metabolites. *I.M.* signifies intermediate metabolites of lesser clinical importance.

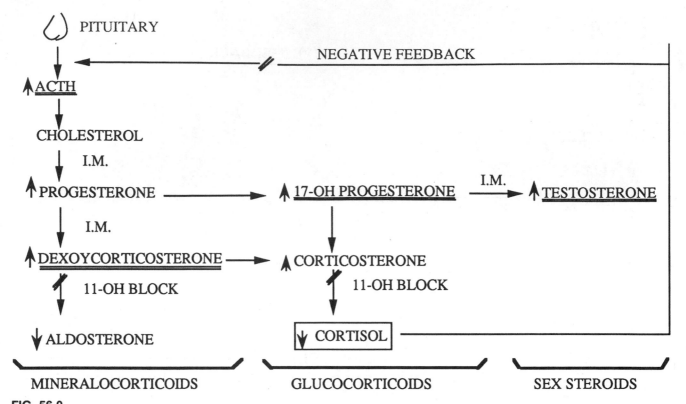

FIG. 56-9

CAH type III: Schematic diagram with emphasis on clinically important metabolites. *I.M.* signifies intermediate metabolites of lesser clinical importance.

important proximal metabolites, the 17-hydroxyprogesterone and the androgen, accumulate. Cortisol deficiency and ACTH excess are features, but there is also an accumulation of a biologically active and very potent mineralocorticoid, deoxycorticosterone (DOC). In affected children, the electrolyte imbalance with hypokalemic acidosis, hypervolemia, and secondary hypertension can be life threatening if left untreated.

Type IV CAH is the only enzyme deficiency that causes CAH and ambiguity in both males and females. The enzymatic block occurs more proximally at the 3β-ol-dehydrogenase level (Fig. 56-4). It is the rarest of the four forms of CAH and, as it is associated with the greatest degree of salt wasting, survival is rare. The principal androgen that accumulates proximal to the block is dehydroepiandrosterone (DHEA), a weak androgen; thus the degree of virilization encountered in affected females is usually not as severe as other types of CAH. Most patients have separate urethral and vaginal orifices. The hormonal deficiencies found are in cortisol and mineralocorticoids, with excess ACTH and severe hyponatremia.

All patients with type I, II, III, or IV CAH require cortisol replacement. Hydrocortisone sodium succinate, 50 mg/m², should be given as a bolus, and another 50 to 100 mg/m² should be added to the infusion of parenteral fluid over the next 24 hours (Conte and Grumbach, 1984). Regular monitoring of serum electrolytes and blood pressure measurements are essential in order to avoid the potential catastrophe of shock or hypokalemic acidosis and hypertension that may occur in most children with female pseudohermaphroditism and mineralocorticoid deficiency or excess, respectively. If profound hypotension and hyperkalemia are present, deoxycorticosterone acetate (DOCA), 1 to 2 mg, should be given intramuscularly over 12 to 14 hours. If the patient is in shock, 20 ml/kg of saline must be given in the first hours of therapy.

Male Pseudohermaphrodites.—Male pseudohermaphrodites constitute by far the most confusing group in the classification of intersex. As defined here, this group is limited to patients presenting with ambiguity in the neonatal period who have a 46,XY karyotype, are chromatin negative, and are H-Y antigen positive. They also have exclusively testicular tissue, and the wolffian system develops while the müllerian system regresses. This group is the most diverse in etiology, with many of the characteristics occurring later in life; these types are therefore considered later. The mechanisms underlying the failure of testosterone synthesis by the testis or the failure of target tissues to respond to circulating testosterone are shown in Figure 56-10. The secretion of testosterone by the fetal testis is influenced by the gonadotrophins, with hypotrophic hypogonadism occur-

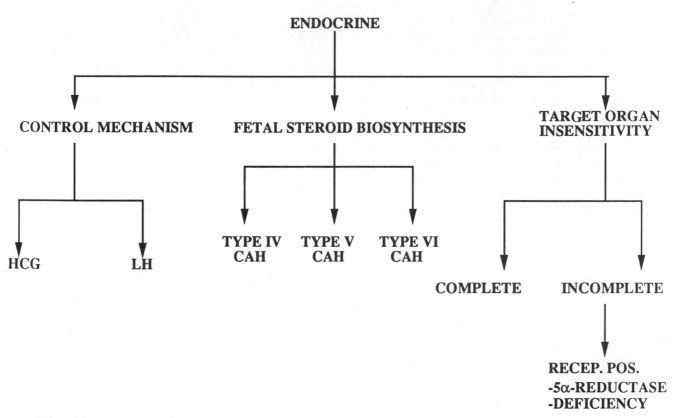

FIG. 56-10
Schematic representation of the different mechanisms implicated in the etiology of male pseudohermaphroditism.

ring where there is deficiency of luteinizing hormone (LH) or of human chorionic gonadotrophin (HCG).

In three enzymes involved in the synthesis of steroid hormones, defects have been identified that result in male pseudohermaphroditism and ambiguous genitalia in the neonate. These enzymes are 20,22-desmolase, 3β-ol-dehydrogenase, and 17, 20-desmolase. All three defects interfere in the cascade production of testosterone or cortisol (see Fig. 56-4). The deficiency in 20,22-desmolase and 3β-ol-dehydrogenase result in death in the majority of affected males. These individuals possess ambiguous external genitalia varying from mild hypospadias to complete failure of masculinization with the presence of a vagina. Most exhibit some element of hypospadias and scrotal fusion. The wolffian ducts are normally developed. These males also have darkly pigmented skin and severe salt wasting. A few patients with the 3β-ol-dehydrogenase deficiency have survived into adulthood and have shown a mixture of partial virilization and gynecomastia at puberty, but no fertility has been reported (Allen, 1985). The virilization phenomena are caused by the accumulation of a weak androgen (DHEA) behind the enzyme block.

A 17,20-desmolase deficiency produces ambiguity with some virilization at the time of puberty. There is no interference with the synthesis of cortisol, no increase in the ACTH drive, and no elevation of pre-cursor steroids behind the block (Allen, 1985); thus there is no CAH. The effect on fertility has not been described in the few cases reported in the literature (Allen, 1985; Zachmann et al., 1982). This syndrome has also been described in one 46,XX female with sexual infantilism (Larrea et al., 1983).

The inability of a target organ to respond to circulating testosterone is the result of androgen insensitivity, which can be complete or partial. Complete androgen insensitivity syndromes (CAIS) are rare, occurring in 1 in 20,000 to 1 in 64,000 male births. The incomplete forms are even rarer, with an incidence one tenth that of the complete form. Since the complete forms do not show ambiguity in the neonatal period, they will be discussed later. Although incomplete forms of androgen insensitivity result in ambiguity in the neonatal period, because their pathophysiology is so closely related to the complete forms they will also be discussed later in this chapter (see Nonambiguous Genitalia in the Neonatal Period).

True Hermaphrodites.—At birth true hermaphrodites display ambiguous genitalia and asymmetry of the gonads. They constitute 10% of the intersex pool (Allen, 1985). A 46,XX karyotype is found in 57% (57% to 80%) of these patients (Lalau-Keraly et al., 1986). The others have a 46,XY pattern (13%) (Luks et al., 1988) or a mosaic with 46,XX/XY (31%). The chromatin is positive in 70%, but the H-Y antigen is also positive in the majority of cases. This is thought to represent a translocation of the testis determinants from the Y chromosome to the X chromosome in patients with 46,XX karyotype.

True hermaphrodites have both ovarian and testicular tissue. This may take the form of an ovary on one side and a testis on the other, or an individual may have both components in the same gonad, representing an ovotestis. Internal duct differentiation follows the appropriate ipsilateral gonad: a fallopian tube develops when an ovary is present, and a vas with the epididymis results when a testis is present. When an ovotestis is present, the differentiation of the ducts is variable. In 1986 Lalau-Keraly reported 10 cases of true hermaphrodites. She documented eight ovotestes by surgical exploration. A fallopian tube was found in 50% of the cases with the ovotestis, a vas was identified in 25%, and in the remaining 25% an "ambiguous duct" was found (Lalau-Keraly et al., 1986). A uterus is almost always present (Lorge et al., 1989) and may be hypoplastic or unicornuate (Allen, 1985).

Although the appearance of the external genitalia may span the spectrum from feminine with slight clitoral prominence to full masculinization, a tendency to maleness with asymmetrically descended gonads and hypospadias occurs in 75% (Lorge et al., 1989). The changes at puberty are variable but generally correlate with the gonadal tissue present. Sex assignment should be made thoughtfully. The presence or absence of an adequate phallus, both functionally and cosmetically, is a cornerstone in the decision process (Table 56-3 and Fig. 56-11).

Three cases of true hermaphroditism and pregnancy have been reported in the literature (Mayou et al., 1978; Narita et al., 1975; Tegenkamp et al., 1979). These three cases constitute the only indication of the potential for fertility in true hermaphrodites. In at least two of the three the karyotype was 46,XX. There is also a report of spermatogenesis in the testis of a true hermaphrodite (Van Niekerk, 1981). All these observations suggest the fertility potential in true hermaphrodites, but further studies are required. It seems certain from observations that at puberty almost half of the true hermaphrodites will have normal menses (Van Niekerk, 1981), and since the reconstructive surgery for sex-assigned females gives by far the better result, it appears logical to preferably assign the true

hermaphrodite the female gender, especially the 46,XX karyotype individual. Assignment of the male gender exposes the individual to many reconstructive procedures, sometimes with poor functional and cosmetic results and inevitably with primary hypogonadism, since in most cases the testes are dysgenetic when adulthood is reached (Lalau-Keraly et al., 1986). Gonadal malignancies have been reported; thus all discordant and dysgenetic tissue should be removed after sex assignment.

Mixed Gonadal Dysgenesis.—Mixed gonadal dysgenesis constitutes the last group presenting in the neonatal period with ambiguous genitalia. The gonads are classically asymmetrical. Most of these patients have a mosaic 46,XY/45,XO karyotype. Their chromatin is negative and their H-Y antigen is positive. Their gonadal composition is characterized by testic-

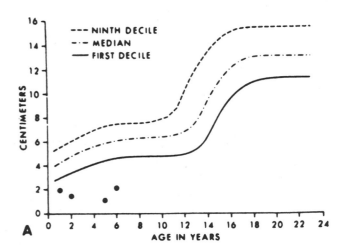

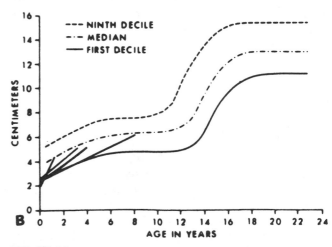

FIG. 56-11

A, Penile length in four children who were seen later than the neonatal period. **B,** Penile length in four neonates who responded to androgen stimulation (neonatal vs. time of study). (From Beheshti M, Hardy BE, Churchill BM, et al: Gender assignment in male pseudohermaphrodite children. *Urology* 1983; 22:604-607. Used by permission.)

TABLE 56-3

Phallus Size

Gestational Age (wk)	Phallic Size (cm)
40	3.5 ± 0.4
35	3.0 ± 0.4
30	2.5 ± 0.4
Average diameter	1.0-1.5

ular tissue on one side and a dysgenetic gonad (streak) on the other. The testis is composed of Sertoli cells and Leydig cells, but no germinal cells are present. The streak gonad appears similar to the ovarian stroma but without oocytes. It occurs most probably secondary to paracrine insufficiency from the testis, and the müllerian duct usually persists unilaterally or bilaterally. The testis is often provided with a fallopian tube rather than a vas and an epididymis. The streak gonad is usually drained by a müllerian duct. A bicornuate or unicornuate uterus is generally present.

Malignancy develops in about 15% to 25% of the streak gonads, usually in the form of gonadoblastomas or dysgerminomas (Lorge et al., 1989). Individuals with a 46,XY karyotype are at a much higher risk than the ones with a mosaic pattern. Individuals tend to virilize and have gynecomastia at the time of puberty. No fertility has been reported so far. Sex assignment should be individualized. The response of the phallus to androgenic stimulation should be assessed in borderline cases, but assignment of the female gender is usually preferred for the following reasons:

1. The development of the phallus is usually inadequate for functional and cosmetic surgical results.
2. The presence of a mosaic pattern with 46,XY/45,XO predisposes these individuals to short stature.
3. These individuals are infertile, and a bilateral gonadectomy is essential in view of the high potential for malignancy of these gonads, particularly those with Y cell–bearing lines.

Patients assigned as female require gonadectomy, clitoroplasty, and vaginoplasty. Those assigned to the male gender usually should undergo removal of any dysgenetic gonadal tissue and repair of the usually severe hypospadias.

Nonambiguous Genitalia in the Neonatal Period

Female Phenotype

Androgen Insensitivity Syndromes.—Androgen insensitivity syndromes represent the lack of response by the different target organs to androgen stimulation. They have in the past been divided in two categories, the complete androgen insensitivity syndromes and the incomplete forms. It is now recognized that the phenotypic spectrum of androgen resistance ranges from 46,XY phenotypic women with the classic syndrome of complete androgen insensitivity, to phenotypic men with mild or focal expressions of subvirilization such as postpubertal gynecomastia with or without impaired spermatogenesis (Griffin, 1992). Between these two extremes is a continuum that includes conditions such as Lubs' syndrome and Reifenstein's syndrome, which were previously classified separately

(see Table 56-2). In addition to the phenotypic expression, the androgen resistance syndromes are now also classified on the basis of abnormalities of the androgen receptor.

Hormonal secretion is totally responsible for the development of the urogenital sinus, the external genitalia, and the secondary sex characteristics along female or male lines depending on the hormonal environment. This process involves normal secretion of steroids or peptides by endocrine glands into the circulation, and normal response of all target organs to that stimulation. In the androgen insensitivity syndromes, the hormonal secretion occurs normally. The deficiency is caused by the lack of response of the target organ to the normally secreted androgen. The defect is thought to be localized at the level of the cytoplasmic androgen receptor of the 5α-reductase enzyme (see Fig. 56-5).

Two major types of defect have been described: quantitative receptor defect (receptor negative, AR−) and qualitative receptor defect (receptor positive, AR+). The receptor-negative syndrome implies that the specific intracellular androgen receptors are undetectable (AR−) in all target organs. Normal levels of androgens are measured in the second variant (AR+). The latter is thought to represent a qualitative defect in the response of the receptor secondary to a structural abnormality of the receptor (Brown et al., 1982). These measurements are usually done by fibroblast culture. There are, in fact, two different 5α-reductase enzymes present in humans; one is most active at a low pH, which is found preferentially in genital skin fibroblasts, and is the deficient enzyme in this disorder. Therefore, use of the genital skin is usually preferable for these studies (Hughes et al., 1988). It is important to understand that the defect is found in all target organs, which include the external genitalia and other urogenital sinus derivatives, and some specific areas such as the pubic and axillary pilosebaceous system, the larynx, and the hypothalamic-pituitary axis.

Clinically, the AR form usually corresponds to complete androgen insensitivity syndrome (CAIS), although some cases of CAIS have been reported with AR+ (Brown et al., 1982). AR+ is probably responsible for the clinically incomplete form with the 5α-reductase deficiency. This pathophysiologic distinction is probably responsible for the different types of presentation encountered with these syndromes.

Indeed, individuals affected by CAIS do not present in the neonatal period with ambiguous genitalia, but rather later in life phenotypically as normal female, a condition best known as the testicular feminization syndrome. CAIS has now been identified as an X-linked mutation that precludes the normal synthesis of the androgen receptor located in the cytosol (Griffin and Wilson, 1980).

The incidence varies from 1 in 20,000 to 1 in 64,000 male births. All patients have a 46,XY karyotype, are chromatin negative, are H-Y antigen positive, and have exclusively testicular tissue (seminiferous tubules with no spermatogenesis and increased numbers of Leydig cells). The internal ducts develop normally as wolffian ducts, and there is regression of all müllerian structures.

These individuals are phenotypically normal, tall, and hairless females with nonambiguous feminine external genitalia and symmetrically undescended gonads. They usually have a shallow vaginal cavity, probably corresponding to a vast prostatic utricle. At the time of puberty, normal breasts develop with axillary and pubic hair absent or scanty. There is slight vulval hair development, and amenorrhea is the rule. Clinically, they present for evaluation of primary amenorrhea usually in the postpubertal period and less often during the prepubertal period because of inguinal herniae.

The gonads are at higher risk for malignancy because of the cryptorchidism in this condition, and gonadectomy is recommended. The timing of gonadectomy must be individualized. Since the testis tumors that can occur rarely develop before puberty, surgical intervention is indicated in the prepubertal period only if the presence of the testis in the labia majora or in the inguinal region results in discomfort or hernia formation. Estrogen therapy will be necessary for individuals who undergo pubertal gonadectomy to ensure normal growth and breast development. When castration is performed postpubertally, estrogen withdrawal symptoms are the rule and estrogen supplements are necessary.

In contrast to CAIS, incomplete androgen insensitivity syndromes including AR+ and 5α-reductase deficiency causes ambiguity in the neonatal period. Although the incidence is about one tenth that of the complete form, innumerable incomplete androgen insensitivity AR+ phenotypes have been described in the literature, and their exhaustive description is beyond the scope of this chapter. The important common characteristics are that the individuals are of 46,XY karyotype, chromatin negative, and H-Y antigen positive. They have exclusively testicular tissue, the internal ducts develop normally and sometimes incompletely (hypoplastic or absent vas) as wolffian ducts, and there is regression of the müllerian structures. There is a minor defect of virilization of the external genitalia consisting of partial fusion of the labioscrotal folds, and some degree of clitoromegaly is present at birth and is responsible for the ambiguity. The gonads are usually symmetrically undescended, and there is a short, blind-ending vagina. At puberty, both some

virilization and some feminization occurs, including the development of normal pubic hair and gynecomastia. Sex assignment should be individualized and made thoughtfully. The same considerations apply as for true hermaphrodites and mixed gonadal dysgenesis. The potential for fertility is usually considered nonexistent. Since some virilization is expected at the time of puberty, in sex-assigned females gonadectomy should be performed during the prepubertal period.

The deficiency in 5α-reductase is a rare syndrome originally described in humans in 1974 (Imperato-McGinley et al., 1974). The deficit is found in the genital sinus and hepatic tissues. A number of cases have been reported in the Dominican Republic, where a recessive trait seems to be the inheritance pattern.

At puberty in the different forms of androgen insensitivity, despite very low affinity of the cytoplasmic receptors for testosterone, some virilization occurs because testosterone is secreted in such excess: the voice deepens, the muscle mass increases, and the phallus lengthens. In 5α-reductase–deficient subjects, basal plasma testosterone levels are normal or elevated, and plasma DHT levels are normal or decreased.

The diagnosis of 5α-reductase deficiency in adults is made by measuring the ratio of testosterone to DHT, which is increased. However, in affected children past infancy, the basal plasma testosterone and DHT are too low for accurate determination of this ratio. This measurement can be made after HCG administration of the Leydig cells. Imperato-McGinley and co-workers (1986) described a new method of diagnosis for this deficiency, which involves measuring the ratio of other C-19 and C-21 steroids and their 5α-reduced urinary metabolites. Of course, the demonstrated inability of the genital skin to convert the testosterone to DHT in tissue culture is the ultimate test for diagnosis (Lorge et al., 1989).

Although hypospadias with or without undescended testes is not usually considered an example of intersexuality, it is obviously closely related. With the progress in understanding the different androgen insensitivity syndromes (Brown et al., 1982; Hughes et al., 1988; Imperato-McGinley et al., 1986), it is reasonable to postulate that if a very isolated resistance to androgen occurs at a critical time during sexual differentiation, it could lead to incomplete virilization phenomena such as hypospadias.

Male Pseudohermaphrodites.—The deficiency of two enzymes in the synthesis of steroid hormones in addition to those described for female pseudohermaphroditism are further causes of male pseudohermaphroditism: 17α-hydroxylase and 17-keto-reductase. These enzyme deficiencies do not cause ambiguity in the neonatal period, and individuals present later in life as amenorrheic phenotypic females. They have 46,XY karyotype, are chromatin negative, and are H-Y antigen positive. In the gonads exclusively testicular tissue is found, with development of the wolffian ducts and regression of the müllerian ducts.

With 17α-hydroxylase deficiency, patients present clinically as phenotypic females with hypogonadism and absence of all secondary sex characteristics. They also have hypertension and hypokalemic alkalosis secondary to the accumulation of deoxycorticosterone (DOC) behind the block (see Fig. 56-4). There is also an excess of ACTH secondary to a virtually undetectable cortisol level (see Fig. 56-4). The aldosterone level is also presumably low secondary to the high plasma DOC level and depressed angiotensin levels. At puberty they remain infantile female although some affected individuals with presumed partial deficiency might develop pathologic gynecomastia. Those individuals with partial deficiency might also present at birth with some ambiguity consisting of varying degrees of hypospadias. This deficiency has been also described in 46,XX subjects who present at puberty with sexual infantilism, amenorrhea, and hypertension.

Males suffering from 17-keto-reductase deficiency have a female phenotype with a blind-ending vagina, but absence of all müllerian derivatives. They usually have bilaterally undescended testes. There is no defect of secretion of cortisol, and thus no excess ACTH production and no CAH (see Fig. 56-4). At puberty, however, because of the increase in LH secretion and some escape through the block, a combination of both virilization and feminization results, with phallic enlargement, pubarche, and a variable degree of breast development.

Pure Gonadal Dysgenesis.—With pure gonadal dysgenesis, there is no ambiguity in the neonatal period, but patients usually present later in life as phenotypic females with sexual infantilism. They have various karyotypes (45,XO, 46,XX, 46,XY) and corresponding chromatin and H-Y antigen. There are bilateral streak gonads, symmetrically undescended, and developed yet hypoplastic müllerian derivatives with regression of the wolffian system. Beyond these similarities, the clinical picture varies depending primarily on chromosomal configuration. Subjects with 45,XO karyotype, for example, exhibit all the stigmata of Turner's syndrome, with short stature, webbed neck, shieldlike chest, and other characteristics. Individuals with 46,XX karyotype are usually normal in height, or even tall, but at puberty display sexual infantilism and amenorrhea. Patients with 46,XY karyotype have similar complaints and appearance, but their streak gonads have a high malignancy potential. Dysgerminoma and gonadoblastoma are particularly common and present clinically as a pelvic

mass or signs of virilization. Bilateral gonadectomy is thus essential at the time of diagnosis for patients with 46,XY karyotype.

Male Phenotype

Klinefelter's Syndrome.—Klinefelter's syndrome was described in 1942 by Klinefelter, Reinstein, and Albright. The original description was of a man with bilaterally small and firm testes, varying degrees of impaired sexual maturation, azoospermia, gynecomastia, and elevated levels of urinary gonadotrophins. Clearly, these patients are not ambiguous at birth.

The karyotype can be 47,XXY, 46,XX/47,XXY, or even 48,XXXY to 49,XXXXY. The chromatin is positive as is the H-Y antigen. They have symmetrically descended testes with normal histology at birth, but in early infancy there is a drastic loss of germ cells, followed by progressive tubular hyalinization during adolescence.

These patients usually seek medical attention at puberty because of sexual infantilism, or later in life because of infertility, which occurs secondary to primary hypogonadism. The syndrome includes a constellation of physical, biochemical, and hormonal abnormalities. The reader is referred to Schwartz and Root (1991).

Hernia Uterine Inguinale.—The persistency of müllerian ducts characterizing hernia uterine inguinale is a rare syndrome resulting from failure of paracrine secretion of AMH by the Sertoli cells or failure of the müllerian ducts to respond to its secretion. Now that AMH has been purified and immunohistochemical techniques are available to stain for AMH, testicular biopsies from these patients can be examined to determine if AMH is present. Out of six patients with this syndrome, AMH was normally expressed in the testicular tissue of two patients. In the other four there was no detectable bioactive or immunoreactive AMH, yet they expressed AMH mRNA with a normal transcription initiation site and in the amount expected for their age (Guerrier et al., 1989). This confirms the heterogeneity of hernia uterine inguinale and suggests that peripheral insensitivity to AMH can be present.

Affected males are not ambiguous at birth and generally present later with symmetrically or asymmetrically undescended testes for orchidopexy or repair of inguinal herniae. They have a 46,XY karyotype, are chromatin negative, and are H-Y antigen positive. The gonadal tissue is exclusively testicular. Both wolffian and müllerian duct derivatives are present, with a vas and epididymis alongside an ipsilateral uterus, fallopian tube, and upper vagina. The external genitalia are nonambiguously male with unilateral or bilateral cryptorchidism. Rare cases of associated hypospadias have been reported.

Several abnormalities in the attachment of the epididymis to the testis in the affected male have been described, as well as some propensity of these testes toward malignancy. It is thus difficult to recommend heroic efforts to salvage all testicular tissue. The fertility potential of these patients can also be compromised when surgery is attempted to remove the müllerian derivatives, as the vas is intimately related to the broad ligament and uterus. However, surgical removal of the müllerian duct derivatives is recommended in this syndrome (Behesti, 1984). To date, no uterine or vaginal malignancies have been reported in these patients. Primary or staged orchidopexy should be attempted, although attaining sufficient length for adequate placement of the testis is difficult with the tethering of the testis to the broad ligament and the passage of the vas through the corpus of the urerus.

XX Male Reversal.—The incidence of XX male reversal is approximately 1 in 20,000 to 1 in 24,000 male births, a rare disorder. The affected individuals are non-ambiguous at birth with normal male phenotype. They have a 46,XX karyotype, are chromatin positive, and may also be H-Y antigen positive. This group of patients have been key in isolating the gene controlling the formation of the testis. By restriction enzyme fragmentation of the X chromosomes and the use of DNA probes, it has been shown that the majority of the XX sex-reversed males contain fragments of DNA from the short arm of the Y chromosome in the distal end of the short arm of the X chromosome (Magenis et al., 1987; Page et al., 1984; Petit et al., 1987). These patients have exclusively testicular tissue and develop the wolffian system while the müllerian ducts regress.

The external genitalia are of nonambiguous male phenotype, very similar to Klinefelter's syndrome, but there is a more frequent association with hypospadias and an average height below normal. The testes are small and firm but bilaterally descended. The penile length is normal or slightly shorter than normal, and these patients also develop gynecomastia and hyalinization of the seminiferous tubules at puberty with incomplete pubarche. Infertility occurs secondary to hypogonadism.

Diagnosis

When the first observation of ambiguous genitalia is made at the time of delivery, the delivery room physicians should seek rapid assistance with two specific goals:

1. Accurate sex assignment
2. Detection of specific underlying endocrinopathies (particularly of the salt-losing variety) that may endanger the infant.

The proposed algorithm for diagnosis of intersex presented in Figures 56-12 and 56-13 allows the clinician to rapidly identify newborns with potential electrolyte imbalance and to make a working diagnosis that will be accurate in 90% of cases.

Only a few adjuncts to this clinical approach are required in order to obtain a correct diagnosis and assign sex to the newborn. The maternal history of androgen exposure, either endogenous or exogenous, is usually very easy to obtain. A family history of neonatal death is a clue for diagnosis of congenital adrenal hyperplasia, although this may be present in an infant with either male or female pseudohermaphroditism. The physical examination will then orient the diagnosis according to whether the gonads are symmetrically or asymmetrically descended. Although ovotestes have been reported to descend completely to the bottom of the labioscrotal folds, generally only testicular material fully descends. If there are palpable inguinal gonads, the diagnoses of a gonadal female, Turner's syndrome, and pure gonadal dysgenesis can be eliminated. Even in what appears to be a fully virilized infant, the presence of impalpable gonads should alert the physician to the possibility of a severely virilized female pseudohermaphrodite with CAH. If the scrotum or labioscrotal folds are rugated with increased pigmentation, the possibility of increased ACTH as part of the adrenogenital syndrome is suggested. The measurement of phallic length and comparison with known nomograms (Behesti et al., 1983) is important, especially with regard to the consideration of penile reconstruction. A rectal examination, ultrasound, or retrograde genitogram may detect the cervix and uterus, confirming müllerian duct structures. This rules out male pseudohermaphrodites, except those with hernia uteri inguinalis and those with dysgenetic gonads. Although the physical examination can be beneficial at the extreme ends of the spectrum, it has limitations in the majority of cases. The establishment of chromosomal sex and measurements of different key biochemical metabolites therefore remains essential.

The chromosomal sex is best determined by karyotyping and can be done within 48 hours with activated T-lymphocytes, but the regular 72-hour lymphocyte culture is preferable. A reliable result can be achieved by microscopy without photography and banding at 3 to 4 days. A complete karyotype with banding and photography can be achieved in 6 to 7 days. The buccal smear is inadequate for definitive sex assignment but is a useful tool (Hughes and Davies, 1980). The buccal smear can be stained with quinacrine dyes and examined by fluorescent microscopy to define the distal end of the long arm of the Y chromosome.

The determination of a raised plasma 17-OH progesterone level is diagnostic of CAH. This measurement should be done after 48 hours of life, as earlier

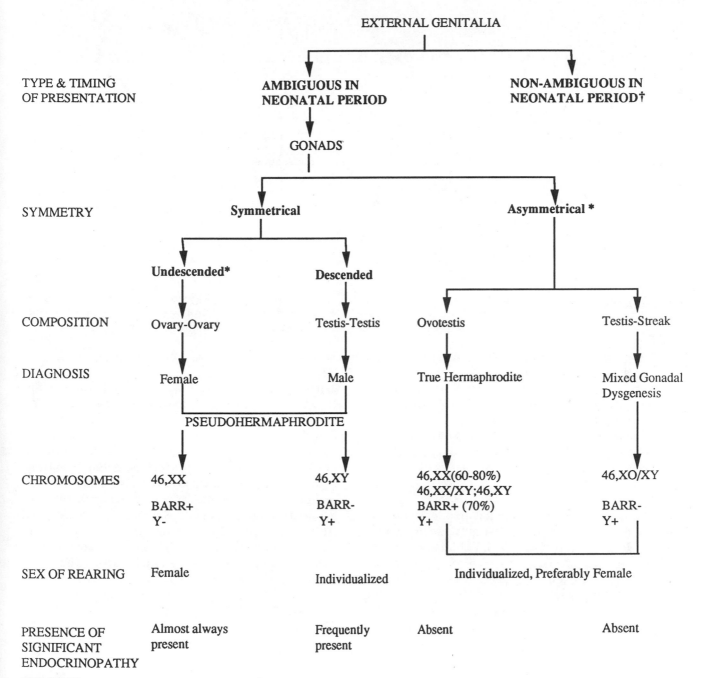

FIG. 56-12
Diagnostic algorithm of intersex. *It is in these categories that a patient with severe hypospadias and bilateral or unilateral cryptorchidism would be classified. This situation underlines the importance of the karyotype, the confirmation of the gonadal composition, and the configuration of the internal ducts in a neonate with ambiguity and asymmetry. †See Fig. 56-13.

levels can reflect the presence of maternal progesterone. The clinical presence of hypokalemic alkalosis or hypertension may reflect underlying deficiencies of cortisol and mineralocorticoids or excess of DOC, requiring urgent correction. Once the diagnosis of CAH is made from elevated levels of 17-OH progesterone, further biochemical measurements of the various precursors can identify the exact enzymatic block.

Additional evaluations are strongly recommended in order to determine the status of the urogenital si-

nus, the ductal system, and gonads by radiology, endoscopy, ultrasonography, laparatomy, and gonadal biopsy (Hughes and Davies, 1980). Only female pseudohermaphrodites and Turner's syndrome (46,XO) do not require gonadal biopsy. All other neonates with ambiguous genitalia should have a biopsy. In the future, the wider dissemination of steroid immunoassays may permit gonadal males with blockage of testosterone production and resultant genital ambiguity to be precisely diagnosed biochemically, as may assays to

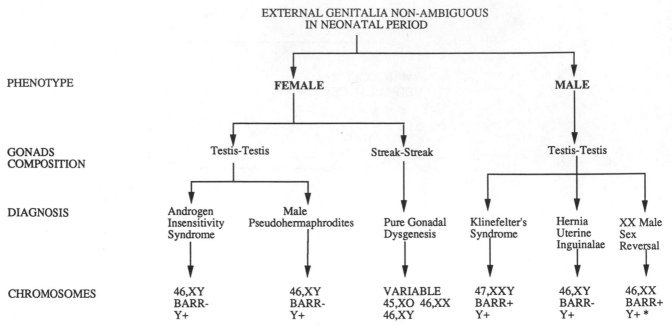

FIG. 56-13
Diagnostic algorithm of intersex. *As detected by the techniques of restriction fragment length polymorphisms.

measure deficiency of 5α-reductase or of androgen binding, without the need for gonadal biopsy.

Once all the relevant information has been obtained, sex assignment should be made thoughtfully. The following considerations are paramount in the decision.

Phallic Size

A comparison of the stretched penile length and corporal body girth with known growth curves must be obtained (Behesti et al., 1983; Feldman and Smith, 1975) (see Fig. 56-11 and Table 56-3). Time-growth response to androgen stimulus can be a key factor in distinguishing borderline cases. This can involve the exogenous administration of testosterone or androgenic stimulation by HCG, with measurement of the phallic response 2 and 4 weeks later. Examples of successful response in four neonates who were raised as males is shown in Figure 56-11, *B.*) This appears to have been the correct decision.

Currently, despite a much improved understanding of the development of sexual identity, phallic size is still believed to be the most significant criterion in gender assignment in the newborn (Behesti et al., 1983; Perlmutter, 1979). Although nomograms are available for penile length, the size of phallus required to avoid male inadequacy is not clearly defined (Behisti et al., 1983).

Fertility Potential and Risk of Gonadal Malignancy

Except for female pseudohermaphrodites and rare cases of true hermaphrodites, the fertility potential is usually considered nonexistent in mixed gonadal dys-genesis, and uncertain in male pseudohermaphroditism. On the other hand, more than 50% of true hermaphrodites will have menses at the time of puberty (Van Niekerk, 1981).

The necessity for gonadectomy for dysgenetic testes must be weighed against the fertility potential in those with Y cell-bearing lines in the decision of sex assignment. Gonadoblastomas are tumors composed of three elements: large germ cells, sex cord derivatives, and stromal elements. Even though gonadoblastomas are not malignant, these tumors frequently contain dysgerminoma elements that can metastasize. The risk of neoplasia in streak gonads with an XY karyotype, as mentioned earlier, is much greater than in streak gonads with XX chromosomes. Cryptorchid testes, even when not associated with intersex, also have an increased risk of malignancy.

Patient or Family Wishes

Family history, culture, and preferences, particularly if based on prior experience, are of major importance. Parental wishes may be very dominant or predetermined in dictating one sex of rearing over the other. This is usually based on long-standing cultural bias and may not be alterable by any medical advice.

The older child with an originally assigned sex of rearing that is inappropriate represents one of the most complex situations in clinical surgery. Raising a female pseudohermaphrodite as a male is an example. Care, extensive psychiatric and endocrinologic consultation, and real communication with the family are of utmost importance.

SURGICAL MANAGEMENT

Surgery for sexual differentiation problems can be classified as follows:

A. Exploratory surgery to obtain biopsy and establish diagnosis
B. Excision of tissue inappropriate to sex of rearing
C. Gonadectomy for high statistical risk of neoplasia or actual presence of neoplasia
D. Surgery designed to feminize the external genitalia, including:
   1. Reconstruction of clitoris
   2. Reconstruction of labial scrotal region
   3. Reconstruction of urogenital sinus and vagina
E. Surgery to masculinize the external genitalia, including:
   1. Hypospadias repair
   2. Scrotal reconstruction
   3. Orchidopexy
   4. Insertion of testicular prosthesis
F. Treatment of gynecomastia

The last two major categories are covered elsewhere in this text and will not be discussed here.

Exploratory Surgery to Obtain Biopsy and Establish Diagnosis

Exploratory surgery is indicated, in our opinion, in most cases of true hermaphrodites, mixed gonadal dysgenesis, and many cases of male pseudohermaphroditism with gender assignment confusion. This involves gonadal biopsy, exploration to determine the nature of the internal ducts, and genital skin biopsy for fibroblast culture in cases of suspected androgen insensitivity. In addition, any endoscopic procedures that would help in obtaining a more precise diagnosis and clarify the nature of the abnormality should be performed at the same time. Laparoscopy can be useful at this stage of evaluation, allowing determination of the nature of the internal ducts as well as localization and biopsy of the nonpalpable gonads when required. Gonadal biopsy is not indicated in female pseudohermaphroditism, which can be accurately diagnosed by other means.

Removal of Inappropriate Tissue

In true hermaphroditism ovarian tissue and müllerian ducts should be removed when the infant is raised as male, with removal of the testes and wolffian ducts in the female. The removal of müllerian structures in patients with failure of AMH is very controversial. The intimate anatomical relationship with the wolffian ducts makes the removal of the müllerian structures technically difficult. It is important to preserve the integrity of the wolffian system and the possibility of fertility in these individuals. The müllerian remnants can usually be removed with meticulous dissection, although a less extensive procedure will result in satifactory orchidopexy in many cases (Behesti et al., 1984). In patients with complete androgen insensitivity syndromes, some (Grumbach and Conte, 1981) prefer prepubertal orchidectomy when the testes are in the inguinal region or labia majora: otherwise, gonadectomy can be done postpubertally to allow a nonmedicated feminization at puberty (see Androgen Insensitivity Syndrome). In mixed gonadal dysgenesis, all testicular and dysgenetic tissue should be removed.

Gonadectomy for Neoplasm or High Risk of Neoplasm

As mentioned earlier, the risk of neoplasia in streak gonads with an XY karyotype is much larger than in streak gonads with XX chromosomes. Malignancy will develop in 15% to 25% of streak gonads, usually in the form of gonadoblastomas or dysgerminomas (Lorger et al., 1989). In one large series of gonadoblastomas, 40% of patients were under 15 years of age and 15% were under 10 years of age (Wilson and Walsh, 1979). Thus early removal of streak gonads is recommended if there is a Y chromosome in the karyotype.

Surgery Designed to Feminize the Partially Masculinized Patient

Feminizing surgery is designed to deal with three structures that have been partially or significantly masculinized in individuals to be reared in the female sex. These structures are the phallus (glans and corporal bodies), labioscrotal folds, and the urogenital sinus.

The exact anatomical diagnosis of the urogenital sinus must be made prior to planning surgery. In our unit, more and more of the reconstructive surgery is being done as a single stage. The exact understanding of the complexity of the abnormality is the most important factor in planning the type and timing of surgery. Virtually all of these patients will require clitoroplasty and reconstruction of the labioscrotal folds, and these two operations go together according to the most recent publications (Donahoe, 1988; Passerini-Glazel, 1989). The key element in this decision-making process is the complexity of the abnormality involving the urogenital sinus and müllerian elements. The criterion of decision-making is the position of the vaginal opening and the presence of a vagina. There are two categories of patients distinguished by the vaginal position (perineal or abnormal) (Fig. 56-14). Those with abnormal vaginal position must be carefully investigated by endoscopic and radiologic techniques to determine the exact anatomy. If the vagina joins the urogenital sinus, the key observation is whether the position of the junction is distal or prox-

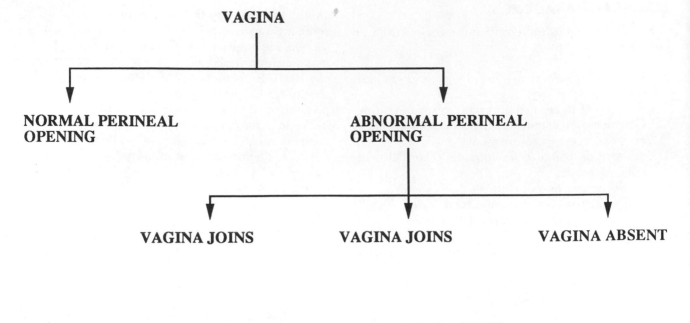

FIG. 56-14
Planning of reconstructive surgery for feminization of partially masculinized patient depending on the position of the vagina and its site of insertion on the urogenital sinus.

imal to the rhabdourinary sphincter. In most patients with type I CAH, mixed gonadal dysgenesis, and true hermaphrodites there is a vaginal opening either in the normal position or joining the urogenital sinus distal to the external urethral sphincter. Cases in this category can be dealt with using a single-stage procedure that combines clitoroplasty, reconstruction of labia minora and posterior perineal (Blandy flap) reconstruction of vaginal introitus. This can be performed at 3 to 6 months of age, and occasionally earlier if significant social factors outweigh the slightly increased risk.

A number of clitoroplasty techniques have been described, some of which are now obsolete. Obsolete techniques include total resection of the clitoris, as originally described by Gross (1966), and clitoroplication with recession of the corporal bodies without resection, as advocated by Lattimer (1961).

The technique originally described by Allen in 1985 (Fig. 56-15) is now the one most commonly performed. This involves complete resection of the corporocavernosal bodies, partial resection of the glans (reduction plasty), meticulous preservation of the dorsal neurovascular bundle and ventral bridge of skin, and complete preservation of the phallic skin with Byar's-like flaps to simultaneously recreate the labia minora, as described by Perlmutter (1979). As indicated previously, this is combined with a posterior-based U-shaped flap if the vagina joins the urogenital sinus in a low position distal to the rhabdourinary sphincter.

In 1982 Allen and co-workers undertook a review at the Hospital of Sick Children in Toronto of 42 patients who had a variety of procedures encompassing these techniques. Satisfactory cosmetic results and normal postoperative clitoral sensation were present

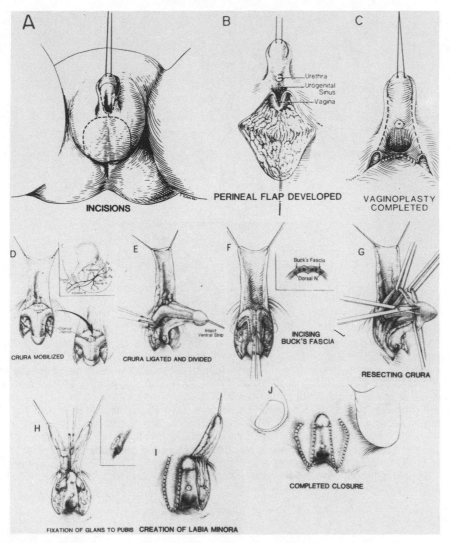

FIG. 56-15
Feminizing clitoroplasty. (From Snyder H, et al: *J Urol* 1983; 129:1025-1026. Used by permission.)

in all patients who had a reduction clitoroplasty and partial resection of the glans (Allen et al., 1982) (see Fig. 56-15). This surgery is best done in the first 3 to 6 months of life to afford a cosmetic appearance consistent with the female sex of rearing, and to allay apprehension on the part of the parents and embarrassment about hiring a babysitter.

Cases where the vagina joins the urogenital sinus proximal to the external sphincter require a significant increase in the complexity of the surgery. As indicated previously, this must be diagnosed prior to planning any surgery.

At the time of initial evaluation, in a small number of children, the vaginal and urethral orifices will be confluent on the perineum. Hendren (1986) has observed that in some of these cases, the vagina joins the urethra proximal to the external urethral sphincter. These children constitute a small minority of the masculinized females, but it is imperative to recognize this and avoid any further injury to the continence

mechanism. This may be deficient, however, and require later bladder neck reconstruction. Hendren and Crawford (1969) advocated an extensive introital reconstruction utilizing a vaginal pull-down technique and perineal-based skin flaps. They noted the need for long-term vaginal dilation using Hagar dilators, with subsequent surgical revision in some cases. The search continues for a more cosmetically acceptable and more functionally successful method of vaginoplasty for these cases. A recent publication by Passerini-Glazel (1989) offers such an option. He described a transvesical approach to accomplish, under direct vision, the separation of the vagina from the urethra. Following this separation, the phallic skin, which has been previously tubularized along with a portion of the urethra, is anastomosed, again under direct vision, to the proximal vaginal stump (see Fig. 56-16 to 56-20). This procedure, although described in only four cases, has the advantage of interposing vascularized genital skin between the introital verge

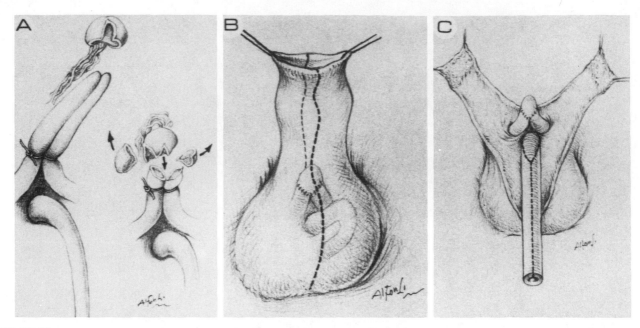

FIG. 56-16

A, Initial stage of clitoral reduction. After the phallus is degloved, a plane of cleavage is developed between the corpora and dorsal neurovascular bundle dorsally and between the corpora and urogenital sinus ventrally. Dissection is continued to separate the tip of the corpora from glandular tissue. The urogenital sinus also is detached from the glans. Neurovascular bundle remains connected to the glans, which appears as the concave cap. Care must be taken to avoid traction on the neurovascular bundle so that vascular spasm does not occur. Should this happen, papaverine may be used to treat it. The glans is then reduced by incising two lateral wedges. The corpora cavernosa are ligated proximally and resected 0.5 cm above the tie. The urogenital sinus is preserved. **B,** After the reduced glans is sutured to the corporal stumps, the phallic cutaneous cylinder is divided dorsally and ventrally. Ventrally the incision is extended to the bottom of the labioscrotal folds where it terminates with a small inserted V flap. Care is taken to preserve the preputial skin. **C,** The urogenital sinus is then incised. A small dorsal flap is created at the proximal end of incision. (From Passerini-Glazel G: A new technique for vaginal reconstruction in severely masculinized female pseudohermaphrodites. *J Urol* 1989; 142(part 2): 565. Used by permission.)

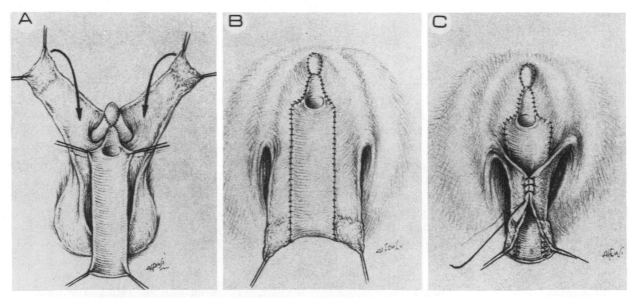

FIG. 56-17

A, The Y urethra is open, and a small "urethral" flap is sutured to the clitoris to create a mucosal lining below the clitoris. **B,** Cutaneous flaps of phallus are then rotated downward and sutured side by side to the urethra so that a mucocutaneous plate is obtained. **C,** Distal portion of the mucocutaneous plate is converted into a cylinder whose inner surface is mucocutaneous. (From Passerini-Glazel G: A new technique for vaginal reconstruction in severely masculinized female pseudohermaphrodites. *J Urol* 1989; 142(part 2): 566. Used by permission.)

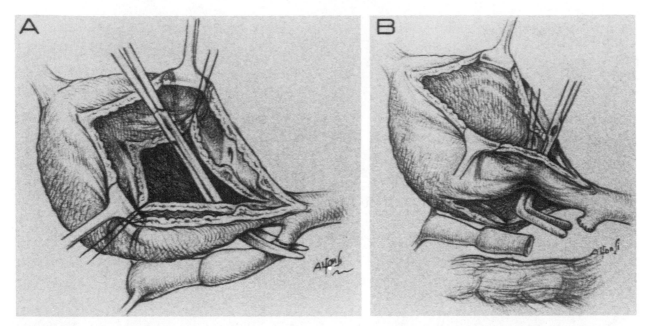

FIG. 56-18
A, If the perineal approach to the vagina seems to be too difficult in cases of high vaginal insertion, one may select to approach the vagina transvesically as suggested by Monfort for the utricle. Posterior incision is carried out through trigone and, if necessary, extended to the bladder neck. The vagina is then easily disconnected from its urethral insertion, with care taken to leave the vaginal stump as short as possible. **B,** The vaginal stump must be sutured. This is done by placing the first stitch at the superior end of the stump and placing continuous suture as disconnection is advanced. Space is then developed from above and between the urethra and rectum. (From Passerini-Glazel G: A new technique for vaginal reconstruction in severely masculinized female pseudohermaphrodites. *J Urol* 1989; 142(part 2):566. Used by permission.)

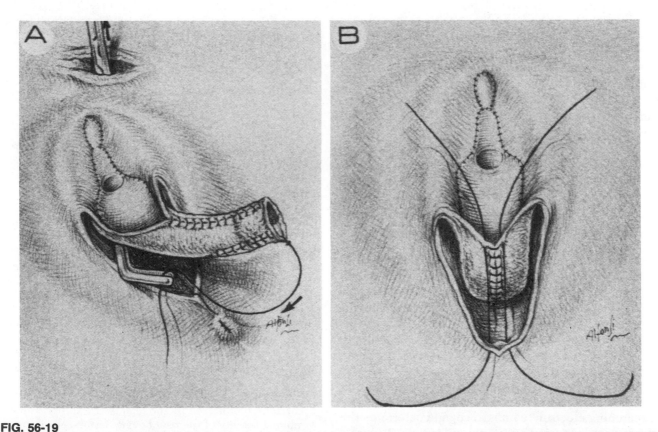

FIG. 56-19
A, If the transtrigonal approach is chosen, the mucocutaneous cylinder is drawn into the interurethral-rectal space and sutured transvesically under direct vision to the detached vagina. **B,** The perineal opening of the vagina is completed by suturing the outer end of the tube to the perineal and "scotal" skin. (From Passerini-Glazel G: A new technique for vaginal reconstruction in severely masculinized female pseudohermaphrodites. *J Urol* 1989; 142(part 2):566. Used by permission.)

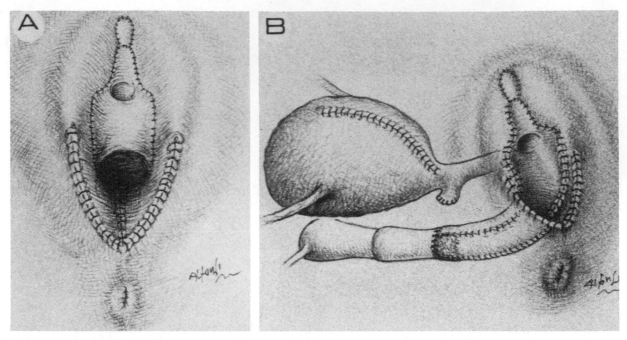

FIG. 56-20
A, Final view of introitus vaginalis. The anterior wall of the reconstructed distal vagina, from the clitoris to its connection with the true vagina, is completely lined by cutaneous surface. **B,** Schema of completed reconstruction. (From Passerini-Glazel G: A new technique for vaginal reconstruction in severely masculinized female pseudohermaphrodites. *J Urol* 1989; 142(part 2):566. Used by permission.)

and the proximal vagina. In these patients the surgical reconstruction is best performed at a later age, around 2 years of age.

An additional subgroup of patients, with more extensive cloacal or urogenital sinus malformations with or without imperforate anus, is also occasionally seen. Surgical repair of these cases is best done using the posterior sagittal approach advocated by Pena (1989) and Hendren (1986). At the time of puberty a number of these children require some form of vaginoplasty to allow normal menses and subsequent sexual intercourse. Many will have had prior perineal surgery, and in such cases a more extensive pull-through vaginoplasty may be required using inlay skin flaps or, if these are insufficient, full- or partial-thickness skin grafts or the interposition of a segment of bowel. The use of a silastic prosthesis is advocated to maintain patency of the newly created vagina in the postoperative period. A vascularized myocutaneous gracilis muscle flap can be used to interpose vascularized tissue for a child requiring an extensive vaginoplasty. This technique may also be successful in the more complex cases.

In summary, it is necessary to establish an exact diagnosis, provide emergency treatment for life-threatening electrolyte imbalance, and determine the optimal sex of rearing, promptly and exactly. This family crisis should be addressed with support and diligent expertise. Specific therapy should be instituted promptly and very careful follow-up maintained for all cases of intersex.

REFERENCES

Allen LE, Hardy BE, Churchill BM: The surgical management of enlarged clitoris. *J Urol* 1982; 128:351.

Allen T: Disorder of sexual differentiation. *Urology* 1976; 7(suppl):1.

Allen T: Disorder of sexual differentiation, in Kelalis PP, King LR, Belman AB (eds): *Clinical Pediatric Urology*, ed 2. Philadelphia, WB Saunders, 1985, pp 904-921.

Barr ML, Bertram EG: A morphological distinction between neurones of male and female, and the behaviour of the nucleolar satellite during acceleration of nucleoprotein synthesis. *Nature* 1949; 163:676.

Beheshti M, Churchill BM, Hardy BE, et al: Gender assignment in male pseudohermaphrodite children. *Urology* 1983; 22:604.

Beheshti M, Churchill BM, Hardy BE, et al: Familial persistant Müllerian duct syndrome. *J Urol* 1984; 131:968.

Behringer RR, Cate RL, Froelick GJ, et al: Abnormal sexual development in transgenic mice chronically expressing Müllerian inhibiting substance. *Nature* 1990; 345:167.

Blanchard MG, Josso N: Source of the anti-Müllerian hormone synthesized by the fetal testis: Müllerian-inhibiting activity of the fetal bovine Sertoli-cells in tissue culture. *Pediatr Res* 1974; 8:968.

Brown TR, Maes M, Rothwell SW, et al: Human complete androgen insensitivity with normal dihydrotestosterone receptor binding capacity in cultured genital skin fibroblasts: evidence for a qualitative abnormality of the receptor. *J Clin Endocrinol Metab* 1982; 55:61.

Bulmer D: The development of the human vagina. *J Anat* 1957; 91:490.

Burgoyne PS, Buehr M, Koopman R, et al: Cell autonomous action of the testis determining gene: Sertoli cells are exclusively XY in XX-XY chimeric mouse testes. *Development* 1988; 102:445.

Byskov AG: Regulation of meiosis in mammals. *Ann Biol Anim Biochim Biophys* 1979; 19:1251-1261.

Byskov AG: Differentiation of mammalian embryonic gonad. *Physiol Rev* 1986; 66:117.

Cohen-Haguenauer O, Picard JY, Mattei MG, et al: Mapping of the gene for anti-müllerian hormone to the short arm of human chromosome 19. *Cytogenet Cell Genet* 1987; 44:2.

Conte FA, Grumbach MM: Abnormalities of sexual differentiation, in Smith DR (ed): *General Urology*. Los Altos, Calif, Lange Medical Publications, 1984, pp 574-597.

de la Chapelle A, Page D, Brown L, et al: The origin of the 45,X males. *Am J Hum Genet* 1986; 38:17.

Donahoe PK: The diagnosis and treatment of infants with intersex abnormalities, in Sheldon CA, Churchill BM (eds): *Pediatric Clinic of North America*. Philadelphia, WB Saunders, 1988, pp 1333-1348.

Donahoe PK, Hendren WH: Intersex abnormalities in the newborn infant, in Holder TF, Ashcraft KW (eds): *Pediatric Surgery*. Philadelphia, WB Saunders, 1980, pp 858-890.

Donahoe PK, Hendren WH: Perineal reconstruction in ambiguous genitalia infants raised as females. *Ann Surg* 1984; 200:363.

Donahoe PK, Ito Y, Price JM, et al: Mullerian-inhibiting substance activity in bovine fetal, newborn and prepubertal testes. *Biol Reprod* 1977; 16:238-243.

Eichwald EJ, Silmser CR: Communication. *Transplantation* 1955; 2:148.

Fajer AB, Schneider J, McCall D, et al: The induction of meiosis by ovaries of newborn hamsters and its relation to the action of the extra-ovarian structures in the mesovarium. *Ann Biol Anim Biochim Biophys* 1979; 19:1273.

Feldman KW, Smith DW: Fetal phallic growth and penile standards for newborn male infants. *J Pediatr* 1975; 86:395.

Feldman SR: Androgen insensitivity syndrome (testicular feminization): a model for understanding steroid hormone receptors. *J Am Acad Dermatol* 1992; 27:615.

Fujimoto T, Ukeshima A, Miyayana Y, et al: The primordial germ cells in amniotes: Their migration in vivo and behaviours in vitro, in Motta PM (ed): *Developments in Ultrastructure of Reproduction*, New York, Alan R Liss, 1988, vol 296.

George FW, Wilson JD: Conversion of androgen to estrogen by the fetal human ovary. *J Clin Endocrinol Metab* 1978b; 47:550.

Glenister TW: The development of the utricle and of the so-called middle lobe or median lobe of the human prostate. *J Anat* 1962; 96:443.

Goodfellow PN: Mapping the Y chromosome. *Development* 1987; 101(suppl):39.

Griffin JE: Androgen resistance: the clinical and molecular spectrum. *N Engl J Med* 1992; 326:611.

Griffin JE, Wilson JD: The syndromes of androgen resistance. *N Engl J Med* 1980; 320:198.

Gross RE, Randolph J, Crigler JF: Clitorestomy for sexual abnormalities, indications and technique. *J Surg* 1966; 59:300.

Gruenwald P: The relation of the growing müllerian duct to the wolffian duct and its importance for the genesis of malformation. *Anat Rec* 1941; 81:1.

Grumbach MM, Conte FA: Disorders of sex differentiation, in Williams RH: *Textbook of Endocrinology*. Philadelphia, WB Saunders, 1981, pp 423.

Grumbach MM, Norishima A, Taylor JH: Human sex chromosome abnormalities in relation to DNA replication and heterochromatinization. *Proc Natl Acad Sci USA* 1963; 49:581.

Guerrier D, Tran D, Vanderwinden JM, et al: The persistent müllerian duct syndrome: a molecular approach. *J Clin Endocrinol Metab* 1989; 68:46.

Hamilton WJ, Mossman HW: The urogenital system, in *Human Embryology: Prenatal Development of Form and Function*, ed 4. New York, Macmillan, 1976.

Hammerton JL: Standardization in human cytogenetics. *Cytogenet Cell Genet* 1975; 15(6):361-2.

Hawkins JR, Taylor A, Goodfellow PN, et al: Mutational analysis of SRY: nonsense and missense mutations in XY sex reversal. *Hum Genet* 1992; 88:471.

Hendren WH: Repair of cloacal anomalies: current techniques. *J Pediatr Surg* 1986; 21:1159.

Hendren WH, Crawford JD: Adrenogenital syndrome: the anatomy of the anomaly and its repair; some new concepts. *J Pediatr Surg* 1969; 4:49.

Hughes IA, Davies PAD: Neonatal endocrine and metabolic emergencies. *Clin Endocrinol Metab* 1980; 9:583.

Hughes IA, Evans BAJ: The fibroblast as a model for androgen resistant states. *J Clin Endocrinol Metab* 1988; 28:565.

Imperato-McGinley J, Gauthier T, Pichardo M, et al: The diagnosis of 5α-reductase deficiency in infancy. *J Clin Endocrinol Metab* 1986; 63:1313.

Imperato-McGinley J, Guerrero L, Gauthier T, et al: Steroid 5α-reductase deficiency in men: an inherited form of male pseudohermaphrodism. *Science* 1974; 186:1213.

Janne OA, Shan LX: Structure and function of the androgen receptor. *Ann N Y Acad Sci* 1992; 626:81-91.

Jost A: The role of fetal hormones in prenatal development. *Harvey Lect* 1960; 55:201.

Jost A: Embryonic sexual differentiation (morphology, physiology, abnormalities), in Jones HW, Scoot WW (eds): *Hermaphroditism, Genital Anomalies and Related Endocrine Disorders*, Baltimore, Williams & Wilkins, 1971, p 16.

Jost A: A new look at the mechanism controlling sex differentiation in mammals. *Johns Hopkins Med J* 1972; 130:38.

Kellklumpu-Lehtinen P: Development of sexual dimorphism in human urogenital sinus complex. *Biol Neonate* 1985; 43:157.

Klinefelter HF Jr, Reinstein EC Jr, Albright F: Syndrome characterized by gynecomastia, aspermatogenesis without A-leydigism, and increased excretion of follicle-stimulating hormone. *J Clin Endocrinol* 1942; 2:615.

Koopman P, Gubbay J, Goodfellow P, et al: Male development of chromosomally female mice transgenic for SRY. *Nature* 1990; 351:117.

Lalau-Keraly J, Amice V, Chaussain JL, et al: L'hermaphrodisme vrai. *Semin Hosp Paris* 1986; 62:2375.

Larrea F, Lisker R, Bañuelos R, et al: Hypergonadotrophic hypogonadism in an XX female subject due to 17, 20 steroid desmolase deficiency. *Acta Endocrinol* 1983; 103:400.

Lattimer JK: Relocation and recession of the enlarged clitoris with preservation of the gland: an alternative to amputation. *J Urol* 1961; 86:113.

Lorge F, Wese FX, Sluysmans TH, et al: L'ambiguité sexuelle: aspects urologiques. *Acta Urol Belg* 1989; 57:647.

Luks FI, Hansbrough F, Klotz DH Jr, et al: Early gender assignment in true hermaphroditism. *J Pediatr Surg* 1988; 23:1122.

Magenis RE, Casanova M, Fellous M, et al: Further cytological evidence for Xp-Yp translocation in XX males using in situ hybridization with Y-derived probe. *Hum Genet* 1987; 75:228.

Mauch RB, Thiedemann KU, Drews U: The vagina is formed by downgrowth of Wolffian and Müllerian ducts. Graphical reconstructions from normal and Tfm mouse embryos. *Anat Embryol (Berl)* 1985; 172:75.

Mayou BG, Armon P, Linderbaum RH: Pregnancy and childbirth in true hermaphrodite following reconstructive surgery. *Br J Obstet Gyncecol* 1978; 85:314.

McLaren A: Controlling events in meiosis. *Symp Soc Exp Biol* 1984; 38:7.

McPhaul MJ, Marcelli M, Tilley WD, et al: Androgen resistance caused by mutations in the androgen receptor gene. *FASEB J* 1991; 5:2910.

Mittwoch U: Males, females and hermaphrodites. *Ann Hum Genet* 1986; 50:103.

Moore CC, Grumbach MM: Sex determination and gonadogenesis: a transcription cascade of sex chromosome and autosome genes. *Semin Perinatol* 1992; 16:266.

Nagai Y, Ciccarese S, Ohno S, et al: The identification of human H-Y antigen and testicular transformation induced by its interaction with the receptor site of bovine fetal ovarian cells. *Differentiation* 1979; 13:155.

Narita O, Manba S, Nakanishi T, et al: *Obstet Gynecol* 1975; 45:593.

Ohno S, Nagai Y, Ciccarese S, et al: Testicular cells lysostripped of H-Y antigen: Dissociation and reorganization experiments of rat gonadal cells. *Cytogenet Cell Genet* 1978; 20:365.

Ohno S, Nagai Y, Ciccarese S: Testis-organizing H-Y antigen and the primary sex-determining mechanism of mammals. *Recent Prog Horm Res* 1979; 35:449.

Ohno S, Stapleton DW: Associative recognition of testis organizing H-Y antigen and immunological confusion. Unpublished findings, 1981.

Page DC, de la Chapelle A: The parental origin of X chromosomes in XX males determined using restriction fragment length polymorphisms. *Am J Hum Genet* 1984; 36:565.

Page DC, Mosher R, Simpson EM, et al: The sex-determining region of the human Y chromosome encodes a finger protein. *Cell* 1987; 51:1091.

Palmer MS, Sinclair AH, Berta P, et al: Genetic evidence that ZFY is not the testis-determining factor. *Nature* 1989; 342:937.

Passerini-Glazel G: A new technique for vaginal reconstruction in severely masculinized female pseudohermaphrodites. *J Urol* 1989; 142(part 2):565.

Pena A: The surgical management of persistent cloaca: results in 54 patients treated with a posterior sagittal approach. *J Pediatr Surg* 1989; 24:590.

Perlmutter AD: Management of intersexuality, in *Campbell's Urology*, ed 4. Philadelphia, WB Saunders, 1979, vol 2, 1535.

Petit C, de al Chapelle A, Levilliers J, et al: An abnormal terminal X-Y interchange accounts for most but not all cases of human XX maleness. *Cell* 1987; 49:595.

Picard JY, Benarous R, Guerrier D, et al: Cloning and expression of cDNA for anti-müllerian hormone. *Proc Natl Acad Sci USA* 1986; 83:5464.

Picard JY, Josso N: Purification of testicular anti-müllerian hormone allowing direct visualization of the pure glycoprotein and determination of yield and purification factor. *Cell Endocrinol* 1984; 35:23.

Rogulska R, Ozdzenski W, Komar A: Behaviour of mouse primordial germ cells in the chick embryo. *J Embryol Exp Morphol* 1971; 25:115.

Schwartz ID, Root AW: The Klinefelter syndrome of testicular dysgenesis. *J Clin Endocrinol Metab* 1991; 20(1): 889-8529.

Sloan WR, Walsh PC: Familial persistent müllerian duct syndrome. *J Urol*, 1976; 115(4):459.

Taketo T, Saeed J, Manganaro T, et al: Müllerian inhibiting substance production associated with loss of oocytes and testicular differentiation in the transplanted mouse XX gonadal primordium. *Biol Reprod* 1993; 49:13.

Tegenkamp TR, Brazzell JW, Tegenkamp I, et al: Pregnancy without benefit of reconstructive surgery in a bisexually active true hermaphrodite. *Am J Obstet Gynecol* 1979; 135:427.

Tho SPT, Layman LC, Lanclos KD, et al: Absence of the testicular determining factor gene SRY in XX true hermaphrodites and presence of this locus in most subjects with gonadal dysgenesis caused by Y aneuploidy. *Am J Obstet Gynecol* 1992; 176:1794.

Tran D, Picard JY, Campargue J, et al: Immunocytochemical detection of anti-müllerian hormone in Sertoli cells of various mammalian species including human. *J Histochem Cytochem* 1987; 35:733.

Van Niekerk WA: True hermaphroditism. *Pediatr Adolesc Endocrinol* 1981; 8:80.

Vigier B, Forest MG, Eychenne B, et al: Anti-Müllerian hormone produces endocrine sex reversal of fetal ovaries. *Proc Natl Acad Sci USA* 1989; 86:3684.

Vigier B, Watrin F, Magre S, et al: Purified bovine AMH induces a characteristic free martin effect in fetal rat prospective ovaries exposed to it in vitro. *Development* 1987; 100:43.

Wartenberg H: Structural aspects of gonadal differentiation in mammals and birds, in Muller U, Franke WW (eds): *Differentiation*. New York, Springer-Verlag, 1982, pp 64-71.

Wilson JD: Sexual differentiation. *Annu Rev Physiol* 1978; 40:279.

Wilson J: Syndromes of androgen resistance. *Biol Reprod* 1992; 46:168.

Wilson JD, Goldstein JL: Classification of hereditary disorders of sexual development, in Bergsma D (ed): *Genetic Forms of Hypogonadism*. Birth Defects Original Article Series, 1975, vol XI, pp 1-16.

Wilson JD, Siiteri PK: Developmental pattern of testosterone synthesis in the fetal gonad of the rabbit. *Endocrinology* 1973; 92:1182.

Wilson JD, Walsh PC: Disorders of sexual differentiation, in Harrison JH, Walsh PC, Gittes RF, et al (eds):

Campbell's Urology, ed 4. Philadelphia, WB Saunders, 1979, vol 2, p 1484.

Winter JSD, Faiman C, Reyes FI: Sex steroid production by the human fetus: its role in morphogenesis and control by gonadotrophins, in Blandau RJ, Bergma D (eds): *Morphogenesis and Malformation of the Genital System*. New York, Alan R Liss, 1977, pp 41-58.

Witschi E: Migration of the germ cells of human embryos from the yolk sac to the primitive gonadal fold. *Contrib Embryol* 1948; 32:67.

Wolfe J: Other genes of the Y chromosome. *Development* 1987; 101(suppl):117.

Zachmann M, Werder EA, Prader A: Two types of male pseudohermaphroditism due to 17,20-desmolase deficiency. *J Clin Endocrinol Metab* 1982; 55:487.

Zamboni L, Upadhyay S, Bezard J, et al: The role of the mesonephros in the development of the sheep testis and its excurrent pathways, in Byskov AG, Peters H (eds): *Development and Function of Reproductive Organs*. Amsterdam, Excerpta Medica, 1981, pp 31-40.

Zenzes MT, et al: Organization in vitro of ovarian cells into testicular structures. *Hum Genet* 1978a; 44:333.

CHAPTER 57

Pediatric Andrology

Stanley Kogan
Faruk Hadziselimovic
Stuart S. Howards
Howard M. Snyder III
Dale Huff

TESTICULAR DEVELOPMENT

Development of the Hypothalamus-Pituitary-Gonadal Axis

Testicular endocrine function is fully established only after puberty. However, even fetal and prepubertal testes function as male endocrine organs. Androgen production of the fetal testis advances the maturation of "gonostat" so that maturity is reached earlier in boys than in girls. At term and after birth mean testosterone levels in plasma are higher in male infants than in female infants. The high levels of luteinizing hormone (LH) and follicle-stimulating hormone (FSH) in the plasma during the first 6 months of life in male infants reach a peak around the second month of life and activate the hypothalamic-pituitary-testicular axis (Forest et al., 1973; Winter et al., 1976). From the seventh month onward and throughout childhood there is a sluggish interim phase during which the interrelationship among the three components of the regulatory axis—namely, the response of the pituitary to gonadotropin-releasing hormone (GnRH), the gonadal response to human chorionic gonadotropin (HCG), and the hypothalamic feedback mechanism—is different from that in adulthood. The plasma sex hormone concentrations are also different from those in the adult.

A peak in urine LH secretion between age 4 and 6 years (Waaler, 1979) parallels the appearance of well-developed juvenile Leydig cells. There is a simultaneous increase in the number of S_b Sertoli cells and B spermatogonia. Primary spermatocytes appear for the first time, indicating a link between the maturation of germ cells, Sertoli cells, and Leydig cells on the one hand and gonadotropin secretion on the other hand (Fig. 57-1).

The male gonad has only an inhibitory effect on the hypothalamus-pituitary-gonadal axis. Existence of the feedback mechanism in prepuberty is suggested by the fact that there is (1) an increase in FSH and compensatory hypertrophy of the descended testis in monorchid and some unilateral cryptorchid patients (Tato et al., 1979) and (2) an augmentation of FSH plasma levels in prepubertal gonadectomized patients (Winter and Faiman, 1972).

The onset of puberty is genetically determined and is related to the maturation of the organism as a whole, particularly of the central nervous system. At the central nervous system level decreasing sensitivity of the hypothalamic "gonostat," increasing stimulatory neurotransmitter production, and pulsatile LH release result in increasing GnRH release (Swerdloff and Heber, 1981). At the pituitary level increasing sensitivity to GnRH and an increasing LH/FSH ratio in response to GnRH occur, resulting in a higher production of gonadotropin, decreased gonad sensitivity to gonadotropin, and changes in androgen biosynthetic pathways (Swerdloff and Heber, 1981). Finally, Sertoli cells mature during this time. As a result of this transformation, testosterone production increases, and production of mature sperm begins.

During puberty in both sexes the LH response increases (Boyar et al., 1974). The FSH response increases similarly in boys but does not increase at puberty in girls.

The main cell types in the prepubertal test are Leydig cells within the interstitium, Sertoli cells and germ cells in the tubules, and fibroblasts surrounding the tubules. Each of these cell types develops differently during the prepubertal period, but there is a clear correlation between the developing stages of each of these cells and the age of the child.

The extensive description of the testicular development is important in understanding the pathophysiologic changes in cryptorchidism, varicocele, and testicular torsion.

Development of Leydig Cells

Immediately after birth numerous Leydig cells can be observed in the interstitium (Hadziselimovic et al., 1975; Hadziselimovic, 1977). Leydig cells are usually

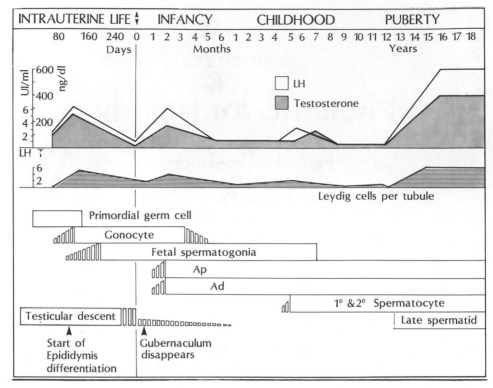

FIG. 57-1
Testicular development. LH and testosterone in relation to age.

arranged around the blood vessels, but no direct contact between Leydig cells and blood vessels is observed in either fetal or prepubertal testes. Well-developed fetal Leydig cells can be observed up to the fourth month of postnatal life, when the number decreases from three to one per tubule and the transformation from the fetal into the juvenile type of Leydig cells occurs (Fig. 57-2 and Fig. 57-3). In puberty, juvenile Leydig cells mature into the adult type (Fig. 57-3). Adult cells are larger than the juvenile Leydig cells. The round nucleus is located eccentrically in the cytoplasm. There is an abundance of smooth endoplasmic reticulum. For the first time crystals of Reinke are present. The number increases to an average of six Leydig cells per tubule (range 3.6 to 7.2 per tubule). Leydig cells are usually located in clusters around the blood vessels, and there is close contact between these cells and the capillaries. Their mitochondria contain the enzyme complex responsible for the conversion of cholesterol to pregnenolone. The smooth endoplasmic reticulum contains the enzyme complex that converts pregnenolone to testosterone. Testosterone concentration in blood plasma may not always reflect actual steroid secretion by the testis because it represents the net effect of production, degradation, and excretion of testosterone (Ewing, 1983). Testosterone levels in plasma increase from 400 mg/dl at age 12 to 17 years to 600 mg/dl in the second or third decade of life (Ewing, 1983). There is evidence suggesting that Leydig cells are a heteroge-

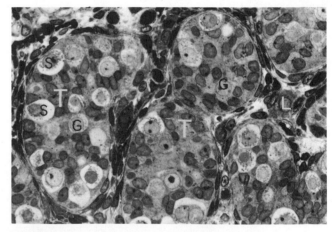

FIG. 57-2
Testicular histology of normal infant testis. Tubules *(T)*, gonocytes *(G)*, fetal spermatogonia *(S)*, and fetal Leydig cells *(L)*.

neous population with distinctly different physical, chemical, and morphologic characteristics (Hadziselimovic, 1977; Payne et al., 1980). These different Leydig cell types represent cells in varying stages of differentiation.

Sertoli Cells
Development

The most common cell found in the seminiferous tubule in the prepubertal period is the Sertoli cell.

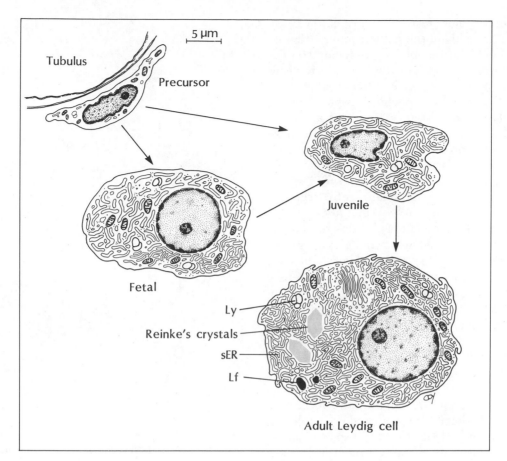

FIG. 57-3
Schematic representation of Leydig cell development.

Four different types can be observed during childhood: S_f, S_a, S_b, and S_c Steroli cells (Fig. 57-4) (Hadziselimovic and Seguchi, 1973; Hadziselimovic, 1976, 1977).

In the first year of life there are mainly two types of Sertoli cells, S_f and S_a. The S_f type is observed predominantly during the first 4 months of life; then there is a switch to the S_a type. This transformation is under hormonal control (Hadziselimovic, 1977). Around the fourth year of life the well-differentiated S_b type appears. With the beginning of puberty, transformation of S_a and S_b types into the S_c type takes place.

The phagocytic function is particularly well developed in fetal and adult Sertoli cells. The phagocytosed degenerating gonocytes or residual cytoplasm is digested by lysosomes that are also involved in the autolysis of degenerating cytoplasmic organelles (Hadziselimovic, 1976). A peculiar structure seen in adult Sertoli cells, the lamellar body, is always associated with lipoid droplets, indicating that this body may have a steroid-producing function as well as enzymatic digestive processes.

The S_f type is believed to produce müllerian-inhibiting substance, thus influencing the regression of the

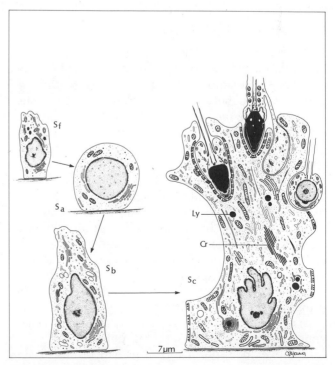

FIG. 57-4
Schematic display of Sertoli cell development.

müllerian duct in males (Jost, 1970; Jost et al., 1973). The S_a type is probably hormonally inactive, whereas the S_b type should be capable of producing steroids because of its well-developed cytoplasm. Sertoli cells are believed to be a target cell for FSH (Tindall et al., 1983). The FSH binds to specific receptors on the Sertoli cell plasma membrane, stimulates adenylate cyclase, activates soluble cyclic adenosine monophosphate–dependent protein kinase, and stimulates ribonucleic acid and protein synthesis (Means and Tindall, 1975; Means and Vaitukaitis, 1972). By affecting these intracellular components, FSH regulates specific protein secretions and cell motility.

FSH influences the production of androgen-binding protein by Sertoli cells. LH also stimulates androgen-binding protein activity to varying degrees in vivo, but this may be caused by its effects on testosterone synthesis (Tindall et al., 1983, 1977). Specific androgen receptors have been demonstrated in Sertoli cells and thus may be involved in testosterone effect on the germ cells (Tindall et al., 1977). When testosterone and FSH are administered together in vivo, an augmentation of androgen-binding protein response above that found with FSH alone is observed (French et al., 1974). γ-Glutamyl transpeptidase (GGTP) is a membrane protein that is also produced in Sertoli cells and may play an important role in transport of amino acids across the plasma membrane (Tindall et al., 1983; Sherins and Hodgen, 1976). FSH stimulates the production of GGTP in human testes (Tindall et al., 1983; Sherins and Hodgen, 1976). Thus the response of GGTP to FSH indicates that the human Sertoli cell is a target cell for FSH (Sherins and Hodgen, 1976).

Development of Germ Cells

The human germ cells are first recognizable among the endodermal cells of the caudal portion of the yolk sac near the allantoic stalk. During week 5 they migrate in an ameboid manner to the angle of the mesentery and the mesonephros (Falin, 1969). The stimulus that triggers the cells to migrate is unknown. The primordial germ cells are observable up to 145 days after conception.

Primordial germ cells differentiate into gonocytes by entering the testicular cords. Some gonocytes come to rest in the center of the seminiferous tubules and are phagocytosed by Sertoli cells. Other gonocytes attach to the basement membrane and give rise to the fetal spermatogonia. Fetal spermatogonia transform into the A type of spermatogonia during the third to fifth month of infancy. The B spermatogonia and the primary spermatocyte first appear during the fourth year of life (Fig. 57-5) (Huff et al., 1993). Spermatogenesis arrests at this stage until puberty (Fig. 57-6). Fully developed spermatogenesis may be observed in 13-year-old boys, and most 15-year-old boys have

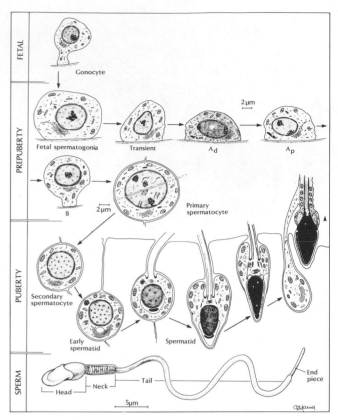

FIG. 57-5
Development and differentiation of germ cells from fetal life until puberty.

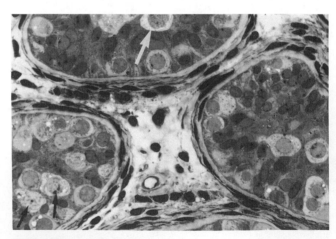

FIG. 57-6
Primary spermatocytes in normal testis of a 6-year-old boy *(arrows)*.

completed spermatogenesis. This period represents a timed event in which spermatogonia develop into spermatozoa. The duration of spermatogenesis in the adult male is suspected to be approximately 74 days (Heller and Clermont, 1964). Because of spermatogonial stem cell renewal, several generations of cells are always seen together in the same area of the seminiferous tubules. This process of differentiation is centripetal so that the more mature cells are found toward the center of the tubules. Six stages of germ cell differentiation are described for the human testis (see Fig. 57-5).

There are five major steps in male germ cell development. At the time of masculinization of the gonad, at 7 to 8 weeks of gestation, primordial germ cells differentiate into gonocytes. At 15 weeks of gestation, gonocytes begin to differentiate into fetal spermatogonia. At 60 to 90 days of postnatal life, gonocytes disappear and adult spermatogonia appear, possibly representing a switch from a fetal to an adult pool of stem cells (Huff et al., 1991). At 4 to 6 years, B spermatogonia and primary spermatocytes abortively appear. At puberty, spermatogenesis begins. Each of these steps is accompanied by surges in gonadotropin and testosterone levels, maturation and increased numbers of Leydig cells, and maturation of Sertoli cells (see Fig. 57-1).

Embryology of Scrotal Development

In embryos in the indifferent stage of sexual development, three protuberances can be observed. The genital tubercle is in front, and the genital swellings are on either side. The genital swellings give rise to the future scrotum. With growth the genital tubercle becomes enlarged and is transformed into the penis. The scrotum is filled with a relatively compact undifferentiated mesenchymal ground substance before testicular descent.

Three layers of spermatic cord are expanded into the scrotal direction (Fig. 57-7). The external spermatic fascia, as well as the cremasteric and internal spermatic fascia, are prolongations of the abdominal fasciae of the three muscle layers. Because the gubernaculum testis is never attached to the wall of the scrotum, the testis and the epididymis together with surrounding fascial sheaths are separated from the tunica dartos of the scrotal wall in the newborn male by a fascial cleft.

The processus vaginalis remains collapsed but patent in 66% of male infants up to 2 weeks of age (Crelin, 1973). The left processus usually becomes obliterated before the right (Crelin, 1973). In 80% of male infants between 10 and 20 days of age, the processus is partially, if not completely, obliterated (Crelin, 1973). After 3 weeks no gubernaculum can be found in the majority of infants with descended testes.

Embryology of Testicular Descent

During the fourth week of intrauterine life the mesonephros is derived from the intermediate mesoderm and extends to the lower cervical region in the posterior body wall down the full length of the embryo around the caudal curve to end at the future site of

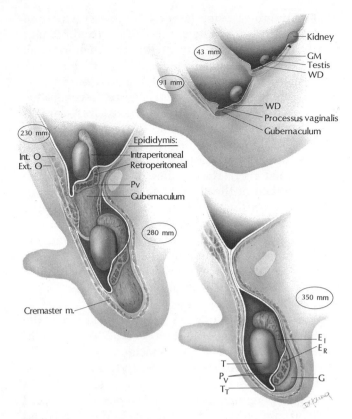

FIG. 57-7

Testicular descent in humans. The wolffian duct *(WD)* differentiates into the epididymis, which is clearly recognizable at 230 mm crown-rump length. The gubernaculum never herniates through the abdominal wall. *Int. O,* internal oblique abdominal muscle; *Ext. O,* external oblique; *Pv,* processus vaginalis; *T,* testis; *TT,* tunica dartos; *EI,* intraperitoneal section of epididymis; *ER,* extraperitoneal section of epididymis; *GM,* gubernaculum.

the internal ring in the inferior-anterior body wall. The gubernaculum and inguinal canal appear in the sixth week (Felix, 1912). With organization of the testis, differentiation and formation of the excretory duct take place by transformation of the wolffian duct and the mesonephric tubules into the epididymis, ductus deferens, and seminal vesicle. Organization of the wolffian duct is dependent on androgen produced by Leydig cells, and the regression of the müllerian duct is dependent on müllerian-inhibiting substance produced by fetal Sertoli cells. In the 43-mm crown-rump human male embryo (10.5 weeks), the mesonephros appears to hold the testis as if within forceps. The processus vaginalis at this time is recognizable as a small invagination at the level of a deep inguinal ring. Two ligaments on each end of the urogenital anlage can be encountered as a continuation of the mesonephros: cranially the diaphragmatic ligament and caudally the gubernaculum. Cranially the gubernaculum inserts onto the wolffian duct, and caudally it extends into the inguinal canal (Hadziselimovic, 1983).

At 90 mm crown-rump (around 14 weeks) important changes occur within the mesonephros. Its upper part is still in continuation with the dorsal abdominal wall over a threadlike elongated diaphragmatic ligament. The cranial portion of the epididymis starts to develop. The coiling of the wolffian duct is clearly recognizable at this stage of development. The processus vaginalis is deeper and broader, whereas the testis has a round shape (Hadziselimovic, 1983). At 17 weeks (125 mm crown-rump) the position of the gonad is deep within the inguinal ring (Hadziselimovic, 1983). With the disappearance of the diaphragmatic ligament the elevation of the long diameter of the testis into the vertical axis has occurred. Three portions of the epididymis are recognizable at this time: the caput, the cauda, and the corpus epididymis (Hadziselimovic, 1983). The epididymis now completely surrounds the testis. The gubernaculum is relatively longer and broader, its diameter equaling that of the gonad. At the peripheral part of the gubernaculum the cremaster muscle fibers are observed. No encroachment into the central gubernaculum substance by the cremaster muscle has occurred. Furthermore, there is no distinct expansion of the gubernaculum outside the inguinal canal. At 26 weeks of embryonal life (230 mm crown-rump) the position of the gonad is still unchanged. The absolute dimensions of both testis and gubernaculum have increased. The epididymis is further developed, and its caput now lies at the entrance to the inguinal canal. At no time during testicular descent does the gubernaculum herniate the abdominal wall; it is always within the testicular coverings. At 40 weeks of gestation, testicular descent is terminated (Hadziselimovic, 1983) (see Fig. 57-7).

Mechanism of Testicular Descent

Role of the Gubernaculum

Since John Hunter's description of testicular descent, there have been ongoing attempts to establish definitively the key role of the gubernaculum in testicular descent, irrespective of the fact that testicular descent occurs in the absence of the gubernaculum. Many theories have been postulated, and the six most recent hypotheses are discussed here.

1. Wensing (1973) described the gubernacular swelling as being a motor of testicular descent. Although testicular descent was originally stated to be androgen independent, recent experiments of his group found that the first part of the descent is androgen dependent, whereas the swelling of gubernaculum, which actively should take the testis down, is dependent on an unknown testicular factor (Wensing, 1973; Baumans et al., 1983). The main evidence against this theory is that if the testis is removed and its tissue replaced by a paraffin ball, descent occurs

after the administration of androgens (Martins, 1938; Backhouse, 1981). Also, no balloonlike swelling has ever been observed in either humans or rats, despite epididymotesticular descent (Hadziselimovic, 1983).

2. In 1981 Elder and co-workers described a gubernaculum of meandering shape during testicular descent in rabbits. This gubernacular configuration is postulated to create a downward force on the testes and epididymides, causing descent into the scrotum, an event under dihydrotestosterone control (Rajfer and Walsh, 1977; Elder et al., 1981). This explanation is not universally accepted because in humans, mice, and rats, there is no meandering-shaped gubernaculum during testicular descent (Hadziselimovic and Kruslin, 1979; Hadziselimovic, 1981; Kruslin, 1981).

3. Between 1979 and 1981 attention was focused on the cremaster muscle, and serious endeavors were made to show that the development of the processus vaginalis and the growth of the cremaster muscle under androgen influence were responsible for epididymotesticular descent (Backhouse, 1981). According to this theory, testicular descent in humans is not associated with any of the contractile forces described by the classical theory of fibromuscular gubernacular traction. Instead there is maintenance of a primitive mesenchymatous core lacking skeletal muscle in the inguinal and scrotal regions that are not encroached by the developing body and scrotal wall structure (Backhouse, 1981). The processus vaginalis, according to this hypothesis, must be adequately developed as a prerequisite for testicular descent. However, from clinical and experimental points of view, it is uncommon to find a deficiency in the growth of the processus vaginalis and cremaster muscle as the only feature of a cryptorchid state unless there is a mechanical barrier to their development (Backhouse, 1981).

4. Recently a "water trap" theory has been advanced to explain downward movement of the epididymotesticular unit (Heynes and DeKlerk, 1985). According to this hypothesis, the marked swelling of the gubernaculum, which dilates the inguinal canal and scrotum, may passively exert traction on the testis by the force of its expansion, which is largely caused by an accumulation of water within the gubernaculum. This process is postulated to be mediated by the intracellular glycosaminoglycans (Heynes and DeKlerk, 1985).

5. Weil's hypothesis of intraabdominal pressure was popular in the period from 1969 to 1975 and has received attention again recently (Weil, 1884; Gier and Marion, 1969; Frey et al., 1983). However, the finding that in boys with omphaloceles testicular descent occurs normally if there are no brain malformations strongly refutes this theory (Hadziselimovic et al., 1987).

6. A biphasic model of testicular descent has been proposed in which an initial phase of transabdominal descent (possibly under the influence of müllerian inhibitory substance) is followed by the final phase of inguinal-scrotal descent effected by active gubernacular undulation and migration (possibly under the influence of calcitonin gene–related peptide released from the genitofemoral nucleus and nerve) (Hutson and Beasley, 1992). However, MIS knock-out mice demonstrate normal testicular descent and normal male germ cell development (Behringer et al., 1994).

In all of the preceding theories, the argument that the gubernaculum has a key role in epididymotesticular descent fails to explain why hormonal treatment, when no gubernaculum exists, induces testicular descent (e.g., prepubertal cryptorchid boys).

However, in mammals with an inguinal canal, the gubernaculum has a definite role in influencing the dilation of the canal and permitting the epididymis to descend, as well as in serving as a guide. No other functions of the gubernaculum in epididymotesticular descent have been proved. The active force in descent in some mammalian species, including humans, is the epididymis pushing, but not pulling, the testis into the scrotum (Hadziselimovic, 1981, 1983).

CRYPTORCHIDISM

Incidence

Cryptorchidism is the most common disorder of the endocrine gland. Available data suggest that the incidence of cryptorchidism in premature boys is 9.2% to 30.0%, whereas the incidence of cryptorchidism in full-term boys is 3.4% to 5.8% (Kleinteich et al., 1979; Scorer and Farrington, 1971). Kleinteich and colleagues (1979) have combined several previous studies and found that after 1 year, 1.82% of 88,526 patients had undescended testes. The percentage remained the same until puberty. Scorer and Farrington (1971), however, found at the end of 12 months that 28 of 3612 babies (0.8%) still had cryptorchidism, and the incidence remained the same up to puberty. These findings underline that after the first year spontaneous descent is unlikely to occur.

Cryptorchidism, or incomplete testicular descent, can be described as unilateral or bilateral, and the position of the testis as abdominal, inguinal, prescrotal, or gliding. The gliding testis is not a retractile testis but rather one that upon being manipulated to the upper portion of the scrotum immediately retracts. However, these testes have the same histology as the cryptorchid testes arrested in their true line of descent, in contrast to true ectopic testes, which have a normal histology. Therefore, the term *ectopic testis* should be used only for those testes that descend normally through the external inguinal ring but are mis-directed in their subsequent descent to perineal, prepenile, transverse scrotal, femoral, or umbilical positions.

One third of boys with true cryptorchidism have bilateral cryptorchid testes; two thirds are unilateral. The right side seems to be more often affected (70%) than the left side (30%) (Kleinteich et al., 1979). Abdominal cryptorchidism has been found in 8%, inguinal cryptorchidism in 72%, and prescrotal cryptorchidism in 20%. In 2.6% (156 of 6127), testicular aplasia or anorchia has been observed (Kleinteich et al., 1979).

Examination Technique

Every general pediatric examination in boys should include examination of the testicular position. The room and the examiner's hands have to be warm, the boy being examined should be given time to relax, and the examination should not be hurried. If cryptorchidism is suspected, the patient should be examined in the cross-legged position (Fig. 57-8). Once the patient is sitting comfortably in this position, most retractile testes descend spontaneously without being manipulated by the examiner. The gonad may be manipulated gently into the scrotum with the thumb and forefinger. Another helpful approach, particularly in older boys, is application of pressure on the femoral artery in the groin. If the testis is retractile, it should immediately descend and remain in the scrotum for a while. Testicular volume can be established by estimating the length and short diameter of the testis or by measuring the testis with an orchidometer. Gonads that do descend into the upper portion of the scrotum but immediately upon release return to the prescrotal position are gliding testes and need to be treated.

High scrotal testes have an increased tendency to glide, and the scrotum may be less developed on the affected side. The management of these high scrotal testes is difficult. Most have normal histology, but in a small proportion considerable damage to the gonad develops with time. Therefore, a careful annual check of the development and position of these gonads is recommended. If any doubt concerning lack of proper growth and position arises, hormonal treatment should be started, particularly if the testis becomes a gliding one.

Indications for Treatment

Once cryptorchidism is diagnosed, early treatment (age 10 months) should be started. The main reasons for early treatment are increased infertility in both unilateral and bilateral cryptorchid patients, increased malignancy rate, and an increased risk of developing testicular torsion. Psychologic problems because of an empty sac are also important. The pediatrician should be able to recognize cryptorchidism and the devel-

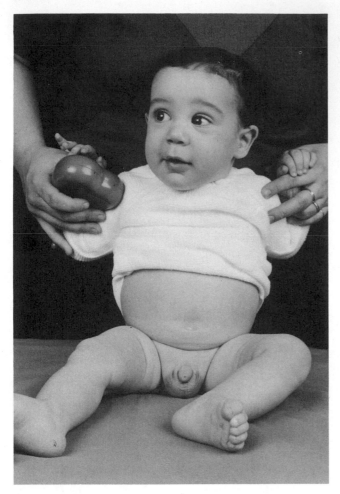

FIG. 57-8
Relaxed patient seated in "cross-legged" position before genital examination.

opment of psychologic difficulties, reassure parents, and commence any necessary treatment.

Histology of the Cryptorchid Testis

The histology of Leydig cells is one of the criteria that enables differentiation between the retractile infant testis and the true cryptorchid testis. In the cryptorchid testis, the number of Leydig cells is diminished and their appearance is atrophic, whereas in boys with retractile testes the number and appearance of Leydig cells are normal. Gonadotropin deficiency in cryptorchid boys stops the transformation from A to B spermatogonia and influences the multiplication of the germ cells to a certain extent. This impairment of transformation of spermatogonia, which is caused by deficient hormone stimulation, becomes apparent if iatrogenic cryptorchidism (after hernia repair) is compared with true cryptorchidism (Hadziselimovic, 1983). Although the iatrogenic cryptorchid testes have the same maldescended position as true cryptorchid testes, transformation from A to B spermatogonia occurs even after years of unfavorable positioning. Be-

fore age 6 years in iatrogenic cryptorchidism, the number of the germ cells is within the normal range.

The difference in germ cell number and differentiation between true cryptorchidism and iatrogenic cryptorchidism in the first 6 years of life is mainly the result of hormonal understimulation, and not of the unfavorable position. However, in iatrogenic cryptorchid testes, early pathologic changes can be observed in the second year of life. Vacuolization of the germ cells takes place, indicating a subtle pathologic change resulting from an unfavorable position.

Furthermore, in cases in which the duration of a secondary cryptorchid state lasts until puberty, atrophy of Sertoli and Leydig cells and impaired transformation of Sertoli cells are evident. This lack of transformation seems to be connected to both the occurrence of complete spermatogenesis and the hormone stimulation. This, however, should not be interpreted as a congenital inability of Sertoli cell to undergo transformation.

Number of Spermatogonia in Cryptorchid Gonads in Relation to Age

The most important observation relating to the germ cell content of cryptorchid testes is that within the first 6 months of life the number of germ cells is within the normal range in all cryptorchid testes. In normally descended testes the number of spermatogonia increases from 50 to 100 germ cells per 50 tubules in the first months after birth. In cryptorchid testes, however, the number of spermatogonia remains low and does not increase with age, although the total number of germ cells is comparable with that in an infant having normally descended testes (Fig. 57-9). This fact gives evidence for the lack of transformation of gonocytes into spermatogonia in the cryptorchid testis. The normal postnatal development of Leydig cells and transformation from gonocytes into spermatogonia parallels the luteinizing hormone (LH) and follicle-stimulating hormone (FSH) increase in the first few months of life. The activation of the gonadal axis not only is responsible for setting the "gonadostat" but also is a prerequisite for adequate testicular development. The latter, however, is lacking in cryptorchid testes.

As early as the second year of life, 38% of unilateral and bilateral cryptorchid testes have completely lost their germ cells as a result of impaired transformation of gonocytes. The development of the germ cells in cryptorchid gonads from the second year of life, in general, remains severely inhibited. The mean number of spermatogonia per tubule remains constant at 0.38 per tubule.

In bilateral cryptorchid testes the mean number of germ cells is 0.25 per tubule on the right side and 0.26 on the left side. There is a positive correlation between the number of germ cells in the left and right

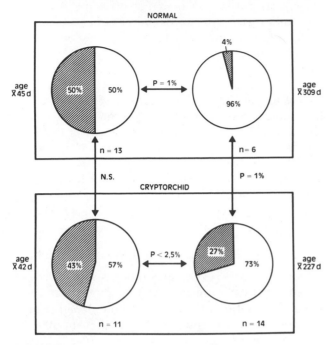

GONOCYTES ▨ / SPERMATOGONIA ▢ RATIO IN NORMAL AND CRYPTORCHID TESTES DURING FIRST 18 mth

FIG. 57-9

Circles show the total number of germ cells in two separate periods of infancy in normal and cryptorchid testes. Mean values of the total number of germ cells for cryptorchid testes [$\bar{x}$ (42) = 215 ± 105], [$\bar{x}$ (227 d) = 82.5 ± 55] and for normal testes [$\bar{x}$ (45 d) = 225 ± 25], [$\bar{x}$ (309 d) = 105 ± 3.9] do not differ significantly. The percentage of gonocytes *(hatched)* and spermatogenia *(blank)* is given for each group. There is significantly impaired transformation of gonocytes into spermatogonia in cryptorchid boys. (Type I error is given in percent per Wilcoxon-Mann-Whitney U test.)

testes (p <0.01). Descended contralateral testes in unilateral cryptorchidism have a germ cell count within the low normal range. Identical correlations are seen in unilateral cryptorchid prepubertal patients and in bilateral cryptorchidism. This correlation is evidence that there is a quantitative but not a qualitative difference between unilateral and bilateral cryptorchidism. The findings also refute the mechanical theory that has been put forward for unilateral cryptorchidism. Moreover, the fact that cryptorchid boys with no germ cells in their testes possess the lowest gonadotropin values supports the premise of hormonal involvement in the cause of cryptorchidism (Hadziselimovic et al., 1979).

There is a significant positive correlation between the number of germ cells in the prepubertal testes and the number of normal sperm and the sperm count after puberty. This correlation indicates that surgery performed in prepuberty has mainly cosmetic value for those boys with no germ cells in their gonads at the time of orchiopexy (Hadziselimovic, 1984b).

Recent successful treatment with buserelin (a

GNRH analog) in this particular group of patients indicates that it is possible to raise the number of germ cells by substituting this hormone for a period of 6 months after surgery (Hadziselimovic et al., 1984a). Therefore, the biopsy during orchiopexy has not only prognostic value but also may have additional therapeutic implications.

Histology in Relation to Position of the Testis

The tubular fertility index (the number of tubules with germ cells) and the number of the spermatogonia per tubule change considerably with the position of the testicles. The higher the testis is located, the worse is its histology (Scorer and Farrington, 1971; Hadziselimovic, 1983). Although an intraabdominally located testis within the first 6 months of life has germ cell numbers in the normal range, before the onset of puberty more than 90% of all intraabdominally located testes completely lose their germ cells. In inguinal and prescrotal testes a total absence of the germ cells was noted in 41% and 20% of the patients, respectively (Hadziselimovic, 1983).

Changes in the Peritubular Connective Tissue Resulting from the Undescended Position of the Testis

The first change in the peritubular connective tissue takes place in the second year, when the collagen fiber layers show an increase in collagen fibers, although the layer is not yet wider than in normal contralateral testes of the same age. The changes in peritubular connective tissue are more pronounced by age 3 years. The collagen fiber layer is broader and more dense than that of the control subjects. The fibers lie close together, and their diameter appears greater than in a normal testis. Collagenization and widening of the tunica propria increase with age in cryptorchid testes. By puberty in cryptorchid testes the collagen fiber layer has become wider, and the collagen fibers are not arranged in an orderly fashion. The six to seven cellular layers around the seminiferous tubules are reduced to two or three. The ring of cells that should entirely surround the tubule is imperfectly formed, the cells being grouped together in clumps. Their processes are only partially developed, and the transformation from fibroblasts into myofibroblasts and the marked fibrosis of peritubular connective tissue make the tubule incapable of contraction. Also, the large mucopolysaccharide deposits induced by fibrosis hinder the exchange of substances between the seminiferous tubules and the interstitium and thereby induce more pathologic changes within the tubules (Hadziselimovic and Seguchi, 1973).

Cryptorchid Testis and Malignant Changes

It has been well documented that there is an increased incidence of malignant disease of the testis associated with cryptorchidism. The combined risk for all cryptorchid males, irrespective of the location of the testes, is 20 to 46 times greater than for patients with normally located testes. The risk of tumor development in patients with cryptorchidism is 48.9 per 100,000 per year, which represents a 22.2-fold increase over the risk in those patients with scrotal testes, in whom the incidence of malignant neoplasm is 2.2 per 100,000 per year. Abdominal undescended testes show a fourfold increased risk over inguinal undescended testes (Cromie, 1983).

In a case-control study of 108 cases of testicular cancer in men younger than age 30 years, cryptorchidism was a major risk factor, with a relative risk (RR) equal to 9.0 (Depue et al., 1983). The multiple factors that affect germ cell development may result in various degrees of atrophy and tubular dysgenesis, which may later result in malignant changes (Cromie, 1983).

Clinical Evidence of Endocrine Dysfunction

The success of hormonal treatment and the increased incidence of cryptorchid testes in congenital hypogonadotrophic hypogonadism and in male pseudohermaphroditism clearly point to hormonal involvement in testicular descent. Based on our study, the overall incidence of cryptorchidism in male infants with omphalocele was 52% (10 of 19). However, analyzing patients according to the occurrence of neural tube defects led to completely different results. All boys with both omphalocele and neural tube defects or malformations of the brain had cryptorchidism, whereas only 2 of 10 boys with omphalocele but no brain malformations had unilateral nondescent. The presence of an omphalocele in a fetus should prevent the normal increase in intraabdominal pressure from occurring. The fact that testicular descent occurred in the group of infants with omphalocele and normal brain development fails to support the theory that normally increasing intraabdominal pressure in the fetuses is the main cause of testicular descent. Moreover, it is well known that cryptorchidism is frequently observed in boys with different kinds of cerebral lesions. Cortada and Kousseff (1984) found that the incidence of cryptorchidism is 33% in hospitalized children with mental retardation. Bilateral cryptorchidism was more common in this group of patients than unilateral cryptorchidism, suggesting that a malfunction of the hypothalamic-pituitary-gonadal axis is the common denominator.

Furthermore, of children with meningomyelocele, 23% (6 of 23) had maldescended testes. When the bony defect was above L2, the incidence was 50%. Whereas 67% of all meningomyelocele children had hydrocephalus, it was present in all meningomyelocele children with cryptorchidism (Kropp and Voeller, 1981).

Biochemical Evidence for Hormonal Involvement

A normal increase in plasma testosterone in the early postnatal period does not occur in most boys with undescended testes (Gendrel et al., 1978). Furthermore, an impaired LH and FSH response to gonadotropin-releasing hormone (GnRH) has been observed in boys with cryptorchidism (Canlorbe et al., 1974). Finally, impaired testicular testosterone response to human chorionic gonadotropin (HCG) has also been noted in cryptorchid boys (Forest, 1971). This deficiency of LH and consequently of testosterone secretion disappears after puberty (Canlorbe et al., 1974). However, according to our study, some of the patients with the most pronounced hypogonadotrophic hypogonadism in prepuberty develop hypergonadotrophic hypogonadism after puberty (Hadziselimovic et al., 1984b).

Experimental Evidence for Hormonal Dysfunction

Evidence from several experiments shows that impaired testicular descent is caused by deficient hormonal stimulation. Estradiol treatment of pregnant mice resulted in cryptorchidism of 90% to 100% of male offspring (Raynaud, 1942). Testicular testosterone and serum testosterone levels were decreased in these animals (Hadziselimovic, 1977). Leydig cell atrophy was marked, and after puberty sterility was commonly found. When these mice were treated simultaneously with HCG, the cryptorchid position was corrected (Hadziselimovic, 1977, 1983; Hadziselimovic et al., 1976). This response indicates that gonadotropins are involved in the regulation of normal testicular descent.

The involvement of epididymis in the process of testicular descent has been shown experimentally by treatment of mutant mice with congenital GnRH deficiency with subcutaneous injection of GnRH for 14 days (Hadziselimovic, 1983). In 60% of mice, testicular descent occurred despite complete absence of any gubernacular swelling or changing within the gubernaculum stump. The originally observed Leydig cell atrophy was corrected with GnRH, and low testicular testosterone levels normalized after treatment. Testicular weights were unchanged after treatment, indicating that testicular weight is not essential for descent (Hadziselimovic, 1983). However, in mice that successfully responded to hormone treatment, the epididymis had a length not significantly different from the control mice, whereas before treatment the length of the epididymis was significantly shorter than in the control mice (Hadziselimovic, 1983).

Additional support for the theory linking the epididymis to epididymotesticular descent can be obtained from mice with testicular feminization. Although these mice have a gubernaculum, testicular descent does not take place because of the lack of wolffian duct structures, and the testes remain at the dorsal abdominal wall throughout life. Further evidence is obtained from experiments with ACI rats. Of adult ACI rats, 12% had a complete lack of epididymis; however, in newborn ACI rats, only 2 of 79 totally lacked an epididymis, indicating that early embryologic mesonephric ductal arrest cannot be solely responsible for agenesis of the epididymis (Hadziselimovic et al., 1984a). Secondary postnatal changes occur and culminate in the total disappearance of the epididymis in the majority of those 12% of adult ACI rats lacking an epididymis. Of special interest is that the degree of transabdominal movement of the testis was proportional to the degree of epididymal differentiation. Newborns completely lacking an epididymis were cryptorchid, whereas those with a partial defect of the epididymis also had impaired testicular descent (Hadziselimovic, 1984). It is important to stress that experimental evidence shows that if the newborn mice or rats have their testes located at the dorsal abdominal wall, they will be cryptorchid in adulthood (Jean, 1973). In most adult ACI rats in which the epididymal defect was encountered, cryptorchidism was associated (9 of 16). The cryptorchid side had a significantly higher rate of epididymal defects compared with the descended side (Hadziselimovic, 1984). This higher rate further supports the observations that an early epididymal developmental arrest results in cryptorchidism and confirms observations on experimentally induced inhibition of wolffian duct development and consequent cryptorchidism because of either vitamin A deficiency, chloraminophen, or E_2B (Dellenbach and Gabriel-Rabez, 1975; Wilson and Warkany, 1948; Raynaud, 1942).

Hormone Treatment

The ultimate aim of all therapeutic approaches to cryptorchidism is to achieve intrascrotally located fertile testes. The intrascrotal position can result from either surgical or hormonal treatment. Until 1975 HCG was the only mode of medical treatment. The largest series of HCG-treated boys was reported by Bergada (1979). He treated 1204 patients and had success in 40% of bilateral cryptorchid boys and in 30% of unilateral cryptorchid boys. However, because of the painful mode of application, psychic alterations, and effect on the growth of genitalia, this treatment is no longer recommended as a therapy of first choice.

Treatment with GnRH nasal spray was introduced in Europe in 1975 and proved successful, although the pathophysiologic background has been questioned, and success rates have been variable. The drug was never released in the United States for this purpose. One of the main objections to the hormonal treatment is that only retractile testes, and not cryptorchid testes, are expected to respond.

Between 1984 and 1986, 79 boys with 91 cryptorchid testes were treated in Europe with a therapy that consisted of a combination of luteinizing hormone releasing hormone (LHRH) nasal spray followed by HCG. Kryptocur (LHRH) was administered as a nasal spray at a dosage of 1.2 mg daily for a period of 14 days. HCG was injected intramuscularly, five times, at 2-day intervals. The dosage was one-half the amount recommended by the WHO. This particular therapeutic strategy was more efficacious than those used previously. During the follow-up 7 years later, 50.5% of the testes were in a scrotal position. The results during a 5-year follow-up of a second study were similar: 67% of the cryptorchid testes were in the scrotum (Waldschmidt et al. 1993)

In 238 boys with cryptorchidism in Switzerland between the ages of 4 and 48 months, LHRH was administered as nasal spray, 1.2 mg/day, for 4 weeks. The nonresponders received HCG, 500 IU, intramuscularly three times a week for 3 weeks. With the combined treatment, 37.8% of testes descended into the scrotum. Testicular descent occurred more often in patients whose testes were located in a lower position. Histological findings indicated a reduction in the number and maturation of germ cells. A clear improvement of germ cell trophism was observed in boys hormonally treated and operated on before the twelfth month of life. Early administered combined treatment with LHRH and HCG is considered by those authors as a substitution for the insufficiency of gonadotropins that is manifested in most cryptorchid infants during the first months of life (Lala et al., 1993).

An analogue of LHRH (Buserelin) was used for treating cryptorchidism. In a double-blind placebo-controlled study, the patients were assigned randomly into three groups: Buserelin treatment ($n = 22$), surgical treatment ($n = 18$), and placebo control group ($n = 19$). The three groups of patients were similar prior to the treatment with regard to testicular position; chronological and bone age; height and weight; LH, FSH, and testosterone levels; and penile size and the volume of the contralateral testis. Buserelin (20 μg) administered daily in a nasal spray significantly induced testicular descent compared with the group treated with a placebo ($p < 0.002$). A normal epididymis was found more often in boys with a successful descent ($p < 0.003$). Boys treated with Buserelin had the highest number and the best maturation index of the germ cells; HCG influenced the descent in both groups but was more efficacious when administered following the treatment with Buserelin, although it had no additional effect on germ cell maturation. None of the boys had retractile testes. Buserelin was capable of inducing testicular descent in addition to simultaneously increasing the number of germ cells and provoking further development of the epididymis (Bica and Hadziselimovic, 1992).

Long-Term Fertility Outcome

In 1960 Charny stated:

> Testicular biopsy in a large number of testes brought into the scrotum by a variety of techniques failed to reveal a single instance of normal spermatogenesis. The prevailing methods of treatment of cryptorchidism are not satisfactory and the operative techniques as practiced by most surgeons yield better cosmetic than functional results. If the surgical technique cannot be improved sufficiently, boys with asymptomatic cryptorchidism without clinically recognized hernia should be spared the hazard and inconvenience of orchiopexy.

Identical observations were promulgated by Mack and colleagues (1961), Canlorbe (1966), and Sizonenko and co-workers (1981). Patients completely lacking germ cells will, in all probability, develop sterility, and even a successful prepubertal orchiopexy cannot significantly improve the number of germ cells in their gonads or their fertility. These observations have been confirmed in prospective studies that reaffirmed the poor fertility prognosis for either unilaterally or bilaterally cryptorchid patients lacking germ cells who underwent orchiopexy during the prepubertal period (Hadziselimovic et al., 1984b). As a consequence of undescended testes, some investigators find infertility rates as high as 32% in unilateral cryptorchid patients and 59% in bilateral cryptorchid patients (Kogan, 1983; Hadziselimovic, 1983). By adulthood, previously cryptorchid testes have only 10% of the germ cells found in the normal population despite prepubertal orchiopexy (Kleinteich et al., 1979). Although some improvement in the germ cell content of cryptorchid testes that were successfully operated on was achieved, biopsy results showed that not a single testis out of 235 (79 unilateral cryptorchid testes, 78 bilateral cryptorchid testes, and 78 contralateral descended testes) that were intrascrotal 1 or several years after surgery achieved the normal level of germ cells (Kleinteich et al., 1979).

ACUTE AND CHRONIC SCROTAL SWELLINGS

Scrotal swellings may result from conditions involving either the scrotal wall or the intrascrotal contents. Scrotal wall swellings occur less frequently than swellings of the intrascrotal contents but may be painful and may simulate the latter. In some cases differential diagnosis may be made only by surgical exploration.

Scrotal Wall Swellings

Acute Idiopathic Scrotal Wall Edema

Acute idiopathic scrotal wall edema is an uncommonly encountered scrotal swelling involving one or both hemiscrotal compartments. The overlying skin may be thickened, edematous, and discolored, with a peculiar violaceous hue (Kaplan, 1977; Evans and Snyder, 1977). In some instances the swelling and erythema may extend onto the abdominal wall or into the perineum. The underlying testis, epididymis, and cord usually are easily palpated, are always nontender, and are not swollen, allowing differentiation from more serious acute intrascrotal conditions. An inflammatory cause has been suggested (e.g., secondary to insect bite or contact), but documentation of these suggested causes is lacking. The actual cause is unknown. Treatment with antibiotics, antihistamines, and cortisteroids has been advocated, but it appears that this condition resolves spontaneously without treatment and without sequelae. Its importance lies in its distinction from the more serious acute intrascrotal catastrophic conditions that it may simulate.

Acute Vasculitis

Acute vasculitis of the scrotal wall from Henoch-Schönlein purpura is uncommon but also simulates an intrascrotal catastrophe. Both the scrotal wall and the testis are involved in up to 15% of patients, and genital findings may precede the onset of the characteristic rash elsewhere (Khan et al., 1977; O'Regan and Robitaille, 1981). The scrotum is purpuric and erythematous and is usually tender, often making examination difficult. The testis, when involved, is often exquisitely tender, is swollen, and may completely mimic the findings seen in spermatic cord torsion. Unfortunately, to further complicate matters, spermatic cord torsion has been reported to occur in Henoch-Schönlein purpura (Loh and Jalan, 1974). A high index of suspicion is needed in making this diagnosis. Adjunctive diagnostic aids, especially isotope scrotal scanning, should be used to ensure the integrity of the testis when the diagnosis is not clear (Stein et al., 1980). This condition resolves with resolution of the generalized condition without genital sequelae.

Idiopathic Fat Necrosis of the Scrotum

Idiopathic fat necrosis of the scrotum is an unusual entity in which the intrascrotal fat undergoes spontaneous necrosis, resulting in a sometimes painful inflammatory swelling. A history of preexisting trauma may be elicited, but this condition often occurs without an antecedent identifiable cause (Donohue and Utley, 1975). This swelling may be unilateral or bilateral and may be diffuse or localized, sometimes presenting as a tumefaction. The testis may be palpated as a distinct entity or may be obscured by the surrounding inflammatory swelling. Scrotal sonography may show the mass to be distinct from the testis, at which time expectant observation may be provided. When the diagnosis is not perfectly clear, however, scrotal exploration to exlude spermatic cord torsion or tumor is indicated.

Spontaneous Gangrene

Spontaneous gangrene of the scrotal wall is a rare but serious cause of scrotal wall swelling in childhood. Swelling, edema, and then frank necrosis progressing to gangrene may occur, resulting in fever and toxemia. Most cases have occurred in neonates and have been associated with an identifiable portal of entry, such as after circumcision (Redman et al., 1979; Woodside, 1980). Treatment consists of intense antibiotic therapy, wet soaks, and sometimes incision or debridement.

Cutaneous Cysts and Tumors

Cutaneous cysts and tumors of the scrotal wall are uncommon in childhood. Sebaceous and epidermoid inclusion cysts are usually easy to identify from their intracutaneous position, completely separate from the underlying intrascrotal contents. Dermoid cysts occur in the scrotum along the midline raphe, similar to their midline position elsewhere in the body, and sometimes are difficult to distinguish from the intrascrotal structures because of their deeper position. Scrotal sonography aids in this diagnosis; operative excision is indicated for confirmation of diagnosis.

Swellings of the Intrascrotal Contents

Swellings of the intrascrotal contents are a commonly encountered problem inpediatric urologic practice and sometimes present a difficult differential diagnostic challenge. Acute swellings resulting from spermatic cord torsion or incarcerated hernia represent surgical emergencies and must be acted on expeditiously, whereas other swellings, such as reducible hernia, hydrocele, and varicocele, represent entities in which proper diagnosis is important in affording appropriate elective treatment. Optimal treatment depends on an exact diagnosis and a clear understanding of the nature of the underlying problem.

Hernias

Hernias and hydroceles result from failure of fusion and obliteration of the processus vaginalis (Fig. 57-10). When the entire processus vaginalis remains patent, as is commonly encountered in infants, a knuckle of bowel may protrude into the lumen of the hernia sac and may incarcerate or strangulate, the latter presenting as an acute painful erythematous scrotal swelling, inguinal swelling, or both. If the distal processus vaginalis is obliterated but the neck remains open, a groin mass rather than a scrotal mass will be encountered. For example, chronic incarceration of omentum may present as a nontender, nonreducible groin swelling, with the testis palpable separately below. A more common occurrence, however, is an intermittently palpable nontender groin swelling representing intermittent prolapse of bowel or omentum into a hernia sac, with spontaneous reduction. Sometimes in these instances the hernia may never be observed by the examining physician, and one must rely only on a good history from the parent to diagnose this condition.

Strangulated hernias require immediate surgical exploration to prevent necrosis of the hernia sac contents. Infants with incarcerated inguinal hernias may be more prone to develop testicular strangulation resulting from the increased pressure on their spermatic cord with resultant testicular atrophy (Murdoch, 1979; Puri et al., 1984). Children with incarcerated hernias should be admitted for observation, sedated and placed in a Trendelenburg position with subsequent attempts at manual reduction. Usually these maneuvers result in successful reduction, but elective hernia repair should be done within a short period thereafter, since reincarceration occurs frequently. Children with asymptomatic reducible inguinal hernias should undergo repair within a reasonable period of time after diagnosis to minimize the risk of incarceration or strangulation. The latter occurs frequently in infants, and surgical repair of inguinal hernias should not be deferred because of the patient's age.

Controversy exists regarding the necessity for exploration of the contralateral inguinal canal. In general, it is believed that closure of the processus vaginalis occurs in most infants during the first several months of age and that a persisting patent processus clinically evident thereafter should be surgically repaired. These figures have led some to believe that routine contralateral inguinal exploration is not advisable, a view based also on the added anesthesia time required for both repairs and the small but definite incidence of testis atrophy, vas injury, and secondary fixation of the testis in an extrascrotal position after inguinal hernia surgery (Hamrick and Williams, 1962). On the other hand, hernias occur in boys who have undergone previous contralateral inguinal hernia repair. A contralateral patent processus vaginalis was found in 59% of boys up to age 16 years who underwent bilateral exploration for a unilateral clinically apparent hernia (Minton and Clatworthy, 1961). These figures are somewhat age dependent, with a greater frequency of clinical hernias present in younger boys, especially those younger than 6 months. McGregor and colleagues (1980) reevaluated 130 patients over a postoperative follow-up period averaging 20 years and found that 29% eventually developed a contralateral inguinal hernia after previous unilateral repair. The chance of contralateral occurrence was found to depend on which side had originally been repaired. If the left side had been repaired formerly, there was a 41% chance of a subsequent right-sided hernia re-

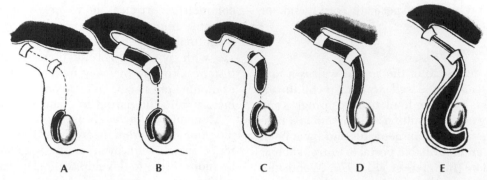

FIG. 57-10
Diagrammatic representation of persisting patent processus vaginalis. **A,** Normal obliteration of patient processus. **B,** Patent processus proximally with inguinal bulge; processus obliterated distally. **C,** Closure proximal and distal with loculated hydrocele of cord. **D,** Complete patency with hernia sac extending into scrotum. **E,** Partial proximal closure, resulting in scrotal hydrocele and proximal patent processus. (From Lewis JE Jr: *Atlas of Infant Surgery.* St Louis, CV Mosby, 1967.)

quiring surgical correction; if the right side was repaired first, there was only 14% chance of a hernia subsequently occurring on the left. Furthermore, nearly one half of the subsequent contralateral hernias occurred within 1 year of the original repair. Despite these observations, they believed that routine contralateral groin exploration was unwarranted since, statistically, two explorations yielding negative findings would be required for every right-sided exploration yielding positive findings, and six left-sided explorations yielding negative findings would be done—an unacceptably high figure in their view (McGregor et al., 1980). However, current opinions diverge somewhat from their conclusions. In a survey of 48 experienced pediatric surgeons, 80% routinely explored the contralateral groin in boys and 90% in females (Rowe and Marchildon, 1981). In general, most surgeons dealing with pediatric hernias believe that the contralateral groin exploration can be done safely and expeditiously (i.e., in the hands of a competent pediatric surgeon); both sides should be explored in cases in which only one hernia is clinically evident in boys younger than age 2 years.

Hydroceles

Hydroceles represent persistence of the processus vaginalis along its course with partial or complete fusion of the processus proximally. In children virtually all hydroceles are communicating (i.e., a narrow persistent processus vaginalis that allows the hydrocele periodically to fill with fluid) and exist proximally, resulting in intermittent enlargement (see Fig. 57-10). Hence a history of a childhood scrotal swelling that intermittently enlarges in the absence of a clinical hernia confirms the presence of a patent processus vaginalis. A related pediatric urologic caveat is, therefore, that boys with hydroceles always be explored

through an inguinal incision rather than through the scrotum to allow for ligation of the coexisting processus vaginalis.

Most infants with a scrotal swelling caused by a hydrocele undergo spontaneous closure of the processus vaginalis with subsequent resolution of the hydrocele. Hence surgical repair is usually reserved for persistent swellings beyond age 2 years, since after this age spontaneous closure of the persisting processus vaginalis occurs far less frequently. Size of the scrotal swelling should not influence a decision regarding early surgical correction, since many of these swellings can be quite large yet will still resolve spontaneously. Observation of a clinical hernia, however, is an indication for prompt surgical repair.

Occasionally an isolated scrotal hydrocele may be encountered in the absence of a proximal patent processus vaginalis. The cause of this may not be obvious but sometimes is the presenting sign of a serious underlying condition (e.g., a testicular tumor or chronic epididymitis). In these instances proximal exploration through an inguinal incision still should be used rather than a scrotal or inguinoscrotal approach, as is commonly used in adults. This incision offers a safe approach, allowing for diagnosis and ligation of an occult patent processus vaginalis and for proximal spermatic cord occlusion if an unsuspected tumor becomes evident.

A loculated hydrocele (hydrocele of the cord) may occur anywhere along the spermatic cord, presenting as a firm groin swelling that is sometimes difficult to distinguish from an incarcerated inguinal hernia or paratesticular rhabdomyosarcoma of the cord. Transillumination of the mass and sonography may aid in this distinction, but most swellings in this location usually require surgical exploration for confirmation of diagnosis and treatment.

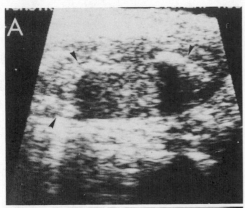

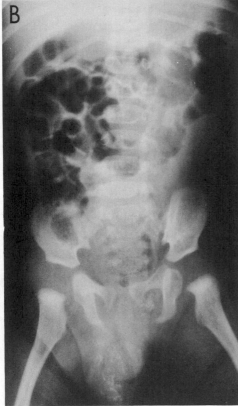

FIG. 57-11
Meconium peritonitis and scrotal mass in a 4-month-old boy.
A, Longitudinal sonogram of right hemiscrotum demonstrating multiple extratesticular echogenic foci *(arrows)* surrounding testis, suggesting calcification. **B,** Plain film indicating multiple calcified areas in scrotum and left inguinal canal along the processus vaginalis.

Antenatal or Postnatal Peritonitis

Antenatal or postnatal peritonitis may present with scrotal findings. An in utero intestinal perforation may heal, but spillage of intraabdominal meconium may track down a patent processus vaginalis into the scrotum, causing an inflammatory mass. As an example, the case shown in Figure 57-11 is a healthy full-term boy who presented with bilateral scrotal hydroceles at birth. As the hydroceles regressed over the first several weeks, a few hard nodular masses were palpated related to the right testis and epididymis, raising the concern of an intrascrotal tumor. Scrotal sonography demonstrated several echogenic foci in both hemiscrotums, suggesting multiple areas of calcification. A plain film subsequently revealed multiple calcified areas in the scrotum and inguinal canal characteristic of meconium peritonitis (Thompson et al., 1973). Similarly, acute appendiceal perforation in boys can track down a patent processus vaginalis and present as an acutely inflamed scrotum with minimal or no intraabdominal or inguinal signs. If pus is encountered in an exploration of an acutely inflamed scrotum, this diagnosis should be considered.

Orchitis

Orchitis as an isolated finding in boys is uncommon and usually results from a concomitant viral infection or as a reactive change to an adjacent epididymitis. The testis is acutely swollen and exquisitely painful, may be surrounded by a reactive hydrocele, and may mimic other acute intrascrotal processes completely. Testicular inflammatory swelling in mumps usually occurs in postpubertal boys and rarely occurs under age 10 years. Estimates of the frequency of mumps orchitis in the literature range from 3% to 100%, but in one carefully analyzed study the frequency was 30%. One third of those having orchitis developed subsequent atrophy (Beard et al., 1977). The risk of infertility is considered to be increased in this group, and there is a questionably increased risk of malignancy developing in these atrophic testes. The treatment is usually supportive, with analgesics, scrotal elevation, and ice packs used in the acute phase.

Epididymitis

Epididymitis is a more common cause of scrotal swelling in childhood than is usually believed. Gierup and colleagues (1975) collected 48 cases over a 25-year period; more recently, Gislason and colleagues (1980) reviewed an additional 25 childhood cases seen over 5 years. Most pediatric urologic referral practices encounter children with epididymitis regularly, since this condition occurs more commonly in boys who have urinary infections, who have structural lesions of the urinary tract, or who undergo reconstructive surgery and who have indwelling urethral catheters. In collating the findings from four series of acute scrotal swellings in boys, epididymitis was noted as the underlying cause in 8% to 41% (Leape, 1967; Kaplan and King, 1970; Moharib and Krahn, 1970; Bourne and Lee, 1975). The peak incidence is usually in adolescence.

Epididymitis may result from an acute urinary tract infection with retrograde spread of infection along the vas deferens. The common embryologic derivation of the ureter, vas deferens, seminal vesicle, and epididymis should be remembered, and in some boys structural abnormalities of the termination of these organs in the trigone and posterior urethra may be present, predisposing them to retrograde vasitis and epididymitis (Fig. 57-12). Indwelling urethral catheters may sometimes precipitate an attack of acute epididymitis in boys with these structural abnormalities without previous urologic symptoms (Fig. 57-13). In older boys epididymitis is a cause of acute, painful scrotal swellings, often in the absence of demonstrable bacterial infection. Numerous studies, including culture of direct epididymal aspirations, have generally failed to demonstrate organisms in these instances. In such cases viral and atypical bacterial infections have been postulated as the cause. Uncommonly epididymitis may be associated with an unusual organism (e.g., *Salmonella, Haemophilus*) in the absence of demonstrable urinary tract infection. In these circumstances direct hematogenous seeding may be the cause. Purulent epididymitis or chronic epididymitis may occur, requiring surgical exploration for diagnosis or drainage of the epididymal abscess.

These findings raise the issue whether radiologic urinary tract screening to detect underlying structural abnormalities is indicated in boys who have epididymitis diagnosed at any age. Some have indicated that infants with epididymitis have an increased likelihood of having underlying structural genitourinary abnormalities and recommend that complete urologic investigations be performed (Williams et al., 1979; Siegel et al., 1987). Others who have reviewed this problem in older children suggest that underlying structural problems are uncommon in this population (Gislason et al., 1980). A selective approach to this problem should be practiced. Boys with epididymitis associated with an acute urinary infection are evaluated with a sonogram and voiding cystourethrogram, just as any other boy with an acute urinary infection. Preadolescent boys with epididymitis having sterile urine have a sonogram and voiding cystourethrogram done as well, though the number of abnormalities found in this group is smaller than in the former. Adolescent boys with epididymitis undergo screening sonography of the kidneys and pelvis to ensure normalcy of the upper urinary tract and to ensure that a rarely encountered wolffian or müllerian duct remnant is not present. Circumcision status seems to play a role: Epididymitis occurs three times as often in uncircumcised boys, regardless of age (Gill et al., 1995).

The diagnosis of epididymitis is made by direct physical examination, with the epididymis found to be enlarged, firm, and exquisitely tender, usually with a normal adjacent testis. In some instances the intrascrotal contents are obscured by a surrounding hydrocele, making the diagnosis difficult. Prehn's sign (relief of pain with elevation of the involved testis) in

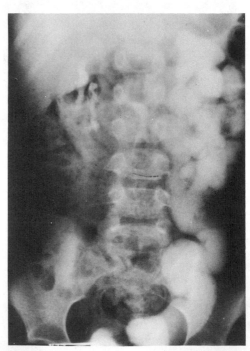

FIG. 57-13
Left epididymitis in a 4-year-old boy who was previously asymptomatic with an indwelling urethral catheter after open-heart surgery. The intravenous pyelogram reveals previously unsuspected horseshoe kidney, gross left hydroureteronephrosis. A Y ureter was found draining the right side and isthmus.

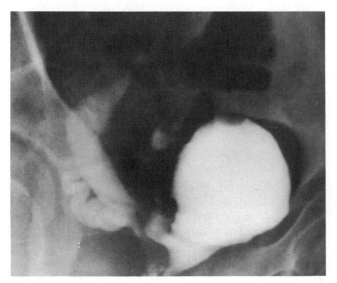

FIG. 57-12
Persistent mesonephric duct in a 6-year-old boy with anorectal anomaly and rectourethral fistula. The voiding cystourethrogram demonstrates reflux into markedly dilated convoluted vas deferens and ureter.

my experience has not proved to be a reliable diagnostic acid in children because of inaccuracies observed with this maneuver and the small size of the pediatric scrotum that naturally draws up the testis. Associated fever, leukocytosis, pyuria, and bacteriuria occur more commonly with epididymitis, helping to distinguish epididymitis from other causes of acute scrotal swelling. These findings, however, should be considered as supportive findings to the general clinical history and examination, rather than as absolute indicators that epididymitis is present. Two studies indicate that although 46% of their patients with epididymitis had pyuria, between 27% and 40% of the patients with spermatic cord torsion also had pyuria (Stage et al., 1981; Abu-Sleiman et al., 1979). Scrotal sonography, isotope scrotal scanning, or both may aid in the difficult case (see later discussion). Treatment with appropriate antibiotics should be provided on the basis of urine culture and sensitivities, as well as on scrotal elevation and restrained physical activity until the acute phase subsides. Worsening swelling and symptoms should raise the issue of a misdiagnosis, such as a missed spermatic cord torsion, and appropriate reevaluation or surgical exploration may then be indicated.

Spermatic Cord Torsion

Scrotal swellings secondary to spermatic cord torsion (Fig. 57-14) represent one of the most serious emergencies encountered in pediatric urology in terms of both urgent management and long-term potential serious sequelae. Urgent accurate diagnosis is needed, followed by surgical exploration and detorsion of the testis. Time is a critical factor, since testis

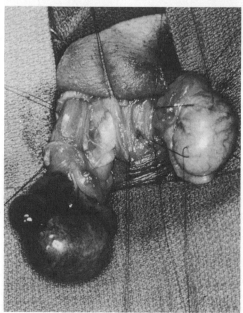

FIG. 57-14
Right spermatic cord torsion in a 12-year-old boy.

survival relates directly to the duration of torsion.

The frequency of spermatic cord torsion has been estimated at 1 in 4000 males younger than age 25 years, making it a realtively common occurrence (Williamson, 1976). This figure probably underestimates the true frequency, since many episodes of missed torsion exist, as well as misdiagnoses with other conditions. Furthermore, evidence now exists that many if not most cases of absent testes result from previous spermatic cord torsion (Kogan et al., 1986a). Though it has been stated that two thirds of cases of spermatic cord torsion occur in boys between ages 12 and 18 years (Williamson, 1976), torsion may occur at any age and has clearly been identified and reported antenatally, neonatally, throughout childhood, and in adulthood (Whitesel, 1971; Kay et al., 1980; Jerkins et al., 1983). An anatomic abnormality in which the peritoneal investiture of the testis inserts high on the spermatic cord rather than on the lower pole allows for poor testicular fixation and extreme testicular mobility (the bell-clapper deformity), predisposing to twisting (Fig. 57-15). Most instances of torsion occur intravaginally (i.e., within this sac); however, in the neonate extravaginal torsion (i.e., a true twist of the entire spermatic cord and testis) is more common. Because this abnormality of the tunica vaginalis is believed to frequently exist bilaterally and because cases of sequential torsion on the opposite side have followed previous unilateral torsion in cases where the uninvolved side was not suture-fixed in place, bilateral suture fixation of the tests is mandatory in any case of unilateral torsion (Harris et al., 1982; Bellinger, 1985).

A historical review of previous publications reveals two key issues concerning the efficacy of management of spermatic cord torsion: confusion in arriving at the proper diagnosis and the effect of delayed diagnosis on testicular survival. Most early series dealing with spermatic cord torsion clearly demonstrate a marked delay in referral and diagnosis and a concomitant high orchiectomy rate necessitated by the frequent finding of testis infarction—estimated overall as high as 90% in the literature before 1966 and 72% in the series of Allan and Brown (1966). Thirty-one percent of testes in the Barker-Raper (1964) series and 42% of testes in the Gartman (1964) series were saved, though many may have had subsequent atrophy. Recognition of these factors led to more expeditious management of this condition and to frequent adoption of the policy of immediate exploration of all cases of acute scrotal inflammation. By 1977 testis survival rates were estimated at approximately 50%, a clear improvement (Williamson, 1976). More recent series using an aggressive approach with rapid scrotal exploration have now achieved testis survival rates close to 90% (Donohue and Utley, 1978; Cass et al., 1980), attesting to the efficacy of this approach.

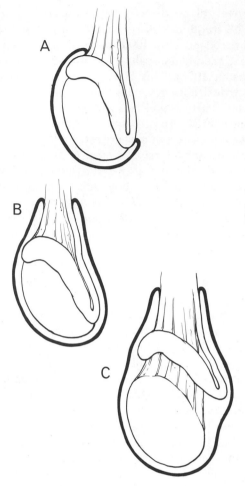

FIG. 57-15
Diagrammatic representation of the anatomy of spermatic cord torsion. **A,** Normal anatomy. Tunica vaginalis does not envelop epididymis. **B,** Bell-clapper deformity. Tunica vaginalis extends high on spermatic cord, enveloping epididymis and allowing testis to twist within. **C,** Testis suspended from epididymis, allowing twist to occur between testis and epididymis.

Just how long can the testis in torsion survive without undergoing irreversible atrophy? Several experimental preparations examining the effects of complete torsion of rat and dog testes reveal that the "save" period for recovery of germinal and tubular epithelium may be somewhere between 4 and 6 hours, though severe, irreversible abnormalities may be seen after even 1 hour (Smith, 1955; Sonda and Lapides, 1961; Cosentino et al., 1984; Turner and Howards, 1985). Leape's (1967) classic article indicated that 17 of 19 boys had their testis saved when operated on within 24 hours of symptom onset, whereas in none of 31 boys operated on after that time was testis salvage feasible. In several additional reviews, maximum survival (70% to 90%) was noted in patients operated on within 12 hours of symptom onset. Survival decreased significantly during the next 12 hours but was still

possible. After 24 hours of torsion in humans, testicular infarction is the rule. The degree of torsion influences survival, since not all torsion result in complete ischemia; 720 degrees of torsion experimentally have been shown to be necessary for complete, irreversible cessation of blood flow (Cosentino et al., 1984; Turner and Howards, 1985). Furthermore, in humans spontaneous incomplete or complete detorsion is not uncommon, explaining the occasional occurrence of testicular salvage after prolonged periods. Nevertheless, these data serve to illustrate graphically the effect of delayed diagnosis on testicular survival.

If time is so critical, why has therapy been delayed so often? Failure to suspect torsion as the underlying cause of the acute scrotal inflammation is the most common reason. In this regard, a lack of uniformity of symptoms and physical findings often suggests alternative diagnoses and has led to a variety of descriptive titles of literature dealing with this subject (Leape, 1967; Williamson, 1977). Many patients do not conform to the classical description of torsion, namely, a sudden onset of hemiscrotal pain, then swelling, acute nausea, and vomiting in the absence of fever and urinary symptoms. The painless swollen testis, which may occur in up to 10% of torsions (most frequently in newborns), is especially confusing, causing delay in diagnosis (Kaplan and King, 1970). Failure to understand that torsion is the leading cause of acute scrotal inflammation in childhood, not epididymitis, also contributes to diagnostic delay.

Conversely, greater than one third of patients with spermatic cord torsion may report previous episodes of severe scrotal pain that remitted spontaneously (Williamson, 1976; Cass et al., 1980). A reliable history of repeated episodes of this nature should be considered sufficient grounds to perform an elective scrotal exploration and testicular fixation with the abnormal anatomy of torsion likely to be encountered.

A further, more recent cause for delay in therapy results from the excessive involvement and blind faith of treating physicians in the newer diagnostic modalities available to distinguish the various cases of scrotal inflammation. Conflict between clinical impressions and diagnostic testing have led to delay in exploration in some and even missed torsion in others. Further discussion of this aspect of management follows in the subsequent section on differential diagnosis of scrotal swellings.

If the recognition of spermatic cord torsion may be somewhat complicated, the management is completely straightforward and noncontroversial. Derotation should be done on an emergent basis. Manual derotation may be done as a temporary maneuver after the patient is given intravenous morphine (0.1 mg/kg of body wight) (Frazier and Bucy, 1975; Betts et al.,

1979). It has been suggested that the anterior portion of each testis torts toward the midline; hence it should be rotated outward to achieve detorsion (Sparks, 1971), though not all agree and attempts can be made in each direction. Successful detorsion is usually associated with marked pain relief immediately and may be documented with Doppler examination. Surgical fixation with nonabsorbable sutures should follow within 24 hours to prevent retorsion, which occurs commonly. Cases have been reported in which retorsion testes has occurred where the previous suture fixation was done with absorbable sutures (Kossow 1980; McNellis and Rabinovitch, 1978; Vorstman and Rothwell, 1982). Simultaneous fixation of the opposite, uninvolved testis is also mandatory, since contralateral sequential torsion has been reported in more than 40% of cases in which the uninvolved testis was not fixed at the time of torsion (Skoglund et al., 1970b; Krarup, 1978).

Neonatal Torsion

Neonatal torsion represents a unique and distinct situation in the management of this condition. The finding of a painless, discolored, hemiscrotal swelling in the neonate is indicative of spermatic cord torsion and should in no circumstances be considered a diagnostic problem. Unfortunately, bilateral synchronous and asynchronous cases may occur. The duration of torsion is difficult to determine in many of these circumstances, and in some instances torsion may begin antenatally. A review of this subject covered approximately 120 previously reported cases in the literature through 1983 (Silber et al., 1984). Attitudes concerning management of this condition were polled among the members of the Society for Pediatric Urology. Most believed that the diagnosis of this condition was self-evident and that exploration was indicated; however, the testicular salvage rate was disappointing. Further controversy over the frequency of contralateral torsion in these instances and the need to suture-fix the contralateral testis existed, since most of these torsions occur extravaginally. This controversy led some to adopt a less aggressive attitude toward emergent exploration.

With increased recognition of this problem, antenatal torsion is similarly being diagnosed with increased frequency. Reports of calcified testes and hypoplastic testes at birth, as well as the unique report of a "free-floating necrotic intra-abdominal testis" found at exploration of a newborn presenting with an acute abdomen and an ipsilateral empty scrotum (Mitchell, 1981) illustrate the spectrum of presentations of this condition. Further investigations indicate that many instances of unilateral absent testes probably result from antenatal torsion (Kogan et al., 1986b; Huff et al., 1991). Unfortunately, testicular salvage after an-

tenatal spermatic cord torsion has not been reported and is unlikely.

The fate of the torted and contralateral untorted testes after correction of spermatic cord torsion has received considerable attention. Salvage rates of "viable" testes have varied, but some series reported atrophy in between one third and two thirds of these testes. A correlation between duration of torsion and subsequent atrophy exists (MacNicol, 1974; Krarup, 1978). These data suggest that in some instances surgeons are preserving poorly viable testes that should have been removed. Furthermore, the incidence of morbidity (prolonged high fever, scrotal abscess, drainage of necrotic tubules through the scrotal incision) is high, approaching 20% in some series (Williamson, 1976).

Additional information strongly suggests that the testis undergoing torsion can adversely affect the contralateral testis by a presumed immunologic process. Various adult rat experimental preparations, beyond the scope of full discussion here, have demonstrated contralateral histologic abnormalities in unilateral torsion (e.g., Cosentino, et al., 1984; Nagler and deVere White, 1982; Kogan et al., 1986b) (Fig. 57-16). Raised antibody titers have been detected in rats and mice in some instances (Harrison et al., 1981; Thomas et al., 1984; Kogan et al., 1986b) but were not detected in rabbits (Cerasaro et al., 1984). Diminished fertility was noted after mating in these circumstances (Merimsky et al., 1984; Nagler and DeVere White, 1982; Cosentino et al., 1984). Orchiectomy (Cosentino et al., 1984), splenectomy and azathioprine administration (Nagler and deVere White, 1982), and corticosteroid administration (Kogan et al., 1986b) have attenuated these adverse findings, further suggesting that an immunologic process is operative. Data suggest that the prepubertal rat testis subjected to torsion does not result in these abnormalities (Nagler, 1985; Kogan et al., 1986b). Human clinical correlates of these experimental findings exist. Eighteen patients who had prolonged prepubertal spermatic cord torsion and who underwent detorsion with replacement of the testis in the scrotum were reviewed 7 to 23 years later. Of the 5 married men, all were fathers. Of the 13 unmarried men, only 3 had abnormal semen analyses. None showed any abnormal sperm autoantibodies. In another study, though, only 9 of 23 adults who had previous spermatic cord torsion had normal semen in their ejaculate (Bartsch et al., 1980; Krarup, 1978). Some of these patients had elevated FSH levels, indicating abnormal testicular function. These studies demonstrate that the contralateral testis can be affected adversely by the torted testis and that orchiectomy should be done if a prolonged period has elaspsed since the onset of symptoms or if a rapid return of blood flow is not seen after detorsion. Leav-

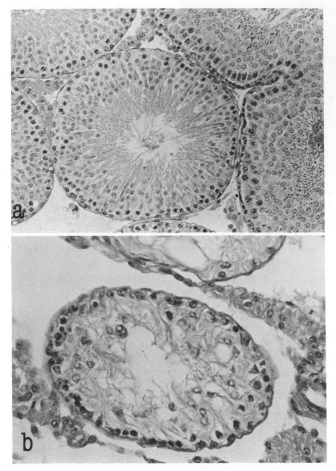

FIG. 57-16
Histologic findings in the contralateral testis of adult rats (age 53 days) 30 days after undergoing chronic unilateral testicular torsion. **A,** Control contralateral testis with normal tubular diameter and spermatogenesis. **B,** Contralateral testis has absent spermatogenesis and reduced tubular diameter. (From Kogan SJ, Owens G, Tarter T, et al: Mechanisms of injury in unilateral testis torsion. *Eur Urol* 1986; 12:184. Used by permission.)

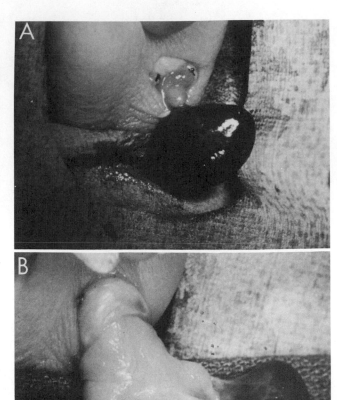

FIG. 57-17
Torsion of the testicular appendage in an 8-year-old boy presenting with 6 hours of acute scrotal pain and inflammation. A large, infarcted intrascrotal mass protrudes **(A),** followed by the testis **(B).** In this unusual case the infarcted appendix testis is as large as the testis.

ing a marginal testis in place probably causes more potential harm than benefit.

Torsion of the Testicular Appendages

Torsion of the testicular appendages occurs frequently and may totally mimic the inflammatory findings of spermatic cord torsion. When an inflammatory, painful hydrocele occurs, obscuring the testis completely and precluding adequate examination, concern must be exercised to exclude spermatic cord torsion. Testicular appendages tend to twist when they are long and pedunculated. Venous engorgement occurs, followed by arterial occlusion and then appendiceal infarction. In some instances the appendage may become strikingly enlarged, sometimes as large the testis (Fig. 57-17). When the appendage in torsion is easily seen and palpated through the scrotal skin (blue-dot sign) and the underlying testis feels normal, spermatic

cord torsion may be excluded with complete confidence despite the surrounding inflammation.

Testicular appendages exist at both the superior and inferior testicular poles (Fig. 57-18), and any may undergo torsion. Clinically the appendix testis is the most frequently encountered appendage, occurring in 92% of one autopsy series, and also is the most common appendage undergoing torsion (Rolnick et al., 1968; Skoglund et al., 1970a). Embryologically this appendage represents the remnant of the cranial part of the müllerian duct. The appendix epididymis represents a remnant of the cranial end of the wolffian duct, as do the paradidymis and vas aberrans.

Though many surgeons advocate emergent exploration of all cases of acute scrotal inflammation, those boys having testicular appendiceal torsion may be spared this inconvenience, providing the diagnosis is made with accuracy (e.g., by clearly palpating a normal testis or finding a blue-dot sign). Virtually all cases of testicular appendiceal torsion resolve sponta-

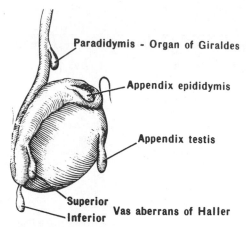

FIG. 57-18
Anatomic distribution of the testicular appendages. (From Rolnick D, Kawanoul S, Szanto P, et al: Anatomical incidence of testicular appendages. *J Urol* 1968; 100:755.)

neously, often with autoinfarction of the appendix. Supportive analgesics are offered, and a follow-up reexamination is important to document resolution of the swelling. The rare instance in which pain is persistent or recurrent after a previous bout has resolved may be dealt with by an ambulatory surgical excision. Though asynchronous contralateral appendiceal torsion occurs, it is uncommon, and most surgeons do not elect to remove both appendages when operating for this condition.

Testicular Tumors

Testicular tumors are an important but infrequent cause of scrotal swellings in children. They may present insidiously and may not be apparent at an initial examination done for nonspecific scrotal pain. Alternatively a tumor may be obscured by a hydrocele of recent onset, making palpation of the tumor mass impossible. Testicular tumors also may have an inflammatory presentation, with chronic erythema and thickening of the overlying skin and underlying swelling. More often, they initially present as a bland, firm, nontender asymptomatic scrotal mass.

Differential Diagnosis

The differential diagnosis of these scrotal swellings requires a thorough working knowledge of the underlying conditions as well as an attempt to characterize the swelling at hand. Evaluation of physical characteristics such as consistency, nodularity, and ability to transilluminate the swelling are helpful in arriving at correct diagnosis. Accurate localization of the swelling to an intratesticular or paratesticular position and determination of reducibility of the mass similarly help to characterize the swelling. The key factor in these instances of scrotal swelling is to determine whether the underlying testis is palpably normal, since testicular swelling usually indicates serious disease. Useful differential diagnostic points are listed in Table 57-1.

Chronic persisting scrotal swellings that cannot be accurately diagnosed clinically should be explored surgically because serious disease often underlies these conditions. When one is dealing with acute swellings, it is helpful conceptually to characterize the swelling as being of either an ischemic or inflammatory nature. This principle has also formed the basis for various noninvasive adjunctive diagnostic tests developed to diagnose these swellings nonoperatively. Radionuclide scrotal scanning with technetium 99m pertechnetate, first introduced in 1973, has gained wide acceptance in this context. Imaging of the scrotum after injection of this agent allows for rapid distinction between inflammatory conditions with an increase in vascularity and ischemic conditions such as torsion, where a cold "hole" in the isotope distribution is noted (Fig. 57-19). The Doppler ultrasonic stethoscope was introduced shortly thereafter based on the same principle. With this instrument in the emergency room, the examiner could make a rapid distinction between torsion (ischemic) and other inflammatory conditions resulting in an increased blood flow. The latter procedure would seem to represent the ideal way to diagnose torsion were it not for a significant incidence of both false-positive and false-negative results (Perri et al., 1976; Nasrallah et al., 1977). A chronically torsive testis often develops a surrounding hyperemic shell of vessels from the spermatic cord, causing a Doppler reading of intact flow. Technique seems to affect the results, and proper probe position and compression of the spermatic cord above (funicular compression test) are important to prevent confusing pulsations from inflamed overlying scrotal skin from blood flow through the spermatic vessels (Haynes et al., 1983).

Radioisotope scrotal scanning has proved highly accurate in trained hands; however, this examination is not readily available in all clinical settings and requires skill in interpreting the images obtained. Proper imaging of the intrascrotal contents is critical; in particular, a pinhole converging collimator should be used to obtain sharp, enlarged images. A recent review of 464 cases of acute scrotal inflammation indicated that in only 4% was an incorrect diagnosis reached (Haynes et al., 1983). False-positive isotope scans, in which torsion is incorrectly believed to be present, may result from overlying hernias or hydroceles and sometimes are seen with epididymitis. False-negative scans may result from abscess formation, from late torsion with surrounding hyperemia, or from recent detorsion-retorsion (see Fig. 57-18). Two reviews contrasted the diagnostic accuracy of isotope scanning and Doppler flowmetry (Rodriguex et al., 1981; Glazier and McGuire, 1980). In the first, the scan findings were correct in 100% of cases, whereas the Doppler

TABLE 57-1

Differential Diagnosis of Acute Scrotal Swelling in Childhood

	Spermatic Cord Torsion	Epididymoorchitis	Appendiceal Torsion
Age	1st yr and adolescence	Adolescence and after	9-12 years
Symptoms and signs			
Pain	Acute, severe onset	Gradual localization to upper or posterior of testis	Usually gradual
	Frequent antecedent similar pains	Uncommon	Occasional
	Localized to testis and radiates to groin and lower abdomen	Usually localized to epididymis and testis, sometimes to groin	Localized to appendix or general scrotal region
Fever	Rare	Common	Rare
Vomiting	Frequent	Rare	Rare
Dysuria	Rare	Common	Rare
Physical examination	Testis may be high-riding, swollen, exquisitely tender	Testis and epididymis are firm, tender, swollen	Testis usually normal; firm mass may be seen and felt at upper pole; distinct from epididymis
Laboratory examination			
Pyuria, urinary infection	Rare	Common	Rare
Blood flow (Doppler, isotope scrotal scan)	Diminished	Increased	Normal or increased

findings were indeterminate in 30% of 20 patients explored for torsion (Rodriguez et al., 1981). In the second, 7 of 32 consecutive patients with an acute scrotum had spermatic cord torsion (Glazier and McGuire, 1980). Five of 7 had the diagnosis confirmed by both modalities; 6 of 7 Doppler studies were consistent with torsion, and 5 of 7 isotope scans were positive. These authors concluded that neither examination was accurate enough to be used individually.

These findings vary somewhat with my personal experience with radioisotope scrotal imaging. My initial experience demonstrated the accuracy of scrotal imaging in correctly diagnosing testicular torsion and the correct scan parameters for predicting that torsion was not present. Since the middle 1970s, our policy has been to explore patients who are believed to have acute spermatic cord torsion without delay, so scrotal imaging has not since been used routinely in these instances. We continue to use the scrotal scan in instances in which the diagnosis is indeterminate, thereby adding objective confirmation to our clinical diagnosis of nontorsion. We reviewed our original 19 patients with this approach, hoping that the normal scan would provide enough information to make surgical exploration unnecessary in these instances (Kogan et al., 1979). In that series and in numerous other instances since, surgical exploration or long-term clinical follow-up of the testis has demonstrated a 100% accuracy in predicting nontorsion. No patient was subsequently found to have torsion or to show evidence of testicular atrophy. In this manner we found the scrotal scan to be extremely helpful in complementing our clinical impressions and in minimizing explora-

tions in all but clear-cut necessary cases. Furthermore, delay from diagnostic testing of strongly suspected cases of torsion has been eliminated by this approach.

By contrast, we subsequently reviewed 45 patients suspected of having torsion who were operated on immediately and found that 40 had torsion at surgical exploration, giving a clinical diagnostic accuracy of 88%. We believed that the 5 patients who underwent an "unnecessary" surgical exploration did not justify routine use of scrotal scanning in this group overall to confirm an already obvious diagnosis (Kogan and Levitt, 1983). This experience has been formulated into an approach that we use in managing boys with acute scrotal inflammation (Fig. 57-20). Those boys whose clinical history and examination strongly indicate spermatic cord torsion undergo surgical exploration without any delay for adjunctive diagnostic testing. In those boys with equivocal findings, a radionuclide scrotal scan is expeditiously obtained. If the scan findings indicate a photopenic central defect compatible with torsion, the patient undergoes immediate surgical exploration, since experience indicates that this finding seldom occurs in other conditions. Different findings (e.g., hyperemia or normal flow) when correlated with the clinical history allow for a more conservative observation approach to be followed with a high degree of certainty that spermatic cord torsion is not present.

Congenital Scrotal Anomalies

Congenital scrotal anomalies occur when normal posteriocaudal migration of the paired labioscrotal folds is impaired. This occurs in intersex conditions,

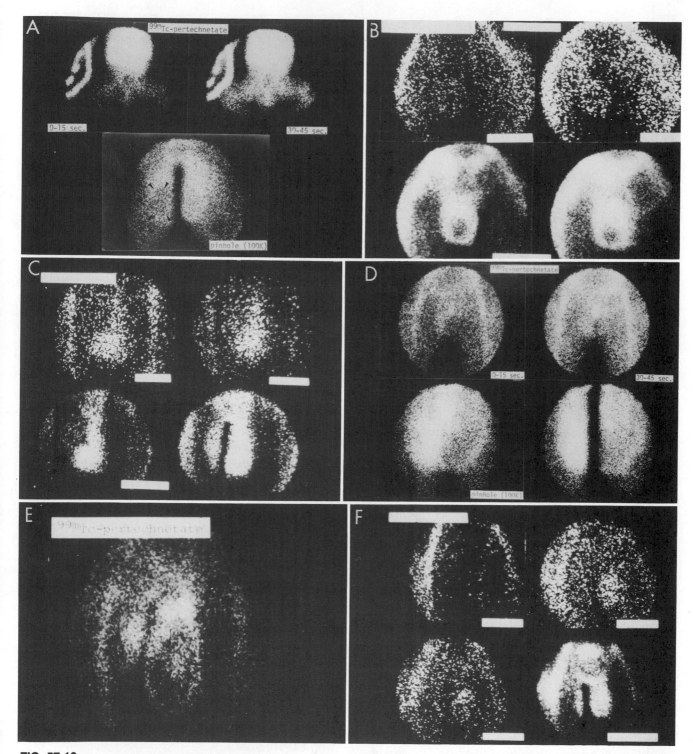

FIG. 57-19

Radionuclide scrotal scanning. **A,** Acute (right) torsion. Cold central photopenic area is evident *(arrowheads).* **B,** Chronic (right) torsion. Central defect is evident with hyperemic surrounding shell of vessels. **C,** Epididymitis (left). Diffusely increased flow on dynamic and static images. **D,** Torsion of (right) testicular appendage. Dynamic imaging may show normal or increased flow; static imaging shows increased flow. **E,** Hernia hydrocele may simulate cold, central defect seen in torsion. **F,** Scrotal abscess may simulate inflammatory changes of epididymitis or sometimes the cold central defect seen in torsion. (**A** and **D** courtesy of Drs. K.J. Chun and D.M. Milstein.)

Clinical Management of the Acutely Inflamed
Scrotum in Childhood

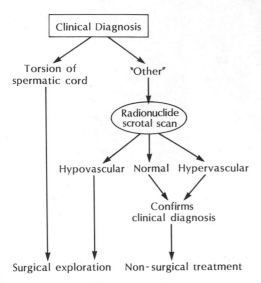

FIG. 57-20
Clinical management of the acutely inflamed scrotum in childhood.

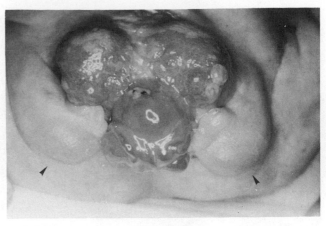

FIG. 57-21
Scrotal ectopia *(arrowheads)* in 46, XY male with cloacal exstrophy.

severe hypospadias, cloacal exstrophy, tail anomalies of the embryo, and sometimes as an isolated defect. These instances suggest that both hormonal and mechanical influences may affect scrotal development.

Scrotal Hypoplasia

Scrotal hypoplasia is seen sometimes in association with cryptorchidism or absent testes. The scrotal skin is often completely flattened and quantitatively deficient. Prominence of the surrounding pubic and perineal skin may suggest a greater overall size to the scrotum, though the consistency and appearance of this skin is different. Scrotal hypoplasia makes orchiopexy or testicular prosthesis placement more difficult. Testes placed dependently at orchiopexy in a hypoplastic scrotum may appear to be in a nondependent position, though over a few years of follow-up the scrotum seems to grow and accommodate the testes. Prostheses sometimes remain high and appear asymmetric when placed in a hypoplastic scrotum, even when the patient is followed through puberty, resulting in an unsatisfactory cosmetic appearance. Pretreatment with testosterone has been suggested to enlarge the hypoplastic scrotum in anorchid boys (Klauber and Sant, 1985).

Scrotal ectopic may occur on the inner thigh, on the perineum, or in the pubic region lateral to the penis. This condition is most commonly seen in males with cloacal exstrophy with diphallus (Fig. 57-21), though I have also encountered it in myelodysplastic boys, Minninberg and Richman (1972) encountered it

in "syndromes," and Lamm and Kaplan (1977) encountered it in otherwise normal children. The testis normally lies within the ectopic scrotum, though it sometimes may be hypoplastic. Treatment usually consists of excision when the ectopic scrotum is distant.

Bifid Scrotum and Penoscrotal Transposition

A bifid scrotum and varying degrees of penoscrotal transposition occur in association with severe hypospadias, intersex conditions, and the latter in association with the caudal regression syndrome (Miller, 1972) (Fig. 57-22). Rarely, either may be seen as an isolated occurrence. Failure of fusion or caudal migration results in separation of the two hemiscrotal compartments in the former instance and envelopment of the penis in the latter. A bifid scrotum is usually corrected naturally as part of a hypospadias repair or feminizing genital reconstruction in intersex. Minor degrees of penoscrotal transposition can be left untreated, though more severe degrees should be corrected with an M to Y type of scrotal recession. Techniques to allow for chordee correction, hypospadias repair, and correction of a coexisting penoscrotal transposition in a single stage have been described (Ehrlich and Scardino, 1981).

Congenital Abnormalities of the Vas Deferens and Epididymis

If one considers the separate embryologic origin of the testis and its excretory system, it should not be surprising that a variety of congenital abnormalities of the epididymis and vas deferens may occur. Once considered a rarity, congenital abnormalities of these organs are now recognized with frequency, especially in situations in which the testes are abnormal, such as infertility and cryptorchidism. Scorer and Farrington (1971) and Marshall and Shermeta (1979) devised

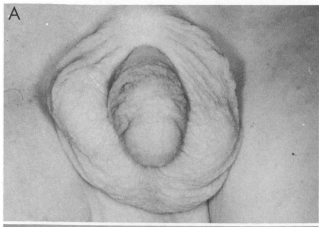
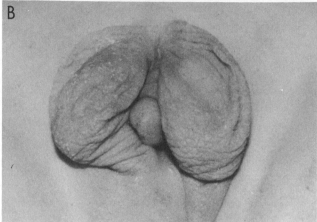

FIG. 57-22
Penoscrotal transportation. **A,** Incomplete. **B,** Complete.

TABLE 57-2

Congenital Anomalies of the Mesonephric Ducts in the Male

I. Agenesis of all mesonephric duct derivatives
II. Epididymis
   A. Agenesis of epididymis
   B. Failure of urogenital union: agenesis or loss of continuity
      1. Nonunion between the head of epididymis and testis
         a. Gross
         b. Microscopic
      2. Agenesis or atresia of the midepididymis
      3. Agenesis or atresia of the tail of epididymis
   C. Elongated or looped epididymis
   D. Epididymal cyst, with or without loss of continuity
III. Vas deferens
   A. Agenesis of vas deferens
      1. Complete
      2. Segmental
   B. Persistent mesonephric duct: ureter entering vas deferens
IV. Seminal vesicle
   A. Agenesis of seminal vesicle
   B. Seminal vesicle cyst
   C. Ureter entering seminal vesicle
V. Ejaculatory duct
   A. Agenesis of ejaculatory duct

classifications of these abnormalities, which have been further revised and addended by Kroovand and Perlmutter (1981), creating a comprehensive working classification of mesonephric duct abnormalities (Table 57-2). In this section abnormalities solely of the vas deferens and epididymis are discussed.

Congenital Unilateral Absence or Atresia of the Vas Deferens

Congenital unilateral absence or atresia of the vas deferens occurs in approximately 0.5% to 1% of the general population (Charny and Gillenwater, 1965; Michelson, 1949; Scorer and Farrington, 1971). The latter has been encountered in 1% of boys undergoing herniorrhaphy (Lukash et al., 1975) and in 20% of boys with congenital rubella undergoing orchiopexy (Priebe et al., 1979). Bilateral absence has been estimated with a frequency of 1% to 10% in azospermatic men (Ithiri and Abulfadl, 1972; O'Conor, 1960). The latter occurs with regularity in boys with cystic fibrosis and may be accompanied by rudimentary development of the entire mesonephric ductal system (Charny and Gillenwater, 1965; Holsclaw and

Perlmutter, 1971). Absence of the vas, in general, is associated with epididymal abnormalities (Michelson, 1949). With bilateral absence the body and tail of the epididymis are usually also absent; the globus major is usually intact (Scorer and Farrington, 1971). An absent vas deferens should also raise the suspicion of a possible upper urinary tract abnormality, since the ureter and vas deferens are both derived from the mesonephric duct (Emery et al., 1974). Ipsilateral renal agenesis may occur more commonly in these instances and may be identified by sonography in these boys. A persistent common mesonephric duct occurs when the terminal excretory duct fails to separate into the ureter and vas deferens, resulting in a persistent common single orifice located somewhere from the trigone to the verumontanum. This is associated with recurrent urinary tract infections and epididymitis and may be diagnosed by voiding cystourethrography (Megalli et al., 1972) (see Fig. 57-12). The ipsilateral seminal vesicle is often cystic, and the ipsilateral kidney is often dysplastic, suggesting total dysplasia of the mesonephric duct and metanephros in these instances (Redman and Sulieman, 1976; Schwarz and Stephens, 1978).

Congenital Abnormalities of the Epididymis

Congenital abnormalities of the epididymis are varied, ranging from total absence, to segmental atresias, to gross structural abnormalities of the intact organ. Most abnormalities of the epididymis have been identified in patients with obstructive azospermia and cryptorchidism. The latter has now been extensively studied in children, and numerous references confirm

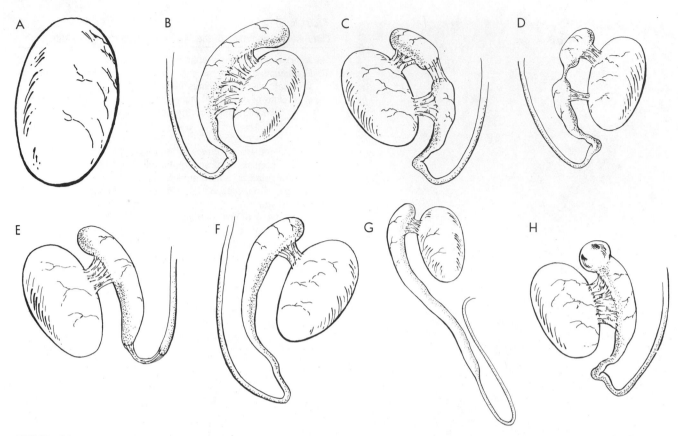

FIG. 57-23
Congenital structural abnormalities of the epididymitis and vas deferens. **A,** Agenesis of all mesonephric duct derivatives. **B,** Nonunion between the globus major of the epididymis and the testis. **C,** Agenesis at the midepididymis. **D,** Atresia at the midepididymis. **E,** Agenesis or atresia at the tail of the epididymis. **F,** Extended or looped epididymis and vas deferens. **G,** Extended or looped epididymis and vas deferens, a more severe abnormality. **H,** Epididymal cyst of globus major. (From Kroovand RL, Perlmutter AD: Congenital anomalies of the vas deferens and epididymis, in Kogan SJ, Hafez ESE (eds): *Pediatric Andrology,* Boston, Martinus Nijhoff, 1981, pp 173-180. Reprinted by permission of Kluwer Academic Publishers.)

a spectrum of epididymal abnormalities in association with this condition. Epididymal abnormalities occur in approximately 33% to 50% of cryptorchid boys (Scorer and Farrington, 1971; Marshall and Shermeta, 1979) and is especially associated with those testes in an intracanalicular or intraabdominal position. The most common abnormality is an extended epididymis (Fig. 57-23) (Kroovand and Perlmutter, 1981). In some instances the looped epididymal tail may be markedly elongated, extending down the entire inguinal canal into the scrotum. In these circumstances the epididymis may be mistaken for a blind-ending spermatic cord or an atrophic testis and may be inadvertently injured or excised, leaving an undiagnosed cryptorchid testis intraabdominally (Fig. 57-24) (Kogan, 1985). Varying degrees of separation of the epididymis from the cryptorchid testis are also common, with the epididymis suspended on a mesentery (Fig. 57-25). Some of these abnormalities may have functional significance, since they may result in occult microscopic ductal obstruction or may affect sperm capacitation.

Epididymal Cysts

Epididymal cysts, though uncommon in the pediatric age group, have received recent attention because of the increased frequency noted in patients with in utero exposure to diethylstilbestrol. These cysts reportedly occur in approximately 5% of normal males and in 21% of males exposed in utero to diethylstilbestrol (Gill et al., 1979). They occur usually in the globus major and rarely may rupture or bleed, causing an acute scrotum (Klauber and Sant, 1985). In general, as accurate diagnosis can be made by palpation, transillumination, and sonograph, surgical exploration is not necessary unless cyst enlargement occurs. The significance of this abnormality on fertility is uncertain.

Congenital Disorders of the Testes

Congenital disorders of the testes in childhood are one of the most common problems dealt with in pediatric urologic practice. In this section they are arbitrarily classified into disorders of number, size, and location.

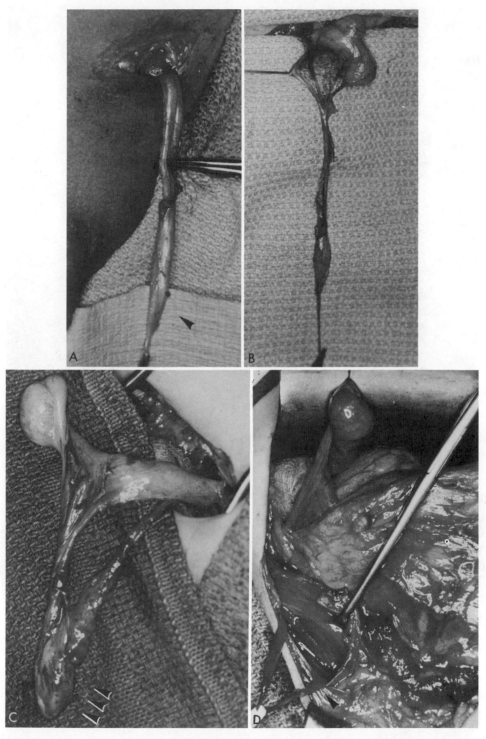

FIG. 57-24
Epididymal structural abnormalities mistaken for blind-ending spermatic cord. **A,** Long-looped vas deferens with nubbin at end *(arrowhead).* The testis lies within the internal ring. **B,** Similar example with long-looped vas deferens and nubbin at end, extending down inguinal canal. The testis was intraabdominal. **C,** Older child with structure mimicking atrophic testis with collapsed surrounding tunica vaginalis at end *(arrowheads)* that had exited through the external inguinal ring. **D,** Blind-ending gubernacularlike structure *(arrowhead)* passing down through inguinal canal. The testis lies above within the abdomen. (From Kogan SJ: Cryptorchidism, in Kelalis PP, King LR, Belman AB (eds): *Clinical Pediatric Urology,* ed 2. Philadelphia, WB Saunders, 1985.)

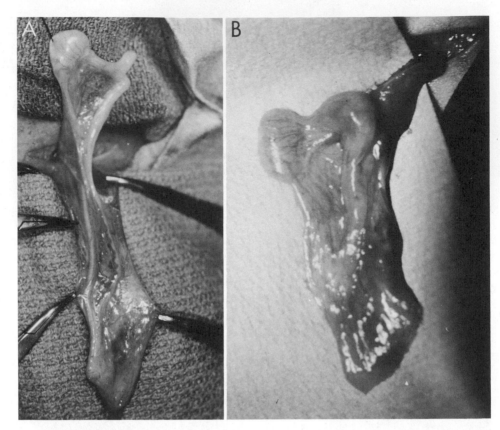

FIG. 57-25
Examples of partial epididymal detachment in cryptorchid testes. **A,** Detachment of the body and tail with long-looped vas deferens. **B,** Virtually complete epididymal detachment with flimsy attachment at epididymal head by a few tubules.

Unilateral Congenital Absence of the Testes

Unilateral congenital absence of the testes occurs uncommonly, with an estimated frequency of 4.0% of the cryptorchid male population. Unilateral congenital absence (monorchia) occurs more commonly (1:25) than bilateral absence or anorchidism (1:20,000) (Levitt et al., 1978b). Absence of the testis may occur from either agenesis (i.e., total development failure of the gonadal ridge) or early deterioration of the testis at some time after initial formation. Because normal fetal testis function is responsible for ipsilateral regression of the müllerian duct and stimulation of the ipsilateral mesonephric duct, examination of these structures gives inferential information about abnormal development of the ipsilateral testis. In this regard, when the testis is found to be absent at surgical exploration, several distinct developmental findings may be encountered: a blind-ending tuft of spermatic vessels, blind-ending ductal structures (epididymis, vas, or both), blind-ending spermatic cord (vas and vessels), or absence of all structures. In our review of 65 cases of surgically diagnosed monorchia, a blind-ending spermatic cord was the most commonly encountered pattern, occurring in 69% (Table 57-3). Absence of all structures, possibly indicating testicular agenesis, was extremely uncommon (14%), and müllerian remnant

TABLE 57-3

Findings in 65 Patients with Unilateral Absent Testes

Findings	Number	Percent
Minispermatic vessels	47	72
Wolffian structures	54	83
Vessels and wolffian structures	45	69
Vessels and vas	20	31
Vessels, vas, and epididymis	12	18
Vessels, vas, epididymis, and terminal nubbin of tissue	13	20
Vas only	9	14
Vessels only	2	3
Absence of vessels and wolffian structures	9	14
TOTAL	**65**	**100**

structures were not seen at surgery (Kogan et al., 1986a). Because the testis is necessary to induce ipsilateral formation of the wolffian (mesonephric) duct and cause regression of the müllerian duct, these surgical findings suggest that testis formation occurred and the testis deteriorated subsequently (i.e., after the fourteenth week, when vas formation is completed). Furthermore, in 20% microscopic examination of a nubbin of tissue at the end of the excised spermatic cord revealed hemosiderin, calcification, or hyalinized tissue compatible with old testicular in-

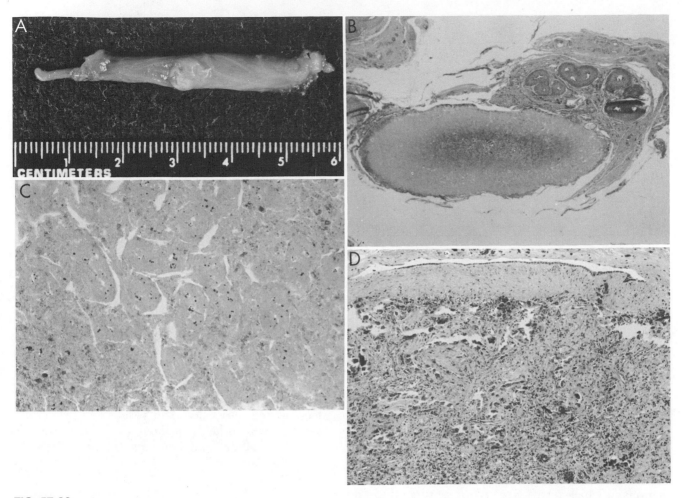

FIG. 57-26
Gross and microscopic findings in congenitally absent testes. **A,** surgical specimen of scrotal nubbin *(arrowhead)* in 3-month-old infant with impalpable testis. **B,** Microscopic view (reduced magnification from × 20) demonstrating necrotic debris with partial calcification in the center with adjacent epididymis. **C,** Higher-power view shows calcification and ghosts of remaining tubules (reduced magnification × 300). **D,** Infarcted testis parenchyma with focal calcification and hemosiderin. Tunica is present along with serosal surface superiorly (reduced magnification × 125). (From Kogan SJ, Gill B, Bennett B, et al: Human monorchidism: a clinicopathological study of unilateral absent testes in 65 boys. *J Urol* 1986; 135:758. Used by permission.)

farction, suggesting that an in utero vascular accident had occurred (i.e., secondary to testicular torsion) (Fig. 57-26). These findings suggest that in utero testicular torsion may be the cause of most cases of congenitally "absent" testes and that most cases of testicular absence result from degeneration of a previously formed testis rather than primary agenesis (Huff et al., 1991)

Bilateral Congenital Absence of the Testes

Similar findings also are encountered in bilateral congenital anorchia, where vasa are usually found at surgical exploration (Levitt et al., 1978a). In this syndrome absent testes are found in an otherwise normal 46,XY phenotypical male. Because testis formation is necessary in utero to stimulate external genital development, these findings imply that the testis deteriorated at some point in time after completion of masculinization (i.e., after the twelfth to fourteenth

week). This syndrome has therefore been appropriately called the "vanishing testis" or "testicular regression syndrome" (Abeyaratne et al., 1969). In situations in which anorchidism is suspected, measurement of basal FSH and LH levels and the response of testosterone secretion to human chorionic gonadotropin (HCG) stimulation have predicted the absence of functioning testicular tissue (Aynsley-Green et al., 1976; Levitt et al., 1978a). Gonadotropin levels in anorchic boys are usually elevated, even early in life (Table 57-4). Even at birth, FSH levels may be elevated, as seen in boys with bilateral neonatal torsion (Kogan, personal observation) and boys with congenital bilateral anorchia. However, LH levels may not elevate until puberty. Testosterone levels in anorchic boys do not rise in response to HCG stimulation; whereas most boys with testes present usually respond to HCG stimulation. When there is a failure to repond to HCG and an elevated FSH (and LH) level, bilateral con-

TABLE 57-4

Endocrine Studies in 10 Anorchic Boys

Age (years)	LH (ng/ml)	FSH (ng/ml)	HCG Stimulation Testosterone	
			Before	After
4	21	318	25	24
5	29	330	31	32
5	29	320	43	41
5.5	61	475	40	40
6	24	308	23	21
7	25	321	25	25
7	27	328	42	44
9	80	900	36	40
10	37	370	44	43
12	180	2100	62	65

genital anorchia may be diagnosed, and surgical exploration for confirmation of diagnosis is not necessary. In these instances, rather than performing an extensive exploratory laparotomy, testicular prostheses are placed through an inguinal incision. When both components of this test are not fulfilled, however (i.e., when a testosterone response to HCG occurs or when gonadotropin levels are not elevated though a testosterone response does not occur), a thorough search must be made because a testis (at least one) lies within.

Confusion regarding the interpretation and diagnostic accuracy of this test has arisen (Kogan, 1978). Three cases with apparently false and misleading evaluations in which testes were found at surgical exploration have been published (Bartone et al., 1984). In these instances, however, careful reading reveals that both components of these strictly defined criteria of a negative test were not fulfilled. The editorial comment after publication also suggested that gonadotropin levels in bilateral anorchics may fall into the normal range between ages 4 and 8 years because of a relatively pituitary-hypothalamic inactivity at this age. Though the latter information was extrapolated from anorchic 45,XO females who demonstrated this phenomenon, and no similar data from anorchic boys were presented, the implication was made that normal gonadotropin levels might occur in the absence of testes. A subsequent review of gonadotropin levels in 30 congenitally anorchic males revealed that one prepubertal patient had normal gonadotropin levels, though the remainder all had elevated levels, indicating that normal levels in prepubertal boys cannot exclude the diagnosis of anorchia. One of two pubertal patients with elevated levels had hypoplastic testes present, indicating that the gonadotropin levels alone cannot diagnose anorchia in the postpubertal male (Jarow et al., 1985). Human chorionic gonadotropin testing alone similarly will not distinguish between anorchia and bilateral impalpable cryptorchidism, since a lack of HCG-in-duced response may occur in hypogonadotropic hypogonadal patients with testes present. Caution must be exercised, therefore, in analyzing data from *post*-pubertal patients, since secondary gonadal failure from damaged testes may be present, resulting (rarely) in elevated gonadotropin levels and failure of response to HCG. In summary, the endocrine diagnosis of bilateral anorchia rests only on demonstration of raised gonadotropin levels *and* a negative testosterone response to HCG. In other circumstances a testis may be present. I am not aware of any cases to date in which this test has not accurately predicted prepubertal bilateral congenital anorchia.

Hormonal testing is not sufficiently accurate to predict unilateral testicular absence. Measurement of FSH and LH levels in 44 patients with monorchia revealed that mean levels were slightly higher than published control values, though too much variation in individual levels existed to make isolated measurements a clinically useful test. In a unique investigation we also contrasted peak-stimulated FSH and LH levels after GnRH stimulation in boys with unilateral impalpable testes who were subsequently found to have a testis present at surgical exploration with those in boys having unilateral absent testes subsequently documented surgically. The results in both groups were indistinguishable, making it an insufficiently accurate clinical discriminatory test (Fig. 57-27) (Kogan et al., 1986a).

Polyorchidism

Polyorchidism is a rare abnormality that probably results from division of the gonadal ridge early in development, since both testes usually have a common proximal blood supply. Occasionally a common vas deferens is present, though usually the epididymis and vas deferens are separate (Mehan et al., 1976). In a review of 53 cases Plender and colleagues (1978) found that in 15% at least one of the ipsilateral testes was cryptorchid. In most instances, therefore, the supernumerary testis is descended and discovered as an asymptomatic swelling in the scrotum. The usual indication for surgical exploration is thus for confirmation of diagnosis. Instances of torsion and malignancy also have been reported.

Abnormalities of Testicular Size

Abnormalities of testicular size are uncommon at birth. Most boys normally have testes measuring about 1 ml at that time. The testes enlarge somewhat during the first few months of life, probably secondary to the postnatal testosterone surge that occurs at 2 months of age, and then decline slightly in size, remaining about 1 to 2 ml until puberty onset (Cassorla et al., 1981). Both hypoplastic and enlarged testes uncommonly occur at birth, the former usually the

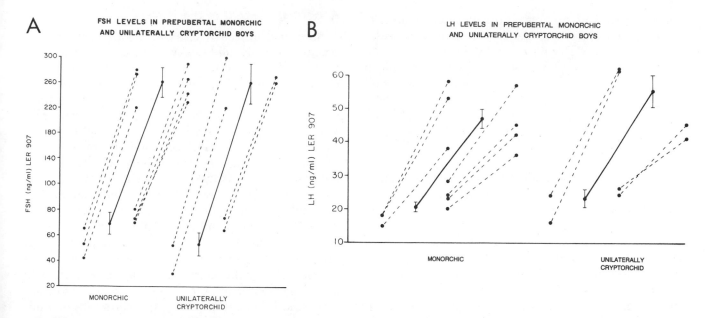

FIG. 57-27
FSH **(A)** and LH **(B)** levels in prepubertal monorchic and unilaterally cryptorchid boys, both with clinically impalpable testes, after GnRH stimulation. *Solid lines* represent mean values; *dotted lines* represent individual values. (From Kogan SJ: Unpublished data.)

result of partial or complete antenatal torsion and the latter as a finding when the contralateral testis is hypoplastic (Huff et al., 1992). Testicular enlargement is the earliest sign of puberty onset in boys, and successive pubertal stages are marked by progressive further testicular enlargement. Abnormalities of testicular size may be noted in both prepubertal and pubertal boys. Measurements of the testes may be accurately done with an orchidometer (Fig. 57-28), with the measured volume compared with published measurements in normal boys at varying ages (Schonfeld and Beebe, 1942).

Microorchidism

Microorchidism may be congenital or may be associated with various syndromes. Najaar and colleagues (1974) described a syndrome of bilateral hypoplastic rudimentary testes and micropenis in siblings in whom the testes were markedly diminished in size and hormonally deficient. The testes are noted to be smaller than expected in Klinefelter's syndrome, even prepubertally (Caldwell and Smith, 1972), and in abnormalities of the hypothalamic-pituitary-gonadal axis (hypogonadotropic hypogonadism). Failure of growth may also result in microorchidism, as is often seen in boys with cryptorchidism and with varicoceles. Smaller than normal testes were seen in 19% of cryptorchid boys at stage P2 puberty, 28.6% at stages P3 and P4, and 38% at stage P5 (Dickerman et al., 1979). Abnormally small ipsilateral testes have been described in between 33% and 50% of boys with vari-

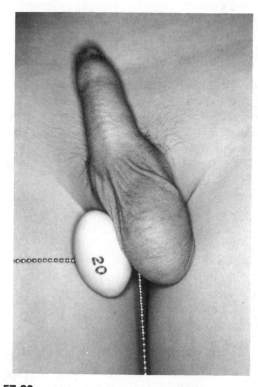

FIG. 57-28
Compensatory hypertrophy of the descended testis of a 12-year-old boy with unilaterally absent contralateral testis. A testis of 20 ml represents the 99th percentile. At age 13 years 2 months, the testis had grown to 50 ml. (From Kogan SJ: Fertility in cryptorchidism, in Hadziselimovic F (ed): *Cryptorchidism: Management and Implications*. New York, Springer-Verlag, 1983, pp 71-82. Used by permission.)

coceles, with this finding occurring more commonly after puberty and in association with large varicoceles (Kass et al., 1987; Lyon et al., 1982; Kogan, 1984). Testicular atrophy also may cause small testes, such as atrophy secondary to previous hernia repair with partial vascular compromise to the testis or testicular torsion. The latter may be a frequent cause of "idiopathic" testis hypoplasia (Kogan et al., 1986a).

Macroorchidism

Unilateral macroorchidism usually results secondarily from a disorder of the contralateral testis, that is, from atrophy or absence, secondary to congenital monorchia or previous torsion (Kogan et al., 1986a; Huff et al, 1992), or from cryptorchidism. Unilateral compensatory hypertrophy was found in 12% of boys with undescended or absent contralateral testes and was associated with FSH hypersecretion. Adult follow-up of seven men revealed oligoaspermia, suggesting that the hypertrophied testis was abnormal as well (Laron et al., 1980). Bilateral testis enlargement is sometimes associated with various syndromes. Precocious puberty, that is, resulting from an intracranial mass, may cause premature skeletal growth and secondary sexual development and testicular enlargement commensurate with the patient's pubertal stage. Hypothyroidism uncommonly causes precocious puberty and bilateral testicular enlargement. Boys with mental retardation have an increased frequency of bilateral macroorchidism. Some have a rare chromosomal disorder in which a small, almost detached portion of the long arm of the X chromosome is seen ("fragile-X syndrome") (Turner et al., 1980). Measurement of testis size in mentally retarded males has been suggested as a simple screening test for this condition. Occasionally a patient is encountered with unilateral or bilateral macroorchidism in the absence of an identifiable cause ("idiopathic") (Lee et al., 1982; Breen et al., 1981). Gonadotropin measurements and a thorough thyroid evaluation should be done, as well as scrotal sonography to exclude a subtle intrascrotal neoplastic process. If these are normal, there is usually no indication for scrotal exploration or biopsy.

Adult-onset, or acquired, congenital adrenal hyperplasia is another rare cause of unilateral testicular enlargement (Chorousos et al., 1981). More commonly in children this condition results in bilateral testicular enlargement, usually with testicular nodularity resulting from islands of benign hyperplastic adrenal tissue within the testis (Kirkland et al., 1977; Newell et al., 1977). The latter conditions are sometimes difficult to distinguish from testicular Leydig cell tumors, which may have similar clinical and endocrinologic manifestations (Waksman, 1981). Serotal sonography is useful in diagnosing 3 conditions and in evaluating potential neoplastic causes of unilateral and bilateral testicular enlargement.

Abnormal Descent of the Testes

Abnormal descent causes the testis to occupy an ectopic or truly undescended position outside the scrotum. Ectopic testes descend normally through the external inguinal ring but are misdirected in the subsequent descent to an extrascrotal position. Fibrous obstruction of the scrotal inlet and gubernacular abnormalities have been described in association with this condition. The most common site of ectopia is the superficial inguinal pouch between the external oblique aponeurosis and the subcutaneous tissue. Perineal, prepenile, transverse scrotal, femoral, and abdominal positions are other, less common sites of ectopia. By contrast, true cryptorchid testes are arrested in their normal line of descent and may occupy an intraabdominal, intracanalicular, or suprascrotal position. Whereas the latter testes may be responsive to hormonal treatment, the former (ectopic) testes are mechanically found in place, therefore requiring operative treatment (Fig 57-29).

Varicoceles

The incidence of varicoceles in boys has been reported to range from 9.0% to 25.8%. A summation of the larger series in the world literature shows a mean of 16.2% in 21,878 boys of ages 10 through 25.

Lyon reported in 1982 (Lyon et al., 1982) that the majority of boys with left varicoceles had small left testes. Pozza and colleagues (1983) found that 74% of 35 boys under the age of 16 with varicoceles had atrophy of the testis and 90% had abnormal testis biopsies. On the other hand, Wyllie found that in 50 normal boys without varicoceles between the ages 10 and 13, there was no significant difference in testis size. Soffer et al. (1988) found that young asymptomatic men with varicoceles had significantly lower testis volume (21.5 ml) and total sperm counts (71 million) than normal controls (30.0 ml; 186 million) and that their testis volume was similar to that for infertile men (21.3 ml; 35 million). Kass and Belman (1987) found that of 20 boys who had varicocele repair 16 were noted to experience an increase in the relative size of the left testis as compared with the right after the repair. Hosli (1988) reported on 20 young men ages 20 to 29 who had had varicoceles repaired at ages 9 to 17. The two testes were equal in size, and the semen quality was better than in an untreated control group. Okuyma and co-workers (1988) studied 40 boys with varicoceles, 24 of whom were treated surgically and 16 of whom refused operation. Testis size improved significantly in the treated boys and deteriorated in the controls. Semen quality was much better in the patients who had surgery. Laven and colleagues (1992) did a randomized study of 88 adolescent males with varicoceles, of whom 33 were observed and 34 were treated. They also studied 21 controls. All patients were followed for a year. The right and left testis vol-

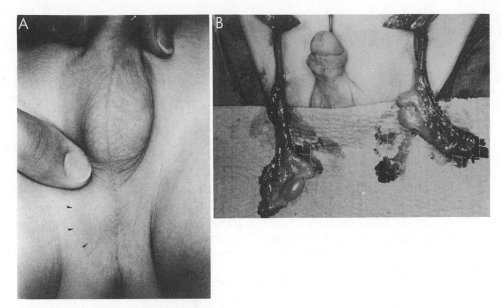

FIG. 57-29
Three-year-old boy with (right) perineal ectopic undescended testis and (left) inguinal cryptorchid testis. **A,** Gross examination reveals perineal bulge *(arrowheads).* **B,** Surgical exposure demonstrates differences in spermatic cord length and in testis size.

ume was smaller in the boys with varicoceles than in the controls. After treatment both left and right testes caught up with the controls, whereas the testes of the untreated group remained smaller than the controls. Similar effects were seen on semen quality. These data strongly suggest that varicoceles can injure the testes in some adolescent boys. In addition, data show that the GnRH infusion test is abnormal in boys with varicoceles.

Most varicoceles appearing in adolescence are asymptomatic. They are usually noticed by a parent or discovered during a routine physical examination. Careful physical examination will often reveal some decrease in size of the left testis compared with the right. This may be difficult to detect unless one uses an orchiometer, calipers, or sonography. We feel that semen analysis should not be routinely done in adolescent boys for two reasons. First, the normal values are variable during development, and second, it is disturbing to some adolescents to be asked to provide a specimen. Semen analysis can be useful in evaluating young men.

There is no consensus as to the indications for varicocele repair in adolescents. We feel that all boys with significant discomfort or atrophy/retarded growth of the left testis should have a varicocele repair. It is much more difficult to reach a firm conclusion relating to boys who have normal testis size bilaterally. The decision in these patients should be individualized. They certainly must be followed, and surgery is recommended at the first sign of decreased growth. In some instances, particularly if the varicocele is large and if the parents, after careful discussion, are agreeable, repair is done. When these young men are older,

they can be followed with yearly semen analyses. Repair is indicated if the semen quality is suboptimal. However, we do feel comfortable recommending varicocele repair, since approximately 20% of these boys will be infertile, and it is not possible to predict which ones.

Recurrences after varicocele repair are not uncommon. The reported recurrence rates in boys are 15% to 16%. Levitt and associates (1987) recently endorsed the recommendation of Sayfen and Adams that intraoperative venography be used to reduce this recurrence rate. Using this technique, they had one recurrence in 28 boys, or a 3.6% recurrence rate. Kass and Marcol (1992) reported respective failure rates of 16%, 11%, and 0 with inguinal repair, high repair sparing the artery, and high repair taking the artery. The last group did not develop testicular atrophy.

Because (1) 15% of couples have a significant fertility problem, (2) in one half of these couples there is a male factor (7.5% of total), (3) 40% of these men have a varicocele (3.0% of total), and (4) the incidence of varicocele is 15%, approximately 20% of adolescent boys with varicocele will require treatment for infertility. The incidence will be higher in those who delay parenthood. Treatment of adult varicoceles is clearly less effective than correction of adolescent varicoceles. Therefore, it is reasonable to fix varicoceles in young men with decreased testis size or reduced semen quality.

Varicoceles can be repaired by high or inguinal open surgery, laparoscopic surgery, or percutaneous radiologic methods. These techniques are discussed in Chapter 34, on infertility.

In summary, varicoceles are quite common anomalies in boys. They may cause testicular injury, including decreased size and histologic abnormalities. These changes may eventually result in infertility. Surgery is recommended for boys in whom injury has been documented or the varicocele is symptomatic. For boys without these findings, the appropriate course is less clear. Certainly, all boys with varicoceles should be followed and careful explanation of the matter should be given to the parents.

Incisions

Access for scrotal and testicular surgery can be provided by either scrotal, inguinal, or abdominal routes. Each particular route has its advantages for performing the specific surgical task at hand. The incisions used for surgery on the testis, scrotum, and cord structures are similar and hence are discussed here in common.

Standard Inguinal Incision

The standard inguinal incision is used for entry into the inguinal canal to perform hernia repair, orchiopexy, varicocelectomy, and so forth, as well as for delivery of the testis from the scrotum to perform hydrocelectomy or radical orchiectomy for tumor. This incision is best placed transversely in the lower abdominal skin crease, where it usually results in a well-healed, indefinable linear scar 1 year or so after treatment. Oblique incisions paralleling the inguinal canal should be avoided, since they do not follow Langer's lines and often result in broad, unsightly scars. The argument that oblique incisions can be used to extend the surgical dissection higher, as in treating high undescended testes, if not founded because in children the same exposure can usually be obtained by using a transverse incision of adequate length.

Following the skin incision, Scarpa's fascia is divided and the external oblique aponeurosis is exposed and opened parallel to the inguinal ligament. Care must be taken to avoid transection of the underlying ilioinguinal nerve, which often hugs the underside of the external oblique fascia, especially in older children. At this point, herniorrhaphy, orchiopexy, or varicocelectomy may be accomplished, as detailed in the following sections. Closure of the external oblique and the subcutaneous tissue is done with an absorbable suture, and the skin is similarly closed with a subcuticular absorbable suture of appropriate size. Bilateral inguinal incisions may be used for simultaneous repair of bilateral defects. In general, these incisions are extremely well tolerated in children and heal without any difficulties.

Suprainguinal Retroperitoneal Muscle-Splitting Incisions

Suprainguinal retroperitoneal muscle-splitting incisions have been described mostly for "high ligation"

of the internal spermatic vein. Some have advocated this approach directly above the internal inguinal ring at a level above the divergence of the vas deferens, since the internal spermatic vein is more likely to be single at this level (Palomo, 1949). A transverse inguinal skin incision is made and then retracted superiorly, and the external oblique aponeurosis is incised, followed by splitting of the underlying muscles to gain entry to the retroperitoneal space. Alternatively, a true lower quadrant or flank incision (Ivanissevich, 1960) may be made to approach the internal spermatic vein higher in the retroperitoneum. In these approaches, care must be taken to identify and protect the adjacent ureter. These muscle-splitting incisions are closed thereafter in layers with absorbable sutures, resulting in a very strong closure.

Lower Abdominal Incisions for Simultaneous Exposure of Both Testes

Various lower abdominal incisions for simultaneous exposure of both testes have been described and are used primarily for orchiopexy when both testes are high or impalpable, when simultaneous separate inguinal incisions may not give adequate exposure for safe dissection. Flynn and King (1971) recommended a midline transperitoneal approach for dissection of the intraabdominal testis, followed by creation of a new inguinal ring just lateral to the pubic tubercle so that the spermatic cord might assume the most direct route into the scrotum (Fig. 57-30). This incision may also be used to approach the testis preperitoneally by dissection along the rectus sheath laterally until the retroperitoneum is entered and then mobilizing the testis and cord at that level (Lipton, 1961; Boley and Kleinhaus, 1966; Hunt et al., 1981). In some instances, especially when an extensive exposure of bilateral intraabdominal testes is necessary, both lower rectus muscles may be totally transected, resulting in wide preperitoneal or intraperitoneal exposure. I favor making a wide transverse skin incision, followed by either a midline entry to the peritoneal cavity or by division of the lower rectus muscles to allow for extensive preperitoneal or intraperitoneal exposure. The latter is the ideal incision to use in boys with prune-belly syndrome undergoing orchiopexy since their lower abdominal muscles are already attenuated.

Incisions into the Scrotum

Incisions into the scrotum are made to allow direct access to the testis and paratesticular structures. In children, the most common indications are for exploration of suspected testicular torsion or torsion of a testicular appendage, or for bilateral testicular biopsy in evaluation of children treated for acute lymphatic leukemia with suspected testicular involvement. Though individual transverse scrotal incisions may be made for direct access to each hemiscrotal compart-

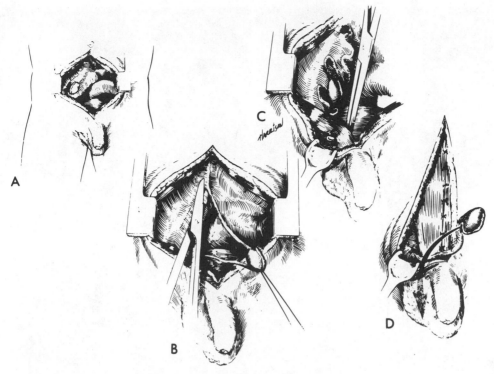

FIG. 57-30

Technique of transabdominal orchiopexy. **A,** Intraabdominal view showing testis intraperitoneally at pelvic brim. **B,** Testicular mobilization from posterior peritoneum and restraining bands. **C,** New external ring created at the level of lateral rectus muscle border and superior pubic ramus. **D,** Testis brought through the opening and placed within the scrotum. (From Kogan SJ: Cryptorchidism, in Kelalis PP, King LR, Belman AB (eds): *Clinical Pediatric Urology,* ed 2. Philadelphia, WB Saunders 1985.)

ment, I prefer a vertical midline raphe incision, since it is simpler and more cosmetic. The midline raphe is incised, with care taken to avoid carrying the incision onto the base of the penis. Following dissection deeper into the dartos, a separate incision is made into each hemiscrotal compartment, through which each testis is delivered separately. Following biopsy or detorsion and suture fixation, each testis is returned, and the separate incisions are closed with interrupted absorbable sutures. The midline raphe incision is then closed separately in one layer with interrupted absorbable sutures. It is important to reemphasize that in children scrotal incisions are not used to perform testicular biopsies when solid tumors are suspected, nor are they used for hydrocelectomy, since invariably an associated processus vaginalis is present that requires ligation superiorly.

Scrotal incisions are also made to fix the testis in place as part of an orchiopexy procedure. The previously described practice of testicular fixation to the contralateral thigh by direct suture or by rubber band traction are not advised, since follow-ups indicated a high frequency of testicular atrophy in these instances. Fixation of the testis into the contralateral hemiscrotal compartment across the midline septum has been described (Ombredanne, 1927) and continues to have its advocates. However, the most popular method of fix-

ation used by child surgeons is the subcutaneous pouch method, with fixation of the testis beneath the skin and above the dartos muscle (Lattimer et al., 1973). Following adequate mobilization of the spermatic cord and testis, a short transverse ipsilateral scrotal incision is made through the skin. A plane is developed between the skin and the underlying dartos with a curved hemostat adequate in size to accommodate the testis and epididymis. An incision of sufficient size to pull the testis within is then made in the underlying dartos with the aid of a previously placed traction suture. The testis is positioned in the pouch, and the traction suture is passed through the dependent scrotal skin and then tied to itself or fastened to a button or gauze pledget. Some prefer to suture the testis directly to the dartos rather than use this dependent suture through the skin. Thereafter, the scrotal incision is closed with interrupted fine chromic sutures in one layer.

Though there have been refinements in the incisions and operations used for orchiopexy, successful surgical placement of the testis within the scrotum continues to depend on the surgical principles first enunciated by Bevan in 1899, namely, adequate mobilization of the testis and spermatic vessels, repair cf the associated hernia, and adequate fixation of the testis within the scrotum. The choice of surgical pro-

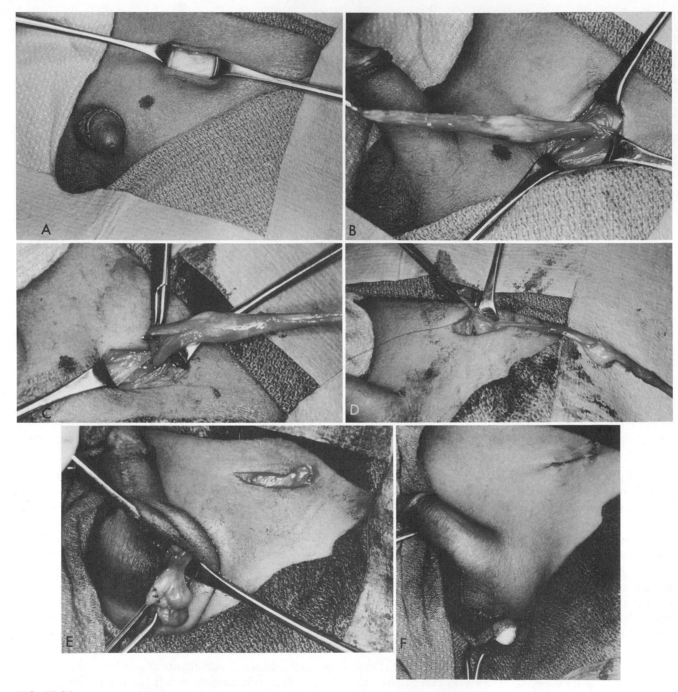

FIG. 57-31
A-F, Technique of orchiopexy for palpable undescended testes (see text for description). (From Kogan SJ: Cryptorchidism, in Kelalis PP, King LR, Belman AB (eds): *Clinical Pediatric Urology,* ed 2. Philadelphia, WB Saunders 1985.

cedure to achieve these goals is determined to a great extent by the location of the testis; therefore, the procedures for palpable and impalpable undescended testes are considered here separately.

Palpable Undescended Testes

Palpable undescended testes are usually located within the superficial ectopic space or within or emerging from the inguinal canal, and therefore are best approached through the standard inguinal incision (Fig. 57-31). The distal attachments to the scrotum are divided sharply, with care taken to avoid a long-looped vas that sometimes extends distally beyond the testis toward the scrotum (see Fig. 57-33). Occasionally these attachments may be ectopic (i.e., extending toward the thigh or pubis). The testis and cord are then sharply dissected up to and into the intestinal inguinal ring (Fig. 57-31, *B*). No attempt is made to dissect within the cord substance, because it does not result in any significant cord lengthening and actually may endanger the spermatic artery. In some instances, as when the undescended testis is quite distal or lies in a superficial ectopic position, no additional dissection is needed; adequate spermatic cord length exists for satisfactory scrotal placement of the testis. Further dissection is necessary in some cases, especially along the lateral attachments of the spermatic cord (lateral spermatic fascia). Anatomic dissections have demonstrated that this extracanalicular dissection can provide up to three fourths of the entire potential length obtainable during orchiopexy, with only one fourth from the intracanalicular dissection (Prentiss et al., 1960). The internal inguinal ring may be opened with the cautery to allow higher dissection within the ring if additional length is needed. This dissection is essentially the mobilization of the spermatic vessels and the vas out of the enveloping endoabdominal fascia. Extending this mobilization allows in most cases sufficient length to the spermatic vessels and vas for even intraabdominal testes to be placed into the scrotum. The hernia sac, which is virtually always present with a true undescended testis and often present in association with an ectopic testis, is sharply dissected proximally off the cord, divided, twisted, doubly ligated at the internal ring with an absorbable suture, and then dropped back into a retroperitoneal position (Fig. 57-31, *C, D*). Occasionally this dissection of the hernia sac may be difficult, resulting in a proximal peritoneal tear extending within the internal ring. In such circumstances the ring must be opened, as described previously, to obtain better visualization and a sound peritoneal closure. A pathway is made into the scrotum with the dissecting finger to ensure that there are no obstructing bands of tissue remaining. Scrotal fixation of the testis is done by the method described previously, and the groin incision is closed (Fig. 57-31, *E, F*).

The important elements, then, in obtaining adequate spermatic cord length for orchiopexy are mobilization up into the internal inguinal ring, division of the lateral spermatic fascia, and division of the hernia sac and dissection of the cord off the posterior peritoneum for an adequate distance. It is often quite surprising how high the spermatic cord can be dissected through the standard inguinal incision, and we have sometimes carried our dissection almost up to the lower pole of the kidney when necessary. The limiting factor in these instances is not the skin incision but rather the internal inguinal ring, which should be opened generously to give adequate exposure. When these maneuvers still do not achieve

adequate spermatic cord length for successful scrotal placement of the testis, the floor of the internal ring may be taken down, dividing the internal epigastric vessels and transversalis fascia, thereby allowing the testis and cord to make a direct path to the pubic tubercle. The floor of the inguinal canal is then closed over the cord, superimposing the internal and external inguinal rings. Skeletization of the vas deferens to achieve additional cord length should not be attempted, because the vas deferens is seldom short enough to be an impediment to successful orchiopexy and because of the inherent dangers to the vas deferens by this manipulation (Shandling and Janik, 1981). Furthermore, this maneuver does not result in any additional cord lengthening.

Laparoscopy

In recent years, the explosive growth of laparoscopic surgery has led to its enthusiastic application to the patient with undescended testis (see Chapter 60). This would appear most appropriate for the approximately 20% of cases where the testis is impalpable. Approximately one quarter to one third of these testes will be found to be intraabdominal. Here one would hope laparoscopy would have its greatest utility. In spite of this enthusiasm, however, how much practical benefit is obtainable remains to be determined.

The diagnostic use of laparoscopy for impalpable testes was suggested by Cortesi and co-workers (1976). In the patient with a unilateral impalpable undescended testis, we have been disinclined to use laparoscopy primarily because in the majority of cases where the testis is absent, we have found that the vas and vessels ended distal to the internal ring (Turek et al., 1994). With our aggressive mobilization of the spermatic vessels by a transperitoneal approach done through the same inguinal incision, we have been able to get almost all intraabdominal testes into the scrotum in a primary operation. Accordingly, we would not exhibit much enthusiasm for the use of laparoscopy in unilateral impalpable testes.

When there are bilateral impalpable testes, however, the situation is different. Here there appears to be a much stronger rationale for the use of initial laparoscopy, as it does indeed let one plan an appropriate strategic approach. We do not feel that the decision concerning the placement of incisions is very critical, as we have consistently been able to deal with all types of undescended testes through a standard inguinal incision with at most a minor lateral extension. This permits the internal ring to be opened, providing excellent exposure for even an extensive mobilization of the spermatic pedicle.

In the boy who is found at laparoscopy to have only

one intraabdominal testis, our approach is to be very conservative concerning the possible loss of that testis, as there continues to be considerable morbidity at present in hormonal replacement in males. Accordingly, we would carry out an open operation, carefully mobilizing the spermatic artery and placing the testis as distal and superficial as possible to permit palpation. If the testis cannot be placed superficial to the external oblique fascia, then it is marked with small metallic clips that permit subsequent ultrasound surveillance with ease (Snyder, 1993). If, at laparoscopy, two intraabdominal testes within 2 cm of the internal ring are located, these should be able to be mobilized to place them in the scrotum without division of the spermatic artery (Peters, 1994, personal communication). This can be accomplished by laparoscopic orchiopexy (Jordan and Winslow, 1994) or by open surgery. In the older boy, a laparoscopic orchiopexy may produce less discomfort than one carried out with two inguinal incisions. In the small boy, however, recovery is so rapid as to make this consideration a minor one. If, at laparoscopy, two very high intraabdominal testes are located, this could perhaps be the most justifiable case for the use of primary laparoscopic approach to orchiopexy. A primary clipping of the spermatic artery will cause the vasal artery to hypertrophy and make a subsequent staged orchiopexy more successful (Bloom, 1991; Caldamone and Amaral, 1994). The experimental work by Pascual and colleagues (1989) provides a good physiologic rationale for this approach. A secondary laparoscopic orchiopexy in this staged fashion has been shown to be highly successful.

The disadvantages of laparoscopy appear to revolve around two primary constraints. Whereas diagnostic laparoscopy can be carried out by one laparoscopic surgeon, for a laparoscopic orchiopexy two well-trained laparoscopic surgeons are needed. As only perhaps one quarter to one third of impalpable testes will need this additional staffing, planning the logistics of a surgical practice could be difficult. Additionally, there is the high initial cost and subsequent expense of maintenance of laparoscopic equipment and supplies. This may double the cost of an orchiopexy over the standard open inguinal approach. For a boy with bilateral intraabdominal testes, this extra expense may be justified, but it would seem to be rarely so for the boy with a unilateral intraabdominal testis. Hinman's suggestion that these unilateral intraabdominal testes may not be worth the salvage in the first place must always be borne in mind (Hinman, 1980).

Impalpable Undescended Testes

Impalpable undescended testes pose special problems in the performance of successful orchiopexy. The choice of incision is different, and the technique of orchiopexy is usually more extensive. Furthermore, since in at least one fourth of these cases the testis will ultimately be discovered to be absent, this surgery must start with a properly planned exploration.

Unilateral Impalpable Testes

Unilateral impalpable testes are explored through a standard inguinal incision, with lateral extension if necessary. If the testis or a small tongue of protruding peritoneum is not encountered within the inguinal canal, the internal inguinal ring is immediately opened, as previously described. This tongue of peritoneum often is the harbinger of an intraabdominal testis within, and futher mobilization of this protrusion often will result in prolapse of the testis out of its intraabdominal position. When the testis is still not evident, no further dissection is done through the internal ring because the vas associated with an intraabdominal testis often runs close by the internal ring, and the vas or the vasal artery may be injured by retroperitoneal dissection. Instead, the peritoneum is opened directly by picking up the peritoneum knuckle that presents at the internal ring. This transperitoneal exposure permits the rapid identification of an intraabdominal testis. Though the testis is a retroperitoneal organ, it is often more easily visualized intraperitoneally, just as the ovary is visualized suspended on its mesentery intraperitonally in the female. Once identified, a suture is taken through the capsule of the testis, and gentle traction is applied to assess the spermatic cord length so that the appropriate method of orchiopexy may then be chosen.

Bilateral Impalpable Testes

When bilateral impalpable testes are present, they can be approached through any one of the previously described transverse lower abdominal skin crease incisions. Since the protruding peritoneal processus or the testis itself is often encountered within the inguinal canal, both canals are opened initially. When no structures are evident, the skin and subcutaneous fascia are dissected superiorly off the rectus fascia, and a midline vertical incision is made, followed by preperitoneal or transperitoneal exposure. Since direct visualization of the proximal spermatic vessels is helpful in these instances, a transperitoneal exposure is preferred.

In the course of exploring for an impalpable testis, it may become evident that the testis is not present. Various anatomic patterns may be found indicating that monorchia exists (see Table 57-3). If structures resembling a blind-ending spermatic cord, vas deferens, or vessels alone are found within the inguinal canal at the onset of exploration, they are traced within the internal ring to the point of divergence of the vas deferens and accompanying vessels, to ensure that the miniature vessels visualized are, in fact, the

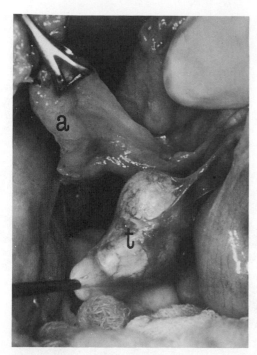

FIG. 57-32
Testis *(t)* located immediately adherent to mesentery of appendix *(a)* medial to cecum. Rudimentary epididymis was present; vas deferens was absent. (From Wu RHK, Kogan SJ, Levitt SB: *Urology* 1966; 27:434.)

spermatic vessels, and are not cremasteric, vasal, or otherwise. This is an extremely important surgical point, since blind-ending spermatic vessels are the sine qua non of testicular absence, and no cases where these vessels were present and a testis was found elsewhere are recorded (Levitt et al., 1978). Identification of the spermatic vessels coursing up the posterior retroperitoneum, therefore, signals the end of the exploration; it is unnecessary to carry the exploration further, provided accurate identification of spermatic vessels is made. If a vas deferens alone is encountered, exploration is carried further as previously indicated, since a wide separation of the vas deferens and the testis is possible with the testis lying within the abdomen (Fig. 57-32). Similarly, absence of all structures demands that the exploration proceed further.

An additional reason for accurately identifying the spermatic vessels within the internal inguinal ring is the frequent misleading appearance of these high undescended testes. Jones (1966) has clearly stated this problem best:

> It should be mentioned that at operation, even when it appears that an atrophic testis had been located, a thorough exploration in the region of the internal ring is still necessary for the macroscopic findings are sometimes bizarre and misleading. Segments of the vas may be absent, a structure resembling the spermatic cord may lay a false scent into the scrotum while the testis

lies in the abdomen. Conversely it is sometimes helpful to invaginate the scrotum into the inguinal incision to inspect the contents before proceeding to further exploration.

The surgical implications of this problem are very clear. Structures within the inguinal canal consisting of a looped epididymis or vas deferens may resemble a blind-ending spermatic cord or atrophic testis and may be mistakenly excised. An absent testis may be misdiagnosed, where the testis may actually lie above, within the abdomen (Marshall and Shermeta, 1979). Occult undescended testes have been discovered within the internal inguinal ring at reexploration after the initial exploration failed to accurately define these structures within the inguinal canal or to include an intraperitoneal exploration (Kogan et al., 1982).

Following completion of this extensive exploration, when the testis is identified, a gentle stretch with a traction suture will allow assessment of spermatic vessel length. If this assessment indicates that adequate length may be achieved by a standard high dissection of the spermatic cord, this approach should be pursued as the most favorable choice. Many surgeons do not appreciate that a conventional high dissection of the spermatic cord will allow for successful orchiopexy of most intraabdominal testes (Fig. 57-33). If the initial assessment reveals that the vessels are too short, precluding satisfactory scrotal placement by this means, a primary orchiopexy by transection of the testicular vessels, with or without microvascular anastomosis, or a staged orchiopexy will be required.

Orchiopexy by Spermatic Vessel Transection

Orchiopexy by spermatic vessel transection was originally described by Bevan in 1903; however, because of poor results, it rapidly fell out of favor until Fowler and Stephens in 1959 better characterized the vascular anatomy of these high undescended testes. Intraoperative angiography was used to demonstrate vascular anastomoses between the vasal and spermatic arteries. They recommended temporarily occluding the internal spermatic vessels to test the capacity of this collateral blood supply (Fowler-Stephens test). Using these principles, they achieved successful scrotal placement of the testis in 8 out of 12 patients. Subsequent success was achieved by Brendler and Wulfson (1967) in all 5 of their patients, and they further refined this procedure by indicating that the spermatic vessels should be ligated high away from the testis, avoiding dissection within the cord itself. In 1972 Clatworthy and colleagues reported on the results of 32 testicular vessel transections, which were divided into those done as a "premeditated" procedure and those done as a "salvage" operation following un-

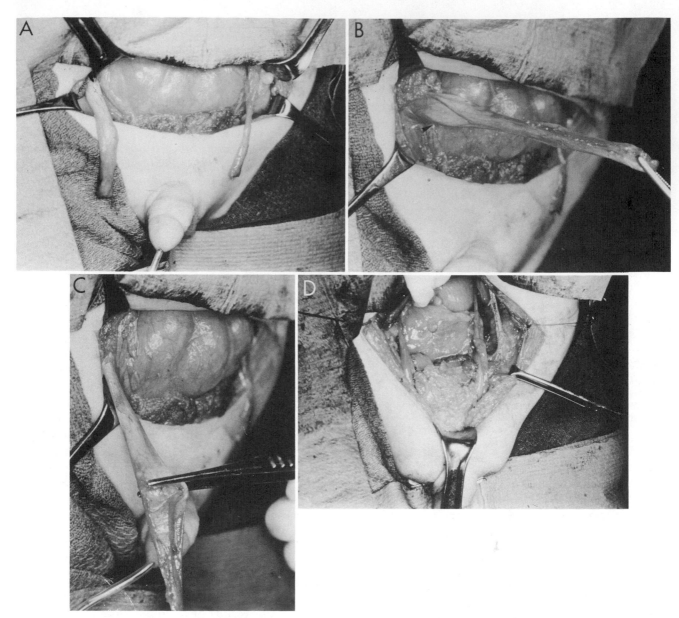

FIG. 57-33
Technique of orchiopexy of impalpable intraabdominal testes by high retroperitoneal dissection. Excellent exposure is provided by complete rectus muscle transection. **A,** Processus vaginalis extending down inguinal canal often indicates higher intraabdominal testis. **B,** Testis extruded from its intraabdominal position into processus. **C,** High retroperitoneal dissection allows for adequate spermatic cord length for testis to reach scrotum. **D,** Direct course of each spermatic cord into scrotum following scrotal fixation.

successful extensive previous cord mobilization. In the former group, 18 or 21 operations were successful; in the latter, only 6 of 11 did not undergo atrophy. These authors recommended leaving the epigastric vessels and floor of the inguinal canal intact, and avoiding mobilization of the posterior wall of the hernia sac off the spermatic cord. Johnston (1977), in discussing orchiopexy of the intraabdominal testis in the prune-belly syndrome, further refined this procedure by indicating that a broad strip of medially based peritoneum along the vas deferens should be left intact,

along with its extensive collateral blood supply (Fig. 57-34). Recent series incorporating these important modifications of the original operation have proved even more successful (Kogan et al., 1989). Gibbons and colleagues (1979) reported success in 22 of 27 patients with intraabdominal testes, with most failures encountered initially when the vessel transection followed extensive spermatic cord mobilization. These authors analyzed retrospectively the possible pitfalls in performing this procedure as (1) failing to leave the wide, medially based peritoneal strip attached to the

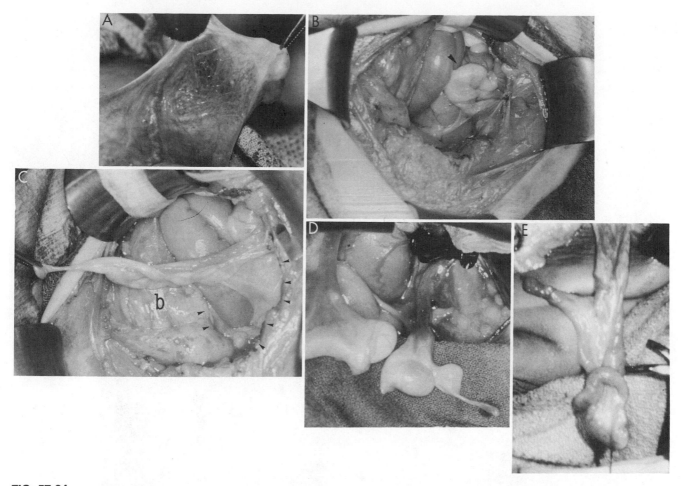

FIG. 57-34

Technique of orchiopexy of intraabdominal testis by testicular vessel transection technique. **A,** Close-up showing collateral vascularity in the peritoneal strip between the spermatic and vasal vessels. **B,** Transabdominal exposure demonstrating high intraabdominal tests *(arrowhead)*. Bladder is at inferior margin of figure. **C,** Left intraabdominal testis, spermatic vessels, and medially based peritoneal strip *(arrowheads)* along the vas deferens. *b,* bladder. **D,** Nontraumatic bulldog clamp applied high on spermatic vessels. **E,** Testis brought down on collateral blood supply within medially based peritoneal strip along vas deferens. (**A** from Kogan SJ: Cryptorchidism, in Kelalis PP, King LR, Belman AB (eds); *Clinical Pediatric Urology* ed 2. Philadelphia, WB Saunders, 1985, pp 864-887. Used by permission.)

vas deferens; (2) doing the procedure as a salvage operation; (3) ligating the internal spermatic vessels too close to the testis; and (4) directly injuring the vasal artery in the course of mobilization.

Woodard and Trulock (1983) have listed the conditions that preclude doing an orchiopexy by testicular vessel transection as (1) the presence of a short, limiting vas deferens; (2) a hypoplastic testis with an uncertain blood supply; (3) segmental vas atresia; and (4) a detached epididymis. In our series we did not encounter either of the last two conditions. Testes with uncertain blood supplies were excluded by the Fowler-Stephens test. Two patients with a short vas deferens had their testes placed in the most dependent position achievable at the time of vessel transection and underwent a successful secondary orchiopexy of these previously transected testes at a later date, indicating that persistence in dealing with these difficult

testes is sometimes necessary. (Kogan et al., 1989).

Ransley and co-workers (1984) have described a novel variation of this operation in which the internal spermatic vessels are first ligated without mobilization at an initial stage. Several months later the vessels are divided, and orchiopexy is completed as described previously. This approach allows for enhanced collateral vessel development and may be more reliable, especially in very small patients. Woodward and Parrott (1978) have also indicated that orchiopexy of the intraabdominal testes found in prune-belly patients may often be done in the neonatal period by mobilization of the intact spermatic pedicle without the need for division of the spermatic vessels.

Microvascular Orchiopexy

Microvascular orchiopexy has given an added dimension to the treatment of intraabdominal testes.

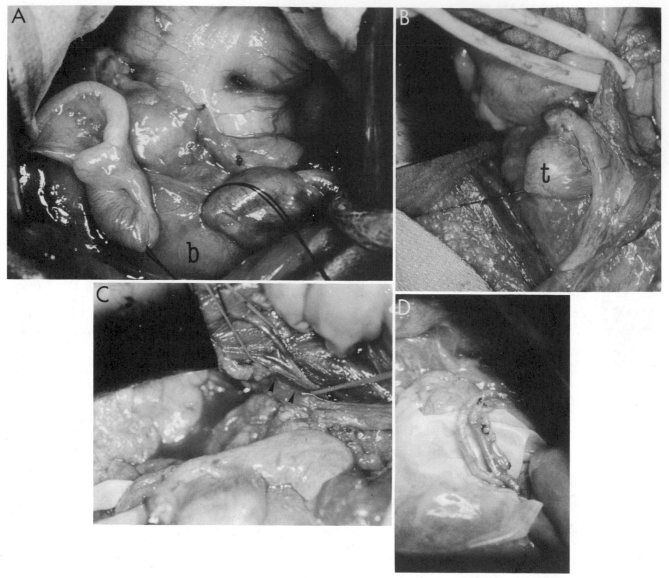

FIG. 57-35
Technique of orchiopexy of intraabdominal testis by microvascular reanastomosis. **A,** Bilateral intraabdominal testes found adjacent to bladder *(b).* **B,** Spermatic vessels (Penrose drain), testis with traction suture *(t),* processus mobilized from within inguinal canal *(lower right).* **C,** Inferior epigastric artery and vein *(arrowheads)* mobilized from under rectus muscle. **D,** Microvascular anastomosis of testicular artery and vein to epigastric vessels. Testis is already positioned inferiorly.

Since the first reported case by Silber and Kelly in 1976, others have reported success using microvascular techniques. The reestablishment of an intact blood supply to the testis by anastomosing the internal spermatic artery to the inferior epigastric artery would seem to offer additional safety beyond reliance on the collateral blood supply accompanying the vas deferens. For microsurgical orchiopexy, the initial exposure and procedure are the same as for testicular vessel transection; however, in this case the internal spermatic vessels are dissected up to their juncture with the aorta or vena cava prior to ligation to ensure as wide a lumen as possible for the anastomosis. This procedure is especially important in younger children,

since these vessels are extremely small. The medial peritoneal pedicle along the vas deferens is developed. The inferior epigastric vessels are exposed by incising the floor of the inguinal canal, with dissection superiorly under the rectus muscle to achieve an adequate length for anastomosis. By use of the operating microscope, following vessel spatulation, the smaller spermatic artery is anastomosed to the larger epigastric artery with an approximating microsurgical clamp and interrupted 10-0 or 11-0 nylon sutures (Fig. 57-35). The vein is done thereafter in a similar manner. Closure of the abdomen and scrotal fixation of the testis are performed as previously described.

Although these initial successful reports are impressive and the surgical technique of microvascular orchiopexy is now well established, it is unlikely that this procedure will be used for routine treatment of these high undescended testes since comparable success rates can be achieved by division of the spermatic vessels without microvascular reanastomosis. Furthermore, though many urologists are now becoming adept with microsurgical techniques, it is uncommon to find the microscope set up and available routinely for surgery of patients with impalpable testes, especially in unilateral cases. Further, more precise follow-up is also needed to determine the failure rate with this procedure when it is used by other operating surgeons, since such failures are often not reported.

Staged Orchiopexy

When neither of the previous procedures is possible or appropriate, a staged orchiopexy may be elected. Estimates describing the need for this operation have ranged form 0.6% (Gross and Jewett, 1956) to 21.5% (Firor, 1971); this discrepancy probably represents the percentage of very high testes present in these series. Two recent series of staged orchiopexies have indicated a success rate between 82% and 90%, testifying to the efficacy of this approach (Zer et al., 1975; Kiesewetter et al., 1981). Following maximal mobilization of the cord and testis, the testis is sutured to its most dependent position obtainable without tension, such as the pubic tubercle, inguinal ligament, or scrotum, with a nonabsorbable suture left long for subsequent identification. The second-stage exploration is done after an interval of at least 1 year. Considerable scarring may be present, and these reoperations are difficult procedures, with a definite risk of vas and vessel injury. This possibility of scarring has led some to advocate wrapping the testis and cord in a sheet of thin Silastic at the first stage (Corkery, 1975). The testis and spermatic cord must again be mobilized completely at the second stage, with the expectation that the time interval has allowed for additional growth and lengthening of the spermatic cord that will result in successful scrotal testicular placement. In a careful, critical review, Redman (1977) suggested that staged orchiopexies represent instances of less-than-complete initial explorations, with a more extensive secondary procedure needed thereafter. He further questioned the concept that further spermatic and cord lengthening occurs after the first procedure. My experience with a select limited number of personal patients on whom I performed both the initial and second stages suggests that this phenomenon of cord lengthening does occur, however, since scrotal testicular placement was always successful following the second stage. With the more extensive dissection that accompanies contemporary orchiopexy techniques as well as selective use of more specialized

techniques for intra-abdominal testes, staged orchiopexies are undertaken far less frequently than was done in the past.

Surgical Complications after Orchiopexy

Surgical complications after orchiopexy have been analyzed in a number of reports (Mengel and Hecker, 1979; Cywes et al., 1981; Lynch et al., 1982; Maizels et al., 1983). Orchiopexy was possible in almost 90% of 207 patients having either palpable or impalpable undescended testes, with 187 patients (also almost 90%) achieving a satisfactory scrotal position. In 6 of these patients undergoing orchiopexy, the testis was in a high scrotal position and was retracted into an inguinal position, and in 13 (7%) postoperative atrophy occurred. Twelve patients in this series of 233 underwent orchiectomy rather than orchiopexy because of dysplastic or primary atrophic appearances. No intraoperative complications were noted (Lynch et al., 1982). In another series of 492 patients, results were graded as "good," "fair," or "poor" according to the testis size, position, consistency, and mobility. Only 60% of testes had a good result, with 22% characterized as poor. Sixteen percent of the overall group were clearly atrophic (Cywes et al., 1981). Of course, postoperative atrophy in undescended testes must be related to the preoperative size of the testis, since some undescended testes are small to begin with; hence, it is likely that some of the "atrophic" testes in this series do not represent surgically induced atrophy. A brighter outlook regarding atrophy is seen in Mengel and Hecker's (1979) series, where a 2% atrophy rate was encountered.

Figures regarding intraoperative injury to the vas deferens are difficult to come by. Mengel and Hecker (1979) cite a 1% to 2% frequency in their series. Vas deferens injury during orchiopexy is completely preventable, and even these figures should be considered excessive.

Maizels and co-workers (1983) examined the reasons for inadequate testis position following orchiopexy in a series of 350 boys, finding a 10% frequency of failure of the initial surgical procedure. Retroperitoneal dissection adequately corrected the initial failure in 58%, whereas local inguinal dissection was adequate in 37%. They concluded that incomplete initial dissection appeared to be the cause of inadequate position after orchiopexy and that aggressive high surgical dissection should prevent inadequate scrotal testicular placement in most instances.

Recently, Cartwright and colleagues (1993) described a successful approach to reoperative orchiopexy that emphasizes the en bloc mobilization of the testis with a strip of the external oblique fascia attached to the underlying vas and spermatic vessels in order to avoid their injury. Using this approach, they report a successful scrotal repositioning of the testis in 24 of 25 cases (Cartwright et al., 1993).

Surgical complications occur more frequently in impalpable undescended testes, and are cited as high as 20% to 50% (Levitt et al., 1978). With the techniques currently available, however, a significantly reduced complication rate should be expected.

Insertion of a Testicular Prosthesis

The preceding descriptions indicate that a plethora of surgical approaches exist to successfully treat the intraabdominal undescended testis. Orchiectomy of the undescended testis is not indicated in the prepubescent child except when there is a major separation of the testis and its ductal structures. In postpubertal boys the testis often is atrophied, is histologically devoid of germ cells, and harbors an increased chance of later malignant degeneration. Orchiectomy is the procedure of choice in these circumstances, even though a successful orchiopexy may be carred out (Martin and Menck, 1975). In these circumstances, insertion of a testicular prosthesis is indicated. Though few studies document the psychologic efficacy and importance of prosthesis placement (Bell, 1974), it is our strong impression that prosthesis placement is important in the monorchic or orchiectomized boy. Testicular prostheses now exist to fit virtually every age and size and are implanted at the same time that these procedures are done, except when a scrotal incision has been made (e.g., for acute spermatic cord torsion). In general, we choose the largest prosthesis that does not look unsightly. Many of our patients do not indicate a desire for replacement with a larger prosthesis after puberty, since the dependency of the existing one often lends a normal cosmetic appearance. Testicular prostheses should never be placed through a scrotal incision since the chance of spontaneous extrusion is significantly increased. Following closure of the abdominal incision, the scrotum is dilated with the aid of the dissecting finger, a moist gauze sponge, or both. The scrotum is inverted, and an absorbable suture is passed through the tab and then carefully through the dartos, with precautions taken that the suture does not penetrate the overlying scrotal skin. If the latter occurs, the suture should be removed and placed again. After the prosthesis is positioned dependently, the neck of the scrotum is closed with two or three absorbable sutures to prevent spontaneous or traumatic upward migration. The wound is irrigated with an antibiotic solution, and a broad-spectrum antibiotic is prescribed for 72 hours. Using these techniques, we have not had a single patient who experienced a scrotal infection following prosthesis placement or had prosthesis extrusion or displacement, and our patients included a few who previously had infected or extruded prostheses elsewhere and

were subsequently reoperated on after appropriate interval treatment.

Controversy has emerged regarding the safety of the silicone components of testicular prostheses, resulting from the medicolegal issues that have surrounded implanted silicone breast prostheses. Whereas most pediatric urologists have not encountered long-term problems with silicone gel-filled testicular prostheses, their safety has not been thoroughly studied. Presently (in 1995) a saline-filled silicone shell prosthesis will be the only model available in the U.S., eliminating the silicone gel or elastomer filling. Ongoing studies and registry of all patients undergoing prosthesis placement will be required.

Surgical Management of Inguinal Hernias and Hydroceles

Inguinal hernias and communicating hydroceles have similar pathologic anatomy in that both involve a patent processus vaginalis. A noncommunicating hydrocele in a child is very rare and, accordingly, the standard approach for treatment should be inguinal. In a small infant, particularly, the delicacy of inguinal surgery should not be underestimated and requires the careful touch of a skilled pediatric surgeon.

A knowledge of anatomy in the inguinal canal helps to keep the surgeon out of trouble. The cremaster muscle is encountered below the fascia of the external oblique and functions as "glue" in the inguinal canal, keeping the cord structures from being elevated. It must be mobilized in order for the processus vaginalis to be dealt with easily. Additionally, since the cremaster is an extension of the internal oblique musculature, its fibers must be teased apart at the level of the internal ring to permit access to the peritoneum through the internal ring. This is how one ensures a high ligation of the processus vaginalis, the essential step in treatment of the pediatric hernia. The other anatomic structure of importance is the internal spermatic fascia. This is a tubular extension of the endoabdominal fascia that extends through the internal ring around the vas, spermatic vessels, and the processus vaginalis. This layer must be opened to allow separation of the processus vaginalis from the vas and vessels. Failure to adequately tease the internal spermatic fascia apart at the level of the internal ring will result in the vas and vessels being pulled into the twist that many surgeons use of the processus vaginalis to ensure that nothing is in the processus prior to its ligature. If the internal spermatic fascia is not adequately divided, the vas and vessels may be pulled into this twist, and it is usually at this level that a urologist later finds evidence of vasal injury following herniorrhaphy.

With these few warnings given, the steps of an inguinal hernia repair or repair of a communicating hydrocele may be outlined. The scrotum is always prepped and draped into the operative field. This is done to permit the surgeon at the end of the procedure to be completely certain about the displacement back into the scrotum of any testis that may be pulled up into the inguinal wound, as occurs so commonly in pediatric hernia surgery. The skin incision is usually just a little longer than the length of the inguinal canal and is placed directly over it. The medial end of the incision may be easily determined by feeling the position of the cord structures as they exit the external ring immediately lateral to the pubic tubercle. Blunt and sharp dissection is carried down to the fascia of the external oblique. The external oblique fascia is cleared at the pubic tubercle to expose the external ring and the cord structures as they exit. This step ensures that the incision made in the external oblique fascia will be properly positioned over the canal. If the external ring is not identified, it is easy to inadvertently place the fascial incision too high or medial, causing the cord structures to be missed. After the external oblique fascia is opened, this fascia incision is continued through the external ring. By doing this, the delivery of an associated hydrocele is much facilitated. The cremaster muscle is mobilized off the undersurface of the external oblique and the transversalis. This permits the cord structures to be raised. By teasing the cremaster fibers off the cord at the internal ring, a small retractor may be inserted later to expose the peritoneum, ensuring a high ligation of the processus vaginalis at its juction with the peritoneum. Following elevation of the structures of the cord and the teasing apart of the cremaster muscle, the next step is to open the internal spermatic fascia. This may be simply accomplished by a very superficial picking up of the tissues over the vas or vessels, as this will prevent injury to the underlying structures. Once the internal spermatic fascia is opened, the processus vaginalis, usually controlled with the placement of a small hemostat, can be separated from the vas and vessels. Before division of the processus vaginalis, it is always wise to check that the vas and vessels are reidentified separate from the processus and that there is nothing in the processus. The processus is then divided between hemostats and dissected up to the internal ring, where it is twisted and doubly ligated at its junction with the peritoneum. If the surgeon has trouble identifying the processus vaginalis, a simple solution is to place a small retractor through the internal ring; then, with gentle traction on the cord structures, the peritoneum can be readily identified. This permits a proximal to distal dissection to identify the processus or confirm its nonpatency.

The surgeon now must deal with the collection of fluid within the tunica vaginalis in a communicating hydrocele. The testis is delivered through gentle traction on the distal end of the processus and the cord structures. The plane of dissection is kept immediately adjacent to the tunica vaginalis, which makes this procedure avascular. If there has been fluid collection in the tunica vaginalis, as is seen in a communicating hydrocele, the tunica vaginalis will be thicker than in an uncomplicated hernia. Here the risk of persistius hydrocele increases if the tunica vaginalis is not widely opened and an opening securely maintained. For this reason, I recommend a wide opening of the tunica vaginalis, which is then turned back behind the cord structures with a single stitch in a bottle technique. There is no need to excise any of the tunica vaginalis. In an inguinal hernia, the tunica vaginalis is often much flimsier, and a wide opening often is adequate to ensure the edges do not recoapt, permitting the formation of a reactive hydrocele postoperatively. A postoperative persisting hydrocele is most unfortunate, as it then appears to the patient's family and referring doctor that the primary problem has not been adequately corrected. After the completion of this step, gentle traction on the scrotum will utilize the gubernaculum and its attachment to the testis to reinvert the testis within the tunica vaginalis and then return the testis to a dependent scrotal position. This should be confirmed by careful palpation of the testis in the scrotum before inguinal closure is begun. If any question exists, the testis should be redelivered inguinally and, if necessary, the gubernaculum divided and the testis sufficiently mobilized to be placed into a subdartos pouch. There is no substitute for a secure scrotal positioning of the testis in the first instance in groin surgery carried out in children. A redo approach is always more arduous. Reconstruction of the inguinal canal is accomplished by reapproximation of the external oblique fascia. However, a good check of the transversalis fascia constituting the floor of the inguinal canal at the internal ring is important. If the internal ring appears to be excessively large, one or two stitches to close the transversalis fascia at this level may prevent a later direct hernia, although this is indeed a rare complication of groin surgery in children.

Scrotal Exploration for Acute Torsion of the Spermatic Cord or Testicular Appendages

Scrotal exploration for acute torsion of the spermatic cord or testicular appendages is accomplished through two separate transverse hemiscrotal incisions or a single midline raphe incision. The successive scrotal layers are incised, and the testis is delivered. Intravaginal torsion may not be evident until the tunica vaginalis is opened (Fig. 57-36). Detorsion and application of warm saline soaks is accomplished, during which time the contralateral testis is delivered. The tunica vaginalis is opened, and suture fixation of the testis is done in at least two places between the testis capsule and the dartos of the scrotum (see

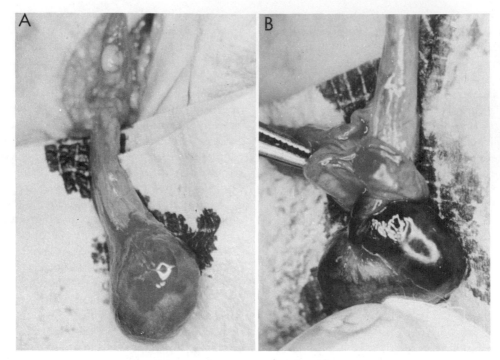

FIG. 57-36
Acute spermatic cord torsion in a 3-year-old boy. **A,** Inflamed testis is delivered, but twist is not evident. **B,** Incision of surrounding tunica vaginalis reveals intravaginal torsion.

Fig. 57-34). A nonabsorbable suture must be used, since both experimental and clinical evidence indicates that torsion may recur after previous suture fixation with absorbable suture material. Thereafter the torsive testis is reassessed, and a decision is made regarding orchiectomy versus preservation and suture fixation. Surgical attitudes have leaned more heavily toward removal of questionably viable testes than previously, in light of current information suggesting that the contralateral testis may be adversely affected by a retained damaged testis. When an appendiceal torsion is encountered, the appendix is ligated or fulgurated carefully and excised. Contralateral excision and suture fixation of the testis are not usually done.

Postsurgical complications of testicular and spermatic cord surgery consist mainly of injury to the vas deferens and spermatic artery and retraction of the testis. Complications following hernia and hydrocele surgery may include any of these. Care must be taken in dissecting the hernia sac off the cord, ensuring that undue traction or pressure is not put on the spermatic vessels. When the internal inguinal ring is narrowed to prevent herniation as part of the repair, an adequate lumen must still be left to allow the spermatic cord to pass without tension. Extreme care must be used to ensure that the testis occupies a dependent scrotal position after hernia repair since secondarily undescended testes can occur after hernia repair, with the testis fixing to the overlying scar. In these circumstances, secondary changes in the testis may occur

similar to those occurring in truly cryptorchid testes as a result of the continued extrascrotal position (Hadziselimovic, 1983). Similar perils may be encountered during the hydrocelectomy, especially when the hydrocele is chronic and thick-walled. In these circumstances, it is better to lay open the hydrocele and suture-evert the sac behind the spermatic cord and testis rather than excise the sac and risk accidental incision of a meandering hidden vas deferens.

REFERENCES

Testicular Development

Backhouse MK: Embryology of the normal and cryptorchid testis, in Fonkalsrud EW, Mengal W (eds): *Undescended Testis*. Chicago, Year Book Medical, 1981, pp 5-29.

Baumans V, Dijkstra G, Wensing CJG: The role of a nonandrogenic testicular factor in the process of testicular descent in the dog. *Int J Androl* 1983; 6:541.

Behringer RR, Finegold MJ, Cate RL: Mullerian inhibiting substance function during mammalian sexual development. *Cell* 1994; 79:415.

Boyar RM, Rosenfeld RS, Kapen S, et al: Human puberty: simultaneous augmented secretions of LH and T during sleep. *J Clin Invest* 1974; 54:609.

Crelin SE: *Functional Anatomy of the Newborn*. New York, Yale University Press, 1973.

Elder SJ, Isaacs TJ, Walsh CP: Androgenic sensitivity of the gubernaculum testis: evidence for hormonal mechanical interactions in testicular descent. *76th Annual Meeting of the AUA*. Boston, May 10-14, 1981.

Ewing LL: Leydig cell, in Lipshultz L, Howards SS (eds): *Infertility in the Male*. New York, Churchill Livingstone, 1983, pp 43-69.

Falin IL: The development of genital glands and the origin of germ cells in human embryogenesis. *Acta Anat* 1969; 72:195.

Felix W: The development of the urogenital organs, in Kiebel F, Mall FP (eds): *Human Embryology*. Philadelphia, Lippincott, 1910, 1912, pp 752-973.

Forest GM, Saez MJ, Bertrand J: Assessment of gonadal function in children. *Pediatrician* 1973; 2:102.

French FS, McLean WS, Smith AR, et al: Androgen transport and receptor mechanisms in testis and epididymis, in Dufau ML, Means AR (eds): *Hormone Binding and Target Cell Activation in the Testis*. New York, Plenum Press, 1974, p 311.

Frey HL, Peng S, Rajfer J: Synergy of abdominal pressure and androgens in testicular descent. *Biol Reprod* 1983; 29:1233.

Gier HT, Marion GB: Development of mammalian testes and genital ducts. *Biol Reprod* 1969 (suppl 1); 1.

Hadziselimovic F: Elektronsko mikrokopska proucavanja promjena na gonocitima djece neposredno poslje rodjenja. *Folia Anat Jugos* 1976; 5:37.

Hadziselimovic F: Cryptorchidism. *Adv Anat Embryol Cell Biol* 1977; 53:3.

Hadziselimovic F: Funktionelle morphologic und pathologie der nebenhoden und ihr einfluss auf den descensus testiculorum. *Morphol Med* 1981; 1:31.

Hadziselimovic F: Cryptorchidism: Management and Implications. New York, Springer-Verlag, 1983.

Hadziselimovic F, Duckett JW, Snyder HM, et al: Omphalocele, cryptorchidism, and brain malformations. *J Pediatr Surg* 1987; 22:854.

Hadziselimovic F, Herzog B, Seguchi J: Surgical correction of cryptorchidism at 2 years: electron microscopic and morphometric investigations. *J Pediatr Surg* 1975; 10:19.

Hadziselimovic F, Kruslin E: The role of epididymis in descended testis and the topographical relationship between the testis and epididymis from the sixth month of pregnancy until after birth. *Anat Embryol (Berl)* 1979; 155:191.

Hadziselimovic F, Seguchi H: Ultramikroskopische untersuchungen am tubulus seminiferous bei kindern von der geburt bis zur pubertat: II. sertoli zellen entwicklung. *Verh Anat Ges* 1973; 68:133.

Heller CG, Clermont Y: Kinetics of the germinal epithelium in man. *Recent Prog Horm Res* 1964; 20:545.

Heynes CF, DeKlerk DP: The gubernaculum testis during testicular descent in the pig fetus. *J Urol* 1985; 133:694.

Huff DS, Hadziselimovic F, Snyder HM, et al: Early postnatal testicular maldevelopment in cryptorchidism. *J Urol* 1991; 146:630.

Huff DS, Hadziselimovic F, Snyder HM, et al: Histologic maldevelopment of unilaterally cryptorchid testes and their descended partner. *Eur J Pediatr* 1993 (Suppl 2); 152:S10.

Hutson JM, Beasley SW: *Descent of the Testis*. London, Edward Arnold, 1992, pp 19-49.

Jost A: Hormonal factors in the sex differentiation of the mammalian fetus. *Philos Trans R Soc Lond Biol* 1970; 259:119.

Jost A, Vigier B, Prepin J, et al: Studies on sex differentiation in mammals. *Recent Prog Horm Res* 1973; 29:1.

Kruslin E: Descensus testis bei der maus mit besonderer berucksichtigung der epididymis und gubernaculumentwicklung (dissertation), Universitat Basel, Basel, Switzerland, 1981.

Martins T: La testosterone peut provoquer la descent de testicules artificiels de paraffine. *CR Soc Biol (Paris)* 1938; 131:299.

Means AR, Tindall DJ: FSH-induction of androgen binding protein in testis of Sertoli cell–only rats, in French FS, Hansson V, Ritzen EM, et al (eds): *Hormonal Regulation of Spermatogenesis*. New York, Plenum Press, 1975, p 383.

Means AR, Vaitukaitis J: Peptide hormone "receptors": specific binding of ^{3}H-FSH to testis. *Endocrinology* 1972; 90:39.

Payne AH, Downing JR, Wong KL: Luteinizing hormone receptors and testosterone synthesis in two distinct populations of Leydig cells. *Endocrinology* 1980; 106:1424.

Rajfer J, Walsh PC: Hormonal regulation of testicular descent: experimental and clinical observations. *J Urol* 1977; 118:985.

Sherins RJ, Hodgen GD: Testicular gamma-glutamyltranspeptidase: an index of Sertoli cells function in man. *J Reprod Fertil* 1976; 48:191.

Swerdloff SR, Heber D: Endocrine control of testicular function from birth to puberty, in Burger H, Kretser D (eds): *The Testis*. New York, Raven Press, 1981, pp 107-126.

Tato L, Mase R, Pinelli L, et al: Monorchidism, in Job JC (ed): *Cryptorchidism: Diagnosis and Treatment*. Basel, Switzerland, S Karger, 1979, pp 148-153.

Tindall DJ, Miller DA, Means AR: Characterization of androgen receptors in Sertoli cell–enriched testis. *Endocrinology* 1977; 101:13.

Tindall JD, Rowley RD, Lipshultz IL: Sertoli cell structure and function in vivo and in vitro, in Lipshultz L, Howards S (eds): *Infertility in the Male*. New York, Churchill Livingstone, 1983.

Waaler PE: Morphometric studies in undescended testes: correlation of morphometric and endocrinological results, in Job JC (ed): *Cryptorchidism: Diagnosis and Treatment, Pediatric Adolescent Endocrinology*. New York, S. Karger, 1979, vol 6, pp 27-36.

Weil C: *Ueber den descensus testiculorum*. Prague, 1884.

Wensing CJG: Testicular descent in some domestic mammals: III. Search for the factors that regulate the gubernacular reaction. *Proc Kon Ned Akad Wetensch C* 1973; 76:196.

Winter JSD, Faiman C: Serum gonadotropin concentrations in agonadal children and adults. *J Clin Endocrinol Metab* 1972; 35:561.

Winter JSD, Hughes IA, Reyes FI, et al: Pituitary-gonadal relations in infancy: 2. Patterns of serum gonadal steroid concentrations in men from birth to two years of age. *J Clin Endocrinol Metab* 1976; 42:673.

Cryptorchidism

Bergada C: Clinical treatment of cryptorchidism, in Bierich JR, Giarola A (eds): *Cryptorchidism*. New York, Academic Press, 1979, pp 367-374.

Bica DTG, Hadziselimovic F: Buserelin treatment of cryptorchidism: a randomized, double-blind, placebo-controlled study. *J Urol* 1992; 148:617.

Canlorbe P: Les cryptorchidies (etude de 145 cas). *Ann Pediatr (Paris)* 1966; 16:249.

Canlorbe P, Toublanc JE, Roger M, et al: Etude de la fonction endocrine dans 125 cas de cryptorchidies. *Ann Med Interne (Paris)* 1974; 125:365.

Charny CW: The spermatogenic potential of the undescended testis before and after treatment. *J Urol* 1960; 83:697.

Cortada X, Kousseff BG: Cryptorchidism in mental retardation. *J Urol* 1984; 131:674.

Cromie WJ: Cryptorchidism and malignant testicular disease, in Hadziselimovic F (ed): *Cryptorchidism: Management and Implications*. New York, Springer-Verlag, 1983, pp 83-92.

Dellenbach P, Gabriel-Rabez O: Malformation genitourinaries, essais de teratogenese experimentale par la chloraminophene. *Rev Fr Gynecol Obstet* 1975; 70:419.

Depue RH, Pike MC, Henderson BE: Estrogen exposure during gestation and risk of testicular cancer. *J Natl Cancer Inst* 1983; 71:6.

Forest GM: Pattern of the response to HCG stimulation in prepubertal cryptorchid boys, in Job JC (ed): *Cryptorchidism: Diagnosis and Treatment. Pediatric Adolescent Endocrinology*. Basal, Switzerland, S Karger, 1971, vol 6, pp 108-120.

Gendrel D, Job JC, Roger M: Reduced postnatal rise of testosterone in plasma of cryptorchid infants. *Acta Endocrinol (Copenh)* 1978; 89:372.

Hadziselimovic F: Cryptorchidism. *Adv Anat Embryol Cell Biol* 1977; 53:3.

Hadziselimovic F: *Cryptorchidism: Management and Implications*. New York, Springer-Verlag, 1983.

Hadziselimovic F: Mechanism of testicular descent. *Urol Res* 1984; 12:155.

Hadziselimovic F, Girard J, Herzog B: Lack of germ cells and endocrinology in cryptorchid boys from one to six years of life, in Bierich RJ, Giarola A (eds): *Cryptorchidism*. New York, Academic Press, 1979, pp 129-134.

Hadziselimovic F, Girard J, Herzog B: Four years' experience with a combined hormonal therapy of cryptorchidism. *Kinderchirurgie* 1984a; 39:324.

Hadziselimovic F, Hecker E, Herzog B: The value of testicular biopsy in cryptorchidism. *Urol Res* 1984b; 12:171.

Hadziselimovic F, Herzog B, Girard J: Impaired intrauterine gonadotropin secretion as an etiological component of cryptorchidism. *Pediatr Res* 1976; 10:883.

Hadziselimovic F, Seguchi H: Elektronenmikroskopische untersuchungen an kinderhoden bei unvollstandigem deszensus. *Acta Anat (Basel)* 1973; 86:474.

Jean C: Croissance et structure des testicules cryptorchides chez les souris nees de meres traitees a l'estradiol pendant la gestation. *Ann Endocrinol (Paris)* 1973; 34:669.

Kleinteich B, Hadziselimovic F, Hesse V, et al: *Kongenitale hodendystopien*. Leipzig, Germany, VEB Georg Thieme, 1979.

Kogan JS: Fertility in cryptorchidism, in Hadziselimovic F (ed): *Cryptorchidism: Management and Implications*. New York, Springer-Verlag, 1983, pp 71-82.

Kropp AK, Voeller KSK: Cryptorchidism in meningomyelocele. *J Pediatr* 1981; 99:110.

Lala R, Matarazzo P, Chiabotto P, et al: Combined therapy with LH-RH and HCG in cryptorchid infants. *Eur J Pediatr* 1993 (Suppl 2); 152:S31.

Mack WC, Scott LS, Gerguson-Smith MA, et al: Ectopic testis and true undescended testis: a histological comparison. *J Pathol* 1961; 82:439.

Raynaud A: *Modification experimentale de la differentiation Sexuelle des Embryons de Souris par Action des Hormones Androgenes et Oestrogenes*. Paris, Herman, 1942.

Scorer CG, Farrington HG: *Congenital Deformities of the Testis and Epididymis*. London, Butterworths, 1971.

Sizonenko CP, Schindler AM, Cuendet A: Clinical evaluation and management of testicular disorders before puberty, in Burger H, Kretser D (eds): *The Testis*. New York, Raven Press, 1981, pp 303-328.

Waldschmidt J, Doede T, Vygen I: The results of 9 years of experience with a combined treatment with LH-RH and HCG for cryptorchidism. *Eur J Pediatr* 1993 (Suppl 2); 152:S34-S36.

Wilson JC, Warkany J: Malformation in the genitourinary tract induced by maternal vitamin A deficiency in rat. *Am J Anat* 1948; 83:357.

Acute and Chronic Scrotal Swellings

Abeyaratne MR, Aherne WE, Scott WS: The vanishing testis. *Lancet* 1969; 2:822.

Abu-Sleiman R, Ho JE, Gregory JG: Scrotal scanning; present value and limits of interpretation. *Urology* 1979; 13:326.

Allan WR, Brown RB: Torsion of the testis: a review of 58 cases. *Br Med J* 1966; 1:1396.

Aynsley-Green A, Zachmann M, Illig R, et al: Congenital bilateral anorchia in childhood: a clinical, endocrine and therapeutic evaluation of twenty-one cases. *Clin Endocrinol* 1976; 5:381.

Barker K, Raper FP: Torsion of the testis. *Br J Urol* 1964; 36:35.

Bartone FF, Huseman CA, Maizels M, et al: Pitfalls in using human chorionic gonadotropin stimulation test to diagnose anorchia. *J Urol* 1984; 132:563.

Bartsch G, Frank S, Marberger H, et al: Testicular torsion: late results with special regard to fertility and endocrine function. *J Urol* 1980; 124:375.

Beard CM, Benson RC, Kelalis PP, et al: The incidence and outcome of mumps orchitis in Rochester, Minnesota 1935 to 1974. *Mayo Clin Proc* 1977; 52:3.

Bellinger MF: The blind-ending vas: the fate of the contralateral testis. *J Urol* 1985; 133:644.

Betts JM, Cromie WJ, Duckett JW Jr: Testicular detorsion: a temporizing manipulation. Paper presented at the American Academy of Pediatrics 48th Annual Meeting, Section on Urology, San Francisco, October 1979.

Bourne HL, Lee RE: Torsion of spermatic cord and testicular appendages. *Urology* 1975; 5:73.

Breen DH, Braunstein GD, Neufeld N, et al: Benign macroorchidism in a pubescent boy. *J Urol* 1981; 125:589.

Caldwell PD, Smith DW: The XXY (Klinefelter's) syndrome in childhood: detection and treatment. *J Pediatr* 1972; 80:250.

Cass AS, Cass BP, Verraraghaven K: Immediate exploration of the unilateral acute scrotum in young male subjects. *J Urol* 1980; 124:829.

Cassorla FG, Golden SM, Johnsonbaugh RE, et al: Testicular volume during early infancy. *J Pediatr* 1981; 99:742.

Cerasaro TS, Nachtsheim DA, Otero F, et al: The effect of testicular torsion on contralateral testis and the production of antisperm antibodies in rabbits. *J Urol* 1984; 132:577.

Charny CW, Gillenwater JY: Congenital absence of vas deferens. *J Urol* 1965: 93:399.

Chorousos GP, Loriaux DL, Sherins RJ, et al: Unilateral testicular enlargement resulting from inapparent 21-hydroxylase deficiency. *J Urol* 1981; 126:127.

Cosentino MJ, Rabinowitz R, Valvo JR, et al: The effect of prepubertal spermatic cord torsion on subsequent fertility in rats. *J Androl* 1984; 5:93.

Dickerman Z, Topper E, Dintsman M, et al: Pituitary-gonadal function, pubertal development and sperm counts in cryptorchidism: a longitudinal study, in Job JC (ed): *Cryptorchidism: Diagnosis and Treatment. Pediatric Adolescent Endocrinology*. Basel, Switzerland, S Karger, 1979, vol 6, pp 167-172.

Donohue R, Utley WLF: Idiopathic fat necrosis in the scrotum. *Br J Urol* 1975; 47:331.

Donahue RE, Utley WLF: Torsion of spermatic cord. *Urology* 1978; 11:33.

Ehrlich RM, Scardino PT: Simultaneous surgical treatment of scrotal transposition and perineal hypospadias, in Duckett JW Jr (ed): *Hypospadias*. Philadelphia, WB Saunders, 1981, vol 8, pp 931-938.

Emery CB, Goldstein AMB, Morrow JW: Congenital absence of vas deferens with ipsilateral urinary anomalies. *Urology* 1974; 4:201.

Evans JP, Snyder M: Idiopathic scrotal edema. *Urology* 1977; 9:549.

Frazier WJ, Bucy JG: Manipulation of torsion of the testicle. *J Urol* 1975; 114:410.

Gartman E: Torsion of the spermatic cord and testicular appendages in adult scrotal testes. *Am J Surg* 1964; 108:802.

Gierup J, von Hedenberg C, Osterman A: Acute nonspecific epididymitis in boys. *Scand J Urol Nephrol* 1975; 9:5.

Gill B, Bennet R, Kogan SJ: Epididymitis in childhood: the circumcision factor? Paper presented at the Annual meeting of the American Academy of Pediatrics, San Francisco, October, 1995.

Gill WB, Schumacher GFB, Bibbo M, et al: Association of diethylstilbestrol exposure in utero with cryptorchidism, testicular hypoplasia and semen abnormalities. *J Urol* 1979; 122:36.

Gislason T, Noronha RFX, Gregory JG: Acute epididymitis in boys: a 5-year retrospective study. *J Urol* 1980; 124:533.

Glazier WB, McGuire EJ: Testicular torsion: comparison of diagnostic modalities. Paper presented at the Annual Meeting of the American Urological Association, San Francisco, 1980.

Hamrick LC, Williams JO: Is contralateral exploration indicated in children with unilateral inguinal herniae? *Am J Surg* 1962; 104:52.

Harris BH, Webb HW, Wilkinson AH Jr, et al: Protection of the solitary testis. *J Pediatr Surg* 1982; 17:950.

Harrison RG, Lewis-Jones DI, de Marval MJ, et al: Mechanism of damage to the contralateral testis in rats with an ischaemic testis. *Lancet* 1981; 2:723.

Haynes BE, Bessen HA, Haynes VE: The diagnosis of testicular torsion. *JAMA* 1983; 249:2522.

Holsclaw DS, Permutter AD: Genital abnormalities in male patients with cystic fibrosis. *J Urol* 1971; 106:568.

Hosli PO: Varicocele results following early treatment of children and adolescents. *Z Kinder* 1988; 43:213.

Huff DS, Snyder HM, Hadziselimovic F, et al: An absent testis is associated with contralateral esticular hypertrophy. *J Urol* 1992; 148:627.

Huff DS, Wu H-Y, Snyder HM, et al: Evidence in favor of the mechanical (intrauterine torsion) theory over the endocrinopathy (cryptorchidism) theory in the pathogenesis of testicular agenesis. *J Urol* 1991; 146:630.

Ithiri A, Abulfadl MAM: Bilateral congenital absence of the vas deferens: diagnostic features of seminal picture in 42 new cases. *J Egypt Med Assoc* 1972; 55:184.

Jarow JP, Berkovitz GD, Migeon CJ, et al: Evaluation of serum gonadotropins establishes the diagnosis of anorchia in bilateral cryptorchid prepubertal boys. Paper presented at the Annual Meeting of the American Academy of Pediatrics, San Antonio, 1985.

Jerkins GR, Noe N, Hollabaugh RS, et al: Spermatic cord torsion in the neonate. *J Urol* 1983; 129:121.

Kaplan GW: Acute idiopathic scrotal edema. *J Pediatr Surg* 1977; 12:647.

Kaplan GW, King LR: Acute scrotal swelling in children. *J Urol* 1970; 104:219.

Kass E J, Belman AB: Reversal of varicocele surgery in adolescents: a comparison of techniques. *J Urol* 1992; 148:694.

Kass EJ, Belman AB, Chandra R: Reversal of testicular growth failure by varicocele ligation in adolescence. *J Urol* 1987; 137:475.

Kay R, Strong DW, Tank ES: Bilateral spermatic cord torsion in the neonate. *J Urol* 1980; 123:293.

Khan AU, Williams TH, Malek RS: Acute scrotal swelling in Henoch-Schönlein syndrome. *Urology* 1977; 10:139.

Kirkland RT, Kirkland JL, Keenan BS: Bilateral testicular tumors in congenital adrenal hyperplasia. *J Clin Endocrinol Metab* 1977; 44:369.

Klauber GT, Sant GR: Disorders of the male external genitalia, in Kelalis PP, King LR, Belman AB (eds): *Clinical Pediatric Urology*. ed 2. Philadelphia, WB Saunders, 1985, pp 825-863.

Kogan SJ: A false negative HCG test? *Soc Pediatr Urol Newsl* Nov 24, 1978.

Kogan SJ: Cryptorchidism, in Kelalis PP, King LR, Belman AB (eds): *Clinical Pediatric Urology*. ed 2. Philadelphia, WB Saunders, 1985, pp 864-887.

Kogan SJ: Pediatric varicoceles: changing concepts, in *Dialogues in Pediatric Urology*, vol 7, no 10. Pearl River, NY, William J. Miller, Oct 1984.

Kogan SJ, Gill B, Bennett B, et al: Human monorchidism: a clinicopathological study of unilateral absent testes in 65 boys. *J Urol* 1986a; 135:758.

Kogan SJ, Levitt SB: Imaging modalities in testicular torsion. *J Urol* 1983; 129:984.

Kogan SJ, Lutzker LG, Perez A, et al: The value of the negative radionuclide scrotal scan in the management of the acutely inflamed scrotum in children. *J Urol* 1979; 122:223.

Kogan SJ, Owens G, Tarter T, et al: Mechanisms of injury in unilateral testis torsion. *Eur Urol* 1986b; 12:184.

Kossow AS: Torsion following orchidopexy. *N Y State J Med* 1980; 80:1136.

Krarup T: The testes after torsion. *Br J Urol* 1978; 50:43.

Kroovand RL, Perlmutter AD: Congenital anomalies of the vas deferens and epididymis, in Kogan SJ, Hafez ESE (eds): *Pediatric Andrology*. Boston, Martinus Nijhoff, 1981, pp 173-180.

Lamm DL, Kaplan GW: Accessory and ectopic scrota. *Urology* 1977; 9:149.

Laron Z, Dickerman Z, Ritterman I, et al: Follow-up of boys with unilateral compensatory hypertrophy. *Fertil Steril* 1980; 33:297.

Laven JS, Haans LCF, Mali WP, et al: Effect of varicocele treatment in adolescents: a randomized study. *Fertil Steril* 1992; 58:756.

Leape LL: Torsion of the testis: invitation to error. *JAMA* 1967; 200:669.

Lee PA, Marshall FF, Greco JM, et al: Unilateral testicular hypertrophy: an apparently benign occurrence without cryptorchidism. *J Urol* 1982; 127:329.

Levitt S, Gill B, Katlowitz N, et al: Routine intraoperative postligation venography in the treatment of the pediatric varicocele. *J Urol* 1987; 137:716.

Levitt SB, Kogan SJ, Engel RM, et al: The impalpable testis: a rational approach to management. *J Urol* 1978a; 120:515.

Levitt SB, Kogan SJ, Schneider KM, et al: Endocrine tests in phenotypic children with bilateral impalpable testes can reliably predict "congenital" anorchism. *Urology* 1978b; 11:11.

Loh HS, Jalan OM: Testicular torsion in Henoch Schoenlein syndrome. *Br Med J* 1974; 2:96.

Lukash F, Zwiren GT, Andrews HG: Significance of absent vas deferens at hernia repair in infants and children. *J Pediatr Surg* 1975; 10:765.

Lyon RP, Marshall S, Scott MP: Varicocele in childhood and adolescence: implications in adulthood infertility? *Urology* 1982; 19:641.

MacNicol MF: Torsion of the testis in childhood. *Br J Surg* 1974; 61:905.

Marshall FF, Shermeta DW: Epididymal abnormalities associated with undescended testis. *J Urol* 1979; 121:341.

McGregor DB, Halverson K, McVay CB: The unilateral pediatric inguinal hernia: should the contralateral side by explored? *J Pediatr Surg* 1980; 15:313.

McNellis DR, Rabinovitch HH: Repeat torsion of "fixed" testis. *Urology* 1978; 16:476.

Megalli M, Gursel E, Lattimer JK: Reflux of urine into ejaculatory ducts as a cause of recurring epididymitis in children. *J Urol* 1972; 108:978.

Mehan DJ, Chehval MJ, Ullah S: Polyorchidism. *J Urol* 1976; 116:530.

Merimsky E, Orni-Wasserlauf R, Yust I: Assessment of immunological mechanism in infertility of the rat after experimental testicular torsion. *Urol Res* 1984; 12:179.

Michelson L: Congenital anomalies of the ductus deferens and epididymis. *J Urol* 1949; 61:384.

Miller SF: Transposition of the external genitalia associated with the syndrome of caudal regression. *J Urol* 1972; 108:818.

Mininberg DT, Richman A: Bilateral scrotal testicular ectopia. *J Urol* 1972; 108:652.

Minton JP, Clatworthy HW: Incidence of patency of the processus vaginalis. *Ohio State Med* 1961; 57:530.

Mitchell ME: Possible missing link in the absent testis syndrome. *Soc Pediatr Urol Newsl* Feb 4, 1981.

Moharib NH, Krahn HP: Acute scrotum in children with emphasis on torsion of spermatic cord. *J Urol* 1970; 104:601.

Murdoch RWG: Testicular strangulation from incarcerated inguinal hernia in infants. *J R Coll Surg Edinb* 1979; 24:97.

Nagler HM: Experimental aspects of testicular torsion. *Dialogues Pediatr Urol* 1985; 8:2.

Nagler HM, DeVere White R: The effect of testicular torsion on the contralateral testis. *J Urol* 1982; 128:1343.

Najaar SS, Takla RJ, Nassar VH: The syndrome of rudimentary testes: occurrence in 5 siblings. *J Pediatr* 1974; 84:119.

Nasrallah PF, Manzone D, King LR: Falsely negative Doppler examinations in testicular torsion. *J Urol* 1977; 118:194.

Newell ME, Lippe BM, Ehrlich RM: Testis tumors associated with congenital adrenal hyperplasia: a continuing diagnostic and therapeutic dilemma. *J Urol* 1977; 117:256.

O'Conor VJ: Surgical correction of male sterility. *Surg Gynecol Obstet* 1960; 110:649.

Okuyma A, Nakamura M, Namiki M, et al: Surgical repair of varicocele at puberty: preventive treatment for fertility improvement. *J Urol* 1988; 139:562.

O'Regan S, Robitaille P: Orchitis mimicking testicular torsion in Henoch-Schönlein's purpura. *J Urol* 1981; 126:834.

Perri AJ, Morales JO, Feldman AE, et al: Necrotic testicle with increased blood flow on Doppler ultrasonic examination. *Urology* 1976; 8:265.

Plender WM, Luna G, Lilly JR: Polyorchidism, case report and literature review. *J Urol* 1978; 119:705.

Pozza D, D'Ottavio G, Masci P, et al: Left varicocele at puberty. *Urology* 1983; 22:271.

Priebe CJ Jr, Holahan JA, Ziring PR: Abnormalities of the vas deferens and epididymis in cryptorchid boys with congenital rubella. *J Pediatr Surg* 1979; 16:834.

Puri P, Guiney EJ, O'Donnell B: Inguinal hernia in infants: the fate of the testis following incarceration. *J Pediatr Surg* 1984; 19:44.

Redman JF, Sulieman JS: Bilateral vasal-ureteral communications. *J Urol* 1976; 116:808.

Redman JF, Yamauchi T, Higginbothom WE: Fournier's gangrene of the scrotum in a child. *J Urol* 1979; 121:827.

Rodriguez DD, Rodriguez WC, Rivera JJ, et al: Doppler ultrasound versus testicular scanning in the evaluation of the acute scrotum. *J Urol* 1981; 125:343.

Rolnick D, Kawanoue S, Szanto P, et al: Anatomical incidence of testicular appendages. *J Urol* 1968; 100:755.

Rowe MI, Marchildon MB: Inguinal hernia and hydrocele in infants and children. *Surg Clin North Am* 1981; 61:1137.

Sayfan J, Soffer Y, Manor H, et al: Varicociles in youth. *Ann Surg* 1988; 207:223.

Schonfeld WA, Beebe GW: Normal growth and variation in the male genitalia from birth to maturity. *J Urol* 1942; 48:759.

Schwarz R, Stephens FD: The persisting mesonephric duct: high junction of vas deferens and ureter. *J Urol* 1978; 120:592.

Scorer CG, Farrington GH: *Congenital Deformities of the Testis and Epididymis*. New York, Appleton-Century-Crofts, 1971, p 136.

Siegel A, Snyder HM, Duckett JW: Epididymitis in infants and boys: underlying urogenital anomalies and efficacy of maging modalities. *J Urol* 1987; 138:1100.

Silber I, Raffel JL, Turk A: Testicular torsion in the newborn: results of national survey of members of the Society for Pediatric Urology and recommendations for future management. Paper presented at the Annual Meeting of the American Academy of Pediatrics, San Francisco, 1984.

Skoglund RW, McRoberts JW, Radge H: Torsion of the testicular appendages: presentation of 43 new cases and a collective review. *J Urol* 1970a; 104:598.

Skoglund RW, McRoberts JW, Radge H: Torsion of the testis: a review of the literature and an analysis of 70 new cases. *J Urol* 1970b; 104:604.

Smith GI: Cellular changes from graded testicular ischaemia. *J Urol* 1955; 73:355.

Sonda LP, Lapides J: Experimental torsion of the spermatic cord. *Surg Forum* 1961; 12:502.

Sparks JP: Torsion of the testis. *Ann R Coll Surg Engl* 1971; 49:77.

Stage KH, Schoenvogal R, Lewis S: Testicular scanning: clinical experience with 72 patients. *J Urol* 1981; 125:334.

Stein BS, Kendall AR, Harke HT, et al: Scrotal imaging in the Henoch-Schönlein syndrome. *J Urol* 1980; 124:568.

Thomas WEG, Cooper MJ, Smith JHF, et al: Sympathetic orchidopathia following acute testicular torsion. *Br J Surg* 1984; 71:380.

Thompson RB, Rosen DI, Gross DM: Healed meconium peritonitis presenting as an inguinal mass. *J Urol* 1973; 110:364.

Turner G, Daniel A, Frost M: X-linked mental retardation, macroorchidism and the Xq27 fragile site. *J Pediatr* 1980; 96:837.

Turner TT, Howards SS: Acute experimental testicular torsion: no effect on the contralateral testis. *J Androl* 1985; 6:65.

Vorstmann B, Rothwell D: Spermatic cord torsion following previous surgical fixation. *J Urol* 1982; 128:823.

Waksman J: Leydig cell tumors and their distinction from testicular tumors associated with congenital adrenal hyperplasia, in Kogan SJ, Hafez ESE (eds): *Pediatric Andrology*. Boston, Martinus Nijhoff, 1981, pp 181-186.

Whitesel JA: Intrauterine and newborn torsion of the spermatic cord. *J Urol* 1971; 106:786.

Williams CB, Litvak AS, McRoberts JW: Epididymitis in infancy. *J Urol* 1979; 121:125.

Williamson RCN: Torsion of the testis and allied conditions. *Br J Surg* 1976; 63:465.

Williamson RCN: Death in the scrotum: testicular torsion. *N Engl J Med* 1977; 196:338.

Woodside JR: Necrotizing fasciitis after neonatal circumcision. *Am J Dis Child* 1980; 134:301.

Wyllie GG: Varicocele and puberty—the critical factor? *Br J Urol* 1985; 57:194.

Surgical Considerations

Bell AI: Psychologic implications of the scrotal sac and testes for the male child. *Clin Pediatr* 1974; 13:838.

Bevan AD: Operation for undescended testicle and congenital inguinal hernia. *JAMA* 1899; 33:773.

Bevan AD: The surgical treatment of undescended testicle: A further contribution. *JAMA* 1903; 41:718.

Bloom DA, Semm K: Advances in genitourinary laparoscopy. *Adv Urol* 1991; 4:167.

Boley SJ, Kleinhaus SA: A place for the Cheatle-Henry approach in pediatric surgery. *J Pediatr Surg* 1966; 1:394.

Brendler H, Wulfson MA: Surgical treatment of high undescended testis. *Surg Gynecol Obstet* 1967; 124:605.

Caldamone AA, Amaral JF: Laparoscopic stage 2 Fowler-Stephens orchiopexy. *J Urol* 1994; 152:1253.

Cartwright PC, Velagapudi S, Snyder HM, et al: A surgical approach to reoperative orchiopexy. *J Urol* 1993; 149:817.

Clatworthy HW Jr, Hollanbaugh RS, Grosfeld JL: The "long loop vas" orchidopexy for high undescended testis. *Am Surg* 1972; 38:69.

Corkery JJ: Staged orhiopexy—a new technique. *J Pediatr Surg* 1975; 10:515.

Cortesi N, Ferrari P, Zambarda E, et al: Diagnosis of bilateral abdominal cryptorchidism by laparoscopy. *Endoscopy* 1976; 8:33.

Cywes S, Retief PJM, Louw JH: Results following orchiopexy, in Fonkalsrud ES, Mengel W: *The Undescended Testis*. Chicago, Year Book Medical, 1981, pp 234-249.

Firor HV: Two-stage orchiopexy. *Arch Surg* 1971; 102:598.

Flynn RA, King LR: Experiences with the midline transabdominal approach in orchiopexy. *Surg Gynecol Obstet* 1971; 131:285.

Fowler R, Stephens FO: The role of testicular vascular anatomy in the salvage of high undescended testes. *Aust N Z J Surg* 1959; 29:92.

Gibbons MD, Cromie WJ, Duckett Jr: Management of the abdominal undesended testicle. *J Urol* 1979; 122:76.

Gross RE, Jewett TC: Surgical experiences from 1,222 operations for undescended testes. *JAMA* 1956; 160:634.

Hadziselimovic F: Histology and ultrastructure of normal and cryptorchid testes, in Hadziselimovic F (ed): *Cryptorchidism: Management and Implications*. New York, Springer-Verlag, 1983, p 53.

Hinman F Jr: Alternatives to orchiopexy. *J Urol* 1980; 123:548.

Hunt JB, Withington R, Smith AM: The midline preperitoneal approach to orchiopexy. *Am Surg* 1981; 47:184.

Ivanissevich O: Left varicocele due to reflux. *J Int Coll Surg* 1960; 34:742.

Johnston JH: Prune belly syndrome, in Eckstein HB, Hohenfellner R, Williams DJ (eds): *Surgical Pediatric Urology*. Philadelphia, WB Saunders, 1977, p 240.

Jones PG: Undescended testes. *Aust Paediatr J* 1966; 2:36.

Jordan GH, Winslow BH: Laparoscopic single stage and staged orchiopexy. *J Urol* 1994; 152:1249.

Kiesewetter WB, Mammen K, Kalyglou M: The rationale and results in two-stage orchiopexies. *J Pediatr Surg* 1981 (suppl); 16:631.

Kogan SJ, Dourmashkin M, Smey P, et al: Occult undescended testes. *N Y State J Med* 1982; 82:1859.

Kogan SJ, Houman BZ, Reda EF, et al: Orchidopexy of the high undescended testis by division of the spermatic vessels: a critical review of 38 selected transections. *J Urol* 1989; 141:1416.

Lattimer JK, Vakili BF, Smith AM, et al: A natural feeling testicular prosthesis. *J Urol* 1973; 110:81.

Levitt SB, Kogan SJ, Engel RM, et al: The impalpable testis: a rational approach to management. *J Urol* 1978; 120:515.

Lipton S: Use of the Cheatle-Henry approach in the treatment of cryptorchidism. *Surgery* 1961; 50:846.

Lynch DF, Brock WA, Kaplan GW: Orchiopexy: experiences at two centers. *Urology* 1982; 19:507.

Maizels M, Gomez F, Firlit CF: Surgical correction of the failed orchiopexy. *J Urol* 1983; 130:955.

Marshall FF, Shermeta DW: Epididymal abnormalities associated with undescended testis. *J Urol* 1979; 121:341.

Martin DC, Menck HR: The undescended testis: management after puberty. *J Urol* 1975; 114:77.

Mengel W, Hecker WC: Cryptorchidism—surgical treatment and its date, in Job JC (ed): *Cryptorchidism: Diagnosis and Treatment. Pediatric and Adolescent Endocrinology*. Basel, Switzerland, S Karger, 1979, vol 6, pp 160-166.

Ombredanne L: Sur l' orchiopexie. *Bull Soc Pediatr (Paris)* 1927; 25:473.

Palomo A: Radical cure of varicocele by a new technique: preliminary report. *J Urol* 1949; 61:604.

Pascual JA, Villaneuva-Meyer J, Salido E, et al: Recovery of testicular blood flow following ligation of testicular vessels. *J Urol* 1989; 142:549.

Prentiss RJ, Weickgenant CJ, Moses JJ, et al: Undescended testis: surgical anatomy of spermatic vessels, spermatic surgical triangles, and lateral spermatic ligament. *J Urol* 1960; 83:686.

Ransley PG, Vordermark JS, Caldamone AA, et al: Preliminary ligation of the gonadal vessels prior to orchidopexy for the intra-abdominal testicle. *World J Urol* 1984; 2:266.

Redman JF: The staged orchiopexy: a critical review of the literature. *J Urol* 1977; 117:113.

Shandling B, Janik JS: The vulnerability of the vas deferens. *J Pediatr Surg* 1981; 16:461.

Silber SJ, Kelly J: Successful autotransplantation of an intraabdominal testis to the scrotum by microvascular technique. *J Urol* 1976; 115:452.

Snyder H III: Bilateral undescended testes. *Eur J Pediatr* 1993 (Suppl 2) 152:S45.

Turek PJ, Ewalt DH, Snyder HM 3d, et al: The absent cryptorchid testis: surgical findings and their implications for diagnosis and etiology. *J Urol* 1994; 151:718.

Winter JS, Faiman C: Serum gonadotropin in concentrations in agonadal children and adults. *J Clin Endocrinal Metab* 1972; 35(4):561.

Woodard JR, Parrott TS: Orchiopexy in the prune belly syndrome. *Br J Urol* 1978; 50:348.

Woodard JR, Trulock TS: Surgical treatment of cryptorchidism, in Hadziselimovic F (ed): *Cryptorchidism: Management and Implications*. New York, Springer-Verlag, 1983, p 121.

Zer M, Wooloch Y, Dintsman M: Staged orchiorraphy: therapeutic procedure in cryptorchid testicle with a short spermatic cord. *Arch Surg* 1975; 110:387.

CHAPTER 58

Pediatric Urologic Oncology

Michael L. Ritchey
Richard J. Andrassy
Panayotis P. Kelalis

WILMS' TUMOR

The treatment of children with Wilms' tumor (WT) is one of the remarkable success stories in pediatric oncology. Renal childhood tumors were described more than 150 years ago, but it was a surgeon, Max Wilms, who proposed that all the various elements of the tumor were derived from the same cell (Zantiga and Coppes, 1992). His thorough review of the literature and careful pathologic description of this tumor in 1899 led to the association of his name with this tumor. At the turn of the century, there were very few long-term survivors. Advances in anesthetic and surgical techniques resulted in an improved survival to 30% to 35% by the late 1930s. Radiation therapy was added to the treatment of these tumors when they were found to be radioresponsive (Priestly and Schulte, 1942), but it was the introduction of effective chemotherapy in the 1950s that led to a marked increase in survival (Farber, 1966). The current excellent outcome in terms of both increased survival and reduced morbidity can be attributed to the randomized trials conducted by cooperative groups such as the National Wilms' Tumor Study and the International Society of Pediatric Oncology. Current management emphasizes reducing the morbidity of treatment for low-risk patients, with more intensive treatment reserved for selected high-risk patients for whom survival remains poor.

Epidemiology

The incidence of Wilms' tumor is 1 in 10,000 children (Young and Miller, 1975), or about 450 to 500 new cases annually in the United States. This tumor represents 5% to 6% of childhood cancers in the United States and is the most common malignant renal tumor of childhood (Breslow et al., 1993). Nephroblastoma is a disease of young children, with a peak incidence of 36.5 months for males and 42.5 months for females with unilateral tumors (Fig. 58-1). The disease occurs nearly equally in girls and boys worldwide, but the frequency is slightly higher among girls in the United States (Breslow et al., 1994). There is some ethnic variation in the incidence of childhood kidney tumors, with slightly lower rates reported for Chinese, Philippino, and Japanese populations compared with the United States and Europe. No evidence has been provided of a consistent association of Wilms' tumor with any parental environmental exposure.

Associated Syndromes

There is a well-known association of Wilms' tumor with certain congenital abnormalities, including sporadic aniridia, hemihypertrophy, and congenital urinary tract malformations (Clericuzio, 1993; Miller et al., 1964). Nephroblastoma occurs with increased frequency in children with the Beckwith-Wiedemann, Denys-Drash, and Perlman syndromes (Beckwith, 1969; Drash et al., 1970; Perlman et al., 1975). The incidence of these conditions for all patients registered to the National Wilms' Tumor Study (NWTS) through 1990 are reported in Table 58-1.

Children with Beckwith-Wiedemann syndrome (BWS) are also at increased risk for the development of Wilms' tumor (Sotelo-Avila et al., 1980). BWS is a rare disorder consisting of developmental anomalies characterized by excess growth at the cellular (adrenal cortical cytomegaly), tissue (pancreatic, renal, pituitary), organ (macroglossia, hepatomegaly), or body segment (hemihypertrophy) level. The incidence of tumor development is 10% to 20% and includes Wilms' tumor, adrenocortical neoplasms, and hepatoblastoma. Although most cases of BWS are sporadic, up to 15% exhibit heritable characteristics with apparent autosomal dominant inheritance.

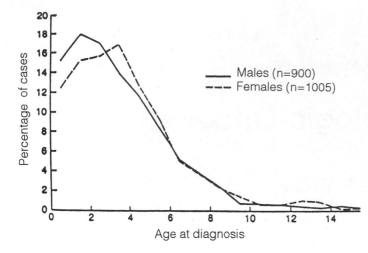

FIG. 58-1

Histogram of age at diagnosis for male and female patients with Wilms' tumor. (With permission from Breslow N, Beckwith JB: Epidemiological features of Wilms' tumors: results of the National Wilms' Tumor Study. *J Natl Cancer Inst* 1982; 68:429.

TABLE 58-1

Incidence of Congenital Anomalies Associated with Wilms' Tumor: Patients Reported to the National Wilms' Tumor Study

Anomaly	Rate (per 1000)
Aniridia	7.6
Beckwith-Wiedemann syndrome	8.4
Hemihypertrophy	33.8
Genitourinary anomalies	
Hypospadias	13.4
Cryptorchidism	37.3
Hypospadias and cryptorchidism	12.0

With or without the stigmata of BWS, patients who develop Wilms' tumor may also be affected by hemihypertrophy (HH), which occurs in 3% of these patients (Breslow et al., 1982). Hemihypertrophy is usually idiopathic, with an incidence in the general population of 1 in 53,000. The risk of WT development in patients with hemihypertrophy is estimated to be on the order of 3% to 5% (Tank and Kay, 1980). Isolated involvement of the leg is the most common manifestation in these patients (Green et al., 1993a) and may not become clinically apparent until after the diagnosis of Wilms' tumor (Boxer and Smith, 1970). Hemihypertrophy may be ipsilateral or contralateral to the tumor. The mean age at diagnosis of WT in the BWS and HH patients is similar to that of the general WT population (Breslow et al., 1988a).

Aniridia is a rare malformation, occurring in 1 in 50,000 persons. There are two forms of aniridia, sporadic and familial. Two thirds of all patients with aniridia have autosomal dominant aniridia, but nephroblastoma almost always occurs in nonfamilial or sporadic aniridia. There has been only one report of Wilms' tumor occurring in a patient with a family history of aniridia (Nelson et al., 1984). The incidence of aniridia in Wilms' tumor patients is 1.1%. Aniridia and Wilms' tumor are most commonly associated in patients with the WAGR syndrome, which is characterized by aniridia, genital anomalies, and mental retardation (Haicken and Miller, 1971). Most affected individuals have a constitutional deletion on chromosome 11, and the incidence of Wilms tumor is 42% (Hittner et al., 1980).

Genitourinary anomalies (hypospadias, cryptorchidism, and other genital anomalies, in addition to renal fusion anomalies) are present in 4.5% of patients with Wilms' tumor, representing a twofold increase over the general population (Breslow et al., 1982). Since many of these disorders are common in children, prospective evaluation for the development of Wilms' tumor is not carried out in most children with genital

anomalies. One specific association of male pseudohermaphroditism, renal mesangial sclerosis, and nephroblastoma was reported independently by Denys and Drash (Drash et al., 1970). Since then over 60 cases have been reported in the literature (Coppes et al., 1993). One should have a high index of suspicion for the development of these conditions in patients with male pseudohermaphroditism (Heppe et al., 1991; Tank and Melvin, 1990). Although XY individuals have been reported most often, the Denys-Drash syndrome has been reported in genotypic/phenotypic females as well as in individuals with gonadal dysgenesis Coppes et al., 1993). Genetic studies indicate that the Denys-Drash syndrome is associated with a specific mutation on chromosome 11, and this marker may help further define this heterogenous group of patients.

An association between Wilms' tumor and horseshoe kidney has been noted (Buntley, 1976; Gay et al., 1983). A review of NWTS patients found that there was a sevenfold increased risk of Wilms' tumor development in patients with a horseshoe kidney (Mesrobian et al., 1985).

Genetics

The genetic epidemiology of Wilms' tumor has produced a number of strong associations leading to hypotheses regarding tumor development. Nephroblastoma was once thought to have a substantial heritable fraction due to the frequency of bilaterality and association with congenital anomalies and specific syndromes. The diagnosis of Wilms' tumor generally occurs at an earlier age in patients with congenital anomalies and also in children with bilateral tumors (Breslow et al., 1982). Bilateral tumors are also observed more frequently in patients with congenital anomalies.

Analysis of these differences between groups of Wilms' tumor patients with regard to age at diagnosis and multicentricity of tumors led to the two-hit mutation theory for Wilms' tumor formation, similar to that proposed for retinoblastoma (Knudson and Strong, 1972a). This model for tumorigenesis predicts that two genetic events are necessary for tumor formation. The first mutation was hypothesized to be either a prezygotic (constitutional) or postzygotic (somatic) event, with the second mutation always occurring postzygotic. When the first mutation was prezygotic, involving all the person's cells, the tumor would be heritable. Since only one additional mutation is required in familial cases, these patients would be expected to have an earlier age of onset and have a greater incidence of multiple tumors. However, it is now recognized that the heritable fraction of Wilms' tumor is small (<1%) (Green et al., 1982). This falls far short of the 30% incidence predicted by the Knudson-Strong model, suggesting that Wilms' tumor formation is more complex than retinoblastoma and may involve more than one genetic locus (Coppes et al., 1994).

The first recognized cytogenetically visible chromosomal abnormality in Wilms' tumor was a constitutional deletion at the short arm of chromosome 11, 11p13, in patients with aniridia, genitourinary abnormalities, and mental retardation (WAGR) syndrome (Riccardi et al., 1978). This provided the first clue to the location of the gene involved in Wilms' tumor development. Subsequent to the cloning and characterization of this gene, designated WT1, deletions and mutations of 11p13 have been shown to occur in tumor DNA from sporadic Wilms' tumors, as well as in the germline of patients with a genetic predisposition to cancer. Approximately 50% of tumors show loss of heterozygosity (LOH) for DNA markers on 11p13 (Huff, 1994; Koufos et al., 1984) implying that these tumors had only one copy of the 11p gene. This suggests that the two genetic events in the two-hit mutation occurred at the same locus. Tumor formation occurred after inactivation of one allele of an 11p13 gene and the subsequent mutation or loss of the homologous allele.

The genetic consequences of WT1 inactivation appear to be restricted to organs that normally express this tumor suppressor gene. WT1 is expressed transiently in the developing kidney and in specific cells of the gonads (Call et al., 1990). Mutations at the WT1 locus, particularly in males, may confer extensive genitourinary defects, most notably male pseudohermaphroditism (Coppes et al., 1992; Pelletier et al., 1991). Of interest is that the affected gonads and kidneys in patients with the Denys-Drash syndrome are heterozygous for germline mutations, implying that the WT1 mutation acts dominantly with respect to genitourinary abnormalities (Huff et al., 1991).

A second Wilms' tumor locus on the short arm of chromosome 11 has been identified, 11p15.5 or WT2, which is distinct from WT1 (Reeve et al., 1989). This locus has been linked to the Beckwith-Wiedemann syndrome (BWS) with the finding of 11p15 triplication in some BWS patients and the mapping of familial BWS to 11p15 (Koufos et al., 1989). It is noted, however, that many types of tumors show LOH in the 11p15 region (Huff, 1994), and the WT2 gene may be important in the development of many different tumor types. BWS is associated with other embryonal neoplasms in addition to Wilms' tumor.

Other molecular genetic abnormalities have been found, including LOH for the long arm of chromosome 16q, which has been noted in approximately 20% of tumors (Maw et al., 1992). This gene is suspected to play a role in tumor progression rather than in the initiation of tumors and will be discussed more extensively later in this chapter. Ultimately, it will be interesting to assess the correlation between the different genetic events with histopathologic features and staging, in order to determine if molecular genetic studies are an additional indicator of clinical behavior and outcome.

Clinical Presentation

Typically, a child with Wilms' tumor presents with an abdominal mass (Fig. 58-2). This is often incidentally discovered by a family member while bathing, clothing, or observing the child. The tumor is palpable on physical examination in over 90% of children. The tumor is generally quite large relative to the size of the child and not always confined to one side of the abdomen. Therefore, this clinical feature cannot be used to distinguish this tumor from neuroblastoma. The outline of a Wilms' tumor on examination is smooth and spherical. Atypical symptoms include general malaise and abdominal pain. A number of tumors have been discovered during exploration for presumed appendicitis. Rupture of the tumor with hemorrhage into the free peritoneal cavity can result in the presentation of an acute abdomen. Hematuria occurs in one fourth of children at diagnosis. Gross hematuria occurs rarely and warrants evaluation to exclude tumor extension into the renal pelvis and ureter.

Hypertension is a well-known clinical manifestation of Wilms' tumor, with an incidence ranging from 25% to 50%. Several explanations have been proposed for hypertension, including production of renin due to ischemia produced by tumor compression directly on the renal artery or within the tumor capsule, arteriovenous fistula formation, or the production of renin by the tumor itself. Elevated plasma renin levels have been reported in Wilms' tumor patients but are not always associated with hypertension (Voute et al., 1971).

The propensity of a Wilms' tumor to grow into the renal vein and inferior vena cava can produce atypical presentations. Varicocele, hepatomegaly due to hepatic vein obstruction, ascites, and congestive heart failure were found in less than 10% of patients with intracaval or atrial tumor extension in NWTS-3 (Ritchey et al., 1988). Fortunately, sudden embolus of a tumor thrombus to the pulmonary artery with its catastrophic consequences is a rare event (Zakowski et al., 1990).

Diagnosis

Imaging

Abdomen.—Preoperative imaging studies are ordered with the intent of obtaining the correct diagnosis prior to surgical exploration, but an equally important

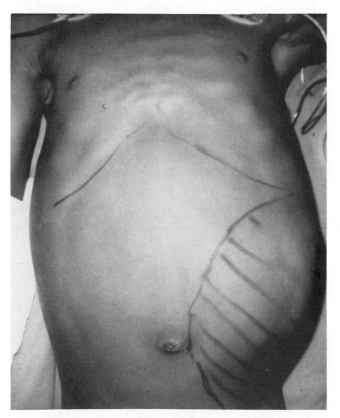

FIG. 58-2
Typical large bulging abdominal mass in a child with nephroblastoma.

goal is to establish that there is a contralateral functioning kidney prior to performing a nephrectomy. There are few distinguishing radiographic features that allow a precise preoperative diagnosis of the histology of a renal mass. However, defining the exact histology is probably not as important as establishing that there is a solid renal tumor present, which will help the surgeon plan for a major cancer operation. There was an incorrect preoperative diagnosis in 2.5% of NWTS-3 patients (i.e., the child had Wilms' tumor, but there was an erroneous diagnosis prior to surgical exploration), and the majority of these patients did not have any preoperative imaging studies performed (Ritchey et al., 1992a). This group of patients was found to have an increased incidence of surgical complications, which underscores the importance of the imaging evaluation.

Classically, the IVP will reveal distortion of the renal contour with splaying of the collecting system (Fig. 58-3, *A*). However, nonopacification of the kidney on IVP in a child with a suspected renal tumor is not uncommon. One review found that tumor obstruction of the collecting system was the most common cause of a nonvisualizing kidney (Nakayama et al., 1988). Complete replacement of the renal parenchyma with neoplasm and intravascular tumor extension were noted less frequently. A review of NWTS patients found that 14% of patients with renal vein extension (Ritchey et al., 1990) and 28% with inferior vena cava (IVC) or atrial extension (Ritchey et al., 1988) have a nonfunctioning kidney on IVP. If vascular invasion is not present, cystoscopy with retrograde pyelography is warranted to exclude ureteral extension in children with a nonfunctioning kidney, particularly if hematuria is present. Recognition of ureteral invasion prior to nephrectomy will facilitate a complete en bloc resection.

Advances in imaging have resulted in ultrasound or computed tomography supplanting the IVP. Ultrasonography is performed routinely in most children with abdominal masses and can distinguish solid and cystic lesions. Ultrasound can generally identify the kidneys and determine if the mass is of renal origin. Ultrasound will demonstrate an echogenic mass, and there may be cystic areas representing hemorrhage or tumor necrosis. Computed tomography (CT) and magnetic resonance imaging (MRI) can further define the extent of the lesion (Fig. 58-3, *B*), but all of the tumors may have a similar appearance (Broecker, 1991; Glass et al., 1991; White and Grossman, 1991).

There is some controversy regarding the utility of CT scans in the preoperative evaluation of children with Wilms' tumor and their role in tumor staging (Cohen, 1993; D'Angio et al., 1993). Accurate staging of children with solid tumors is essential to define tumor extent prior to initiating treatment. This is especially true for children with Wilms' tumor where outcome is highly correlated with stage and histology (D'Angio et al., 1989). However, these data are most accurately derived from the findings at surgery as confirmed by pathologic examination. Preoperative CT can suggest extension into the adjacent perirenal fat and evidence of regional adenopathy, which can then be confirmed at surgical exploration. However, prospective correlation with pathologic findings to validate the utility of CT staging has not been done. Enlarged retroperitoneal benign lymph nodes are common in children and can create significant diagnostic error. Correlation between pathologic findings and lymph node evaluation at surgical exploration in Wilms' tumor patients have found false-positive and false-negative error rates of 18% and 31%, respectively (Othersen et al., 1990). Current imaging modalities should not be expected to achieve greater accuracy. A new application using positron emission tomography with the glucose analog 2-deoxy-2-fluoro-D-glucose has been reported that does show promise in imaging of renal tumors (Wahl et al., 1991). This technique can provide anatomical imaging of both the primary tumor and metastatic disease, but at present experience in childhood malignancies is limited.

Liver invasion by right-sided tumors is particularly difficult to assess by CT. Dynamic scanning of the liver after bolus injection is recommended to obtain the best information. Ng and colleagues (1991) noted that the majority of children identified as having probable or possible invasion of the liver on CT later proved to be negative at surgical exploration. CT did have a 100% predictive value for absence of liver invasion, but deep-seated liver metastases that would not be visible at surgery are uncommon (Thomas et al., 1991).

An important role for ultrasound is to exclude tumor extension into the IVC, which occurs in 4% of Wilms'

tumor patients (Ritchey et al., 1988). Real-time ultrasonography can document the presence of tumor thrombi in the inferior vena cava (Fig. 58-4). CT visualization of the IVC is often hindered because of compression of the cava by a large tumor or an inadequate bolus injection of contrast. Although inferior venacavography is now used sparingly, there are few false-negative findings (Ritchey et al., 1988). MRI is the newest imaging modality for evaluation of the IVC, and early reports suggest that it is superior to CT and ultrasound (Weese et al., 1991). In a series of 26 adult patients with renal cell carcinoma, MRI revealed the IVC thrombus in 13 out of 13 patients and was able to identify renal vein extension in 88% (Roubidoux et al., 1992). The latter finding is quite impressive, as renal vein extension is rarely identified preoperatively in Wilms' tumor patients (Ritchey et al. 1990). In a report of four children with intracaval extension of Wilms' tumor, Weese et al., (1991) found that both ultrasound and MRI were able to diagnose the IVC thrombus. However, MRI was more effective in defining the extent of intravascular tumor extension, including those with intracardiac extension.

Contralateral Kidney.—Standard procedure during exploration in Wilms' tumor patients is to open Gerota's fascia to allow both palpation and inspection of all surfaces of the contralateral kidney. Identifying patients with bilateral involvement is important, as therapeutic recommendations are different for this subset of patients (Blute et al., 1987; Montgomery et al., 1991). It has been suggested that improved imaging capabilities should enable accurate assessment of the contralateral kidney, obviating formal exploration (Goleta-Dy et al., 1992; Koo et al., 1990). However, a recent review of 122 patients with synchronous bilateral Wilms' tumor enrolled in NWTS-4 noted that 7% of bilateral lesions were missed by the preopera-

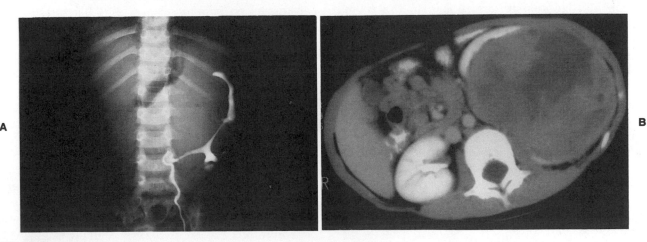

FIG. 58-3
A, Retrograde pyelogram demonstrates distortion of the collecting system from the intrarenal mass. (Photograph courtesy of Dr. Stanford Goldman.) **B,** Computed tomographic scan of a large left Wilms' tumor with a small rim of functioning renal parenchyma.

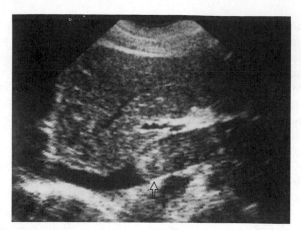

FIG. 58-4
Ultrasound depicting intracaval thrombus *(arrow).*

tive imaging studies (Ritchey et al., 1995). CT was more sensitive than ultrasound in detecting bilaterality, but not a single study was able to detect more than 50% of lesions less than 1 cm in diameter. CT and MRI may have an advantage in detecting intrarenal lesions that arise deep in the kidney from intralobar nephrogenic rests (Beckwith et al., 1990), but the incidence of such lesions is unknown. Until a more reliable indicator of bilateral disease is found, exploration of the contralateral kidney continues to be recommended by the NWTS.

Metastatic Disease.—The lungs are the most common site of metastasis for all malignant renal tumors, and therefore a search for pulmonary lesions is essential in all patients. The majority of these lesions can be identified on routine chest x-ray films. If the patient is documented to have metastases on chest radiographs, chest CT will add little to the evaluation. Additional, smaller metastases will often be discovered, but CT findings will not alter the adjuvant treatment required for Wilms' tumor patients (whole lung irradiation and addition of doxorubicin to the chemotherapy regimen). There is debate on the need for a chest CT in children with negative chest x-ray films and whether those patients discovered to have lesions on CT alone need additional treatment (Cohen, 1994; Green et al., 1991; Wilimas et al., 1988). One advantage of obtaining plain chest radiographs alone is there will be a lower false-positive error rate than with CT scans of the chest (Hidalgo et al., 1983). Because of its increased sensitivity, CT can detect a number of benign lesions that may require surgical resection for confirmation.

Another concern is whether those patients found to have very small metastases require additional treatment. Green and co-workers (1991) reviewed 32 children enrolled in NWTS-3 who had a negative chest roentgenogram but in whom metastatic lesions were identified on a chest CT. In patients treated according to the extent of the abdominal disease alone, the survival was not worsened by omitting pulmonary irradiation. The small number of patients studied, however, precluded a definitive statement regarding management. One study using decision analysis of the clinical value of chest CT concluded that it was unnecessary at diagnosis for patients with favorable-histology Wilms' tumor (Hutchinson, 1991). A different conclusion was reached by Wilimas and colleagues (1988), who reported that 40% of favorable-histology patients with pulmonary densities detected on CT alone developed recurrent disease when pulmonary irradiation was omitted. Clearly, further information is needed to define the proper management of this select group of patients.

Additional imaging studies are recommended to detect the presence of metastases in selected renal tumors with unfavorable histology (D'Angio et al., 1993). Clear cell sarcoma of the kidney (CCSK) and renal cell carcinoma have a propensity to metastasize to the skeleton. Skeletal surveys and bone scans are both recommended after the histologic diagnosis is confirmed. Rhabdoid tumor of the kidney (RTK) and CCSK are associated with brain metastases, and MRI of the brain should be obtained in the early postoperative period.

Screening of High-Risk Patients.—Children with hemihypertrophy, Beckwith-Wiedemann syndrome, and aniridia have an increased risk of developing Wilms' tumor. It has been recommended that screening studies be performed periodically for the detection of new renal tumors. The expectation is that the tumor will then be discovered at an earlier stage. A review of such patients reported to the NWTS did find that there were more stage I tumors in patients whose tumors were detected radiographically (Green et al., 1993a). There were not enough patients in this retrospective review to determine if early detection had an impact on patient survival. Another question regarding screening studies concerns the optimal interval between examinations. The report by Green and associates noted that in patients with aniridia, there was a median interval of 182 days between the last negative screening examination and the diagnosis of the mass. The shortest interval was 79 days. The current recommendations for screening of high-risk patients are listed in Table 58-2.

Differential Diagnosis

There are few distinguishing radiographic features that will allow a precise preoperative diagnosis of the histology of a renal mass. Nephroblastoma accounts for over 90% of renal tumors in children. RTK and CCSK are distinct from Wilms' tumor and comprise 5% of pediatric renal tumors. CCSK frequently will involve skeletal metastases, and both

TABLE 58-2

Selection of Imaging Studies for Follow-up of Children with Renal Neoplasms of Proven Histology and Free of Metastases at Diagnosis

Tumor Type	Study	Schedule Following Primary Therapy
Favorable-histology Wilms' tumor	Chest films	6 wk and 3 mo postop; then q3 mo × 5, q6 mos. × 3, yearly × 2
Stage I anaplastic Wilms' tumor		
Irradiated patients only	Irradiated bony structures*	Yearly to full growth, then q5 yr indefinitely†
Without nephrogenic rests, stages I and II	Abdominal ultrasound	Yearly × 3
Without nephrogenic rests, stage III	Abdominal ultrasound	As for chest films
With nephrogenic rests, any stage‡	Abdominal ultrasound	q3 mo × 10, q6 mo × 5, yearly × 5
Stage II and III anaplastic	Chest films	As for favorable histology
	Abdominal ultrasound	q3 mo × 4; q6 mo × 4
Renal cell carcinoma	Chest films	As for favorable histology
	Skeletal survey and bone scan	As for CCSK
Clear cell sarcoma (CCSK)	Brain MRI and/or opacified CT	When CCSK is established; then q6 mo × 10
	Skeletal survey and bone scan	As for favorable histology
	Chest films	
Rhabdoid tumor	Brain MRI and/or opacified CT	As for CCSK
	Chest films	As for favorable histology
Mesoblastic nephroma§	Abdominal ultrasound	q3 mo × 6

Modified, with permission, from D'Angio GJ, Rosenberg H, Sharples K, et al: Position paper: Imaging methods for primary renal tumors of childhood: cost versus benefits. *Med Pediatr Oncol* 1993; 21:205.
*To include any irradiated osseous structures.
†To detect second neoplasms, benign (osteochondromas) or malignant.
‡The panelists at the first International Conference on Molecular and Clinical Genetics of Childhood Renal Tumors, Albuquerque, New Mexico, May 1992, recommended a variation: q3 mo for 5 yr or until age 7, whichever comes first.
§Data from the files of Dr. J.B. Beckwith reveal that 20 of 293 MN patients (7%) relapsed or had metastases at diagnosis—4 of the 20 in the lungs, 1 of the 4 at diagnosis. All but 1 of the 19 relapses occurred within 1 year. Chest films for MN patients may be elected on a schedule such as q3 mo × 4, q6 mo × 2.

CCSK and RTK can metastasize to brain. The presence of these tumors should be considered in patients who present with metastases in these locations. Congenital mesoblastic nephroma (CMN) is found predominantly in infants and is generally a benign lesion, although there have been reports of local recurrence and occasional metastases (Gormley et al., 1989; Heidelberger et al., 1993; Joshi et al., 1986). CMN is found in approximately 2% of childhood renal tumors. Renal cell carcinoma (RCC) is indistinguishable from the tumor found in adults and is the least common renal malignancy in children (Broecker, 1991).

Other clinical parameters will aid the clinician in narrowing the diagnostic possibilities in a child with a renal mass. Beckwith (1991) has noted that patient age is useful in that congenital mesoblastic nephroma is far more common in children less than 6 months of age at diagnosis. However, favorable-histology Wilms' tumor and rhabdoid tumor of the kidney can also present in the first few months of life. A renal tumor that develops in a child known to have aniridia, hemihypertrophy, or other syndromes associated with an increased incidence of nephroblastoma can safely be assumed to be a Wilms' tumor. Bilateralism or multicentricity is more typical of Wilms' tumor, but renal lymphoma can also present in this fashion.

Pathology

The gross appearance of Wilms' tumor is that of a spherical mass (Fig. 58-5) with a light gray or tan color on cross-section. Most tumors are soft and friable, and hemorrhagic or necrotic areas are generally noted. Cysts are common and may be a dominant feature. The adjacent normal renal parenchyma is usually compressed by the tumor and its pseudocapsule, composed of compressed, atrophic renal tissues.

The microscopic features of Wilms' tumor are variable. The classic triphasic pattern includes blastemal, stromal, and epithelial cells (Fig. 58-6). Tumors that consist predominantly of one or two of these elements are commonly encountered. The stromal component can differentiate into striated muscle, cartilage, or fat. The primitive blastermal cells usually show distinctive patterns that allow their recognition by experienced pathologists.

Prognostic Factors

Analysis of early NWTS patients identified a group of tumors with "unfavorable" histologic features that were associated with increased rates of relapse and death (Beckwith and Palmer, 1978). These characteristics included tumors of extreme nuclear atypia (anaplasia) and monomorphic sarcomatous-appearing tumors. The latter tumors have been reclassified as the rhabdoid tumor and clear cell sarcoma of the kidney

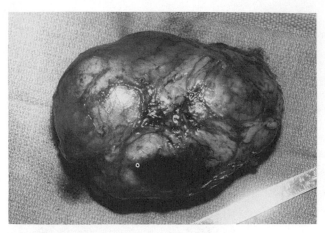

FIG. 58-5
Gross specimen of a Wilms' tumor.

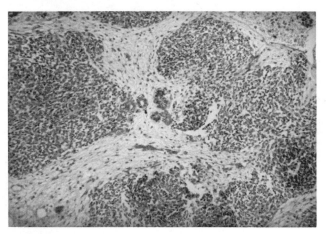

FIG. 58-6
Photomicrograph of typical Wilms' tumor demonstrating the classic triphasic pattern, which includes blastemal, stromal, and epithelial cells.

and are now considered to be distinct entities from Wilms' tumors. These unfavorable features occurred in approximately 10% of patients but accounted for almost half of the tumor deaths in early NWTS studies (Breslow et al., 1985). Identification of these high-risk patients allows stratification of patients, with greater treatment intensity reserved for those with a poor prognosis.

Anaplasia.—The cytopathologic features of anaplasia are threefold or greater nuclear enlargement, hyperchromasia of enlarged nuclei, and increased mitotic figures. Anaplasia was present in 4% of cases enrolled in NWTS-3. It is rare in the first 2 years of life, but the incidence increases to 13% in children age 5 years or older (Bonadio et al., 1985). Anaplastic features can occur focally, so thorough sampling of the primary tumor is necessary to avoid missing this poor prognostic feature. There has recently been a reclassification of patients with focal and diffuse anaplasia, with a change in the definition of focal anaplasia. Pre-

viously, anaplasia was considered focal when present in fewer than 10% of the high-power fields examined and diffuse when present in more than 10% of the tumor (Beckwith and Palmer, 1978). Recently, a new classification of anaplasia has been devised (Faria and Beckwith, 1993). The new definition of focal anaplasia is based on a topographical principle, requiring that the anaplastic nuclear changes be confined to a specified region of the primary tumor and absent from the surrounding portions of the lesion. Diffuse anaplasia is diagnosed when anaplasia is present in more than one portion of the tumor or found in any extrarenal or metastatic site. This definition is much more restrictive than the original one, and the implications in terms of therapy are discussed later.

Clear Cell Sarcoma of the Kidney.—This tumor is also known as the "bone-metastasizing renal tumor of childhood" because of its predilection for these sites (Marsden, 1980; Beckwith, 1983). CCSK accounts for 3% of renal tumors reported to the NWTS. Although it is not currently considered a variant of Wilms' tumor, the age at diagnosis and location are the same as for nephroblastoma. Since CCSK is associated with a much higher rate of relapse and death, its recognition is quite important in order that the appropriate therapy be instituted. Unlike tumors with anaplasia, even stage I CCSK lesions are associated with increased rates of relapse; five of seven such patients in NWTS-2 relapsed and died with tumor. Recent studies have demonstrated that the use of doxorubicin is associated with a significant improvement in outcome for these children (D'Angio et al., 1989).

Rhabdoid Tumor of the Kidney.—RTK is a highly malignant tumor of the kidney and accounts for 2% of renal tumors registered to the NWTS. RTK is now considered a sarcoma of the kidney, and not of metanephric origin (D'Angio et al., 1989). This tumor is typically seen in infants and very young children, with a mean age of 13 months. RTK metastasizes to the brain, which is exceedingly uncommon for Wilms' tumor. In several cases primary neuroectodermal tumors of the brain have occurred separately in children with RTK (Bonnin et al., 1984). The prognosis of RTK remains dismal with conventional chemotherapeutic regimens, and new treatment strategies are being developed for management of these children.

Congenital Mesoblastic Nephroma

Congenital mesoblastic nephroma (CMN) was first described as a separate clinical and pathologic entity by Bolande et al., who reported eight cases of the tumor (Bolande et al., 1967). In CMN, tumor induction is postulated to occur at a time when the multipotent blastema is predominantly stromagenic (Snyder et al., 1981; Tomlinson et al., 1992). There have been no cytogenetic or molecular markers discovered

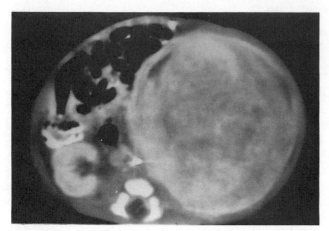

FIG. 58-7
Computed tomographic scan of a large congenital mesoblastic nephroma in a 2-day-old infant that was detected on antenatal ultrasound.

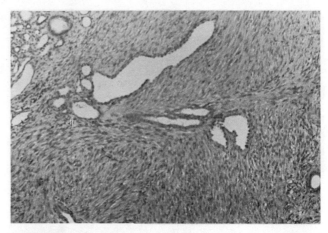

FIG. 58-8
Microscopic view of typical congenital mesoblastic nephroma with interlacing sheets of mature connective tissue cells (hematoxylin and eosin, ×100).

that are unique to CMN. WT1 and N-myc are not expressed in this tumor (Tomlinson et al., 1992). It is the most common renal tumor in infants, with a mean age at diagnosis of 3.5 months, but CMN has been reported in an adult (Howell et al., 1982; Levin et al., 1980). The tumor occurs more commonly in males and is usually unilateral. The typical form of presentation is a newborn with an abdominal mass, but in recent years a number of cases have been recognized prenatally (Fig. 58-7) (Ohmichi et al., 1989). There is a frequent association with polyhydramnios (Blank et al., 1978; Ohmichi et al., 1989). Fourteen percent of children with congenital mesoblastic nephromas have had other congenital anomalies, which is comparable to the incidence found in Wilms' tumor patients (Howell et al., 1982). Imaging studies cannot reliably distinguish CMN from other renal mass lesions. Distortion of the collecting system from an intrarenal mass is noted on excretory urography. Abdominal CT shows a heterogeneous solid mass arising from the kidney.

Congenital mesoblastic nephroma is a very firm tumor on gross examination, and the cut surface has the yellowish-gray trabeculated appearance of a leiomyoma. The tumor tends to demonstrate local infiltration into the surrounding perirenal connective tissue, lacking the pseudocapsule typically seen in Wilms' tumor (Fig. 58-8). The neoplasm is histologically distinct from Wilms' tumor. The cell population is characterized by interlacing sheets of connective cells. An atypical or cellular variant has been reported (Gormley et al., 1989; Johsi et al., 1986). This lesion is characterized by a high mitotic index and dense cellularity, but these features are present in 25% of CMN specimens (Beckwith, 1986).

Complete excision is curative for most patients with CMN. The growth pattern is one of local invasion and extension through the capsule (Howell et al., 1982).

Local recurrence has been reported in several patients with a cellular variant of CMN. Adequacy of surgical resection and age at diagnosis in these patients appear to be more important predictors of relapse than is histology (Beckwith, 1986). The risk of recurrence is thought to be less in children under 3 months of age at diagnosis, but metastases have been reported in a few infants (Heidelberger et al., 1993). Neither chemotherapy nor radiation therapy is routinely recommended (Howell et al., 1982), but adjuvant treatment should be considered for patients with cellular variants that are incompletely resected (Gormley et al., 1989).

Solitary Multilocular Cyst

Solitary multilocular cyst, also known as multilocular cystic nephroma, is an uncommon, benign renal tumor with a bimodal incidence. Fifty percent of the multilocular cysts reported in the literature have been found in young children, usually boys. The second peak incidence occurs in adults, usually, unlike the pediatric cases, in women (Banner et al., 1981; Johnson et al., 1973).

The most common presenting feature of multilocular cyst of the kidney is an abdominal or renal mass found on routine physical examination. All cases of multilocular cystic renal disease have been unilateral. The gross appearance of the tumor is its most distinguishing feature (Fig. 58-9). The cut surfaces reveal a well-circumscribed multilocular tumor composed of cysts ranging from several millimeters to several centimeters in greatest diameter. The tumor is well encapsulated, compressing the surrounding renal parenchyma.

Multilocular cyst is a benign lesion that is cured by nephrectomy; there have been no reports of tumor recurrence or metastases. Some of the smaller lesions can be managed by partial excision, salvaging a portion

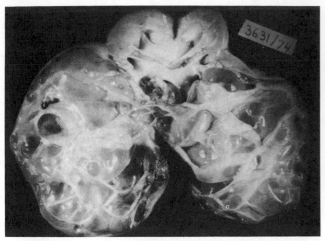

FIG. 58-9
Gross nephrectomy specimen. Note the well-circumscribed, predominantly cystic tumor. Cysts near the hilus prolapse into the renal pelvis but do not communicate with it. A small portion of the remaining renal parenchyma is seen at the upper pole. (From Joshi W, Banerjee AK, Yadav K, et al: *Cancer* 1977; 40:789. Used by permission.)

of the kidney. If partial nephrectomy is considered, use of frozen section is indicated to exclude cystic, partially differentiated nephroblastoma (Joshi and Beckwith, 1989). This tumor has a similar gross appearance but has elements typical of Wilms' tumor within the septa. These tumors are best managed by nephrectomy.

Precursor Lesions of Wilms' Tumor

Lesions apparently representing Wilms' tumor precursors have been recognized for many years. They have been found in 1% of kidneys in infants on postmortem exam (Bennington and Beckwith, 1975) and in 30% to 40% of kidneys removed for Wilms' tumor (Bove and McAdams, 1976). The terminology for these lesions has been confusing as it has evolved over the years. These lesions were previously termed *persistent nodular renal blastema*, *Wilms' tumorlet*, or *nephroblastomatosis* if there were diffuse lesions. The currently preferred term is *nephrogenic rest*, which is defined as foci of abnormally persistent nephrogenic cells that can form a Wilms' tumor (Beckwith et al., 1990). Two distinct categories of nephrogenic rests have been identified: perilobar nephrogenic rest (PLNR) and intralobar nephrogenic rest (ILNR). This classification is based on the position of these lesions within the renal lobe. The developing renal lobe matures in a centrifugal fashion, with each generation of nephrons added sequentially to the periphery (Beckwith, 1993). PLNRs are found in the periphery, and ILNRs can be found anywhere within the renal lobe (Fig. 58-10). It is inferred that ILNRs situated deep in the renal lobe reflect an earlier developmental

event. The presence of multiple or diffuse nephrogenic rests will lead to the diagnosis of nephroblastomatosis.

Nephrogenic rests display a variety of appearances. Hyperplasia of the rest can occur and be easily mistaken for a small Wilms' tumor. Given that the incidence of nephrogenic rests is much greater than that of Wilms' tumor, it is not surprising that regression of the rests is common. Sclerosing ILNR can be indistinguishable from focal renal dysplasia (Beckwith, 1993). There has been much concern regarding the occasional discovery of nephrogenic rests in multicystic dysplastic kidneys (Dimmick et al., 1989; Noe et al., 1989). Beckwith has estimated that approximately 1 in 80 nephrogenic rests will develop into nephroblastoma. Assuming a 5% prevalence of nephrogenic rests in multicystic kidneys, the removal of over 1500 kidneys would be necessary to prevent the formation of one Wilms' tumor (Beckwith, 1992).

ILNR and PLNR differ in a number of epidemiologic characteristics. These are summarized in Table 58-3. The age at diagnosis is lower for Wilms' tumor arising in association with ILNR, and children with WAGR and Drash syndromes are more likely to have ILNR. In contrast, there is a higher prevalence of PLNR in hemihypertrophy and in the Beckwith-Wiedemann syndrome. The presence of multiple rests in one kidney usually implies that nephrogenic rests are also present in the other kidney, making this an extremely important pathologic feature for identifying patients at risk for metachronous Wilms' tumor. These patients need careful imaging follow-up to detect contralateral recurrence (see Table 58-2). Both types of nephrogenic rests are associated with bilateral Wilms' tumor, where the incidence of nephrogenic rests is much higher than that seen in unilateral Wilms' tumor.

In summary, several clinical implications can be drawn from the data on nephrogenic rests (Beckwith, 1993): (1) Wilms' tumors can occur without any identifiable precursor lesions. (2) Hyperplastic nephrogenic rests can be mistaken for Wilms' tumor, and the exact criteria for distinguishing these two lesions remain to be defined. (3) If nephrogenic rests are present in the normal kidney adjacent to a unilateral tumor, the patient is at risk for a metachronous tumor. (4) Since metachronous Wilms' tumor does occur in patients previously treated with conventional chemotherapeutic regimens, nephrogenic rests cannot always be eradicated. We do not know the impact of therapy on nephrogenic rests or whether it decreases their oncogenic potential.

Biologic Parameters

The excellent survival of most patients with favorable-histology Wilms' tumor makes it increasingly dif-

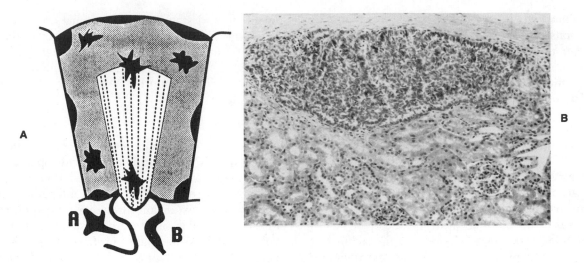

FIG. 58-10
A, Illustration of the renal lobe showing characteristic locations of intralobar nephrogenic rests *(dark gray)* and perilobar nephrogenic rests *(black)*. (With permission from Beckwith JB: Precursor lesions of Wilms tumor: clinical and biological implications. *Med Pediatr Oncol* 1993; 21:158.) **B,** Perilobar nephrogenic rest composed of blastemal cells just beneath the renal capsule (hematoxylin and eosin, × 40) (Photo courtesy of Dr. Jeff Bonadio).

TABLE 58-3

Approximate Prevalence of Nephrogenic Rests

Patient Population	PLNR (%)	ILNR (%)
Infant autopsies	1	0.01
Renal dysplasia	3.5	Unknown
Unilateral Wilms' tumor	25	15
Synchronous bilateral Wilms' tumor	74-79	34-41
Metachronous bilateral Wilms' tumor	42	63-75
Beckwith-Wiedemann, hemihypertrophy	70-77	47-56
Aniridia	12/20	84-100
Drash syndrome	11	78

Adapted from Beckwith JB: Precursor lesions of Wilms tumor: clinical and biological implications. *Med Pediatr Oncol* 1993; 21:158.

ficult to find any particular histologic feature of a given tumor that will predict the risk of relapse. If a method could be identified to further stratify favorable-histology Wilms' tumor patients into low- and high-risk groups for relapse, this would allow a reduction in treatment intensity for a large number of patients.

Tumor Markers.—The criteria for an ideal tumor marker are that the substance can be readily assayed, the assay must be sensitive and the marker must be specific for the tumor type, levels must return to normal following treatment, and subsequent elevation must correlate with evidence of tumor recurrence (Johnston et al., 1991). Several biologic markers for Wilms' tumor are under investigation, including serum renin, neuron-specific enolase, hyaluronic acid, hyaluronidase, and hyaluronic acid–stimulating activity (Coppes, 1993). The latter markers are of particular interest in that hyaluronic acid metabolism may be associated with tumorigenesis and angiogenesis. Elevated levels of hyaluronic acid and hyaluronic acid–

stimulating activity were reported in both urine and serum of five Wilms' tumor patients (Stern et al., 1991). Following surgical removal of the tumor, the levels returned to normal. A subsequent report of urine hyaluronic acid in 100 patients with nephroblastoma confirmed these findings and also noted that patients with persistent disease or relapse had significantly higher levels 1 to 6 months after surgery (Lin et al., 1994). Further studies are being conducted prospectively by the Children's Cancer Group to determine if these biologic markers can assess response of the tumor to treatment or detect tumor recurrence.

Elevated plasma renin levels have been reported in Wilms' tumor patients, and following treatment a reduction in plasma levels occurs (Carachi et al., 1987; Voute et al., 1971). There has been no clear correlation with systemic blood pressure, which has been attributed to the elevation of an inactive precursor of renin—prorenin—rather than active renin. Recently, elevated plasma renin levels were noted in four children with relapse of Wilms' tumor (Johnston et al., 1991). In all cases, the renin level decreased after initial tumor excision and subsequently became elevated. The development of a radioimmunoassay using monoclonal antibodies specific for both active and inactive renin should allow further studies to be conducted of this potential biological marker (Tsuchida et al., 1993).

DNA Content.—Flow cytometry has been utilized in a number of tumor systems. Flow cytometry is used to measure DNA content and to estimate the proliferative rate of populations of cells composing solid malignancies. A major advance has been the ability to measure DNA content on paraffin-embedded specimens. Flow cytometry attempts to identify aggressive populations of tumor cells, which may predict which low-stage tumors are at risk for metastatic disease. Normal somatic cells have a diploid DNA content, cells in mitosis are tetraploid, and tumor cells with gross karyotypic abnormalities in number are labeled aneuploid. An analysis of 47 Wilms' tumor patients found that those with a diploid or aneuploid DNA histogram had a 100% survival at 5 years (Rainwater et al., 1987). Those with tetraploid patterns had a 69% 5-year survival. Stage III and IV patients with tetraploid patterns fared significantly worse, with a 25% 5-year survival. However, others have found that DNA ploidy was not a more accurate predictor of survival than histology and stage (Layfield et al., 1989).

Nuclear Morphometry.—Nuclear morphometric techniques have been used in various urologic solid tumors to predict clinical outcome (Mohler et al., 1988). This technology has also been applied to the investigation of Wilms' tumor (Partin et al., 1990). With this technique, the nuclei of the tumor are visualized on a computer monitor. Image analysis is performed, and 16 shape descriptors of the nuclei are analyzed with mathematical equations. No single shape descriptor has been found to predict response of the tumor to therapy. In an initial review of 27 favorable-histology Wilms' tumor patients, multivariate analysis found a combination of three shape descriptors that could be used to separate patients with a poor prognosis (Gearhart et al., 1992). A subsequent report of 108 Wilms' tumor patients with favorable histology identified two shape factors that could identify patients with an unfavorable outcome (Partin et al., 1993). However, only one of these factors had proven to be predictive of outcome in the prior report. Further studies are ongoing to determine if this technique will prove to be a reliable and reproducible method of predicting response to therapy.

Chromosomal Abnormalities.—Wilms' tumor specimens have been noted to have numerous karyotypic abnormalities on cytogenetic examination. This led to the discovery of genes on chromosome 11 believed to be responsible for the induction of Wilms' tumor. Investigation for other sites of DNA gain or loss have found a LOH for a portion of chromosome 16q in 20% of Wilms' tumor patients (Maw et al., 1992). This was not found to be a germline mutation, suggesting that this region may play a role in tumor progression rather than tumor initiation. A prospective study of 232 patients registered on the NWTS found LOH for 16q in 17% of the tumors (Grundy et al., 1994). Patients with tumor-specific LOH for chromosome 16q had statistically significantly poorer 2-year relapse-free and overall survival rates than for those patients without LOH for chromosome 16q. This difference in outcome persisted after adjustment for

histology and stage. If this information is confirmed in a larger prospective study, molecular markers may serve to further stratify Wilms' tumor patients for treatment. Patients identified with unfavorable molecular findings could be selected for alternate forms of therapy.

Patterns of Spread

The most important determinants of outcome in children with Wilms' tumor are the histopathology and tumor stage. Determination of local tumor stage is the responsibility of both the surgeon and pathologist. Examination for extension through the capsule, residual disease, vascular involvement, and lymph node involvement are essential to properly assess the extent of the tumor. Stage I tumors are limited to the kidney and are completely resected. However, evidence for tumor extension can be subtle. The first signs of spread outside the kidney are in the renal sinus and lymphatic vessels. Penetration through the renal capsule is the next most common site of extrarenal spread. Tumors that penetrate the renal capsule are considered stage II lesions. Clear demonstration of tumor cells in the perirenal fat is required for documenting capsular penetration. Tumor extension into the renal sinus that does not occur beyond the hilar plane of the kidney is considered stage I.

The NWTS pathologists have identified several variables predictive of tumor relapse that could be used to stratify stage I tumors (Weeks et al., 1987). These "microsubstaging" variables are invasion of the tumor capsule, presence of an inflammatory pseudocapsule, renal sinus invasion, and tumor in the intrarenal vessels. Capsular invasion is defined as the presence of tumor cells in the outer half of the tumor capsule. An inflammatory pseudocapsule is postulated to be secondary to undetected focal tumor rupture or transcapsular tumor spread. Analysis of these variables found that one or more of these features were present in 24 stage I favorable-histology patients from NWTS-3 who developed tumor relapse (Weeks et al., 1987). In a control group of 48 stage I patients in whom all four microsubstaging variables were negative, none had relapse. Approximately 40% of stage I patients would meet these criteria. It was suggested that this group of patients might be potential candidates for a treatment with nephrectomy alone. Omission of postoperative adjuvant therapy has been proposed for small stage I tumors of favorable histology that occur in children under 2 years of age (Cassady tumor) (Green and Jaffe, 1979; Larsen et al., 1990).

A subsequent study of NWTS-4 favorable-histology stage I patients found that the 2-year relapse-free survival rate was 96.5% if all microsubstaging variables were negative (Green et al., 1994a). In the same study, the 2-year relapse-free survival for patients under age

2 years and tumor weights under 550 g was 95.5%. There was good correlation between patients meeting these criteria and negative microsubstaging variables. Therefore, it was concluded that the variables of age and weight could be more easily applied in clinical practice to stratify patients for treatment, as they are easily determined (Green et al., 1993b).

Surgical Management

The early improvements in survival of Wilms' tumor patients were brought about by improved surgical management. Today complete removal of the tumor continues to be an essential part of management, not only in terms of patient survival but also in decreasing the intensity of adjuvant treatment necessary. After a child is discovered to have an abdominal mass, the imaging evaluation and preparation of the patient for surgery can be completed in 48 hours in most major medical centers. Unless there is evidence of active bleeding, emergent operation is not necessary. All patients should be explored through a generous transperitoneal incision. This will afford excellent exposure and allow ready access to the contralateral kidney. A thoracoabdominal incision is only occasionally needed and is associated with an increased incidence of surgical complications (Ritchey et al., 1992a).

Thorough exploration of the abdominal cavity is carried out initially to exclude liver metastases, lymph node involvement, or other evidence of tumor spread. Exploration of the contralateral kidney should be performed prior to nephrectomy if technically feasible. The colon is reflected and Gerota's fascia opened so that the kidney can be palpated and inspected on all surfaces. Any abnormalities of the opposite kidney should be biopsied to exclude occult Wilms' tumor or the presence of nephrogenic rests. As noted previously, one cannot rely entirely on the preoperative imaging studies to rule out bilateral disease (Ritchey et al., 1995). The finding of bilateral involvement is a contraindication to primary nephrectomy, and therefore it is essential that this be investigated at the outset (Montgomery et al., 1991). Patients with bilateral tumors are best managed with biopsy followed by chemotherapy, without attempts at primary resection.

Radical nephrectomy is performed with sampling of regional lymph nodes, as gross inspection of the lymph nodes can be unreliable, but formal lymph node dissection is not required (Othersen et al., 1990). Gentle handling of the tumor throughout the procedure is mandatory to avoid tumor spillage. This is very important because NWTS-3 patients with intraoperative spill had a six-fold increase in local abdominal relapse despite the lack of significant difference in eventual outcome (D'Angio et al., 1989). Ligation of the renal vessels is performed prior to mobilization of the tumor, but only if exposure is adequate. More important, the surgeon should ascertain that the contralateral renal vessels, aorta, and iliac or superior mesenteric arteries have not been mistakenly ligated (Ritchey et al., 1992b).

Palpation of the renal vein and IVC should be performed to exclude intravascular tumor extension prior to vessel ligation. Renal vein involvement (extrarenal) is found in 11.3% of patients (Ritchey et al., 1990), and further propagation into the IVC or atrium occurs in an additional 4% (Nakayama et al., 1986; Ritchey et al., 1988). Identification of intracaval extension on the preoperative imaging studies will allow the surgical team to adequately prepare for the operative procedure. A review of NWTS-3 patients found that the diagnosis of intracaval and atrial tumor extension was correctly made in only 62% of children (Ritchey et al., 1988). Certain operative findings may suggest intravascular extension when it has not been correctly diagnosed preoperatively. Excessive bleeding from dilated superficial and retroperitoneal collaterals is a clue to obstruction of the vena cava. More ominous is the finding of sudden unexplained hypotension, which can result from embolization of the tumor thrombus.

For vena caval involvement below the level of the hepatic veins, the caval thrombus can be removed via cavotomy after proximal and distal vascular control is obtained. Generally the thrombus will be free-floating, but if there is adherence of the thrombus to the caval wall, the thrombus can often be delivered with the passage of a Fogarty or Foley balloon catheter. Caval resection may be necessary when there is direct invasion of the vena cava wall. Measurement of renal vein pressures can verify satisfactory collateral venous outflow for the contralateral kidney (Gonzalez et al., 1983). Patients with atrial extension may require cardiopulmonary bypass for thrombus removal (Nakayama et al., 1986).

Recent reports have suggested that patients with extensive intracaval or atrial extension of tumor can be managed with preoperative chemotherapy to shrink the tumor and thrombus (Dykes et al., 1991; Oberholzer et al., 1992; Ritchey et al., 1993a). This will facilitate complete removal of the tumor with decreased morbidity. There has been one report of tumor embolus during chemotherapy (Borden, 1992), but this complication can also occur prior to or during surgical removal of the tumor (Shurin et al., 1982; Zakowski et al., 1990).

In some patients the tumor may be quite massive, precluding primary resection. Biopsy of the tumor can be followed by chemotherapy and/or radiation therapy. This approach will generally result in a significant reduction of the tumor burden, allowing subsequent tumor resection (Bracken et al., 1982; Ritchey et al,. 1993a). Radical en bloc resection of the tumor is probably not justified in most children, as this is associated with increased surgical morbidity. Nephroblastomas are large tumors that often compress and adhere to adjacent structures without frank invasion. The gross appearance of the tumor at the time of surgery can be misleading in interpreting tumor extent, and in the majority of cases tumor invasion is not confirmed after the adjacent visceral organs are removed (Ritchey et al., 1992a). There may still be circumstances, however, when removal of other organs is justified. In a patient known to have extracapsular extension, resection of a small portion of liver or tail of the pancreas to avoid leaving residual tumor, for example, may eliminate the need for radiation therapy and allow a reduction in the amount of chemotherapy. Even if the tumor is confined to the kidney, en bloc resection of nonessential structures may also prevent violation of the tumor capsule and obviate tumor rupture or spill during nephrectomy. Therefore, there is a trade-off between the added surgical morbidity of en bloc resection and a potential reduction in long-term complications of adjuvant treatment. One should not overlook the morbidity of surgery, which can produce both acute and late complications. A review of NWTS-3 patients undergoing primary nephrectomy found a 20% incidence of surgical complications (Ritchey et al., 1992a). The most common complications were intestinal obstruction (Ritchey et al., 1993b) and hemorrhage. Factors associated with an increased rate of complications were incorrect preoperative diagnosis, higher local tumor stage, intravascular extension, and en bloc resection of other visceral organs. In some children with Wilms' tumor, the increased bleeding might be attributed to an acquired von Willebrand disease, which has been found in 8% of newly diagnosed Wilms' tumor patients (Coppes et al., 1993b). Children with nephroblastoma should be screened for these defects, as they can be reversed with the administration of DDAVP.

NWTS Trials

Since the inception of the NWTS there have been many significant advancements in the understanding and treatment of nephroblastoma. Important results of the early clinical trials included the findings that combination chemotherapy was more effective than single agents alone, the identification of unfavorable histologic features of Wilms' tumor, and the identification of prognostic factors that allowed refinement of the staging system to stratify patients into high-risk and low-risk treatment groups (Farewell et al., 1981). Several important prognostic factors were identified over the course of the NWTS trials. After the completion of NWTS-1 and NWTS-2, it was recognized that the presence of lymph node metastases had an adverse outcome on survival. This underscores the importance of adequate lymph node sampling during the course of removal of a nephrob-

TABLE 58-4

Staging System of the National Wilms' Tumor Study

Stage	
I	Tumor limited to the kidney and completely excised. The renal capsule is intact, and the tumor was not ruptured prior to removal. There is no residual tumor.
II	Tumor extends through the perirenal capsule but is completely excised. There may be local spillage of tumor confined to the flank, or the tumor may have been biopsied. Extrarenal vessels may contain tumor thrombus or be infiltrated by tumor.
III	Residual nonhematogenous tumor confined to the abdomen: lymph node involvement, diffuse peritoneal spillage, peritoneal implants, tumor beyond surgical margin either grossly or microscopically, or tumor not completely removed.
IV	Hematogenous metastases to lung, liver, bone, brain, etc.
V	Bilateral renal involvement at diagnosis.

lastoma. Local tumor extension is another important factor in identifying risk of tumor relapse. Patients with diffuse tumor spill were found to be at increased risk of abdominal relapse and therefore considered stage III and given whole abdominal irradiation. Recent data show that more subtle signs of local tumor aggressiveness can be responsible for increased risk of relapse in patients with apparently localized tumors (Weeks et al., 1987). The ability to stratify patients into different treatment groups has allowed a reduction in the intensity of therapy for the majority of patients while maintaining overall survival. This is very important in that the treatment of nephroblastomas can be associated with significant morbidity, and all Wilms' tumor patients should be carefully followed long-term to detect treatment-related complications (see Late Effects).

The current staging system employed by the NWTS is summarized in Table 58-4. For NWTS-3, the distribution by stage of favorable-histology tumors was stage I, 47%; stage II, 22%; stage III, 22%; and stage IV, 9% (D'Angio et al., 1989). Patients with anaplastic tumors are twice as likely to present with stage IV disease than those with favorable-histology tumors (Green et al., 1994b).

Identification of unfavorable-histology tumors is of paramount importance since these tumors are responsible for 50% of tumor deaths but occur in only 10% of patients (Breslow et al., 1985). As noted previously, CCSK and RTK account for 5% of childhood renal tumors. These are highly malignant tumors with a very poor prognosis that do not respond to conventional Wilms' tumor treatment. In NWTS-3, it was noted that the addition of doxorubicin (DOX) increased the survival of patients with CCSK. Currently all children with CCSK receive vincristine (VCR), dactinomycin (AMD), and DOX. All of these patients receive irradiation of the local tumor bed. The current chemotherapeutic regimen for patients with RTK in-

TABLE 58-5

Protocol for National Wilms' Tumor Study 4

	Radiotherapy	Chemotherapy
Stage I, II FH and anaplasia	None	EE-4A—*pulse*-intensive AMD plus VCR (18 wk)
Stage III, IV FH and focal anaplasia II-IV	1,080cGy	DD-4A—*pulse*-intensive AMD, VCR and DOX (24 wk)
Stage II-IV diffuse anaplasia CCSK	Yes*	Regimen I†
Stage I-IV Rhabdoid tumor of the kidney	Yes*	Regimen RTK‡

AMD, actinomycin-D; *VCR*, vincristine; *DOX*, doxorubicin; *FH*, favorable histology; *UH*, unfavorable histology.
*Radiation therapy is given to all clear cell sarcoma patients. Stage IV/FH patients are given radiation based on the local tumor stage. Consult protocol for specific treatment.
†Regimen I: AMD, VCR, DOX, cyclophosphamide and etoposide.
‡Regimen RTK: Carboplatin, etopsoide and cyclophosphamide.

cludes cyclophosphamide, carboplatinum, and etoposide. These children also receive irradiation of the local tumor bed.

As noted above, there has recently been a reclassification of patients with focal and diffuse anaplasia with a change in the definition of focal anaplasia (Faria and Beckwith, 1993). This has allowed therapy to be individualized for another segment of the unfavorable-histology tumors. In NWTS-4, children with stage I anaplastic tumors have been treated in a similar fashion to those with favorable histology. Patients with stage II-IV focal anaplasia are treated with AMD, VCR, and DOX and receive irradiation to the tumor bed. If there is evidence of diffuse anaplasia, stage II-III patients should also receive cyclophosphamide. Stage IV patients with diffuse anaplasia should be considered for the same regimen recommended for rhabdoid tumor of the kidney.

Lessons learned from the early NWTS trials were incorporated into the last intergroup study, NWTS-4 (Table 58-5), which was recently closed for patient entry. The goals of NWTS-4 were to decrease treatment intensity for patients with favorable prognosis while trying to maintain their excellent survival. In addition, a pulse-intensive regimen was employed to try and decrease the number of days of hospitalization required for administration of chemotherapy and hence the cost of cancer treatment. At the time of publication, only limited results were available for NWTS-4. The study found that the pulse-intensive regimens produce less hematologic toxicity than the standard regimens, and that the administered drug dose intensity is greater for the pulse-intensive regimens (Green et al., 1994c). Survival was equivalent for both the pulse-intensive and standard chemotherapy regimen (unpublished data from the NWTS.) A report from the Brazilian Wilms' tumor study has shown that the pulse-intensive chemotherapy regimen is equally as effective, in terms of patient survival, as the standard regimen (de Camargo et al., 1993). It is too early at this time to determine if there is a survival advantage for long versus short courses (Table 58-5) of chemotherapy.

Patients with stage I favorable histology Wilms' tumor can be treated successfully with a 10-week regimen of vincristine (VCR) and dactinomycin (AMD). The 4-year relapse-free survival in NWTS-3 was 89%, and the overall survival was 95.6%. NWTS-3 stage II favorable histology patients treated with AMD and VCR without postoperative radiation therapy (XRT) had an equivalent survival, 4-year overall survival of 91.1%, patients that received doxorubicin and XRT. Stage III favorable histology patients continue to receive abdominal irradiation XRT, but the dosage has been reduced to 1000 cGy. This was shown to be as effective as 2000 cGy in preventing abdominal relapse if doxorubicin (DOX) is also given in addition to VCR and AMD. Four-year relapse-free survival was 82% in NWTS-3, and the 4-year overall survival was 90.9%. Patients with stage IV favorable histology tumors receive abdominal irradiation based on the local tumor stage and also receive 1200 cGy to both lungs. In NWTS-3 the combination of VCR, AMD, and DOX produced a 4-year relapse-free survival of 71.9%, and the overall survival was 78.4%.

Future Directions

The next intergroup cooperative Wilms' tumor study, NWTS-5, is now open for patient entry. This study will include treatment of selected stage I patients, age <2 years and tumor weight <550 g, with surgery alone (Table 58-5). The study will focus on the evaluation of biologic prognostic factors for Wilms' tumor. These factors could help further stratify patients for treatment with the goal of decreasing the amount of therapy for children with tumors at low risk for relapse, while intensifying treatment for high risk patients. All children with the same tumor stage will be treated with a uniform treatment regimen. Patients with diffuse anaplasia and rhabdoid tumor of the kidney will be treated with more aggressive chemotherapy regimens to try and improve the dismal survival rate for this group of patients. Preoperative chemotherapy is recommended for all patients with bilateral tumors, inoperable tumors, and patients with extensive inferior vena caval extension. Lastly, a uniform retrieval protocol is available for patients with tumor relapse.

Radiation Therapy

Radiation therapy used to be an integral part of therapy for all Wilms' tumor patients. In NWTS-1, it was shown that there is no need for routine radiation therapy in patients under 2 years of age with stage I tumors if they receive routine postoperative AMD (D'Angio et al., 1976). Results from NWTS-2 and NWTS-3 found that the combination of VCR and AMD was effective in treating some micrometastases and that radiation therapy could be omitted for all stage I and stage II tumors (D'Angio et al., 1989). In addition, a lower dose of radiation, 1080 cGy, was found to be effective for stage III favorable-histology tumors. Currently, only 24% of children entered in NWTS-4 receive postoperative abdominal irradiation (Green et al., 1992).

Radiation therapy is usually begun within the first week after surgery. The radiation fields vary according to the extent of disease. Except in patients with diffuse intraabdominal spill, the radiation portals are confined to the tumor bed. If there is bulky residual disease, additional boosts of radiation are given to these areas. All metastatic sites also receive irradiation. The dosages are adjusted according to age because of the recognition that radiation injury to normal tissues is greater in younger children.

Special Considerations
Bilateral Disease

Synchronous bilateral nephroblastoma occurs in about 5% of children, with metachronous lesions developing in only 1% (Blute et al., 1987; Montgomery et al., 1991). The importance of intraoperative examination of the contralateral kidney was addressed earlier. In the past, bilateral Wilms' tumor patients were managed with a primary surgical approach. A nephrectomy of the more involved kidney was performed followed by partial excision of the contralateral tumor, if feasible. One problem with this approach was that the majority of patients had residual disease after the initial operation, although overall survival was quite good. In a review of 145 NWTS-2 and NWTS-3 patients, Blute et al., (1987) found that survival was comparable between patients treated with primary surgical resection and patients treated with biopsy only followed by preoperative chemotherapy. International Society of Pediatric Oncology (SIOP) investigators have also reported good overall survival in patients treated with preoperative chemotherapy, with a decrease in the incidence of residual disease (Coppes et al., 1989). One advantage of the latter approach is that more renal units will be spared if surgery is deferred until after the tumor burden is reduced (Montgomery et al., 1991; Shaul et al., 1992). This is important because renal failure has been reported in as many as 5% of bilateral tumor patients (Ritchey et al., 1994b).

Therefore, the preferred approach for patients with bilateral Wilms' tumor is initial biopsy followed by preoperative chemotherapy. Radical excision of the tumor should not be performed at the initial operation. Partial nephrectomy or wedge excision should be employed at the initial operation only if all tumor can be removed with preservation of two thirds or more of the renal parenchyma *on both sides*. Bilateral biopsies should be obtained to confirm the presence of Wilms' tumor in both kidneys and to define the histologic type. Suspicious lymph nodes should be biopsied and a surgical stage assigned. Patients are then given chemotherapy to reduce the tumor burden. Surgical exploration with definitive resection is deferred until there has been a significant reduction in tumor burden. A second-look operation should be performed following the completion of the initial course of chemotherapy, usually in 8 to 10 weeks. Preoperative CT should be used to assess the reduction in tumor volume and to assess the feasibility of partial resection. At the time of the second-look procedure, partial nephrectomies or wedge excisions of the tumors are performed. This should be done only if it will not compromise tumor resection and negative margins can be obtained. If there is extensive tumor involvement precluding partial resection, complete excision of tumor from the least involved kidney is performed. If this leaves a viable kidney, then nephrectomy of the other kidney is carried out.

Some patients may not have a measurable response to preoperative chemotherapy. Serial imaging evaluation is helpful to assess response, but radiographic evidence of persistent disease can occasionally be misleading. Failure of the tumor to shrink could be due to predominance of skeletal muscle or benign elements, and a second-look procedure to confirm persistent viable tumor may be necessary (Zuppan et al., 1991). Patients with persistent viable tumor should be changed to a different chemotherapeutic regimen. The patient should be examined after an additional 12 weeks to assess the feasibility of resection. If there is a possibility that the remaining kidney can be salvaged, partial nephrectomy or wedge excision of the tumor is performed. If there is extensive tumor involvement precluding partial resection in one kidney, complete excision of the tumor from the least involved kidney is performed. If this procedure leaves a viable and functioning kidney, then radical nephrectomy is performed to remove the kidney with extensive tumor involvement.

Bilateral nephrectomy and dialysis may be required if the tumors fail to respond to chemotherapy and radiation therapy. The most common cause of renal failure in NWTS patients is bilateral nephrectomy for persistent tumor (Ritchey et al., 1994b). If transplantation is later considered, a waiting period of 2 years is recommended to ensure that the patient does not develop metastatic disease (Penn, 1979). However, bilateral Wilms' tumor patients need long-term follow-up, as relapses have occurred as late as 4 years post-treatment (Coppes et al., 1989).

Preoperative Therapy

Preoperative treatment has been under study for decades. This has been employed electively in patients with large Wilms' tumors judged to be unresectable or those involving vital structures that preclude primary excision (Bracken et al., 1982). Radiotherapy alone was the first preoperative treatment utilized, and later dactinomycin and vincristine were used for preoperative treatment because of their demonstrated activity against Wilms' tumor. Preoperative treatment can produce a dramatic reduction in the size of the primary tumor, facilitating surgical excision (Fig. 58-11). SIOP began to evaluate the role of preoperative treatment for Wilms' tumor in the early 1970s, and their initial studies demonstrated that preoperative radiation therapy would decrease the incidence of tumor rupture (Lemerle et al., 1976). Later SIOP trials demonstrated that preoperative chemotherapy with dactinomycin and vincristine was as effective as radiotherapy in preventing tumor rupture (Lemerle et al., 1983). It should be noted that there was no survival advantage over the primary surgical approach. A significant number of patients are "downstaged" after chemotherapy, and the latter stage determines the amount of postoperative therapy in the SIOP trials. This postchemotherapy stage may inadequately define the risk of intraabdominal recurrence in unirradiated patients. In SIOP-6, patients who were postchemotherapy stage II were randomized to receive or not receive abdominal irradiation. Investigators found that there was an unacceptable increase in the number of intraabdominal recurrences in non-irradiated patients (Tournade et al., 1993). As a result, these patients are now given an anthracycline as part of the chemotherapy regimen (Green et al., 1993c). The added chemotherapy could increase the incidence of late complications, particularly congestive heart failure, which currently are quite low in the NWTS. This raises some concern regarding the utility of post-chemotherapy staging as opposed to staging at initial surgery, used by NWTS, to predict tumor behavior. If one looks carefully at both NWTS and SIOP data, the two groups show similar results with respect to their attempts to decrease the number of patients receiving postoperative XRT. For favorable-histology patients, only 24% of children enrolled in NWTS-4 are given XRT, compared with 16% of SIOP patients (Green et al., 1992).

Another potential difficulty of preoperative chemotherapy is the inability to classify the tumor by histologic subtype and stage following treatment. The SIOP studies found that histologic patterns could still be recognized after chemotherapy, whereas preoperative radiation caused far more tumor destruction (Burger et al., 1985). This problem has also been addressed by Zuppan et al., (1991) in their review of inoperable NWTS-3 patients who received preoperative chemotherapy. Anaplastic elements were still recognizable after preoperative chemotherapy. In patients with favorable histology, the viability of the tumor after treatment appeared to correlate with treatment outcome. Patients with no viable tumor at the time of resection were thought to have a favorable histologic type, as none of these children had died of tumor progression.

The NWTS continues to recommend primary surgical treatment of Wilms' tumor. This will allow precise staging of patients with modulation of treatment for each individual, thereby decreasing the intensity of treatment when possible while maintaining excellent overall survival. The current recommendations from the NWTS are that preoperative chemotherapy is of benefit to patients with bilateral involvement

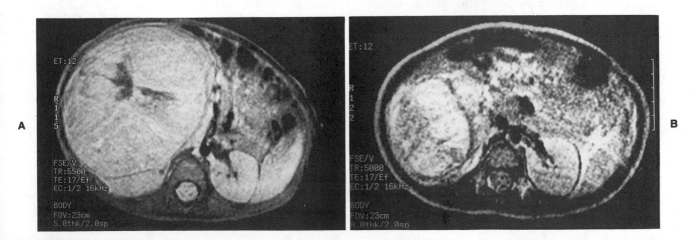

FIG. 58-11
A, Magnetic resonance imaging scan of a large, inoperable Wilms' tumor. **B,** After 6 weeks of chemotherapy the same tumor has dramatically decreased in size.

(Blute et al., 1987), patients who are inoperable at surgical exploration (Ritchey et al., 1994c), and patients with IVC extension above the hepatic veins (Ritchey et al., 1993a). All other patients should undergo primary nephrectomy.

Inoperable Tumors

There are some patients with massive tumors judged by the surgeons to pose too great a risk for surgical removal. Past experience in NWTS (Ritchey et al., 1994c) and SIOP (Tournade et al., 1993) has shown that pretreatment with chemotherapy almost always reduces the bulk of the tumor and renders it resectable. However, this method does not result in improved survival rates and does result in the loss of important staging information. Patients who are determined to have unresectable tumors should be considered stage III and treated accordingly (Ritchey et al., 1994c). Once there is an adequate reduction in the size of the tumor to facilitate nephrectomy, then definitive resection should be completed. In general, the operative procedure can be performed within 6 weeks of initiation of treatment. Serial imaging evaluation is helpful in assessing response. Patients who fail to respond can be considered for preoperative irradiation as this may produce enough shrinkage to facilitate nephrectomy. If the tumor remains inoperable, biopsy of both the primary tumor and accessible metastatic lesions should be performed. Patients with progressive disease have a very poor prognosis and require treatment with a different chemotherapeutic regimen (Ritchey et al., 1994c).

Treatment of Relapses

Results from NWTS-3 demonstrate that the risk of tumor relapse at 3 years is 9.6%, 11.8%, 22%, and 22%, respectively, for stages I through IV. Relapses occurred in 36% and 45% of unfavorable-histology patients stages I-III and IV, respectively (D'Angio et al., 1989). Children with Wilms' tumor relapse have a variable prognosis, depending on the initial stage, site of relapse, time from initial diagnosis to relapse, and prior therapy. Adverse prognostic factors include previous treatment that included doxirubicin, relapse less than 12 months after diagnosis, and intraabdominal relapse in previously abdominal-irradiated patients (Grundy et al., 1989). Treatment of these patients has been highly individualized. A prospective intergroup study using a uniform treatment for relapsed Wilms' tumor is currently being conducted by the Children's Cancer Group and The Pediatric Oncology Group. This protocol will evaluate a more aggressive approach, including the use of autologous bone marrow transplantation, particularly for those patients with adverse prognostic factors at the time of relapse.

Late Effects

As survival of Wilms' tumor patients has increased dramatically over the past 35 years, there has been an ever-increasing cohort of long-term survivors of therapy. NWTS patients who survive 5 years after completion of therapy are asked to participate in a late-effects study. Numerous organ systems are subject to the late sequela of anticancer therapy. Clinicians must now become familiar with the spectrum of problems that face these children as they grow into adulthood. An early report of 608 NWTS patients followed more than 5 years found that musculoskeletal problems such as scoliosis were seven times more common in children treated with radiation (Evans et al., 1991). It should be noted that these patients were from NWTS-1 and NWTS-2, where treatment intensity was much greater than is currently recommended (75% of the children enrolled in NWTS-1 received XRT compared with 25% currently).

Damage to reproductive systems can lead to problems with hormonal dysfunction or infertility. Gonadal radiation in males can result in temporary azospermia and hypogonadism (Kinsella et al., 1989). The severity of damage to the testis is dependent on the dose of radiation. Female Wilms' tumor patients who received abdominal radiation have a 12% incidence of ovarian failure (Stillman et al., 1987). In addition, women with prior abdominal radiation have the potential for adverse pregnancy outcomes. Perinatal mortality rates are higher, and infants are more likely to have low birth weights (Li et al., 1987).

Congestive heart failure is a well-known complication of treatment with anthracycline, and the incidence is dose related (Gilladoga et al., 1976). In addition to the acute cardiotoxicity, reports are surfacing of cardiac failure up to 20 years after treatment (Steinherz et al., 1991). In a preliminary review of patients entered in the first three NWTS groups, the frequency of congestive heart failure was 1.7% among doxorubicin-treated patients (Green et al., 1994d). The risk was increased if the patient received whole-lung irradiation. In light of these findings, all children who undergo treatment with these modalities should undergo periodic reevaluation.

Children treated for Wilms' tumor are at increased risk for second malignant neoplasms, (SMNs). Alkylating agents have been implicated in chemotherapy-induced second tumors (Harris, 1976). Two studies in Wilms' tumor survivors have noted a 1% cumulative incidence at 10 years postdiagnosis, and a rising incidence thereafter (Breslow et al., 1988b; Li et al., 1983). All but 2 of 26 SMNs in the two studies occurred in irradiated patients, most often in the radiation field. All children who developed hepatocellular carcinoma had received flank irradiation (Kovalic et al., 1991).

Recently there has been concern about the late occurrence of renal dysfunction in children who have undergone nephrectomy. There is both clinical and experimental evidence of hyperfiltration damage of remnant nephrons after a loss of renal mass (Anderson et al., 1985). Most experimental studies involve a loss of more than three quarters of the total renal mass, but there are only limited data concerning long-term renal function in children following unilateral nephrectomy (Argueso et al., 1992; Robitaille et al., 1989).

This concern of renal dysfunction has led some surgeons to recommend parenchyma-sparing procedures for unilateral tumors (McLorie et al., 1991). The majority of Wilms' tumors are too large for a partial nephrectomy at initial presentation. After preoperative chemotherapy, 10% of patients may be amenable to partial nephrectomy. Disadvantages of such an approach include the potential for increased surgical complications and the possibility of local recurrence. The use of partial nephrectomy is probably a sound idea for those with solitary kidneys, renal insufficiency, or a genetic predisposition to bilateral tumors such as Beckwith-Wiedemann syndrome, but for the majority of patients with unilateral Wilms' tumor the indication is less clear. The incidence of renal failure in unilateral Wilm's tumor patients reported to NWTS is less than 0.2%, and the majority of these had Drash syndrome, which is associated with end-stage renal disease (Ritchey et al. 1994b).

Future Directions

The next intergroup cooperative Wilms' tumor study is now being planned. Concepts under consideration are the treatment of selected stage I patients with surgery alone, preoperative therapy for patients with inoperable tumors and patients with extensive inferior vena caval extension, more aggressive chemotherapy regimens for patients with diffuse anaplasia and rhabdoid tumor of the kidney, and a retrieval protocol for patients with tumor relapse. A very important part of the next study will be the evaluation of biologic prognostic factors for Wilms' tumor. These factors could help further stratify patients for treatment, with the goal of decreasing the amount of therapy for children with tumors at low risk for relapse and intensifying treatment for high-risk patients.

Other Renal Tumors

Renal cell carcinoma is the most common non-Wilm's renal tumor of childhood. Only 5 percent of renal cell carcinomas occur in children (Broecker, 1991; Hartman et al., 1982). Patients with these tumors generally present after age 5 years, and it is the most common malignancy in the second decade of life. It has been reported in infants under 1 year of age (Pochedly et al., 1971), and in these patients, there is

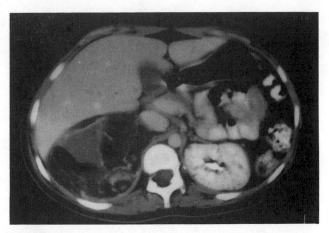

FIG. 58-12
Angiomyolipoma of the right kidney in a patient with tuberous sclerosis.

no sex predilection, contrasting with the male predominance seen in adult patients. The signs and symptoms are similar to those of other solid renal tumors, with an abdominal mass being the most common presentation in a child. Hematuria is more common in renal cell carcinoma than in Wilms' tumor (Broecker, 1991). Imaging studies cannot differentiate renal cell carcinomas from other solid renal tumors.

Survival of children with renal cell carcinoma is dependent on the ability to completely resect the tumor. Raney et al. found that all children with stage I lesions survived, and others have reported 64% to 80% survival for stage I and II tumors (Castellanos et al., 1974; Dehner et al., 1970; Raney et al., 1983). Overall survival was about 50%. Age is also a prognostic factor, with improved survival in children younger than 11 years (Raney et al., 1983). These tumors do not appear to be responsive to chemotherapy or radiation therapy.

Renal angiomyolipoma is a hamartomatous lesion that is only rarely seen in childhood. There is a clear association with tuberous sclerosis, and this tumor is more often bilateral in these patients (Blute et al., 1988). Although these vascular tumors are prone to hemorrhage, symptomatic cases are rare in children (Hendren and Monfort, 1987). The presence of this tumor may be suspected based on the demonstration of fat within the lesion by CT scan (Fig. 58-12). Small asymptomatic lesions, less than 3 cm, that are discovered incidentally can be observed without surgery (Blute et al., 1988).

Tumors of the renal collecting system are also very uncommon in childhood. Transitional cell carcinoma of the renal pelvis has been reported, and these lesions are managed with nephroureterectomy (Hudson et al., 1981). Fortunately, most filling defects of the upper collecting system represent benign lesions. The most common lesion is a fibroepithelial polyp (Gleason

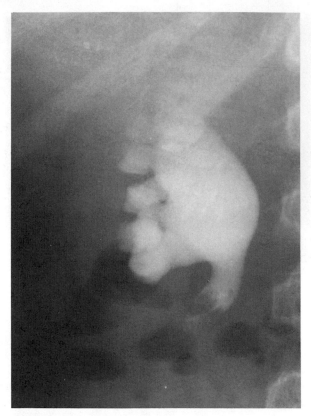

FIG. 58-13
Fibroepithelial polyp at the ureteropelvic junction, causing intermittent obstruction of the right kidney.

and Kramer, 1994). These patients typically present with symptoms secondary to obstruction (Fig. 58-13). Management consists of segmental resection and reconstruction of the urinary tract.

NEUROBLASTOMA

Neuroblastoma was first described by Virchow in 1864 (Virchow, 1864). Herxheimer in 1914 showed that neuroblastoma shared staining characteristics with neural tissues, which suggested its origin (Herxheimer, 1914). Neuroblastoma is known to arise from cells of the neural crest that form the adrenal medulla and sympathetic ganglia. Tumors derived from the sympathetic nervous system are differentiated along two lines: the pheochromocytoma line and the sympathoblastoma line. The latter includes neuroblastoma, ganglioneuroblastoma, and ganglioneuroma.

Genetics

It is suggested that 20% of neuroblastoma cases occur in patients with an inheritable mutation (Knudson and Strong, 1972b). The familial cases reported are postulated to represent an autosomal dominant pattern of inheritance. The median age at diagnosis of unselected patients with neuroblastoma is 21 months, contrasting with the median age of 9 months in familial cases of neuroblastoma (Kushner et al., 1986). Twenty

percent of patients with familial neuroblastomas have bilateral or multifocal primary tumors. The risk of neuroblastoma developing in a sibling or offspring of a patient with neuroblastoma is less than 6% (Kushner et al., 1986). Some of the difficulties in detecting the incidence and penetrance of an inheritable susceptibility to neuroblastoma is due to the frequent spontaneous regression and maturation of the tumor, the high mortality rate, and the complications of therapy, which preclude reproduction of multigenerational pedigrees for evaluation.

Numerous karyotypic abnormalities have been found in neuroblastoma. These changes occur in the forms of chromosomal deletions, translocations, and cytogenetic evidence of gene amplification. Deletion of the short arm of chromosome 1 is found in 70% to 80% of neuroblastomas (Brodeur, 1980). This deletion is thought to represent the loss of a gene, the putative neuroblastoma suppressor gene, that prevents tumor development. Unlike the WT1 gene associated with Wilms' tumor, there has been no evidence of constitutional deletions of this gene in neuroblastoma patients or of any chromosome 1p deletion syndromes.

Spontaneous Regression

Neuroblastoma and ganglioneuroblastoma are remarkable neoplasms and are most notable for the occurrence of spontaneous complete regression or maturation. The proclivity of neuroblastoma to transfer into benign ganglioneuroblastoma and ganglioneuroma was first reported in 1927 (Cushing and Wolbach, 1927). The incidence of spontaneous regression in childhood neuroblastoma has been reported to be 1% to 2% (Everson and Cole, 1966). Most cases of regression or maturation of neuroblastoma occur in the first year of life.

In addition to maturation of clinically evident cases of neuroblastoma, spontaneous regression of "in situ" neuroblastoma may occur far more often. Beckwith and Perrin coined this term in 1963 for small nodules of neuroblastoma cells found incidentally within the adrenal gland that histologically are indistinguishable from neuroblastoma (Beckwith and Perrin, 1963). In infants less than 3 months of age undergoing postmortem exam, neuroblastoma in situ was found in 1 per 224 infants. This represents an incidence of in situ neuroblastoma about 40 to 45 times greater than the incidence of clinical tumors. If these lesions clearly are neoplastic, then the majority undergo spontaneous involution, mature, or remain clinically occult. Notably, there have been no known instances of in situ neuroblastoma identified in an extraadrenal site. Neuroblastic nodules are considered a normal part of the fetal adrenal gland. In the developing fetus, the adrenal goes through a stage in which clusters of neuroblasts are seen that resemble neuroblastoma in situ. This reaches a peak level at 18 to 20 weeks of gestation (Turkel and Itabashi, 1974). There is some difficulty in distinguishing in situ neuroblastoma from nodules of neuroblast cells that linger into early infancy. The relationship of neuroblastic nodules to in situ neuroblastoma is unclear.

Pathology

Neuroblastoma

The gross morphology in neuroblastoma can vary considerably. Small adrenal tumors usually appear well encapsulated. The adrenal gland may be draped over the tumor, but larger tumors generally preclude precise identification of the anatomic site of origin. On cross-section, the tumor will vary in appearance and consistency depending on the degree of stromal elements. The tumor may rupture during removal, spilling out friable and hemorrhagic tumor. Cystic degeneration may be a prominent feature.

Neuroblastoma is the prototypical small "blue-cell" tumor of childhood (Fig. 58-14). The most common histologic pattern is that of lobular growth, but it may have a more diffuse or solid pattern. Neuroblastoma can be confused with lymphoma, Ewing's sarcoma or embryonal sarcoma. A characteristic feature of this tumor is the arrangement of the nuclei into pseudorosettes (Wright, 1910). The nuclei are separated by fibrils, which can appear as a meshwork. The nuclei vary in size and have a stippled nuclear chromatin pattern. Ganglion cell differentiation in neuroblastoma is evidence of maturation. Special staining may help characterize neuroblastoma cells. Neuron-specific enolase staining of the tumor is reported to be specific for neuroblastoma (Odelstad et al., 1982). Neuroblastoma usually lacks glycogen, which will help differentiate it from some of the sarcomas.

Before the modern techniques of immunohistochemistry were available, electron microscopy was important for the diagnosis of neuroblastoma. The ultrastructural features closely reflect the histologic findings of light microscopy (Romansky et al., 1978). There are interdigitating and back-to-back cytoplasmic neurites present with abundant neurofibrils. Neurosecretory granules are also readily found in thetumor representing accumulations of catecholamines.

A variety of antibodies are used to detect the presence of certain structural products, cellular products, and membrane-associated antigens. Most antibodies used are monoclonal. Although no specific neuroblastoma monoclonal antibody is available, a battery of antibodies can be used in the diagnostic evaluation of neuroblastoma or a similar-appearing neoplasm (Kleihues et al., 1987). Although these immunohistochemical stains have some limitations, they can help dif-

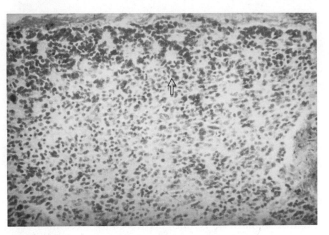

FIG. 58-14
Microscopic hematoxylin and eosin view of neuroblastoma demonstrating pseudorosette formation *(arrow)*.

ferentiate neuroblastomas from other small blue-cell tumors of childhood.

Ganglioneuroma

A ganglioneuroma is a histologically benign neoplasm and is quite rare compared with other benign neural tumors such as neurofibromas and schwannomas. Most ganglioneuromas are diagnosed in older children and are usually located in the posterior mediastinum and retroperitoneum, with only a small number arising in the adrenal glands (Enzinger and Weiss, 1988). Due to their site of origin, the ganglioneuromas tend to have a paravertebral location. In the retroperitoneum the presacral space is the most common site. Ganglioneuromas generally grow to a very large size before they cause symptoms due to compression of adjacent structures (Benjamin et al., 1972). Catecholamine excretion is elevated in 20% of patients and appears to increase as a function of tumor size (Lucas et al., 1994).

The pathology of ganglioneuroma is that of a well-circumscribed tumor with a fibrous pseudocapsule. These tumors are very firm and rubbery in consistency on cross-section. Careful examination of a ganglioneuroma is necessary to exclude ganglioneuroblastoma, which can have a similar gross appearance. On microscopic examination, mature ganglion cells with abundant cytoplasm are scattered throughout a mature Schwann cell matrix.

It is unclear whether a ganglioneuroma arises de novo or by maturation of a preexisting neuroblastoma or ganglioneuroblastoma. Cases of metastatic lesions that have been observed to develop the histology of mature ganglioneuromas support the latter theory (Hayes et al., 1989). In rare cases a ganglioneuroma has undergone malignant transformation into a malignant peripheral nerve sheath tumor or malignant schwannoma. In some of these patients there has been antecedent abdominal radiation (Keller et al., 1984).

Ganglioneuroblastoma

Ganglioneuroblastoma is intermediate between neuroblastoma and ganglioneuroma. It is difficult to determine where neuroblastoma ends and ganglioneuroblastoma begins. A grading classification of neuroblastoma introduced in 1984 has helped to define subtypes of ganglioneuroblastoma (Shimada et al., 1984).

Incidence

Neuroblastoma is one of the more common solid tumors, accounting for 7% to 8% of all childhood malignancies (Young et al., 1986). In the United States the annual incidence is 10 per 1 million live births. There are no sex-related differences in incidence rates. It is the most common malignant tumor of infancy, with 50% of cases occurring under age 2 years and 75% noted by the fourth year of life (Fortner et al., 1968). Neuroblastomas and ganglioneuroblastomas are occasionally seen in adults (Aleshire et al., 1985). There are few associated congenital anomalies. An association with neurofibromatosis has been reported (Knudson and Amromin, 1966), and there is

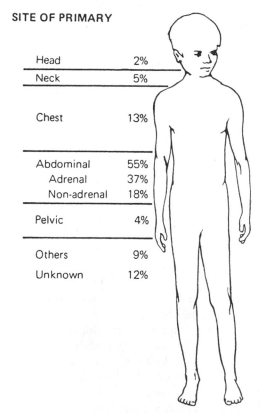

SITE OF PRIMARY

Head	2%
Neck	5%
Chest	13%
Abdominal	55%
Adrenal	37%
Non-adrenal	18%
Pelvic	4%
Others	9%
Unknown	12%

FIG. 58-15
Anatomic sites of origin of neuroblastoma. (Modified from Williams TE, Donaldson MH: Neuroblastoma, in Sutow WW, Vietti TJ, Fernabach DJ (eds): *Clinical Pediatric Oncology.* St Louis, CV Mosby, 1973, p 388.)

an increased incidence of brain and skull defects (Miller et al., 1968).

Clinical Presentation

The clinical manifestations of neuroblastoma vary widely with the site of the primary tumor, the presence of metastases, and secretion of biochemical products. More than one-half of neuroblastomas originate in the abdomen, and two-thirds of these arise in the adrenal gland (Fig. 58-15). Patients with an abdominal tumor may present with an abdominal mass, pain, or weight loss. The mass is typically hard and irregular, often extending across the midline. Pelvic neuroblastoma accounts for only 4% of tumors. Extrinsic compression of the bowel and bladder produces symptoms of urinary retention and constipation. Mediastinal and paraspinal retroperitoneal tumors that arise from sympathetic ganglia have a propensity to grow into the intervertebral foramen in a dumbbell configuration. A presentation of extradural spinal cord compression is more common for thoracic neuroblastoma than other locations (Adams et al., 1993; Akwari et al., 1978). Unilateral Horner's syndrome may develop in cervical or upper mediastinal tumors. There may also be asymmetric coloration of the iris, as the sympathetic nervous system is involved in iris pigmentation (Jaffe et al., 1975). About half of the mediastinal tumors are diagnosed incidentally (Adams et al., 1993).

Metastases are present in 70% of neuroblastoma patients at diagnosis and can be responsible for a variety of the clinical signs and symptoms of presentation (Gross et al., 1959). Fever, lethargy, weight loss, and bony pain are among these findings. The skull and long bones are most commonly involved. Radiographs will reveal lytic lesions that are frequently bilateral and asymmetric. More than 50% of patients with neuroblastoma will have involvement of the bone marrow (Finkelstein et al., 1970), and anemia is found in over one third of children.

Retrobulbar soft tissue involvement can result in another unique presentation of metastatic neuroblastoma. The tumor produces proptosis and periorbital ecchymosis. Subcutaneous nodules are common in infants with metastatic disease (Shown and Durfee, 1970). These have been described to have the appearance of blueberry muffins because of their bluish color.

Neuroblastoma is a biochemically active tumor with catecholamine secretion by over 90% of tumors. Symptoms may mimic pheochromocytoma, with paroxysmal hypertension, palpitation, flushing, and headache. Secretion of vasoactive intestinal peptide (VIP) by the tumor can produce severe watery diarrhea and hypokalemia (Cooney et al., 1982). Another unusual presentation of neuroblastoma is acute myoclonic encephalopathy (Farrelly et al.,

1984; Senelick et al., 1973). These patients develop myoclonus, rapid multidirectional eye movements (opsoclonus), and ataxia. The etiology is unclear but is thought to be secondary to catecholamine catabolites. Tumors associated with this syndrome generally have a good prognosis.

Diagnosis

Laboratory Evaluation

A complete blood count is essential. Anemia is noted in children with widespread bone marrow involvement. Coagulation abnormalities may be present due to massive liver metastases. Bone marrow aspiration is performed in all children with suspected neuroblastoma. Metastatic tumor to the bone marrow can occur in the absence of skeletal metastases (Finkelstein et al., 1970).

Twenty-four-hour urine collection will detect elevated levels of the two major metabolites of catecholamine production, vanillylmandelic acid (VMA) and homovanillic acid (HVA) in 90% of tumors (Williams and Greer, 1963). It is surprising that hypertension is not more common in neuroblastoma patients, but increased serum levels of norepinephrine are not present in neuroblastoma. This is attributed to breakdown of the catecholamines in the tumor. It has been noted that catecholamine storage vesicles are relatively lacking in patients with neuroblastoma as compared with patients with pheochromocytoma (Page and Jacoby, 1964). Since these storage vesicles protect the catecholamines from degradative enzymes, norepinephrine and epinephrine concentrations are much higher in pheochromocytoma, leading to the clinical symptoms. Another explanation for the lack of clinical signs and symptoms related to catecholamines could be the absence of periodic massive catecholamine release by tumor vesicles in neuroblastoma patients.

Urinary levels of HVA and VMA can be monitored throughout treatment. Therapy with various modalities has been shown to produce a reduction in catecholamine metabolite excretion in the majority of patients (Gerson and Koop, 1974). These metabolites can also be followed to detect tumor relapse. Biochemical evidence of relapse has been found before clinical evidence of a recurrent mass or other symptoms.

Another clinical marker is neuron-specific enolase, which is elevated in more than 90% of patients with metastatic disease (Zeltzer et al., 1983). Elevated serum ferritin levels are found in 40% to 50% of patients with advanced stage neuroblastoma (Hann et al., 1985). This can be followed during treatment, and it returns to normal during periods of remission.

Imaging

Imaging studies play an important role in the evaluation of a child with neuroblastoma. The diagnosis is suggested on excretory urography, which reveals inferior displacement of the kidney by a suprarenal mass. The kidney generally lacks the calyceal distortion typically seen with Wilms' tumor. Invasion of the renal parenchyma is not uncommon and can be detected radiographically by CT (Albregts et al., 1994). A speckled pattern of calcification is noted in 50% of cases on plain abdominal films. An even greater percentage of patients will have calcifications noted on CT (Fig. 58-16). Ultrasound and CT will both demonstrate the solid nature of the mass and the location of the tumor. Examination of the the liver for metastases is accomplished with either of these studies. Ultrasound is not as helpful for defining anatomic relationships of the tumor, particularly in extraabdominal sites. Prenatal diagnosis of neuroblastoma is possible with ultrasound (Jennings et al., 1993). MRI has advantages over CT in the evaluation of intraspinal tumor extension (Azizhkan and Haase, 1993). MRI can also define involvement of the major vessels and central nervous system.

A skeletal survey is routine to exclude associated metastases. These lesions are found most commonly in the long bones and skull. If the skeletal films are negative, a radionuclide bone scan may detect earlier metastases. A newer method of imaging both the tumor and metastatic sites is with radiolabeled ^{123}I metaiodobenzylguanidine (MIBG) (Geatti et al., 1985; Horne et al., 1986). MIBG bears structural similarity to norepinephrine and is taken up by the adrenergic secretory vesicles of the tumor cells both in the primary and in metastatic sites. MIBG scintigraphy can be used to determine the extent of disease and also to detect recurrence of tumor after completion of therapy (Geatti et al., 1985). Not all tumors have uptake of MIBG, and false negatives occur. It appears that maturation of the neuroblastoma to more mature forms such as ganglioneuroma also results in the loss of an ability to concentrate MIBG.

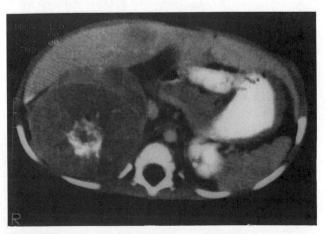

FIG. 58-16
Neuroblastoma arising from the right adrenal gland.

Screening

Mass population screening for neuroblastoma has been advocated to detect disease at an earlier stage and thus improve survival. This was initiated in Kyoto, Japan, in 1974 (Sawada et al., 1984) and has been widely used in Japan since 1985 (Nishi et al., 1987). Screening is generally performed at 6 months of age. Initially, a VMA spot test was performed using the LaBrosse method (LaBrosse, 1968). Although this method is quite economical, costing only 50 to 80 cents per sample, the test has a low sensitivity and specificity. In addition, many compounds other than VMA will react positively to the spot test. Because of these problems, many centers have switched to using high-performance liquid chromatography (HPLC) (Nishi et al., 1987). This test has a much lower false-positive rate and is more sensitive, but costs about $6 per sample. Some of the centers in Japan continue to use the spot test method of screening and then perform the HPLC technique or a quantitative HVA and VMA analysis, if the spot test is positive. An increased number of infants less than 1 year of age have been diagnosed with the mass screening program (Ishimoto et al., 1990), and the majority of these patients have lower-stage tumors (Sawada, 1992). Before mass screening started, 20% were diagnosed under 1 year of age, whereas 55% were diagnosed under 1 year of age after mass screening was instituted. A decrease in the percentage of primary adrenal gland tumors has been noted in the postscreening era. This suggests an increase in the diagnosis of tumors at other sites that could possibly have regressed undetected if screening had not been instituted.

An unanswered question is whether early detection of tumors will have an overall impact on survival (Naito et al., 1990). It is clear that patients diagnosed under 1 year of age with low-stage tumors have a better outlook (Breslow and McCann, 1971). In addition, tumors diagnosed by screening have other striking biologic differences from tumors that are detected clinically (Hayashi et al., 1992). In a review of 48 cases discovered by screening, none were observed to have amplified N-myc oncogene expression (see Prognostic Factors) (Ishimoto et al., 1991). In addition, 80% had a diploid chromosome pattern, which is associated with a favorable prognosis. All 48 patients were still alive without tumor. Altogether there have been 357 patients from Kyoto diagnosed by mass screening, and the overall survival is 97% (Sawada, 1992). Given the favorable biologic characteristics of tumors discovered by screening, it is possible that these patients would have the same excellent survival if they were discovered later in life due to clinical symptoms. There is also some concern that many of the unfavorable-histology tumors destined to present clinically at an older age go undetected by mass screening (Suita et al., 1994).

TABLE 58-6

Staging System for Neuroblastoma

Stage 0	Neuroblastoma in situ
Stage I	Tumors confined to the organ or structure of origin
Stage II	Tumors extending in continuity beyond the organ or structure of origin but not crossing the midline; the regional lymph nodes on the ipsilateral side may be involved
Stage III	Tumors extending in continuity beyond the midline; regional lymph nodes may be involved bilaterally
Stage IV	Distant metastases involving bones, bone marrow, brain, skin, liver, lung, soft tissues, or distant lymph node groups
Stage IV-S	Patients who would otherwise be classified with stage I or II disease but who have remote spread of tumor confined to one or more of the following sites: liver, skin, or bone marrow (without radiographic evidence of bony metastases on complete skeletal survey)

Staging

As with most solid tumors, staging of neuroblastoma patients is an important aspect of management, as the stage of the disease is a significant prognostic variable. Of the different staging classifications, the one proposed by Evans is the most widely used clinically (Table 58-6) (Evans et al., 1971). This system relies more on anatomic staging based on clinical assessment, imaging studies, and histopathological information. Other proposed classifications have included the resectability of the tumor, which is another important prognostic factor (Brodeur et al., 1988).

Prognostic Factors

There are many variables that have an impact on the prognosis of neuroblastoma. The site of origin is of significance. Nonadrenal primary tumors are associated with better survival than those that originate from the adrenal. The majority of children with thoracic neuroblastoma present at a younger age with localized disease and have an improved survival, even with correction for age and stage (Adams et al., 1993). Overall survival was 88% at 4 years in 96 patients with thoracic neuroblastoma studied by the Pediatric Oncology Group.

Age at diagnosis is another powerful prognostic indicator. Survival is inversely correlated with age at diagnosis. Children under 1 year of age have a far better survival than those diagnosed later in life (Breslow and McCann, 1971). This may be attributed to more favorable biologic parameters in tumors diagnosed at this age. Spontaneous regression is also more likely to occur in children less than 6 months of age.

Stage of the disease is also an important prognostic factor. Virtually all stage I patients with complete resection of the primary tumor will survive. Stage II patients also have a more favorable survival, even though there may be incomplete excision (Matthay et al., 1989). Advanced regional disease, stage III and stage IV, fares less well and requires more aggressive treatment. Clearly, tumors that can be completely resected have a more favorable prognosis. Whether this is independent of biologic factors is unclear.

In 1984 an age-linked histopathologic classification of neuroblastoma was introduced with definition of subtypes of ganglioneuroblastoma (Shimada et al., 1984). One of the important aspects of the Shimada classification is determining whether the tumor is stroma poor or stroma rich. Stroma-rich tumors can be separated into three subgroups: nodular, intermixed, and well differentiated. The last category consisted of tumors that more closely resemble ganglioneuroblastomas or immature ganglioneuromas. The survival of stroma-rich patients was as follows: well-differentiated, 100%; intermixed, 92%; and nodular, 18%.

The stroma-poor tumors can be divided into favorable and unfavorable subgroups based on the patient's age at diagnosis, degree of maturation, and the mitosis-karyorrhexis index (MKI). This index is based on a differential count of the mitoses in the tumor. Patients with stroma-poor tumors with unfavorable histopathologic features (higher MKI, higher age, undifferentiated histology) have a very poor prognosis, with less than 10% survival. Patients with stroma-poor favorable tumors have an excellent survival rate (>90%) (Shimada et al., 1984). Using the Shimada classification, all stage IV-S neuroblastomas studied by Hachitanda et al. were in a favorable-prognosis group of stroma-poor tumors (Hachitanda et al., 1991).

DNA content of tumor cells and ploidy number have been reported to have prognostic value. Studies of DNA content measured by flow cytometry showed that DNA aneuploidy correlated with better prognostic factors (age <1 year; stage I, II, or IV-S) and a good outcome (Look et al., 1984; Kusafuka et al., 1994). DNA diploidy and tetraploidy were associated with poor prognostic indicators (age >1 year and advanced clinical studies) and decreased survival.

A number of cytogenetic abnormalities have been identified in neuroblastomas, with the most consistent structural abnormalities noted on the short arm of chromosome 1 (Brodeur and Fong, 1989). Loss of heterozygosity for chromosome 1 is found in the majority of children with neuroblastoma but does not correlate as well as other prognostic factors with advanced stage of disease (Fong et al., 1990). Also noted in about one third of neuroblastoma tumors was the presence of homogeneously staining regions (HSRs) and double minute chromosomes (DMs) (Brodeur et al., 1977). These abnormalities are cytogenetic manifestations of gene amplification that led to the investigation of tumor oncogenes in neuroblastoma. DMs and HSRs are found in approximately 30% of neuroblastomas, and it was subsequently found that the N-myc oncogene was mapped to these regions. Amplification of the N-myc oncogene has been recognized in approximately one third of patients (Brodeur et al., 1984). The association of N-myc amplification with the pathogenesis of neuroblastoma is unclear, but the level of expression and amplification of the oncogene is quite important in determining prognosis (Seeger et al., 1985).

N-myc amplification is associated with a poor prognosis independent of patient age or stage of disease at presentation, and appears to remain constant regardless of therapy or tumor status. Children with multiple copies or genomic amplification of the N-myc tumor oncogene generally present with clinically advanced tumors that progress rapidly and respond poorly to therapy. In a recent study of stage I and IV-S tumors, none of the patients was found to have multiple copies of N-myc, and the tumors were associated with a good prognosis (Hachitanda et al., 1991). On the other hand, 50% of patients with stage III or IV disease have N-myc amplification (Azizkhan and Haase, 1993). There was an 18-month progression-free survival of 70% when there was no genomic amplification, compared with 30% in those patients with 3 to 10 copies of N-myc and only 5% in those with more than 10 copies of the oncogene. Many advanced-stage tumors lack N-myc amplification at diagnosis, and recurrence or progressive disease develops in the majority of these patients. Therefore, it is important that other prognostic factors involved in the pathogenesis of neuroblastoma be identified.

Several other biologic markers have prognostic value. Elevated levels of serum ferritin have been found in patients with neuroblastoma (Hann et al., 1985). Serum ferritin levels are elevated in 40% to 50% of patients with stage III or IV disease. Only 4% of Evans stage IV patients with levels above 140 ng/ml survive 2 years, compared with 30% survival in children with levels less than 75 ng/ml. If the serum ferritin is not elevated in stage III disease, survival is markedly better (76% vs. 23% 2-year disease-free survival). Patients can also be subdivided based on age and serum ferritin levels. Patients with normal serum ferritin and age less than 2 years have a 93% 2-year survival, patients older than 2 years of age with normal serum ferritin levels have 38% 2-year survival, and patients of any age with abnormal serum ferritin levels have a 19% 2-year survival (Hann et al., 1985). Neurone-specific enolase (NSE) is another biologic marker that has been noted to be elevated in over 90% of patients with metastatic neuroblastoma at diagnosis (Zeltzer et al., 1983). In infants less than 1 year of age, the survival rate was only 25% with high NSE levels compared with almost 100% survival in those infants in whom NSE was less than 190 g/ml. However, NSE is more difficult to assay, which has limited its widespread application.

Stage IV-S

Stage IV-S (S = special) comprises a distinct group of infants with distant liver, skin, and bone marrow metastases without radiologic evidence of bone metastases (Evans et al., 1980). Eight to 12% of all children with neuroblastoma present with this stage of disease. These children typically have a small intraabdominal adrenal primary, but in 10% of cases no primary can be identified. The median age of these infants is about 3 months, but occasionally they present after 1 year of age. This group of patients has an overall good prognosis, ranging from 80% to 87% (Stephenson et al., 1986). Many of these tumors undergo spontaneous regression (Evans et al., 1987; Haas et al., 1986). This regression can occur without treatment even in patients with a significant tumor burden. It is suggested that these patients do not have metastases but simply have collections of nonmalignant neural crest cells in these other sites. Studies of children with stage IV-S neuroblastoma have not revealed significant cytogenetic abnormalities or other adverse prognostic findings, such as N-myc oncogene amplification or elevated serum ferritin typically seen in children with stage IV neuroblastoma (Hachitanda et al., 1991; Hann et al., 1981).

Treatment

Surgical treatment of neuroblastoma was the only means to effect a cure at the beginning of this century. The first reported successful excision was by Bartlett in 1916 (Lehman, 1917). When radiotherapy became available, it was utilized in the treatment of this disease. However, survival remained dismal, with the best overall cure rates no better than 25% to 35% (Gross et al., 1959). It wasn't until an appropriate staging system was available that patients could be separated into groups for stratification of treatment (Evans et al., 1971). The addition of biologic and prognostic factors has allowed further separation of patients into favorable and unfavorable categories of tumors.

Favorable Disease (Stage I, II or IV-S)

Localized neuroblastoma can be treated by surgical excision alone with excellent results. Stage I patients with complete excision have an excellent prognosis. (O'Neill et al., 1985). The Pediatric Oncology Group reviewed 101 children with localized neuroblastoma who had complete gross excision of the primary tumor (Nitschke et al., 1988). The overall disease-free survival rate at 2 years was 89%. Nine patients developed relapses, but six were salvaged with chemotherapy. Stage II tumors can usually be completely resected. Radical resection is probably not justified in this group of patients. Radical lymph nodes dissection is not necessary, but diagnosis of contralateral lymph nodes is an important aspect of staging (Evans et al., 1971).

Radiation of the local tumor bed has been advocated for treatment of residual disease in Stage II patients. A report of 156 patients with stage II neuroblastoma found a 90% 6-year progression-free survival whether or not radiotherapy was used (Matthay et al., 1989). Therefore, surgical excision alone probably constitutes adequate therapy for the majority of stage II tumors.

In stage IV-S tumors, resection of the primary is not mandatory. A retrospective review of 37 patients did demonstrate that removal of the primary can be safely accomplished (Martinez et al., 1992), and after resection a 95% survival rate was noted. However, information regarding histologic prognostic factors was not available for all of these patients. Others have found that stage IV-S patients do very well whether or not their primary tumors are resected or they are given chemotherapy (Evans et al., 1987; Nickerson et al., 1985). However, patients with extensive metastatic disease who are N-myc positive represent a high-risk group (Martinez et al., 1992). These patients should be considered for a more aggressive treatment with multimodal therapy. Treatment of symptomatic infants with massive hepatic involvement using radiation therapy or chemotherapy can initiate tumor regression (Evans et al., 1980).

Unfavorable Group (Stage III or IV)

Advanced tumors require multimodal treatment. There is some debate on the intensity of the surgical resection required for stage III lesions. A report of 58 patients with stage III disease found that 8 out of 12 with initial complete excision and 12 of 14 with subsequent resection of the primary tumor were long-term survivors (Haase et al., 1989). This contrasts with only 9 of 32 survivors among patients in whom complete tumor excision could not be accomplished. There was significant morbidity reported in association with the surgical procedures, with 21 major complications. Nephrectomy was also required for complete excision in 6 of the patients. In a retrospective review, Kieley compared the results of radical tumor resection versus more conventional surgery (Kieley, 1994). In a large group of stage III and IV patients, he found no difference in survival of 46 patients treated with radical surgical procedures versus 34 patients treated with more conventional surgery. Both groups had 30% long-term survival rate.

Usually the safest approach for advanced tumors is to defer tumor resection until after initial chemotherapy. There is no clear advantage to debulking or cytoreductive surgery in this disease (Shochat, 1992). Neuroblastoma is a highly vascular tumor but does respond to chemotherapy. After chemotherapy, the tumors are smaller and firmer with less risk of rupture and hemorrhage. Timing of surgery is generally 13 to 18 weeks after initiation of chemotherapy (Azizkhan and Haase, 1993). Many children with bulky unresectable tumors or with widespread metastases at diagnosis can benefit from delayed attempts at surgery. This is particularly true in regard to debulking patients prior to bone marrow transplantation. Other attempts at local tumor control for unresectable diseases have included the use of intraoperative radiation therapy. This technique has the advantage of delivering a higher dose of radiation to the operative field while sparing normal adjacent tissues. Intraoperative radiation therapy has been used at Denver Children's Hospital in 30 children with neuroblastoma (Haase et al., 1993). Nine of 14 with advanced disease remain alive at a mean of 40 months.

Chemotherapy

A number of different agents have been employed in the treatment of neuroblastoma. However, the long-term survival in patients greater than 1 year of age with metastatic disease remains poor. Response of neuroblastoma to chemotherapy is believed to be reduced due to a large number of nonproliferating tumor cells (Kushner et al., 1987). Most regimens now employ a combination of nonspecific and cell cycle–specific drugs. Although there is often a good initial response, relapse continues to be a major problem, with 4-year overall-survival at 20% in stage IV disease (Haase et al., 1991; Ikeda et al., 1989).

Autologous bone marrow transplantation following sublethal chemotherapy or total body irradiation has resulted in complete remission in up to 50% of patients with recurrent stage IV disease (Dinndorf et al., 1992; Haase et al., 1993; Seeger et al., 1991). One problem that is becoming apparent with this treatment, though, is the late risk of relapse. The presence of bulky disease results in increased failure. Tumor debulking with surgery or radiation therapy is warranted prior to autologous bone marrow transplantation. Toxicity of bone marrow transplantation can be lethal, but these risks are necessary given that long-term survival is difficult to achieve in these patients.

Another option in the treatment of metastatic neuroblastoma is the use of ^{131}I MIBG (Hutchinson et al., 1992). The finding that both the primary tumor and metastatic areas take up this radiotracer suggested the possibility that therapeutic doses can be delivered to the tumor. Preliminary analysis indicates that objective responses do occur in terms of reduction of tumor volume. Little toxicity and few side effects have been reported.

TESTICULAR TUMORS

Testicular tumors account for 1% to 2% of all pediatric solid tumors. The peak incidence of childhood testicular tumors is at 2 years of age (Li and Fraumeni, 1972). The incidence tapers after age 4 years, but then

TABLE 58-7

Classification of Prepubertal Testicular Tumors

Germ cell tumors
  Yolk sac
  Teratoma
  Mixed germ cell
  Seminoma
Gonadal stromal tumors
  Leydig cell
  Sertoli cell
  Juvenile granulosa cell
  Mixed
Gonadoblastoma
Tumors of supporting tissues
  Fibroma
  Leiomyoma
  Hemangioma
Lymphomas and leukemias
Tumorlike lesions
  Epidermoid cyst
  Hyperplastic nodule secondary to congenital adrenal hyperplasia
Secondary tumors
Tumors of the adnexa

From Kay R: Prepubertal testicular tumor registry. *J Urol* 1993; 150:671.

begins to rise again at puberty. The incidence of germ cell tumors is not as high as in adults, accounting for only 65% of prepubertal testicular tumors. A greater percentage of benign testicular lesions occur in children (Table 58-7). Testis tumors are rare in black and Asian children. The etiology of testicular cancer is unknown. There is clearly a link between cryptorchidism and germ cell tumors of the testis (Campbell, 1959), but these are quite rare in childhood (Kay, 1993).

Clinical Presentation and Diagnosis

The most common presentation of patients with testicular tumors is a painless scrotal mass. The mass is typically nontender and does not transilluminate. Disorders that must be excluded are epididymitis, hernia, hydrocele, and torsion. There is often a delay of 7 months from first recognition of the scrotal swelling by the parents and initiation of treatment (Brosman, 1979). Some patients with hormonally active tumors may have small intratesticular lesions that are not palpable on physical examination. Tumors that develop in abdominal undescended testes are prone to torsion (Fig. 58-17) and can present with acute abdominal pain.

Imaging

Ultrasound is very helpful in the evaluation of testicular abnormalities. Hydrocele fluid around the testicle may prevent palpation of the testes. Ultrasound can detect small lesions not palpable on exam and identify cystic components of a teratoma of testis or epidermoid cyst (Fig. 58-18). If a benign lesion such

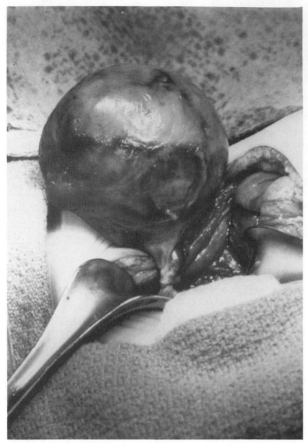

FIG. 58-17
Teratoma arising from an abdominal undescended testis. The patient presented with acute abdominal pain.

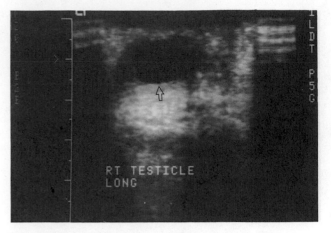

FIG. 58-18
Testicular ultrasound demonstrating cystic lesion *(arrow)* that proved to be a teratoma of the testicle. The patient underwent a testis-sparing procedure.

as teratoma or epidermoid cyst is suspected preoperatively, a testicular sparing procedure can be considered (Grunert et al., 1992; Rushton et al., 1990). Color Doppler ultrasound has been reported to be more effective than gray-scale ultrasound in detecting intratesticular neoplasms in the pediatric population (Luker and Siegel, 1994). Very small functioning Leydig cell tumors that are not evident on ultrasound have been detected with MRI (Kaufman et al., 1990).

Examination of the retroperitoneum for metastatic disease is indicated in patients with malignant tumors. Abdominal CT is most commonly employed. Chest x-ray or chest CT is mandatory to exclude pulmonary metastases.

Tumor Markers

Alpha-fetoprotein (AFP) is a single-chain glycoprotein produced by the fetal yolk sac, liver, and gastrointestinal tract. Various benign and malignant conditions can produce elevations of AFP, including yolk sac tumors of the testis. AFP has a half-life of 5 days, and degradation curves can be followed after orchiectomy to assess for residual disease. The age of the patient must be taken into consideration when monitoring serum levels of AFP, as the normal adult reference lab values do not apply to young children (Brewer and Tank, 1993; Lahdenne et al., 1991; Wu et al., 1981). Reference normal values for infants have now been established (Table 58-8) (Wu et al., 1981). Normal adult levels (<10 mg/ml) are not reached until 8 months of age. Recognition of this may avoid unfounded concern regarding residual disease following orchiectomy for yolk sac tumor in a young infant. Levels are monitored to detect tumor recurrence.

The beta subunit of human chorionic gonadotropin (B-HCG) is a glycoprotein that is produced by embryonal carcinoma and mixed teratomas. The normal value for B-HCG is less than 5 IU/L. The half-life of B-HCG is approximately 24 hours.

Carcinoma in Situ

Carcinoma in situ (CIS) occurs in the majority of patients with testicular tumors, suggesting that it is a precursor to the development of invasive germ cell tumor (Skakkebaek, 1975). There is an increased incidence of CIS in subgroups of patients known to be at high risk for the development of germ cell tumors. These include patients with cryptorchidism and intersex disorders (Muller et al., 1985). The diagnosis of CIS is determined by histologic examination of the testis. Screening programs using open testicular biopsy in adults who have previously undergone orchidopexy reveal an incidence of 1.7% (Giwercman et al., 1989). In the prepubertal patient, identification of CIS is more difficult. Biopsies at the time of orchidopexy in prepubertal children have only rarely demonstrated CIS (Hadziselimovic et al., 1984). The prepubertal patient with CIS should be followed with a repeat biopsy after puberty because the natural history of the disease in younger patients is unknown

TABLE 58-8

Average Normal Serum Alpha-Fetoprotein of Infants at Various Ages

Age	Number	Mean ± SD (ng/ml)
Premature	11	134,734 ± 41,444
Newborn	55	48,406 ± 34,718
Newborn-2 wk	16	33,113 ± 32,503
Newborn-1 mo	43	9452 ± 12,610
2 wk-1 mo	12	2654 ± 3080
2 mo	40	323 ± 278
3 mo	5	88 ± 87
4 mo	31	74 ± 56
5 mo	6	46.5 ± 19
6 mo	9	12.5 ± 9.8
7 mo	5	9.7 ± 7.1
8 mo	3	8.5 ± 5.5

From Wu J, Book L, Sudark: Serum alpha-fetoprotein (AFP) levels in normal infants. *Pediatr Res* 1981; 15:50.

TABLE 58-9

Intergroup Staging System for Testicular Germ Cell Tumors

Stage	Extent of Disease
I	Limited to testis (testes), completely resected by high inguinal orchiectomy; no clinical, radiographic, or histologic evidence of disease beyond the testes; tumor markers normal after appropriate half-life decline (AFP, 5 days; B-HCG, 16 hours). Patients with normal or unknown tumor markers at diagnosis must have a negative ipsilateral retroperitoneal node sampling to confirm stage I disease.
II	Transcrotal orchiectomy; microscopic disease in scrotum or high in spermatic cord (≤5 cm from proximal end); retroperitoneal lymph node involvement (≤2 cm) and/or persistently elevated or increased tumor markers.
III	Retroperitoneal lymph node involvement (≤2 cm), but no visceral or extraabdominal involvement. *Not eligible for this protocol.*
IV	Distant metastases, including liver. *Not eligible for this protocol.*

(Giwercman et al., 1988). An exception is the patient with androgen insensitivity or dysgenetic gonads.

Germ Cell Tumors

Yolk sac tumor is the most common prepubertal testicular tumor, accounting for 60% of all tumors (Kay, 1993). Over 75% of childhood yolk sac tumors occur in the first 2 years of life. It is known by a number of other eponyms, including endodermal sinus tumor, embryonal adenocarcinoma, infantile adenocarcinoma of the testis, orchidoblastoma, and Teilum's tumor. These tumors are believed to arise from the yolk sac elements. Grossly, the tumor is firm and yellow-white on cross-section, and hemorrhage is unusual. The characteristic histologic finding in yolk sac tumors are Schiller-Duval bodies (Wold et al., 1984). Eosinophilic cytoplasmic inclusions are common, and specialized staining techniques demonstrate the presence of AFP.

The clinical behavior of yolk sac tumor is quite at variance with its adult counterpart, embryonal carcinoma, despite the histologic similarities. Unlike adult tumors, spread to the retroperitoneal lymph nodes is quite uncommon, with an incidence of only 4% to 6% (Bracken et al., 1978; Brosman, 1979; Exelby, 1980). When distant metastases do occur, they are most likely to be hematogenous metastases to the lung, which are found in 20% of patients.

Radical inguinal orchiectomy is the standard initial therapy for all children with yolk sac tumors. There has been controversy regarding the need for retroperitoneal lymph node dissection (RPLND) both for staging and treatment. Historically, the addition of RPLND has been associated with increased survival. Staubitz et al., (1965) reported that patients with retroperitoneal disease could be cured with orchiectomy and RPLND. Hopkins et al. (1978) found a better

survival with orchiectomy and RPLND compared with orchiectomy alone (84% vs. 50%). However, all of these patients were given adjuvant chemotherapy and radiation therapy if there were involved nodes. Others reported a similar survival advantage for node dissection plus orchiectomy in comparison with orchiectomy alone (Drago et al., 1978; Jeffs, 1972). Treatment options considered for retroperitoneal disease included radiation therapy and chemotherapy. A radiation dose of 2000 to 3000 cGy has achieved an 84% survival rate (Ise et al., 1976). Adjuvant chemotherapy has also been advocated to prevent relapse, but this has not been performed prospectively in a large number of patients.

The need for RPLND began to be questioned based on the low incidence of metastases to retroperitoneal lymph nodes, improved imaging of the retroperitoneum for staging purposes, and the availability of a reliable tumor marker for the presence of residual or metastatic disease. It is interesting that most authors who reported improved survival with retroperitoneal lymph node dissection did not find evidence of nodal disease (Hopkins et al., 1978). CT imaging of the retroperitoneum can identify most patients with lymph node metastases, but there is a 15% to 20% false-negative rate (Pizzocara et al., 1987). Another justification for omitting RPLND was the development of effective combination chemotherapy that allows salvage of relapsed patients with clinical stage I disease (Kramer et al., 1984; Mann et al., 1989).

There is currently an intergroup study (Children's Cancer Group and Pediatric Oncology Group) on the treatment of localized and advanced germ cell tumors in children. The staging system is presented in Table 58-9. AFP levels are determined at diagnosis and monitored after radical inguinal orchiectomy to determine if there is an appropriate half-life decline. CT scans of the retroperitoneum and chest are obtained to exclude metastatic lesions.

Clinical stage I patients do not receive additional adjuvant treatment after radical orchiectomy. Chest x-ray, CT, or MRI of the retroperitoneum is recommended monthly for 3 months, again 3 months later, and then every 6 months. This surveillance is continued up to 36 months posttreatment. Tumor markers and physical examination are performed at more frequent intervals. Patients with normal or unknown tumor marker levels at diagnosis (marker negative) undergo ipsilateral retroperitoneal lymph node sampling rather than formal node dissection.

Patients who have undergone prior scrotal biopsy or transcrotal orchiectomy are considered stage II and undergo ipsilateral hemiscrotectomy. This approach has proven to be of benefit in adult patients with gross contamination during removal of germ cell tumors (Giguere et al., 1988). Patients with persistent elevation of AFP undergo retroperitoneal lymph node sampling. All stage II patients are given chemotherapy (bleomycin, cisplatin, and etoposide). At 12 weeks, patients with evidence of recurrent disease or elevation of tumor markers will undergo surgery. Residual retroperitoneal masses postchemotherapy are uncommon (Uehling and Phillips, 1994) but warrant resection to establish a histologic diagnosis. Patients with persistent viable tumor are then switched to another treatment regimen.

Children with stage III and IV germ cell tumors initially undergo retroperitoneal lymph node sampling. Those patients that develop relapse after initial treatment of a stage I tumor should also undergo biopsy for histologic confirmation. All patients with stage III and IV germ cell tumors receive chemotherapy. Patients with elevated tumor markers or clinically evident retroperitoneal disease after chemotherapy undergo biopsy and/or resection. Radiation therapy is not a routine part of the protocol for treatment of yolk sac tumors. A similar regimen has been employed by the United Kingdom Children's Cancer Study Group (Mann et al., 1989). Survival in patients with stage III and IV germ cell tumors was 83% and 67%, respectively. However, overall survival for 68 patients with yolk sac tumors was 99%.

Teratoma is a germ cell tumor with recognizable elements of more than one germ cell layer: endoderm, ectoderm, and mesoderm. The incidence of teratoma is lower in children than in adults, but it is the second most common testis tumor in children (Brosman, 1979). These tumors generally appear well encapsulated on gross examination. There are multiple cysts present, but consistency on cross-section varies with the amount of solid tissue present between the cysts. The microscopic appearance varies with the relative amounts of tissue derived from the different germ layers and the degree of maturation (Mostofi and Price, 1973). Cartilage, bone, mucous glands, or muscle may be evident.

Prepubertal teratomas have a benign clinical course, in contrast to the clinical behavior of teratomas in adults, which have the propensity to metastasize (Mostofi and Price, 1973). In past years, the majority of these tumors have been managed with radical orchiectomy. However, ultrasound of the testis can demonstrate the cystic nature of this lesion, suggesting the diagnosis of teratoma. Other cystic lesions of the testis such as simple cysts or epidermoid cysts must be considered in the differential diagnosis. The latter lesions generally have a hyperechoic center surrounded by an outer hypoechoic rim (Maxwell and Mantora, 1990). Teratomas appear more as complex hypoechoic areas surrounded by highly echogenic signals (Krone and Carroll, 1985). If the preoperative evaluation suggests a benign intratesticular lesion, then a testicular sparing procedure can be considered. (Altadonna et al., 1988; Dodat et al., 1986; Haas et al., 1986; Marshall et al., 1983; Rushton et al., 1990). Although only a limited number of patients have been treated with enucleation of the tumor, there have been no recurrences reported to date (Rushton et al., 1990). Theoretical concerns include tumor seeding, incorrect diagnosis, and multifocal microscopic disease within the testis. However, frozen section diagnosis of teratoma is straightforward due to the characteristic histologic features of the tumor. In addition, a detailed review of 21 cases of prepubertal teratoma at the Armed Forces Institute of Pathology did not reveal evidence of multifocal disease or carcinoma in situ of the adjacent testis (Rushton et al., 1990).

Gonadal Stromal Tumors

Gonadal stromal tumors are the most common nongerminal testicular tumors in children. Leydig cell tumors are the most common gonadal stromal tumors in both children and adults. The peak incidence is age 4 to 5 years. Leydig cells produce testosterone, and the tumor may continue production of the hormone, resulting in precocious puberty. Leydig cell tumors account for approximately 10% of all cases of precocious puberty in boys (Urban et al., 1978). In addition, the boys may have accelerated skeletal and muscle development, which may not resolve after removal of the tumor (Mengel and Knorr, 1983). Other hormones produced by Leydig cell tumors include estrogens, progesterone, and corticosteroids. These can be responsible for the production of gynecomastia, which occurs more often in adults with Leydig cell tumors (Johnstone, 1967).

Differential diagnosis of precocious puberty includes pituitary lesions, which can be excluded by the finding of prepubertal LH and FSH levels with an increased serum testosterone. Leydig cell tumors also must be differentiated from Leydig cell hyperplasia, tumors of adrenal rest tissue, and hyperplastic testicular nodules that develop in boys with poorly controlled congenital adrenal hyperplasia (CAH) (Fig. 58-19) (Cunnah et al., 1989; Srikath et al., 1992; Wilson and Netzloff, 1983). Leydig cell hyperplasia can be distinguished by normal levels of urinary 17-ketosteroids. Testicular nodules in CAH often present in the second decade of life. These lesions tend to occur bilaterally, but there have also been reports of bilateral Leydig cell tumors (Bokemeyer et al., 1993). A family history of CAH is helpful in making the diagnosis. The hyperplastic nodules that develop in CAH resemble Leydig cells histologically but behave biochemically like adrenal cortical cells (Radfar et al., 1977). Urinary ketosteroids are elevated in patients with 21-hydroxylase deficiency, and serum levels of 17-hydroxy progesterone are elevated. Urinary pregnanetriol levels are absent in Leydig cell tumors. Glucocorticoid replacement in CAH will generally produce regression of the hyperplastic nodules, but this is not universal (Srikath et al., 1992). This may be due to the presence of fibrosis or calcification in the nodule.

Leydig cell tumors appear well encapsulated, with compression of the adjacent testicular tissue. They appear yellow to brown on cross-section, reflecting the steroid production by the tumor. The pathognomonic histologic feature of Leydig cell tumor, Reinke's crystals, are present in only about 40% of tumors (Mostofi and Price, 1973). Increased mitotic figures or other features suggestive of malignancy are absent in prepubertal Leydig cell tumors. Since malignancy has not been reported in children, orchiectomy is adequate treatment (Brosman, 1979).

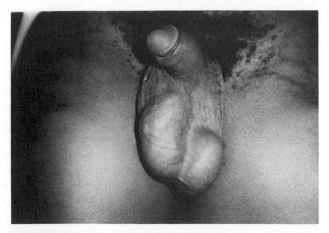

FIG. 58-19
Precocious puberty in an 11-year-old boy due to hyperplastic Leydig cell nodules. (Photograph courtesy of Dr. David Bloom.)

Sertoli cell tumors are the next most common gonadal stromal tumor in children. These tumors are not as metabolically active as Leydig cell tumors, but gynecomastia has been reported (Gabrilove et al., 1980). The typical presentation is usually a painless testicular mass, and these tumors present at an earlier age than Leydig cell tumors. Treatment is orchiectomy, but examination of the retroperitoneum is warranted, as there has been one report of retroperitoneal spread (Rosvoll and Woodard, 1968).

Gonadoblastomas occur in children with dysgenetic gonads and are associated with the presence of a Y chromosome in karyotype (Manuel et al., 1976). Gonadoblastomas are small benign tumors that are bilateral in up to one third of cases. The tumor is composed of germ cells, sex cord derivatives resembling immature granulosa and Sertoli cells, and occasionally stromal elements. These are the most common tumors found in association with intersex disorders. The risk of tumor formation in patients with mixed gonadal dysgenesis is 25% (Schellas, 1974), and the incidence increases with age (Manuel et al., 1976). The germ cell component of gonadoblastoma is prone to malignant degeneration into seminoma and nonseminomatous tumors. It has been recommended that all streak gonads in patients with gonadal dysgenesis be removed (Aarskog, 1970). Patients with gonadal dysgenesis raised as females should have the gonads removed at diagnosis (Gourlay et al., 1994; Olsen et al., 1988). In addition, all undescended testes should be removed, but scrotal testes can be preserved, as they are less prone to tumor development. Early gonadectomy is advocated, as tumors have been reported in children under the age of 5 years (Gourlay et al., 1994; Olsen et al., 1988). Carcinoma in situ has been demonstrated in gonadal biopsies of children with gonadal dysgenesis, and this has been suggested as a means of identifying those at risk for development of malignant germ cell tumors (Muller et al., 1985). However, recognition of carcinoma in situ in prepubertal gonadal biopsies can be difficult, and a negative biopsy does not preclude the later development of a germ cell tumor.

Secondary Tumors

Leukemia and lymphoma are the most common malignancies to spread to the testicle in children. Occult testicular involvement has been found in up to 20% of patients with acute lymphoblastic leukemia (Askin et al., 1981; Braren et al., 1980). This may be an early indication of relapsed or persistent disease. The testis acts as a sanctuary, and it is postulated that the blood-testis barrier prevents the chemotherapeutic agents from reaching the malignant cells. Some centers routinely perform open-wedge biopsies of the testis prior to discontinuing treatment, but there is concern about a significant false-negative rate (Pui et al., 1985). Patients with leukemic infiltrates can be salvaged with further chemotherapy and radiation to the testes (Askin et al., 1981). Testicular involvement occurs in 4% of boys with Burkitt's lymphoma and may be the initial clinical presentation (Lamm and Kaplan, 1974).

GENITOURINARY RHABDOMYOSARCOMA IN CHILDHOOD

Rhabdomyosarcoma (RMS) is the most common soft tissue sarcoma in infants and children. RMS accounts for approximately half of all pediatric soft tissue sarcomas and 15% of all pediatric solid tumors. RMS can arise from almost any site and has peak incidence between the ages of 2 and 5 years. Genitourinary RMS accounts for approximately 20% of these tumors (Maurer et al., 1988). The most common genitourinary sites are the prostate, bladder, and vagina. Survival varies with the site, and special sites such as the vagina and paratesticular region have a better prognosis than bladder/prostate primaries (Crist et al., 1990; Rodary et al., 1988). There is a male predominance for genitourinary RMS (Maurer et al., 1977).

The etiology of RMS is unknown, but subgroups of children with a genetic predisposition have been identified. The Li-Fraumeni syndrome associates childhood sarcomas with mothers who have an excess of premenopausal breast cancer and with siblings who have an increased risk of cancer (Li and Fraumeni, 1969). A mutation of the p53 tumor suppressor gene was found in the tumors in all patients with this syndrome (Malkin et al., 1990). An increased incidence of RMS has been found in association with neurofibromatosis (McKeen et al., 1978).

Pathology

There are several histologic variants of RMS. Embryonal RMS is the most common subtype seen in children and accounts for more than 60% of genitourinary tumors (Maurer et al., 1977). This may occur in solid form arising in muscle groups such as the trunk and extremities or as the so-called sarcoma botyroides, a polypoid variety that occurs in hollow organs or body cavities such as the bladder, vagina, nasopharynx, or biliary tree. The Intergroup Rhabdomyosarcoma Study (IRS) has reported that more than 90% of genitourinary tumors in children are embryonal (Newton et al., 1988).

The second most common form is alveolar, which occurs more commonly in extremity lesions than genitourinary sites and has a worse prognosis (Hays et al., 1983; Newton et al., 1988). Alveolar RMS also has a higher rate of spread to regional lymph nodes, local recurrence, bone marrow involvement, and distant spread.

A less common subtype in children is pleomorphic RMS. This tumor is no longer considered to be a separate entity, but rather an anaplastic variant of the more common embryonal or alveolar RMS (Kodet et al., 1993). Anaplastic histology is associated with an unfavorable prognosis. Monomorphous round cell RMS is another unfavorable histologic variant. The diagnosis of rhabdomyosarcoma by conventional histologic techniques can be difficult. In difficult cases, histology may be combined with a number of other studies, including electron microscopy, cytogenetics, immunohistochemistry, and DNA flow cytometry (Shapiro et al., 1991).

Metastatic spread of RMS is usually to the lungs. Regional lymph node metastases are fairly common and vary with site of the primary tumor. Positive regional nodes may be treated with radiation to prevent nodal recurrence.

Clinical Staging

The outcome of treatment is most dependent on the stage at diagnosis (Lawrence et al., 1987). Clinical grouping was employed in the early IRS studies; this classification is shown in Table 58-10. One of the difficulties inherent in this system is that the stage is dependent to a large extent on the completeness of surgical excision. As the treatment of RMS has evolved, more patients are undergoing biopsy only at the initial surgical procedure, leaving gross residual disease. This results in the shifting of more patients from group I to group III. Biologically equivalent tumors could end up in different categories depending on the aggressiveness of the initial surgical resection. A clinical staging system was devised for IRS-IV (Table 58-11) (Lawrence et al., 1987a). This classification relies on clinical findings from physical examination, and laboratory and imaging studies. Tumor site, size, regional nodal involvement, and distant metastasis were most predictive of survival. The preclinical staging is also more predictive of outcome than the clinical grouping system.

TABLE 58-10

IRS Clinical Grouping Classification

Group I	Localized disease completely resected
	Confined to organ of origin
	Contiguous involvement
Group II	Total gross resection with evidence of regional spread
	Microscopic residual
	Positive nodes but no microscopic residual
	Positive nodes but microscopic residual in nodes or margins
Group III	Complete resection with gross residual disease
	After biopsy only
	After gross or major resection of the primary (>50%)
Group IV	Distant metastasis at diagnosis (lung, liver, bones, bone marrow, brain, and nonregional nodes)
	Positive cytology in CSF, pleural, or peritoneal fluid or implants on pleural or peritoneal surfaces are regarded as stage IV

TABLE 58-11

IRS Pretreatment TGNM Clinical Staging Based on Clinical, Radiographic, and Laboratory Examination and Histology of Biopsy

Stage A:	Favorable site, nonmetastatic
Stage B:	Unfavorable, small, negative nodes, nonmetastatic
Stage C:	Unfavorable, big and/or positive nodes, nonmetastatic
Stage D:	Any site, metastatic
Tumor:	$T_{site\,1}$—Confined to site of origin
	$T_{site\,2}$—Fixation to surrounding tissues
	<5 cm in size
	>5 cm in size
Histology:	G_1—Favorable histology (mixed, embryonal botryoid, other)
	G_2—Unfavorable histology (alveolar)
Regional lymph nodes:	N_0—regional lymph nodes not clinically involved
	N_1—regional lymph nodes clinically involved
Metastases:	M_0—No distant metastases
	M_{1site}—Metastases present

Treatment: General Principles

Radical surgical excision was the first effective treatment for RMS. For pelvic genitourinary tumors, this consisted of total pelvic exenteration. It was later noted that RMS was radiosensitive (Stobbe and Dargeon, 1950), but high doses were required for local tumor control. In the 1960s, contribution therapy was employed with the use of chemotherapy and radiation therapy following attempts at complete surgical excision (Pinkel and Pickren, 1961). These efforts showed that survival was significantly enhanced if chemotherapy was routinely administered after surgery (Heyn et al., 1974).

Due to the small number of patients encountered at any single institution, a cooperative effort was initiated to study the different therapeutic efforts for RMS (Maurer et al., 1977). Over the last 20 years there has been a progressive increase in survival among children with RMS. The major factor in this success has been the multimodal approach, which includes chemotherapy, radiation therapy, and surgery. During the early years of the IRS (1972 to 1978), radical surgical intervention prior to chemotherapy with or without radiation was standard. Once it was demonstrated that most patients would survive the disease, investigators explored the utilization of primary chemotherapy and radiation therapy to avoid the exenterative surgery employed for genitourinary RMS (Ortega, 1979; Voute et al., 1981). A major aim of the protocols for patients with primary tumors in these sites in IRS-II (1978 to 1984) was the preservation of a functional distal urinary tract with maintenance of the high survival rates achieved in IRS-I (Raney et al., 1990). Unfortunately, primary chemotherapy with VAC (vincristine, dactinomycin, cyclophosphamide)

did not obviate the need for radiation therapy or radical surgery for patients with pelvic RMS. The percentage of patients alive after 3 years was the same for IRS-II as for IRS-I (Hays, 1993). In IRS-III (1985 to 1992), more intensive chemotherapy was used—VAC plus doxorubicin and cisplatinum—and radiation therapy was initiated sooner. With the intensification of treatment for pelvic RMS in IRS-III, there has been an increased rate of salvage of functional bladders with overall survival maintained (Hays, 1993).

A number of therapeutic and nontherapeutic advances have been made during the IRS studies. Some of these specifically related to the surgical aspects of genitourinary RMS include: (1) identification of histology, site, and extent of disease as prognostic factors (Lawrence et al., 1987); (2) reduced need for radical surgery; (3) increased bladder salvage from 25% to 60% along with increased survival (Hays et al., 1982); (4) partial cystectomy affording comparable survival with satisfactory bladder function (Hays et al., 1990a); (5) demonstration of the benefit of primary tumor reexcision for microscopic residual after initial nondefinitive excision; (6) second-look surgery to determine pathologic state while increasing complete response rate and possibly survival (Hays et al., 1990b); (7) elimination of "routine" lymphadenectomy for localized paratesticular RMS (Weiner et al., 1994); and (8) reduction or elimination of radiation therapy for special groups or sites.

Specific Sites
Bladder and Prostate Tumors

A common clinical presentation of RMS of the bladder or prostate is urinary obstruction. Tumors of the bladder usually occur as a botryoid form and grow intraluminally, usually at or near the trigone (Hays, 1982). Prostatic RMS tends to present as a solid mass rather than the botryoid form seen in the bladder. Extension into the bladder neck results in bladder outlet obstruction. Determining the actual site of origin of some pelvic tumors can be difficult. Signs and symptoms include urinary frequency, stranguria, acute urinary retention, and hematuria. On physical examination an abdominal mass from either tumor or a distended bladder is often present. Contrast studies reveal filling defects within the bladder or elevation of the bladder base in prostatic RMS (Fig. 58-20). Ultrasound or CT shows the extent of tumor and evaluates the retroperitoneal and pelvic nodes. Cystoscopic evaluation establishes the diagnosis, and transurethral biopsies can be obtained.

As previously mentioned, the use of surgical intervention has become more conservative during the past 20 years. Biopsy, chemotherapy, and bladder salvage are the mainstays of treatment today. Although conservative surgical therapy for bladder tumors has not

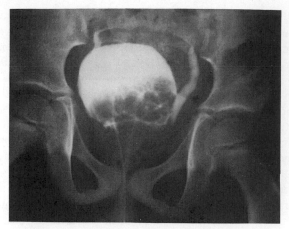

FIG. 58-20
Excretory urogram demonstrating filling defects in the bladder due to rhabdomyosarcoma. (Photograph courtesy of Dr. Stanford Goldman.)

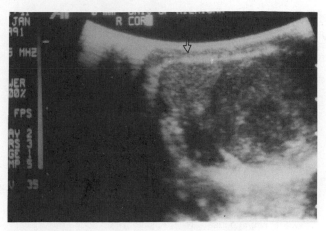

FIG. 58-21
Scrotal ultrasound of a young boy presenting with a painless mass that shows compression of the testicular parenchyma *(arrow)* by the paratesticular rhabdomyosarcoma.

been as successful as for vaginal primaries, the bladder salvage rate has increased (Hays, 1993; Hays et al., 1990a). With the intensification of treatment for pelvic RMS in IRS-III, there has been an increased rate of salvage of functional bladders with maintenance of overall survival. Currently, 60% of patients retain a functional bladder 4 years from diagnosis, and overall survival exceeds 85% (Hays, 1993).

Initial anterior pelvic exenteration is no longer considered the initial therapy for pelvic RMS (Raney et al., 1993). Partial resection of the bladder wall for primary tumors affecting the dome or sides of the bladder distant from the trigone is recommended either as initial therapy or as a delayed procedure after chemotherapy. This has been employed in 40 patients reported to the IRS, with an overall survival of 80% (Hays, 1993). Of the 32 long-term survivors, 75% have no bladder-related symptoms. Bladder augmentation or substitution has been utilized in some of these patients with good functional results (Hicks et al., 1993).

Unfortunately, a large percentage of these tumors arise from the trigonal area of prostate and are not amenable to local or partial resection. Local recurrence is high if adequate resection is not accomplished. If chemotherapy does not result in adequate shrinkage to allow partial resection, then radical cystectomy may be necessary. Pelvic exenteration is also employed for relapsed tumors (Hays, 1993). Prostatectomy without cystectomy has been performed in selected patients with persistent disease or local relapse (Hays, 1993; McLorie et al., 1989). However, local relapses have occurred in 40% of these patients. The completeness of surgical resection may be difficult to determine by frozen section, which can lead to local recurrence (McLorie et al., 1989).

Paratesticular RMS

Paratesticular RMS arises in the distal portion of the spermatic cord and may invade the testis or surrounding tissues. Of all primary genitourinary tumors, 7% are located in the paratesticular area (Bruce and Gough, 1991). Over 90% of paratesticular RMSs are embryonal in histology and have a good prognosis. The peak age of presentation is between 1 and 5 years (Weiner et al., 1994).

Presentation is often a unilateral painless scrotal swelling or mass above the testis. On physical examination, a firm mass is found that is usually distinct from the testis. Ultrasound can confirm the solid nature of the lesion (Fig. 58-21).

Radical inguinal orchiectomy is recommended for initial treatment. Performance of a prior transcrotal procedure increases the risk of local recurrence and nonregional lymph node spread. If cord elements remain, an inguinal exploration with removal of the remaining spermatic cord and a partial hemiscrotectomy including the prior scrotal incision are performed. In a review of 14 hemiscrotectomy specimens at Memorial Sloan-Kettering Cancer Center, 29% had residual tumor identified (LaQuaglia, 1989).

Prior to the advent of effective systemic therapy, surgery alone produced a 50% relapse-free survival at 2 years (Sutow et al., 1970). With the introduction of multimodal treatment, chemotherapy, and radiation therapy for selected patients, survival rates of 90% are expected (Hamilton et al., 1989; Weiner et al., 1994). A metastatic evaluation is performed at diagnosis. CT imaging of the retroperitoneum to identify nodal metastases is mandatory, as lymphatic spread is present in 28% to 40% of children (Lawrence et al., 1987; Raney et al., 1978). The initial use of RPLND for paratesticular RMS was based on the management of non-RMS testicular malignancies and the high incidence of retroperitoneal lymph node involvement. It was thought that the node dissection itself was not of therapeutic value, but was indicated to stage the disease (Banowsky and Shultz, 1970). A unilateral dissection was recommended with sampling of the contralateral nodal chain. Patients found to have positive lymph nodes receive radiation therapy to the involved areas.

The role of RPLND in paratesticular rhabdomyosarcoma is controversial (Olive et al., 1984; Rodary et al., 1992; Weiner et al., 1994). Arguments against its routine use are that grossly involved retroperitoneal nodes can be detected by preoperative imaging studies, microscopic nodal disease can be effectively treated by chemotherapy, and there is significant morbidity associated with RPLND. Heyn and associates (1992) reported a 10% incidence of intestinal obstruction, 8% incidence of ejaculatory dysfunction, and 5% incidence of edema of the lower extremities in patients who had undergone RPLND for paratesticular RMS. This series involved patients reported to the first IRS study, with the majority undergoing bilateral node dissection. A modified unilateral node dissection is appropriate for staging and with the addition of nerve-sparing techniques may avoid some of the reported morbidity of node dissection (LaQuaglia et al., 1989; Donohue et al., 1990). It is clear that even with the current advances in imaging there is a significant false-negative rate of CT—14% for IRS-III patients—for identifying retroperitoneal lymph nodes in patients with paratesticular RMS (Wiener et al., 1994). The ability of laparoscopy to identify retroperitoneal nodal disease in this setting remains to be evaluated, but may offer a less morbid alternative to RPLND.

Olive and colleagues (1984) reported on a group of 19 children with paratesticular RMS who had no clinical evidence of retroperitoneal nodal involvement. Nodal recurrence developed in two patients (10.5%), but both survived after salvage therapy. In a subsequent report of the SIOP experience with 46 children with completely excised tumors and negative CT or lymphangiogram treated with intensive chemotherapy alone, again all children survived (Olive-Sommelet, 1989). However, it should be noted that the vast majority of children did receive doxorubicin, which has potential for adverse late effects.

In a review of 121 children with paratesticular RMS undergoing RPLND reported to IRS-III, 14% of patients with clinically negative nodes were found to have positive lymph nodes on pathologic evaluations (Wiener et al., 1994). There were two cases of nodal relapse, one of which had a prior negative RPLND. This suggests a small risk of nodal relapse in these patients, if regional radiation therapy and appropriate chemotherapy are received. The overall 5-year survival for the 98 patients with clinically negative nodes

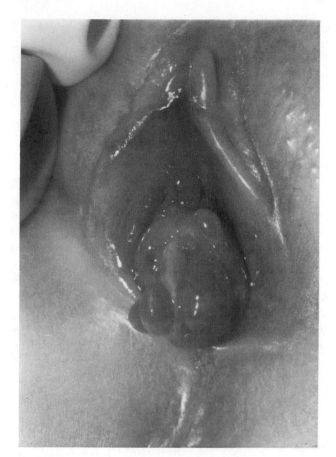

FIG. 58-22
Mass protruding from the vaginal introitus in a young girl with vaginal rhabdomyosarcoma.

was 96%, but less than 10% of patients received doxorubicin. Although the finding of positive retroperitoneal lymph nodes did identify a group of patients with decreased survival, it is now recommended that patients with clinically negative nodes undergo treatment with primary chemotherapy alone (Rodary et al., 1992). One exception may be the child over 10 years of age, as this group of patients has a significantly worse prognosis (Wiener et al., 1994).

Vaginal/Vulvar RMS

Vaginal RMS originates mainly from the anterior vaginal wall in the middle or distal third of the vagina (Andrassy et al., 1995). Vaginal tumors may invade the vesicovaginal septum or bladder wall due to its proximity. Cystoscopy is warranted during initial evaluation and at intervals during follow-up (Andrassy et al., 1995). The clinical presentation can be quite striking if there is prolapse of the mass from the vaginal introitus (Fig. 58-22). Vaginal bleeding or discharge is also common. The diagnosis is made by vaginoscopy and biopsy of the lesion.

Treatment used to consist of anterior pelvic exenteration, but since this tumor was found to be very chemosensitive, definitive surgery is delayed until after an initial course of therapy (Hays et al., 1988). Delayed tumor resection may consist of partial vaginectomy or vaginectomy with hysterectomy. More recently, these patients have been treated with primary chemotherapy and repeat biopsies with primary chemotherapy and repeat biopsies unless there is persistence of disease (Andrassy et al., 1995).

Uterine RMS

Previous studies have suggested that uterine RMS represents a distinct group of patients who present at an older age and have less response to treatment and thus poorer prognosis compared with vaginal RMS (Hays et al., 1981; Hays et al., 1985). However, a recent review of patients in IRS-III and pilot IRS-IV treated by primary chemotherapy and delayed resection suggests that these previously held beliefs may not be true (Corpron et al., 1995). Patients with uterine RMS in these more recent clinical trials were of the same age group as the vaginal RMA patients and responded well to chemotherapy and conservative surgical intervention. With this approach it may be possible to salvage the uterus and vagina as well as the bladder in many of these patients (Corpron et al., 1995).

Other Tumors of the Lower Urinary Tract

Benign polyps of the prostatic urethra are the most common benign lesions of the prostate. Obstruction is the most common presentation (Gleason and Kramer, 1994). These fibroepithelial polyps arise from a stalk near the verumontanum. On histologic examination these lesions are covered by normal transitional epithelium. There have been no reports of recurrence when these lesions have been completely excised.

Transitional cell carcinoma of the bladder is extremely rare in the first 2 decades of life (Javadpour and Mostofi, 1969; Kurz et al., 1987). Most of these tumors are of low grade and stage and can be managed endoscopically. Another bladder tumor occasionally found in children is nephrogenic adenoma (Ritchey et al., 1984). These lesions appear to arise as a metaplastic response to chronic inflammation in the bladder. Transurethral excision is all that is needed in most patients, but periodic endoscopic surveillance is recommended because of reports of recurrence.

REFERENCES

Aarskog D: Clinical and cytogenetic studies in hypospadias. *Acta Paediatr Scand Suppl* 1970; 203:1.

Adams GA, Shochat SJ, Smith EI, et al: Thoracic neuroblastoma: a Pediatric Oncology Group study. *J Pediatr Surg* 1993; 28:372.

Akwari OE, Payne WS, Onofrio BM, et al: Dumbbell neurogenic tumors of the mediastinum: diagnosis and management. *Mayo Clin Proc* 1978; 53:353.

Albregts AE, Cohen MD, Galliani CA: Neuroblastoma invading the kidney. *J Pediatr Surg* 1994; 29:930.

Aleshire SL, Glick AD, Cruz VE, et al: Neuroblastoma in adults: pathologic findings and clinical outcome. *Arch Pathol Lab Med* 1985; 109:352.

Altadonna VM, Snyder HM, Rosenberg HK, et al: Simple cysts of the testis in children: preoperative diagnosis by ultrasound and excision with testicular preservation. *J Urol* 1988; 140:1505.

Anderson S, Meyer TW, Brenner BM: The role of hemodynamic factors in the initiation and progression of renal disease. *J Urol* 1985; 133:363.

Andrassy RJ, Hays DM, Raney RB, et al: Conservative surgical management of vaginal and vulvar pediatric rhabdomyosarcoma: a report from the Intergroup Rhabdomyosarcoma Study III. *J Pediatr Surg* 1995 (in press).

Argueso LR, Ritchey ML, Boyle ET Jr, et al: Prognosis of the solitary kidney after unilateral nephrectomy in childhood. *J Urol* 1992; 148:747.

Askin FB, Land VJ, Sullivan MP, et al: Occult testicular leukemia: testicular biopsy at three years continuous complete remission of childhood leukemia; a Southwest Oncology Group Study. *Cancer* 1981; 47:470.

Azizkhan RG, Haase GM: Current biologic and therapeutic implications in the surgery of neuroblastoma. *Semin Surg Oncol* 1993; 9:493.

Banner MP, Pollack HM, Chatten J, et al: Multilocular renal cysts: radiologic-pathologic correlation. *AJR* 1981; 136:239.

Banowsky LH, Shultz GN: Sarcoma of the spermatic cord and tunics: review of the literature, case report and discussion of the role of retroperitoneal lymph node dissection. *J Urol* 1970; 103:628.

Beckwith JB: Macroglossia, omphalocele, adrenal cytomegaly, gigantism and hyperplastic visceromegaly. *Birth Defects* 1969; 5:188.

Beckwith JB: Wilms tumor and other renal tumors of childhood: a selective review from the National Wilms' Tumor Study Pathology Center. *Hum Pathol* 1983; 14:481.

Beckwith JB: Congenital mesoblastic nephroma. When should we worry? *Arch Pathol Lab Med* 1986; 110:98.

Beckwith JB: A pathologist's perspective on biopsies in pediatric renal tumor management. *Dial Pediatr Urol* 1991; 14:2.

Beckwith JB: Should asymptomatic unilateral multicystic dysplastic kidneys be removed because of the future risk of neoplasia? *Pediatr Nephrol* 1992; 6:511.

Beckwith JB: Precursor lesions of Wilms tumor: clinical and biological implications. *Med Pediatr Oncol* 1993; 21:158.

Beckwith JB, Kiviat NB, Bonadio JF: Nephrogenic rests, nephroblastomatosis, and the pathogenesis of Wilms' tumor. *Pediatr Pathol* 1990; 10:1.

Beckwith JB, Palmer NF: Histopathology and prognosis of Wilms' tumor: results from the National Wilms' Tumor Study. *Cancer* 1978; 41:1937.

Beckwith JB, Perrin EV: In situ neuroblastomas: a contribution to the natural history of neural crest tumors. *Am J Pathol* 1963; 43:1089.

Benjamin SP, McCormack LJ, Effler DB, et al: Primary tumors of the mediastinum. *Chest* 1972; 62:297.

Bennington JL, Beckwith JB: Tumors of the kidney, renal pelvis, and ureter, in *Atlas of Tumor Pathology*, series 2, fasc. 12. Bethesda, Armed Forces Institute of Pathology, 1975.

Blank E, Neerhout RC, Burry KA: Congenital mesoblastic nephroma and polyhydramnios. *JAMA* 1978; 240:1504.

Blute ML, Kelalis PP, Offord KP, et al: Bilateral Wilms' tumor. *J Urol* 1987; 138:968.

Blute ML, Malek RS, Segura JW: Angiomyolipoma: a clinical metamorphosis and concepts for management. *J Urol* 1988; 139:20.

Bokemeyer C, Kuczyk M, Schoffski P, et al: Familial occurrence of Leydig cell tumors: a report of a case in a father and his adult son. *J Urol* 1993; 150:1509.

Bolande RP, Brough AJ, Izant RJ Jr: Congenital mesoblastic nephroma of infancy: a report of eight cases and the relationship to Wilms' tumor. *Pediatrics* 1967; 40:272.

Bonadio JF, Storer B, Norkool P, et al: Anaplastic Wilms' tumor: clinical and pathological studies. *J Clin Oncol* 1985; 3:513.

Bonnin JM, Rubenstein IJ, Palmer NJ, et al: The association of embryonal tumors originating in the kidney and the brain. *Cancer* 1984; 54:2137.

Borden TA: Wilms tumor and pulmonary embolism. *Soc Pediatr Urol Newsletter* 1992; 27.

Bove KE, McAdams AJ: The nephroblastomatosis complex and its relationship to Wilms' tumor: a clinicopathologic treatise. *Perspect Pediatr Pathol* 1976; 3:185.

Boxer LA, Smith DL: Wilms' tumor prior to onset of hemihypertrophy. *Am J Dis Child* 1970; 120:564.

Bracken RB, Johnson DE, Cangir A, et al: Regional lymph nodes in infants with embryonal carcinoma of testis. *Urology* 1978; 11:376.

Bracken RB, Sutow WW, Jaffe N, et al: Preoperative chemotherapy for Wilms' tumor. *Urology* 1982; 19:55.

Braren V, Lukens JN, Stroup SL, et al: Testicular infiltrate in childhood acute lymphocytic leukemia: the need for biopsy in suspected relapse. *Urology* 1980; 16:370.

Breslow NE, Beckwith JB: Epidemiological features of Wilms' tumor: results of the National Wilms' Tumor Study. *J Natl Cancer Inst* 1982; 68:429.

Breslow NE, Beckwith JB, Ciol M, et al: Age distribution of Wilms tumor: report from the National Wilms' Tumor Study. *Cancer Res* 1988a; 48:1653.

Breslow NE, Churchill G, Beckwith JB, et al: Prognosis for Wilms' tumor patients with nonmetastatic disease at diagnosis: results of the Second National Wilms' Tumor Study. *J Clin Oncol* 1985; 3:521.

Breslow N, McCann B: Statistical estimation of prognosis for children with neuroblastoma. *Cancer Res* 1971; 31:2098.

Breslow NE, Norkool PA, Olshan A, et al: Second malignant neoplasm in survivors of Wilms' tumor: a report from the National Wilms' Tumor Study. *J Natl Cancer Inst* 1988b; 80:592.

Breslow N, Olshan A, Beckwith JB, et al: Epidemiology of Wilms' tumor. *Med Pediatr Oncol* 1993; 21:172.

Breslow N, Olshan A, Beckwith JB, et al: Ethnic variation in the incidence, diagnosis, prognosis and follow-up of children with Wilms' tumor. *J Natl Cancer Inst* 1994; 86:49.

Brewer JA, Tank ES: Yolk sac tumors and alpha-fetoprotein in first year of life. *Urology* 1993; 42:79.

Brodeur GM, Fong CT: Molecular biology and genetics of human neuroblastoma. *Cancer Genet Cytogenet* 1989; 41:153.

Brodeur GM, Green AA, Hayes FA: Cytogenetic studies of primary human neuroblastomas. *Prog Cancer Res Ther* 1980; 12:73.

Brodeur GM, Seeger RC, Barrett A, et al: International criteria for diagnosis, staging and response to treatment in patients with neuroblastoma. *J Clin Oncol* 1988; 6:1874.

Brodeur GM, Seeger RC, Schwab M, et al: Amplification of N-myc in untreated human neuroblastomas correlates with advanced disease stage. *Science* 1984; 224:1121.

Brodeur GM, Sekhon GS, Goldstein MN: Specific chromosomal aberration in human neuroblastoma. *Am J Hum Genet* 1975; 27:20A.

Brodeur GM, Sekhon GS, Goldstein MN: Chromosomal aberrations in human neuroblastomas. *Cancer* 1977; 40:2256.

Broecker B: Renal cell carcinoma in children. *Urology* 1991; 38:54.

Brosman SA: Testicular tumors in prepubertal children. *Urology* 1979; 13:581.

Bruce J, Gough DCS: Long-term follow-up of children with testicular tumours: surgical issues. *Br J Urol* 1991; 67:429.

Buntley D: Malignancy associated with horseshoe kidney. *Urology* 1976; 8:146.

Burger D, Moorman-Voestermans CGM, Mildenberger H, et al: The advantages of preoperative therapy in Wilms' tumor: a summarized report on clinical trials conducted by the International Society of Pediatric Oncology (SIOP). *Z Kinderchir* 1985; 40:170.

Call KM, Glaser T, Ito CY, et al: Isolation and characterization of a zinc finger polypeptide gene at the human chromosome 11 Wilms' tumor locus. *Cell* 1990; 60:509.

Campbell HE: The incidence of malignant growth of the undescended testicle: a reply and re-evaluation. *J Urol* 1959; 81:663.

Carachi R, Lindop GBM, Leckie BJ: Inactive renin: a tumor marker in neuroblastoma. *J Pediatr Surg* 1987; 22:278.

Castellanos RD, Aron BS, Evans AT: Renal adenocarcinoma in children: incidence, therapy and prognosis. *J Urol* 1974; 111:534.

Clericuzio CL: Clinical phenotypes and Wilms tumor. *Med Pediatr Oncol* 1993; 21:182.

Cohen MD: Staging of Wilms' tumor. *Clin Radiol* 1993; 47:77.

Cohen MD: Current controversy: is CT scan of the chest needed in patients with Wilms' tumor? *J Pediatr Hematol Oncol* 1994; 16:191.

Cooney DR, Voorhess ML, Fisher HE, et al: Vasoactive intestinal peptide producing neuroblastoma. *J Pediatr Surg* 1982; 17:821.

Coppes MJ: Serum biological markers and paraneoplastic syndromes in Wilms' tumor. *Med Pediatr Oncol* 1993; 21:213.

Coppes MJ, deKraker J, vanKijken PJ, et al: Bilateral Wilms' tumor: long-term survival and some epidemiological features. *J Clin Oncol* 1989; 7:310.

Coppes MJ, Liefers GJ, Higuchi M, et al: Inherited WT1 mutations in Denys-Drash syndrome. *Cancer Res* 1992; 52:6125.

Coppes MJ, Haber DA, Grundy P: Genetic events in the development of Wilms' tumor: current concepts. *N Engl J Med* 1994; 331:586.

Coppes MJ, Huff V, Pelletier J: Denys-Drash syndrome: relating a clinical disorder to genetic alterations in the tumor suppressor gene WT1. *J Pediatr* 1993a; 123:673.

Coppes MJ, Zandvoort SWH, Sparling CR, et al: Acquired von Willebrand disease in Wilms' tumor patients. *J Clin Oncol* 1993b; 10:1.

Corpron C, Andrassy RJ, Raney RB, et al: Conservative management of uterine rhabdomyosarcoma: a report from the Intergroup Rhabdomyosarcoma Studies III and IV Pilot. *J Pediatr Surg* 1995.

Crist WM, Garnsey L, Beltangady MS, et al: Prognostic factors in children with rhabdomyosarcoma: a report of the Intergroup Rhabdomyosarcoma Studies I and II. *J Clin Oncol* 1990; 8:443.

Cunnah D, Perry L, Dacie JA, et al: Bilateral testicular tumours in congenital adrenal hyperplasia: a continuing diagnostic and therapeutic dilemma. *Clin Endocrinol (Oxf)* 1989; 30:141.

Cushing H, Wolbach SB: The transformation of a malignant paravertebral sympathicoblastoma into a benign ganglioneuroma. *Am J Pathol* 1927; 3:203.

D'Angio GJ, Breslow N, Beckwith JB, et al: Treatment of Wilms' tumor: results of the Third National Wilms' Tumor Study. *Cancer* 1989; 64:349.

D'Angio GJ, Evans AE, Breslow N, et al: The treatment of Wilms' tumor: results of the National Wilms' Tumor Study. *Cancer* 1976; 38:633.

D'Angio GJ, Evans, A, Breslow N, et al: The treatment of Wilms' tumor: results of the Second National Wilms' Tumor Study. *Cancer* 1981; 47:2302.

D'Angio GJ, Rosenberg H, Sharples K, et al: Position paper: imaging methods for primary renal tumors of childhood: cost versus benefits. *Med Pediatr Oncol* 1993; 21:205.

de Camargo B, Franco EL: A randomized clinical trial of single-dose versus fractionated-dose dactinomycin in the treatment of Wilms' tumor: results after extended follow-up. *Cancer* 1993; 73:3081.

Dehner LP, Leestma JE, Price EB Jr: Renal cell carcinoma in children: a clinicopathologic study of 15 cases and review of the literature. *J Pediatr* 1970; 76:358.

Dimmick JE, Johnson HW, Coleman GU, et al: Wilms' tumorlet, nodular renal blastema and multicystic renal dysplasia. *J Urol* 1989; 142:484.

Dinndorf P, Johnson L, Gaynon P, et al: Outcome of autologous (auto) vs. allogeneic (allo) bone marrow trans-

plantation in 25 children with neuroblastoma (nb) and unfavorable features (UPF). *J Cell Biochem* 1992; 16A(suppl):201 (abstract).

Dodat J, Chavrier Y, Dyon JF, et al: Tumeurs testiculaires primitives de l'enfant. *Chir Ped* 1986; 27:1.

Donohue JP, Foster RS, Rowland RG, et al: Nerve-sparing retroperitoneal lymphadenectomy with preservation of ejaculation. *J Urol* 1990; 144:287.

Drago JR, Nelson RP, Palmer JM: Childhood embryonal carcinoma of testes. *Urology* 1978; 12:499.

Drash A, Sherman F, Hartmann WH, et al: A syndrome of pseudohermaphroditism, Wilms' tumor, hypertension and degenerative renal disease. *J Pediatr* 1970; 76:585.

Dykes EH, Marwaha RK, Dicks-Mireaux C, et al: Risks and benefits of percutaneous biopsy and primary chemotherapy in advanced Wilms' tumour. *J Pediatr Surg* 1991; 26:610.

Enzinger FM, Weiss SW: *Soft Tissue Tumors*. St Louis, Mosby, 1988, pp 828-831.

Evans AE, D'Angio GJ, Randolph R: A proposed staging for children with neuroblastoma. *Cancer* 1971; 27:374.

Evans AE, Chatten J, D'Angio GJ, et al: A review of 17 IV-S neuroblastoma patients at the Children's Hospital of Philadelphia. *Cancer* 1980; 45:833.

Evans AE, D'Angio GJ, Propert K, et al: Prognostic factors in neuroblastoma. *Cancer* 1987; 59:1853.

Evans AE, Norkool P, Evans I, et al: Late effects of treatment for Wilms' tumor: a report from the National Wilms' Tumor Study Group. *Cancer* 1991; 67:331.

Everson TC, Cole WH: *Spontaneous Regression of Cancer*. Philadelphia, WB Saunders 1966, pp 88-163.

Exelby PR: Testicular cancer in children. *Cancer* 1980; 45(suppl):1803.

Farber S: Chemotherapy in the treatment of leukemia and Wilms' tumor. *JAMA* 1966; 198:826.

Farewell VT, D'Angio GJ, Breslow N, et al: Retrospective validation of a new staging system for Wilms' tumor. *Cancer Clin Trials* 1981; 4:167.

Faria P, Beckwith JB: A new definition of focal anaplasia (FA) in Wilms' tumor identifies cases with good outcome: a report from the National Wilms Tumor Study: *Mod Pathol* 1993; 6:3p (abstract).

Farrelly C, Daneman A, Chan HSL, et al: Occult neuroblastoma presenting with opsomyoclonus: utility of computed tomography. *AJR Am J Roentgenol* 1984; 142:807.

Finklestein JZ, Eckert H, Isaacs H, et al: Bone marrow metastases in children with solid tumors. *Am J Dis Child* 1970; 119:49.

Fong CT, Dracopoli NC, White PS, et al: Loss of heterozygosity for chromosome 1p in human neuroblastomas: correlation with n-myc amplification. *Proc Natl Acad Sci USA* 1989; 86:3753.

Fortner J, Nicastri A, Murphy ML: Neuroblastoma: natural history and results of treating 133 cases. *Ann Surg* 1968; 167:132.

Gabrilove JL, Freiberg EK, Leiter E, et al: Feminizing and nonfeminizing Sertoli cell tumors. *J Urol* 1980; 124:757.

Gay BB Jr, Dawes RK, Atkinson GD Jr, et al: Wilms' tumor in horseshoe kidneys: radiologic diagnosis. *Radiology* 1983; 146:693.

Gearhart JP, Partin AW, Leventhal B, et al: The use of nuclear morphometry to predict response to therapy in Wilms' tumor. *Cancer* 1992; 69:806.

Geatti O, Shapiro B, Sisson J, et al: Iodine-131 metaoidobenzylguanidine scintigraphy for the location of neuroblastoma: preliminary experience in ten cases. *J Nucl Med* 1985; 26:736.

Gerson JM, Koop CE: Neuroblastoma. *Semin Oncol* 1974; 11:35.

Giguere JK, Stablein DM, Spaulding JT, et al: The clinical significance of unconventional orchiectomy approaches in testicular cancer: a report from the testicular cancer intergroup study. *J Urol* 1988; 139:1225.

Gilladoga AC, Manuel C, Tan CT, et al: The cardiotoxicity of adriamycin and daunomycin in children. *Cancer* 1976; 37:1070.

Giwercman A, Bruun E, Frimont-Moller C, et al: Prevalence of carcinoma in situ and other histopathological abnormalities in testes of men with a history of cryptorchidism. *J Urol* 1989; 142:998.

Giwercman A, Muller J, Skakkebaek NE: Cryptorchidism and testicular neoplasia. *Horm Res* 1988; 30:157.

Glass RBJ, Davidson AJ, Fernbach SK: Clear cell sarcoma of the kidney: CT, sonographic and pathologic correlation. *Radiology* 1991; 180:715.

Gleason PE, Kramer SA: Genitourinary polyps in children. *Urology* 1994; 44:106.

Goleta-Dy A, Shaw PJ, Stevens MM: Re: The necessity of contralateral surgical exploration in Wilms' tumor with modern noninvasive imaging technique: a reassessment. *J Urol* 1992; 147:171 (letter).

Gonzalez R, Clayman RV, Sheldon CA: Management of intravascular nephroblastoma to avoid complications. *Urol Clin North Am* 1983; 10:407.

Gormley TS, Skoog SJ, Jones RV, et al: Cellular congenital mesoblastic nephroma: what are the options? *J Urol* 1989; 142:479.

Gourlay WA, Johnson HW, Pantzar JT, et al: Gonadal tumors in disorders of sexual differentiation. *Urology* 1994; 43:537.

Green DM, Beckwith JB, Breslow NB, et al: The treatment of children with stage II-IV anaplastic Wilms' tumor: a report from the National Wilms' Tumor Study. *J Clin Oncol* 1994b; 12:2126.

Green DM, Beckwith JB, Weeks DA, et al: The relationship between microsubstaging variables, tumor weight and age at diagnosis of children with stage I/favorable histology Wilms' tumor: a report from the National Wilms' Tumor Study. *J Clin Oncol* 1994a; 74:1817.

Green DM, Breslow NE, Beckwith JB, et al : Screening of children with hemihypertrophy, aniridia, and Beckwith-Wiedemann syndrome in patients with Wilms' tumor: a report from the National Wilms' Tumor Study. *Med Pediatr Oncol* 1993; 21:188.

Green DM, Breslow NE, Beckwith JB, et al: Treatment outcomes in patients less than two years of age with small, stage I/favorable histology Wilms' tumors: a report from the National Wilms' Tumor Study. *J Clin Oncol* 1993b; 11:91.

Green DM, Breslow NE, D'Angio GJ: The treatment of children with unilateral Wilms' tumor. *J Clin Oncol* 1993c; 11:1009.

Green DM, Breslow NE, Evan I, et al: Effect of dose intensity of chemotherapy on the hematological toxicity of the treatment of Wilms' tumor: a report from the National Wilms' Tumor Study. *Am J Pediatr Hematol Oncol* 1994c; 16:207.

Green DM, Breslow NE, Moksness J, et al: Congestive failure following initial therapy for Wilms' tumor: a report from the National Wilms' Tumor Study. *Pediatr Res* 1994d; 35:161A (abstract).

Green DM, D'Angio GJ, Kelalis P, et al: The risks associated with prenephrectomy chemotherapy for unilateral Wilms' tumor patients. *Dial Ped Urol* 1992; 15:7.

Green DM, Fernbach DJ, Norkool P, et al: The treatment of Wilms' tumor patients with pulmonary metastases detected only with computed tomography. A report from the National Wilms' Tumor Study. *J Clin Oncol* 1991; 9:1776.

Green DM, Fine NE, Li FP: Offspring of patients treated for unilateral Wilms' tumor in childhood. *Cancer* 1982; 49:2285.

Green DM, Jaffe N: The role of chemotherapy in the treatment of Wilms' tumor. *Cancer* 1979; 4:52.

Gross RE, Farber S, Martin LW: Neuroblastoma sympatheticum: a study and report of 217 cases. *Pediatrics* 1959; 23:1179.

Grundy P, Breslow N, Green DM, et al: Prognostic factors for children with recurrent Wilms' tumor: results from the Second and Third National Wilms' Tumor Study. *J Clin Oncol* 1989; 7:638.

Grundy PE, Telzerow PE, Breslow N, et al: Loss of heterozygosity for chromosomes 16q and 1p in Wilms' tumor predicts an adverse outcome. *Cancer Res* 1994; 54:2331.

Grunert RT, Van Every MJ, Uehling DT: Bilateral epidermoid cysts of the testicle, *J Urol* 1992; 147:1599.

Haas D, Ablin AR, Miller C, et al: Complete pathologic maturation and regression of stage IV-S neuroblastoma without treatment. *Cancer* 1990; 62:2572.

Haas GP, Shumaker BP, Cerny JC: The high incidence of benign testicular tumors. *J Urol* 1986; 136:1219.

Haase GM, Hays DM, LaQuaglia MP, et al: Abdominal solid tumors, in Donellan W, Kimura K, Soper RT (eds): *Abdominal Surgery in Infancy and Childhood.* Reading, Harwood Academic, 1995.

Haase GM, O'Leary MC, Ramsay N, et al: Aggressive surgery combined with intensive chemotherapy improves survival in poor risk neuroblastoma. *J Pediatr Surg* 1991; 26:1119.

Haase GM, Wong KY, de Lorimier AA, et al: Improvement in survival after excision of primary tumor in stage III neuroblastoma. *J Pediatr Surg* 1989; 24:194.

Hachitanda Y, Ishimoto K, Shimada H: Stage IVS neuroblastoma: histopathology of 27 cases compared with conventional neuroblastomas. *Lab Invest* 1991; 64:5P.

Hadziselimovic F, Hecker E, Herzog B: The value of testicular biopsy in cryptorchidism. *Urol Res* 1984; 12:171.

Haicken BN, Miller DR: Simultaneous occurrence of congenital aniridia, hamartoma, and Wilms' tumor. *J Pediatr* 1971; 78:497.

Hamilton CR, Pinkerton R, Horwich A: The management of paratesticular rhabdomyosarcoma. *Clin Radiol* 1989; 40:314.

Hann H, Evans A, Siegel S, et al: Biologic differences between neuroblastoma stages IV-S and IV neuroblastoma: measurement of serum ferritin and E-rosette inhibition in 30 children. *N Engl J Med* 1981; 305:425.

Hann HW, Evans AE, Siegel S, et al: Prognostic importance of serum ferritin in patients with stage III and IV neuroblastoma: the CCSG experience. *Cancer Res* 1985; 45:2843.

Harris CC: The carcinogenicity of anticancer drugs: a hazard in man. *Cancer* 1976; 37:1014.

Hartman D, Davis C, Madewell J, et al: Primary malignant tumors in the second decade of life: Wilms' tumor versus renal cell carcinoma. *J Urol* 1982; 127:888.

Hayashi Y, Hanada R, Yamamoto K: Biology of neuroblastomas in Japan found by screening. *Am J Pediatr Hematol Oncol* 1992; 14:342.

Hayes FA, Green AA, Rao BN: Clinical manifestations of ganglioneuroma. *Cancer* 1989; 63:1211.

Hays DM: Bladder/prostate rhabdomyosarcoma: results of the multi-institutional trials of the Intergroup Rhabdomyosarcoma Study: *Semin Surg Oncol* 1993; 9:520.

Hays DM, Lawrence W, Crist W, et al: Partial cystectomy in the management of rhabdomyosarcoma of the bladder: a report from the Intergroup Rhabdomyosarcoma Study (IRS). *J Pediatr Surg* 1990a; 25:719.

Hays DM, Newton W Jr, Soule E, et al: Mortality among children with rhabdomyosarcoma of the alveolar histologic subtypes. *J Pediatr Surg* 1983; 18:412.

Hays DM, Raney RB, Crist W, et al: Secondary surgical procedures to evaluate primary tumor status in patients with chemotherapy responsive stage III-IV sarcomas. *J Pediatr Surg* 1990b; 25:1100.

Hays DM, Raney RB, Lawrence W, et al: Rhabdomyosarcoma of the female urogenital tract. *J Pediatr Surg* 1981; 16:828.

Hays DM, Raney RB, Lawrence W, et al: Primary chemotherapy in the treatment of children with bladder-prostate tumors in the Intergroup Rhabdomyosarcoma Study (IRS-II). *J Pediatr Surg* 1982; 17:812.

Hays DM, Shimada H, Raney RB, et al: Sarcomas of the vagina and uterus: the Intergroup Rhabdomyosarcoma Study. *J Pediatr Surg* 1985; 20:718.

Hays DM, Shimada H, Raney RB Jr, et al: Clinical staging and treatment results in rhabdomyosarcoma of the female genital tract among children and adolescents. *Cancer* 1988; 61:1893.

Heidelberger KP, Ritchey ML, Dauser RC, et al: Congenital mesoblastic nephroma metastatic to the brain. *Cancer* 1993; 72:2499.

Hendren WG, Monfort GJ: Symptomatic bilateral renal angiomyolipomas in a child, *J Urol* 1987; 137:256.

Heppe RK, Koyle MA, Beckwith JB: Nephrogenic rests in Wilms tumor patients with the Drash syndrome. *J Urol* 1991; 145:1225.

Herxheimer G: Ueber tumoren des nebennierenmarkes, insbesondere das neuroblastoma sympaticum. *Beitr Pathol Anat* 1914; 57:112.

Heyn RM, Holland R, Newton WA Jr, et al: The role of combined chemotherapy in the treatment of rhabdomyosarcoma in children. *Cancer* 1974; 34:2128.

Heyn RM, Raney B, Hayes D, et al: Late effects of therapy in patients with paratesticular rhabdomyosarcoma: for the Intergroup Rhabdomyosarcoma Study Committee. *J Clin Oncol* 1992; 10:614.

Hicks BA, Hensle TW, Burbige KA, et al: Bladder management in children with genitourinary sarcomas. *J Pediatr Surg* 1993; 28:1019.

Hidalgo H, Korobkin M, Kinney TR, et al: The problem of benign pulmonary nodules in children receiving cytotoxic chemotherapy. *AJR Am J Roentgenol* 1983; 140:21.

Hittner HM, Riccardi VM, Ferrell RE, et al: Genetic heterogeneity of aniridia: negative linkage data. *Metab Pediatr Syst Ophthalmol* 1980; 4:179.

Hopkins TB, Jaffe N, Colodny A, et al: The management of testicular tumors in children. *J Urol* 1978; 120:96.

Horne T, Granowska M, Dicks-Mireaux C, et al: Neuroblastoma imaged with ^{123}I-metaiodobenzylguanidine and with ^{123}I-labelled monoclonal antibody, UJI3A, against neural tissue. *Br J Radiol* 1985; 58:476.

Howell CJ, Othersen HB, Kiviat NE, et al: Therapy and outcome in 51 children with mesoblastic nephroma: a report of the National Wilms' Tumor Study. *J Pediatr Surg* 1982; 17:826.

Hudson HC, Kramer SA, Tatum AH, et al: Transitional cell carcinoma of renal pelvis: rare occurrence in young male. *Urology* 1981; 18:284.

Huff V: Inheritance and functionality of Wilms' tumor genes. *Cancer Bull* 1994; 46:255.

Huff V, Villalba F, Riccardi VM, et al: Alteration of the WT1 gene in patients with Wilms' tumor and genitourinary anomalies. *Am J Hum Genet* 1991; 49:44 (abstract).

Hutchinson RJ: Decision analysis of the expected clinical value of chest computed tomography in children with favorable histology Wilms' tumor. *Pediatr Res* 1991; 29:4 (abstract).

Hutchinson RJ, Sisson JC, Shapiro B, et al: I^{131}-metaiodobenzylguanidine treatment in patients with refractory advanced neuroblastoma. *Am J Clin Oncol* 1992; 15:226.

Ikeda K, Nakagawara A, Yano H, et al: Improved survival rate in children over one year of age with stage III or IV neuroblastoma following an intensive chemotherapeutic regimen. *J Pediatr Surg* 1989; 24:189.

Ise T, Ohtsuki H, Matsumoto K, et al: Management of malignant testicular tumors in children. *Cancer* 1976; 37:1539.

Ishimoto K, Kiyokawa N, Fujita H, et al: Problems of mass screening for neuroblastoma: analysis of false-negative cases. *J Pediatr Surg* 1990; 25:398.

Ishimoto K, Kiyokawa N, Fujita H, et al: Biological analysis of neuroblastoma in mass screened negative cases, in Evans AE, D'Angio GJ, Knudson AG, et al. (eds): *Advances in neuroblastoma Research*, vol. 3. 1991; pp 602-608.

Jaffe N, Cassady R, Filler RM: Heterochromia and Horner's syndrome associated with cervical and mediastinal neuroblastoma. *J Pediatr* 1975; 87:75.

Javadpour N Mostofi FK: Primary epithelial tumors of the bladder in th first two decades of life. *J Urol* 1969; 101:706.

Jeffs RD: Management of embryonal adenocarcinoma of the testis in childhood: an analysis of 164 cases, in Godden JO (ed): *Cancer in Childhood: The 17th Clinical Conference of the Ontario Cancer Treatment and Research Foundation.* New York, Plenum Press, 1973, p 63.

Jennings RW, LaQuaglia MP, Leong K, et al: Fetal neuroblastoma: prenatal diagnosis and natural history. *J Pediatr Surg* 1993; 28:1168.

Johnson DE, Ayala AG, Medellin H, et al: Multilocular renal cystic disease in children. *J Urol* 1973; 109:101.

Johnston MA, Carachi R, Lindop GBM, et al: Inactive renin levels in recurrent neuroblastoma. *J Pediatr Surg* 1991; 26:613.

Johnstone G: Prepubertal gynecomastia in association with an interstitial cell tumor of the testis. *Br J Urol* 1967; 39:211.

Joshi VV, Beckwith JB: Multilocular cyst of the kidney (cystic nephroma) and cystic, partially differentiated nephroblastoma: terminology and criteria for diagnosis. *Cancer* 1989; 64:466.

Joshi VV, Kasznica J, Walters TR: Atypical mesoblastic nephroma: pathologic characterization of a potentially aggressive variant of conventional congenital mesoblastic nephroma. *Arch Pathol Lab Med* 1986; 110:100.

Kaufman E, Akiya F, Foucar E, et al: Virilization due to Leydig cell tumor diagnosis by magnetic resonance imaging. *Clin Pediatr* 1990; 29:414.

Kay R: Prepubertal testicular tumor registry. *J Urol* 1993; 150:671.

Keller SM, Papzoglou S, McKeever P, et al: Late occurrence of malignancy in a ganglioneuroma 19 years following radiation therapy to a neuroblastoma. *J Surg Oncol* 1984; 25:227.

Kiely EM: The surgical challenge of neuroblastoma. *J Pediatr Surg* 1994; 29:128.

Kinsella TJ, Trivette G, Rowland J, et al: Long-term follow-up of testicular function following radiation for early-stage Hodgkin's disease. *J Clin Oncol* 1989; 7:718.

Kleihues P, Kiessling M, Janzer RC: Morphologic markers in neuro-oncology. *Curr Top Pathol* 1987; 77:307.

Knudson AG Jr, Amromin GD: Neuroblastoma and ganglioneuroma in a child with multiple neurofibromatosis. *Cancer* 1966; 19:1032.

Knudson AG Jr, Strong LC: Mutation and cancer: a model for Wilms' tumor of the kidney. *J Natl Cancer Inst* 1972a; 48:313.

Knudson AG Jr, Strong LC: Mutation and cancer: neuroblastoma and pheochromocytoma. *Man J Hum Genet* 1972b; 24:514.

Kodet R, Newton WA Jr, Hamoudi AB, et al: Childhood rhabdomyosarcoma with anaplastic (pleomorphic) features. *Am J Surg Pathol* 1993; 17:443.

Koo AS, Koyle MA, Hurwitz RS, et al: The necessity of contralateral surgical exploration in Wilms' tumor with modern noninvasive imaging technique: a reassessment. *J Urol* 1990; 144:416.

Koufos A, Grundy P, Morgan K, et al: Familial Wiedemann-Beckwith syndrome and a second Wilms' tumor locus both map to 11p15.5. *Am J Hum Genet* 1989; 44:711.

Koufos A, Hansen MF, Lampkin BC, et al: Loss of alleles at loci on human chromosome 11 during genesis of Wilms' tumor. *Nature* 1984; 309:170.

Kovalic JJ, Thomas PRM, Beckwith JB, et al: Hepatocellular carcinoma as second malignant neoplasms in successfully treated Wilms' tumor patients. *Cancer* 1991; 67:342.

Kramer SA, Wold LE, Gilchrist GS, et al: Yolk sac carcinoma: an immunohistochemical and clinicopathological review: *J Urol* 1984; 131:315.

Krone KD, Carroll BA: Scrotal ultrasound. *Rad Clin North Am* 1985; 23:121.

Kurz KR, Pitts WR, Vaughan ED: The natural history of patients less than 40 years old with bladder tumors. *J Urol* 1987; 137:395.

Kusafuka T, Fukuzawa M, Oue T, et al: DNA flow cytometric analysis of neuroblastoma: distinction of tetraploidy subset. *J Pediatr Surg* 1994; 29:543.

Kushner BH, Gilbert F, Helson L: Familial neuroblastoma: case reports, literature review and etiologic considerations. *Cancer* 1986; 57:1887.

Kushner BH, Helson L: Coordinated sequentially escalated cyclophosphamide and cell cycle specific chemotherapy (N4SE protocol) for advanced neuroblastoma: Experience with 100 patients. *J Clin Oncol* 1987; 5:1746.

LaBrosse EH: Biochemical diagnosis of neuroblastoma: use of a urine spot test. *Proc Am Assoc Cancer Res* 1968; 9:39 (abstract).

Lahdenne P, Kuusela P, Siimes MA, et al: Biphasic reduction and concanavalin A binding properties of serum alpha-fetoprotein in preterm and term infants. *J Pediatr* 1991; 118:272.

Lamm DL, Kaplan GW: Urologic manifestations of Burkitt's lymphoma. *J Urol* 1974; 112:402.

Larsen E, Perez-Atayde A, Greene DM, et al: Surgery only for the treatment of patients with stage I (Cassady) Wilms' tumor. *Cancer* 1990; 66:264.

LaQuaglia M, Ghavimi F, Heller G, et al: Mortality in pediatric paratesticular rhabdomyosarcoma: a multivariate analysis. *J Urol* 1989; 142:473.

Lawrence W, Gehan EA, Hays DM, et al: Prognostic significance of staging factors of the UICC staging system in childhood rhabdomyosarcoma: a report from the Intergroup Rhabdomyosarcoma Study (IRS-II). *J Clin Oncol* 1987b; 5:46.

Lawrence W Jr, Hays DM, Heyn R, et al: Lymphatic metastasis with childhood rhabdomyosarcoma. *Cancer* 1987a; 60:910.

Layfield LJ, Ritchie AWS, Ehrlich R: The relationship of deoxyribonucleic acid content to conventional prognostic factors in Wilms' tumor. *J Urol* 1989; 142:1040.

Lehman EP: Neuroblastoma: with report of a case. *J Med Res* 1917; 36:309.

Lemerle J, Voute PA, Tournade MF, et al: Preoperative versus postoperative radiotherapy, single versus multiple courses of actinomycin D, in the treatment of

Wilms' tumor: preliminary results of a controlled clinical trial conducted by the International Society of Paediatric Oncology (SIOP). *Cancer* 1976; 38:647.

Lemerle J, Voute PA, Tournade MF, et al: Effectiveness of preoperative chemotherapy in Wilms' tumor: results of an International Society of Paediatric Oncology (SIOP) clinical trial. *J Clin Oncol* 1983; 1:604.

Levin NP, Damajanov I, Depillis VJ: Mesoblastic nephroma in an adult patient. Recurrence 21 years after removal of the primary. *Cancer* 1982; 49:573.

Li FP, Fraumeni JF Jr: Soft-tissue sarcomas, breast cancer and other neoplasms: a familial syndrome? *Ann Intern Med* 1969; 71:747.

Li FP, Fraumeni JF Jr: Testicular cancers in children: epidemiologic characteristics. *J Natl Cancer Inst* 1972; 48:1575.

Li FP, Gimbrere K, Gelber RD, et al: Outcome of pregnancy in survivors of Wilms' tumor. *JAMA* 1987; 257:216.

Li FP, Yan JC, Sallan S, et al: Second neoplasms after Wilms' tumor in childhood. *J Natl Cancer Inst* 1983; 71:1205.

Lin RY, Argent PA, Sullivan KM, et al: Urinary hyaluronic acid is a Wilms' tumor marker. American Pediatric Surgical Association 25th Annual Meeting, 1994 (abstract 29).

Look AT, Hayes FA, Nitschke R, et al: Cellular DNA content as a predictor of response to chemotherapy in infants with unresectable neuroblastoma. *N Engl J Med* 1984; 311:231.

Lucas K, Gula MJ, Knisely AS, et al: Catecholamine metabolites in ganglioneuroma. *Med Pediatr Oncol* 1994; 22:240.

Luker GD, Siegel MJ: Pediatric testicular tumors: evaluation with gray-scale and color Doppler US. *Radiology* 1994; 191:561.

Malkin D, Li FP, Strong LC, et al: Germ line p53 mutations in familial syndrome of breast cancer, sarcomas, and other neoplasms. *Science* 1990; 250:1233.

Mann JR, Pearson D, Barrett A, et al: Results of the United Kingdom Children's Cancer Study Groups' malignant germ cell tumor studies. *Cancer* 1989; 63:1657.

Manuel M, Kayatama K, Jones HW Jr: The age of occurrence of gonadal tumors in intersex patients with a Y-chromosome. *Am J Obstet Gynecol* 1976; 124:293.

Marsden HB, Lawler W: Bone metastasizing renal tumour of childhood. Histopathological and clinical review of 38 cases. *Virchows Arch* 1980; 387:341.

Marshall S, Lyon RP, Scott MP: A conservative approach to testicular tumors in children: 12 cases and their management. *J Urol* 1983; 129:350.

Martinez DA, King DR, Ginn-Pease ME, et al: Resection of the primary tumor is appropriate for children with the stage IV-S neuroblastoma: an analysis of 37 patients. *J Pediatr Surg* 1992; 27:1016.

Matthay KK, Sather HM, Seeger RC, et al: Excellent outcome of stage II neuroblastoma is independent of residual disease and radiation therapy. *J Clin Oncol* 1989; 7:236.

Maurer HM, Beltangady M, Gehan EA, et al: The Intergroup Rhabdomyosarcoma Study—I. A final report. *Cancer* 1988; 61:209.

Maurer HM, Moon T, Donaldson M, et al: The Intergroup Rhabdomyosarcoma Study: a preliminary report. *Cancer* 1977; 40:2015.

Maw MA, Grundy PE, Millow LJ, et al: A third Wilms' tumor locus on chromosome 16q. *Cancer Res* 1992; 52:3094.

Maxwell AJ, Mantora H: Sonographic appearance of epidermoid cyst of the testis. *J Clin Ultrasound* 1990; 18:188.

McKeen EA, Bodurtha J, Meadows AT, et al: Rhabdomyosarcomas complicating multiple neurofibromatosis. *J Pediatr* 1978; 93:992.

McLorie GA, Abara OE, Churchill BM, et al: Rhabdomyosarcoma of the prostate in childhood: current challenges. *J Pediatr Surg* 1989; 24:977.

McLorie GA, McKenna PH, Greenburg M, et al: Reduction in tumor burden allowing partial nephrectomy following preoperative chemotherapy in biopsy proved Wilms' tumor. *J Urol* 1991; 146:509.

Mengel W, Knorr D: Leydig cell tumours in childhood. *Prog Pediatr Surg* 1983; 16:133.

Mesrobian H-G, Kelalis PP, Hrabovsky E, et al: Wilms' tumor in horseshoe kidneys. *J Urol* 1985; 133:1002.

Miller RW, Fraumeni JF, Hill JA: Neuroblastoma: epidemiologic approach to its origin. *Am J Dis Child* 1968; 115:253.

Miller RW, Fraumeni JF, Manning MD: Association of Wilms tumor with aniridia, hemihypertrophy and other congenital malformations. *N Engl J Med* 1964; 270:922.

Mohler JL, Partin AW, Epstein JI, et al: Nuclear roundness factor measurement for assessment of prognosis of patients with prostate carcinoma. *J Urol* 1988; 139:1080.

Montgomery BT, Kelalis PP, Blute ML, et al: Extended follow-up of bilateral Wilms' tumor: results of the National Wilms' Tumor Study. *J Urol* 1991; 146:514.

Mostofi FK, Price EB: Tumors of the male genital system, in *Atlas of Tumor Pathology*, ser 2, fasc 8, Washington, DC, Armed Forces Institute of Pathology, 1973.

Muller J, Skakkebaek NE, Ritzen M, et al: Carcinoma in situ of the testis in children with 45,X/46,XY gonadal dysgenesis. *J Pediatr* 1985; 106:431.

Naito H, Sasaki M, Yamashiro K, et al: Improvement in prognosis of neuroblastoma through mass population screening. *J Pediatr Surg* 1990; 25:245.

Nakayama DK, deLorimier AA, O'Neill JA Jr, et al: Intracardiac extension of Wilms' tumor: a report of the National Wilms' Tumor Study. *Ann Surg* 1986; 204:693.

Nakayama DK, Ortega W, D'Angio GJ, et al: The nonopacified kidney with Wilms' tumor. *J Pediatr Surg* 1988; 23:152.

Nelson LB, Spaeth GL, Nowinski TS, et al: Aniridia: a review. *Surv Ophthalmol* 1984; 28:621.

Newton W, Soule EH, Hamoude A, et al: Histopathology of childhood sarcomas, Intergroup Rhabdomyosarcoma Studies I and II: clinicopathologic classification. *J Clin Oncol* 1988; 6:67.

Ng YY, Hall-Craggs MA, Dicks-Mireaux C, et al: Wilms' tumour: pre- and post-chemotherapy CT appearances. *Clin Radiol* 1991; 43:255.

Nickerson HJ, Nesbit ME, Grosfeld JL, et al: Comparison of stage IV and IV-S neuroblastoma in the first year of life. *Med Pediatr Oncol* 1985; 13:261.

Nishi M, Miyake H, Takeda T, et al: Mass screening of neuroblastoma in Sapporo City, Japan, *Am J Pediatr Hematol Oncol* 1992; 14:327.

Nitschke R, Smith EI, Schochat S, et al: Localized neuroblastoma treated by surgery: a Pediatric Oncology Group Study. *J Clin Oncol* 1988; 6:1271.

Noe HN, Marshall JH, Edwards OP: Nodular renal blastema in the multicystic kidney. *J Urol* 1989; 142:486.

Oberholzer HF, Falkson G, DeJager LC: Successful management of inferior vena cava and right atrial neuroblastoma tumor thrombus with preoperative chemotherapy. *Med Pediatr Oncol* 1992; 20:61.

Odelstad L, Pahlma S, Lackgren EL, et al: Neuron specific enolase: a marker for differential diagnosis of neuroblastoma and Wilms' tumor. *J Pediatr Surg* 1982; 17:381.

Ohmichi M, Tasaka K, Sugita N, et al: Hydramnios associated with congenital mesoblastic nephroma: a case report. *Obstet Gynecol* 1989; 74:469.

Olive D, Flamant F, Zucker JM, et al: Paraaortic lymphadenectomy is not necessary in the treatment of localized paratesticular rhabdomyosarcoma. *Cancer* 1984; 54:1283.

Olive-Sommelet D: Paratesticular rhabdomyosarcoma: International Society of Pediatric Oncology Protocol. *Dial Pediatr Urol* 1989; 12:4.

Olsen MM, Caldamone AA, Jackson CL, et al: Gonadoblastoma in infancy: indications for early gonadectomy in 46XY gonadal dysgenesis. *J Pediatr Surg* 1988; 23:270.

O'Neill JA, Littman P, Blitzer P, et al: The role of surgery in localized neuroblastoma. *J Pediatr Surg* 1985; 20:708.

Ortega JA: A therapeutic approach to childhood pelvic rhabdomyosarcoma without pelvic exenteration. *J Pediatr* 1979; 94:205.

Othersen HB Jr, DeLorimer A, Hrabovsky E, et al: Surgical evaluation of lymph node metastases in Wilms' tumor. *J Pediatr Surg* 1990; 25:1.

Page LB, Jacoby GA: Catecholamine metabolism and storage granules in pheochromocytoma and neuroblastoma. *Medicine* 1964; 43:379.

Partin AW, Gearhart JP, Leonard MP, et al: The use of nuclear morphometry to predict prognosis in pediatric urologic malignancies: a review: *Med Pediatr Oncol* 1993; 21:222.

Partin AW, Walsh AC, Epstein JI, et al: Nuclear morphometry as a predictor of response to therapy in Wilms' tumor: a preliminary report. *J Urol* 1990; 144:1222.

Pelletier J, Bruening W, Kashtan CE, et al: Germline mutations in the Wilms' tumor suppressor gene are associated with abnormal urogenital development in Denys-Drash syndrome. *Cell* 1991; 67:437.

Penn I: Renal transplantation for Wilms' tumor: report of 20 cases. *J Urol* 1979; 122:793.

Perlman M, Levin M, Wittels B: Syndrome of fetal gigantism, renal hamartomas, and neuroblastomatosis with Wilms' tumor. *Cancer* 1975; 35:1212.

Pinkel D, Pickren J: Rhabdomyosarcoma in children. *JAMA* 1961; 175:293.

Pizzocara G, Zanoni F, Salvioni R, et al: Difficulties of a surveillance study omitting retroperitoneal lymphadenectomy in clinical stage I nonseminomatous germ cell tumors of the testis. *J Urol* 1987; 138:1393.

Pochedly C, Suwansirikul S, Penzer P: Renal cell carcinoma with extrarenal manifestations in a 10 month child. *Am J Dis Child* 1971; 121:528.

Priestly JT, Schulte TL: The treatment of Wilms' tumor. *Urology* 1942; 47:7.

Pui C-H, Dahl GB, Bowman WP, et al: Elective testicular biopsy during chemotherapy for childhood leukemia is of no clinical value. *Lancet* 1985; 2:410.

Radfar N, Bartter FC, Easley T, et al: Evidence for endogenous LH suppression in a man with bilateral testicular tumors and congenital adrenal hyperplasia. *J Clin Endocrinol Metab* 1977; 45:1194.

Rainwater LM, Hosaka Y, Farrow GM, et al: Wilms tumors: relationship of nuclear deoxyribonucleic acid ploidy to patient survival. *J Urol* 1987; 138:974.

Raney RB Jr, Gehan EA, Hays DM, et al: Primary chemotherapy with or without radiation therapy and or surgery for children with localized sarcoma of the bladder, prostate, vagina, uterus, and cervix. *Cancer* 1990; 66:2072.

Raney RB Jr, Hay DM, Lawrence W Jr, et al: Paratesticular rhabdomyosarcoma in children. *Cancer* 1978; 42:729.

Raney RB Jr, Heyn D, Hays MD, et al: Sequelae of treatment in 109 patients followed for 5 to 15 years after diagnosis of sarcoma of the bladder and prostate. *Cancer* 1993; 71:2387.

Raney RB Jr, Palmer N, Sutow WW, et al: Renal cell carcinoma in children. *Med Pediatr Oncol* 1983; 11:91.

Raney RB Jr, Tefft M, Lawrence W Jr, et al: Paratesticular sarcoma in childhood and adolescence: a report from the Intergroup Rhabdomyosarcoma studies I and II, 1973-1983. *Cancer* 1987; 60:2337.

Reeve AE, Sih SA, Raizis AM, et al: Loss of allelic heterozygosity at a second locus on chromosome 11 in sporadic Wilms' tumor cells. *Mol Cell Biol* 1989; 44:711.

Riccardi VM, Sujansky E, Smith AC, et al: Chromosomal imbalance in the aniridia-Wilms' tumor association: 11p interstitial deletion. *Pediatrics* 1978; 61:604.

Ritchey ML, Green DM, Breslow NE, et al: Accuracy of current imaging modalities in the diagnosis of synchronous bilateral Wilms' tumor. *Cancer* 1995; 75:600.

Ritchey ML, Green DM, Thomas P, et al: Renal failure in Wilms' tumor. Proceedings of SIOP, 25th Annual Meeting. *Med Pediatr Oncol* 1994b (abstract) 23:264.

Ritchey ML, Kelalis PP, Breslow N, et al: Surgical complications following nephrectomy for Wilms' tumor: a report of National Wilms' Tumor Study-3. *Surg Gynecol Obstet* 1992a; 175:507.

Ritchey ML, Kelalis P, Breslow N, et al: Small bowel obstruction following nephrectomy for Wilms' tumor. *Ann Surg* 1993b; 218:654.

Ritchey ML, Kelalis PP, Breslow N, et al: Intracaval and atrial involvement with neuroblastoma: review of National Wilms' Tumor Study-3. *J Urol* 1988; 140:1113.

Ritchey ML, Kelalis PP, Haase GM, et al: Preoperative therapy for intracaval and atrial extension of Wilms' tumor. *Cancer* 1993a; 71:4104.

Ritchey ML, Lally KP, Haase GM, et al: Superior mesenteric artery injury during nephrectomy for Wilms' tumor. *J Pediatr Surg* 1992b; 27:612.

Ritchey ML, Novicki DE, Schultenover SJ: Nephrogenic adenoma of bladder: a report of 8 cases. *J Urol* 1984; 131:537.

Ritchey ML, Othersen HB Jr, deLorimier AA, et al: Renal vein involvement with neuroblastoma: a report of National Wilms' Tumor Study-3. *Eur Urol* 1990; 17:139.

Ritchey ML, Pringle K, Breslow N, et al: Management and outcome of inoperable Wilms' tumor: a report of National Wilms' Tumor Study. *Ann Surg* 1994c; 220:683.

Robitaille P, Mongeau JG, Lortie L, et al: Long-term follow-up of patients who underwent nephrectomy in childhood. *Lancet* 1985; 1:1297.

Rodary C, Flamant F, Maurer H, et al: Initial lymphadenectomy is not necessary in localized and completely resected paratesticular rhabdomyosarcoma. *Med Pediatr Oncol* 1992; 20:430 (abstract).

Rodary C, Rey A, Olive D, et al: Prognostic factors in 281 children with non-metastatic rhabdomyosarcoma (RMS) at diagnosis. *Med Pediatr Oncol* 1988; 16:71.

Romansky SG, Crocker W, Shaw KNF: Ultrastructural studies on neuroblastoma: evaluation of cytodifferentiation. *Cancer* 1978; 42:2392.

Rosvoll RV, Woodward JR: Malignant Sertoli cell tumor of the testis. *Cancer* 1968; 22:8.

Roubidoux MA, Dunnick NR, Sostman HD, et al: Renal carcinoma: detection of venous extension with gradient-echo MR imaging. *Radiology* 1992; 182:269.

Rushton G, Belman AG, Sesterhenn et al: Testicular sparing surgery for prepubertal teratoma of the testis: a clinical and pathological study. *J Urol* 1990; 144:726.

Sawada T, Kidowaki T, Sakamoto I, et al: Neuroblastoma: mass screening for early detection and its prognosis. *Cancer* 1984; 53:2731.

Sawada T: Past and future of neuroblastoma screening in Japan. *Am J Pediatr Hematol Oncol* 1992; 14:320.

Schellas HF: Malignant potential of the dysgenetic gonad, I and II. *Obstet Gynecol* 1974; 44:298.

Seeger RC, Brodeur GM, Sather H, et al: Association of multiple copies of the N-myc oncogene with rapid progression of neuroblastoma. *N Engl J Med* 1985; 313:1111.

Seege RC, Villablanca JG, Matthay KK, et al: Intensive chemoradiotherapy and autologous bone marrow transplantation for poor prognosis neuroblastoma. *Prog Clin Biol Res* 1991; 366:527.

Senelick RC, Bray PF, Lahey ME, et al: Neuroblastomas and myoclonic encephalopathy: two cases and a review of the literature. *J Pediatr Surg* 1973; 8:623.

Shapiro DM, Parham DM, Douglas EC, et al: Relationship of tumor-cell ploidy to histologic subtype and treatment outcome in children and adolescents with unresectable rhabdomyosarcoma. *J Clin Oncol* 1991; 9:159.

Shaul DB, Srikanth M, Ortega JA, et al: Treatment of bilateral Wilms' tumor: comparison of initial biopsy and chemotherapy to initial surgical resection in the preservation of renal mass and function. *J Pediatr Surg* 1992; 27:1009.

Shimada H, Chatten J, Newton WA Jr, et al: Histopathologic prognostic factors in neuroblastic tumors: definition of subtypes of ganglioneuroblastoma and an age-linked classification of neuroblastomaa. *J Natl Cancer Inst* 1984; 73:405.

Shochat SJ: Update on solid tumor management in childhood. *Surg Clin Amer* 1992; 72:1417.

Shown TE, Durfee MF: Blueberry muffin baby: Neonatal neuroblastoma with subcutaneous metastases. *J Urol* 1970; 140:193.

Shurin SB, Gauderer MWL, Dahms BB, et al: Fatal intraoperative pulmonary embolization of Wilms tumor. *J Pediatr* 1982; 101:559.

Skakkebaek NE: Atypical germ cells in the adjacent "normal" tissue of testicular tumors. *Acta Pathol Microbiol Scand* 1975; 83:127.

Snyder HM III, Lack EE, Chetty-Baktovizian A, et al: Congenital mesoblastic nephroma: relationship to other renal tumors of infancy. *J Urol* 1981; 126:513.

Sotelo-Avila C, Gonzalez-Crussi F, Fowler JW: Complete and incomplete forms of Beckwith-Wiedemann syndrome: their oncogenic potential. *J Pediatr* 1980; 96:47.

Srikath MS, West BR, Ishitani M, et al: Benign testicular tumors in children with congenital adrenal hyperplasia. *J Pediatr Surg* 1992; 27:639.

Staubitz WJ, Jewett TC Jr, Magoss IV, et al: Management of testicular tumors in children. *J Urol* 1965; 94:683.

Steinherz LJ, Steinherz PG, Tan CTC, et al: Cardiac toxicity 4 to 20 years after anthracycline therapy. *JAMA* 1991; 266:1672.

Stephenson SR, Cook BA, Mease AD, et al: The prognostic significance of age and pattern of metastases in stage IV-S neuroblastoma. *Cancer* 1986; 58:372.

Stern M, Longaker MT, Adzick NS, et al: Hyaluronidase levels in urine from Wilms' tumor patients. *J Natl Cancer Inst* 1991; 83:1569.

Stillman RJ, Schinfeld JS, Schiff I, et al: Ovarian failure in long term survivors of childhood malignancy. *Am J Obstet Gynecol* 1987; 139:62.

Stobbe GC, Dargeon H: Embryonal rhabdomyosarcoma of the head and neck in children and adolescents. *Cancer* 1950; 3:826.

Suita S, Zaizen Y, Yano H, et al: How to deal with advanced cases of neuroblastoma detected by mass screening: a report from the Pediatric Oncology Study Group of the Kyushu area of Japan. *J Pediatr Surg* 1994; 29:599.

Sutow WW, Sullivan MP, Ried HL, et al: Prognosis in childhood rhabdomyosarcoma. *Cancer* 1970; 25:1385.

Tank ES, Kay R: Neoplasms associated with hemihypertrophy, Beckwith-Weidemann syndrome and aniridia. *J Urol* 1980; 124:266.

Tank ES, Melvin T: The association of Wilms' tumor with nephrologic disease. *J Pediatr Surg* 1990; 25:724.

Thomas PRM, Shochat SJ, Norkool P, et al: Prognostic

implications of hepatic adhesion, invasion, and metastases at diagnosis of Wilms' tumor. *Cancer* 1991; 68:2486.

Tomlinson GE, Argyle JC, Velasco S, et al: Molecular characterization of congenital mesoblastic nephroma and its distinction from Wilms tumor. *Cancer* 1992; 70:2358.

Tournade MF, Com-Nougue C, Voute PA, et al: Results of the sixth International Society of Pediatric Oncology Wilms' tumor trial and study: a risk-adapted therapeutic approach in Wilms' tumor. *J Clin Oncol* 1993; 11:1014.

Tsuchida Y, Yokomori K, Nishiura M, et al: Total renin as a marker for paediatric tumours. *Med Pediatr Oncol* 1993; 21:603 (abstract).

Turkel SB, Itabashi HH: The natural history of neuroblastic cells in the fetal adrenal gland. *Am J Pathol* 1974; 76:225.

Uehling DT, Phillips E: Residual retroperitoneal mass following chemotherapy for infantile yolk sac tumor. *J Urol* 1994; 152:185.

Urban MD, Lee PA, Plotnick LP, et al: The diagnosis of Leydig cell tumors in childhood. *Am J Dis Child* 1978; 132:494.

Virchow R: *Die Krankenhaften Geschwulste*. Berlin, Hirschwald 11:149, 1864.

Voute PA, Van Der Meer J, Staugaard-Kloosterziel W: Plasma renin activity in Wilms' tumour. *Acta Endocrinol (Copenh)* 1971; 67:197.

Voute PA, Vos A, deKraker J, et al: Rhabdomyosarcoma: chemotherapy and limited supplementary treatment to avoid mutilation. *Monogr Natl Cancer Inst* 1981; 56:121.

Wahl RL, Harney J, Hutchins G, et al: Imaging of renal cancer using positron emission tomography with 2-deoxy-2-fluoro-d-glucose: pilot animal and human studies. *J Urol* 1991; 146:1470.

Weeks DA, Beckwith JB: Relapse-associated variables in stage I, favorable histology Wilms' tumor. *Cancer* 1987; 60:1204.

Weese DL, Applebaum H, Taber P: Mapping intravascular extension of Wilms' tumor with magnetic resonance imaging. *J Pediatr Surg* 1991; 26:64.

Weiner ES, Lawrence S, Hays D, et al: Retroperitoneal node biopsy in childhood paratesticular rhabdomyosarcoma. *J Pediatr Surg* 1994; 29:171.

White KS, Grossman H: Wilms' and associated renal tumors of childhood. *Pediatr Radiol* 1991; 21:81.

Wilimas J, Douglass EC, Magill HL, et al: Significance of pulmonary computed tomography at diagnosis in Wilms' tumor. *J Clin Oncol* 1988; 6:1144.

Williams CM, Greer M: Homovanillic acid and vanillylmandelic acid in diagnosis of neuroblastoma. *JAMA* 1963; 183:836.

Wilson BE, Netzloff ML: Primary testicular abnormalities causing precocious puberty Leydig cell tumor, Leydig cell hyperplasia, and adrenal rest tumor. *Ann Clin Lab Sci* 1983; 13:315.

Wold LE, Kramer SA, Farrow GM: Testicular yolk sac and embryonal carcinomas in pediatric patients: comparative immunohistochemical and clincopathologic study. *Am J Clin Pathol* 1984; 81:427.

Wright JH: Neurocytoma or neuroblastoma, a kind of tumor not generally recognized. *J Exp Med* 1910; 12:556.

Wu JT, Book L, Sudar K: Serum alpha-fetoprotein (AFP) levels in normal infants. *Pediatr Res* 1981; 15:50.

Young JL, Miller RW: Incidence of malignant tumors in U.S. children. *J Pediatr* 1975; 86:254.

Young JL, Ries LG, Silverberg E: Cancer incidence, survival, and mortality for children younger than age 15 years. *Cancer* 1986; 58:598.

Zakowski MF, Edwards RH, McDonough ET: Wilms' tumor presenting as sudden death due to tumor embolism. *Arch Pathol Lab Med* 1990; 144:605.

Zantiga AR, Coppes MJ: Max Wilms (1867-1918): the man behind the eponym. *Med Pediatr Oncol* 1992; 20:515.

Zeltzer P, Parma A, Dalton A, et al: Raised neuron-specific enolase in serum of children with metastatic neuroblastoma. *Lancet* 1983; 2:361.

Zuppan CW, Beckwith JB, Weeks DA, et al: The effect of preoperative therapy on the histologic features of Wilms' tumor: an analysis of cases from the Third National Wilms' Tumor Study. *Cancer* 1991; 68:385.

CHAPTER 59

Outpatient Pediatric Urology

Anthony A. Caldamone
Seth Schulman
Ronald Rabinowitz

HISTORICAL FACTORS

Pediatric urology is a natural evolutionary end point of the progressive specialization of medical care. Although Hippocrates did not distinguish between medical and surgical treatment, there were specialists in Egypt in antiquity and in Greece by the first century. The divisions between medicine and surgery became more clearly delineated in the Middle Ages. In the United States, the full-time limited practice of surgery began in the late nineteenth century (Wangensteen and Wangensteen, 1978). It also was becoming apparent that the surgical care of children was different from that of the adult. In the second decade of the twentieth century, the surgeons at the Boston Children's Hospital progressively limited their practice to the surgery of children (Ladd and Gross, 1941).

Urology also had its origins in antiquity with stone disease and abnormalities of the urine. In 1877, Max Nitze constructed the first incandescent cystoscope, an event that was to make urology a specialty apart from general surgery (Murphy, 1972), the American Urological Association was founded in 1902. The presidential address to the annual meeting in 1911 was entitled "Is Urology Entitled To Be Regarded As a Specialty?" (Cabot, 1911). Just as Ladd limited his surgical practice to children, Meredith Campbell was the first to limit his urologic practice to infants and children and is thus regarded as the father of pediatric urology. He published the first text of pediatric urology in 1937 (Campbell, 1937) and later reported his experience of 33 years in the private practice of pediatric urology in New York City in his monumental book *Clinical Pediatric Urology* (Campbell, 1951). Pediatric general surgeons also included urologic diseases as part of their specialty. At the 1974 annual meeting of the American Surgical Association, Dr. J. Hartwell Harrison asked, "Is it time for children's hospitals to have divisions of urology?" Dr. W. Hardy Hendren responded that pediatric urology constituted approximately one third of pediatric surgery and that there was "great need for a number of men throughout the country to take special interest in this field. . . . I believe we must gear our residency programs to train those surgeons who are interested in this field, whether they come from parent programs in urology or from pediatric surgery" (Ravitch, 1981).

The Society for Pediatric Urology was founded in 1951, the first president being Dr. Meredith Campbell. In 1960, the Urologic Section of the American Academy of Pediatrics was founded with 16 members. This small group of urologists whose practice was limited to pediatric urology was initially chaired by Dr. John K. Latimer (Bicknell, 1980) and has now grown to more than 100 members. With progressive specialization culminating in the specialty of pediatric urology, along with improvements in surgical techniques and anesthesia, much of the modern practice of pediatric urology now takes place in the office and the ambulatory surgery center.

THE PEDIATRIC UROLOGIC OFFICE

The pediatric urologic office is primarily a place for the practitioner to see and examine children. It incorporates aspects of a pediatric office, a pediatric surgical office, and an urologic office. Since the object of concern is the child, an effort must be made to have the child feel relaxed and comfortable in the office and examination room surroundings. Even young children participate in history taking, and many questions can be directed to them. The pediatric urologist gains the child's trust by making him or her a participant. The office and examination rooms, along with the waiting areas, should be bright and cheery, even with cartoon wallpaper. Toys, puzzles, and children's books all serve to put the child at ease. The ambient temperature in the examination rooms should be warm so that the undressed child will feel comfortable and the thermolabile neonate will not become cold. A warm examination room also greatly assists in the examination of boys for testicular descent, for instance.

Relatively little equipment is required for the pediatric urologic office. Small metal sounds, catheters, feeding tubes (3.5, 5, and 8 F), and ⅛-oz ophthalmic ointment tubes of Lacri-Lube S.O.P., Cortisporin, Neosporin, or Polysporin are necessary. Also needed are suture trays, suture removal kits, fine hemostats, mosquito clamps, fine scissors, fine absorbable sutures and ties, cotton swabs, lubricant, urine and wound culture containers, needles and syringes, and local anesthetic.

PATIENT POPULATION

History

The pediatric urologic office is commonly the sight of the initial history. Aspects of the history were well described years ago by Campbell (1951). He emphasized the importance of including the child in the history-taking process, because it tended to calm the child and also gave the practitioner the opportunity to observe the child. Indeed, Campbell (1951) stated that older children "can usually give a satisfactory history and I have found it more reliable than that given by the parents. . . . " The child may give the chief complaint and history in his or her own words, which may be extremely valuable. Obviously, the family also is required; they will add to the present history and give additional information regarding the past history and family history. In 1951, Campbell stated that "heredity is rarely a factor in urologic disease in the young. . . " and "despite the occasional occurrence of urologic disease in several siblings. . . hereditary influence in general may be disregarded." As pediatric urology has progressed, the family history and hereditary aspects have become more important in renal disease, cryptorchidism, reflux, and hypospadias.

The office population and conditions referred to the urologist have not changed significantly over the past decades. They continue to include urinary abnormalities, including infections, abdominal masses, voiding dysfunctions, genital abnormalities, and structural anomalies of the urinary tract. In 1962, Tudor and associates published a 10-year review of the children seen in their general urologic practice. Two thirds of these 2403 children were girls, and almost 60% were referred because of urinary infection. Almost 1200 intravenous (IV) pyelograms were obtained, 7.5% being abnormal. Ten percent of the almost 300 girls who had cystograms had vesicoureteral reflux. Seventy-one renal anomalies were seen, including 37 ureteropelvic junction obstructions. Genital abnormalities predominated in the boys. One hundred sixty-six were re-

ferred for meatal stenosis, 31 had urethral strictures, 69 had hypospadias, and 80 had an undescended testis, hernia, or hydrocele.

More recently, Kroovand and Perlmutter reviewed their combined practice in 1981 (Kroovand, 1982), and Rabinowitz reviewed his own practice in 1982 (Rabinowitz and Caldamone, 1985). In one year, Rabinowitz saw 1574 children (56% boys), and Kroovand and Perlmutter saw 2395 children (64% boys). Kroovand's group saw 682 new children, of whom 297 had voiding dysfunction, urinary tract infection, or both. Similarly, 256 of the 533 new patients in Rabinowitz's practice had these signs or symptoms. Of the 183 new patients with urinary infections, 44% had reflux in Kroovand's group, and 41% of 179 new patients with urinary infections has reflux in Rabinowitz's practice. Of the new patients seen, Kroovand and Perlmutter saw 102 boys with hypospadias, 109 with undescended testis, hernia, or hydrocele, and 34 with meatal stenosis during 1 year. Rabinowitz saw 71 with hypospadias, 82 with cryptorchidism, hernia, or hydrocele, and 32 with meatal stenosis in 1982. Over 1 year, Rabinowitz operated on 21% of the total number of children seen that year (72% were boys). Similarly, Kroovand and Perlmutter operated on 29% of the total number of children seen during 1971, and 79% of these were boys. The patterns of referral also were reviewed in both practices. Pediatricians or family practitioners accounted for 77% of the new referrals to Kroovand and Perlmutter and 86% of the new referrals to Rabinowitz. Other urologists accounted for 8% of Kroovand-Perlmutter's new patients compared with 5% of Rabinowitz's. Pediatric surgeons referred 5% of Rabinowitz's new patients and 3% of those seen by Kroovand and Perlmutter. Patient's families accounted for 12% of the new patients in the Kroovand-Perlmutter practice and 4% in Rabinowitz's practice. When follow-up studies were assessed, Kroovand and Perlmutter obtained 562 follow-up IV urograms, 350 voiding cystourethrograms, 3 renal scans, and 131 ultrasounds. In 1982, follow-up studies in Rabinowitz's practice included 267 excretory urograms, 387 voiding cystourethrograms, 86 renal scans, 55 nuclear cystograms, and 84 ultrasounds. Since that time, there have been progressively decreasing numbers of IV urograms and increasing numbers of renal scans (Bueschen and Witten, 1979; Majd and Belman, 1979) and ultrasound examinations (Kangarloo et al., 1985; Mason, 1984).

Physical Examination

The physical examination in the urologic office begins with observations while taking the history. The physical characteristics, alertness, dexterity, and any signs of nonurologic abnormality are noted. Children like to climb, and most older than infants prefer to climb onto the examination table themselves. This allows the examiner to assess many physical characteristics and gross motor ability. Facial, chest, abdominal, and spinal abnormalities may be observed. In the warm examining room, the male genitalia and testes may relax, and the retractile testis may be visualized in the scrotum even before palpation confirms the absence of true cryptorchidism. Infants are commonly examined while they are feeding or sucking on a pacifier, often in the lap of a parent. Examination of the abdomen and scrotal contents should be complete, yet very gentle. Gentle compression of the base of the penis commonly elicits an erection in boys being examined for hypospadias and chordee. The adolescent male should be examined in the erect and supine position for varicocele. The importance of the rectal examination to the pediatric urologic physical examination was emphasized many years ago by Campbell (1951).

CONDITIONS REFERRED

Urinary Tract Infections

Urinary tract infection is extremely common in children and the most common mode of representation of an internal structural urologic anomaly. It represents the second most common infection in children after respiratory tract infections. The documentation of urinary tract infection makes evaluation mandatory.

The child may be seen in the pediatric urologic office with the signs and symptoms of urinary infection or after the infection has been treated. Since approximately two thirds of boys and one third of girls who have a documented urinary infection will have an underlying structural urologic anomaly, and since more than three fourths of girls with infection will have a recurrence, all children should be evaluated after the first documented infection (Burbige et al., 1984; Fair et al., 1974; Kunin, 1970; Parkkulainen and Kosunen, 1977; Savage et al., 1969; Smellie et al., 1975). However, one must first document the infection. Valid urine specimens are often obtained with voided urine or urine collection bag. Sterile catheterization using an infant feeding tube and suprapubic bladder aspiration are simple office techniques for obtaining urine under sterile conditions for culture documentation. If the child presents to the urologist with an infection, treatment decisions must be made. If there are minimal or absent symptoms, one can await culture documentation and sensitivity results before prescribing an oral antibiotic. If there are significant lower tract symptoms, treatment with oral antibiotics is initiated before the final culture report is available. If the child is systemically ill, hospitalization may be required for parenteral fluid and antibiotic therapy. In these instances, once the systemic symptoms have resolved, if parenteral antibiotics are still necessary, they can be administerd on an outpatient basis, similar to home parenteral nutrition and dialysis, with the assistance of health care officials. This can avoid prolonged hospitalization once the child in clinically well but still in need of completion of eradication of infection (Poretz et al., 1982).

It is mandatory that children with documented urinary infection undergo evaluation in view of the high incidence of structural urologic anomalies, the very high recurrence rate, and the belief that many of these children have had previous unrecognized or undocumented urinary infections (Kunin, 1970; Savage et al, 1969; Smellie et al., 1975).

If the child responds promptly to treatment, evaluation can be performed in 4 to 6 weeks, allowing for resolution of infection-induced edema and inflammation that might distort the radiographic interpretation (Grana et al., 1965; Pais and Retik, 1975; vanGool and Tanagho, 1977). If the child was initially ill and febrile, in view of the high incidence of vesicoureteral reflux and the high incidence of recurrence, these children are maintained on antibiotic prophylaxis in the interim between treatment of the infection and investigation (Belman, 1980). In some children with severe infection, clinical response is delayed. In these instances, one must rule out urinary tract obstruction. This is most easily accomplished with a voiding cystourethrogram under antibiotic coverage in boys to rule out urethral valves and a renal ultrasound in boys and girls to rule out significant upper tract obstruction.

The standard evaluation of the child with urinary tract infection has been the voiding cystourethrogram and excretory urogram. With progressive refining and greater experience with renal ultrasonography, the radiographic evaluation of these children can be tailored to obtain the maximum information with a minimal amount of irradiation. Because the most common structural anomaly found in these children is vesicoureteral reflux, the initial study must be a voiding cystourethrogram. This is an extremely well-tolerated procedure when performed by experienced personnel sensitive to children's needs. The use of general anesthesia to perform an expression cystogram is not warranted because this study is less sensitive than the awake study and does involve the risk of anesthesia (Vlahakis et al., 1971). If the voiding cystourethrogram is normal, and if the child's symptoms are limited to the lower urinary tract, the kidneys can be evaluated with ultrasonography (Kangarloo et al., 1985; Leonides et al, 1985; Mason, 1984). It is most important to emphasize that to substitute renal sonography in place of excretory urography, one must have interested, experienced, and expert pediatric ultrasonographers. Unlike excretory urography, one must often be present while ultrasonography is being performed to have a total picture. If the voiding cystourethrogram is abnormal, if the renal ultrasound is abnormal, or if there are signs or symptoms of upper tract involvement with the infection, a nuclear renal parencymal scan (DMSA or ghicoeptovate) or an excretory urogram is necessary. Cystoscopy is not indicated in the evaluation of the child with urinary tract infections. In addition, it plays only a selected role in the evaluation of those children with urinary tract infections found to have vesicoureteral reflux and is thus not routinely indicated (Johnson et al., 1980; Walther and Kaplan, 1979).

Hematuria

Hematuria in childhood most commonly originates in the kidney, and the etiology is most commonly nephrologic (Chan, 1978). However, the presence of hematuria is an indication for an excretory urogram with a voiding film of the urethra to obviate a formal voiding cystourethrogram. The structurally abnormal kidney is at significantly increased risk for bleeding secondary to trauma, even minor trauma (Malek, 1980; Mertz et al., 1963). Much less commonly, renal or bladder tumor can present with hematuria and should be readily discovered with excretory urography.

Perineal, pelvic, or genital trauma resulting in hematuria, or bloody drainage per urethra is indication for lower tract uroradiographic investigation in the form of a retrograde or voiding cystourethrogram. The presence of bloody urethral discharge may be secondary to straddle injury and needs similar radiographic investigation. Again, an excretory urogram with a voiding view of the urethra suffices. Blood spotting, or urethrorrhagia, is rarely associated with significant urinary tract pathology and is most often self-limited. The temptation for endoscopy should be curtailed except for associated other symptoms (Kaplan and Brock, 1982). Hematuria in association with red blood cell casts, or an inappropriate degree of proteinuria warrants further nephrologic workup, including C3 and ASO titers.

In the absence of an abnormality on excretory urogram or evidence of glomerulonephritis, hypercalciuria should be ruled out. This can easily be done with a spot urinary calcium to creatinine ratio or a 24-hour urine collection for calcium (Kalia et al., 1981; Stapleton et al., 1984). If no uroradiographic abnormality is identified, the need for cystocopy in children with hematuria rarely is indicated (Johnson et al., 1980; Kaplan and Brock, 1982; Walther and Kaplan, 1979).

Urethrorrhagia

Urethrorrhagia occurs in males and consists of terminal hematuria or blood staining on the underwear, which may be without discomfort or associated with mild dysuria. This condition generally causes great anxiety for parents and pediatricians. In the past, this condition was evaluated with a workup that included an excretory urogram and cystoscopy. However, studies have indicated that the yield of positive findings is extremely low. In a study by Kaplan and Brock (1982), radiographic evaluation with excretory urogram and voiding cystourethrogram was normal in all 21 boys studied. In addition, cystoscopy in 15 of those patients revealed nonspecific findings, most consistently hyperemia of the prostrate urethra. The symptoms usually are intermittent and may be prolonged lasting up to a year or longer in some boys. In the study by Kaplan and Brock, the mean duration of symptoms was 17 months.

The diagnosis of urethrorrhagia is made by history and confirmed by a normal physical examination. The urinalysis will often show microscopic hematuria without proteinuria or casts and a negative urine culture. It may be helpful to perform a fractionated urinalysis to determine the site of the red blood cells. Evaluation should start with an ultrasound of the kidneys and bladder to exclude a structural abnormality. Some clinicians prefer an excretory urogram with a voiding urethrogram when the bladder fills with contrast from the kidneys. Cystoscopy is rarely indicated unless there is total hematuria, or the history is not pure for urethrorrhagia. Although there is no evidence to support cystoscopic evaluation, many clinicians may perform a VCUG or cystoscopy if the symptoms persists beyond 6 months (Zderic and Duckett, 1994).

Abdominal Mass

The urinary tract is the most common origin of an abdominal mass in infants. Most neonatal masses are discovered before newborn discharge from the hospital. After the neonatal period, the two most common renal masses are the obstructed kidney and tumor. Initial evaluation of the child with an abdominal mass includes percussion, gentle palpation, and fiberoptic transillumination. The history must include questions regarding trauma, voiding dysfunction, and recurrent abdominal pain. Ultrasonography is the initial study of choice in the child with an abdominal mass (Shkolnik, 1980). This study usually will localize the mass to an organ of origin and also distinguish between solid (neoplastic) and cystic lesions. Further workup is dictated by this study. The solid renal lesion may be evaluated by excretory urography, computed tomography, or magnetic resonance imaging (Ehrlich and Kangarloo, 1985; Kuhn and Berger, 1981). The cystic renal mass would be evaluated for structure with an IV urogram and voiding cystourethrogram and for function and obstruction with differential and diuretic renal scan (Powers et al., 1981; Thrall et al., 1981).

If the abdominal mass is associated with bladder or

prostrate, further staging and management would be dictated by the radiographic findings.

Wetting

The child who wets is often referred for urologic investigation, but not all children who wet should undergo such investigation. Indeed, many children who wet have only nocturnal enuresis. If these children have no daytime urinary symptoms and an otherwise normal history and physical examination, urologic investigation is not indicated (Perlmutter, 1979). These children and their families should be reassured of the benign and self-limited nature of nocturnal enuresis. If the family seeks reassurance that no structural abnormality is present, ultrasonography of the urinary tract can be carried out, including prevoid and postvoid views of the urinary bladder. If the child or family, having been reassured, is highly motivated to intervene and treat, this can be carried out using conditioning with an enuresis alarm or use of pharmacologic agents.

Functional incontinence attributable to bladder/sphincter dysfunction is an entity assigned to children with urinary incontinence when organic causes (i.e., anatomic and neurogenic) have been excluded. Unfortunately, there is confusion secondary to the misuse of medical terminology and an inability to strictly define the subsets of functional incontinence: urge syndrome and dysfunctional voiding. For the purposes of this chapter we define *enuresis* as normal voiding at an inappropriate time when urinary control is expected. Enuresis differs from *incontinence*, which is a failure of voluntary control of bladder and/or urethral muscle activity, with constant or frequent involuntary passage of urine. Hence, enuretic children usually empty their bladders and incontinent ones simply leak.

The complex of dysfunctional voiding and recurrent urinary tract infections (UTI) is an established clinical entity seen in school age children, especially in girls. Among 7-year-old Swedish school children the prevalence of this condition is 8.4% in girls and 1.7% in boys. In this study the mutual association between dysfunctional voiding and UTIs, already known from retrospective clinical studies, was documented epidemiologically. Textbooks and editorials treat the two parts of the complex separately leading to separate treatment of the individual UTI and the primary symptom of dysfunctional voiding, wetting. Equally confusing is the improper treatment of children with nocturnal enuresis with behavior modification and pharmacotherapy when, in fact, some of these children have symptoms suggestive or urge incontinence or dysfunctional voiding. There is evidence that dysfunctional voiding is associated with vesicoureteral reflux; hence there is the potential for reflux nephrop-

athy and a social stigma. School-age children consider wetting in school the third worst stress following the death of a parent and going blind.

Physiology and Maturation of Normal Voiding

Bladder storage and emptying involve several complex processes and depend on an intact nervous system, including the cerebral cortex, midbrain, spinal cord, and peripheral nerves. The somatic and autonomic nervous systems (sympathetic and parasympathetic) are both responsible for effective lower urinary tract function. The somatic component innervates the external sphincter. The parasympathetic branch of the autonomic nervous system is primarily responsible for bladder emptying. The preganglionic nerves arise from the sacral area of the spinal cord (S2, S3, S4) and synapse close to the bladder. The major neurotransmitter is acetylcholine and its receptors are located throughout the bladder fundus and at the posterior urethra. Stimulation causes a detrusor contraction. The sympathetic branch of the autonomic nervous system arises from the thoracolumbar area of the spinal cord (T10, T11, T12, L1) with ganglia near the cord; they function to facilitate the storage/filling phase of micturition. Norepinephrine is the primary neurotransmitter. Alpha receptors, primarily located in the bladder neck and posterior urethra, respond to stimulation by contracting, thereby increasing resistance. Beta receptors, primarily located at the bladder fundus, respond to stimulation by relaxing the detrusor muscle.

The micturition reflex pathways involve afferent nerves carrying impulses secondary to bladder distension reaching the sacral spinal cord. Spinal tract neurons carry impulses to the brainstem. The cortex communicates with the brainstem either permitting or inhibiting micturition. When normal voiding occurs there is both contraction of the detrusor and relaxation of the sphincter. Interruption of the higher pathways still allows reflex detrusor contraction but in an uncoordinated fashion, with improper relaxation of the sphincter causing dyssynergy. More detail can be found elsewhere in this text.

Maturation of these pathways allows the child to progress toward toilet training. The infants bladder serves as a reservoir with intermittent and coordinated emptying. Eventually the child develops an appreciation of bladder distension; however, voiding is inhibited by consciously contracting the sphincter during a detrusor contraction until he or she is able to reach the toilet. Further maturation involves cortical inhibition of the contractions, allowing the child more time to wait before "needing" to void. Ultimately by 4 to 5 years of age the child can voluntarily choose to void prior to any sensation of bladder fullness.

Clinical Characteristics of Dysfunctional Voiding

Urge Syndrome and Urge Incontinence.—Urge syndrome and urge incontinence are characterized by frequent attacks of imperative urge to void, countered by hold maneuvers, such as squatting. Urge incontinence, when present, usually peaks in the afternoon, and consists of small quantities of urine loss. Many children do not express their urine loss, choosing instead to use techniques to camouflage their wetting. Parents of these children know the location of every toilet outside the home. Urge incontinence may have a nocturnal component, again in the form of slight loss of urine, which may or may not wake up the child. The symptoms and signs are caused by uninhibit detrusor contractions countered by voluntary contraction of the pelvic floor. The functional capacity of the bladder is small for the child's age. Micturition is normal with complete relaxation of the pelvic floor in many cases, although some children may prematurely contract their sphincter, resulting in incomplete emptying. This habit of inhibiting urge with voluntary pelvic floor contraction leads to postponement of defecation, leading to constipation and fecal soiling, not to be confused with the encopresis of children with behavioral problems.

Dysfunctional Voiding.—*Staccato voiding* often is termed dyssynergic voiding, in analogy to the true detrusor-sphincter dyssynergy in neuropathic bladder-sphincter dysfunction. Sometimes it is combined with urge syndrome; sometimes children with urge syndrome only have a history of urge syndrome. This peculiar voiding pattern is caused by periodic bursts of pelvic floor activity during voiding, resulting in peaks of bladder pressure coinciding with dips in urine flow rate. Flow time is prolonged and often incomplete, increasing the child's risk of developing UTIs.

Fractionated, incomplete *voiding* is characterized by infrequent voiding with micturition occurring in several small fractions. This usually is associated with incomplete bladder emptying, thus postvoid residuals. The bladder is large for age secondary to a hypoactive bladder, and urge is inhibited easily. Micturition occurs in fractions secondary to unsustained bladder contractions with abdominal pressure necessary to shorten the flow time. The flow rate is highly irregular because of reflex activity of the pelvic floor muscles, triggered by increases in abdominal pressure. Ostensibly, wetting in this form of dysfunctional voiding is secondary to overflow incontinence.

Other Forms.—The *lazy bladder syndrome* is the net result of long-standing fractionated and incomplete voiding. Abdominal pressure is the primary driving force for voiding and detrusor contractions are virtually absent. These children void infrequently and leave large postvoid residuals, subjecting them to an increased risk of developing UTIs. This should not be confused with pure *diurnal enuresis* an entity associated with normal, albeit infrequent, voiding usually seen in boys who simple delay emptying until it becomes too late.

The *Hinman syndrome* (nonneurogenic neurogenic bladder), first elaborated by Hinman may represent the right-most end of the natural history of dysfunctional voiding, characterized first by detrusor overactivity followed by bladder-sphincter dyssynergy and ultimately lazy bladder syndrome. Radiographs show thick, trabeculated bladder walls, vesicoureteral reflux, and reflux nephropathy. Initially, severe psychological disturbance was postulated as the etiology in these patients, and hypnotherapy was recommended. Surgical treatment prior to correcting this imbalance is discouraged.

History and Physical Examination

A complete history and physical examination are essential to help identify children with neurogenic bladders and to distinguish between classifications of enuresis and the different forms of functional incontinence. Daytime wetting is usually the hallmark of dysfunctional voiding. The wetting is usually in small amounts, causing damp spots on the underwear. The wetting is most prevalent in the afternoon because during school, children are most anxious about remaining dry. Children with advanced stages of dysfunctional voiding will wet as well but tend to skip early-morning voiding. The nocturnal component usually involves losses of small amounts of urine with some children awakening. This is in contrast to nocturnal enuresis where voiding is complete and unnoticed until the morning.

Voiding frequency should be charted by the child for at least 2 weeks in a diary. Children with urge syndrome usually void at least seven times a day; those with infrequent voiding empty only one to three times a day and may strain or use manual pressure to assist in complete emptying. A staccato flow is a reliable sign of sphincter overactivity during voiding.

Sudden and imperative sensations of urge numerous times a day are characteristic of urge syndrome. Most children with urge syndrome have adopted typical hold maneuvers to prevent wetting with each contraction. Despite this they are not successful and dampen their pants. Children with lazy bladder syndrome never demonstrate urge. Finally, children with classical diurnal enuresis deny urge and ignore uncontrolled voiding.

Other features include obtaining a history of recurrent urinary tract infections, which points to dysfunctional voiding associated with incomplete bladder emptying as the etiology. Incontinence in conjunction with stress may be seen in children with urge syndrome when increasing abdominal pressure provokes a detrusor contraction as opposed to pure stress incontinence, which is caused by structural incompetence of the ureteral closure mechanism. Likewise, incontinence associated with laughing may, in some cases, represent children with urge syndrome with detrusor instability exacerbated by increased abdominal pressure in contrast to true giggle micturition defined as sudden, involuntary, uncontrollable and complete emptying of the bladder upon giggling in otherwise normal children. Finally, constipation is associated with dysfunctional voiding.

The physical examination should focus on findings that might lead one to suspect an occult neuropathic bladder. These include lipomeningocele, sacral dimple, cafe-au-lait spots, lipoma, and a hairy tuft at the sacrum. An absent or asymmetrical gluteal cleft suggests sacral agenesis. The neurologic examination includes careful attention to the lower extremity including tone, strength, sensation and reflexes. Anal tone and the child's gait should be assessed.

Urodynamics

We and others believe that urodynamic studies, by showing the interaction between detrusor and sphincter activity, are an essential adjunct to the diagnosis and therapy of children with functional incontinence in most patients because they help reveal the pathophysiological patterns behind the signs and symptoms of the condition.

Careful review of the literature supports the idea that most urodynamic patterns fit into two categories of bladder/sphincter overactivity. One category is characterized by strong uninhibited detrusor contractions early in the filling phase, countered by voluntary pelvic floor activity giving rise to frequency, urgency, hold maneuvers, and urge incontinence with essentially normal voiding parameters. The other is characterized by incomplete relaxation (or frank overactivity) of striated pelvic floor muscles during actual voiding, causing a staccato or fractionated flow associated with incomplete emptying despite a normal filling phase. One should note that the clinical patterns, urge syndrome and dysfunctional voiding (staccato or fractionated pattern), to which may be added the lazy bladder syndrome, may not be the distinct entities they seem and probably represent different stages in the natural history of nonneurogenic bladder/sphincter dyssynergy in children.

Radiologic Findings

All children with daytime wetting should have an ultrasound of the kidneys and bladder to exclude anatomic abnormalities responsible for incontinence. In addition, a voiding cystourethrogram (VCUG) is performed in the subject with UTIs. Not surprisingly, children with dysfunctional voiding will show the ab-

normalities on VCUG, ultrasound, and intravenous urography that are characteristic for the pediatric population with recurrent UTIs, such as vesicoureteral reflux (VUR) and reflux nephropathy, with the prevalence known from studies on recurrent UTIs in schoolage children.

Some patients demonstrate a peculiar anomaly found at VCUG; the so-called spinning top configuration of the urethra. Seen during filling or voiding whenever a girl or boy with urge syndrome tries to inhibit imperative urge by contracting the pelvic floor, the force of the detrusor contraction will dilate the proximal urethra down to the closed external sphincter.

The detrusor muscle contracting against a tightly closed urethra generates high pressures explaining the variability in grade of VUR in children with urge syndrome and recurrent UTIs. Traditionally VUR is graded on the appearance of the refluxing urinary tract on one or more static images taken during filling and micturition. Elevated bladder pressures will momentarily dilate a refluxing urinary tract making VUR a dynamic event difficult to grade consistently on a static VCUG. As a consequence, the incidence of reflux nephropathy in children with dysfunctional voiding and recurrent UTIs does not show the expected correlation with the grade of VUR.

Therapy

Only a proportion of children with functional incontinence will become free of symptoms with traditional methods of treatment (i.e., careful explanation of the problem, voiding instructions, and control of recurrent UTIs). Children may remain incontinent despite treatment under the auspices of a urotherapist in a structurally organized out-patient program. The primary treatment modalities we provide include antibiotic prophylaxis, anticholinergics, and biofeedback with psychological counselling when indicated.

Long-term chemoprophylaxis has a definite place in the management of children with recurrent UTIs and functional incontinence. If recurrences can be avoided for a period of at least 6 months, signs and symptoms may diminish appreciably, breaking the dysuria-tentative (dysfunctional) voiding-UTI cycle.

Children with urge syndrome respond to therapy with anticholinergic drugs aimed specifically at reducing the number of overactive detrusor contractions and restoring the reduced functional bladder capacity. This has, in some cases, reduced the degree of vesicoureteral reflux. However, results are often unpredictable and not long lasting. The best results with anticholinergic treatment are obtained in combination with a well organized traditional treatment program; one might postulate that the general measures of the program itself are more essential to success than the anticholinergic medication.

Children with urge syndrome must learn how to recognize the first sensations of urge and how to suppress these sensations by normal central inhibition, instead of emergency procedures, such as urethral compression. Children with dysfunctional voiding must learn to void with a relaxed pelvic floor. A program aimed at retraining the child to remain continent and empty effectively would be the best approach to manage these children, assuming the child has sufficient cognitive ability to understand what they are being taught and provided that an element of feedback can be incorporated into the retraining process. Biofeedback, a term coined by Miller, is defined as the use of modern instrumentation to give a person better moment-to-moment information about a specific physiological process that is under control of the central nervous system, but not clearly or accurately perceived. Urodynamic signals, such as urine flow rate, pelvic floor electromyogram, or detrusor pressure, are perfectly suited for biofeedback. The success rate of such programs, estimated to be as great at 70% in uncontrolled studies, underlies the importance of the physiological concept behind the clinical complex of bladder/sphincter dyssynergy and recurrent UTIs.

Other forms of therapy have been suggested for the child with daytime wetting. Severing the filum terminale has been recommended by some, especially in the presence of spina bifida occulta, but has been discouraged by others. Neuromodulation and acupuncture also have been advocated although the mechanisms leading to successful treatment have yet to been elucidated. Schneider and colleagues taught children with voiding dysfunction the Kegel exercise and found considerable improvement in the incidence of incontinence. Empirically this seems counterintuitive as most children with urge syndrome or dysfunctional voiding, in our experience, already overutilize their pelvic floor musculature.

Primary Nocturnal Enuresis

Primary nocturnal enuresis is a heterogenous condition that affects between 5% to 8% of children 7 years of age, with a spontaneous resolution rate of 15% per year. Because the vast majority of cases do resolve spontaneously, some physicians choose to ignore the problem. Although enuresis does not cause physical harm to children, it can cause emotional disturbances and poor self-esteem. Some parents feel as though they have failed, and often both the children and their parents choose to keep enuresis a family secret.

Etiology

After excluding structural and neurogenic causes, systemic diseases, and functional incontinence, usually after obtaining a thorough history and physical examination, there is no single etiology to explain en-

uresis in every child. Clearly genetics plays an important role, since 40% of offspring will be enuretic if one parent has the condition, and 70% will be enuretic if both parents are affected. Some investigators have found small functional bladder capacities in children with nocturnal enuresis created by the development of detrusor contractions during sleep. These children may fall into our categorization of urge syndrome, especially when symptoms are associated with daytime frequency, urgency, and wetting. Others feel that children with nocturnal enuresis are unusually heavy sleepers although sleep studies have failed to show a clear difference between children with enuresis and children who can remain dry. In addition, most children able to remain dry at night do so without awakening, suggesting more than a dyssomnia as the etiology.

A deficiency of antidiuretic hormone, first reported by Nørgaard and Rittig, has been used to explain enuresis, especially in young adolescents. Thus, these children are prone to produce more urine than their functional bladder capacity will allow at night. This theory is inconsistent when one considers that approximately half of children with diseases causing resistance to antidiuretic hormone, such as sickle cell disease, can remain dry at night.

Evaluation

Little more than a complete history and physical examination is necessary when evaluating children with nocturnal enuresis. Careful attention to daytime voiding behavior is important to exclude bladder-sphincter dysfunction. Children with a history of urinary tract infections should be evaluated with imaging studies. Constipation can cause enuresis and should be treated. The physical examination should include emphasis on normal growth and blood pressure to exclude chronic renal failure, and neurological examination to exclude an occult neuropathic bladder. A urinalysis should be performed to look for proteinuria, hematuria, and normal concentrating ability. Imaging studies are not necessary if history, physical examination, and urinalysis are normal.

Therapy

The treatment for nocturnal enuresis should be directed in a manner that is age appropriate and is either behavioral or pharmacological. Usually it is best for younger children to have a motivationally based program, with medications used in older children and adolescents. Many studies have shown improvement in nocturnal enuresis when compared to placebo, but few, if any, compare one therapy to another.

Behavioral therapy in the form of self-awakening can be used by having the child pretend that his bladder is full and trying to awaken him. Others recommend self-hypnosis with the posthypnotic suggestion that the child will use the bathroom at night. Dry-bed training involves the parents more and teaches the child to self-awaken by going through a series of programmed awakenings over several days until the child becomes independent. A high cure rate (92%) has been reported with a relapse rate of 20%.

Enuresis alarms are very popular and, if the family and child are motivated, can be quite successful (approximately 70%). Most commercially available alarms are easy to use, free of risk, inexpensive, and relatively comfortable. Their disadvantages include the time commitment necessary until they can be discontinued. They are not very helpful if the alarm is triggered several times per night secondary to either decreased bladder capacity or polyuria.

Three medications are currently available for treatment of nocturnal enuresis, oxybutynin, imipramine, and desmopressin acetate (DDAVP). Oxybutynin may be useful for the nocturnal component in children with urge syndrome, but it has not been proven beneficial in children with primary isolated nocturnal enuresis. Imipramine has been used extensively for nocturnal enuresis and seems to exert both an anticholinergic effect aimed at increasing bladder capacity and a central effect that decreases the amount of time spent in rapid-eye movement sleep. Imipramine when taken in a dose of 50 to 75 mg at bedtime had a positive effect in 10% to 60% of patients, with some children relapsing after withdrawal. Imipramine can cause nausea, anxiety, and malaise, with some children experiencing personality changes, cardiac arrhythmias or sleep disorders. It must be kept out of the reach of small children because of its potentially lethal effects when taken at inappropriately high doses.

In 1985, Nørgaard and associates suggested that a component of nocturnal enuresis may be caused by a deficiency of the normal surge of antidiuretic hormone usually seen in children able to remain dry at night. Hence DDAVP, at a dose of 20 to 40 μg/night intranasally, would appear useful because it would reduce a child's urine output such that he could remain dry prior to needing to void. DDAVP seems to be more effective in children where there is a family history of nocturnal enuresis (91%) as compared to 7% where a family history was not observed. Moffatt evaluated 18 randomized controlled trials and determined that DDAVPs effect produces complete dryness in only a minority of patients for a short period of time and suggested than an enuresis alarm should be primary therapy. Water intoxication has been observed extremely infrequently with more common side effects including nasal stuffiness, epistaxis, and mild abdominal pain. DDAVP is recently available in oral formulation with comparable results to intranasal dosing.

It is essential that one recognize that isolated primary nocturnal enuresis should not be confused with other forms of wetting described above. Children who do not respond to conventional therapy may have diurnal enuresis, which is a complex behavioral problem, urge syndrome, or dysfunctional voiding.

Undescended Testis

A common referral to the pediatric urologist is the boy with known or suspected cryptorchidism. Surgery for this condition is generally regarded as the most common pediatric urologic surgical procedure. However, many boys referred for cryptorchidism simply have a retractile testis. Aspects of the physical examination are thus extremely important in making an accurate diagnosis. Both the examiner's hands and the ambient temperature in the office should be warm. The child should be made to feel comfortable in the office surroundings, and, at the time of physical examination, attention should not be immediately focused to the genitalia. The child may begin to relax during the initial portion of the examination, and, while performing cardiac auscultation or the like, one may observe retractile testes descending. The retractile testis is often palpable in the inguinal canal and can be gently "milked" into the dependent portion of the scrotum, where it remains without immediate retraction. In these boys, the hemiscrotum is well developed, rather than the small, empty scrotum of cryptorchidism. Sometimes the retractile testis is best identified with the boy in the sitting cross-legged position. Having the boy blow up a balloon may also assist in cremasteric muscle relaxation and testicular descent. If one is still suspicious of a retractile testis but cannot confirm this entity, human chorionic gonadotropin (HCG) stimulation is helpful in distinguishing the retractile from the true cryptorchid testis. At times the diagnosis is made under anesthesia before orchiopexy.

The use of HCG-stimulation studies in the boy with bilateral nonpalpable testes is diagnostic of anorchia if the testosterone levels are low and nonresponding, along with elevated baseline levels of luteinizing hormone and follicle-stimulating hormone (Levitt et al, 1978). There have been reports, however, in which the HCG stimulation testing has been falsely negative in the presence of testes (Bartone et al., 1984). In this report, the authors noted no testosterone response to HCG in two patients with testes present at exploration. Curiously, the baseline levels of gonadotropin were not elevated, which may distinguish this group from the true anorchic patient.

Therefore, a modicum of caution should be used in interpretation of HCG testing. The occurrence of cryptorchidism in association with hypospadias, especially the more severe degrees, should alert the physician to the presence of an abnormality of sexual differentiation, and chromosomal analysis is indicated (Rajfer and Walsh, 1976).

Scrotal Mass

The presence of a scrotal mass is a common referral to the pediatric urologist. Similar to the examination for cryptorchidism, warm examiner hands, a warm office, and a relaxed child make the examination much easier and more accurate. Historical factors of importance include the presence or absence of symptoms and changes in the character of scrotal swelling over relatively short durations of time or with activity. The inguinal canal is examined for thickening of the spermatic cord, as this would suggest the presence of a patent processus vaginalis. Transillumination distinguishes the cystic vs. solid nature of the intrascrotal components. Communicating hydroceles can often be gently milked dry of their fluid, only to observe the hemiscrotum refill when the child increases the intraabdominal pressure by coughing, crying, or blowing up a balloon. However, the history of changes in the size of the hydrocele with activity is often diagnostic of a communication.

Although testis tumors are uncommon in childhood, testis tumors commonly present as a painless enlargement. Scrotal ultrasonography is extremely helpful in preoperative diagnosis.

The adolescent with a scrotal mass must be examined in both the supine and erect positions. A left scrotal mass in the adolescent is commonly a varicocele and this empties completely in the supine position. It is important to measure respective testicular volume, and this can be easily and reproducibly performed using a series of punched-out plates (Rabinowitz et al., 1984). If the varicocele-associated testis is small compared with the right one, ligation of the varicocele may result in reversal of testicular growth retardation (Belman and Kass, 1981).

Hypospadias

Penile anomalies, the most common of which is hypospadias, are often referred to the pediatric urologist for evaluation and treatment. Some of these boys may have been circumcised. The urethral meatus is identified, and an attempt is made to determine any degree of curvature or chordee. An erection is commonly elicited by gently squeezing the base of the penis. Demonstrating the anatomy to the parents, explaining the embryology in laymen's terms, explaining the final position of the urethral meatus following correction of chordee, and outlining and diagramming the anticipated technique of repair is usually very helpful in the long-term management of these boys. The review and the explanation of the anatomy and reconstruction allow preparation for a simple or complex repair with relatively low complication rates. The majority of these reconstructions are performed at a single stage. Follow-up postoperative visits may entail urethral calibration. The issue of uroradiographic evaluation in patients with hypospadias has been addressed (Khuri et al., 1981; Shelton and Noe, 1985). It appears that those cases of proximal hypospadias (penoscrotal or more proximal) or hypospadias in association with other anomalies or a history of urinary tract infection warrant at least a minimal evaluation with abdominal ultrasound.

Meatal Stenosis

Boys who have been circumcised are at risk for the development of meatal stenosis, usually secondary to trauma or meatitis. Many boys referred for meatal stenosis have a normal meatal caliber (Litvak et al., 1976). Therefore, one must observe the urinary stream for caliber, deflection, and straining. If the stream is indeed pinpoint width, if the child takes an inordinate amount of time to empty the bladder, if there is obvious straining, and if there is deflection of the urinary stream, intervention is indicated. Often, this can be carried out in the office, especially if the meatal scarring is thin. The tip of a ⅛-oz tube of ophthalmic ointment or the tip of a small mosquito hemostat can often, with gentle pressure, restore normal meatal caliber. When the meatal scarring is quite thick, a more formal clamp and incision meatotomy is necessary. In some boys, this can be performed with local anesthetic, but the child and parents must be assessed to see how well this would be tolerated. Rather than lose the child's confidence, the procedure can be performed under a brief general anesthetic. Following meatotomy, the tip of an ophthalmic ointment tube is inserted into the meatus once or twice daily for a few weeks until healing is complete to ensure an adequate caliber orifice.

Redundant Foreskin

Over the past decade, many pediatricians and pediatric urologists have recognized that "routine" neonatal circumcision is unnecessary in the majority (Rombert, 1985; Wallerstein, 1980). Pediatric urologists are rarely involved in the parental decision regarding newborn circumcision, however. When a boy is referred to the office because of redundant foreskin, there is usually a genital anomaly, such as hypospadias, penile torsion, or chordee. In some boys whose parents had originally intended them to be circumcised, prematurity or an associated severe neonatal illness prevented circumcision. Sometimes an older infant or child is being adopted, and the new parents are seeking consultation. If the foreskin is still adherent, it should be explained that this phimosis is physiologic and not an indication for circumcision. Most foreskins should be easily retractable by 4 years of age, but some do not become freely retractable until late childhood. The practice of forcible foreskin retraction is not only painful but is contraindicated, because it may promote secondary scarring and acquired phimosis. Some parents may request (and pediatricians may recommend) circumcision because of the accumulation of "pus" between the glans and foreskin. These collections usually represent an accumulation of shed epithelial cells between the inner prepuce and the glans. The accumulation of these "pearls," also called smegma, is simply part of the physiologic retraction of the foreskin. These usually spontaneously progress to the junction of foreskin and glans, and in doing so resolve the physiologic adhesions (Kaluber et al, 1982). In a few boys, the adhesions to the foreskin become very thick and scarred. In these instances, circumcision may be necessary.

If the boy has been circumcised and there is residual foreskin adherent to the glans, this is most likely secondary to incomplete separation of glans and foreskin at the time of the neonatal procedure, and these adhesions should gradually and spontaneously lyse without intervention. If the foreskin had been completely freed at the time of circumcision and a segment of shaft skin reattaches to an area of denuded glans, a thick skin bridge may form that cannot be bluntly lysed. These require surgical excision in which the glans end must be suture closed for hemostasis (Klauber and Boyle, 1974).

Labial Adhesions

On occasion the labia minora may be fused in the midline, congenitally or following an inflammatory process. If these adhesions are mild or asymptomatic, no intervention is necessary. However, long adhesions, associated local symptoms, vaginal voiding, and urinary stasis may necessitate lysis of the fused area, which is usually easily performed with gentle pressure on the fused midline using a lubricated cotton swab. Readhesion may be prevented by applying estrogen cream to the denuded labial edges. Alternatively, the application of estrogen cream on a daily basis for 5 to 7 days may induce lysis as well.

USE OF LOCAL ANESTHETICS IN THE OFFICE SETTING

There are several procedures that can be performed in the office depending on the cooperation of the child. Meatotomy, division of bridges from the penile shaft to the glans, and lysis of labial adhesions commonly are managed in the office setting in appropriate children. These procedures require local anesthesia and cooperation of both the child and the parents. The subcutaneous infiltration of lidocaine, bupivacaine, or a combination of the two has been the traditional method of local anesthesia. More recently the use of the eutectic mixture of lidocaine and prilocaine hydrochloride in a 1:1 oil/water mixture, EMLA has been shown to be an effective local superficial anesthetic.

It can be used as the sole anesthetic for meatotomy, division of skin bridges, or lysis of labial adhesions, or it may be used as a topical anesthetic for IV insertion or deeper subcutaneous local infiltration. EMLA cream is slow acting and requires placement 1 hour prior to the procedure. It should be covered with an occlusive nonabsorptive dressing to ensure its locally concentrated effect.

AMBULATORY SURGERY IN PEDIATRIC UROLOGY

History of Ambulatory Surgery

Ambulatory medical care was provided in temples in Egypt 5000 years ago, as the ill came to these houses of healing. Fractures and lacerations were cared for. Indian hospitals more than 2000 years ago also cared for patients on an outpatient basis. Similarly, the Greeks and Romans used the temples for both inpatient and outpatient care. Although there were few hospitals in the Middle Ages, some had outpatient facilities (Schultz, 1979).

In the United States, Dr. Benjamin Waterhouse, physician in charge of the Marine Hospital at Boston, developed the first outpatient service in 1808. Because of the unusually large number of hospital patients, "I have instituted what we call 'out-patient,' that is given advice and medicine to numbers. . . and thereby prevent them from becoming boarders." (Thurm, 1972). The first outpatient department opened 10 years later at the Massachusetts General Hospital. These clinics functioned mainly as dispensaries and provided little surgical care (Schultz, 1979).

With improved techniques of anesthesia and surgical techniques, the surgery of children seemed appropriate for the outpatient setting. In 1909, James Nicoll reported that surgery of children on an outpatient basis was safe, successful, and cost effective. In reporting on more than 7000 pediatric surgical procedures, he stated:

> I have no alternative to the opinion that the treatment of a large number of the cases at present treated indoor constitutes a waste of the resources of a children's hospital or a children's ward. The results obtained in the outpatient department at a tithe of the cost are equally good. . . . Infants and young children in a ward are noisy, and not infrequently malodorous. The main idea in their admission is the supposed benefit of 'trained' nursing. That benefit is largely wasted on them. . .Continuous quiet rest on the back on the part of a young child in pain is a pretty idea, rarely obtainable, and not specially necessary after such operations. After operation in an outpatient room, such young children with their wounds closed with collodion or rubber plaster are easily carried home in their mothers' arms and rest there more quietly, on the whole, than anywhere else.

Herzfeld (1938) and Farquharson (1955) reported great success with outpatient pediatric herniorrhaphy and the lack of need for postoperative restrictions. In the 1960s, outpatient surgery programs were initially hospital based (Cohen and Dillon, 1966; Levy and Coakley, 1968). Free-standing ambulatory surgery centers followed shortly thereafter, the model being the Phoenix Surgicenter (Cloud et al., 1972; Reed, 1982; Reed and Ford, 1976). The U.S. military has also set up ambulatory surgery units (Lenneville and Steinbruckner, 1982).

In the past decade, ambulatory surgery programs have rapidly expanded. In 1982, 18% of all hospital surgery was performed on an ambulatory basis (Haug and Chupack, 1985). In 1980, more than 70% of non-federal hospitals in the United States offered ambulatory surgery (Detmer and Buchanan-Davidson, 1982). As early as 1972, it was estimated that 20% to 40% of inpatient surgical procedures could be performed as an outpatient (Davis and Detmer, 1972). More recently, it is thought that more than half of all surgical procedures can be carried out in an ambulatory care unit (American Medical Association Socioeconomic Monitoring System, 1982). Ambulatory surgery has been one of the most rapidly expanding areas of health care. It includes day surgery, outpatient surgery, and in-and-out surgery in hospitals, hospital-based ambulatory surgery centers, and free-standing ambulatory surgery centers.

Design of Ambulatory Surgery Center for Pediatric Patients

Since a significant percentage of ambulatory surgery patients are children, the design and running of the ambulatory surgery center must take into account the special needs of the pediatric patient. Whether the ambulatory surgery unit is free-standing or hospital-based, the waiting area should have a large play area for children. This should include safe toys and children's books. Except in those instances in which there is a long traveling distance, the child should have a preadmission blood count and tour of the facility a few days prior to the scheduled surgery. If indicated, preanesthesia consultation is carried at the same time. These preadmission tours significantly reduce the anxiety level among the children and their parents. The surroundings become familiar and both the child and parents are given the opportunity to ask questions.

Prior to the ambulatory surgical procedure, detailed written instructions are sent. Older children are given nothing by mouth after midnight prior to the procedure and younger children are given nothing by mouth for approximately 6 hours prior to the scheduled time of surgery.

On the day of the procedure, parents or guardians are with the child while vital signs are checked. The anesthesiologist meets the family and the child is given a choice of anesthetic technique. The younger child is generally accompanied by a favorite toy or doll to the operating room. In many institutions a parent is allowed to be present during induction. Once the child has sufficiently recovered from anesthesia, the parents are returned to the child in the recovery room. Several units have experimented successfully with having parents present for anesthetic induction and in the recovery room. This has been found to ease the management of the very anxious child and parents in selected cases.

At the time of discharge from the ambulatory surgery unit, detailed written postoperative instructions are given. This includes information regarding dietary and activity restriction, bathing, and the management of postoperative discomfort and fever. Instructions regarding postoperative follow-up and emergency telephone numbers are included. All families are contacted the day following the procedure by the ambulatory surgery center, the physician's office, or both.

Conditions Cared for in Ambulatory Surgery Center

As time has progressed, the number and types of surgical procedures in children amenable to surgical correction without the need for overnight hospitalization has increased significantly. In pediatric urology, cystoscopy, circumcision, herniorrhaphy and hydrocelectomy, and meatotomy were part of the original list of surgical procedures amenable to ambulatory repair. This list has been expanded significantly to include unilateral and bilateral orchiopexy, varicocelectomy, internal optical urethrotomy, resection of urethral valves, repair of urethral fistula, and both simple and complex hypospadias repairs (Caldamone and Rabinowitz, 1982; Nadelson et al., 1984; Rabinowitz, 1988; Reed and Dawson, 1979; Shepard et al., 1984; Siegel et al., 1986). These pediatric procedures account for approximately one third of the total number of pediatric patients using ambulatory surgical care (Cloud, 1982; Cohen et al., 1980; Kroovand, 1982; Kroovand and Perlmutter, 1978). As the list of pediatric procedures amenable to outpatient performance has expanded, outpatient surgery has become a major proportion of pediatric urologic practice. In 1981, Kroovand reported that 48% of their surgical procedures were performed on an outpatient basis (Kroovand, 1982). Rabinowitz (1982) reported 58% of his pediatric urologic procedures performed as outpatient. More recently, Siegel and colleagues (1986) reported that 62% of the urologic surgical procedures at Children's Hospital in Philadelphia were performed on an outpatient basis. Rabinowitz (1990) now reports that 77% of his surgical procedures in 1988 and 1989 were performed on an outpatient basis.

In the early days of ambulatory surgery, most pediatric candidates were very healthy, had no preexisting medical conditions, and were scheduled to have only a brief surgical procedure. These indications have been vastly expanded. The presence of major preexisting medical conditions is no longer a contraindication for ambulatory surgery. It is most important that the anesthesiologist be informed of any preexisting medical condition, and this sometimes necessitates a preoperative anesthesia consultation. With these factors in mind, preexisting cardiac anomalies and stable neurologic conditions are no longer contraindications for ambulatory surgery (Rabinowitz, 1982). Likewise, multiple surgical procedures under the same anesthetic or reoperative surgery is also amenable to the ambulatory setting. If a prolonged anesthetic or an extensive dissection is anticipated, the family should be prepared for the increased possibility of overnight hospitalization. However, multiple operative procedures by one or more surgeons and reoperative procedures, such as repeat orchiopexy, are performed safely on an outpatient basis (Caldamone and Rabinowitz, 1982).

Anesthesia and Postoperative Analgesia

The anesthesiologist is a full partner in the ambulatory pediatric urologic surgery. As part of the history and physical examination, information regarding previous anesthetics, family history of anesthesia, and any preexisting medical condition must be made known to the anesthesiologist. Preoperative anesthesia consultation may be necessary (Dimino, 1979). In general, premedication is not used; atopine may be given intramuscularly following induction of anesthesia, and inhalation agents are used (Cloud, 1982; Steward, 1980). When the anesthesiologist meets the child and family, the child participates in the decision regarding technique of induction. Many older children prefer IV induction. The younger children usually prefer mask inhalation. In those instances, the unpleasant smell of the rubber mask is hidden by a flavored extract painted or rubbed on the inside of the mask. It is helpful to have many flavors available so that the child can choose his or her favorite. Many children who undergo short anesthetics (cystoscopy, meatotomy, circumcision, herniorrhaphy/hydrocelectomy, unilateral orchiopexy) are ambulating, retaining oral fluids, and are ready for discharge within 2 hours following completion of their anesthetic (Dawson, 1979). If these children are otherwise healthy, they should not require IV fluids (Cloud, 1982). However, with longer anesthetics (hypospadias repair, bilateral orchiopexy, reoperative surgery), IV fluids are given both intraoperatively and postoperatively. This as-

sures adequate hydration in a child who may have some nausea and vomiting following 1.5 to 2 hours of anesthesia. In addition, IV hydration assures prompt voiding in hypospadias reconstructions where catheters are not used postoperatively.

The decision regarding endotracheal intubation is left to the anesthesiologist. Although some anesthesiologists are reluctant to intubate a child and send that child home the same day (Cohen et al., 1980; Morse, 1972; Smith, 1980), endotracheal intubation has not affected the outcome, resulted in increased complications, or increased the risk for overnight hospitalization (Caldamone and Rabinowitz, 1982; Dawson, 1979; Jones and Smith, 1980; Steward, 1973). Rabinowitz reported endotracheal intubation in 15%, Cloud (1982) in 35%, and Hertzler (1981) in 80%.

Recovery and return to normal activity are hastened by freedom from postoperative pain. In many older children intramuscular meperidine given during the operative procedure may eliminate the need for postoperative narcotic analgesia (Cloud, 1982). In addition, peripheral nerve blockage for inguinal and penile surgery is highly effective. Bupivacaine is a long-acting anesthetic with a duration of action of 3 to 6 hours. However, the onset of action is 10 to 20 minutes. Therefore, this agent should be administered well before the child awakens to ensure maximum effect (Scott and Cousins, 1980; Shandling and Steward, 1980).

It has recently been shown that the irrigation of an inguinoscrotal surgical wound with bupivacaine prior to closure was effective in reducing postoperative pain and narcotic requirement (Shefield et al., 1995). Shenfield and coworkers (1995) found that 97% of children receiving wound irrigation with bupivacaine required no postoperative narcotic administration.

Regional anesthesia via a caudal block is used commonly as an adjunct to general anesthesia in pediatric patients undergoing inguinal, scrotal, or genital surgery. It allows for a lighter degree of general anesthesia and postoperative pain relief. In addition, it has been suggested that the use of caudal block reduces blood loss during hypospadias surgery (Gunter, 1990). In a comparison of caudal and general anesthesia versus general anesthesia alone, Blaise and Roy (1986) found that children undergoing hypospadias repair were more comfortable and less agitated in the recovery room. A caudal block is given by administering a local anesthetic into the sacral canal, which is contiguous with the epidural space. This is administered through the sacral hiatus, which is a midline depression between the sacral cornua.

The administration can vary depending on the length of the surgical procedure. The caudal may be given as a simple injection at the start of the operation for those operations that are 2 hours or less. Alternatively, an indwelling short intravenous catheter can be placed in the sacral canal at the start of the procedure which can facilitate redosing at the conclusion of the longer operation.

Lidocaine or bupivacaine are used most commonly for caudal block. This can be used with epinephrine-added preparations to increase the duration of activity. Bupivacaine is also effective in reducing bladder spasms postoperatively in patients who have had bladder surgery or who have an indwelling bladder catheter postoperatively. The duration of analgesic effect from bupivacaine is 4 to 8 hours. Reported complications from the use of caudal blockade are rare. They include intravascular or interosseous injection leading to systemic toxicity, subarachnoid injection leading to spinal anesthesia, perforation of pelvic viscera or vessels, hypotension, and urinary retention (Reynolds 1990). Of 750 caudal blocks, Dalens and Hasnaoui (1989) reported no complications.

Complications

The ambulatory setting for performance of surgical procedures has not resulted in an increased complication rate, nor has it affected the surgical results. At the Phoenix Surgicenter, more than 70,000 surgical procedures have been performed without a death or cardiac arrest (Cloud, 1982; Dawson, 1979). Natof (1980) reported a single postoperative fatality of more than 13,000 ambulatory surgical patients over 5 years. Of the greater than 17,000 children operated on at the Phoenix Surgicenter, the postoperative hospitalization rate was 0.2%. An additional 0.1% of patients were seen for a postoperative problem in the hospital emergency room (Cloud, 1982). Of course, some procedures constitute a higher risk for postoperative complications than others. The most extensive the dissection and the longer the anesthetic, the greater the risk for delay in recovery and necessity for overnight hospitalization (Fahy and Marshall, 1969). Shepard and co-workers (1984) reported that all children undergoing ambulatory surgical procedures that were hospitalized were discharged the following day. Those children who will require overnight hospitalization are recognized before discharge. Fisher (1981) reported one child requiring hospitalization for postoperative complications following discharge from the ambulatory unit during a 10-year experience. Cloud (1982) reported no surgical or anesthesia-related complication requiring readmission in the vast Surgicenter experience. Siegel and colleagues (1986) reported no re-hospitalizations following 420 outpatient pediatric urologic procedures, including 130 hypospadias repairs. Over a 1-year period, Kroovand and Perlmutter (1978) reported a similar experience in more than 300 outpatient pediatric urologic procedures. Like-wise, Rabinowtiz (1982) reported no readmissions for 4 years of outpatient orchiopexies. Caldamone and Rabinowitz (1982) found no difference in the complication rate of outpatient vs. inpatient orchiopexy, even though many of the outpatients require extensive dissection. Only 5% remained overnight, and all were discharged the following day.

Benefits

Ambulatory pediatric urologic surgery is safe, surgically successful, phychologically less detrimental than inpatient surgery, and highly cost effective.

Ambulatory pediatric surgery was first shown to be very safe and highly successful more than 75 years ago (Nicoll, 1909). Modern widespread experience has confirmed Nicoll's early recommendation for outpatient surgery in the pediatric urologic practice (Cloud, 1982; Kroovand, 1982; Rabinowtiz, 1982; Shepard et al, 1984; Siegel et al., 1986). Both the anesthesiologist and the pediatric urologic surgeon must be even more careful and precise in the handling of the child. Precise application of anesthesia without premedication, with minimal amount of anesthetic, and with local supplementation by the surgeon contribute to rapid recovery and early mobilization. Meticulous hemostasis and tissue handling by the surgeon are imperative. Othersen and Clatworthy (1968) have confirmed the significantly lower incidence of acquisition of nosocomial infection in the outpatient, undoubtedly attributable to the limited duration of time spent in the hospital and lesser number of contacts. The more rapid recovery from anesthetic and earlier discharge has meant early mobilization. This has not impaired the surgical results in herniorrhaphy (Othersen and Clatworthy, 1968) or orchiopexy (Caldamone and Rabinowitz, 1982).

There is significant psychologic benefit for children having their surgery as an outpatient as opposed to an inpatient. Vaughan (1957) showed that children less than 4 years of age were more phychologically stressed than older children by their hospitalization. At this age, children are extremely close to their mothers (Vernon et al., 1966) and at age 2 years, separation anxiety and stranger anxiety are greatest (Petrillo and Sanger, 1972). The more time spent by parents with their hospitalized child, the lesser the psychological stress and postoperative behavioral disturbances. (Prugh et al., 1953). In 1971, Cloud, a pediatric surgeon affiliated with the Surgicenter in Phoenix, stated (Holton, 1971):

> When you take children out of a hospital setting and send them home immediately after surgery, you seem to relieve a lot of their apprehension. In most hospital cases, we have orders for pain killers to be available, and frequently they are used. When we send a child home from Surgicenter, he will occasionally need aspirin but that is all . . . [I] have observed that children

are happier, less frightened, and therefore seem to recover more smoothly.

Ambulatory surgery limits the duration of hospital stay, minimizes the separation between parent and child, limits the contact with strangers, and is significantly less psychologically detrimental to the child. "Children accept short-stay surgery with an amazing amount of adaptability and grace" (Hertzler, 1981).

It is estimated that approximately one fourth of the cost of health care in the United States is for surgical care (Wolcott, 1981). The per diem cost of hospital care is the largest single contributing factor to increased costs of health care (Schultz, 1979). When costs are compared for the same procedure performed as an inpatient vs. an outpatient, the outpatient savings in charges are approximately 50% (Caldamone and Rabinowitz 1982; Fraley, 1985; Hoffmann, 1981; Reed and Dawson, 1979; Shepard et al., 1984). This significant cost savings does not include additional significant savings, which are hidden. Ambulatory surgery results in a significant reduction of the need for utilization of hospital beds. Each procedure performed on an ambulatory basis frees two or more in-hospital beds per procedure. There is significantly less money spent on laboratory fees, in-hospital studies, and medications. There is a significant decrease in the need for hospital personnel from the laboratory and nursing standpoint. Around the clock nursing is not required, and one trained ambulatory surgery nurse can care for more than twice the number of patients when compared to the in-hospital setting (Caldamone and Rabinowitz, 1982). Thus, ambulatory pediatric urologic surgery is cost effective when compared to the in-hospital bill. There is additional cost reduction from the standpoint of decreased personnel required, decreased laboratory cost, and decreased in-hospital bed utilization. Further financial benefit results from the more rapid return to normal of each individual family. Parents are often able to return to work the day following the procedure, and the limitation of emotional stress results in additional savings.

Ambulatory surgery has changed the nature of the practice of pediatric urology. It has allowed for an increased efficiency in the practice of pediatric urology, while improving the care of children. It has been shown to be safe, successful, beneficial, and cost effective.

REFERENCES

Bartone FF, Huseman CA, Maizels M, et al: Pitfalls in using human chorionic gonadotropin stimulation test to diagnose anorchia. *Urol* 1984; 132:563

Belman AB: Office pediatric urology. *Url Clin North Am* 1980; 7:64.

Belman AB, Kass EJ: Reversal of testicular growth failure by varicocele ligation. *Soc Pediatr Urol Newslett* 1981; 4:64.

Bicknell FB: Pediatric urology. In *The History of urology*. AUA-Roche, 1980.

Blaise G, Roy WL: Postoperative pain relief after hypospadias repair in pediatric patients: regional anesthesia versus systemic analgesics. *Anesthesiology* 1986; 65(1):84.

Bueschen AJ, Witten DM: Radionuclide evaluation of renal function. *Urol Clin North Am* 1979; 6:307.

Burbige KA, Retik AB, Colody AH, et al: Urinary tract infection in boys. *J Urol* 1984:132-541.

Cabot H: Is urology entitled to be regarded as a specialty? *Trans Am Urol Assoc* 1911; 5:1.

Caldamone AA, Rabinowitz R: Outpatient orchiopexy. *J Urol* 1982; 127:286.

Campbell M: *Clinical Pediatric Urology*. Philadelphia, WB Saunders Co, 1951.

Campbell MF: *Pediatric Urology*. New York, Macmillan Publishing Co, 1937.

Chan JCM: Hematuria and proteinuria in pediatric patients. Diagnostic approach. *Urology* 1978; 11:205.

Cloud DT: Outpatient pediatric surgery: a surgeon's view. *Int Anesthesiol Clin* 1982; 20:99.

Cloud DT, Reed WA, Ford JL, et al: The surgicenter: a fresh concept in outpatient pediatric surgery. *J Pediatr Surg* 1972; 7:206.

Cohen D, Keneally J, Black A, et al: Experience with day stay surgery. *J Pediatr Surg* 1980; 15:21.

Cohen DD, Dillon JB: Anesthesia for outpatient surgery. *JAMA* 1966: 196:1114.

Dalens B, Hasnaoui A: Caudalanesthesia in pediatric surgery: success rate and adverse effects in 750 consecutive patients. *Anesth Analg* 1989; 68(2):83.

Davis JE, Detmer DE: The ambulatory surgical unit. *An Surg* 1972; 175:856.

Dawson B: Anesthetic management. In Schultz RC (ed): *Outpatient Surgery*. Philadelphia, Lea & Febiger, 1979, pp 29-44.

Detmer DE, Buchanan-Davidson DJ: Ambulatory surgery. *Surg Clin North Am* 1982; 62:685.

Dimino ER: Preparation of patients for short stay surgery at CHNMC: assessment and recommendations. *Clin Proc Child Hosp Natl Med Cent* 1979; 38:310.

Ehrlich RM, Kangarloo H: The use of MRI in pediatric urology. *Soc Pediatr Urol Newslett* 1985; 7:28.

Fahy A, Marshall M: Postanaesthetic morbidity in outpatients. *Br J Anaesth* 1969; 41:433.

Fair WR, Govan DE, Friedland GW, et al: Urinary tract infections in children: I. Young girls with nonrefluxing ureters. *West J Med* 1974; 121:366.

Farquharson EL: Early ambulation with special reference to herniorhaphy as an outpatient procedure. *Lancet* 1955; 2:517.

Fisher CG: Outpatient surgery. *Dial Pediatr Urol* 1981; 4(12):6.

Fraley GL: Financial considerations. In Kaye KW (ed): *Outpatient Urologic Surgery*. Philadelphia, Lea & Febiger, 1985, pp 48-51.

Grana L, Kidd J, Idriss F, et al: Effect of chronic urinary tract infection on ureteral peristalsis. *J Urol* 1965; 94:652.

Gunter JB, Forestiner JE, Manley CB: Caudal epidural anesthesia reduces blood loss during hypospadias repair. *J Urol* 1990; 144:517.

Haug JN, Chupack NK: *Socio-economic Fact Book for Surgery—1985*. American College of Surgeons, 1985.

Hertzler J: Effectively dealing with the problems of pediatric patients. In *Successful Management of Ambulatory Surgery Programs*. Atlanta, American Health Consultants, 1981, pp 277-292.

Herzfeld G: Hernia in infancy. *Am J Surg* 1938; 39:422.

Hoffmann GL: Quality control in ambulatory surgery. *Bull Am Coll Surg* 1981; 66:6.

Holton FA: Surgicenter: new way to cut hospital costs. *Physician's Management*, December 1971, p 23.

Johnson DK, Kroovand RL, Perlmutter AD: The changing role of cystoscopy in the pediatric patient. *J Urol* 1980; 123:232.

Jones SEF, Smith BAC: Anesthesia for pediatric day-surgery. *J Pediatr Surg* 1980; 15:31.

Kalia A, Travis LB, Brouhard BH: The association of idiopathic hypercalciuria and asymptomatic gross hemoruria. *J Pediatr* 1981; 99:716.

Kangarloo H, Gold RH, Fine RN, et al: Urinary tract infection in infants and children evaluated by ultrasound. *Radiology* 1985; 154:367.

Kaplan GW, Brock WA: Idiopathic urethrorrhagia in boys. *J Urol* 1982, 128:1001.

Khuri FJ, Hardy BE, Churchill BM: Urologic anomalies associated with hypospadias. *Urol Clin North Am* 1981; 8:565.

Klauber GT, Boyle J: Preputial skin-bridging—complication of circumcision. *Urology* 1974; 3:722.

Klauber GT, Mutter AZ, King LR, et al: Neonatal circumcision. *Dial Pediatr Urol* 1982; 5(12):2.

Kroovand RL: Update on outpatient pediatric urology. *Dial Pediatr Urol* 1982; 5(8):2.

Kroovand RL, Perlmutter AD: Short stay surgery in pediatric urology. *J Urol* 1978; 120:483.

Kuhn JP, Berger PE: Computed tomography of the kidney in infancy and childhood. *Radiol Clin North Am* 1981; 19:445.

Kunin GM: The natural history of recurrent bacteriuria in school girls. *N Engl J Med*. 1970; 282:1443.

Ladd WF, Gross RE: *Abdominal Surgery of Infancy and Childhood*. Philadelphia, WB Saunders Co. 1941.

Lenneville MW, Steinbruckner KP: Marketing of a military ambulatory surgical center. *Milit Med* 1982, 147:963.

Leonidas JC, McCauley RGK, Klauber GC, et al: Sonography as a substitute for excretory urography in children with urinary tract infection. *Am J Radiol* 1985; 144:851.

Levitt SB, Kogan SJ, Schneider KM, et al: Endocrine tests in phenotypic children with bilateral impalpable testes can reliably predict 'congenital' anorchism. *Urology* 1978; 11:11.

Levy ML, Coakley CS: Survey of "in and out surgery"—first year. *South Med J* 1968; 61:995.

Latvak AS, Morris JA, McRoberts JW: Normal size of the urethral meatus in boys. *J Urol* 1976; 115:736.

Majd M, Belman AB: Nuclear cystography in infants and children. *Urol Clin North Am* 1979; 6:395.

Malek RS: Renal trauma. *Dial Pediatr Urol* 1980; 3(5):6.

Mason WG: Urinary tract infections in children: renal ultrasound evaluation. *Radiology* 1984; 153:109.

Mertz JHO, Widhard WN, Nourse MH, et al: Injury of the kidney in children. *JAMA* 1963; 183:730.

Morse TS: Pediatric outpatient surgery. *J Pediatr Surg* 1972; 7:283.

Murphy LJT: *The History of Urology*. Springfield, Ill, Charles C Thomas Publisher, 1972.

Nadelson EJ, Cohen M, Warner R, et al: Update: varicocelectomy—safe outpatient procedure. *Urology* 1984; 24:259.

Natof HE: Complications associated with ambulatory surgery. *JAMA* 1980; 244:1116.

Nicoll JH: The surgery of infancy. *Br Med J (Clin Res)* 1909; 2:753.

Othersen HB Jr, Clatworthy HW Jr: Outpatient herniorrhaphy for infants. *Am J Dis Child* 1968; 116:78.

Pais VM, Retik AB: Reversible hydronephrosis in the neonate with urinary sepsis. *N Engl J Med* 1975; 292:465.

Parkkulainen KV, Kosunen TU: Follow-up of female children treated for chronic or recurrent urinary tract infection. *Birth Defects* 1977; 13:409.

Perlmutter AD: Enuresis. In Harrison JH, Gittes RG, Perlmutter AD, et al (eds): *Campbell's Urology*. Philadelphia, WB Saunders Co, 1979, pp 1823-1834.

Petrillo M, Sanger S: *Emotional Care of Hospitalized Children*. Philadelphia, JB Lippincott Co, 1972, pp 19-33.

Poretz DM, Eron LJ, Goldenberg RI, et al: Intravenous antibiotic therapy in an outpatient setting. *JAMA* 1982; 248:336.

Powers TA, Stone WJ, Grove RB, et al: Radionuclide measurement of differential glomerular filtration rate. *Invest Radiol* 1981; 16:59.

Prugh DG, Staub EM, Sands HH, et al: A study of the emotional reactions of children and families to hospitalization and illness. *Am J Orthopsychiatry* 1953; 23:70.

Rabinowitz R: Update on outpatient pediatric urology. *Dial Pediatr Urol* 1982; 5(S):5.

Rabinowitz R: Outpatient management of hypospadias and the complications of repair. *Probs Urol* 1988; 2:109.

Rabinowitz R: Personal communication, 1990.

Rabinowitz R, Caldamone AA: Office and outpatient pediatric urology. In Kelalis PP, King LR, Belman AB (eds): *Clinical Pediatric Urology* ed 2. Philadelphia, WB Saunders Co. 1985, p 28.

Rabinowitz R, Takihara H, Consentino MJ, et al: Testicular volume measurement using a punched out elliptical orchiometer. *Soc Pediatr Urol Newslett* 1984; 7:4.

Rajfer J, Walsh PC: The incidence of intersexuality in patients with hypospadias and cryptorchidism. *J Urol* 1976; 116:769.

Ravitch MM: *A Century of Surgery*. Philadelphia, JB Lippincott Co, 1981.

Reed WA: The surgicenter experience. *Contemp Surg* 1982, 20:66.

Reed WA, Dawson B: The ambulatory surgical facility. In Schultz RC (ed): *Outpatient Surgery,* Philadelphia, Lea & Febiger, 1979, pp 15-24.

Reed WA, Ford JL: Development of an independent outpatient surgical center. *Int Anesth Clin* 1976; 14:113.

Reynolds PI, Rosen DA: Perioperative options in anesthesia: caudal analgesia for pediatric urologic procedures. *Dial in Pediatric Urol* 1990; 13(12):6-7.

Romberg R: *Circumcision: The Painful Dilemma.* South Hadley, Mass, Bergin and Garvey Publishers Inc, 1985.

Savage DCL, Wilson MI, Ross EM, et al: Asymptomatic bacteriuria in girl entrants to Dundee primary schools. *Br Med J (Clin Res)* 1969; 3:75.

Schultz RC: Outpatient surgery from antiquity to the present. In Schultz RC (ed): *Outpatient Surgery* Philadelphia, Lea & Febiger, 1979, pp 5-14.

Scott DB, Cousins MJ: Clinical pharmacology of local anesthetic agents. In Cousins MJ, Bridenbaugh PO (eds): *Neural Blockage in Clinical Anesthesia and Management of Pain.* Philadelphia, JB Lippincott Co, 1980, pp 86-121.

Shandling B, Steward DJ: Regional analgesia for postoperative pain in pediatric outpatient surgery. *J Pediatr Surg* 1980; 15:477.

Shelton TB, Noe HN: The role of excretory urography in patients with hypospadias. *J Urol* 1985; 134:97.

Shenfield O, Eldar L, Lotan G et al: Intraopeative irrigation with bupinvacaine for analgesic after orchidopexy and herniorrhapy in children. *J Urol* 1995, 153:185.

Shepard B, Hensle TW, Burbige KA, et al: Outpatient surgery in pediatric urology patient. *Urology* 1984; 24:581.

Shkolnk A: The role of ultrasound in pediatrics. *Pediatr Ann* 1980; 9:27.

Siegel AL, Snyder HM, Duckett JW: Outpatient pediatric urological surgery: techniques for a successful and cost-effective practice. *J Urol* 1986; 136:879.

Smellie J, Edwards D. Hunter N, et al: Vesico-ureteric reflux and renal scarring. *Kidney Int* 1975, 8(suppl 4):5.

Smith RM: Anesthesia for outpatient and emergency surgery. In *Anesthesia for Infants and Children,* ed 4. St Louis, Mosby, 1980, pp 510-521.

Stapleton FB, Roy S III, Noe HN, et al: Hypercalciuria in children with hematuria. *N Engl J Med* 1984; 310:1345.

Steward DJ: Experiences with an outpatient anesthesia service for children. *Anesth Analg* 1973; 52:877.

Steward DJ: Anaesthesia for paediatric out-patients. *Can Anaesth Sco J* 1980, 27:412.

Thrall JH, Kof SA, Keyes JW Jr: Diuretic radionuclide urography and scintigraphy in the differential diagnosis of hydronephrosis. *Semin Nucl Med* 1981, 11:89.

Thurm RH: Doctor Benjamin Waterhouse and the Boston Marine Hospital. *Ann Intern Med* 1972; 76:801.

Tudor JM, Carter OW, McClellan RE, et al: An analysis of 2403 consecutive pediatric urological consultations. *J Urol* 1962; 87:68.

vanGool J, Tanagho EA: External sphincter activity and recurrent urinary tract infections in girls. *Urology* 1977; 10:348.

Vaughan GF: Children in hospital. *Lancet* 1957; 1:1117.

Vernon DTA, Schulman JL, Foley JM: Changes in children's behavior after hospitalization: some dimensions of response and their correlates. *Am J Dis Child* 1966; 111:581.

Vlahakis E, Hartman GW, Kelalis PP: Comparison of voiding cystourethrography and expression cystourethrography. *J Urol* 1971; 106:414.

Wallerstein E: *Circumcision: An American Health Fallacy.* New York, Springer Publishing Co, 1980.

Walther PC, Kaplan GW: Cystoscopy in children: indications for its use in common urologic problems. *J Urol* 1979; 122:717.

Wangensteen OH, Wangensteen SD: *The Rise of Surgery from Empiric Craft to Scientific Discipline.* Minneapolis, University of Minnesota Press, 1978.

Wolcott MW (ed): *Ambulatory Surgery and the Basics of Emergency Surgical Care.* Philadelphia, JB Lippincott Co, 1981.

Zderic SA, Duckett JW: Adolescent urology. *AUA Update Series* 1994; 13(19):150.

CHAPTER 60

Pediatric Endourology

Gary J. Faerber
David A. Bloom

The Greek term endon, meaning *within,* is the source for *endo,* a nearly ubiquitous prefix in modern medical practice. Endourology is thus the operative manipulation of genitourinary structures within the body, in the absence of incisional access, using natural passageways (i.e., the urethra) or direct percutaneous techniques. Catheters, needles, electrical energy, and complex instruments are manipulated externally but function within the body. Endourology is viewed as a relatively recent technology, yet in reality urologic surgery, if not interventional medicine itself, most likely had its origins well before recorded medical history with endourologic access to a bladder obstructed by stone or stricture (Bloom et al., 1994). Upper tract endourology was performed repeatedly by Hillier begining in 1864 in a child with congenital hydronephrosis, but this brave intervention was hidden in the archives of the past century until recent resurrection (Bloom et al., 1989).

Cystoscopy

Max Nitze and Milhelm Diecke invented the first practical light cystoscope in Dresden, Germany, in 1877. From these humble beginnings to the present, great strides in technology have resulted in fiberoptics, miniaturization, flexible endoscopy, and video capabilities that have allowed the endoscopist to perform ever more diagnostic and therapeutic procedures which previously would have required open surgical intervention.

In the adult, cystourethroscopy is an essential tool in the evaluation of lower urinary tract pathology and its role is well defined. In children the role of cystourethroscopy in the evaluation and management of the lower urinary system is less well defined and has diminished as less invasive techniques have been developed.

Traditional pediatric cystoscopes with conventional lens telescopes are available in sizes from 7 F up to 13.5 F and are accompanied by various accessories such as grasping and biopsy forceps as well as electrodes for cautery, which can be placed through the working ports. Fiberoptic technology has produced infant and pediatric flexible cystoscopes with 7 F and 9 F outer diameters that have steerable distal tips that allow for easier and less traumatic visualization of the anterior bladder and dome. Neonatal and pediatric resectoscopes as small as 8.5 F can be fitted with various shaped cutting and cautery electrodes. These electrodes are used primarily in the endoscopic treatment of posterior urethral valves. In addition, various shaped cold cutting knives have been designed for the endoscopic treatment of urethral strictures.

Although pediatric cystourethroscopy technique is similar to that in the adult, certain caveats should be kept in mind. The urethra is so fragile and delicate that minimal trauma will easily result in injury and subsequent stricture. All instruments should be well lubricated, and negotiation of the urethra is best performed under direct visualization. If the cystoscope is passed with the obturator in place, it must be guided and not forced.

Pediatric cystoscopy usually requires general anesthesia. Infants can be placed in frog leg posture, whereas older children are placed in standard dorsolithotomy position. In addition to the endoscopic evaluation, the anesthetized child presents an opportunity for careful examination of the lower abdomen, the genital area (including vaginoscopy), and rectum.

Each age group has a normal range of urethral calibers. The male neonatal urethra will usually accept an 8 F or a 10 F instrument, whereas preadolescent boys can accept instruments of 13 F to 14 F. The urethral meatus is usually the narrowest portion of the male urethra (Allen et al., 1972; Litvak et al., 1976). The distal urethra is often overlooked, and therefore it is important to visualize the entire urethra either at the beginning of cystoscopy or at the termination of the procedure. Note should be made of any abnormalities such as lacuna magna, stricture, diverticulum, or polyp. Anterior valves in the fossa navicularis may cause strangury and stream disturbance. Visual inspection of the external sphincter and bladder neck should be carried out, and note should be made whether they are open or closed. The configuration of the verumontanum and prostatic utricle should also be appreciated. In males, inspection for urethral valves should be performed both with retrograde and antegrade flow of irrigant. In females, larger diameter instruments can be used because of the inherent elasticity and distensibility of the female urethra (Immergut and Wahman, 1968). Nevertheless, the smallest instrument necessary for adequate visualization should be passed. Once in the bladder note should be made of the characteristics of the content of the bladder (urine characteristics, presence of blood, calculi, foreign bodies), the appearance of the epithelium, configuration of the trigone, position, configuration and length of the ureteral orifices, and the approximate bladder capacity (Berger et al., 1983). One must be aggressive in looking for duplex orifices, even if unsuspected. Effluxing urine from the orifices should be also be observed.

Complications of cystourethroscopy are few. Infection is the most common, and therefore instrumented children are given preoperative antimicrobials. Infected urine is a relative contraindication to cystoscopy. Urethral injury (laceration, perforation, or formation of a false passage) is the result of traumatic instrumentation. Stricture formation can present early with stranguria, split stream, or decreased force of stream, or symptoms may not become apparent until years later. Bladder perforation from direct trauma from the cystoscope or because of overdistention of the bladder is uncommon. Irrigant fluid pressure should not exceed 60 cm H_2O. Bladder overdistention in small children has also been associated with arrhythmias and oxygen desaturation.

The relative indications for cystoscopy in children can be categorized into: urinary tract infection, vesicoureteral reflux, voiding dysfunction, and hematuria (Johnson et al., 1980; Walther and Kaplan, 1979). Gross hematuria in adults always warrants cystoscopic evaluation, but bloody urethral spotting or urethrorrhagia in children does not necessarily require cystoscopic evaluation (Kaplan and Brock, 1982). Urethrorrhagia lasting longer than 6 months, gross and microscopic hematuria of greater than 10 RBCs/HPF in the absence of infection, trauma, calculus disease, or other obvious causes should be evaluated (Brock, 1994). Recently we discovered a stage I transitional cell carcinoma in a 17-year-old boy with a history of gross hematuria. He also gave a history of regular marijuana use and had significant household exposure to cigarette smoke. We also discovered a transitional cell papilloma in a 7-year-old with bloody spotting.

Hensle described a bulbar urethral stricture in a 7-year-old boy who was asymptomatic with the exception of bloody spotting (Bloom and Hensle, 1992).

Children with uncomplicated urinary tract infection with both normal intravenous pyelogram or ultrasound and voiding cystourethrogram do not generally require cystoscopic evaluation. In some children with recurrent infections cystoscopy may be indicated. Routine cystoscopy to evaluate ureteral orifices in management of vesicoureteral reflux is no longer common practice. Recent studies indicate that lateral displacement and golf-hole configuration was the only significant prognostic indicator on cystoscopy. This finding was present in only 15% of grade IV VUR, therefore suggesting that cystoscopy looking at ureteric orifice configuration has no predictive value (Bellinger and Duckett, 1984; Mulcahy and Kelalis, 1978).

ENDOSCOPIC MANAGEMENT OF SPECIFIC LOWER GENITOURINARY PROBLEMS

The pediatric endoscopic equipment available today has improved substantially over the equipment available as recently as 15 years ago. It is, however, ironic that as instrumentation improved the indications for cystoscopy have diminished. Nonetheless specific conditions require not only cystoscopic evaluation but also the use of specially designed endoscopic equipment manufactured specifically for the treatment of these pathologic conditions. Pediatric resectoscopes have enabled primary early incision of posterior valves, thereby obviating vesicostomy or supravesical diversion. Several techniques are used, but all consist of incision of the valves with either a hook knife, a small Bugbee electrode, or a laser probe. Although usually performed retrograde via the urethra, endoscopic antegrade ablation via a suprapubic puncture can also be performed (Zaontz and Gibbons, 1984) (Fig. 60-1). This is especially useful for valve ablation in neonates with very small urethras in whom urethroscopy could result in subsequent stricture formation.

Urethral Stricture

Direct vision urethrotomy is the procedure of choice in the treatment of short discreet urethral stricture disease (Scherz and Kaplan, 1990; Scherz et al., 1988). Cold-knife internal urethrotomy is effective for short, weblike stricture disease. Faerber and associates successfully used a contact-tipped Nd:YAG laser to treat recurrent urethral strictures in a group of 12 boys who failed previous cold-knife internal urethrotomy (Faerber et al., 1994). Of the 12 boys, 10 have remained asymptomatic with no evidence of stricture recurrence. More extensive stricture disease has also been managed successfully by a combination of endoscopic incision and subsequent intermittent obturation (Noe, 1983).

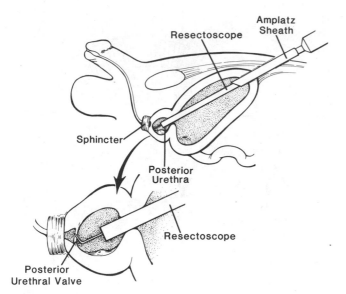

FIG. 60-1
Percutaneous antegrade approach to posterior urethral valves. This method is preferred in neonates with very narrow urethras through which urethroscopy is not possible.

Endoscopic Treatment of Vesicoureteral Reflux

Vesicoureteral reflux is present in 0.4% of the normal population (Bailey RR, 1988). Certain groups are at higher risk of having or developing VUR: dysfunctional voiders, neurogenic bladders, children with familial history of reflux, and patients with radiation or chemical cystitis (Chappel et al., 1990; Duckett, 1981; Kaplan, 1990; van Gool et al., 1992). At present results from the International Reflux Study for Children fail to show clear superiority of either medical or surgical management in dilating grades of reflux (Duckett, 1993). Surgical treatment might be preferred over medical therapy in younger children, noncompliant children, and in those children who because of geographic factors cannot be adequately followed. The standard open surgical treatments for vesicoureteral reflux all attempt correction of VUR by increasing the length of the intramural portion of the affected ureter. The same principle applies to the subureteral endoscopic injection of either polytetrafluoroethylene particles or collagen paste. Matouschek, in 1981, was the first to report use of Teflon for adults with vesicoureteral reflux (Matouschek, 1981). O'Donnell and Puri, and others, described successful use of Teflon to treat children with vesicoureteral reflux (Michael et al., 1993; O'Donnell and Puri, 1984; Walker, 1989). Recently, Puri and associates reported on the multicenter European study involving 4166 children with 6216 refluxing ureters who were treated with Teflon for vesicoureteral reflux. With more than 90% of the children with follow-up greater than 2 years, 95% of all ureters were cured or improved after two injections. Less than 0.3% of the treated ureters developed

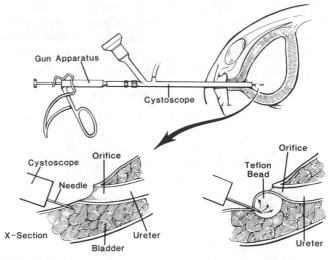

FIG. 60-2
Technique of submucosal Teflon injection to correct vesicoureteral reflux.

vesicoureteric obstruction requiring open reimplantation (Puri et al., 1995) (Fig. 60-2).

Polytef is a viscous suspension of Teflon particles in a glycerol solution and requiring the use of a special injection pistol and a 5 F Puri needle placed through a cystoscope with an offset lens. The needle is placed subepithelialy into the lamina propria at a position just proximal to the ureteral orifice. The Teflon paste is injected until the ureteral orifice is elevated and is deformed into a slitlike configuration. Correct needle placement is vital; if the needle is placed too deeply into the detrusor, no deformity will occur. If the needle is placed too superficially, the paste will rupture through the epithelium.

Although Teflon injection has proven efficacious, its safety has been questioned because of reports of local inflammatory tissue responses and suspected distant particle migration in experimental studies in which it has been injected into the urethras of monkeys and dogs (Malizia et al., 1984). Cross-linked bovine collagen is another injection agent of the treatment of vesicoureteral reflux. Unlike Teflon, glutaraldehyde-treated collagen paste is not nearly as viscous and is easily injected without the need for an injection pistol. Comparable results have been achieved with collagen, although long-term studies have not been completed (Borwka, 1991; Frey et al, 1992; Gearhart, 1990; Leonard et al., 1991). Unlike Teflon, collagen does not elicit the same granulomatous response in animals as Teflon (Canning et al., 1988). Gearhart performed a histologic evaluation of seven patients who underwent surgical reimplantation after failed endoscopic correction with collagen. There was only minimal inflammation and no evidence of a granulomatous response. More important, the presence of the collagen implant did not interfere with the subsequent ureterneocystostomy (Gearhart, 1990). The collagen implant was encapsulated by a fibrous capsule, and endogenous fibroblasts were found to be active in replacing the implant with human type I and III collagen (Frey et al., 1992).

Transurethral Incision of Ureterocele

Single and duplex ureteroceles can be successfully managed endoscopically (Fig. 60-3). This technique is particularly advantageous in the neonate who may require immediate decompression. Tank reported on 40 patients who underwent transurethral unroofing of a ureterocele, and of the 40, half demonstrated improved function, while only four patients developed reflux requiring surgical correction (Tank, 1986). Blyth and associates reported successful decompression and preservation of upper pole function in greater than 95% of children who underwent endoscopic incision of intravesical ureteroceles. Incision of extravesical ureteroceles resulted in decompression and preservation of upper pole function approximately half the time. Reflux resulted in approximately 50% of the incised extravesical ureteroceles necessitating a secondary procedure (Blyth et al., 1993).

Endoscopic Injection Therapy for Urinary Incontinence

Murless in 1938 first described sclerosing agent injection into the anterior vaginal wall of incontinent women to develop an inflammatory response that would compress the incompetent urethra (Murless, 1938). Since that time several other injectable agents have been used for female stress urinary incontinence. Injectable materials are thought to work by increasing outflow resistance and urethral coaptation. Politano and others reported successful outcomes with the periurethral injection of Teflon (Lockhart et al., 1988; Politano, 1978; Vessey et al., 1988). Vorstman and associates reported on 11 children ages 6 months to 16 years with urinary incontinence who were treated with Teflon injection (Vorstman et al., 1985). With a mean follow-up of 5 years, eight of the 11 showed cure or improvement. The only complication was a perineal abscess requiring incision and drainage. The complications of granuloma formation and alleged metastatic particle migration have limited the widespread use of Teflon (Claes et al., 1989). Shortliffe and associates and others have demonstrated the effectiveness of periurethral collagen for female stress urinary incontinence (Appel, 1990; McGuire et al., 1990; Shortliffe et al., 1989). McGuire postulated that collagen injection therapy would be effective for any patient with intrinsic sphincter deficiency (McGuire, 1990). Wan and colleagues reported on the use of collagen in eight children with incontinence. All had neurogenic bladders and dysfunctional bladder necks and were treated

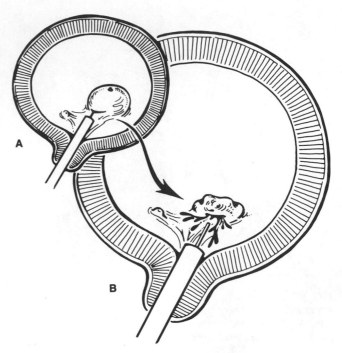

FIG. 60-3
A and **B,** Technique of endoscopic incision of ureterocele for decompression of ipsilateral hydronephrosis.

with intermittent catheterization (Wan et al., 1992). With a relatively short median follow-up of less than a year, five were cured, and two were improved for an overall success rate of 88%. Reports of long-term follow-up of patients treated with collagen for stress incontinence are lacking; however, Faerber and colleagues reported that women treated with collagen for stress incontinence appeared to retain their immediate posttreatment continence even after a median follow-up of more than 3 years (Faerber et al., 1994). This late failure might be anticipated due to resorption of the collagen and/or the carrier medium or shifting of the collagen once placed. The latter explanation coincides with our disappointing results in the pediatric myelomeningocele patients who are on intermittent catheterization. Repeated catheterization results in deformation of the collagen implant and decreased coaptation. Another explanation for late failures may be secondary to extrusion of the collagen paste from the injection site. Extrusion of the implant via the injection sites has occurred as late as a month postinjection. The development of newer types of implantable collagen will hopefully obviate these problems.

PERCUTANEOUS NEPHROSTOMY

Although Goodwin in 1995 was credited with the first therapeutic percutaneous nephrostomy, the earliest report of successful therapeutic puncture of a hydronephrotic kidney should be credited to Thomas

TABLE 60-1

Indications for Percutaneous Nephrostomy in Children

Antegrade Imaging
Pressure-perfusion testing (Whitaker)
Decompression of obstructed kidney
Percutaneous manipulation (e.g., extraction of renal calculi, incision of ureteropelvic junction obstruction, dilation of ureteral stricture)
Antegrade irrigation (fungus ball, chemolysis of upper tract stones)

From Doucnias R, Smith AD, Brock WA: Urol Clin North Am 17:419, 1990.

Hillier in 1864 (Bloom et al., 1989; Goodwin et al., 1955). Regardless of when percutaneous nephrostomy was described, it has now become a vital and commonplace method for the treatment of upper tract pathology. Percutaneous nephrostomy has been successfully performed in the pediatric age group from the fetus through the adolescent (Elder, 1990; Elder and Duckett, 1988; Stanley and Diament, 1986). The indications for percutaneous nephrostomy tubes are listed (Table 60-1). By far the most common indication for percutaneous catheter placement is temporary decompression of an obstructed kidney.

General anesthesia is required for infants and children, and access can be obtained with the aid of fluoroscopy or ultrasound. Stanley and Diament recommend 8 F pigtail catheters for children older than 2 years of age and a 6 F catheter for children less than 2 years of age (Stanley and Diament, 1986). They also recommended that infants be drained with 4 F tubes, but we find these smaller tubes are more likely to kink, obstruct, or become dislodged. All tubes in children regardless of age should be secured adequately, which includes suturing the catheter directly to the skin. Larger tubes may be necessary to ensure adequate drainage if the urine is purulent, bloody, or particulate.

The complication rate of percutaneous nephrostomy in the pediatric population is approximately 4%, which is similar to that seen in the adult population (Ball et al., 1986; Pfister et al., 1983; Stanley and Diament, 1986). Bleeding and sepsis were the most common and composed more than half of the major complications. Tube displacement is a particular problem in infants and small children, and special attention to securing the tube is necessary to prevent this complication (Riedy and Lebowitz, 1986).

Whitaker Test (Pressure-flow Study)

Since Whitaker introduced the pressure-flow study in 1973 to assess obstruction in hydronephrotic kidneys, it has become a valuable aid in the evaluation of equivocal urinary tract obstruction (Whitaker, 1973, 1978). Bladder pressure must be measured simulta-

neously and the intravesical pressures subtracted from the renal pelvic pressures to prevent a false-positive result (Mayo and Ansell, 1980). Optimally, bladder pressure can be negated by performing the study with an indwelling Foley catheter.

PERCUTANEOUS NEPHROLITHOTRIPSY

The first to perform percutaneous nephrolithotomy in children was Woodside and associates in 1985 (Woodside et al., 1985). They described the successful removal of renal stones in seven children between the ages of 5 and 18 years employing the same techniques used in adults. Since that time numerous others have documented their experience with percutaneous stone removal in children. Success rates defined as stonefree ranged from 67% to 100% with complication rates similar to those seen in adult series of percutaneous nephrolithotomy. The technique of percutaneous access in children is essentially the same as that used in adults.

PERCUTANEOUS ENDOPYELOTOMY

Surgical correction of ureteropelvic junction obstruction has primarily consisted of open pyeloplasty employing several different surgical techniques to reconfigure the UPJ. Scardino and Scardino reviewed the results of greater than 20 series of pyeloplasties in children and reported a success rate greater than 90% (Scardino and Scardino, 1981). Currently the most popular open technique is the one decribed by Anderson and Hynes (Anderson and Hynes, 1949). With the advent of percutaneous technique several authors described incision of an ureteropelvic junction obstruction performed in conjunction with nephrolithotomy (Segura, 1984; Wickham and Kellet, 1983; Witfield et al., 1983). The rationale for endoscopic incision of a ureteropelvic junction obstruction is based on the pioneering work of Davis. He observed with a longitudinal strip of ureter containing all components of the ureter would result in complete full-thickness regeneration around a stenting catheter (Davis, 1958; Davis et al., 1948). Endopyelotomy is essentially a Davis intubated ureterotomy (Davis, 1943). The earliest series of endopyelotomies were performed on adults with success rates from 60% to 100% (Badlani et al., 1986; Brannan et al., 1988; Korth et al., 1988; Ramsay et al., 1984; Van Cangh et al., 1989). In 1984 King and associates were the first to describe endopyelotomy in children (King et al., 1984). Several others have reported results with endopyelotomy in children as young as 11 weeks of age. Success rates ranged from 50% to 83% (Table 60-2). Secondary strictures or primary strictures that are short in length appear to be more successfully managed by endopyelotomy than do long strictures or secondary strictures present for more than 7 months.

TABLE 60-2

Results of Pediatric Endopyelotomy

Authors	Patients (age range)	Success	Follow-up
King et al., 1984	2 (1 year-4 year)	1/2 (50%)	18 months
Kavoussi et al., 1991	4 (6.5 weeks-5.5 years)	4/4 (100%)	18-36 months
Towbin et al., 1987	3 (11-18 years)	2/3 (67%)	10-27 months
Faerber et al., in press	5 (11 months-4 years)	4/5 (80%)	2.5 years
Rich and Smith, 1991	10 (11 weeks-18 years)	8/10 (80%)	—
Tan et al., 1993	17 (4 months-16 years)	13/17 (77%)	15 months
Total	41	32/41 (78%)	

King LR, et al: *J Urol* 1984; 131:1167.
Kavoussi LR, et al: *J Urol* 1991; 145:345.
Towbin RB, et al: *Radiology* 1987; 163:381.
Faerber GJ, et al: *J Urol*, in press.
Rich MA and Smith AD: Pediatric endourology In Gillenwater JY, Grayhack JT, Howards SS, Duckett JW (eds.): *Adult and pediatric urology*. Mosby–Year Book, St. Louis, MO 1991; 2343-2366.
Tan HL, et al: *Eur Urol* 1993; 24:84.

Complications from endopyelotomy include bleeding, either secondary to access or inadvertent incision of an unidentified aberrant crossing vessel at the UPJ, urinary tract infection, or restricture. Although restricture formation usually occurs early after removal of the stent, Tan and associates reported restenosis 6 months following endopyelotomy (Tan et al., 1993). Factors implicated in failure include high insertion, presence of a crossing lower pole vessel, long strictures, and a redundant renal pelvis (Carson, 1992; Van Cangh et al., 1989).

Endopyelotomy in the pediatric age group appears to have a limited role. Open pyeloplasty can be performed through a small cosmetically appearing incision, this time not warranted in the young child with primary UPJ obstruction, especially because open pyeloplasty is so successful. Antegrade endopyelotomy may play a role in treatment of secondary UPJ obstruction after a failed open pyeloplasty in the infant or young child (Faerber et al., 1995). In the adolescent endopyelotomy may be considered as a viable treatment alternative even for primary ureteropelvic junction obstruction. Time, however, will tell us whether this new endourologic technique can stand up to the rigors of clinical trials and experience.

PEDIATRIC URETEROSCOPY

In 1929 Young reported the first case of ureteroscopy in a child with posterior urethral valves (Young and McKay, 1929). Employing the standard cystoscopic equipment of the day, he was easily able to negotiate the patulous ureteral orifices and advance the cystoscope up the dilated ureter. Beginning in the mid 1980s and continuing to the present, refinements in instrumentation have allowed ureteroscopy to become commonplace in adult urology. Ureteroscopy in the pediatric age group is less common of a procedure, because the main indication for ureteroscopy, ureteral

calculus disease, is less common. Ritchey and associates reported the first successful lithotripsy and removal of a distal ureteral calculus in a 4-year-old boy using an 8.5 F ureteroscope (Ritchey et al., 1988). Since then, others have described their experience with ureteroscope stone extraction in children. Approximately 90% of cases resulted in successful treatment of the ureteral calculus (Caione et al., 1990; Itill et al., 1990; Thomas et al., 1993) (Tables 60-3 and 60-4).

Complications related to ureteroscopy in the pediatric age group are similar to those reported in the adult population, with ureteral perforation and avulsion being the most common. The ureteral musculature is less developed in children than in adults, and therefore great attention to technique is paramount to prevent ureteral perforation during endoscopic manipulation (Fig. 60-4). Also, the possibility of avulsion at the UPJ is theoretically higher in children than in adults because of the relative paucity of ureteral muscle bulk in this area, and therefore ureteroscopy of the upper third of the ureter should be performed only by experienced ureteroscopists.

Urinary tract infection, while accounting for as much as 25% of the complications reported in adult series, has not been shown to be a common complication of pediatric ureteroscopy (Sosa and Vaughan, 1988). Ureteral stricture following ureteroscopy has also been reported in adults, but this sequelae of ureteroscopy has not been reported in children (Banner et al., 1983). Another potential complication is injury to the urethra in small boys and the subsequent formation of urethral stricture. While Thomas and associates reported no adverse sequelae (vesicoureteral reflux, ureteral stricture) after dilation of the ureter to 15 F prior to ureteroscopy, others have cautioned against dilation for fear of inducing reflux (Caione et al., 1990; Hill et al., 1990; Thomas et al., 1993). Low-

TABLE 60-3

Small-Diameter Rigid Ureteroscopes Suitable for Pediatric Ureteroscopy

Company	Size of Tip (F)	Length of Endoscope (cm)	Accessory Channel (F)	Lens (degrees)
Circon ACMI	6.9	33 or 41	3.4, 2.3	5
Karl Storz Endoscopy-America	7	34 or 43	3.5	0
	9.5	34 or 43	2, 5	0
	12.5	43	6	6
Olympus Corp.	6.6	40	2.1, 2.1	0
	8	40	2.1, 3.6	0
	10.9	35	5.5	7
	11.9	35	4.5, 3.5	7
Wolf Corp.	6	32.5 or 42.5	3.3	0
	7	43	4.8	5
	7.5	32.5 or 42.5	4	10
Applied Urology, Inc.	5.5	33	2.3	5
	6.9	33	3.7	5
Candela Laser Corp.	7.2	41	3.2, 1.8	5
Bard Urological Division	8.3	35	4	0

Circon ACMI, Stamford, CT.
Karl Storz Endoscopy-America, Culver City, CA.
Olympus Corp., Lake Success, NY.
Wolf Corp., Chicago, IL.
Applied Urology, Inc., Laguna Hills, CA.
Candela Laser Corp., Wayland, MA.
Bard Urological Division, Covington, GA.

TABLE 60-4

Summary of Results of Ureteroscopic Stone Extraction in Children

Number of children	27
Age range (years)	3-14
Location of stone	
Mid ureter	5
Distal ureter	22
Ureteroscope used	
8.5 F	6 procedures
11.5 F	13 procedures
7.5 F	9 procedures
Method used to treat calculus	
Basket retrievel	13
Basket + EHL	2
Basket + laser	1
Ultrasonic lithotripsy	8
EHL + Ultrasonic lithotrispy	4
Technically able to perform ureteroscopy	27/27 (100%)
Technically able to treat calculus	24*/27 (89%)
Complications	
Vesicoureteral reflux	1 patient

*One patient had proximal migration of stone and subsequently underwent ESWL, two procedures were aborted secondary to equipment malfunction.
Caione P, et al: *J Urol* 1990; 144:484-485.
Thomas R, et al: *J Urol* 1993; 149:1082-1084.
Hill DE, et al: *J Urol* 1990; 144:481-483.

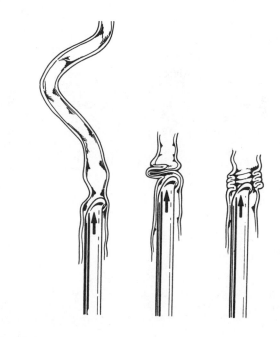

FIG. 60-4
The intrinsically smaller diameter lumen of the ureter in a child increases the risk of perforation or avulsion if the endoscopist attempts to force the scope beyond a narrowed portion in the ureter. (From Carson CC III: Complications of ureteroscopy. In Paulson DF, Carson CC, (eds): *Problems in urology.* JB Lippincott, Philadelphia, PA, 1992; 6:307-322.)

grade reflux has been reported even by experienced endoscopists who did not predilate (Hill, 1990; Hill et al., 1990).

With the development of extracorporeal shock wave lithotripsy (ESWL) and its high success rates of treating in situ distal ureteral stones, controversy now exists as to what is the optimal therapy for distal ureteral stones in adults: ureteroscopic stone removal or ESWL. The same dilemma exists when discussing optimal therapy for distal ureteral stones in children. ESWL is less invasive, often times does not require the use of a stent, is less time-consuming, less technically demanding, but has a slightly higher failure rate than ureteroscopy. Both procedures in children require general anesthesia regardless of whether ESWL is performed with an HM3 lithotriptor or any of the newer so-called anesthesia-free machines. Ureteroscopy in children with urolithiasis may be best reserved for mid or distal ureteral calculi that have not been successfully treated initially with ESWL.

PEDIATRIC ESWL

Although by definition ESWL is not an endourologic technique, it could be described as the ultimate in "minimally-invasive surgery" and has certainly revolutionized the surgical treatment of urolithiasis.

Christian Chaussy in 1980 reported the first successful fragmentation of a stone using electrically generated, focused shock waves (Chaussy et al., 1982). Thus was born the era of extracorporeal shock wave lithotripsy. A multitude of studies revealed that ESWL was a safe and efficacious method of treating urolithiasis in the adult population. It was not until later that several investigators found that ESWL in children appeared to be safe and effective as it was in the adult population (see Table 60-5) (Bohle et al., 1989; Frick et al., 1988; Kramolowsky et al., 1987; Krovand et al., 1987; Marberger et al., 1989; Nijman et al., 1989; Mininberg et al., 1988; Newman et al., 1986; Sigman et al., 1987; Wilbert et al., 1988).

Virtually all children require general anesthesia regardless of whether they are being treated on an older generation lithotriptor or one of the newer so-called anesthesia-free machines. Modification of the gantry or the use of a Stryker frame is usually necessary to treat all but the oldest of children (Kroovand et al., 1987; Wiatrak et al., 1991).

Complications from EWSL for renal or ureteral lithiasis in children have been few. The theoretic problem of passing fragments through the smaller diameter urinary system has not been realized. In fact, children seem to pass their fragments more easily than adults. Whereas almost all children will develop skin bruis-

TABLE 60-5

Summary of ESWL Results in Children

	Number of Pts	Age (years)	Number of Treatments	Stone Free at 3 Months	Shock Waves (Average)	Kv
Kramalowsky (HM3)	14	3-17	16 (2 bilat)	11/14	600-2400 (1250)	
Kroovand (HM3)	18	3-20	28 (2 bilat) (6 retreat.)	15/18	700-2850 (1800)	18-24 (21)
Sigman (HM3)	38	1-16		27/38	268-2000 (1295)	15-24 (18)
Mininberg (HM3)	17	3-17	19 (1 bilat) (1 retreat.)	9/17	600-2000 (1720)	18-24
Newman (HM3)	15	3-17	18 (3 bilat)	10/15	250-2000 (960)	18-24
Frick (HM3)	14	2-14	18	12/14	300-1000 (840)	15-18
Wilbert (HM3)	21	6-18	24		(1020)	18-23
Bohle (HM3)	24	3-16		22/24	330-2000 (950)	16
Nijman (HM3)	73	2-18	111	58/73		
Wilbert (Lithostar)	13	2-16	16		(1330)	16-20
Marberger	22	4 mo.-14	42	21/22	200-10,800	
Overall	235			185/235 (79%)		

ing, perirenal hematoma formation is very rare. Newman found no correlation between hematoma formation and the number of shock waves delivered or the applied energy (Newman, 1987). Permanent renal injury, while a theoretic risk, has not been substantiated in humans. Early reports of ESWL-induced hypertension in adults have not been substantiated (Lingeman and Kulb, 1987). Hypertension in children has not been reported, although early reports of ESWL in children did not specifically address this issue. Marberger, however, witnessed no hypertension in 22 children treated with the piezoelectric lithotriptor (Marberger et al., 1989). Thomas and colleagues found that no significant effect on renal function or renal growth in children treated with ESWL (Thomas et al., 1992). Most investigators advocate decreasing applied energy delivered by decreasing the kilovoltage. Two potential concerns regarding treatment of distal ureteral calculi with ESWL are the effects of shock waves on the female reproductive system and on developing bone. McCullough and associates found no deleterious structural or functional effects of shock waves on rat ovaries (McCullough et al., 1989). Vieweg and associates retrospectively studied 84 females treated with ESWL for distal ureteral calculi. They found no adverse effect on female fertility and no increased teratogenic risk (Vieweg et al., 1992). Longitudinal studies comparing fertility rates of women who were treated with ESWL for distal ureteral calculi while premenarcheal with controls will be required to answer the question of whether there is an adverse effect on developing ovaries in female children. Yeaman studied the effects of shock waves on the structure and growth of the immature rat epiphysis and found significant growth plate dysplasia and in some cases cessation of bone growth (Yeaman et al., 1989), while Kroovand found no adverse effects in experimental animals (Kroovand, 1992). ESWL appears to be a safe, noninvasive, and effective modality for the treatment of upper urinary calculi in the treatment of childhood urolithiasis. Although extensive data are not yet available there appear to be few significant long-term sequelae in children treated with this technique.

ENDOSCOPIC MANAGEMENT OF CONTINENT POUCH CALCULI

Calculus formation following creation of a continent urinary diversion is a well-known complication with a reported incidence ranging from 3% to 33% (Burbige and Hensle, 1986; Hendren and Hendren, 1990; Skinner et al., 1984). The majority of stones found within a reservoir are composed of struvite and typically form on the surface of exposed nonabsorbable staples used to create the reservoir (Hensle and Dean, 1991).

Most stones in patients with continent diversions can be managed endoscopically. Small stones less than 5 mm in size can be grasped and removed intact. Larger stones often require fragmentation using either ultrasonic, electrohydraulic, or laser lithotripsy prior to removal. It is imperative that all the fragments be removed to prevent subsequent regrowth of these calculi.

Appendiceal or ureteral conduits limit the size of instrument that can be placed into the reservoir via the efferent limb to treat reservoir calculi (Cendron and Gearhart, 1991). Faerber and associates reported successful removal of stones from a continent ileocecocystoplasty urinary reservoir via supravesicle percutaneous tract (Faerber et al., 1992). A suprapubic tract was created and subseqently dilated so that a nephroscope could be used to ultrasonically fragment and remove all the calculi. The tract closed within 7 days of its creation with no subsequent complication. Others have also reported successful percutaneous extraction of bladder calculi from augmented bladders in which the urethra was closed (Colberg et al., 1993). Successful percutaneous removal of large calculi from continent colonic neobladders has also been described (Sutherland et al., 1993; Seaman et al., 1994). Large calculi may still require open surgical removal (Blyth et al., 1992).

PEDIATRIC LAPAROSCOPY

Laparoscopy and peritoneoscopy describe the intracorporeal examination and manipulation of visceral structures with instruments controlled extracorporeally. Nitze's cystoscope of 1877 and Edison's incandescent lamp of 1880 was combined in a device that made endoscopy and laparoscopy feasible. Kelling in 1901 described the technique of celioscopy, whereby in dogs he inspected the abdominal viscera using a cystoscope after having insufflated the abdominal cavity with air (Kelling, 1923). In 1910, Jacobaeus utilized a cystoscope for thoracoscopy and peritoneoscopy with air insufflation in more than 40 patients with cirrhosis, tuberculosis, and various neoplasms (Ruddock, 1937; Winfield et al., 1991). Not until 1976 when Cortesi described the location of nonpalpable testes by peritoneoscopy, as he preferred to call it, did laparoscopy find a role in the treatment of urologic disease (Cortesi et al., 1976). Nonetheless, aside from gynecologic application, laparoscopy remained a peripheral modality until its role in cholecystectomy proved it as safe and efficacious as open surgery. Simultaneously, an explosion of new laparoscopic instrumentation facilitated the interest in this and other minimally invasive methods of surgery.

Indications for Pediatric Laparoscopy

In 1991 Winfield and colleagues recognized more than 20 urologic applications of laparoscopic surgery

(Winfield et al., 1991). Whereas many open surgical procedures can be performed laparoscopically, it is contestable which urologic conditions are best served by laparoscopy. The real and potential advantages of laparoscopy over open surgery appear to be shortened hospital stay, less postoperative morbidity and pain, and quicker return to normal activity. Children, however, require less postoperative analgesia, have shorter hospital stays, and return to normal activity faster than adults having the same surgical procedure.

Technique of Pediatric Laparoscopy

Laparoscopy is performed with the patient under general anesthesia with the abdomen, groin, scrotum, and upper thigh regions prepped to facilitate laparotomy, if necessary. The bladder is emptied prior to laparoscopy to prevent inadvertent bladder injury. An indwelling urethral catheter is necessary for prolonged procedures. An orogastric tube decompresses the stomach prior the needle placement and peritoneal insufflation. The arms are tucked at the side to prevent brachial plexus injury. The field is prepared widely enough for open abdominal exploration. It is important that the child be firmly affixed to the table to prevent inadvertent shifting during movement of the table.

A small semilunar incision is made along the inferior or superior border of the umbilicus and the fascia scored. The periumbilical skin is grasped and held upward while the needle is advanced at 45 degrees angled caudad. With proper placement of the needle, there is a slight "pop" as the needle pierces the fascia and then another less pronounced one as the peritoneum is entered. Once the needle is placed, proper positioning is verified by instilling a few milliliters of saline solution through the needle. No resistance to injection and no return of the saline solution with aspiration indicates proper placement. Another effective method of verifying proper position is placing a drop of saline solution in the hub of the Veress needle. With opening of the stopcock or lifting of the abdominal wall, the drop should flow into the abdominal cavity. If there is resistance to injection, return of saline solution with aspiration, or if the drop test is negative, improper needle placement is suspected and the needle repositioned. An alternative to using the Veress needle is the open Hasson technique, whereby a small peritonotomy is made and, under direct vision, the trocar is introduced into the abdominal cavity (Hasson, 1974). Opening insufflation pressures are usually less than 5 mm Hg, but if one encounters higher pressures or there is an abrupt rise of pressure during filling, insufflation should be terminated immediately. The needle should be repositioned and rechecked. Tympany over the liver in the right upper quadrant is a reliable sign that proper insufflation is occurring. The abdominal cavity should distend symmetrically. Insufflation with CO_2 is continued until the intraabdominal pressure is 15 to 20 mm Hg, at which time the Verres needle is removed and the appropriate sized trocar and laparoscope is inserted. In most children 1.5 to 3.0 L is required for insufflation. A 5 mm laparoscope is usually sufficient for diagnosis laparoscopy; however, a larger trocar and scope and additional ports are necessary if more complicated procedures are anticipated. Children are more esthenic than adults, and therefore the retroperitoneal structures are in closer proximity to the anterior abdominal wall. The pediatric laparoscopist should be cognizant of the potential for inadvertent trocar-related injury to retroperitoneal structures, and strict attention is maintained with needle and trocar placement (Fig.

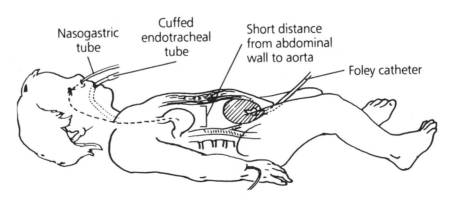

FIG. 60-5
Pediatric laparoscopy. Nasogastric tube placed for gastric decompression and Foley catheter allows for drainage of the bladder. Proper Veress needle placement is very important in children because of the close proximity of the aorta to the anterior abdominal wall. (From Kavoussi LR: Pediatric applications of laparoscopy. In Clayman RV, McDougall EM (eds): *Laparoscopic urology.* Quality Medical Publishing, St. Louis, MO 1993, pp 209-224.)

60-5). Elevation of the abdominal wall can be further facilitated by placing sutures in the fascia and holding onto these sutures as each trocar is introduced. Also, it is helpful to make a small nick in the fascia prior to placement of the trocar. Once placed, a telescope is inserted and the intraabdominal contents inspected. A video monitoring system allows visualization for the other members of the operating room team. Diagnostic laparoscopy usually requires approximately 10 mm Hg pressure, but more complex procedures require higher intraabdominal pressures and flow rates that are more easily obtained with a 10/11 mm cannula. If working ports are necessary, they are placed under direct vision.

At the completion of diagnostic or operative laparoscopy, the intraabdominal pressure is lowered and the surgical sites and port sites inspected carefully for bleeding. Trocar sheaths are removed sequentially under vision and fascial defects closed with absorbable interrupted sutures. The skin is closed with subcuticular sutures.

Hernia

Whereas laparoscopic hernia repair in adults has some justification, routine laparoscopic hernia repair in children has little to recommend it. Conventional pediatric herniorrhaphy is minimally invasive as it is and can be performed quickly, safely, and accurately. Endoscopy still may have a place in this condition as Chu and colleagues reported in 1993. They reported laparoscopic inspection of the contralateral internal inguinal ring through the patent procesus vaginalis of the operated side. This technique allowed accurate determination of whether to explore the asymptomatic opposite side in patients with inguinal hernias (Chu, 1993).

Nonpalpable testicle

Cryptorchid testes occur in approximately 3% to 5% of newborn boys (Berkokwitz et al., 1985). Prematurity, low birth weight, small size for gestational age, familial history of cryptorchidism, and concomitant associated abnormalities such as hypospadias, myelomeningocele, and midline neurofacial defects are associated with higher incidence of cryptorchid testes (Czeizel et al., 1981; Grossman and Pire, 1968; Kropp and Voeller, 1981). The majority of undescended testes are in the superficial inguinal pouch or canalicular. The term nonpalpable testis should be reserved only when the gonad remains impalpable despite a deliberate set of diagnostic maneuvers: examination in a warm room under calm conditions, milking the testicle down from the internal ring, and using lubricating jelly or soap to reduce tactile friction. Nonpalpable testes comprise from 5% to 28% of undescended

testes. The optimal method of diagnosis has been the subject of debate (Bloom, 1992; Saw et al., 1992; Walker, 1992). Radiologic localization employing ultrasonography, computed tomography, or magnetic resonance imaging of a nonpalpable testis incurs significant cost without significant enhancement of the treatment of cryptorchid boys (Hrebinko and Bellinger, 1993). Venography is successful in localization of a nonpalpable testis for 75% of patients but requires sedation or anesthesia and is technically demanding. Laparoscopy alone or in conjunction with inguinal exploration is a reliable method for localization of a nonpalpable testis (Table 60-6 and Fig. 60-6) (Jordan, 1993; Walker, 1993).

Diagnostic laparoscopy for nonpalpable testis is performed through a 5 mm sheath. The median umbilical ligament is identified. The vas deferens is found where it crosses the ligament, and it is then followed laterally to the internal inguinal ring (Fig. 60-7). If the vas deferens and the spermatic vessels enter the inguinal ring, one can conclude that a testis had descended at some point in time. A normal testis or an atretic remnant will probably be present distally (Fig. 60-8). In either case inguinal exploration is indicated; a viable testis is brought down into a dependent portion of the ipsilateral hemiscrotum, or gonadal remnants are removed (Jordan and Bloom, 1994). When spermatic cord structures enter into the inguinal ring, inguinal exploration is warranted regardless of whether the ring is open or closed. Germ cells were found in 9% to 13% of boys explored who were found at the time of inguinal exploration to have gonadal remnants (Rozanski et al., in press; Scherz and Kaplan, 1994).

If the vas deferens and spermatic vessels terminate in a scar prior to entering the internal ring, this is consistent with the vanished testis syndrome. The laparoscopic procedure can be terminated, and subsequent inguinal exploration is not necessary. A canalicular or "peeping" testis is identified by placing gentle pressure on the external canal and can usually

TABLE 60-6

Laparoscopic Findings in 115 Patients at the University of Michigan

	Number of Patients	Right	Left	Bilateral
Attenuated vessels	52	16	30	6
Missed low testes	25	10	10	5
Abdominal testes	31	11	12	8
No vessels	5	—	5	—
Transverse testicular ectopia	2	1	1	—

(From Jordan GH, Bloom DA: Laparoendoscopic Genitourinary Surgery in Children. In Laparoscopic Surgery. Gomella LG, Kozminski M, Winfield HN, (eds), New York, 1994, Raven Press.)

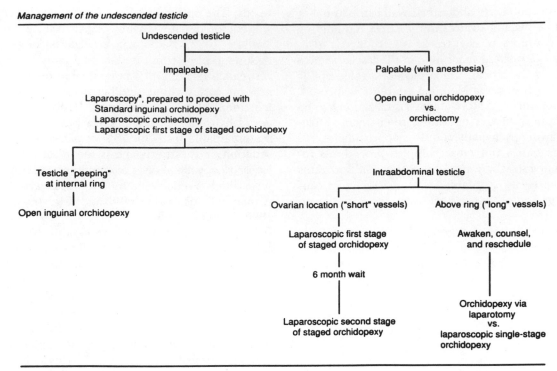

Management of the undescended testicle

* If testicle grossly abnormal at laparoscopy, proceed with laparoscopic orchiectomy.

FIG. 60-6
Algorithm for the Management of the Undescended Testicle. From Jordan GH, Bloom DA: Laparoendoscopic Genitourinary Surgery in Children. In Gomella LG, Kozminski M, Winfield HN (eds): *Laparoscopic surgery,* 1994.

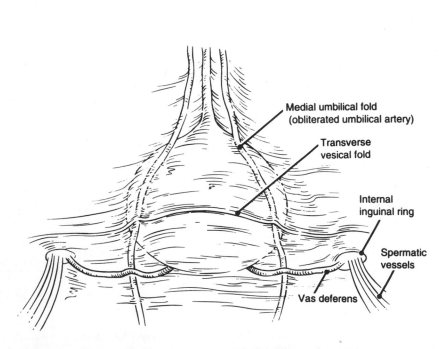

FIG. 60-7
View of the pediatric male pelvis during diagnostic laparoscopy and the important landmarks that should be readily identified. (From Bloom DA, Ritchey ML, Manzoni G: Laparoscopy for the nonpalpable testis. In Holcomb GW III (ed): *Pediatric endoscopic surgery.* Appleton and Lange, Norwalk, Conn., 1994, pp 41-50.)

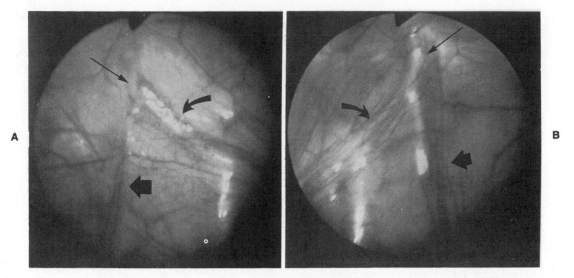

FIG. 60-8
Blind-ending spermatic vessels on the left side in a boy with a nonpalpable left testis and a normal right testis. **A,** Left side: Spermatic vessels *(short thick arrow)* end above the closed internal inguinal ring *(thin arrow)*. Normal vas deferens *(curved arrow)*. **B,** Right side: Normal spermatic vessels *(short thick arrow)* cross into internal ring *(thin arrow)* adjacent to vas deferens *(curved arrow)*. (From Bloom DA, Ritchey ML, Manzoni G: Laparoscopy for the nonpalpable testis. In Holcomb GW III (ed): *Pediatric endoscopic surgery.* Appleton and Lange, Norwalk, Conn., 1994, pp 41-50.)

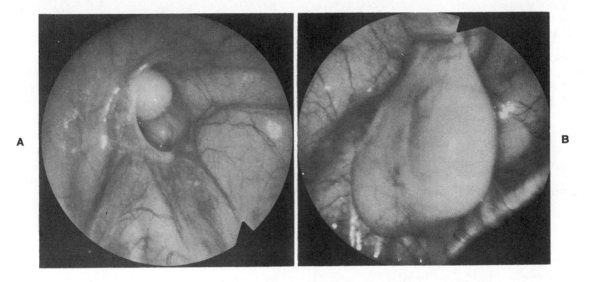

FIG. 60-9
A, A "peeping testis" at the internal ring. Laparoscopic demonstration of a peeping testis can be elicited by slight external compression of the inguinal canal. **B,** Laparoscopic view of a true intraabdominal testis. (From Bloom DA, Ritchey ML, Manzoni G: Laparoscopy for the nonpalpable testis. In Ed Holcomb GW III (ed): *Pediatric endoscopic surgery.* Appleton and Lange, Norwalk, Conn., 1994, pp 41-50.)

be managed with standard inguinal orchiopexy (Fig. 60-9). True intraabdominal testes may require several different approaches depending on the normalcy of the testis, the length of the cord structures, and the mobility of the testis. Orchiectomy is a logical choice in postpubertal boys or when the testis is grossly abnormal. Laparoscopic orchiectomy may be performed at the time of initial diagnostic laparoscopy (Castilho

et al., 1992; Jordan and Bloom, 1994). Laparoscopically assisted staged Fowler-Stevens orchiopexy has been described where the spermatic vessels are clipped. After an interval of 6 months or more, the testis is mobilized on its vasoperitoneal pedicle and brought down into a scrotal position (Bloom, 1991). Jordan described primary laparoscopic orchiopexy whereby the gubernaculum is divided, the spermatic

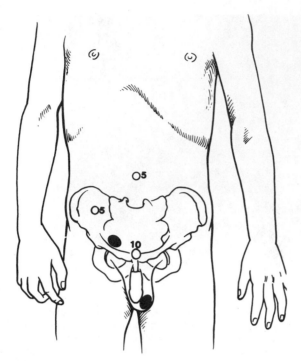

FIG. 60-10
Laparoscopic clip ligation of the testicular vessels as the first stage of a two-stage orchidopexy requires a 10 mm port through which an endoclip applier can be passed. A third 5 mm port in the ipsilateral lower quadrant is necessary for laparoscopic orchiectomy. (From Bloom DA, Ritchey ML, Manzoni G: Laparoscopy for the nonpalpable testis. In Holcomb GW III (ed): *Pediatric endoscopic surgery.* Appleton and Lange, Norwalk, Conn., 1994, pp 41-50.)

vessels are mobilized, and the mobilized testis is brought into the scrotum via a trans-scrotal trocar (Fig. 60-10) (Jordan et al., 1992).

Evaluation of ambiguous genitalia

Laparoscopy is useful in evaluation and treatment of children with ambiguous genitalia (Droesch et al., 1990; Wolfman and Kreutner, 1984). Wilson and associates successfully removed a gonadoblastoma-containing dysgenetic gonad laparoscopically, and McDougall and associates reported successful removal of bilateral intraabdominal testes in a patient with testicular feminization syndrome (McDougall and Clayman, 1994; Wilson et al., 1992).

Varicocele ligation

Debate exists regarding the need for intervention and its timing in adolescent boys with varicocele. Varicocele ligation is usually recommended for older teenagers with abnormal semen parameters. In young adolescents or in those in whom a semen analysis cannot be obtained, loss of testicular volume ipsilateral to the varicocele may be an indication for varicocele ligation.

Laparoscopic transabdominal varicocele ligation in adults was reported by Donovan and Winfield and

TABLE 60-7

Indications for Pediatric Laparoscopic Nephrectomy

Recurrent pyelonephritis in a poorly functioning kidney
End-stage kidney failure associated with protein-losing nephropathy
Renal hypertension
Symptomatic atrophic or hypoplastic kidney
Multicystic, dysplastic kidney

(Adapted from Kerbl K, Clayman RV, Kavoussi LR: Laparoscopic Nephrectomy. In *Pediatric Endoscopic Surgery.* Holcomb, GW III, (ed), Appleton and Lange, Norwalk, Conn., 1994, 94.)

Hagood and associates in 1992 (Donovan and Winfield, 1992; Hagood, 1992). Sparing of the testicular artery, shorter convalescence, favorable cosmesis, and a low varix recurrence rate were felt to make laparoscopic varicocelectomy a preferred method compared with traditional open procedures (retroperitoneal, inguinal). At present, there have been no reports specifically describing laparoscopic varicocele ligation in the pediatric age group; the advantages of laparoscopic varicocelectomy in adults cannot necessarily be translated to the pediatric/adolescent age group.

Kidney

Although retroperitoneal, the kidney can be accessed laparoscopically via a transabdominal approach. Clayman and associates were the first to perform laparoscopic nephrectomy in adults (Clayman et al., 1991). Since that time, successful partial nephrectomy, pyeloplasty, renal biopsy, renal cyst decortication, and pyelolithotomy have been described (Table 60-7) (Gaur et al., 1994; Kerbl and Clayman, 1994). In adults laparoscopic renal surgery results in longer intraoperative times but shorter hospitalization, less analgesia, and shorter convalescence than traditional open approaches. In the pediatric population hospitalization stay and convalescence, while shorter after laparoscopy, should not be the overriding issues when it comes to deciding between laparoscopy versus traditional open renal surgery. Soon after the first adult laparoscopic nephrectomy, Koyle and Kavoussi reported on the successful laparoscopic removal of a multicystic kidney in an 8-month-old child (Koyle et al., 1993). This was performed via a transabdominal approach requiring less than 1 hour operative time, and the patient was discharged later that same day. Several other investigators reported on their successful experience with laparoscopic nephrectomy (Ehrlich et al., 192; Suzuki et al., 1993). Operative time was in most cases significantly longer than when compared with open simple nephrectomy, hospital stay was less, the amount of analgesics required was minimal, and the return to normal activity was less than a week.

The most common indications for laparoscopic nephrectomy in children appear to be multicystic dysplastic kidneys or poorly functioning kidneys secondary to reflux nephropathy. Aspiration of the fluid contents from large cysts may be necessary to facilitate removal of the kidney specimen from the abdominal cavity. Laparoscopic heminephrectomy of nonfunctioning dysplastic segments has also been performed. Hemostasis during amputation of the polar segment is accomplished by laser, electro-coagulation, endostapler, or argon beam coagulator (Ehrlich et al., 1993; Janetschek et al., 1994). One major criticism of laparoscopic renal surgery has been the transabdominal approach, thereby placing at risk intraperitoneal organs that otherwise would not be in jeopardy with standard open retroperitoneal approaches. Gaur described a dissecting balloon that has facilitated retroperitonoscopy, thereby making it possible to avoid the intraperitoneal contents while performing renal surgery. Simple nephrectomy, renal biopsy, and ureterolithotomy have all been performed using this method (Gaur et al., 1993, 1994).

Ureterolithotomy

Raboy and colleagues first described laparoscopic ureterolithotomy in an adult in 1992 (Raboy et al., 1992). Using a four-port transabdominal approach, an obstructing ureteral calculus was removed with a laparoscopic grasping forceps. A stent was placed, and there was no attempt at suturing the ureterotomy. Extracorporeal shock wave lithotripsy and the availability of pediatric endoscopic instruments, which allow for safe passage of instruments even in the pediatric ureter, would preclude the need for laparoscopic ureteral surgery in almost all cases of pediatric stone disease.

Bladder auto-augmentation

Autoaugmentation was first described by Snow and Cartwright as an alternative to enterocystoplasty to attain a large-capacity, low-pressure reservoir (Cartwright and Snow, 1989). In essence a large bladder diverticulum is created by partially excising the detrusor muscle. Ehrlich and Gershman described laparoscopic seromyotomy via a transabdominal approach in an 8-year-old child with incontinence secondary to nonneurogenic neurogenic bladder (Ehrlich and Gershman, 1993). Four trocars were placed, and the seromyotomy extended from the cul-de-sac posterior to the fusion of the bladder and peritoneal reflection superiorly. Postoperatively the patient developed a small intraperitoneal urine leak requiring temporary percutaneous suprapubic drainage. McDougall and associates described autoaugmentation via a retropubic approach (McDougall et al., 1995). Dissection of the retropubic space was facilitated by the use of an inflatable balloon inserted through a small incision made in the midline midway between the symphysis pubis and the umbilicus and then inflated with 60 ml saline solution. The seromyotomy was performed employing four ports and was more anterior than that described by Ehrlich and Gershman. The advantage of retropubic seromyotomy is that a urine leak which may occur in the immediate postoperative period would be contained to the retroperitoneum, and the risk of intraabdominal urine leak and peritonitis avoided. The disadvantage of retropubic autoaugmentation compared with intraabdominal autoaugmentation is the increase in operative time (6.5 hours vs. 70 minutes). Long-term follow-up studies will be necessary to determine first whether autoaugmentation is a better alternative to conventional enterocystoplasty and second whether laparoscopic autoaugmentation is better than an open approach.

Ureterolysis

Ureterolysis was first performed laparoscopically by Kavoussi and associates in 1992 on a 15-year-old girl with unilateral retroperitoneal fibrosis in 1992 (Kavoussi et al., 1992). Localization of the involved ureter was enhanced by prior placement of an external ureteral catheter. The ureter was intraperitonealized, and titanium clips were used to reapproximate the previously incised peritoneal edges. Operative time was more than 5 hours, and hospitalization was 6 days. Postoperative renal scintigraphy at 8 months revealed no evidence of obstruction. Since then others have reported successful transabdominal laparoscopic ureterolysis.

Ileal loop diversion

In 1992 Kozminski and colleagues reported the first successful laparoscopic ileal loop urinary diversion (Kozminski and Partamian, 1992). The bowel anastomoses were performed extracorporeally, although in later patients the bowel anastomosis was performed intracorporally utilizing laparoscopic stapling devices. Kozminski utilized laparoscopy for the ureteral enteric anastomosis in a subsequent patient, thereby achieving complete laparoscopic ileal conduit diversion. Laparoscopic bowel procedures such as colonic resections and total proctocolectomies have been reported in the general surgery literature (Cooperman and Zucker, 1991). Although the need for urinary diversion in children is less than that of adults, there exists the potential for a future role for laparoscopic urinary diversion, such as the creation of continent urinary reservoirs or bladder augmentation in children with lower urinary tract dysfunction. The limitations are mainly those of existing equipment and the competence, patience, and perseverance of the laparoscopic surgeon.

Complications

Complications for nongynecologic laparoscopy are approximately 5% for minor and 0.6% to 2.5% for major complications with mortality rates approaching zero (Cuschieri, 1980; Kane and Kreijs, 1984). Early complication rates of urologic laparoscopy dealt mainly with those complications related to laparoscopic pelvic lymphadenectomy for staging of prostatic carcinoma. Major complications ranged from 8% to 20% with minor complications ranging from 12% to 33% (Capelouto and Kavoussi, 1993; Kozminski et al., 1992; Winfield, et al., 1991). Complications from laparoscopy can be divided into anesthetic, intraoperative, and postoperative problems (Scherz and Kaplan, 1994). Anesthetic complications vary from nuisances (difficulty in mechanical ventilation secondary to increased intraperitoneal pressure and decreased diaphragmatic excursion) to crises (hypercarbia and acidosis, hypertension, hypotension, arrhythmias, CO_2 embolus with cardiovascular collapse). Fortunately anesthetic-related complications are rare in children. If CO_2 embolus is suspected, insufflation should be immediately stopped and the patient placed in Trendelenberg position with the right side up, and attempts at aspiration of the embolus should be attempted via central venous access.

Intraoperative complications can be subdivided further into those that occur at the time of pneumoperitoneum, at insertion of the trocar(s), during surgical intervention, and at the time of trocar removal. Placement of the Veress needle and trocar insertion are the most hazardous steps in laparoscopy. Strict attention to detail will minimize the potential risks. Special care must be used in children when placing needle and trocar because of the relative proximity of the posterior retroperitoneal structures. Placement of the child in 15 degree Trendelenberg position and pulling the abdominal wall forward greatly enhances the chances of proper intraabdominal placement of the Veress needle. Open placement of a Hasson type trocar obviates the need for a Veress needle. Injuries to the bladder or bowel with a Veress needle require removal of the needle and decompression of the involved viscus. Aspiration of blood through Veress needle denotes vascular injury and usually requires conversion to an open procedure. Trocar insertion is another dangerous technical aspect of laparoscopy, but several steps minimize the risk of trocar insertion-related injury. A sharp trocar point is important to allow for the least amount of force necessary to enter the intraabdominal cavity. Epigastric vessel injury is the most common vascular injury. This usually occurs during placement of accessory lateral trocars. Epigastric vessel injury may be managed by placement of a figure-of-eight sutures adjacent to the offending trocar. Vascular injuries to the aorta or iliac vessels during trocar placement require immediate open surgical exploration and repair. Major vascular injury to the aorta and common iliac vessels has an incidence of 0.3 to 0.9 per 1000 cases (Capelouto and Kavoussi, 1993). Be cognizant that in some thin adults and in children the aorta may lie only 2 to 3 cm from the skin (Malinak et al., 1988).

Trocar insertion into small and large intestine occurs in 1 to 2.7 per 1000 cases. Lacerations to the liver, spleen, and mesentery have been reported to a lesser degree. Open repair of hollow viscus organs is usually required, and major colonic injuries to unprepped bowel should be accompanied by a diverting colostomy. The most common complications occurring during surgical intervention is inadvertent thermal injury during electrocautery. Switching from monopolar to bipolar cautery may minimize the occurrence of this injury, but strict attention to technique is the best method of avoiding this serious complication. The most common complication occurring during removal of the trocars is bleeding from the trocar sites. All the trocar sites should be visualized during removal and the CO_2 insufflation pressure reduced to 5 mm Hg. Bleeding vessels can be managed via several steps previously outlined. Finally, all the CO_2 should be evacuated to prevent shoulder pain referred secondary to subdiaphragmatic irritation. Postoperative problems specifically related to laparoscopy are the formation of incisional hernias. Bloom and Ehrlich reported two instances of omental evisceration through fascial defects caused by improper closure of the trocar sites (Bloom DA, Ehrlich RM, 1993).

REFERENCES

Allen JS, Summers JL, Wilkerson JE: Meatal calibration of newborn boys. *J Urol* 1972; 107:498.

Anderson JC, Hynes W: Retrocaval ureter: a case diagnosed preoperatively and treated successfully by plastic operation. *Br J Urol* 1949; 21:209.

Appel RA: Injectables for urethral incompetence. *World J Urol* 1990; 8:208.

Badlani G, Eshghi M, Smith A: Percutaneous surgery for ureteropelvic junction obstruction (endopyelotomy): technique and early results. *J Urol* 1986; 135:26.

Bailey RR: Vesicoureteral reflux and reflux nephropathy. In Schrier RW, Gottschalk CW (eds): *Diseases of kidney,* 1988; 747-783.

Ball WS Jr, Towbin RB, Strife JL, et al: Interventional genitourinary radiology in children: review of 61 procedures. *AJR* 1986; 147:791.

Banner MP, Pollack HM, Ring EJ, et al: Catheter dilation of benign strictures. *Radiology* 1983; 147:427.

Bellinger MF, Duckett JW: Vesico ureteral reflux: a comparison of non-surgical and surgical management. In Hodson J (ed): *Reflux nephropathy update, contributions to nephrology.* S Karger Publishers, 1984, pp 81-93.

Bennett AH, Colodny AH: Urinary tract calculi in children. *J Urol* 1973; 109:318.

Berger RM, et al: Bladder capacity (ounces) equals age (years) plus 2 predicts normal bladder capacity and aids in diagnosis of abnormal voiding patterns. *J Urol* 1983; 129:347.

Berkokwitz GS, Lapinski RH, Dolgin SE, et al: Prevalence and natural history of cryptorchidism. *Pediatrics* 1993; 92:44.

Bloom DA: Two-step orchiopexy with pelviscopic clip ligation of the spermatic vessels. *J Urol* 1991; 145:1030.

Bloom DA: Symposium. What is the best approach to the nonpalpable testis? *Contemp Urology* 1992; 4:39.

Bloom DA, Ehrlich RM: Omental evisceration through a small laparotomy port site. *J Endourol* 1993; 7:31-32.

Bloom DA, Hensle TW: Genitourinary endoscopy. In Ritchey M, Gonzalez R, (eds): *Dialogues in pediatric urology*. 1992; Vol. 15, pp 1-3.

Bloom DA, McGuire EJ, Lapides JA: A brief history of urethral catheterization *J Urol* 1994; 151:317.

Bloom DA, Morgan RJ, Scardinao PL: Thomas Hillier and percutaneous nephrostomy. *Urology* 1989; 23:346.

Blute ML, Segura JW, Patterson DE: Ureteroscopy. *J Urol* 1988; 139:510.

Blyth B, Ewald DH, Duckett JW, et al: Lithogenic properties of enterocystoplasty. *J Urol* 1992; 148:575.

Blyth B, Passerini-Glazel G, Camuffo C, et al: Endoscopic incision of ureteroceles: intravesical versus ectopic. *J Urol* 1993; 149:556.

Bohle A, Knipper A, Thomas S: Extracorporeal shock wave lithotripsy in paediatric patients. *Scand J Urol Nephrol* 1989; 23:137.

Borgman V, Nagel R: Urolithiasis in childhood: a study of 181 cases. *Urol Int* 1982; 37:198.

Borwka A, Hanecki R, Kuzaka B, et al: Early results of endoscopic treatment of vesico-ureteral reflux in children. *Urolog* 1991; 30:264.

Boyd SD, Everett RW, Schiff Wm, et al: Treatment of unusual Kock pouch urinary calculi with extracorporeal shock wave lithotripsy. *J Urol* 1988; 139:805.

Brannan GE, Bush WH, Lewis GP: Endopyelotomy for primary repair of ureteropelvic junctio obstructio. *J Urol* 1988; 139:29.

Brock JW III: Endourology. In Holcomb GW (ed): *Pediatric endoscopic surgery*, Appleton and Lange, Norwalk, Conn., 1994; p. 147.

Burbige KA, Hensle TW: The complications of urinary tract reconstruction. *J Urol* 1986; 136:292.

Caione P, DeGennaro M, Capozza N, et al: Endoscopic manipulation of ureteral calculi in children by rigid operative ureterorenoscopy. *J Urol* 1990; 144:484.

Canning D, Peters C, Gearhart J, et al: Local tissue response to glutaraldehyde cross-linked collagen in the rabbit bladder. *J Urol* 1988; 139:258.

Capelouto CC, Kavoussi LR: Complications of laparoscopic surgery. *Urology* 1993; 42:2-12.

Cartwright PC, Snow BW: Bladder autoaugmentation: early clinical experience. *J Urol* 1989; 142:505.

Castilho LN, Ferreira V, Netto NR Jr, et al: Laparoscopic pediatric orchiectomy. *J Endourol* 1992; 6:155-157.

Cendron M, Gearhart JP: The Mitrofanoff principle: technique and application in continent urinary diversion. *Urol Clinic North Am* 1991; 18:615.

Chappel CR, Christmas TJ, Turner-Warwick RT: VUR in the adult male. *Br J Urol* 1990; 65:144.

Chaussy C, Schmidt E, Jocham D, et al: First clinical experience with extracorporeally induced destruction of kidney stones by shock waves. *J Urol* 1982; 127:417.

Choi H, Snyder HM III, Duckett JW: Urolithiasis in childhood: current management. *J Ped Surg* 1987; 22:158.

Chu C, Chu C, Hsu T, et al: Intraoperative laparoscopy in unilateral hernia repair to detect a contralateral patent processus vaginalis. *Pediatr Surg Int* 1993; 8:385.

Claes H, Stroobants D, Van Meerbeek J, et al: Pulmonary migration following periurethral polytetrafluoroethylene injection for urinary incontinence. *J Urol* 1989; 142:821.

Clayman RV, Kavoussi LR, Soper NJ, et al: Laparoscopic nephrectomy: initial case report. *J Urol* 1991; 146:278.

Colberg J, Keetch D, Basler JW: Percutaneous method for bladder stone removal from augmented bladders. *(Abst 409)* 88th Annual Mtg, AUA, San Antonio, TX, 1993; 315A.

Cooperman AM, Zucker KA: Laparoscopic guided intestinal surgery. *Surgical Laparoscopy* 1991; 205:310.

Cortesi N, Ferrari P, Zambarda E, et al: Diagnosis of bilateral abdominal cryptorchidism by laparoscopy. *Endoscopy* 1976; 8:33.

Culley CC: Endopyelotomy for ureteropelvic junction obstruction. In Paulson DF (ed): Problems in Urology. 1992; Vol 6, p. 355.

Cuschieri A: Laparoscopy in general surgery and gastroenterology *Br J Hosp Med* 1980; 24:252.

Czeizel A, Erodi E, Joth J: Genetics of undescended testis. *J Urol* 1981; 126:528.

Davis DM: Intubated ureteotomy: a new operation for ureteral and ureteropelvic stricture. *Surg Gynecol Obstet* 1943; 76:513.

Davis DM: The process of ureteral repair: a recapitulation of the splinting question. *J Urol* 1958; 79:215.

Davis DM, Strong GH, Drake WM: Intubated ureterotomy: experimental work and clinical results. *J Urol* 1948; 59:851.

Donovan JF Jr, Winfield HN: Laparoscopic varix ligation with Nd:YAG laser. *J Endourol* 1992; 6:165.

Donovan JF, Winfield HN: Laparoscopic varix ligation *J Urol* 1992; 147:77.

Droesch K, Droesch J, Chumas J, et al: Laparoscopic gonadectomy for gonadal dysgenesis. *Fertil Steril* 1990; 53:360.

Duckett JW: Ureterovesical junction and aquired vesicoureteral reflux. *J Urol* 1981; 127:249.

Duckett JW: Update on vesicoureteral reflux. *AUA Updates* 1993; 12:34.

Ehrlich RM, Gershman A: Laparoscopic seromyotomy (auto-augmentation) for non-neurogenic neurogenic bladder in a child: initial case report. *Urology* 1993; 42:175.

Ehrlich RM, Gershman A, Fuchs G: Laparoscopic renal surgery in children. Presented at the Society for Pediatric Urology Annual Meeting. San Antonio, Tex., May, 1993.

Ehrlich RM, Gershman A, Mee S, et al: Laparoscopic nephrectomy in a child: expanding horizons for laparoscopy in pediatric urology. *J Endourol* 1992; 6:463.

Elder JS: Intrauterine intervention for obstructive uropathy. *Kidney* 1990; 22:19.

Elder JS, Duckett JM: Management of the fetus and neonate with hydronephrosis detected by prenatal ultrasonography. *Pediatr Ann* 1988; 17:19.

Faerber GJ, Kennelly M, Richardson T: Long-term results of endoscopic injection of Gax-collagen for the treatment of female Type III stress urinary incontinence. NIDDK Symposium on Women's Urological Health Research. Bethesda, Maryland, March, 1994.

Faerber GJ, Park J, Bloom DA: Treatment of pediatric urethral stricture disease with the Nd:YAG laser. *Urology* 1994; 144:264.

Faerber GJ, Ritchey ML, Bloom DA: Percutaneous endopyelotomy in infants and children after failed pyeloplasty. *J Urol* 1995.

Faerber GJ, Wan J, Bloom DA, et al: Percutaneous extraction of calculi from continent augmentation cystoplasty. *J Endourol* 1992; 6:417.

Frey P, Berger D, Jenny P, et al: Subureteral collagen injection for the endoscopic treatment of vesicoureteral reflux in children: follow-up study of 97 treatedureters and histological analysis of collagen implants. *J Urol* 1992; 148:718.

Frick J, Kohle R, Kunit G: Experience with extracorporeal shock wave lithotripsy in children. *Eur Urol* 1988; 14:181.

Gaur DD, Agarwal DK, Khochikar MV, et al: Laparoscopic renal biopsy via retroperitoneal approach. *J Urol* 1994; 151:925.

Gaur DD, Agarwal DK, Purohit KC: Retroperitoneal laparoscopic nephrectomy: initial case report. *J Urol* 1993; 149:103.

Gaur DD, Agarwal DK, Purohit KC: Retroperitoneal laparoscopic ureterolithotomy and renal biopsy. *J Urol* 1993; 149:408A.

Gearhart JP: Endoscopic management of vesicoureteral reflux. In Kramer SA (ed), *Problems in urology: recent advances in urology*. 1990; Vol. 4, p. 639.

Goodwin WE, Casey WC, Woolf W: Percutaneous trocar (needle) nephrostomy in hydronephrosis. *JAMA* 1955; 157:891.

Grossman H, Pirie D: The incidence of urinary tract anomalies in cryptorchid boys. *Am J Roentgenol* 1968; 103:210.

Hagood PG, Mehan DJ, Worischeck JH, et al: Laparoscopic varicocelectomy: preliminary report of a new technique *J Urol* 1992; 147:73.

Hasson HM: Open laparoscopy: a report of 150 cases. *J Reprod Med* 1974; 12:234.

Hill DE: Ureteroscopy and extracorporeal shock wave lithotripsy in children. In Kramer SA, Paulson DF (eds): *Problems in urology: recent advances in pediatric urology*. Vol. 4, p. 727.

Hill DE, Segura JW, Patterson DE, et al: Ureteroscopy in children. *J Urol* 1990; 144:481.

Hrebinko RL, Bellinger MF: The limited role of imaging techniques in managing children with undescended testes. *J Urol* 1993; 150:458.

Immergut MA, Wahman GE: The urethral caliber of female children with recurrent urinary tract infections. *J Urol* 1968; 99:189.

Janetschek G, Reissigl A, Bartsch G: Laparoscopic heminephroureterectomy in an infant. *J Endourol* 1994; 8:V3-107A.

Johnson DK, Kroovand RL, Perlmutter AD: The changing role of cystoscopy in the pediatric patient. *J Urol* 1980; 123:232.

Jordan GH: Management of the abdominal nonpalpable undescended testicle. *Atlas Urol Clin North Am* 1993; 1:49.

Jordan GH, Bloom DA: Laparoscopic genitourinary surgery in children. In Gomella LG, Kozminski M, Winfield HN, (ed): *Laparoscopic urologic surgery*. New York, Raven Press, 1994; pp 223-246.

Jordan GH, Robey EL, Winslow BH: Laparoendoscopic surgical management of the abdominal/transinguinal undescended testicle. *J Endourol* 1992; 6:157.

Kane MG, Kreijs GJ: Complications of diagnostic laparoscopy in Dallas: a 7-year prospective study. *Gastrointest Endosc* 1984; 30:237.

Kaplan GW, Brock WA: Idiopathic urethrorrhagia in boys. *J Urol* 1982; 128:1001.

Kaplan WE: Early evaluation and Treatment of children with meningomyelocele. In Kramer SA (ed): *Problems in urology: recent advances in pediatric urology*. 1990; 4 p 676.

Kavoussi LR, Clayman RV, Brunt LM, et al: Laparoscopic ureterolysis. *J Urol* 1992; 147:426.

Kelling G: Zur Colioskopie. *Arch Klin Chir* 1923; 126:226.

Kerbl K, Clayman RV: Advances in laparoscopic renal and ureteral surgery. *Eur Urol* 1994; 25:1.

Kerbl K, Clayman RV, Kavoussi LR: Laparoscopic Neproctomy. In Pediatric Endoscopic Surgery. Holcomb GW III (ed). Appleton and Lange, Norwalk, Conn., 1994, p. 94.

Kerfoot WF, Carson CC: The surgical anatomy of the ureter. In Carson CC, Paulson DF (eds), Vol 6, 1992; p. 234.

King LR, Coughlin PWF, Ford KK, et al: Initial experience with percutaneous and transurethral ablation of post-operative ureteral strictures in children. *J Urol* 1984; 131:1167.

Kogan SJ: Cryptorchidism. In Kelalis PP, King LR, Belman AB (eds): *Clinical pediatric urology*, 2nd ed. WB Saunders Co., Philadelphia, 1985 p. 868.

Korth K, Kuenkel M, Erschig M: Percutaneous pyeloplasty. *Urology* 1988; 31:503.

Koyle MA, Woo HH, Kavoussi LR: Laparoscopic nephrectomy in the first year of life. *J Pediatric Surg*

Kozminski M, Gomella L, Stone N, et al: Laparoscopic urologic surgery: outcome assessment. *J Urol* 1992; 147:245A.

Kozminski M, Partamian KO: Case report of laparoscopic ileal loop conduit. *J Endourol* 1992; 6:147.

Kramolowsky EV, Willoughby BL, Loening SA: Extracorporeal shock wave lithotripsy in children. *J Urol* 1987; 137:939.

Kroovand RL: Stones in pregnancy and in children. *J Urol* 1992; 148:1076.

Kroovand RL, Harrison LH, McCullough DL: Extracorporeal shock wave lithotripsy in childhood. *J Urol* 1987; 138:1106.

Kropp KA, Voeller KSK: Cryptorchidism in meningomyelocele. *J Pediatr* 1981; 99:110.

Kruyt RH, Kums JJ: Kock pouch urinary diversion: followup by ultrasound. *Br J Radiol* 1988; 61:811.

Leonard MP, Canning DA, Peters CA, et al: Endoscopic injection of glutaraldehyde cross-linked bovine dermal collagen for correction of vesicoureteral reflux. *J Urol* 1991; 145:115.

Lingeman JE, Kulb TB: Hypertension following extracorporeal shock wave lithotripsy. *J Urol* 1987; 137:45A.

LiPuma JP, Haaga JR, Bryan PJ, et al: Percutaneous nephrostomy in neonates and infants *J Urol* 1984; 132, 722.

Litvak AS, Morris JD, McRoberts JW: Normal size of the urethral meatus in male children. *J Urol* 1976; 115:736.

Lockhart JL, Walker RD, Vorstman B, et al: Periurethral polytetraflouroethylene injection following urethral reconstruction in female patients with urinary incontinence. *J Urol* 1988; 140:51.

Lyon ES, Kyker JS, Schoenberg HW: Transurethral ureteroscopy in women: a ready addition to the urological armamentarium. *J Urol* 1978; 119:35.

Malek RS: Urolithiasis. In Kelalais PP, King LR, Belman AB (eds): *Clinical pediatric urology*, 2nd ed. Philadelphia, WB Saunders Co., 1985; Vol 2, p. 1093.

Malinak LR, Wheeler JM, Simolke G: Vascular injuries at laparoscopy. In Nichols DH (ed), *Clinical problems, injuries, and complications of gynecologic surgery*. Williams and Wilkins, 1988, pp 58-61.

Malizia A, Reiman H, Myers R, et al: Migration and granulomatous reaction after periurethral injection of polytef (Teflon). *JAMA* 1984; 251:3277.

Marberger M, Turk C, Steinkogler I: Piezoelectric extracorporeal shock wave lithotripsy in children. *J Urol* 1989; 142:349.

Matouschek E. Treatment of vesicoureteral reflux by transurethral Teflon injection. *Urologe* 1981; 20:263.

Mayo ME, Ansell JS: The effect of bladder function on the dynamics of the ureterovesical junction. *J Urol* 1980; 123:229.

McCullough DL, Yeaman LD, Bo WJ, et al: Effects of shock waves on the rat ovary. *J Urol* 1989; 141:666.

McDougall EM, Clayman RV: Advances in laparoscopic urology. Part 1. History and development of procedures. *Urology* 1994; 43:420.

McDougall EM, Clayman RV, Figenshau RS, et al: Laparoscopic retropubic auto-augmentation of the bladder. *J Urol* 1995; 153:123.

McGuire EJ: Urinary incontinence: clinical correlations. AUA Updates 1990; 9:37.

McGuire EJ, Wang SC, Appell R, et al: Treatment of urethral incontinence by collagen injection-one year followup. *J Urol* 1990; 143:224A, abstract 142.

Michael V, Davaris P, Arhontakis A, et al: Effects of submucosal Teflon paste injection in vesicoureteric reflux:

results with 1 and 2 year follow-up data. *Eur Urol* 1993; 23:379.

Mininberg DT, Steckler R, Riehle RA Jr: Extracorporeal shock wave lithotripsy for children. *Am J Dis Child* 1988; 142:279.

Minkov N, Konstantinov D, Goster G: Urolithiasis in children. *Eur Urol* 1981; 7:132.

Mulcahy JJ, Kelalis PP: Non-operative treatment of vesicoureteric reflux. *J Urol* 1978; 120:336.

Murless BC: The injection treatment of stress incontinence. *J Obst Gynec Brit Commonw* 1938; 45:67.

Newman DM, Coury TA, Lingeman JE, et al: Extracorporeal shock wave lithotripsy experience in children. *J Urol* 1986; 136:238.

Newman RC: Clinical and experimental effects associated with EDWL. In Riehle RA (ed): *Principles of extracorporeal shock wave lithotripsy*. New York, Churchill-Livingstone, 1987; p. 31.

Nijman RJM, Ackaert K, Scholtmeijer RJ, et al: Long term results of extracorporeal shock wave lithotripsy in children. *J Urol* 1989; 142:609.

Noe HN: Complications and management of childhood urethral stricture disease. *Urol Clin North Am* 1983; 10:531.

Noe HN, Stapleton FB, Jerkins, GR et al: Clinical experience with pediatric urolithiasis. *J Urol* 1903; 129:1166.

O'Donnell B, Puri P: Treatment of vesicoureteral reflux by endoscopic injection of Teflon. *Br Med J* 1984; 289:7.

O'Donnell B, Puri P: Endoscopic treatment of primary vesicoureteral reflux. *Br J Urol* 1986; 58:601.

Pfister RC, Newhouse JH: Interventional percutaneous pyelourethral techniques: II-percutaneous nephrostomy and other procedures. *Radilo Clin North Am* 1979; 17:351.

Pfister RC, Newhouse JH, Yoder IC, et al: Complications of pediatric percutaneous renal procedures: incidence and observations. *Urol Clin North Am* 1983; 19:563.

Politano VA: Periurethral Teflon injection for urinary incontinence. *Urol Clin North Am* 1978; 5:415.

Puri P, Ninan GK, Surana R: Subureteric Teflon injection (STING). *Eur Urol* 1995; 27:71.

Raboy A, Ferzli GS, Ioffreda R, et al: Laparoscopic ureterolithotomy. *Urology* 1992; 39:223.

Ralls PW, Barakos JA, Skinner DG, et al: Imaging of the Kock continent ileal urinary reservoir. *Radiology* 1986; 161:477.

Ramsay JWA, Miller RA, Kellett MJ, et al: Percutaneous pyelolysis: indications, complications and results. *Br J Urol* 1984; 56:586.

Riedy MJ, Lebowitz RL: Percutaneous studies of the upper urinary tract in children, with special emphasis on infants. *Radiology* 1986; 160:231.

Ritchey M, Patterson DE, Kelalis PP, et al: A case of pediatric ureteroscopic lasertripsy. *J Urol* 1988; 139:1272.

Rozanski T, Wojno K, Bloom DA: The remnant orchiectomy. *J Urol* (in press).

Ruddock JC: Peritoneoscopy. *Surg Gynecol Obstet* 1937; 65:623.

Saw KC, Eardley I, Dennis MJS, et al: Surgical outcomes of orchiopexy in previously unoperated testes. *Br J Urol* 1992; 70:90.

Scardino PT, Scardino PL: Obstruction at the ureteropelvic junction. In H Bergman (ed): *The ureter*, 2nd ed. New York, Springer-Verlag, 1981, p. 697.

Scherz HC, Kaplan GW: Etiology, diagnosis and management of urethral strictures in children. *Urol Clin North Am* 1990; 17:389.

Scherz HC, Kaplan GW: Pediatric laparoscopy. *AUA Updates* 1994; 13:158-163.

Scherz HC, Kaplan GW, Packer MG, et al: Post-hypospadias repair of urethral strictures: a review of 30 cases. *J Urol* 1988; 140:1253.

Seaman EK, Benson MC, Shabsigh R: Percutaneous approach to treatment of Indiana pouch stones. *J Urol* 1994; 151:690.

Segura JW: Endourology. *J Urol* 1984; 132:1079.

Segura JW: Ureteroscopy for lower ureteral stones. *Urology* 1993; 42:356.

Shortliffe LM, Freiha FS, Kessler R, et al: Treatment of urinary incontinence by the peri-urethral implantation of glutaraldehyde cross-linked collagen. *J Urol* 1989; 141:538.

Sigman M, Laudone VP, Jenkins AD, et al: Initial experience with extracorporeal shock wave lithotripsy in children. *J Urol* 1987; 138:839.

Skinner DG, Boyd SD, Lieskovsky G: Clinical experience with the Kock continent ileal reservoir for urinary diversion. *J Urol* 1984; 132:1101.

Sosa RE, Vaughan ED: Complications of ureteroscopy. *AUA Updates* 1988; 7:275.

Stables DP: Percutaneous nephrostomy: techniques, indications and results. *Urol Clin North Am* 1982; 9:15.

Stanley PS, Diament MJ: Pediatric percutaneous nephrostomy: experience with 50 patients. *J Urol* 1986; 135:1223.

Suatengco DE, Bloom DA, Oshima K, et al: Correction of vesicoureteral reflux by intravesical injection of collagen in a canine model. *J d'Urol* 1991; 97:51.

Sutherland RW, Barada JH, Kaufman RP, et al: Percutaneous puncture of continent urinary reservoirs for stone manipulation. *(Abst 743)* 88th Annual Mtg, AUA, San Antonio, Tex, 1993; 398A.

Suzuki K, Ihara H, Kurita Y, et al: Laparoscopic nephrectomy for atrophic kidney associated with ectopic ureter in a child. *Eur Urol* 1993; 23:463.

Tan HL, Najmaldin A, Webb DR: Endopyelotomy for pelvi-ureteric junction obstruction in children. *Eur Urol* 1993; 24:84.

Tank ES: Experience with endoscopic incision and open unroofing of ureteroceles. *J Urol* 1986; 136:241.

Thomas R, Frentz JM, Harmon E, et al: Effect of extracorporeal shock wave lithotripsy on renal function and body height in pediatric patients. *J Urol* 1992; 148:1064.

Thomas R, Ortenberg J, Lee BR, et al: Safety and efficacy of pediatric ureteroscopy for management of calculus disease. *J Urol* 1993; 149:1082.

Van Cangh PJ, Jorian JL, Wese FX, et al: Endoureteropyelotomy: percutaneous treatment of ureteropelvic junction obstruction. *J Urol* 1989; 141:1317.

van Gool JD, Hjalmas K, Tamminen-Mobius T, et al.: Historical clues to the complex of dysfunctional voiding, urinary tract infection and vesicoureteral reflux *J Urol*, 1992.

Vessey SG, Rivett A, O'Boyle PJ: Teflon injection in female stress incontinence. Effect on urethral pressure profile and flow rate. *Br J Urol* 1988; 62:39.

Vieweg J, Weber HM, Miller K, et al: Female fertility following extracorporeal lithotripsy of distal ureteral calculi. *J Urol* 1992; 148:1007.

Vorstman B, Lockhart J, Kaufman MR, et al: Polytetrafluoroethylene injection for urinary incontinence in children. *J Urol* 1985; 133:248.

Walker RD: The injection of Teflon paste to correct urinary incontinence and vesicoureteral reflux. *AUA Update Series* 1989; 8:154.

Walker RD: Diagnosis and management of the nonpalpable undescended testicle. *AUA Update Series* 1992; 11:153.

Walther PC, Kaplan GW: Cystoscopy in children: indications for its use in common urologic problems. *J Urol* 1979; 122:717.

Wan J, McGuire EJ, Bloom DA, et al: The treatment of urinary incontinence in children using glutaraldehyde cross-linked collagen. *J Urol* 1992; 148:127.

Webb DR, Tan HL, Kelly S, et al: Paediatric endourology. *Br J Urol* 1988; 62:474.

Whitaker RH: Methods of assessing obstruction in dilated ureters. *Br J Urol* 1973; 50:76.

Whitaker RH: Clinical assessment of pelvic and ureteral function. *Urology* 1978; 12:146.

Wiatrak M, Ohl DA, Sonda LP III: Stryker frame gantry modification for extracorporeal shock wave lithotripsy to circumvent positioning problems. *J Urol* 1991; 146:283.

Wickham JEA, Kellet MJ: Percutaneous pyelolysis. *Eur Urol* 1983; 9:122.

Wilbert DM, Schofer O, Reidmiller H: Treatment of pediatric urolithiasis by extracorporeal shock wave lithotripsy. *Eur J Pediatr* 1988; 147:579.

Wilson EE, Vuitch F, Carr BR: Laparoscopic removal of dysgenic gonads containing a gonadoblastoma in a patient with Swyer syndrome. *Obstet Gynecol* 1992; 79:842.

Winfield WN, Donovan JF, See WA, et al: Urological laparoscopic surgery. *J Urol* 1991; 146:941.

Witfield HN, Mills V, Miller RA, et al: Percutaneous pyelolysis: an alternative to pyeloplasty. *Br J Urol* 1983; (suppl):93.

Wolfman WL, Kreutner K: Laparoscopy in children and adolescents. *J Adolesc Health Care* 1984; 5:261.

Woodside JR, Stevens GF, Stark GL, et al: Percutaneous stone removal in children. *J Urol* 1985; 134:1166-67.

Yeaman LD, Jerome CP, McCullough DL: Effects of shock waves on the structure and growth of the immature rat epiphysis. *J Urol* 1989; 141:670.

Young HH, McKay RW: Congenital valvular obstruction of the prostatic urethra. *Surg Gynecol Obstet* 1929; 48:409.

Young PR, Weinerth JL: Endoscopic management of calculi in Kock pouch continent urinary diversion. *Problems in Urology* 1992; 6:392.

Index